T0406404

Principles and Practice of Clinical Trials

Steven Piantadosi • Curtis L. Meinert
Editors

Principles and Practice of Clinical Trials

Volume 2

With 241 Figures and 191 Tables

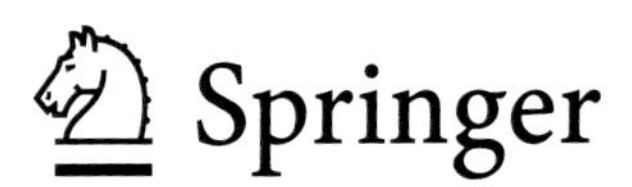

Editors
Steven Piantadosi
Department of Surgery
Division of Surgical Oncology
Brigham and Women's Hospital
Harvard Medical School
Boston, MA, USA

Curtis L. Meinert
Department of Epidemiology
School of Public Health
Johns Hopkins University
Baltimore, MD, USA

ISBN 978-3-319-52635-5 ISBN 978-3-319-52636-2 (eBook)
https://doi.org/10.1007/978-3-319-52636-2

© Springer Nature Switzerland AG 2022
This work is subject to copyright. All rights are reserved by the Publisher, whether the whole or part of the material is concerned, specifically the rights of translation, reprinting, reuse of illustrations, recitation, broadcasting, reproduction on microfilms or in any other physical way, and transmission or information storage and retrieval, electronic adaptation, computer software, or by similar or dissimilar methodology now known or hereafter developed.
The use of general descriptive names, registered names, trademarks, service marks, etc. in this publication does not imply, even in the absence of a specific statement, that such names are exempt from the relevant protective laws and regulations and therefore free for general use.
The publisher, the authors, and the editors are safe to assume that the advice and information in this book are believed to be true and accurate at the date of publication. Neither the publisher nor the authors or the editors give a warranty, expressed or implied, with respect to the material contained herein or for any errors or omissions that may have been made. The publisher remains neutral with regard to jurisdictional claims in published maps and institutional affiliations.

This Springer imprint is published by the registered company Springer Nature Switzerland AG.
The registered company address is: Gewerbestrasse 11, 6330 Cham, Switzerland

In memory of
Lulu, Champ, and Dudley

A Foreword to the Principles and Practice of Clinical Trials

Trying to identify the effects of treatments is not new. The *Book of Daniel* (verses 12–15) describes a test of the effects King Nebuchadnezzar's meat:

> *Prove thy servants, I beseech thee, ten days; and let them give us pulse to eat, and water to drink. Then let our countenances be looked upon before thee, and the countenance of the children that eat of the portion of the King's meat: and as thou seest, deal with thy servants. So he consented to them in this matter, and proved them ten days. And at the end of ten days their countenances appeared fairer and fatter in flesh than all the children which did eat the portion of the King's meat.*

The requirement of comparison in identifying treatment effects was recognized in the tenth century by Abu Bakr Muhammad ibn Zakariya al-Razi (Persian physician):

> *When the dullness (thiqal) and the pain in the head and neck continue for three and four and five days or more, and the vision shuns light, and watering of the eyes is abundant, yawning and stretching are great, insomnia is severe, and extreme exhaustion occurs, then the patient after that will progress to meningitis (sirsâm)... If the dullness in the head is greater than the pain, and there is no insomnia, but rather sleep, then the fever will abate, but the throbbing will be immense but not frequent and he will progress into a stupor (lîthûrghas). So when you see these symptoms, then proceed with bloodletting. For I once saved one group [of patients] by it, while I intentionally neglected [to bleed] another group. By doing that, I wished to reach a conclusion (ra'y). And so all of these [latter] contracted meningitis.* (Tibi 2006)

But it was not until the beginning of the eighteenth century before the importance of treatment comparisons was broadly acknowledged, for example, as in chances of contracting smallpox among people inoculated with smallpox lymph versus those who caught smallpox disease naturally (Bird 2018).

By the middle of the eighteenth century there were examples of tests with comparison groups, for example, as described by James Lind in relation to his scurvy experiment on board the HMS Salisbury at sea:

> *On the 20th of May 1747, I took twelve patients in the scurvy, on board the Salisbury at sea. Their cases were as similar as I could have them. They all in general had putrid gums, the spots and lassitude, with weakness of their knees. They lay together in one place, being a proper apartment for the sick in the fore-hold; and had one diet common to all, viz., watergruel sweetened with sugar in the morning; fresh mutton-broth often times for dinner;*

at other times puddings, boiled biscuit with sugar, etc; and for supper, barley and raisins, rice and currants, sago and wine, or the like. Two of these were ordered each a quart of cyder a-day. Two others took twenty-five gutts of elixir vitriol three times a day, upon an empty stomach; using a gargle strongly acidulated with it for their mouths. Two others took two spoonfuls of vinegar three times a day, upon an empty stomach; having their gruels and their other food well acidulated with it, as also the gargle for their mouth. Two of the worst patients, with the tendons in the ham rigid, (a symptom none of the rest had), were put under a course of seawater. Of this they drank half a pint every day, and sometimes more or less as it operated, by way of gentle physic. Two others had each two oranges and one lemon given them every day. These they eat with greediness, at different times, upon an empty stomach. They continued but six days under this course, having consumed the quantity that could be spared. The two remaining patients, took the bigness of a nutmeg three times a-day, of an electuary recommended by an hospital surgeon, made of garlic, mustard-seed, rad raphan, balsam of Peru, and gum myrrh; using for common drink, barley-water well acidulated with tamarinds; by a decoction of which, with the addition of cremor tartar, they were gently purged three or four times during the course.

* * *

The consequence was, that the most sudden and visible good effects were perceived from the use of the oranges and lemons; one of those who had taken them, being at the end of six days fit for duty. (Lind 1753)

Lind did not make clear how his 12 sailors were assigned to the treatments in his experiment. During the late nineteenth and early twentieth century, alternation (and sometimes randomization) became used to create study comparison groups that differed only by chance (Chalmers et al. 2011).

In 1937 assignment was discussed in Hill's book, *Principles of Medical Statistics*, in which he emphasized the importance of strictly observing the allocation schedule. Implementation of this principle was reflected in concealment of allocation schedules in two important clinical trials designed for the UK Medical Research Council in the 1940s (Medical Research Council 1944; 1948). Sir Austin Bradford Hill's 1937 book went into 12 editions, and his other writings, such as *Statistical Methods in Clinical and Preventive Medicine*, helped propel the upward methodological progression.

The United States Congress passed the Kefauver-Harris Amendments to the Food, Drug, and Cosmetic Act of 1938 in 1962. The amendments revolutionized drug development by requiring drug manufacturers to prove that a drug was safe and effective. A feature of the amendments was language spelling out the nature of scientific evidence required for a drug to be approved:

The term "substantial evidence" means evidence consisting of adequate and well-controlled investigations, including clinical investigations, by experts qualified by scientific training and experience to evaluate the effectiveness of the drug involved, on the basis of which it could fairly and responsibly be concluded by such experts that the drug will have the effect it purports or is represented to have under the conditions of its use prescribed, recommended, or suggested in the labeling or proposed labeling thereof. (United States Congress 1962)

Post World War II prosperity brought sizeable increases in government funding for training and research. The National Institutes of Health played a major role in training biostatisticians in the 1960s and 1970s with its fellowship programs. By the

1980s clinical trial courses started showing up in syllabi of academic institutions. By the 1990s academic institutions started offering PhDs focused on design and conduct of trials with a few now offering PhD training in clinical trials.

The clinical trial enterprise is huge. There were over 25,000 trials registered on CT.gov starting in 2019. That number, assuming CT.gov registrations account for 70% of all registered trials, translates to 38,000 trials. That amounts to 2.3 million people studied when those trials are finished assuming a median sample size of 60 per trial.

Lind did his trial before IRBs and consents, before requirements for written protocols, before investigator certifications, before the Health Insurance Portability and Accountability Act (HIPAA), before data sharing, before data monitoring committees, before site visiting, and before requirements for posting results within 1 year of completion. Trials moved from the backroom of obscurity to front and center with trials seen as forms of public trust.

The act of trying progressed from efforts involving a single investigator to efforts involving cadres of investigators with training in medicine, biostatistics, epidemiology, programming, data processing, and in regulations and ethics underlying trials.

The size of the research team increases with the size and complexities of the trials. Multicenter trials may involve investigatorships numbering in the hundreds.

Enter trialists – persons with training and experience in the design, organization, conduct, and analysis of trials. Presently trialists are scattered, located in various departments in medical schools and schools of public health. They have no academic home.

The scattering works to the disadvantage of the art and science of trials in that it stymies communications and development of curricula relevant to trials. One of our motivations in undertaking this work is hope of speeding development of such homes.

The blessing of online publications is that works can be updated at will. The curse is that the work is never done. We hope to advance the science of trials by providing the trials world with a comprehensive work from leaders in the field covering the waterfront of clinical trials serving as a reference resource for novices and experts in trials for use in designing, conducting, and analyzing them.

13 May 2020 Steven Piantadosi and Curtis L. Meinert
Editors

Postscript

When we started this effort, there was no COVID-19. Now we are living through a pandemic caused by the virus leading us to proclaim in regard to trials, as Charles Dickens did in his *A Tale of Two Cities* in a different context, "the best of times, the worst of times."

"The best of times" because never before has there been more interest and attention directed to trials, even from the President. Everybody wants to know when there will be a vaccine to protect us from COVID-19.

"The worst of times" because of the chaos caused by the pandemic in mounting and doing trials and the impact of "social distancing" on the way trials are done now.

It is a given that the pandemic will change how we do trials, but whatever those changes will be, trials will remain humankind's best and most enduring answer to addressing the conditions and maladies that affect us.

Acknowledgment
We are indebted to Sir Iain Chalmers for his review and critical input in reviewing this piece. Dr. Chalmers is founder of the Cochrane Collaboration and first coordinator of the James Lind Library.

Events in the Development of Clinical Trials

Date	Author/source	Event
1747	Lind	Experiment with untreated control group (Lind 1953)
1799	Haygarth	Use of sham procedure (Haggard 1932)
1800	Waterhouse	Smallpox trial (Waterhouse 1802, 1800)
1863	Gull	Use of placebo treatment (Sutton 1865)
1918		First department of biostatistics; Johns Hopkins University, https://www.jhsph.edu/departments/biostatistics/about-us/history/
1923	Fisher	Application of randomization to experimentation (Fisher and MacKenzie 1923)
1931		Committee on clinical trials created by the Medical Research Council of Great Britain (Medical Research Council 1931)
1931	Amberson	Random assignment of treatment to groups of patients (Amberson et al. 1931)
1937	NIH	Start of NIH grant support with creation of the National Cancer Institute (National Institutes of Health 1981)
1944		Publication of multicenter trial on treatment for common cold (Patulin Clinical Trials Committee 1944)
1946		Nüremberg Code for Human Experimentation (Curran and Shapiro 1970) https://history.nih.gov/research/downloads/nuremberg.pdf
1948	MRC	Streptomycin TB multicenter trial published; BMJ: 30 Oct, 1948 (Medical Research Council 1948)
1962	Hill	Book: *Statistical Methods in Clinical and Preventive Medicine* (Hill 1962)
1962	Kefauver, Harris	Amendments to the Food, Drug, and Cosmetic Act of 1938 (United States Congress 1962)

Date	Author/source	Event
1964	NLM	MEDLARS® (MEDical Literature Analysis and Retrieval System) of the National Library of Medicine initiated
1966; 8 Feb	USPHS	Memo from Surgeon General of USPHS informing recipients of NIH funding of requirement for informed consent as condition for funding henceforth (Stewart 1966), https://history.nih.gov/research/downloads/surgeongeneraldirective1966.pdf
1966	Levine	Publication of U.S. Public Health Service regulations leading to creation of Institutional Review Boards for research involving humans (Levine 1988)
1966; 6 Sep	US govt	Freedom of Information Act (FOIA) signed into law by Lyndon Johnson 6 September 1966 (Public Law 89-554, 80 Statue 383); Act specifies US Governmental Agencies records subject to disclosure under the Act; amended and extended in 1996, 2002, and 2007, https://www.justice.gov/oip/foia_guide09/foia-final.pdf; 5 September 2009
1967	Tom Chalmers	Structure for separating the treatment monitoring and treatment administration process (Coronary Drug Project Research Group: 1973)
1974; 12 July	US govt	Creation of U.S. National Commission for the Protection of Human Subjects of Biomedical and Behavioral Research; part of the National Research Act (Public Law No. 93-348, § 202, 88 Stat. 342)
1974	US govt	US Code of Federal Regulations promulgated establishing Institutional Review Boards, https://www.hhs.gov/ohrp/humansubjects/guidance/45cfr46
1979	OPRR	Belmont Report (Ethical Principles and Guidelines for the Protection of Human Subjects of Research); product of the National Commission for the Protection of Human Subjects of Biomedical and Behavioral Research (Office for Protection from Research Risks Belmont Report 1979)
1979	Gorden	NIH Clinical Trials Committee (chaired by Robert Gorden) recommends that "every clinical trial should have provisions for data and safety monitoring" (National Institutes of Health 1979)
1979		Society for Clinical Trials established
1980		First issue of *Controlled Clinical Trials* (Meinert and Tonascia 1998)
1981	Friedman	Book: *Fundamentals of Clinical Trials* (Friedman et al. 1981)

Date	Author/source	Event
1983	Pocock	Book: *Clinical Trials: A Practical Approach* (Pocock 1983)
1986	Meinert	Book: *Clinical Trials: Design, Conduct, and Analysis* (Meinert and Tonascia 1986)
1990	ICH	International Conference on Harmonisation (ICH) formed (European Union, Japan, and the United States) (Vozeh 1995)
1990		Initiation of PhD training program in clinical trials at Johns Hopkins University
1992	FDA	Prescription Drug User Fee Act (PDUFA) enacted; allows FDA to collect fees for review of New Drug Applications (Public Law 102-571; 102 Congress; https://www.fda.gov/ForIndustry/UserFees/PrescriptionDrugUserFee/ucm200361.htm; 2002)
1993	US govt	Mandate regarding valid analysis for gender and ethnic origin treatment interactions (United States Congress 1993)
1993	UK	Cochrane Collaboration founded under leadership of Iain Chalmers; developed in response to Archie Cochrane's call for up-to-date, systematic reviews of all relevant trials in the healthcare field
1996	HIPAA	Health Insurance Portability and Accountability Act (HIPAA) enacted (Public Law 104-191; 104th US Congress; https://aspe.hhs.gov/admnsimp/pL10419.htm)
1996	NLM	PubMed (search engine for MEDLINE) made free to public
1996		Consolidated Standards of Reporting Trials (CONSORT) (Begg et al. 1996)
1997	US govt	US public law calling for registration of trials; Food and Drug Administration Modernization Act of 1997; Public Law 105-115; Nov 21, 1997 (https://www.govinfo.gov/content/pkg/PLAW-105publ115/pdf/PLAW-105publ115.pdf)
1997	Piantadosi	Book: *Clinical Trials: A Methodologic Perspective* (Piantadosi 1997)
2000	NIH	ClinicalTrials.gov registration website launched (Zarin et al. 2007)
2003	NIH	NIH statement on data sharing (National Institutes of Health 2003)
2003	UK	Launch of James Lind Library; marking 250th anniversary of the publication of James Lind's Treatise of the Scurvy (https://www.jameslindlibrary.org/search/)

Date	Author/source	Event
2004	ICMJE	Requirement of registration of trials in public registries as condition for publication for trials starting enrollment after 1 July 2005 by member journals of the International Committee of Medical Journal Editors (ICMJE) (DeAngelis et al. 2004)
2004; 3 Sep	NIH	NIH notice NOT-OD-04-064 (Enhanced Public Access to NIH Research Information) required "its grantees and supported Principal Investigators provide the NIH with electronic copies of all final version manuscripts upon acceptance for publication if the research was supported in whole or in part by NIH funding" for deposit in PubMed Central within six months after publication
2006	WHO	World Health Organization (WHO) launch of International Clinical Trials Registry Platform (ICTRP) (https://www.who.int/ictrp/en/)
2007	FDA	Requirement for investigators to post tabular results of trials covered under FDA regulations on ClinicalTrials.gov within one year of completion [Food and Drug Administration Amendments Act of 2007 (FDAAA)]
2007		Wiley Encyclopedia of Clinical Trials (4 vols) (D'Agostino et al. 2007)
2013		Standard Protocol Items: Recommendations for Interventional Trials (SPIRIT) (Chan et al. 2013)
2016	NIH	Final NIH policy on single institutional review board for multi-site research (NOT-OD-16-094)
2017	FDA	2007 requirement for posting results extended to all trials, whether or not subject to FDA regulations (81 FR64983)
2017	ICMJE	ICMJE requirement for data sharing in clinical trials (Ann Intern Med doi: 10.7326/M17-1028) (Taichman et al. 2017)

References

Amberson JB Jr, McMahon BT, Pinner M (1931) A clinical trial of sanocrysin in pulmonary tuberculosis. Am Rev Tuberc 24:401–435

Begg C, Cho M, Eastwood S, Horton R, Moher D, Olkin I, Pitkin R, Rennie D, Schulz KF, Simel D, Stroup DF (1996) Improving the quality of reporting of randomized controlled trials. The CONSORT statement. JAMA 276(8):637–639

Bird A (2018) James Jurin and the avoidance of bias in collecting and assessing evidence on the effects of variolation. JLL Bulletin: Commentaries on the history of treatment evaluation. https://www.jameslindlibrary.org/articles/james-jurin-

and-the-avoidance-of-bias-in-collecting-and-assessing-evidence-on-the-effects-of-variolation/
Chalmers I, Dukan E, Podolsky SH, Davey Smith G (2011) The advent of fair treatment allocation schedules in clinical trials during the 19th and early 20th centuries. JLL Bulletin: Commentaries on the history of treatment evaluation. https://www.jameslindlibrary.org/articles/the-advent-of-fair-treatment-allocation-schedules-in-clinical-trials-during-the-19th-and-early-20th-centuries/
Chan AW, Tetzlaff JM, Altman DG, Laupacis A, Gøtzsche PC, Krleža-Jeric K, Hróbjartsson A, Mann H, Dickersin K, Berlin JA, Doré CJ, Parulekar WR, Summerskill WSM, Groves T, Schulz KF, Sox HC, Rockhold FW, Drummond R, Moher D (2013) SPIRIT 2013 statement: defining standard protocol items for clinical trials. Ann Intern Med 158(3):200–207
Coronary Drug Project Research Group (1973) The Coronary Drug Project: design, methods, and baseline results. Circulation 47(Suppl I):I-1-I-50
Curran WJ, Shapiro ED (1970) Law, medicine, and forensic science, 2nd edn. Little, Brown, Boston
D'Agostino R, Sullivan LM, Massaro J (eds) (2007) Wiley encyclopedia of clinical trials, 4 vols. Wiley, New York
DeAngelis CD, Drazen JM, Frizelle FA, Haug C, Hoey J, Horton R, Kotzin S, Laine C, Marusic A, Overbeke AJPM, Schroeder TV, Sox HC, Van Der Weyden MB (2004) Clinical Trial Registration: A statement from the International Committee of Medical Journal Editors. JAMA 292:1363–1364
Fisher RA, MacKenzie WA (1923) Studies in crop variation: II. The manurial response of different potato varieties. J Agric Sci 13:311–320
Friedman LM, Furberg CD, DeMets DR (1981) Fundamentals of clinical trials, 5th edn, [2015]. Springer, New York
Haggard HW (1932) The Lame, the Halt, and the Blind: the vital role of medicine in the history of civilization. Harper and Brothers, New York
Hill AB (1937) Principles of medical statistics. Lancet
Hill AB (1962) Statistical methods in clinical and preventive medicine. Oxford University Press, New York
Levine RJ (1988) Ethics and regulation of clinical research, 2nd edn. Yale University Press, New Haven
Lind J (1753) A treatise of the scurvy (reprinted in Lind's treatise on scurvy, edited by CP Stewart, D Guthrie, Edinburgh University Press, Edinburgh, 1953). Sands, Murray, Cochran, Edinburgh
Medical Research Council (1931) Clinical trials of new remedies (annotations). Lancet 2:304
Medical Research Council (1944) Clinical trial of patulin in the common cold. Lancet 16:373–375
Medical Research Council (1948) Streptomycin treatment of pulmonary tuberculosis: a Medical Research Council investigation. Br Med J 2:769–782
Meinert CL, Tonascia S (1986) Clinical trials: design, conduct, and analysis. Oxford University Press, New York (2nd edn, 2012)
Meinert CL, Tonascia S (1998) Controlled Clinical Trials. Encyclopedia of biostatistics, vol 1. Wiley, New York, pp 929–931

National Institutes of Health (1979) Clinical trials activity (NIH Clinical Trials Committee; RS Gordon Jr, Chair). NIH Guide Grants Contracts 8 (# 8):29

National Institutes of Health (1981) NIH Almanac. Publ no 81-5. Division of Public Information, Bethesda

National Institutes of Health (2003) NIH data sharing policy and implementation guidance. http://grants.nih.gov/grants/policy/data_sharing/data_sharing_guidance.htm

Office for Protection from Research Risks (1979) The Belmont Report. Ethical principles and guidelines for the protection of human subjects of research, 18 April 1979

Patulin Clinical Trials Committee (of the Medical Research Council) (1944) Clinical trial of Patulin in the common cold. Lancet 2:373–375

Piantadosi S (1997) Clinical trials: a methodologic perspective. Wiley, Hoboken (3rd edn, 2017)

Pocock SJ (1983) Clinical trials: a practical approach. Wiley, New York

Stewart WH (1966) Surgeon general's directives on human experimentation. https://history.nih.gov/research/downloads/surgeongeneraldirective1966.pdf

Sutton HG (1865) Cases of rheumatic fever. Guy's Hosp Rep 11:392–428

Taichman DB, Sahni P, Pinborg A, Peiperl L, Laine C, James A, Hong ST, Haileamlak A, Gollogly L, Godlee F, Frizelle FA, Florenzano F, Drazen JM, Bauchner H, Baethge C, Backus J (2017) Data sharing statements for clinical trials: a requirement of the International Committee of Medical Journal Editors. Ann Intern Med 167(1):63–65

Tibi S (2006) Al-Razi and Islamic medicine in the 9th century; J R Soc Med 99(4): 206–207

United States Congress (103rd; 1st session): NIH Revitalization Act of 1993, 42 USC § 131 (1993); Clinical research equity regarding women and minorities; part I: women and minorities as subjects in clinical research, 1993

United States Congress (87th): Drug Amendments of 1962, Public Law 87-781, S 1522. Washington, Oct 10, 1962

Vozeh S (1995) The International Conference on Harmonisation. Eur J Clin Pharmacol 48:173–175

Waterhouse B (1800) A prospect of exterminating the small pox. Cambridge Press, Cambridge

Waterhouse B (1802) A prospect of exterminating the small pox (part II). University Press, Cambridge

Zarin DA, Ide NC, Tse T, Harlan WR, West JC, Lindberg DAB (2007) Issues in the registration of clinical trials. JAMA 297:2112–2120

Preface

The two of us have spent our professional lives doing trials; writing textbooks on how to do them, teaching about them, and sitting on advisory groups responsible for trials. We are pleased to say that over our lifetime trials have moved up the scale of importance to now where people feel cheated if denied enrollment.

Clinical trials are admixtures of disciplines: Medicine, behavioral sciences, biostatistics, epidemiology, ethics, quality control, and regulatory sciences to name the principal ones, making it difficult to cover the field in any textbook on the subject. This reality is the reason we campaigned (principally SP) for a collective work designed to cover the waterfront of trials. We are pleased to have been able to do this in conjunction with Springer Nature, both as print and e-books.

There has long been a need for a comprehensive clinical trials text written at a level accessible to both technical and nontechnical readers. The perspective is the same as that in many other fields where the scope of a "principles and practice" textbook has been defining and instructive to those learning the discipline. Accordingly, the intent of *Principles and Practice of Clinical Trials* has been to cover, define, and explicate the field in ways that are approachable to trialists of all types. The work is intended to be comprehensive, but not encyclopedic.

Boston, USA	Steven Piantadosi
Baltimore, USA	Curtis L. Meinert
April 2022	Editors

Acknowledgments

The work involved nine subject sections and appendices.

Section	Section editor	Affiliation
1 Perspectives on clinical trials	Steven N. Goodman Karen A. Robinson	Stanford University; Professor Johns Hopkins University; Professor
2 Conduct and management	Eleanor McFadden	Managing Director; Frontier Science (Scotland)
3 Regulation and oversight	Winifred Werther	Amgen; Epidemiologist
4 Bias control and precision	O. Dale Williams	Florida International University; Retired
5 Basics of trial design	Christopher S. Coffey	University of Iowa; Professor
6 Advanced topics in trial design	Babak Choodari-Oskooei Mahesh K. B. Parmar	University College London; Senior Research Associate University College London; Professor
7 Analysis	Stephen L. George	Duke University; Professor Emeritus
8 Publication and related issues	Tianjing Li	University of Colorado; Associate Professor
9 Special topics	Lawrence Friedman Nancy L. Geller	NIH:NHLBI; Retired NIH:NHLBI; Director, Office of Biostatistics Research
10 Appendices	Gillian Gresham	Cedars-Sinai Medical Center (Los Angeles); Assistant Professor

We are most grateful to the section editors in producing this work.

Thanks to Springer Nature in making this work possible.

Thanks for the guidance and council provided by Alexa Steele, editor, Springer Nature, and for the help and guidance provided by Rukmani Parameswaran and Swetha Varadharajan in shepherding this work to completion.

A special thanks to Gillian Gresham for her production of the appendices and her efforts as Senior Associate Editor.

Steven Piantadosi and Curtis L. Meinert
Editors

Contents

Volume 1

About the Editors

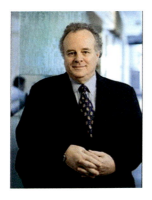

Steven Piantadosi, MD, PhD, is a clinical trialist with 40 years' experience in research, teaching, and healthcare leadership. He has worked on clinical trials of all types, including multicenter and international trials, academic portfolios, and regulatory trials. Most of his work has been in cancer; he also works in other disciplines such as neurodegenerative and cardiovascular diseases.

Dr. Piantadosi began his career in clinical trials early during an intramural Staff Fellowship at the National Cancer Institute's Clinical and Diagnostic Trials Section from 1982 to 1987. That group focused on theory, methodology, and applications with the NCI-sponsored *Lung Cancer Study Group*. Collaborative work included studies of bias induced by missing covariates, factorial clinical trials, and the ecological fallacy. In the latter years, the Branch was focused on Cancer Prevention, including design of the PLCO Trial, which would conclude 30 years later.

In 1987, Dr. Piantadosi joined the Johns Hopkins Oncology Center (now the Johns Hopkins Sidney Kimmel Comprehensive Cancer Center) as the first Director of Biostatistics and the CC Shared Resource. He also carried appointments in the Department of Biostatistics, and in the Johns Hopkins Center for Clinical Trials in the Department of Epidemiology in the School of Public Health (now the Johns Hopkins Bloomberg School). The division he founded became well diversified in cancer research and peer reviewed support, including the CCSG, 6 SPORE grants, PPGs, R01s, and many other grants. A program in Bioinformatics was begun jointly with the Biostatistics Department in Public Health, which would eventually develop into its own funded CCSG Shared Resource. The Biostatistics Division also had key responsibilities in Cancer Center teaching, the Protocol Review and Monitoring Committee, Clinical Research Office, Clinical Informatics, and Research Data Systems and Informatics.

From 1987 onward Dr. Piantadosi's work involved nearly every type of cancer, but especially bone marrow transplant, lung cancer, brain tumors, and drug development. In 1994, he helped to found the New Approaches to Brian Tumor Therapy Consortium (now the *Adult Brian Tumor Consortium*, ABTC), focused on early developmental trials of new agents. This group was funded by NCI for 25 years, was one of the first to accomplish multicenter phase I trials, and was an early implementer of the Continual Reassessment Method (CRM) for dose-finding.

Collaborations at Johns Hopkins extended well beyond the Oncology Department and included Epidemiology (Multi-Center AIDS Cohort Study), Biostatistics, Surgery, Medicine, Anesthesiology, Urology, and Neurosurgery. His work on design and analysis of brain tumor trials through the Department of Neurosurgery led to the FDA approval of BCNU-impregnated biodegradable polymers (Gliadel) for treatment of glioblastoma. He also maintained important external collaborations such as with the *Parkinson's Study Group*, based at the University of Rochester. He ran the Coordinating Center for the *National Emphysema Treatment Trial (NETT)* sponsored by NHLBI and CMS. Numerous important findings emerged from this trial, not the least of which was sharpened indications for risks, benefits, and efficacy of lung volume reduction surgery for emphysema. Dr. Piantadosi also participated actively in prevention trials such as the Alzheimer's Disease Anti-Inflammatory Prevention Trial (ADAPT) and the Chemoprevention for Barrett's Esophagus Trial, both employing NSAIDs and concluding that they were ineffective preventives. He worked with FDA, serving on the *Oncologic Drugs Advisory Committee*, and afterwards on various review panels, and as advisor to industry.

From 2007 to 2017, Dr. Piantadosi was the inaugural Director of the Samuel Oschin Cancer Institute at Cedars Sinai, a UCLA teaching hospital, Professor of Medicine, and Professor of Biomathematics and

Medicine at UCLA. Cedars is the largest hospital in the western USA and treats over 5000 new cancer cases each year, using full-time faculty, in-network oncologists, and private practitioners. Broadly applied work continued with activities in the *Long-Term Oxygen Treatment Trial* (LOTT), dose-finding designs for cancer drug combinations, neurodegenerative disease trial design, and support of the UCLA multi-campus CTSA. During this interval, numerous clinicians and researchers were recruited. Peer-reviewed funding increased from ~$1M to over $20M annually. A clinical trialist is an unusual choice for a Cancer Center director, but it represented an opportunity to improve cancer care in Los Angeles, strengthen the academics at the institution using the NCI P30 model, and serve as a role model for clinical trialists.

In 2018, Dr. Piantadosi joined the Division of Surgical Oncology at Brigham and Women's Hospital, as Professor in Residence, Harvard Medical School. Work at BWH, HMS, includes roles on the *Alliance* NCTN group Executive Committee as the Associate Group Chair for Strategic Initiatives and Innovation, as well as mentoring in the Alliance Statistics Office. He is currently course Co-director for Methods in Clinical Research at DFCI and Course Director for Advanced Clinical Trials (CI 726) in the Master of Medical Sciences in Clinical Investigation Program at Harvard Medical School.

Teaching and Education: In 1988, while at Hopkins Dr. Piantadosi began teaching Experimental Design followed by advanced Clinical Trials. This work formed the foundation for the textbook *Clinical Trials: A Methodologic Perspective*, first published in 1997 and now in its 3rd edition. His course was a staple for students in Biostatistics, Epidemiology, and the Graduate Training Program in Clinical Investigation, where he also taught a research seminar. Subsequently, he mentored numerous PhD graduate students and fellows and served on many doctoral committees. At UCLA, he continued to teach Clinical Trials in their Specialty Training and Research Program.

Dr. Piantadosi has also taught extensively in national workshops focused on training of clinical investigators in cancer, biostatistics, and neurologic disease. This began with the start of the well-known Vail Workshop, and similar venues in Europe and Australia. He was also the Director of several similarly structured courses solely for biostatisticians sponsored by AACR. Independent of those workshops, he taught extensively in Japan, Holland, and Italy.

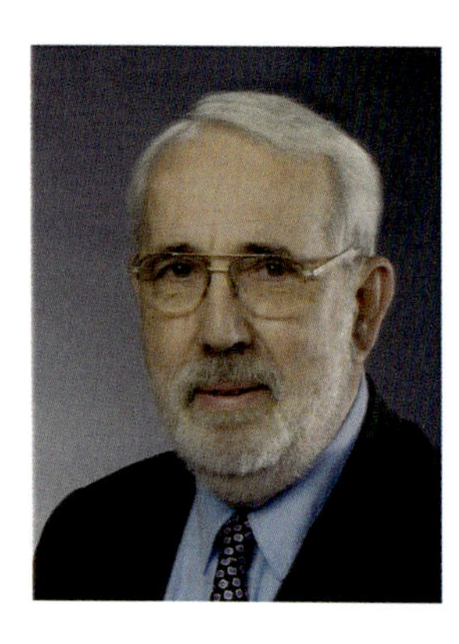

Curtis L. Meinert
Department of Epidemiology
School of Public Health
Johns Hopkins University
Baltimore, MD, USA

Professor Emeritus (Retired 30 June 2019)

I was born 30 June 1934 on a farm four miles west of Sleepy Eye, Minnesota.

My birthday was the first day of a three-day rampage orchestrated by Adolf Hitler known as the Night of the Long Knives. Ominous foreboding of events to come.

My first 6 years of schooling was in a country school located near the Chicago and Northwestern railroad line. There was no studying when freight trains got stuck making the grade past the school.

As was the custom of my parents, all four of us were sent to St John's Lutheran School in Sleepy Eye for our seventh and eighth years of schooling for modicums of religious training. After Lutheran School it was Sleepy Eye Public School, and after that it was the University of Minnesota.

Bachelor of Arts in psychology (1956)

Masters of Science in biostatistics (1959)

Doctor of Philosophy in biostatistics (1964) (Dissertation: Quantitation of the isotope displacement insulin immunoassay)

My sojourn in trials started when I was a graduate student at the University of Minnesota. It started when I signed on to work with Chris Klimt looking for someone to work with him developing what was to become the University Group Diabetes Program (UGDP).

Dr. Klimt decided to move to Baltimore in 1962 to take an appointment in the University of Maryland Medical School. He wanted me to move with him. I did, albeit reluctantly because I wanted to stay and finish my PhD dissertation.

Being Midwestern, Baltimore seemed foreign. People said we talked with an accent, but in our mind it was they who had the accents. A few days after we unpacked I told my wife we would stay a little while, but that I did not want to wake up dead in Baltimore. That surely now is my fate with all my daughters and grand children living here.

The UGDP begat the Coronary Drug Project (CDP; 1966) and it begat others.

I moved across town in 1979 to accept an appointment in the Department of Epidemiology, School of Public Health, Johns Hopkins University. The move led to classroom teaching, mentoring passels of doctoral students, several text books, and a blog site trialsmeinertsway.com.

It was Abe Lilienfeld, after I arrived at Hopkins, who rekindled my "textbook fire." I had taken a sabbatical a few years back while at Maryland to write a text on design and conduct of trials and produced nothing! The good news was that the "textbook bug" was gone – that is until Abe got a hold of me at Hopkins.

Trials became my life with the creation of the Center for Clinical Trials (now the Center for Clinical Trials and Evidence Synthesis) established in 1990 with the urging and help of Al Sommer, then dean of the school. The Center has done dozens and dozens of trials since its creation.

I lost my wife 20 February 2015. I met her at a Tupperware party on Washington's birthday in 1954. We married a year and half later. She was born and raised in Sioux Falls, South Dakota. Being 5′9″ inches tall she was happy to be able to wear her 3″ heels when we went out on the town and still be 6 in. shorter than her escort. Height has its advantages, but not when you are in the middle seat flying sardine!

I came to know Steve Piantadosi after he arrived at Hopkins in 1987. He started talking about a collective work as we are now involved in long before it had a name. For years I ignored his talk, but the "smooth talking North Carolinian" can be insidious and convincing.

So here I am, with Steve joined at the hip, trying to shepherd this work to the finish line.

About the Section Editors

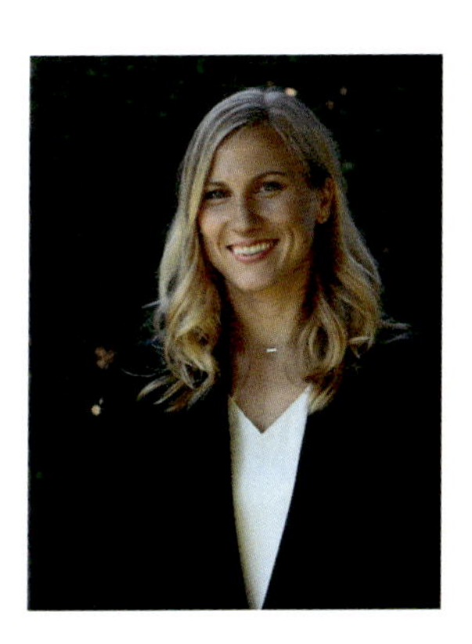

Gillian Gresham
Department of Medicine
Cedars-Sinai Medical Center
Los Angeles, CA, USA

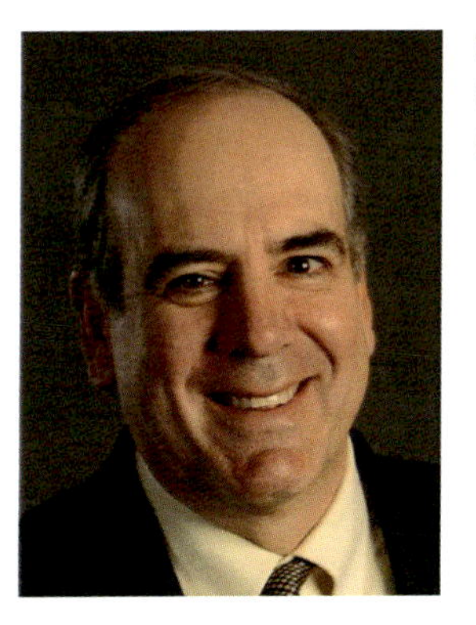

Steven N. Goodman
Stanford University School of Medicine
Stanford, CA, USA

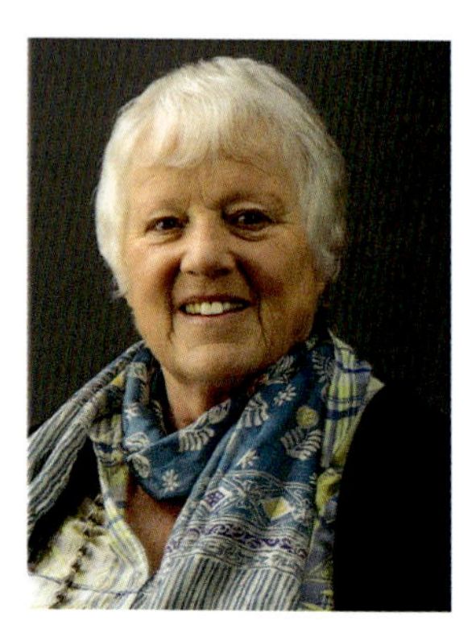

Eleanor McFadden
Frontier Science (Scotland) Ltd.
Kincraig, Scotland

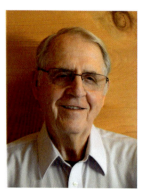

O. Dale Williams
University of North Carolina at Chapel Hill
Chapel Hill, NC, USA

University of Alabama at Birmingham
Birmingham, AL, USA

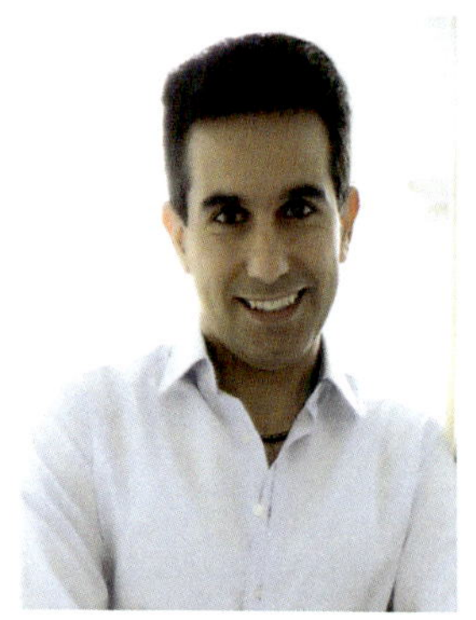

Babak Choodari-Oskooei
MRC Clinical Trials Unit at UCL
Institute of Clinical Trials and Methodology, UCL
London, UK

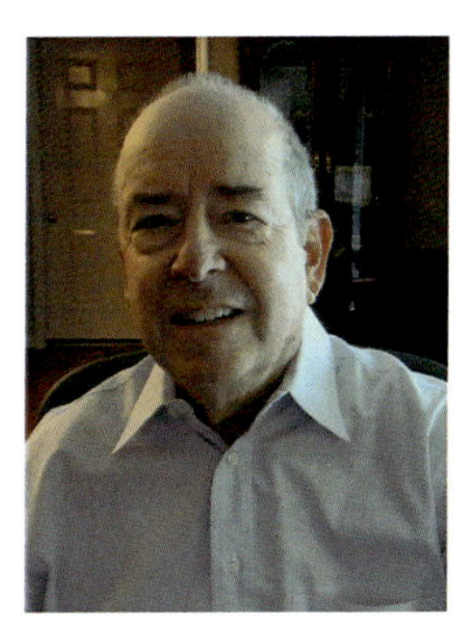

Stephen L. George
Department of Biostatistics and Bioinformatics
Duke University School of Medicine
Durham, NC, USA

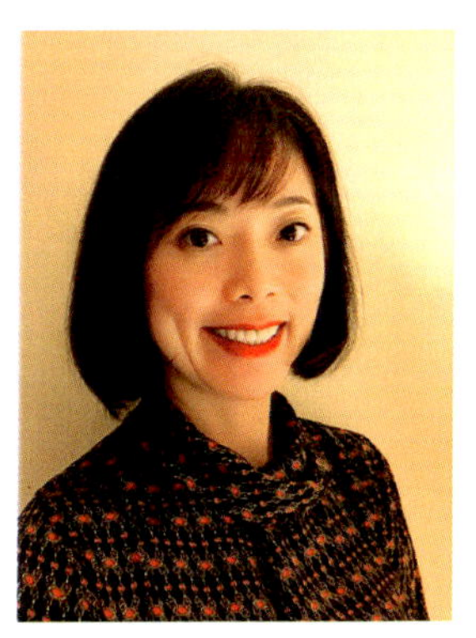

Tianjing Li
Department of Ophthalmology
School of Medicine
University of Colorado Anschutz Medical Campus
Colorado School of Public Health
Aurora, CO, USA

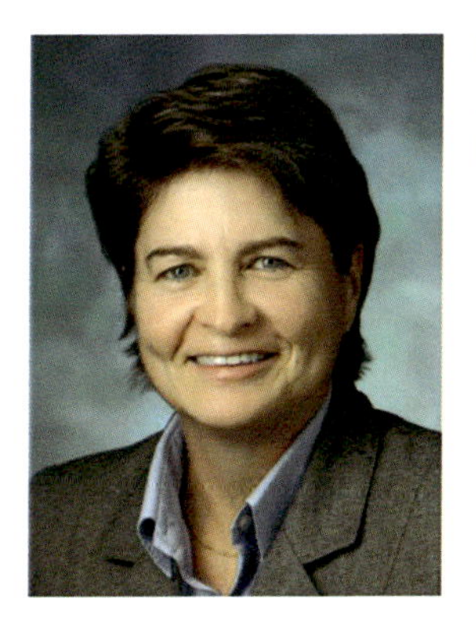

Karen A. Robinson
Johns Hopkins University
Baltimore, MD, USA

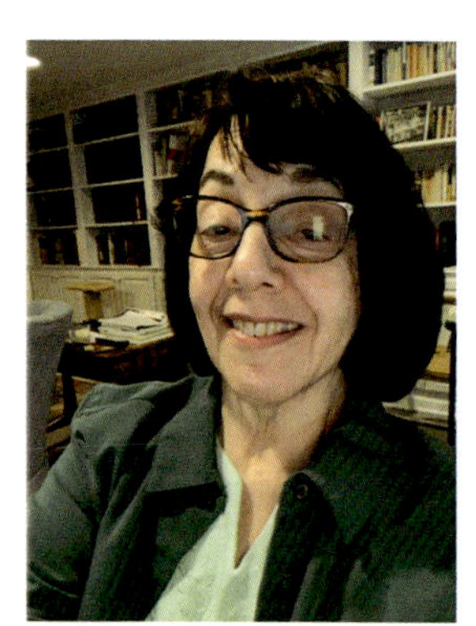

Nancy L. Geller
Office of Biostatistics Research
NHLBI
Bethesda, MD, USA

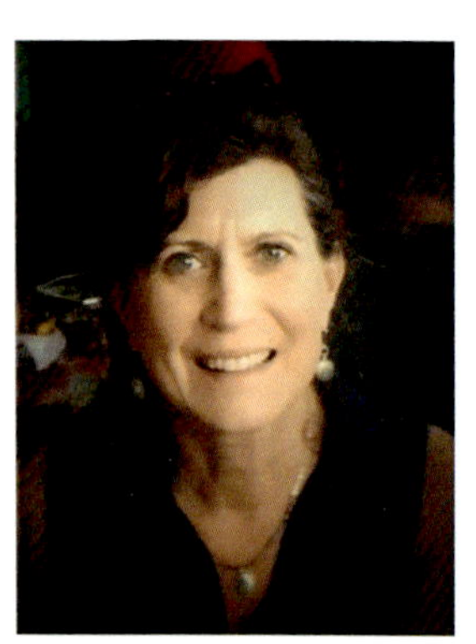

Winifred Werther
Amgen Inc.
South San Francisco, CA, USA

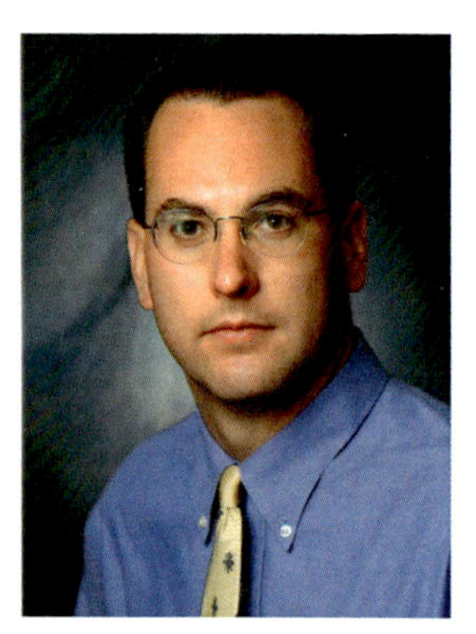

Christopher S. Coffey
University of Iowa
Iowa City, IA, USA

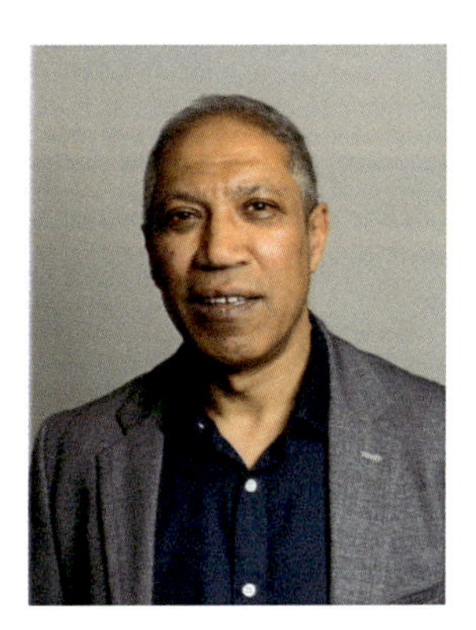

Mahesh K. B. Parmar
University College of London
London, England

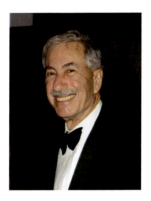

Lawrence Friedman
Rockville, MD, USA

Contributors

Inmaculada Aban Department of Biostatistics, University of Alabama at Birmingham, Birmingham, AL, USA

Trinidad Ajazi Alliance for Clinical Trials in Oncology, University of Chicago, Chicago, IL, USA

Andrew S. Allen Department of Biostatistics and Bioinformatics, Duke University, School of Medicine, Durham, NC, USA

Daniel Almirall University of Michigan, Ann Arbor, MI, USA

Suresh Ankolekar Cytel Inc, Cambridge, MA, USA

Maastricht School of Management, Maastricht, Netherlands

M. Antoniou F. Hoffmann-La Roche Ltd, Basel, Switzerland

Gillian Armstrong GSK, Slaoui Center for Vaccines Research, Rockville, MD, USA

Sheriza Baksh Johns Hopkins Bloomberg School of Public Health, Baltimore, MD, USA

Bruce A. Barton Department of Population and Quantitative Health Sciences, University of Massachusetts Medical School, Worcester, MA, USA

Emine O. Bayman University of Iowa, Iowa City, IA, USA

Vance W. Berger Biometry Research Group, National Cancer Institute, Rockville, MD, USA

Kate Bickett Emmes, Rockville, MD, USA

Lynette Blacher Frontier Science Amherst, Amherst, NY, USA

Gillian Booth Leeds Institute of Clinical Trials Research, University of Leeds, Leeds, UK

Laura E. Bothwell Worcester State University, Worcester, MA, USA

Anne-Laure Boulesteix Institute for Medical Information Processing, Biometry, and Epidemiology, LMU Munich, Munich, Germany

Isabelle Boutron Epidemiology and Biostatistics Research Center (CRESS), Inserm UMR1153, Université de Paris, Paris, France

Otis W. Brawley Johns Hopkins School of Medicine, and Johns Hopkins Bloomberg School of Public Health, Baltimore, MD, USA

L. C. Brown MRC Clinical Trials Unit, UCL Institute of Clinical Trials and Methodology, London, UK

Carolyn Burke The Emmes Company, LLC, Rockville, MD, USA

Kristin M. Burns National Heart, Lung, and Blood Institute, National Institutes of Health, Bethesda, MD, USA

Marc Buyse International Drug Development Institute (IDDI) Inc., San Francisco, CA, USA

CluePoints S.A., Louvain-la-Neuve, Belgium and I-BioStat, University of Hasselt, Louvain-la-Neuve, Belgium

Interuniversity Institute for Biostatistics and Statistical Bioinformatics (I-BioStat), Hasselt University, Hasselt, Belgium

Samantha-Jo Caetano Department of Mathematics and Statistics, McMaster University, Hamilton, ON, Canada

Steve Canham European Clinical Research Infrastructure Network (ECRIN), Paris, France

Ashley Case Emmes, Rockville, MD, USA

Anna Chaimani Université de Paris, Research Center of Epidemiology and Statistics (CRESS-U1153), INSERM, Paris, France

Cochrane France, Paris, France

Bingshu E. Chen Canadian Cancer Trials Group, Queen's University, Kingston, ON, Canada

Victoria Chia Amgen Inc., Thousand Oaks, CA, USA

Emmanuel Chigutsa Pharmacometrics, Eli Lilly and Company, Zionsville, IN, USA

Babak Choodari-Oskooei MRC Clinical Trials Unit at UCL, Institute of Clinical Trials and Methodology, London, UK

Joan B. Cobb Pettit Johns Hopkins Bloomberg School of Public Health, Baltimore, MD, USA

Graham A. Colditz Division of Public Health Sciences, Department of Surgery, Washington University School of Medicine, Saint Louis, MO, USA

Alan Colley Amgen, Ltd, Cambridge, UK

Julia Collins The Emmes Company, LLC, Rockville, MD, USA

Mark R. Conaway University of Virginia Health System, Charlottesville, VA, USA

David Couper Department of Biostatistics, Gillings School of Global Public Health, University of North Carolina, Chapel Hill, NC, USA

Gary R. Cutter Department of Biostatistics, University of Alabama at Birmingham, Birmingham, AL, USA

John J. DeBoy Covington & Burling LLP, Washington, DC, USA

James J. Dignam Department of Public Health Sciences, The University of Chicago, Chicago, IL, USA

Márcio A. Diniz Biostatistics and Bioinfomatics Research Center, Samuel Oschin Cancer Center, Cedars Sinai Medical Center, Los Angeles, CA, USA

Damien Drubay INSERM U1018, CESP, Paris-Saclay University, UVSQ, Villejuif, France

Gustave Roussy, Service de Biostatistique et d'Epidémiologie, Villejuif, France

Lea Drye Office of Clinical Affairs, Blue Cross Blue Shield Association, Chicago, IL, USA

Amylou C. Dueck Division of Biomedical Statistics and Informatics, Department of Health Sciences Research, Mayo Clinic, Scottsdale, AZ, USA

Keren R. Dunn Office of Research Compliance and Quality Improvement, Cedars-Sinai Medical Center, Los Angeles, CA, USA

Richard Emsley Department of Biostatistics and Health Informatics, King's College London, London, UK

Katrina Epnere WCG Statistics Collaborative, Washington, DC, USA

Ann-Margret Ervin Johns Hopkins Bloomberg School of Public Health, Baltimore, MD, USA

The Johns Hopkins Center for Clinical Trials and Evidence Synthesis, Johns Hopkins University, Baltimore, MD, USA

Theodoros Evrenoglou Université de Paris, Research Center of Epidemiology and Statistics (CRESS-U1153), INSERM, Paris, France

Valerii V. Fedorov ICON, North Wales, PA, USA

Bart Ferket Ichan School of Medicine at Mount Sinai, New York, NY, USA

Maria Figueroa The Emmes Company, LLC, Rockville, MD, USA

Jane Forrest Frontier Science (Scotland) Ltd, Grampian View, Kincraig, UK

Boris Freidlin Biometric Research Program, Division of Cancer Treatment and Diagnosis, National Cancer Institute, Bethesda, MD, USA

Patricia A. Ganz Jonsson Comprehensive Cancer Center, University of California at Los Angeles, Los Angeles, CA, USA

Elizabeth Garrett-Mayer American Society of Clinical Oncology, Alexandria, VA, USA

Jennifer J. Gassman Department of Quantitative Health Sciences, Cleveland Clinic, Cleveland, OH, USA

Nancy L. Geller National Heart, Lung and Blood Institute, National Institutes of Health, Bethesda, MD, USA

Stephen L. George Department of Biostatistics and Bioinformatics, Basic Science Division, Duke University School of Medicine, Durham, NC, USA

Bruce J. Giantonio The ECOG-ACRIN Cancer Research Group, Philadelphia, PA, USA

Massachusetts General Hospital, Boston, MA, USA

Department of Medical Oncology, University of Pretoria, Pretoria, South Africa

David V. Glidden Department of Epidemiology and Biostatistics, University of California San Francisco, San Francisco, CA, USA

Ekkehard Glimm Novartis Pharma AG, Basel, Switzerland

Jogarao V. Gobburu Center for Translational Medicine, University of Maryland School of Pharmacy, Baltimore, MD, USA

Judith D. Goldberg Department of Population Health and Environmental Medicine, New York University School of Medicine, New York, NY, USA

Benjamin A. Goldstein Department of Biostatistics and Bioinformatics, Duke Clinical Research Institute, Duke University Medical Center, Durham, NC, USA

Julie D. Gottlieb Johns Hopkins University School of Medicine, Baltimore, MD, USA

Stephen J. Greene Duke Clinical Research Institute, Durham, NC, USA

Division of Cardiology, Duke University School of Medicine, Durham, NC, USA

Gillian Gresham Samuel Oschin Comprehensive Cancer Institute, Cedars-Sinai Medical Center, Los Angeles, CA, USA

Jeff Jianfei Guo Division of Pharmacy Practice and Administrative Sciences, University of Cincinnati College of Pharmacy, Cincinnati, OH, USA

Gordon H. Guyatt McMaster University, Hamilton, ON, Canada

Olivia Hackworth University of Michigan, Ann Arbor, MI, USA

Tarek Haddad Medtronic Inc, Minneapolis, MN, USA

Susan Halabi Department of Biostatistics and Bioinformatics, Duke University Medical Center, Durham, NC, USA

Eric Hardter The Emmes Company, LLC, Rockville, MD, USA

Barbara S. Hawkins Johns Hopkins School of Medicine and Bloomberg School of Public Health, The Johns Hopkins University, Baltimore, MD, USA

Richard J. Hayes Faculty of Epidemiology and Population Health, London School of Hygiene and Tropical Medicine, London, UK

Adrian F. Hernandez Duke Clinical Research Institute, Durham, NC, USA

Division of Cardiology, Duke University School of Medicine, Durham, NC, USA

Sally Hopewell Centre for Statistics in Medicine, Nuffield Department of Orthopaedics, Rheumatology and Musculoskeletal Sciences, University of Oxford, Oxford, UK

George Howard Department of Biostatistics, University of Alabama at Birmingham, Birmingham, AL, USA

Asbjørn Hróbjartsson Cochrane Denmark and Centre for Evidence-Based Medicine Odense, University of Southern Denmark, Odense, Denmark

Sam Hsiao Cytel Inc, Cambridge, MA, USA

Jason C. Hsu Department of Statistics, The Ohio State University, Columbus, OH, USA

Julie Jackson Frontier Science (Scotland) Ltd, Grampian View, Kincraig, UK

Shu Jiang Division of Public Health Sciences, Department of Surgery, Washington University School of Medicine, Saint Louis, MO, USA

Byron Jones Novartis Pharma AG, Basel, Switzerland

David S. Jones Harvard University, Cambridge, MA, USA

A. L. Jorgensen Department of Health Data Science, University of Liverpool, Liverpool, UK

John A. Kairalla University of Florida, Gainesville, FL, USA

Eloise Kaizar The Ohio State University, Columbus, OH, USA

Shamir N. Kalaria Center for Translational Medicine, University of Maryland School of Pharmacy, Baltimore, MD, USA

Michael Kelsh Amgen Inc., Thousand Oaks, CA, USA

Siyoen Kil LSK Global Pharmaceutical Services, Seoul, Republic of Korea

Christopher Kim Amgen Inc., Thousand Oaks, CA, USA

Jonathan Kimmelman Biomedical Ethics Unit, McGill University, Montreal, QC, Canada

Kristin Knust Emmes, Rockville, MD, USA

Edward L. Korn Biometric Research Program, Division of Cancer Treatment and Diagnosis, National Cancer Institute, Bethesda, MD, USA

Richard Kravitz University of California Davis, Davis, CA, USA

Wen-Hua Kuo National Yang-Ming University, Taipei City, Taiwan

Sabine Landau Department of Biostatistics and Health Informatics, King's College London, London, UK

Jimmy Le National Eye Institute, Bethesda, MD, USA

Justin M. Leach Department of Biostatistics, University of Alabama at Birmingham, Birmingham, AL, USA

Michael LeBlanc SWOG Statistical Center, Fred Hutchinson Cancer Research Center, Seattle, WA, USA

J. Jack Lee Department of Biostatistics, University of Texas MD Anderson Cancer Center, Houston, TX, USA

Shing M. Lee Department of Biostatistics, Mailman School of Public Health, Columbia University, New York, NY, USA

Cheng-Shiun Leu Department of Biostatistics, Mailman School of Public Health, Columbia University, New York, NY, USA

Bruce Levin Department of Biostatistics, Mailman School of Public Health, Columbia University, New York, NY, USA

Fan Li Department of Biostatistics, Yale University, School of Public Health, New Haven, CT, USA

Heng Li Center for Devices and Radiological Health, U.S. Food and Drug Administration, Silver Spring, MD, USA

Liang Li Department of Biostatistics, The University of Texas MD Anderson Cancer Center, Houston, TX, USA

Tianjing Li Department of Ophthalmology, University of Colorado Anschutz Medical Campus, Aurora, CO, USA

Amanda Lilley-Kelly Clinical Trials Research Unit, Leeds Institute of Clinical Trials Research, University of Leeds, Leeds, UK

Yuliya Lokhnygina Department of Biostatistics and Bioinformatics, Duke University, Durham, NC, USA

James P. Long Department of Biostatistics, University of Texas MD Anderson Cancer Center, Houston, TX, USA

Anita M. Loughlin Corrona LLC, Waltham, MA, USA

Zheng Lu Clinical Pharmacology and Exploratory Development, Astellas Pharma, Northbrook, IL, USA

Tiago M. Magalhães Department of Statistics, Institute of Exact Sciences, Federal University of Juiz de Fora, Juiz de Fora, Minas Gerais, Brazil

Adrian P. Mander Centre for Trials Research, Cardiff University, Cardiff, UK

Linda Marillo Frontier Science Amherst, Amherst, NY, USA

Barbara K. Martin Administrative Director, Research Institute, Penn Medicine Lancaster General Health, Lancaster, PA, USA

J. Rosser Matthews General Dynamics Health Solutions, Defense and Veterans Brain Injury Center, Silver Spring, MD, USA

Madhu Mazumdar Director of Institute for Healthcare Delivery Science, Mount Sinai Health System, NY, USA

Gina L. Mazza Division of Biomedical Statistics and Informatics, Department of Health Sciences Research, Mayo Clinic, Scottsdale, AZ, USA

Michael P. McDermott Department of Biostatistics and Computational Biology, University of Rochester Medical Center, Rochester, NY, USA

Eleanor McFadden Frontier Science (Scotland) Ltd., Kincraig, Scotland, UK

Katie Meadmore University of Southampton, Southampton, UK

Cyrus Mehta Cytel Inc, Cambridge, MA, USA

Harvard T.H. Chan School of Public Health, Boston, MA, USA

Curtis L. Meinert Department of Epidemiology, School of Public Health, Johns Hopkins University, Baltimore, MD, USA

Catherine A. Meldrum University of Michigan, Ann Arbor, MI, USA

Sreelatha Meleth RTI International, Atlanta, GA, USA

Diana Merino Friends of Cancer Research, Washington, DC, USA

Peter Mesenbrink Novartis Pharmaceuticals Corporation, East Hannover, NJ, USA

Silvia Metelli Université de Paris, Research Center of Epidemiology and Statistics (CRESS-U1153), INSERM, Paris, France

Assistance Publique - Hôpitaux de Paris (APHP), Paris, France

Catherine M. Meyers Office of Clinical and Regulatory Affairs, National Institutes of Health, National Center for Complementary and Integrative Health, Bethesda, MD, USA

Stefan Michiels INSERM U1018, CESP, Paris-Saclay University, UVSQ, Villejuif, France

Gustave Roussy, Service de Biostatistique et d'Epidémiologie, Villejuif, France

Johanna Mielke Novartis Pharma AG, Basel, Switzerland

J. Philip Miller Division of Biostatistics, Washington University School of Medicine in St. Louis, St. Louis, MO, USA

Reza D. Mirza Department of Medicine, McMaster University, Hamilton, ON, Canada

David Moher Centre for Journaology, Clinical Epidemiology Program, Ottawa Hospital Research Institute, Canadian EQUATOR centre, Ottawa, ON, Canada

Lawrence H. Moulton Departments of International Health and Biostatistics, Johns Hopkins Bloomberg School of Public Health, Baltimore, MD, USA

Rajat Mukherjee Cytel Inc, Cambridge, MA, USA

Patrick Onghena Faculty of Psychology and Educational Sciences, KU Leuven, Leuven, Belgium

Jamie B. Oughton Clinical Trials Research Unit, Leeds Institute of Clinical Trials Research, University of Leeds, Leeds, UK

Matthew J. Page School of Public Health and Preventive Medicine, Monash University, Melbourne, VIC, Australia

Yuko Y. Palesch Data Coordination Unit, Department of Public Health Sciences, Medical University of South Carolina, Charleston, SC, USA

Olympia Papachristofi London School of Hygiene and Tropical Medicine, London, UK

Clinical Development and Analytics, Novartis Pharma AG, Basel, Switzerland

Mahesh K. B. Parmar MRC Clinical Trials Unit at UCL, Institute of Clinical Trials and Methodology, London, UK

Wendy R. Parulekar Canadian Cancer Trials Group, Queen's University, Kingston, ON, Canada

Gail D. Pearson National Heart, Lung, and Blood Institute, National Institutes of Health, Bethesda, MD, USA

Victoria L. Pemberton National Heart, Lung, and Blood Institute, National Institutes of Health, Bethesda, MD, USA

Michelle Pernice Dynavax Technologies Corporation, Emeryville, CA, USA

Julien Peron CNRS, UMR 5558, Laboratoire de Biométrie et Biologie Evolutive, Université Lyon 1, France

Departments of Biostatistics and Medical Oncology, Centre Hospitalier Lyon-Sud, Institut de Cancérologie des Hospices Civils de Lyon, Lyon, France

Gina R. Petroni Translational Research and Applied Statistics, Public Health Sciences, University of Virginia Health System, Charlottesville, VA, USA

David Petullo Division of Biometrics II, Office of Biostatistics Office of Translational Sciences, Center for Drug Evaluation and Research, U.S. Food and Drug Administration, Silver Spring, MD, USA

Patrick P. J. Phillips UCSF Center for Tuberculosis, University of California San Francisco, San Francisco, CA, USA

Department of Epidemiology and Biostatistics, University of California San Francisco, San Francisco, CA, USA

Steven Piantadosi Department of Surgery, Division of Surgical Oncology, Brigham and Women's Hospital, Harvard Medical School, Boston, MA, USA

Scott H. Podolsky Harvard Medical School, Boston, MA, USA

Gregory R. Pond Department of Oncology, McMaster University, Hamilton, ON, Canada

Ontario Institute for Cancer Research, Toronto, ON, Canada

Philip C. Prorok Division of Cancer Prevention, National Cancer Institute, Bethesda, MD, USA

Michael A. Proschan National Institute of Allergy and Infectious Diseases, Bethesda, MD, USA

Eric Riley Frontier Science (Scotland) Ltd., Kincraig, Scotland, UK

Karen A. Robinson Department of Medicine, Johns Hopkins University, Baltimore, MD, USA

Emily Robison Optum Labs, Las Vegas, NV, USA

Frank W. Rockhold Department of Biostatistics and Bioinformatics, Duke Clinical Research Institute, Duke University Medical Center, Durham, NC, USA

Sergei Romashkan National Institutes of Health, National Institute on Aging, Bethesda, MD, USA

Wayne Rosamond Department of Epidemiology, Gillings School of Global Public Health, University of North Carolina, Chapel Hill, NC, USA

William F. Rosenberger Biostatistics Center, The George Washington University, Rockville, MD, USA

Patrick Royston MRC Clinical Trials Unit at UCL, Institute of Clinical Trials and Methodology, London, UK

Estelle Russek-Cohen Office of Biostatistics, Center for Drug Evaluation and Research, U.S. Food and Drug Administration, Silver Spring, MD, USA

Laurie Ryan National Institutes of Health, National Institute on Aging, Bethesda, MD, USA

Anna Sadura Canadian Cancer Trials Group, Queen's University, Kingston, ON, Canada

Ian J. Saldanha Department of Health Services, Policy, and Practice and Department of Epidemiology, Brown University School of Public Health, Providence, RI, USA

Amber Salter Division of Biostatistics, Washington University School of Medicine in St. Louis, St. Louis, MO, USA

Marc D. Samsky Duke Clinical Research Institute, Durham, NC, USA

Division of Cardiology, Duke University School of Medicine, Durham, NC, USA

Frank J. Sasinowski University of Rochester School of Medicine, Department of Neurology, Rochester, NY, USA

Willi Sauerbrei Institute of Medical Biometry and Statistics, Faculty of Medicine and Medical Center - University of Freiburg, Freiburg, Germany

Roberta W. Scherer Department of Epidemiology, Johns Hopkins Bloomberg School of Public Health, Baltimore, MD, USA

Pamela E. Scott Office of the Commissioner, U.S. Food and Drug Administration, Silver Spring, MD, USA

Nicholas J. Seewald University of Michigan, Ann Arbor, MI, USA

Praharsh Shah University of Pennsylvania, Philadelphia, PA, USA

Linda Sharples London School of Hygiene and Tropical Medicine, London, UK

Pamela A. Shaw University of Pennsylvania Perelman School of Medicine, Philadelphia, PA, USA

Dikla Shmueli-Blumberg The Emmes Company, LLC, Rockville, MD, USA

Ellen Sigal Friends of Cancer Research, Washington, DC, USA

Ida Sim Division of General Internal Medicine, University of California San Francisco, San Francisco, CA, USA

Richard Simon R Simon Consulting, Potomac, MD, USA

Jennifer Smith Sunesis Pharmaceuticals Inc, San Francisco, CA, USA

Alfred Sommer Johns Hopkins Bloomberg School of Public Health, Baltimore, MD, USA

Mark Stewart Friends of Cancer Research, Washington, DC, USA

Inna Strakovsky University of Pennsylvania, Philadelphia, PA, USA

Oleksandr Sverdlov Novartis Pharmaceuticals Corporation, East Hannover, NJ, USA

Michael J. Sweeting Department of Health Sciences, University of Leicester, Leicester, UK

Department of Public Health and Primary Care, University of Cambridge, Cambridge, UK

Matthew R. Sydes MRC Clinical Trials Unit at UCL, Institute of Clinical Trials and Methodology, London, UK

Szu-Yu Tang Roche Tissue Diagnostics, Oro Valley, AZ, USA

Catherine Tangen SWOG Statistical Center, Fred Hutchinson Cancer Research Center, Seattle, WA, USA

Mourad Tighiouart Cedars-Sinai Medical Center, Los Angeles, CA, USA

Guangyu Tong Department of Sociology, Duke University, Durham, NC, USA

Xiao Tong Clinical Pharmacology, Biogen, Boston, MA, USA

Alison Urton Canadian Cancer Trials Group, Queen's University, Kingston, ON, Canada

Diane Uschner Department of Statistics, George Mason University, Fairfax, VA, USA

James E. Valentine University of Maryland Carey School of Law, Baltimore, MD, USA

Ben Van Calster Department of Development and Regeneration, KU Leuven, Leuven, Belgium

Department of Biomedical Data Sciences, Leiden University Medical Center, Leiden, The Netherlands

S. Swaroop Vedula Malone Center for Engineering in Healthcare, Whiting School of Engineering, The Johns Hopkins University, Baltimore, MD, USA

Jenifer H. Voeks Department of Neurology, Medical University of South Carolina, Charleston, SC, USA

Sunita Vohra University of Alberta, Edmonton, AB, Canada

Annie X. Wang Covington & Burling LLP, Washington, DC, USA

Hechuan Wang Center for Translational Medicine, University of Maryland School of Pharmacy, Baltimore, MD, USA

J. Wason Population Health Sciences Institute, Newcastle University, Newcastle upon Tyne, UK

MRC Biostatistics Unit, University of Cambridge, Cambridge, UK

Claire Weber Excellence Consulting, LLC, Moraga, CA, USA

Heidi L. Weiss Biostatistics and Bioinformatics Shared Resource Facility, Markey Cancer Center, University of Kentucky, Lexington, KY, USA

Pascale Wermuth Basel, Switzerland

Winifred Werther Center for Observational Research, Amgen Inc, South San Francisco, CA, USA

Matthew Westmore University of Southampton, Southampton, UK

Graham M. Wheeler Imperial Clinical Trials Unit, Imperial College London, London, UK

Cancer Research UK & UCL Cancer Trials Centre, University College London, London, UK

O. Dale Williams Department of Biostatistics, University of North Carolina, Chapel Hill, NC, USA

Department of Medicine, University of Alabama at Birmingham, Birmingham, AL, USA

Janet Wittes Statistics Collaborative, Inc, Washington, DC, USA

Jianrong Wu Biostatistics and Bioinformatics Shared Resource Facility, Markey Cancer Center, University of Kentucky, Lexington, KY, USA

Samuel S. Wu University of Florida, Gainesville, FL, USA

Sharon D. Yeatts Data Coordination Unit, Department of Public Health Sciences, Medical University of South Carolina, Charleston, SC, USA

Lauren Yesko Emmes, Rockville, MD, USA

Gui-Shuang Ying Center for Preventive Ophthalmology and Biostatistics, Department of Ophthalmology, Perelman School of Medicine, University of Pennsylvania, Philadelphia, PA, USA

Jessica L. Yoos University of Pennsylvania, Philadelphia, PA, USA

Qilu Yu Office of Clinical and Regulatory Affairs, National Institutes of Health, National Center for Complementary and Integrative Health, Bethesda, MD, USA

Fan-fan Yu Statistics Collaborative, Inc., Washington, DC, USA

Lilly Q. Yue Center for Devices and Radiological Health, U.S. Food and Drug Administration, Silver Spring, MD, USA

Rachel Zahigian Vertex Pharmaceuticals, Boston, MA, USA

Lijuan Zeng Statistics Collaborative, Inc., Washington, DC, USA

Xiaobo Zhong Ichan School of Medicine at Mount Sinai, New York, NY, USA

Tracy Ziolek University of Pennsylvania, Philadelphia, PA, USA

Part IV

Bias Control and Precision

Controlling for Multiplicity, Eligibility, and Exclusions

39

Amber Salter and J. Philip Miller

Contents

Abstract

Multiple comparison procedures play an important role in controlling the accuracy of clinical trial results while trial eligibility and exclusions have the potential to introduce bias and reduce external validity. This chapter introduces the issues and sources of multiplicity and provides a description of the many different procedures that can be used to address multiplicity primarily used in the confirmatory clinical trial setting. Additionally, trial inclusion/exclusion criteria and enrichment strategies are reviewed.

A. Salter (✉) · J. P. Miller
Division of Biostatistics, Washington University School of Medicine in St. Louis, St. Louis, MO, USA
e-mail: amber@wustl.edu; jphilipmiller@wustl.edu

© Springer Nature Switzerland AG 2022

S. Piantadosi, C. L. Meinert (eds.), *Principles and Practice of Clinical Trials*,
https://doi.org/10.1007/978-3-319-52636-2_210

Keywords

Multiple comparison procedures · Inclusion/exclusion criteria · Enrichment strategies

Introduction

Clinical trial design continues to evolve and become increasingly complex due, in part, to efforts on making evaluation of new treatments more efficient. The use of multiple outcomes, dose levels, and/or populations results in challenges for decision-making, especially concern over making incorrect conclusions about the efficacy or safety of a treatment. As the multiplicity increases, the probability of making a false conclusion increases. Multiple strategies have been developed recently to maintain strong control over the error rate in clinical trials. Regulatory bodies such as the Federal Drug Administration (FDA) and European Medical Agency (EMA) have both recognized this issue and provided guidance on aspects of multiplicity in confirmatory clinical trials. In addition to issues of multiplicity, eligibility criteria and exclusions have the potential to add bias and reduce the external validity of a clinical trial.

Multiplicity

Introduction

Multiplicity problems in clinical trials results from conducting many comparisons within a single trial. Scenarios include evaluating multiple outcomes, dose levels, or patient populations. The chances of making incorrect conclusions regarding the hypotheses being tested increase as the multiplicity increases. Phase III trials are primarily used to demonstrate specific efficacy and safety claims of a drug, treatment, or device. In this setting, there is a need to control the increased probability of making an error. The consequence of this type of error in this confirmatory phase of treatment development could lead to adoption of a treatment with no beneficial effect.

Confirmatory clinical trials are designed primarily to establish evidence that a drug, treatment, or device is effective and safe. Most clinical trials make decisions about the success of the trial by constructing a hypothesis to test predetermined objectives. The hypothesis testing framework is traditionally associated with two types of error: type I (α) and type II (β) errors. Type I error, or rejecting a true null hypothesis, is controlled at a prespecified level; however, in the multiplicity setting, this error for each test has the potential to be inflate the trial level error rate when no adjustments are made for multiple comparisons. For confirmatory clinical trials, the type I error mandated by most regulatory agencies is a two-sided 5% level. Conventionally, the power ($1-\beta$) of a trial is set at 0.8 or above. While multiplicity increases the type I error in hypothesis testing, the statistical methods to control multiplicity may differentially affect the power of a trial. The effects on power should be examined in the trial planning stages.

Recognition for the importance of controlling multiplicity is increasing. While not every confirmatory trial is conducted to obtain regulatory approval, the EMA published a guidance document on multiplicity in clinical trials (EMA (European Medicines Agency) 2017) and the FDA released guidance on multiple outcomes in clinical trials in 2017 (FDA (U.S. Food and Drug Administration) 2017). The development of these guidance documents was partly a result of sponsors increased efforts to improve the efficiency of clinical trials. This efficiency can be gained by having a trial evaluate more than one outcome or more than one population. However, the need to control multiplicity in this setting is critical to maintain scientific rigor.

Safety measures are an important component in clinical trials, and specific safety outcomes or concerns are based on experiences in earlier phase trials. Specific safety outcomes are one type of safety measure and may be a specific outcome to be tested in a Phase III trial in conjunction with an efficacy outcome. Other safety measures, such as adverse events, may be considered more descriptive or exploratory in nature (Dmitrienko and D'Agostino 2018). If adverse event data is compared between groups, this could be considered a multiplicity issue which has the potential to identify false positive safety concerns. Application of methods such as the double false discovery rate has been proposed to more rigorously evaluate adverse events (Mehrotra and Heyse 2004) and reduce the complexity of safety profiles, especially in large drug or vaccine trials.

Statistical adjustment for multiplicity is not always necessary in the multiplicity setting. The objectives of the analysis need to be considered and scenarios which do not require adjustments for multiplicity exist. For instance, the use of co-primary outcomes where success of the trial depends on all outcomes being less than the significance level or when supplemental analyses are conducted (adjusting for covariates or a per-protocol analyses) for a single outcome (FDA (U.S. Food and Drug Administration) 2017; Proschan and Waclawiw 2000). While scenarios, such as co-primary outcomes, may not affect the type I error rate, their possible effect on power needs to be addressed in the design stage.

Sources of Multiplicity

Multiplicity problems arise in clinical trials from a variety of sources, such as evaluating treatment effects for several outcomes, for multiple dose levels, testing a prespecified set of potential moderator variables on subgroups or for multiple component outcomes. Interim analyses are another source of multiplicity. Statistical methods developed specifically for this issue are addressed in ▶ Chap. 59, "Interim Analysis in Clinical Trials." Clinical trials with just one multiplicity factor present are considered to have a single source multiplicity while those with more than one factor have a multiple source multiplicity. An example of multiple source multiplicity is a trial evaluating several dose levels in a general population and a targeted subgroup of the population.

Different methods are used for single and multiple sources of multiplicity. Choice of adjustment procedure utilizes clinical and statistical information to decide which method to implement. The multiplicity procedure chosen should be in line with the clinical trial objectives and investigate the effect of the method on statistical power. Simulations are often used to evaluate the effect of the procedures on power.

Adjustment for Single Sources of Multiplicity

For single sources of multiplicity, adjustment methods fall into two main categories: single step and hypothesis ordered methods. Single step methods test all hypotheses simultaneously, while ordered methods test hypotheses in a stepwise manner with the order based on the data (size of p-values) or are prespecified based on strong clinical information or prior studies. These methods can step-up or step-down where the significance level changes as the procedure progresses through the set of null hypotheses being tested due to the error rate being transferred from rejection of the prior null hypothesis. The step-up procedure will order the hypotheses from largest to smallest according to the p-values. The step-down procedures in data-driven hypotheses ordering will arrange the hypotheses from smallest to largest based on their associated p-values, and the testing ceases when a hypothesis fails to be rejected. Within these categories of adjustment methods, distributional information about the hypothesis tests is relevant to the choice of multiplicity method. Increased knowledge regarding the joint distribution of the test statistics among the hypotheses being tested leads to more powerful procedures being chosen (Dmitrienko and D'Agostino 2013). Nonparametric procedures make no assumptions regarding the joint distribution while semiparametric procedures assume the hypothesis tests follow a distribution but have an unknown correlation structure (Dmitrienko et al. 2013). Additionally, there are parametric procedures, such as the Dunnett's test (Dunnett 1955), which assume an explicit distribution for the joint distribution of hypothesis tests and are associated with classical regression and analysis of variance and covariance models.

Single step procedures control the error rate using simple decision rules in order to adjust the significance level. The Bonferroni correction is a classic example of a single step nonparametric multiplicity adjustment where the overall error rate is divided by the number of tests being tested to obtain an adjusted significance level for all tests (α/m) (Dunn 1961). For example, if the overall error rate is 0.05 and three tests are being conducted, the adjusted significance level for all three tests is 0.0167. The Bonferroni method can also be applied by assigning prespecified weights to different tests to account for clinical importance or other factors in the multiplicity adjustment (FDA (U.S. Food and Drug Administration) 2017).

Other single step procedures include the Simes and Šidák semiparametric multiplicity adjustment methods (Šidák 1967; Simes 1986). Both are uniformly more powerful than the Bonferroni. The Simes procedure is a global null hypothesis test, similar to the omnibus F test in an analysis of variance (ANOVA). While the procedure is able to identify if at least one null hypothesis is false, it does not identify which of the specific hypotheses is false. The Šidák procedure adjusts the significance level (p_i) using the number of hypotheses tested (m) at the overall error level (α) by $p_i \leq 1 - (1-\alpha)^{1/m}$. As in the example for the Bonferroni correction, if there are three tests being conducted at an overall error rate of 0.05, the adjusted significance level using the Šidák procedure is $1 - (1–0.05)^{1/3} = 0.0170$.

While the single step procedures have the advantage of simplicity and relative ease of implementation, stepwise procedures are more powerful procedures. The Simes and Šidák procedures can be utilized as stepwise procedures with data-driven hypothesis ordering and have increased power compared to the single step procedure. The step-down Šidák procedure tests each hypothesis sequentially according to ordered p-values (smallest to largest). The first $i = 1 \ldots m-1$ hypotheses have an adjusted significance level of $p_i \leq 1 - (1-\alpha)^{1/(m - i + 1)}$ where subsequent hypotheses are only tested if the ith hypothesis is rejected. The final m hypothesis is tested at a significance level of 0.05. Thus, if there are three hypotheses being tested at an overall error rate of 0.05, the first hypothesis would be tested at an adjusted significance level of 0.0170, the second hypothesis would be tested at 0.0253, and the third hypothesis tested at 0.05.

Other stepwise procedures include the nonparametric Holm procedure (Holm 1979) and the semiparametric Hochberg and Hommel procedures (Hochberg 1988; Hommel 1988). The Holm procedure is a step-up procedure utilizing the Bonferroni procedure where the mth hypothesis is adjusted for the remaining hypotheses to be tested. To illustrate for a set of three hypotheses at a significance level of 0.05, the first hypothesis is tested at the 0.0167 ($\alpha/3$), the second hypothesis is tested at 0.025 ($\alpha/2$), and the third hypothesis is tested at 0.05 ($\alpha/1$). The Hochberg and Hommel procedures are stepwise extensions of the Simes' procedure based on step-up algorithms. Starting with the largest p-value, the Hochberg procedure compares the hypothesis p-value to the adjusted significance level determined by $p_{(m - i + 1)} \leq \alpha/i$, and if the hypothesis is rejected, then all m hypotheses are rejected. Otherwise, the next hypotheses are tested in a similar manner until a hypothesis is rejected or the final m hypothesis is reached. At the mth hypothesis, the adjusted significance level is $p_m \leq \alpha/m$. With three hypotheses being tested at the 0.05 significance level, the first hypothesis with the largest p-value is tested at the 0.05 significance level, the second and third hypotheses are tested at the 0.025 and 0.0167 levels, respectively. The Hommel procedure is similar to the Hochberg procedure; however, instead of depending only on the p-value associated with the null hypothesis being tested as is the case with the Hochberg, the Hommel procedure adds other conditions when a hypothesis fails to be rejected to increase the number of hypotheses rejected. The Hommel procedure incorporates the preceding hypothesis to reject the current null hypothesis (Dmitrienko et al. 2013).

Multiple testing procedures used for prespecified hypothesis ordering, such as the nonparametric fixed-sequence or fallback procedures, incorporate prior clinical and logical information. The order in which the hypotheses will be tested is defined before the trial begins. The fixed-sequence method places the more important hypotheses to be tested first and is tested at the trial significance level. If the hypothesis is rejected, then the next hypothesis is tested; however, if the hypothesis fails to be rejected, the testing ceases and the remaining hypotheses fail to be rejected. The fallback procedure is a more flexible approach to prespecified ordering that allows for other hypotheses to be tested in the event the preceding hypothesis fails to be rejected (FDA (U.S. Food and Drug Administration) 2017; Wiens 2003). The fixed sequence of hypotheses are maintained, but the type I error is divided up between the hypothesis being tested. The division of the significance level uses weights (w_i) which are nonnegative and sum to 1. The first hypothesis is tested at the adjusted significance level determined by $p_i \leq \alpha w_i$, and if the hypothesis fails to be rejected, the second hypothesis is tested at $p_i \leq \alpha w_i$. However, if the first hypothesis is rejected, then second hypothesis is tested at the overall error rate as the unused alpha is passed on to the next test in the sequence.

Adjustments for Multiple Sources of Multiplicity

The procedures used for multiple sources of multiplicity have an additional complexity inherent in that the multiple sources of multiplicity need to be addressed. A common manifestation of having multiple sources of multiplicity is having multiple families of hypotheses in the form of hierarchy in clinical trial objectives (primary, secondary, and tertiary objectives). The strategy usually employed for this setting is called a gatekeeping procedure and tests the hypotheses in the first (primary objectives) family with a single source adjustment method. The second family of hypotheses is tested with a multiplicity adjustment only if the primary family has demonstrated statistical success. The first family of hypothesis tests acts as a gatekeeper to testing the second family of hypotheses. The gatekeepers can be designed to be serial or parallel where serial gatekeepers require all hypotheses in the first family to be rejected before proceeding to the second family of hypotheses, while parallel gatekeepers only require at least one hypothesis to be rejected. These procedures allow for the error rate to be transferred to subsequent families of testing. These approaches can be further extended to allow for retesting to occur by transferring error back from the subsequent families to previous families (second family of hypothesis back to the first family). The choice of procedure again depends on the clinical objectives of the trial. Trials which have used these procedures include the lurasidone trial in schizophrenia and CLEAN-TAVI in severe aortic stenosis (Haussig et al. 2016; Meltzer et al. 2011).

Software

Software implementation of these procedures is found in SAS and R software. SAS has a procedure PROC MULTTEST to compute the adjusted p-values for the more common procedures. R packages have been developed to implement many of the multiple testing procedures, such as multcomp and multxpert (Dmitrienko and D’Agostino 2013).

Summary

Multiplicity issues arise from various sources in clinical trials and are defined as the evaluation of different aspects of treatment efficacy simultaneously (Dmitrienko et al. 2013). The more commonly encountered multiplicity problems are found in the use of multiple outcomes, composite outcomes and their components, multiple doses, and multiple subgroups or populations. One or a combination of these may be found in a clinical trial, and as the number of multiple comparisons increases, the probability of making a false conclusion, or type 1 error, increases. This inflation of the type 1 error has the consequence of incorrectly concluding that a treatment is efficacious or safe. Multiple methods for controlling for multiplicity have recently been developed (Dmitrienko et al. 2013). These methods range from simple to complex where there is a need to handle multiple sources of multiplicity in a clinical trial. The choice of adjustment to be used should be based on clinical and statistical information and predefined in the statistical analysis plan for a clinical trial (Gamble et al. 2017).

Eligibility and Exclusion

A clinical trial aims to have a sample which is representative of the population that would have the treatment applied clinically if the trial is positive. The selection of individuals for inclusion into a clinical trial is based on predefined eligibility criteria. Criteria in clinical trials may be used to limit the heterogeneity of the trial population, limit inference for obtaining the outcome measure (e.g., individuals with a comorbidities at high risk of dying for an unrelated cause prior to the outcome assessment), and related to safety concerns (e.g., pregnant women or individuals at increased risk of an adverse outcome). Yet, the potential consequences of eligibility criteria are to create selection bias in the study population and reduced external validity for the trial. One of the primary ways to control selection bias is through randomization and allocation concealment. By using randomization to assign individuals to a treatment or intervention, there will be balance in the known and unknown factors, on average, between the groups. Yet, randomization alone does not completely eliminate selection bias. There is still a chance for individuals to be selectively enrolled in a trial should those in charge of recruitment know what the next treatment allocation will be. Without concealment, those enrolling patients may take eligible individuals which they perceive may do worse and randomize them when they know a placebo assignment is likely. It is established that clinical trial populations differ from the larger clinical population. The eligibility criteria often create a highly selected population that can limit the external validity of the trial. Recommendations to improve the reporting of the eligibility criteria are encouraged in order to increase awareness among clinicians reading the findings to more appropriately assess who the results apply to.

Run-in periods, placebo or treatment, or implementing enrichment strategies are examples of exclusion criteria in clinical trials. These occur prior to randomization and are utilized to select or exclude individuals from a trial. Using a run-in period can help reduce the number of noncompliant individuals who are randomized or excluding those who experience adverse events (Rothwell 2005). Enrichment strategies focus on recruiting individuals who are likely to respond well in a trial such as nonresponders to a previous treatment. These exclusion criteria have the potential to reduce the external validity of the study.

Summary and Conclusion

There is a need for inclusion/exclusion criteria in clinical trials, but their use may result in potential bias or lack of generalizability of the study results. Enrichment strategies are useful in limiting individuals who may discontinue participation in a trial or not respond well to a treatment. While these strategies may result in more subjects (and consequently more power), the external validity of the trial may be compromised.

Key Facts

- Awareness is increasing for the need to identify and address multiplicity issues in confirmatory clinical trials.
- There are many procedures which control the type I error inflation resulting from multiplicity issues in clinical trials. The choice of procedure should be based on clinical and statistical information and determined during the design phase of a clinical trial.
- Eligibility criteria and exclusion strategies may be necessary to implement in a clinical trial; however, careful review of the potential biases as a result should be conducted.

Cross-References

▶ Confident Statistical Inference with Multiple Outcomes, Subgroups, and Other Issues of Multiplicity
▶ Interim Analysis in Clinical Trials

References

Dmitrienko A, D'Agostino R (2013) Traditional multiplicity adjustment methods in clinical trials. Stat Med 32(29):5172–5218. https://doi.org/10.1002/sim.5990

Dmitrienko A, D'Agostino RB (2018) Multiplicity considerations in clinical trials. N Engl J Med 378(22):2115–2122. https://doi.org/10.1056/NEJMra1709701

Dmitrienko A, D'Agostino RB Sr, Huque MF (2013) Key multiplicity issues in clinical drug development. Stat Med 32(7):1079–1111. https://doi.org/10.1002/sim.5642

Dunn OJ (1961) Multiple comparisons among means. J Am Stat Assoc 56(293):52–64. https://doi.org/10.1080/01621459.1961.10482090
Dunnett CW (1955) A multiple comparison procedure for comparing several treatments with a control. J Am Stat Assoc 50(272):1096–1121. https://doi.org/10.1080/01621459.1955.10501294
EMA (European MedicinesAgency) (2017) Guideline on multiplicity issues in clinical trials. Retrieved from www.ema.europa.eu/contact
FDA (U.S. Food and Drug Administration) (2017) Multiple endpoints in clinical trials: guidance for industry. Retrieved from http://www.fda.gov/Drugs/GuidanceComplianceRegulatoryInformation/Guidances/default.htm
Gamble C, Krishan A, Stocken D, Lewis S, Juszczak E, Doré C, . . . Loder E (2017) Guidelines for the content of statistical analysis plans in clinical trials. JAMA 318(23): 2337. https://doi.org/10.1001/jama.2017.18556
Haussig S, Mangner N, Dwyer MG, Lehmkuhl L, Lücke C, Woitek F, . . . Linke A (2016). Effect of a cerebral protection device on brain lesions following transcatheter aortic valve implantation in patients with severe aortic stenosis. JAMA 316(6): 592. https://doi.org/10.1001/jama.2016.10302
Hochberg Y (1988) A sharper Bonferroni procedure for multiple tests of significance. Biometrika 75(4):800–802. https://doi.org/10.1093/biomet/75.4.800
Holm S (1979) A simple sequentially rejective multiple test procedure. Scand J Stat 6(2):65–70. Retrieved from https://www.jstor.org/stable/pdf/4615733.pdf?refreqid=excelsior%3Ab73e56d22a17fe5eebc22397ada28121
Hommel G (1988) A stagewise rejective multiple test procedure based on a modified Bonferroni test. Biometrika 75(2):383–386. https://doi.org/10.1093/biomet/75.2.383
Mehrotra DV, Heyse JF (2004) Use of the false discovery rate for evaluating clinical safety data. Stat Methods Med Res 13(3):227–238. https://doi.org/10.1191/0962280204sm363ra
Meltzer HY, Cucchiaro J, Silva R, Ogasa M, Phillips D, Xu J, . . . Loebel A (2011) Lurasidone in the treatment of schizophrenia: a randomized, double-blind, placebo- and olanzapine-controlled study. Am J Psychiatry 168(9): 957–967. https://doi.org/10.1176/appi.ajp.2011.10060907
Proschan MA, Waclawiw MA (2000) Practical guidelines for multiplicity adjustment in clinical trials. Control Clin Trials 21(6):527–539. https://doi.org/10.1016/S0197-2456(00)00106-9
Rothwell PM (2005) External validity of randomised controlled trials: "to whom do the results of this trial apply?". Lancet 365(9453):82–93. https://doi.org/10.1016/S0140-6736(04)17670-8
Šidák Z (1967) Rectangular confidence regions for the means of multivariate normal distributions. J Am Stat Assoc 62(318):626–633. https://doi.org/10.1080/01621459.1967.10482935
Simes RJ (1986) An improved Bonferroni procedure for multiple tests of significance. Biometrika 73(3):751–754. https://doi.org/10.1093/biomet/73.3.751
Wiens BL (2003) A fixed sequence Bonferroni procedure for testing multiple endpoints. Pharm Stat 2(3):211–215. https://doi.org/10.1002/pst.064

Principles of Clinical Trials: Bias and Precision Control

40

Randomization, Stratification, and Minimization

Fan-fan Yu

Contents

Abstract

The fundamental difference distinguishing observational studies from clinical trials is randomization. This chapter provides a practical guide to concepts of randomization that are widely used in clinical trials. It starts by describing bias and potential confounding arising from allocating people to treatment groups in a predictable way. It then presents the concept of randomization, starting from a simple coin flip, and sequentially introduces methods with additional restrictions

F.-f. Yu (✉)
Statistics Collaborative, Inc., Washington, DC, USA
e-mail: fan-fan.yu@statcollab.com

© Springer Nature Switzerland AG 2022
S. Piantadosi, C. L. Meinert (eds.), *Principles and Practice of Clinical Trials*,
https://doi.org/10.1007/978-3-319-52636-2_211

to account for better balance of the groups with respect to known (measured) and unknown (unmeasured) variables. These include descriptions and examples of complete randomization and permuted block designs. The text briefly describes biased coin designs that extend this family of designs. Stratification is introduced as a way to provide treatment balance on specific covariates and covariate combinations, and an adaptive counterpart of biased coin designs, minimization, is described. The chapter concludes with some practical considerations when creating and implementing randomization schedules.

By the chapter's end, statistician or clinicians designing a trial may distinguish generally what assignment methods may fit the needs of their trial and whether or not stratifying by prognostic variables may be appropriate. The statistical properties of the methods are left to the individual references at the end.

Keywords

Selection bias · Assignment bias · Randomization · Allocation concealment · Random assignment · Permuted block · Biased coin · Stratification · Minimization · Covariate-adaptive randomization

Introduction

An apple a day keeps the doctor away.

How does one test this hypothesis? Researchers conducting an observational cohort trial might gather a group of like individuals, follow them for a period of time, and record whether they made non-wellness visits to their primary care physician. The analysis would look at the relationship between this outcome and whether or not those with and without the outcome ate apples or not. Investigators of a clinical trial, however, would approach this differently by preemptively assigning apples to one group of people, no apples to another, and then observe whether they made non-wellness visits to their physician. This approach directly tests whether an apple-eating lifestyle affects health. Alternatively, a clinical trial could hone in on the vitamin C in apples and give participants a dose equivalent to apples to one group and placebo to another.

The long-standing lure of a miracle health benefit from everyday foods still drives medical research. Such was the case not for apples, but carrots: observational studies in the early 1990s showed evidence that people who consumed more fruits and vegetables rich in beta-carotene had lower rates of heart disease and cancer. It was not clear, however, whether health benefits were the direct result of beta-carotene, antioxidant vitamins and other nutrients in beta-carotene-rich foods, dietary habits in general, or other behaviors. A series of long-term, large-scale, randomized, clinical trials followed to provide direct tests of the benefits of beta-carotene on these health outcomes.

In a "classic" parallel-group clinical trial, people are assigned one of two different therapies, often to compare a new treatment intervention to placebo or standard of care. In the case of beta-carotene, one trial, the Physicians' Health Study, randomized two groups of men to a 12-year supplementation regimen of either beta-carotene or beta-carotene placebo (Hennekens et al. 1996). The outcome for such a trial is compared between the groups, with the goal of obtaining an estimate of treatment effect that is free of bias and confounding (which will be addressed later in this chapter).

In an observational trial, the adjustment of the exposure effect between groups of people often occurs in the analysis through a stratified analysis or by including potential confounders in a regression model. Although a clinical trial analysis can apply the same adjustment methods, designers of a clinical trial can control bias and confounding at the start of the trial. One way to do so is through randomization, the process of assigning individuals to treatment groups using principles of chance for assignment. Because the presence of bias can greatly affect the interpretation and generalizability of a clinical trial, many aspects in trial design, including randomization, exist to ensure its minimization.

Randomization is the fundamental difference distinguishing observational studies from clinical trials. In controlling for biases and confounding, randomization forms the basis for valid inference. Careful thought should be given to its elements, described in this chapter (block size, strata, assignment ratio, and others) and, naturally, discussed between statisticians and a trial's clinical leadership.

Assignment Without Chance: A Motivating Example

To begin, consider two examples, more generic in nature, of nonrandom assignment for a multicenter trial enrolling participants. Investigators are aware of the assignment process but are masked to treatment:

1. Assign the first 50 people who consent to the trial to treatment A and the next 50 to treatment B.
2. Assign alternating treatments: odd-numbered participants receive A and even-numbered participants receive B.

These approaches are simple and systematic but with drawbacks. In the first approach, there is a high likelihood that participants within groups are more alike than those in opposing groups. This could occur if Dr. X had all the earlier appointments and Dr. Y the later ones.

In the second approach, the pattern is predictable. From observing the previous set of participants, the caring Dr. Compassion has figured out that A is the novel, active treatment. A patient he has known for many years has been very sick, and Dr. Compassion believes that this patient may benefit from the experimental therapy in the trial. The patient would be tenth in line and therefore slated to receive B, the control therapy. Dr. Compassion – whether consciously or unconsciously – decides to hold his patient back in the enrollment order, so that the patient receives the active treatment A instead.

Bias

These situations show two examples of bias that could easily occur during assignment of treatment groups. In both cases, the treatment schedule is predictable. If the trial is unmasked, or if the novel treatment is obvious despite masking, then, like Dr. Compassion, investigators may manipulate the timing of participant enrollment so that certain participants receive certain treatments. Both cases are prone to selection bias. This bias occurs when investigators have knowledge of the treatment assignment and the selection of a participant for a trial is based on that knowledge. Such selection could occur in an unmasked trial or if the randomization scheme's assignment pattern is predictable.

This issue of predictability raises the importance of *allocation concealment*. The risk of investigator-influenced assignments and selection bias can be minimized if the investigators do not know what the next assignment will be. Note that this is different from blinding or masking, which seeks to conceal the treatment altogether. Two easy ways to conceal assignments before they are handed out are (1) avoiding easy assignment patterns and (2) avoiding publicly available lists, such as the notorious example of one tacked up on the nurses' station bulletin board. Allocation concealment is possible in an unmasked trial, as long as investigators are unaware of the assignment before a participant receives the intervention.

In the first case, the participants who enroll early may share certain baseline characteristics that differ from those of participants who enroll later. These baseline characteristics are often prognostic factors for the disease of trial. For trials enrolling over long periods of time, demographic shifts do occur. The characteristics of participants, which sometimes reflect changed and improved standards of care, may differ temporally depending on when they enter the trial. Byar et al. (1976) described the Veterans' Administration Cooperative Urological Research Group trial in participants with prostate cancer. Earlier recruited participants had shorter survival than those who entered later. A similar contrast arises with prevalent versus incident cases of disease. Those available at first might have had the disease for a long time; incident cases that arise during the trial may be more rapidly (or more slowly) progressive. When the assignment results in prognostic factors that are unequally distributed across the treatment groups, then the effect of the treatment on the final outcome may be confounded with the effect of the factor. This is an example of assignment bias.

Mitigating bias results in more accurate estimates of treatment differences. To see this mathematically, consider a hypothetical trial in diabetic children as presented in Matthews (2000). Hemoglobin A1c is a measure of average blood glucose levels over the past 2–3 months. HbA1c levels tend to be higher in adolescents (9–10%) than in young children (6–7%). Consider a trial comparing active treatment (A) to placebo (B) showing no treatment effect. Matthews nicely shows how assignment bias with respect to age grouping affects the treatment difference. Assuming there is no treatment difference, the expected value of HbA1c is μ_1 for children and μ_2 for adolescents. The mean HbA1c in group A may be expressed as the sum of all n_A children's observations plus the sum of all $(N - n_A)$ adolescent observations:

$$\overline{H}_A = \frac{\sum_{i=1}^{n_A} X_i + \sum_{i=n_A+1}^{N} X_i}{N}$$

The mean for group B is similarly calculated. The expected HbA1c in each group is

$$E\left(\overline{H}_A\right) = \frac{n_A\mu_1 + (N - n_A)\mu_2}{N}, E\left(\overline{H}_B\right) = \frac{n_B\mu_1 + (N - n_B)\mu_2}{N}$$

Mathematically, the expected treatment effect can then be expressed as the difference between the expected response in children μ_1 and adolescents μ_2, multiplied by a factor dependent on the number of children in each group, n_A and n_B:

$$E\left(\overline{H}_A\right) - E\left(\overline{H}_B\right) = \frac{(n_A - n_B)}{N}(\mu_1 - \mu_2)$$

Recall that there is no actual treatment effect; thus the expected difference above equals 0.

Since children and adolescents have different HbA1c levels, $\mu 1 < \mu 2$. If the number of children in groups A and B is balanced ($n_A = n_B$), then the above equation is also to 0. The balancing of the prognostic factor, age, provides an unbiased estimate of the treatment effect. If the number of children in groups A and B are not balanced ($n_A \neq n_B$), the treatment effect is non-zero. The treatment effect is biased, showing a treatment difference when there actually is none.

Randomization may help to avoid this type of bias, making sure the two groups are similar. In that way, the observable difference between the two groups is the result of the treatment.

Methods of Randomization

Simple randomization, as described below, may produce treatment groups of different sizes. Blocking and stratification, which are methods of randomization, address the problems of imbalance in important covariates.

Simple Randomization

Synonyms: Complete Randomization, Fair Coin Flip

The simplest example of randomization is the fair coin flip. Each participant who is in the queue to participate is randomized independently to one treatment or another with 50% probability. The electronic equivalent of the coin flip – more efficient, current, and most importantly reproducible – would be a generated random probability assignment for each person, who receives treatment A if the probability assignment is less than 0.5 and treatment B if it's more. Reproducibility of experiments is important for scientific validity. It allows corroboration of trial methods and results and protects against fraud.

A pre-generated, formalized randomization *list (synonyms: randomization schedule, randomization scheme)* would pre-generate each assignment so that one can refer to the next entry on the list rather than flipping a coin for each assignment. As participants are enrolled, their place in the queue corresponds with a specific assignment to A or B in the list. One way to do this would be to:

(a) First, generate a sequence of numbers from 1 to n, where n is the total sample size.
(b) Then, perform an independent coin flip (probability 0.5 for each treatment) for each number in sequence. For example, in the R software, use the command rbinom(n, 1, 0.5) to generate the probabilities, and assign treatment A or B depending on whether the probability is less or more than 0.5.

Note that this process introduces no selection bias, because each successive participant's assignment is completely random and independent of each other.

A graphical depiction of simple randomization appears in Fig. 1, which uses a game-board spinner to depict the coin probabilities.

Fun fact. A computer-generated coin flip is actually *pseudorandom*, as it's the result of algorithm-based number generator which makes the result reproducible given an initial number or "seed." A series of ideal coin flips is randomness in its purest form, but it is not reproducible.

Because a coin flip is binomial, the large sample theory of binomial distributions applies. An assignment of 50% in each group becomes more likely as the number of coin flips, or trials, increases. With smaller sample sizes, the assignment of people to one group or another is likely to be unequal for some period of time.

Clinical trials aiming for a 1:1 assignment seek to attain equal experience with both treatments. As discussed above, using simple randomization may not guarantee that assignment when the sample size is small. In reality, however, the assignment from simple randomization will not be far from 1:1; the larger the sample size, the greater the likelihood of balance. Lachin (1988b) states one need not worry about the imbalance for trials of more than 200 people.

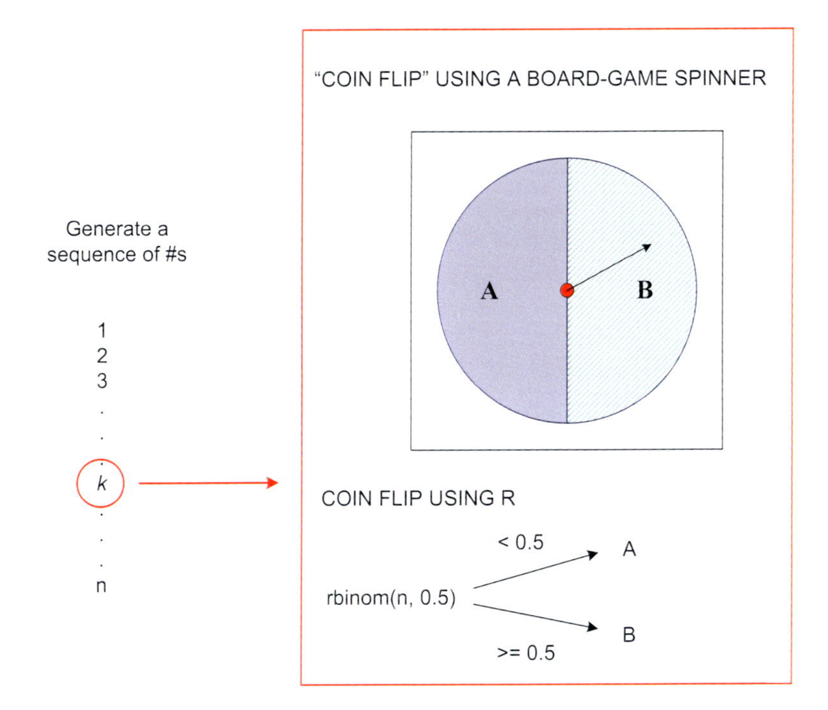

Fig. 1 Simple randomization. A graphical depiction of simple randomization

Restricted Randomization

An alternative to avoiding imbalance in participant numbers in each group is to consider putting restrictions on the randomization process. For trials under 200 participants, additional conditions on the randomization procedure may ensure more equal assignment of participants between the two treatment groups. As discussed below, these conditions in *restricted randomization* also extend to better balance of prognostic variables between the two treatment groups.

Random Assignment

A step beyond simple randomization's fair coin flip is random assignment. An analogy is a typical American elementary school game of musical chairs, modernized so that no one is eliminated and everyone wins: for an equal number of boys and girls (1:1 assignment of treatments A and B) and the same number of chairs, music plays while the children dance freely inside the circle of chairs (randomization placement); after the music stops, the children scramble to find a new chair, forming a new seating arrangement (random assignment of treatments). More formally, for a 1:1 assignment, this procedure pre-specifies the exact sample size in advance and then restricts the randomization to half the participants receiving

Table 1 Random assignment

a) 5 As and 5 Bs		b) Scramble	And reorder			
Sequence number	Group	Sort variable using SAS function RANUNI (465)	Sort variable in ascending order	Sequence number	Group	Final randomization order
001	A	0.0075949673	0.0075949673	001	A	1
002	A	0.0912527778	0.0912527778	002	A	2
003	A	0.9183023315	0.1542221867	009	B	3
004	A	0.6203701001	0.236651111	008	B	4
005	A	0.5451987076	0.4853155145	007	B	5
006	B	0.7139676347	0.5451987076	005	A	6
007	B	0.4853155145	0.6203701001	004	A	7
008	B	0.236651111	0.7139676347	006	B	8
009	B	0.1542221867	0.9183023315	003	A	9
010	B	0.9534464944	0.9534464944	010	B	10

A and the other half receiving B. Then, true to the method's name, it randomly allocates each participant's placement in the list sequence. A list constructed programmatically could do the following for 100 planned assignments:

(a) List 100 sequence numbers: 1–50 as A and 51–100 as B.
(b) Scramble the numbers by using a random number generator to assign a random number to each of the 100 assignments, and then sort the list by the order of the random numbers. The RANUNI function in SAS is useful for this.

The schema below (Table 1) illustrates the process on a smaller scale for 10 assignments, using a seed number of 465 with the SAS RANUNI function for the reordering.

In practice, pre-generated randomization lists provide more assignments than the planned sample size in order to account for higher-than-expected enrollment, potential errors, and other just-in-case scenarios.

Fun fact. Random assignment is the simplest form of a permuted block design – it's a single block of size n.

Permuted Block Designs

One concern with random assignment is the possibility of a long run of a single treatment – for example, treatment B occurring many times in a row. Another problem may be unbalanced group sizes at some time during the randomization. One way to address these issues is to use blocking, a concept that puts restrictions on the allocated numbers of participants within each group by permuting the assignment sequence in smaller subgroupings (blocks). This method achieves treatment balance within each block rather than over half the subjects in the trial.

Blocks, then, are assignment groups of predetermined sizes, and treatments are allocated within a block, sitting like shelves in a bookcase. With the last block as a base and the first block on top, the blocks are then "stacked" to produce a tower, which comprises the randomization list.

In the simplest case, 1:1 assignments use even block sizes, while 2:1 randomizations use multiples of 3.

How does one build the tower of blocks? First, figure out the different sequences for particular block sizes. For instance, a block size of 2 has only two sequence options:

Sequence option number	1	2
Sequence	AB	BA

Then, decide on the number of assignments – typically a multiple of the block size chosen. To produce a randomization list of 100 assignments, first generate a random list comprised of 50 numbers. Each number is either 1 or 2 (sampling with replacement), representing the two block types above. An example for the first ten participants would be a sequence of 1, 1, 2, 1, 2. This corresponds to a randomization list of AB|AB|BA|AB|BA. The first person randomized is assigned treatment A, the second treatment B, the third treatment A, etc.

A block size of 4 has six block sequence options:

Sequence number	1	2	3	4	5	6
Sequence	AABB	BBAA	ABAB	BABA	ABBA	BAAB

A list of 100 assignments using a block size of 4 would produce a list of 25 randomly selected block sequence numbers. Each of those 25 numbers corresponds to one of the six block types above.

Example. A trial with two treatments (A and B) and a 1:1 assignment uses a permuted block design for randomization. The block size is 4. Although the design of the trial specifies enrolling 80 participants, the randomization list generates 100 assignments to be "on the safe side." A partial list of the first 20 assignments appears below in Table 2. The program generates 25 block numbers with replacement from the block sequence list {1, 2, 3, 4, 5, 6}. The selected block sequence numbers appear in the second column. The corresponding assignment sequences of As and Bs appear in the third column. A unique randomization number appears in the fourth column. This number can serve either as the participant ID or maps uniquely to a separate participant ID.

Choosing Block Sizes

The choice of block size for a randomization list depends on the trial size and specific features of the trial. Ideally, a well-chosen block size can lower the ability to predict future treatments by lowering the predictability of patterns and therefore protecting the masking of treatment groups. The decision of block size should also consider the longest acceptable "run" of a single treatment. An example appears above in Table 2 between the consecutive block sequence numbers of 1 and 2. As seen here, the longest run of a single treatment using blocks of size 4 is four in a row.

Table 2 First 20 assignments for a permuted block design (block size of 4)

Block number	Sequence number	Assignment group	Randomization number
1	4	B	1001
		A	1002
		B	1003
		A	1004
2	3	A	1005
		B	1006
		A	1007
		B	1008
3	1	A	1009
		A	1010
		B	1011
		B	1012
4	2	B	1013
		B	1014
		A	1015
		A	1016
5	5	A	1017
		B	1018
		B	1019
		A	1020
...			
25	Etc.	Etc.	Etc.

In many studies, randomization is stratified by trial site. If many sites are expected to enroll few subjects, or if a trial is small, a smaller block size may be appropriate. This helps to ensure better assignment of treatment within a block and prevents the majority of participants from receiving a single treatment at one site. Larger studies with many randomized at each site are able to accommodate larger block sizes.

Example. A trial of 100 people has 10 sites but expects enrollment to occur at the 2 main sites located in major metropolitan areas. Trial coordinators at the smaller sites expect few enrollees. The randomization, which stratifies by trial site, uses a block size of 8. The first block in the randomization list for one of the smaller sites has assignment sequence AAAABBBB. Only four participants enroll at this site; all four therefore receive treatment A. The analysis of the outcome cannot disentangle the effect of this site from the effect of treatment. Because the effect of treatment is potentially confounded with the effect of site, a smaller block size would be appropriate here.

As a rule of thumb: block sizes of 4 to 6 are typical for studies with sites that are expected to enroll only a few participants, 2 is a small block, and 8 is considered large. Block sizes greater than 8 need careful consideration in relation to the size of the trial. They are not recommended for small studies. Long runs, such as AAAABBBB|BBBBAAAA, may occur with a block size of 8, and a block may not fill completely as seen in the example above. In the case of a 12-participant trial with this randomization, the trial would actually be a 2:1 randomization instead of the intended 1:1. This defeats the purpose of blocking to achieve better balance between treatment groups. While this example may be extreme, it is still an important consideration within blocks and for a stratified randomization (more on this later in section "Stratified Randomization").

For trials with more than two treatment groups, the block size should be a multiple of the number of treatment groups if the assignment is 1:1. A trial with three treatment groups and block sizes of 2 and 4 make less sense than a trial with block sizes of 3 and 6.

Keeping the Block Size Secret

In certain situations, investigators like Dr. Compassion, whom we met earlier in the chapter's introduction, may be able to predict, with a fair degree of accuracy, the next treatment in the assignment sequence if they know the block size.

Example. In a placebo-controlled masked trial, an investigator has noticed the telltale effects of the active group, a prostanoid therapy: symptoms of nausea and diarrhea, jaw pain, and flushing. By observing participants, she has noticed that the sequence thus far at her site is likely to have been placebo, active, active. Knowing that the block size is 4, she can predict with certainty that fourth participant will be assigned the active treatment. Similarly, if investigators know that the block size is 2, then it is easy to predict all of the even-numbered assignments.

Similar situations could arise with larger block sizes; the probability of predicting the treatment increases at the ends of blocks. Thus, one important aspect of permuted block designs is to limit knowledge of the block size to a select few, preferably to the statisticians at the data coordinating center who generate the randomization and who may have access to unmasked data during the trial. Keeping the blocking information from investigators decreases the potential for selection bias (Lachin et al. 1988). In the absence of this measure, the potential for selection bias decreases as a function of the block size unless random blocks are used in the randomization scheme (Matts and Lachin 1988; see section "Mix It Up: Using Random Permuted Blocks with Unequal Block Sizes").

This issue of keeping the block size hush is especially important in unmasked studies, which have a greater potential for selection bias if investigators are able to guess the ordering of assignment assignments. Investigators may be more susceptible to influencing who gets which assignment if the randomization uses permuted blocks and the block size is known. Below are several other methods to reduce the predictability of treatments within a permuted block design.

Use, or Add On, Block Sizes of 2

Block sizes of 2 are considered small and not always ideal because of the predictability of assignment. In some situations, however, particularly in stratified randomizations (see section "Stratified Randomization"), block sizes of 2 help to minimize the possibility that participants within a stratum are randomized to the same treatment:

- A trial has several centers but only a few enrollees per center are expected. Initiation of sites often occurs in groups and sequentially over time. Thus, enrollment at certain times in the trial – for example, in the first few months – may occur only at a few sites. To minimize the chance that sites enroll participants from the same treatment group, consider a block size of 2.
- A small trial has multiple sites with anywhere from four to eight participants expected per site. Randomization will be stratified by site. Use a block size of 2 first to guarantee treatment balance for the first two randomized, and then mix it with block sizes of 4.
- A block size of 6 may run the risk of having this assignment: AAABBB| BBBAAA, a run of 6 Bs in a row at a single site. Rather than using a block size of 6, mix block sizes within a randomization; for example, combine a block size of 4 with a block size of 2. For continuous runs such as AABB|BA, the maximum run of any one treatment in this case is 3.

An alternative for a larger trial is to mix more than two block sizes – for example, sizes of 2, 4, and 6.

Mix It Up: Using Random Permuted Blocks with Unequal Block Sizes

A way to address the selection bias that may occur by predicting treatment assignments at the ends of blocks is to mix up the block sizes and use random block sizes rather than fixed ones. Rather than choosing among the six possible blocks of size 4, one could choose among blocks of size 4 or 2. For a list of 100 numbers,

1. First generate a list of number corresponding to a block length of either 2 or 4.
2. For each block generate a number within that block type.
3. Select the sequence corresponding to the block type.

An example of the random block length sequence is 4, 2, 4, 4, 2. The sequence numbers within each block type is 6, 2, 3, 1, 1. Recall the list of six sequence options defined earlier for a block of size 4:

Sequence number	1	2	3	4	5	6
Sequence	AABB	BBAA	ABAB	BABA	ABBA	BAAB

and the two sequence options for a block size of 2:

Sequence option number	1	2
Sequence	AB	BA

The corresponding randomization assignments for the first 16 participants is

BAAB | BA | BABA | AABB | AB

Random block length sequence	4	2	4	4	2
Sequence number	6	2	3	1	1
Randomization assignment	BAAB	BA	BABA	AABB	AB

Urn-Adaptive Randomization Designs

Synonyms: Adaptive Randomization, Dynamic Randomization

A trial sponsor may want to have treatment balance during a trial in real time rather than just at the end, for example, when the trial has staggered entry of participants and when the total number of participants is not entirely known. Enter urn-adaptive randomization designs, extensions of restricted randomized designs. The general principle is this: rather than using a fair coin toss as described earlier, urn-adaptive designs use a biased coin. For now, say this coin has a heavier tail side and is weighted 30:70 heads/tails. When a new participant is enrolled, look to see which treatment group has fewer people, and then flip the coin. If it lands tails (and remember, this is a 70% chance of this), then the person goes to the group with fewer people. If it lands heads, then the person goes to the group with more people.

This is an example of *Efron's biased coin design*, where the first participant, or first several participants, is randomized by simple randomization. Generalizing the above (where $p = 0.70$), for the k-th participant, consider the difference in the number of people between the groups, A–B.

If A–B < 0 (more Bs), randomize to A with probability p, where $p > 0.5$.
If A–B > 0 (more As), randomize to A with probability 1- p.
If A–B $= 0$, randomize to A with probability 0.5.

Note that p is constant even when there is imbalance. The design is summarized visually in Fig. 2, again using a game-board spinner instead of a coin for illustration purposes.

Two other designs are Wei's urn design (1978) and its generalization, Smith's generalized biased coin design. Wei's urn design is similar to Efron's except that p fluctuates depending upon the balance between the two groups. Both are urn models with n balls labeled A and n balls labeled B. For Wei's urn design, when the k-th person is randomized, a "ball" is picked from the urn. If the ball is labeled A, then:

- The person is randomized to group A.
- The A ball is returned to the urn.
- m balls labeled B are added to the urn.
- Repeat for the $(k + 1)$st person randomized.

Fun fact. Complete randomization is the situation if no B ball is added to the urn.

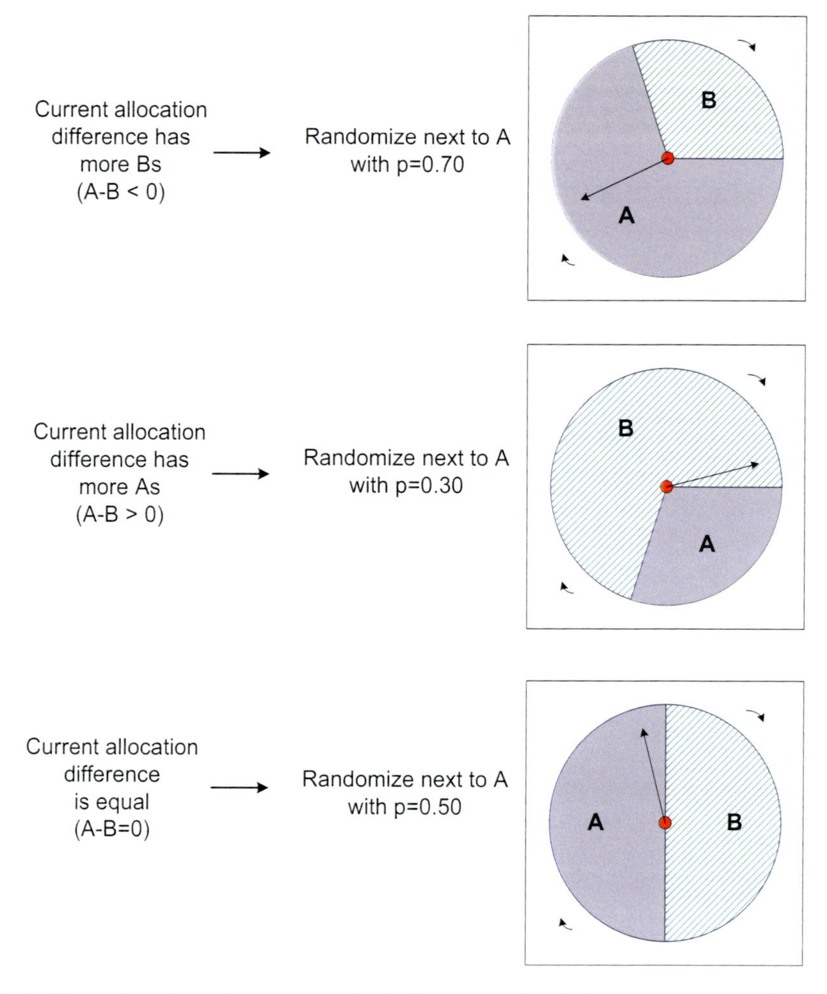

Fig. 2 Efron's biased coin design, using a 30:70 "biased coin" as depicted by a game-board spinner

Because the probability of assignment is biased toward the group with fewer assignments, urn-adaptive designs adapt the probability of choosing the next treatment on the basis of the assignment ratio thus far. This helps maintain balance as the trial is ongoing, but doesn't guarantee complete balance at the end of trial. In terms of bias, the procedure reduces the predictability of the assignments and thereby reduces the bias associated with that. For smaller trials, urn designs provide balance along the way and behave more like complete randomization as the sample size gets large.

Stratified Randomization

Let's return to the earlier example of a trial of diabetic children, where HbA1c tends to be higher in adolescents as compared to young children. An imbalance in the number of children in group A versus group B could occur using the randomization methods just described and could lead to a biased treatment effect. An alternative is to achieve treatment balance within each age grouping, rather than achieving balance between treatments over all participants. This method, stratified randomization, achieves balance within pre-chosen strata (young children vs. adolescents) defined by important prognostic factors (age grouping), whose levels may affect the outcome (HbA1c). In the simplest case of a two-strata factor, the randomization list is essentially two lists, one for each stratum.

One major goal of stratification is to minimize the chances of one treatment occurring primarily within a single factor – for instance, the majority of adolescent trial participants receiving treatment B – such that the analysis cannot disentangle the effect of the factor from the effect of treatment. This helps avoid correlation between predictors (for factors not associated with the outcome) and confounding (for factors associated with the outcome).

A trial with two two-level factors, such as age and gender, has four strata: male pediatric, male adult, female pediatric, and female adult. Statisticians will often picture this as a 2 by 2 table and refer to each stratum as a "cell." A trial with two treatment groups will therefore have eight cells. This trial will have four separate randomization lists, one for each stratum. Within each stratum, randomization may occur using random assignment or permuted blocks.

Fun fact. For random assignment, stratification may be viewed as blocking, with each stratum acting as one large block using simple randomization.

A real challenge in designing stratified trials is selecting the most important strata on which to achieve balance. A true story is a discussion among researchers who were planning a trial. Each clinician felt very strongly about a prognostic factor whose levels would affect the outcome. The list grew to include gender, baseline disease status, age category, a disease-specific clinical characteristic, and a biomarker. When the trial statistician pointed out that there were now at least 32 strata, and therefore 64 cells, for a 100-person trial, the researchers had to step back to re-prioritize as a group.

As seen in Table 3, the number of strata quickly multiplies as the number of prognostic variables increases. A risk of including so many factors is that numerous strata may result in certain "cells" having few or no people. Having empty cells, or many cells with a single person, not only goes against achieving balance but also

Table 3 Number of prognostic factors and strata for a trial with two treatment groups

Two-level factors	*Example*	*Number of strata*	*Number of cells*
1	Gender	2	4
2	Gender, age (pediatric vs. adult)	4	8
3	Gender, age, baseline disease status (WHO class I/II vs. III/IV)	8	16
4	Gender, age, baseline disease status, genetic biomarker	16	32
N		2^N	2^{N+1}

presents problems when analyzing the data. For the analysis, many trial teams choose to pool strata that have only one or two people randomized.

Another operational consideration for limiting the number of strata is the possibility for mis-stratification. Investigators are humans; they may enter the wrong stratum criterion when randomizing a participant. Deciding how to handle mis-stratifications then becomes a challenge in the conduct and interpretation of an analysis. For example, if a woman is stratified as a man, should she be analyzed as a man, to reflect the actual randomization, or as a woman, because that is what she is?

There is some debate as to whether, and when, studies should stratify. Lachin et al. (1988) recommend stratification for trials with fewer than 100 participants. For larger trials, the advantages are negligible for efficiency; they recommend stratifying by center but not by other prognostic factors. Others argue that investigators may want to stratify for other scientific reasons – such as characteristics of a disease – that may affect trial outcome. An example is the breast cancer trial in Table 5, which stratified by first- versus second-line therapy. With an outcome of progression-free survival, it was important to monitor that the randomization obtained balance between those who were farther along in their treatment (second-line therapy) than those who were not.

A special consideration is stratification by clinical site, which was addressed earlier in the discussion of block sizes in section "Permuted Block Designs." Because of the sequential nature of site initiation in a trial and the similarities in patient care within a site, many studies will stratify randomization by site. This helps to avoid confounding of the treatment effect by site and ensures balance within site.

Because blocking is usually employed within site, unmasked studies should probably avoid stratifying by site. The prediction of treatment patterns at the ends of blocks is much easier in this setting.

Minimization

Synonyms: Covariate-Adaptive Randomization, Dynamic Randomization, Strict Minimization

When a trial has many prognostic factors needing balancing, minimization may provide a good assignment alternative compared to more traditional randomization methods. Recall the trial mentioned earlier with the five different two-level prognostic variables and the resulting problematic 64 cells for 100 people. That trial may have been a candidate for minimization if the clinicians decided that each of the five variables was equally important for stratification.

Minimization refers to minimizing the treatment imbalance over several covariates by the use of a dynamic, primarily nonrandom method. As an alternative to stratified block randomization, minimization allows balancing on many prognostic variables in real time. The method uses information on prognostic factors – the stratification variables used with the randomization methods above – to determine

Table 4 Participants randomized to two groups, by strata

		After 15 participants		
Factor	Stratum	Group A	Group B	A–B
Gender	Female	4	2	2
	Male	5	4	1
Age	<18	3	3	0
	18+	3	6	−3

where the imbalance is. Then, generally, the method chooses the arm that best minimizes the imbalance and assigns the next participant to that arm. Similar to biased coin designs, the next assignment is partially determined by the treatment group with fewer people. Here, the assignment is done by defining a weighted metric that combines the treatment differences *across all the strata* for a covariate. This weighted metric then determines the assignment probability to assignment of that arm. The goal of minimization, like urn-adaptive randomization, is to ensure a small absolute difference between the numbers randomized in each treatment group. The difference between urn-adaptive methods and minimization is that minimization uses stratum-specific differences to minimize the differences between treatment groups.

First introduced by Taves (1974), a deterministic version of the method with the four strata in Table 4 would randomize the first set of participants using complete randomization (Table 3). Within each stratum, calculate the differences for A-B as seen in the last column of the table; positive values indicate more participants in A and vice versa. To determine the assignment for the 16th participant, add the differences for the subject-specific strata.

If sum < 0 (more Bs), randomize to A.
If sum > 0 (more As), randomize to B.
If sum $= 0$ (equal assignment), randomize to A with probability $= 0.5$.

Example: In Table 3, 15 people have been randomized. The 16th subject is a pediatric female. To determine this person's assignment, add the differences A-B for these two strata, $2 + 0 = 2$. This indicates that because currently A has more people for this combination of factors, this person receives treatment B. Update the table using this person's information, and then allocate the next person.

Pocock and Simon (1975) independently proposed a similar method but used a probability $p > 0.5$ for assigning participants to a specific arm. Proschan et al. (2011) refer to Taves' deterministic method as strict minimization, and Pocock and Simon's method as minimization.

If sum < 0, randomize to A with probability p.
If sum > 0, randomize to B with probability p.
If sum $= 0$, randomize to A with probability $= 0.5$.

A p of 0.8 gives a relatively high probability for receiving the treatment currently in "deficit." Pocock and Simon generally prefer a p of 0.75.

This method balances marginally over all covariates rather than within stratum as for stratification using permuted block designs. While the method achieves better balance in real time on the selected factors, unlike conventional randomization methods, it does not guarantee balance on unspecified factors. It works best in small trials (e.g., trials of <100 people). Pocock and Simon have generalized this method to three or more groups, which is not covered here (Fig. 3).

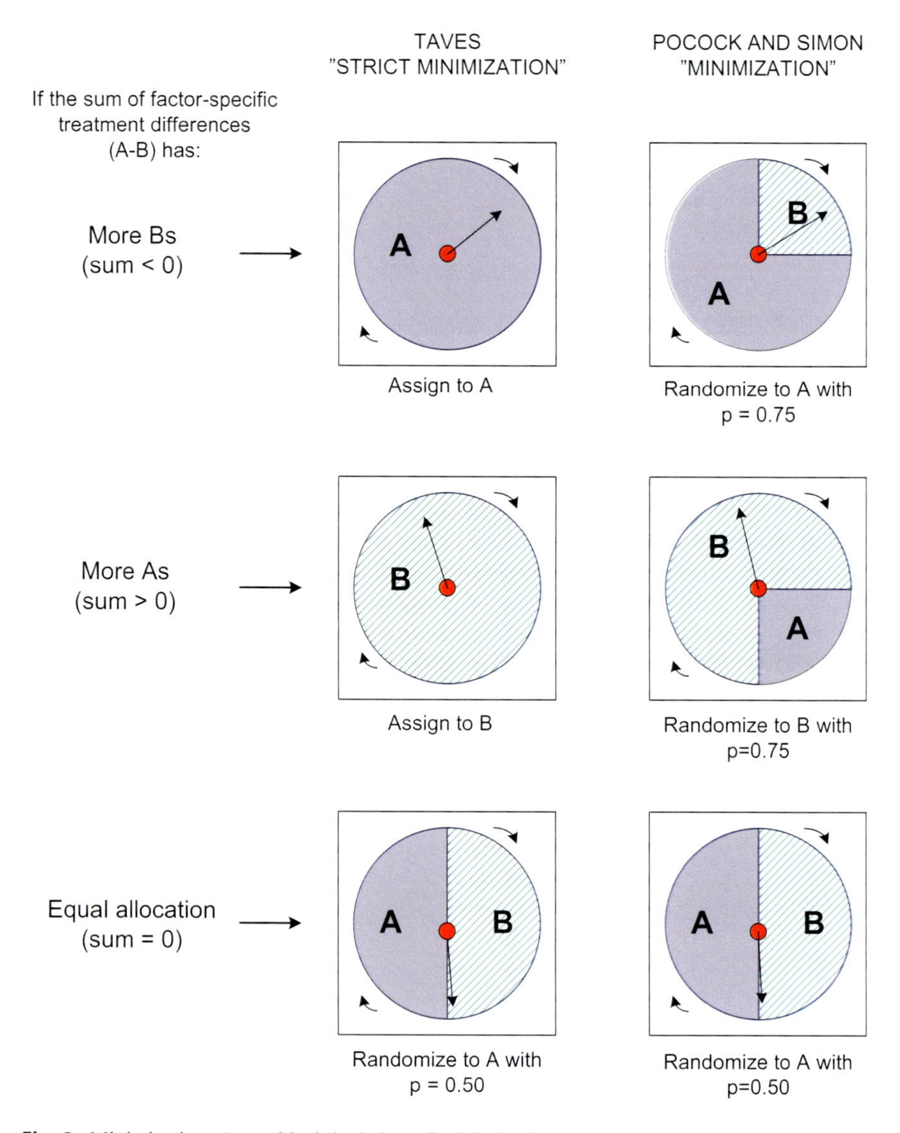

Fig. 3 Minimization. A graphical depiction of minimization

One disadvantage to dynamic randomization is its computational complexity. Unlike conventional randomization, a pre-generated list prior to trial start is not feasible. Although a list of probabilities for p may be pre-generated, dynamic methods require real-time monitoring of the strata and current imbalance for each participant enrolled and "randomized." In more complicated methods, such as urn designs with dynamic p, several lists for p will need pre-generation. The added complexity introduces the potential for computational error and, if implemented incorrectly, may counter the intention for increased real-time balance.

Other Methods

Additional approaches to randomization models include urn models where the distribution of treatment "balls" within urns is based on the responses observed so far. These response-adaptive randomizations include randomized play the winner (Wei and Durham 1978) and drop the loser (Ivanova 2003), among others. The basic premise is that if one treatment is showing better response than the other, then the assignment probabilities can favor the better treatment. This type of randomization is more suitable with trials where responses are viewed quickly and addresses ethical concerns about participants exposing themselves to treatment groups that may not be effective. This chapter does not address these methods further.

Practicalities and Implementation

Unequal Allocation

Although this chapter focused on 1:1 assignments, some trials may choose to use other assignment ratios. A common alternative is 2:1, which in some cases has less power than its 1:1 counterpart. Figure 4 displays the total sample size needed for a continuous, normally distributed outcome represented by $\Phi\left[\frac{\Delta}{\sigma}\frac{1}{\sqrt{\frac{1}{n_1}+\frac{1}{n_2}}}-1.96\right]$, where $\frac{\Delta}{\sigma}=0.65$ and power of 80%, 90%, and 95%.

For an often small loss in power (or increase in sample size), however (Fig. 4), in some trials investigators will prefer to have unequal allocation because of nonstatistical reasons. Some trials may face high-cost issues for obtaining the control treatment from sponsors. In rare diseases, it allows more people access to the novel treatment, and a single trial will therefore have more experience with the novel treatment.

An example of unequal allocation comes from a trial of a novel gene therapy, delivered by subretinal injection to the eye, which had a promise to restore vision to blind participants who had a particular mutation. The sponsor and investigators did not want to burden control participants with a sham injection procedure, especially when many participants would be children. As a result, masking the treatment groups was not possible. With the potential to regain vision from blindness or to stop the path

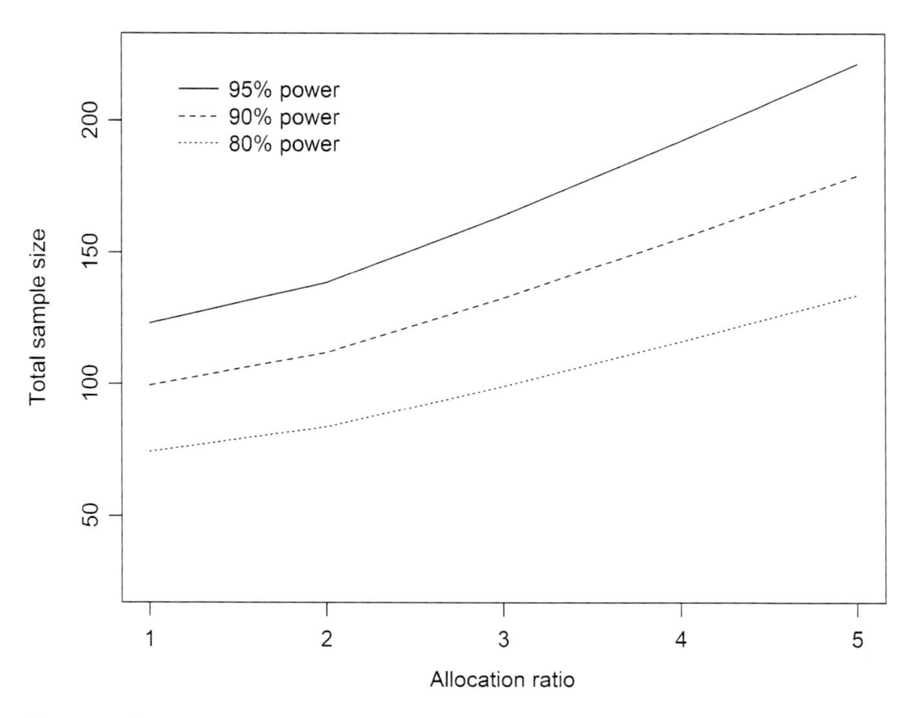

Fig. 4 Total sample size as a function of the assignment ratio for 80%, 85%, and 90% power

toward blindness, everyone recruited was keen on receiving the novel treatment in a rare disease population where finding patients was already difficult. The final design used a 2:1 randomization with an extension period. Despite a small loss in power compared to a 1:1 randomization in an already small trial, this design limited the number of control participants, and the extension period allowed the opportunity for controls to receive treatment after a year on the main trial (Russell et al. 2017).

Checks on the Actual Randomization Schedule

Prior to finalizing a complete or permuted block randomization scheme for a trial, a statistician should run a series of checks on the schedule using the intended final seed. If the seed number is 8675309, then prior to calling pseudorandom number generator functions, one can use *set.seed*(8675309) in R and *call streaminit* (8675309) in SAS. Other functions, such as *ranuni* in SAS, also have seed as the main argument. The final randomization scheme should be checked for what randomization strives to achieve: balance and desired assignment of treatment groups overall, within blocks, and within strata.

Ideally, a randomization schedule should be reproducible when using the same seed as the original schedule. The seed and the block size are best kept from the sponsors, sites, and investigators as discussed in section "Permuted Block Designs." A few checks may include:

- Check for patterns to ensure that the distribution of possible block permutations is not unusual. An example is to ensure that all A–B blocks do not all occur early in the list and all B–A blocks at the end. Another is to avoid a long string of Bs occurring such as a block size of 6; a run of AAABBB|BBBAAA|AAABBB gives two long runs of As and Bs, respectively. One might want to consider a different seed to achieve runs that alternate more between the treatment groups.
- Check to see if the distribution of the position of treatment assignment within blocks is well-balanced. For example, for blocks of size 6, As occur more often in position 5/6.
- Check to see there are no patterns of transitions between treatment assignments. For example, across all blocks, there are more A–B transitions than B–A.
- If there is an abbreviated treatment group identifier (A, B or 1, 2), then a variable should have the decoded variable ("active," "placebo").

Assessing Balance of Prognostic Factors

Reports of randomized and unrandomized studies typically present a table of demographic and baseline characteristics as part of the overall summary of the trial analysis. The table shows the distributions of participant characteristics to see how comparable or "balanced" the groups are. "Balanced" means that important characteristics are distributed similarly in each treatment group. Table 5 displays a subset of the demographic and baseline characteristics from a large breast cancer trial comparing the effects of epoetin alfa to the best standard of care among participants who develop anemia during chemotherapy (Leyland et al. 2016). Because the trial randomized a large number of women, 2000, one would expect that randomization would result in similar distributions of prognostic factors in the two groups. As seen in Table 5, this is the case.

Fun fact. An interesting aspect of baseline tables is that people often request a p-value to provide formal comparisons of differences between treatments for each variable summarized. A p-value is the probability that the observed differences are the result of chance alone. Randomization is a mechanism assigning people by chance to one group or another. Therefore, the p-value for each of the differences in a baseline table of a *randomized* trial, by definition, is 1 (of course, unless the process of randomization was flawed).

For randomized clinical trials, tables of baseline characteristics also help show whether randomization is doing its job. Data and Safety Monitoring Boards (DSMBs), who review interim data of ongoing trials, will use such tables to monitor imbalances of important prognostic factors partway through ongoing trials and whether the trend persists over time. They will also monitor to see if the trial's baseline population reflects the target population. If not, a DSMB may encourage the trial sponsor to further its efforts to recruit particular types of subjects.

For the final analysis of a trial, such a table helps describe the trial population to evaluate how generalizable the trial results are to the larger population.

Table 5 A typical demographics/ baseline characteristics table

	Best standard of care *N = 1,048*	*Epoetin alfa* *N = 1,050*
Age, years		
Median	52.0	52.0
Range (min, max)	23, 81	24, 79
Race, n (%)		
White	724 (69.1)	692 (65.9)
Asian	304 (29.0)	335 (31.9)
Black	4 (0.4)	4 (0.4)
Weight, kg		
Mean (SD)	67.0 (16.08)	67.6 (16.56)
BMI, kg/m^2		
Mean (SD)	26.3 (5.35)	26.4 (5.64)
Stage at initial diagnosis, n (%)		
I	58/1036 (6)	52/1029 (5)
II	323 (31)	331 (32)
III	303 (29)	325 (32)
IV	336 (32)	306 (30)
Unknown	16 (2)	15 (2)
Line of chemotherapy, n (%)		
First line	828/1048 (79)	837/1050 (80)
Second line	220 (21)	213 (20)
Baseline tumor-related characteristics, n (%)		
HER2−/neu-positive	407/1044 (39)	405/1048 (39)
Had prior surgery	740/1048 (71)	753/1050 (72)
Had prior chemotherapy	851/1048 (81)	849/1050 (81)

Taken from Leyland-Jones et al. (2016), American Society of Clinical Oncology

Accounting for the Randomization in Analyses

Models Underlying Randomization and Inference

The analysis of data includes making certain assumptions about the underlying distributions. This is relevant because the underlying distributions form the basis for statistical tests, which inform inference. Although the clinical trial populations are treated in analyses as if they were true random samples from the larger population, sometimes they are not. The three main theoretical models for the underlying population of a trial sample (Lachin 1988a) are briefly described below.

The population model. This is the idea that any sample drawn randomly for the trial, including the treatment groups resulting from randomization, is a representative sample from an infinitely larger population. All samples can all have the same underlying distribution, and clinical responses among individual people in the sample are independent.

A homogeneous population model assumes that the people in the sample satisfy the same inclusion and exclusion criteria. In this model, the assignment of treatments does not affect the type I error rate or power of a test. A heterogeneous population model assumes that people differ in terms of their (baseline) characteristics and are sampled from multiple populations. The underlying distribution of participant responses is a function of the participant's characteristics.

The invoked population model. Randomized groups may be similar with respect to baseline variables, but each group may not necessarily be a perfect sampling distribution from the larger population. The reality is that recruitment for a trial's trial population is far from a random sampling procedure of an infinitely large population. In fact, much of it is nonrandom, targeting specific hospitals and communities and selecting participants who satisfy certain eligibility criteria. The only random element comes from the act of randomization itself (Rosenberger et al. 2018). The data are still analyzed as if they were a random sample representative of the infinitely larger population. While the randomized participants may be somewhat representative of the larger population, this belief still requires a leap of faith and is appropriately called the invoked population model (Lachin 1988a). It invokes the assumption that the analysis and inferences are from samples of the larger, homogeneous population where the underlying distributions are the same.

The randomization model. Another approach is to say that the underlying distributions of the treatment groups are not expected to be similar or are unknown. In fact, there is no way ever to know the underlying distribution or to even make assumptions about them under the invoked population model. Although this sounds philosophical, this situation is tangible in the real-world setting of a small trial. Here, the sample size may be too small to assume normality, which is the basis of many tests. An alternative is to make no assumptions about the underlying distributions, and therefore tests of treatment differences do not rely on those assumptions. Instead, the test solely compares whether the outcome is related to the treatment.

In a randomization test, the basic idea is to assume that treatment label has nothing to do with a person's outcome. The null hypothesis is that the participant's responses are unaffected by the treatment. The observed difference, then, is only the result of how the participants were allocated. The test is actually multiple rounds of reshuffling and is sometimes referred to as "re-randomization." To perform the test,

- Randomize the assignment of treatment label to the participant; participants keep their outcomes but jumble their treatment labels.
- Repeat the analysis with the new labels 10,000 times or so, without replacement. This process is really sampling from the distribution of randomization permutations.
- Next, calculate the test statistic and/or the p-value from the model.
- Then line up all the p-values in order, and see if the original result observed in the first place is one of the extreme outcomes.
- The randomization test p-value is the proportion of new p-values that are as or more extreme than the original observed in the actual dataset.

If the two groups were really not different, the reassignments are unlikely to produce significant differences.

The benefit of the randomization test is that it requires no distributional assumptions; the disadvantage is that the computationally intensive process can be time-consuming and complex programmatically.

Fun fact. A randomization test is often referred to as a permutation test, but they are not technically the same thing. A permutation test assumes that the data are exchangeable and that all outcomes in the permutation have the same likelihood. Rosenberger et al. show that this may be the case for random assignment, but not under other randomization designs.

Randomization Method

Earlier parts of the chapter reference adjusting for prognostic factors when the treatment groups are not balanced. In most cases, the analysis needs to account for the randomization in order to account for the type I error properly.

In a stratified randomization, many statisticians advocate including the stratification factors as covariates in the analysis. One reason for this is that in stratifying, participants within a stratum are more alike; the stratification induces correlation among those participants (Kahan and Morris 2012). This affects the variances of the treatment difference. If the analysis ignores the stratification, and therefore the correlation, then the standard error of the treatment difference is larger than the truth. This in turn affects both power (lower than accounting for stratification) and p-values (smaller than accounting for stratification).

If one is performing a permutation or randomization test for the analysis, then re-randomization should use the same method for the original randomization. For example, if assignment occurred using a permuted block design, then re-randomization should use the same in order for the tests to have the proper type I error rate.

For a trial where assignment is determined using minimization, the method of analysis is less clearly defined. Taves advocated including the factors used for minimization as covariates in the analysis. Others have argued for a randomization test to control alpha, although conducting one may be complicated. Re-randomization for trials using minimization may have issues if there is unequal allocation (Proschan et al.) and may also be unnecessary, producing similar results as a t-test or test of proportions (Buyse 2000). Further review of this discussion appears in Scott et al. (2002).

Randomization Errors: FAQs

Q What if someone is misrandomized?

A In an intent-to-treat (ITT) analysis [covered in another chapter], use the randomized treatment group. In an as-treated analysis situation, use the actual treatment group. (Note that some people do not accept as-treated analyses as valid.)

Q What if someone is mis-stratified?

A If randomization used a permuted block design, use the individual's actual (correct) stratification in the analysis. If someone is mis-stratified as a male when she is really female, then use female in the analysis. (Note that some people maintain that the person should remain mis-stratified).

Q For treatment errors: what if someone is randomized to A but receives B?

A In a true ITT analysis, the analysis uses the randomized assignment. Receiving the wrong treatment could be receiving the wrong, one-time treatment, which would be different from receiving one wrong dose out of many doses. The philosophy, especially in a Phase 3 setting, is that the assigned treatment regimen is the main comparison. A sensible extra analysis would analyze the data using the actual treatment received.

Conclusion and Key Facts

The choice of randomization method depends on, of course, the size and needs of the trial, with input from the trial sponsor and investigators. The table below (Table 6) summarizes considerations for the different types of assignment methods discussed in this chapter.

Table 6 Randomization properties and methods

	Simple randomization	Random assignment	Permuted block	Stratification	Urn-adaptive	Minimization
Treatment balance at trial's end for N > 200	✓	✓	✓	✓	✓	
N ≤ 200		✓	✓			
Possible treatment imbalance during assignment process	✓	✓				
Treatment balance during assignment process in real time			✓		✓	
Pre-generated assignment list	✓	✓	✓	✓		
Treatment balance within unspecified factors	✓	✓	✓	✓		
Treatment balance within 1–3 specified factors			✓	✓	✓	
Treatment balance within >3 specified factors						✓
Special recommendations for N < 100				✓		✓
Dynamic					✓	✓
Complex programming					✓	✓
Allocation concealment in unmasked trial	✓	✓				✓
With random/ mixed blocks only			✓			

Cross-References

▶ Randomization and Permutation Tests

References

Buyse M (2000) Centralized treatment allocation in comparative clinical trials. Applied Clinical Trials 9:32–37

Byar D, Simon R, Friendewald W, Schlesselman J, DeMets D, Ellenberg J, Gail M, Ware J (1976) Randomized clinical trials – perspectives on some recent ideas. N Engl J Med 295:74–80

Hennekens C, Buring J, Manson J, Stampfer M, Rosner B, Cook NR, Belanger C, LaMotte F, Gaziano J, Ridker P, Willett W, Peto R (1996) Lack of effect of long-term supplementation with beta carotene on the incidence of malignant neoplasms and cardiovascular disease. N Engl J Med 334:1145–1149

Ivanova A (2003) A play-the-winner type urn model with reduced variability. Metrika 58:1–13

Kahan B, Morris T (2012) Improper analysis of trials randomized using stratified blocks or minimisation. Stat Med 31:328–340

Lachin J (1988a) Statistical properties of randomization in clinical trials. Control Clin Trials 9:289–311

Lachin J (1988b) Properties of simple randomization in clinical trials. Control Clin Trials 9:312–326

Lachin JM, Matts JP, Wei LJ (1988) Randomization in clinical trials: Conclusions and recommendations. Control Clin Trials 9(4):365–374

Leyland-Jones B, Bondarenko I, Nemsadze G, Smirnov V, Litvin I, Kokhreidze I, Abshilava L, Janjalia M, Li R, Lakshmaiah KC, Samkharadze B, Tarasova O, Mohapatra RK, Sparyk Y, Polenkov S, Vladimirov V, Xiu L, Zhu E, Kimelblatt B, Deprince K, Safonov I, Bowers P, Vercammen E (2016) A randomized, open-label, multicenter, phase III study of epoetin alfa versus best standard of care in anemic patients with metastatic breast cancer receiving standard chemotherapy. J Clin Oncol 34:1197–1207

Matthews J (2000) An introduction to randomized controlled clinical trials. Oxford University Press, Inc., New York

Matts J, Lachin J (1988) Properties of permuted-block randomization in clinical trials. Control Clin Trials 9:345–364

Pocock S, Simon R (1975) Sequential treatment assignment with balancing for prognostic factors in the controlled clinical trial. Biometrics 31:103–115

Proschan M, Brittain E, Kammerman L (2011) Minimize the use of minimization with unequal allocation. Biometrics 67(3):1135–1141. https://doi.org/10.1111/j.1541-0420.2010.01545.x

Rosenberger W, Uschner D, Wang Y (2018) Randomization: the forgotten component of the randomized clinical trial. Stat Med 38(1):1–12

Russell S, Bennett J, Wellman J, Chung D, Yu Z, Tillman A, Wittes J, Pappas J, Elci O, McCague S, Cross D, Marshall K, Walshire J, Kehoe T, Reichert H, Davis M, Raffini L, Lindsey G, Hudson F, Dingfield L, Zhu X, Haller J, Sohn E, Mahajin V, Pfeifer W, Weckmann M, Johnson C, Gewaily D, Drack A, Stone E, Wachtel K, Simonelli F, Leroy B, Wright J, High K, Maguire A (2017) Efficacy and safety of voretigene neparvovec (AAV2-hRPE65v2) in patients with

REP65-mediated inherited retinal dystrophy: a randomised, controlled, open-label, phase 3 trial. Lancet 390:849–860
Scott N, McPherson G, Ramsay C (2002) The method of minimization for allocation to clinical trials: a review. Control Clin Trials 23:662–674
Taves DR (1974) Minimization: a new method of assigning patients to treatment and control groups. Clin Pharmacol Ther 15:443–453
Wei L, Durham S (1978) The randomized play-the-winner rule in medical trials. J Am Stat Assoc 73(364):840–843

Power and Sample Size

41

Elizabeth Garrett-Mayer

Contents

Abstract

A critical component of clinical trial design is determining the appropriate sample size. Because clinical trials are planned in advance and require substantial resources per patient, the number of patients to be enrolled can be selected to

E. Garrett-Mayer (✉)
American Society of Clinical Oncology, Alexandria, VA, USA
e-mail: liz.garrett-mayer@asco.org

© Springer Nature Switzerland AG 2022

S. Piantadosi, C. L. Meinert (eds.), *Principles and Practice of Clinical Trials*,
https://doi.org/10.1007/978-3-319-52636-2_213

ensure that enough patients are enrolled to adequately address the research objectives and that unnecessary resources are not spent by enrolling too many patients. The most common approach for determining the optimal sample size in clinical trials is power calculation. Approaches for power calculations depend on trial characteristics, including the type of outcome measure and the number of treatment groups. Practical considerations such as trial budget, accrual rates, and drop-out rates also affect the study team's plan for determining the planned sample size for a trial. These aspects of sample size determination are discussed in addition.

Keywords

Power · Sample size · Type I error · Type II error · Clinically meaningful · Effect size

Introduction

A critical component of clinical trial design is determining the appropriate sample size. Because clinical trials are planned in advance and require substantial resources per patient, the number of patients to be enrolled can be selected to ensure that enough patients are enrolled to adequately address the research objectives and that unnecessary resources are not spent by enrolling too many patients. The most common approach for determining the optimal sample size in clinical trials is power calculation. In clinical trials evaluating a new treatment regimen relative to a standard treatment, power is the probability of concluding that the new treatment is superior to the standard treatment if the new treatment *really is* superior to the standard treatment. In designing a trial, the research team wants to ensure that the power of the trial is sufficiently high. If the trial does not have sufficient power, the team is likely to incorrectly conclude that a promising treatment has low efficacy.

The concept of power is based on hypothesis testing, a method used in most phase II and phase III clinical trials. As an example, consider a randomized trial with two treatment groups, an experimental treatment and a standard-of-care treatment, and assume that the outcome of interest is a binary indicator of response (i.e., a patient responds or does not respond to the assigned treatment). When a research team embarks on a trial, they have a hypothesis about the level of response for the treatment under study that would be considered "a success" relative to the control group. If the researchers are treating a condition where the standard treatment leads to a 10% response rate in patients, then perhaps a 25% response rate would be considered sufficiently high in the experimental treatment to pursue further study. In this example, to design the trial, the known information and assumptions regarding response rates in the standard of care and new treatment are used to set up the hypothesis test with two hypotheses: the null hypothesis (H_0) and the alternative hypothesis (H_1). H_0 represents the response rate if the new treatment is no better than the standard of care; H_1 represents the response rate if the new treatment is better

Table 1 Possible results of a clinical trial designed using hypothesis testing

		Truth	
		H_0	H_1
Hypothesis selected based on trial results	H_0	✓	Type II error
	H_1	Type I error	✓

than the standard of care. When developing a power calculation, these are usually written in the format

$$H_0 : p_1 = 0.10;\ p_2 = 0.10$$

$$H_1 : p_1 = 0.10;\ p_2 = 0.25,$$

where p_1 is the assumed response rate (or response probability) in the standard treatment and p_2 is the assumed response rate in the experimental treatment.

Type I and Type II Errors

In our hypothesis testing example assuming one of the two hypotheses is true, at the end of the trial, the research team will either choose the correct or the incorrect hypothesis. If the null hypothesis is true, but the data collected lead the research team to choose the alternative hypothesis, then the team has made a type I error. If the alternative hypothesis is true, but the data lead the research team to choose the null hypothesis, then the team has made a type II error. Table 1 shows the possible outcomes that a research team can make.

When designing a clinical trial, the research team wants to minimize making errors and sets the type I and II error rates to relatively low levels. Traditionally, type I error rates are set to values between 2.5% and 10%; type II errors are usually in the range of 10–20%. Note that the type I error rate is also called the alpha (α) level of the hypothesis test and the type II error rate the beta (β) level of the test. Power is 1 minus beta ($1-\beta$). Because it is desirable to keep the type II error relatively low ($\leq$20% in most trials), the power is usually at least 80% in well-designed studies.

In our example, there are four elements to include to calculate our optimal sample size: (1) the response rate under the null hypothesis, (2) the response rate under the alternative hypothesis, (3) the type I error rate, and (4) the type II error rate. As will be seen in later sections, when you have other types of outcomes, you may need additional information to perform the power calculation (e.g., the assumed variance if the outcome is a continuous variable).

Illustrations of Power

Graphical displays to illustrate power are shown in Fig. 1. In panel A, there are two bell curves (i.e., distributions) where the x-axis is the difference in proportions from

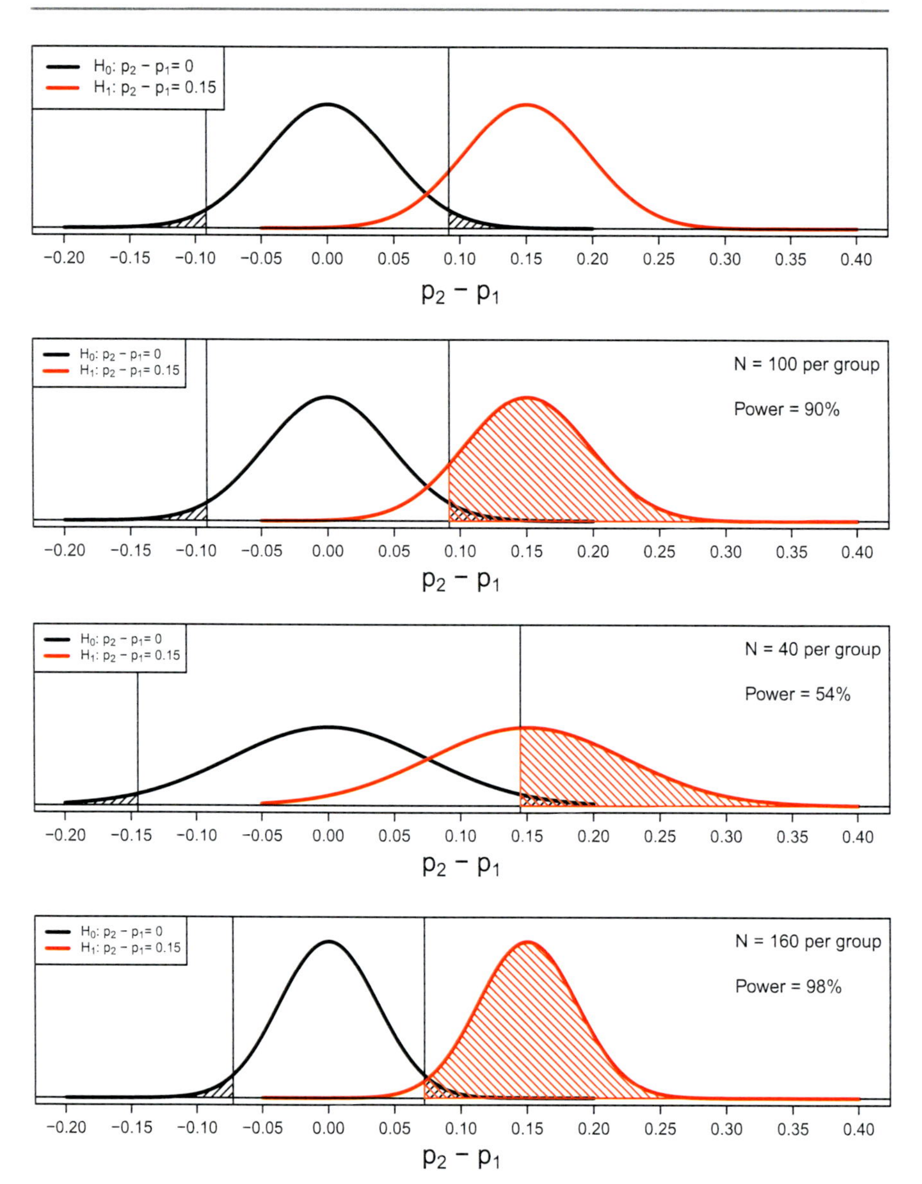

Fig. 1 Illustration of power and alpha levels for varying sample sizes with response rate as the outcome in a randomized trial with two treatment groups. Panels a, b, c and d are ordered vertically from top to bottom

our example. Each curve represents the response rate in the experimental group minus the response rate in the control group under one of our hypotheses. The black distribution represents the null hypothesis, where the difference in response rates is 0 (i.e., the response rate in both groups is 0.10 if the null hypothesis is true); the red distribution represents the alternative hypothesis where the difference in response rates is 0.15 (i.e., a 0.25 response rate in the experimental group minus a 0.10 response rate in the control group). These curves demonstrate the distributions of expected differences in response rates. For the black curve, it is very likely we will see a difference in response rate in the range of −0.05 to 0.05, given the height of the curve over that range. However, if the alternative is true, it is rather unlikely that we will see differences in that range, noted by the low height of the red curve in the region of −0.05 to 0.05.

Although there is not substantial overlap in the red and black curves in Fig. 1a, there is some overlap, suggesting there are some resulting observed differences in response rates that are similarly consistent with both hypotheses. For example, if the trial is completed and the difference in response rates is 0.07, this difference is about equally well-supported by both H_0 and H_1 as can be seen by the height of the curves at 0.07 on the x-axis. It is in this region where type I and II errors are likely to be made. In Fig. 1a, the black hashed sections represent the tails of the null distribution curve and, more specifically, the tails of the curve that correspond to the alpha level. In this example, the alpha level has been set to 0.05 (or 5%), meaning that each tail has 2.5% of the area under the curve. If the difference in response rates lies in one of these tails, then the null hypothesis is rejected, as it is considered relatively unlikely if the null hypothesis is true. Thus, the vertical black lines in Fig. 1a define the rejection regions: if the difference in proportions is outside the vertical black lines, then the null hypothesis is rejected because the data collected are inconsistent with H_0, relative to H_1.

Focusing on the alternative distribution now, the area under the red curve to the right of the rejection threshold line represents the power, which is the probability of rejecting the null hypothesis if the alternative hypothesis is true. This is illustrated in Fig. 1b where the red shaded area shows the power. Thus, in our example in Fig. 1a, b, the vertical lines define the rejection region; the black hashed areas show the alpha level of the trial and the red shaded region the power of the trial.

A critical aspect of the trial characteristics shown in Fig. 1a, b is the sample size. In Fig. 1a, b, the sample size in each group is 100. Fixing alpha at 0.05, this leads to a power of 90% (and, thus, a type II error of 10%). Figure 1c, d shows the effects on the shapes of the distributions that represent our trial when we change the sample size and the effects on power. In Fig. 1c, the sample size per group is 40. This leads to wider distributions and more overlap in the distributions. Assuming that alpha is maintained at 0.05 (i.e., 2.5% of the area in each tail defines the rejection region), the power drops to 54% (i.e., 54% of the area under the red curve is to the right of vertical rejection region threshold). This suggests that enrolling 40 patients per group is not enough: with only 40 patients per group, if the experimental treatment is better than the control treatment, we only have a 54% chance of making that conclusion at the end of the trial, even if the observed differences in response rates are close to the hypothesized difference of 0.15. We call this an "underpowered" trial because the power is too low.

Figure 1d shows a trial that is "overpowered." With a sample size of 160 per group, there is almost no overlap in the curves. Fixing the alpha again at 0.05, there is almost no region of the red curve that is to the left of the rejection threshold, and the power is 98%. While the research team will be pleased to know that they have a high chance of finding a significant difference in treatments if the treatments are different, many would argue that this trial is wasteful because it utilizes too many resources and could be completed without enrolling so many patients.

Trade-Offs in Power Calculations

From the previous section, there were four quantities that were specified to calculate the power of the trial: (1) the response rates under H_0; (2) the response rates under H_1; (3) the alpha level; and (4) the sample size. (As noted above, with other outcomes, the assumed variance may also be required.) In theory, one can specify the power and solve for any of the other four quantities. However, in most trials the null hypothesis and the alpha level are prespecified. Ideally, the research team would solve for the sample size based on the other quantities, but due to resource constraints, many trials have an upper limit on a feasible sample size, and thus power or the alternative hypothesis is determined based on the sample size limitations.

Clinically Meaningful Effect Sizes and Sample Size

It is important to ensure that the alternative hypothesis represents a *clinically meaningful difference* or *clinically meaningful effect size*. That is, the difference in response rates should represent a difference that would lead experts in the area to conclude that the experimental treatment represents a meaningful improvement in response and worthy of either further study or should be used regularly in clinical practice (depending on the phase of the trial and other supporting evidence). Additionally, the alternative hypothesis should not be unrealistic: it is not useful to assert a very large effect size as the alternative hypothesis if it is not likely attainable. The sample size will be small, but the trial is likely to fail to find a difference, and even a moderately large observed difference would not lead to rejection of the null hypothesis. If the alternative hypothesis in our example was set to difference in response rates of 0.50 (i.e., the assumed response rate in the experimental group is 0.60 under the alternative hypothesis), the required sample size would only be 42 patients (21 per treatment), but the observed difference in response rates would have to be relatively large to reject the null hypothesis. Looking back after the trial, if the research team had seen a response rate of 33% in the experimental group and 10% in the control group, the team might be disappointed to conclude that they cannot reject the null even though the difference in response rates was 23%; the p-value for this result would be 0.13 using a Fisher's exact test.

Similarly, research teams should be discouraged from seeking small differences, as they may not be clinically meaningful. This has been addressed in cancer clinical trials by numerous authors, concerned that anticancer therapies may be approved for use in cancer patients due to statistical significance, but may not confer any meaningful improvement in survival (Sobrero and Bruzzi 2009). Studies like this led to efforts to define clinically meaningful differences in cancer clinical trials, with the goal of ensuring that trials would be designed with appropriate levels of power and sample size to ensure that detectable effect sizes would be clinically meaningful (Ellis et al. 2014).

Choosing Alpha and Beta (or Power) Levels

There are conventions in clinical trials that have been used for many decades, leading to almost no consideration given to appropriate selection of alpha and beta levels. Most commonly, one will see alpha set to 5% and beta set to 20% (i.e., power set to 80%). These are not *correct* levels, but are the most commonly chosen. Strident arguments can be made that setting alpha low for a phase III trial is appropriate: making a type I error when deciding whether or not to approve an experimental agent is a very serious error. That is, a type I error would lead to approving an agent when the agent is not better as compared to the control group. From an approval standpoint, making a type II error is less grievous; not approving an effective treatment is less worrisome than approving ineffective treatments. Thus, for trials that are intended to provide direct evidence for approval of the agent, setting alpha substantially lower than beta may be sensible. However, in earlier phase trials, setting alpha and beta to similar levels may be a better strategy. In many early efficacy trials in cancer research, alpha and beta are both set to 10%, suggesting that each type of error has equally bad implications. In this setting, the research team is more willing to take an ineffective agent to the next phase of research (higher alpha), but less willing to discard an effective agent (lower beta).

Power Calculations for Common Trial Designs

Different areas of medical research tend to use different primary outcomes in their trials, leading to differences in test statistics used in hypothesis tests and thus in how power calculations are performed. Most outcomes fall into one of the three categories: continuous, binary, or time-to-event outcomes. The example in the previous section was based on a comparison of response rates and a binary outcome. In the following sections, comparative and single-treatment studies are reviewed for each of these outcomes.

Comparative Studies

Binary Outcomes

A randomized trial with a binary outcome example was developed in section "Introduction." For binary outcomes, there are various options and assumptions that can be used in power calculations. In Fig. 1, a normal approximation was used, which is simple to calculate and works well when the response probabilities are not close to 0 or

Table 2 Differences in power using different power calculation approaches for a randomized trial with a binary indicator of response as the outcome, assuming response probabilities of 0.10 and 0.25 in the control and experimental treatments under the alternative hypotheses, respectively

Power calculation type	Sample size per treatment	Power (%)
Normal test, approximation 1	40	54
Normal test, approximation 2	40	31
Chi-square test	40	42
Fisher's exact test	40	33
Normal approximation 1	100	90
Normal approximation 2	100	80
Chi-square test	100	83
Fisher's exact test	100	76
Normal approximation 1	160	98
Normal approximation 2	160	93
Chi-square test	160	96
Fisher's exact test	160	94

1 in either group, and the sample size is relatively large. Other normal approximations are also used which differ in their approach for estimating the denominator of the test statistic (i.e., the standard error of the difference in proportions). Depending on the sample size and the assumed response rates, the power estimates may be very similar or dissimilar depending on the approximation used. When planning a trial, the approach used to calculate the power or sample size should be consistent with the approach used to analyze the data at the end of the trial (Table 2).

Continuous Outcomes

In the previous example with a binary outcome, in addition to knowing the power and alpha, one only needed to know the expected response rates under the null and alternative hypotheses. When the outcome of the trial is a continuous variable, and the goal is to compare the means between two groups, the research team must set null and alternative hypotheses for the means in the groups, and they must also make an assumption about the variance of the outcome. For example, assume that a trial is being planned to evaluate the efficacy of vitamin D supplementation in individuals with vitamin D deficiency where individuals are randomized to a low dose of vitamin D (400 IU) in one group and a high dose in another group (2000 IU). The outcome is 25(OH)D, which is a measure of vitamin D in the blood. The research team assumes (based on their previous research) that the standard deviation of 25 (OH)D is approximately 14 ng/mL in individuals who do not have deficiency. The research team plans to compare 25(OH)D levels between the two groups after 6 months of supplementation using a two-sample t-test.

In the previous example, the width of the curves that determined power (Fig. 1) was determined based on the both assumed response rates in the null and alternative hypotheses and the sample sizes in each group. When using a continuous outcome, the means in the null and alternative hypotheses and the

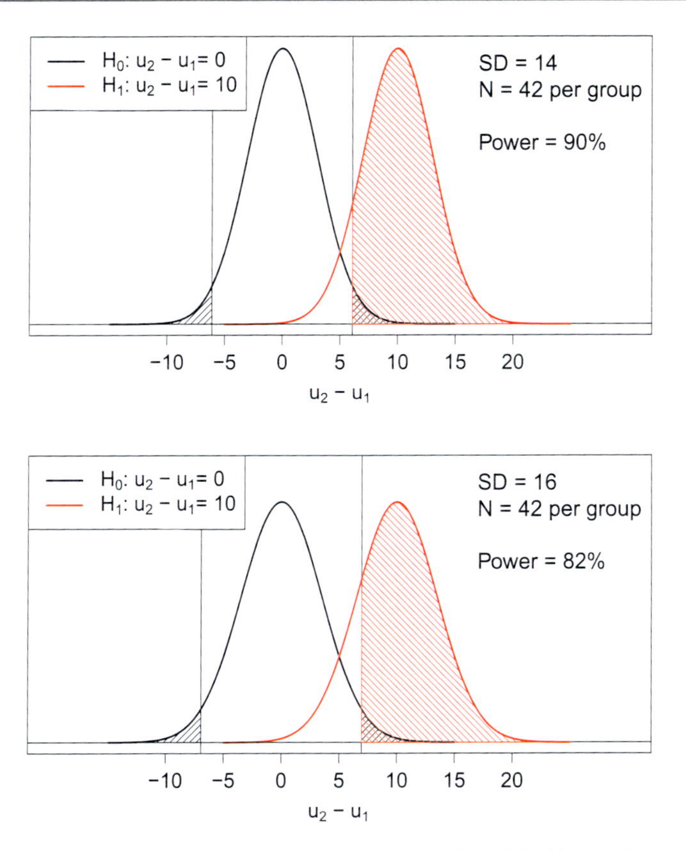

Fig. 2 Illustration of effect of the standard deviation on power in a trial with a continuous outcome. Panels a is on the top; panel b is on the bottom

sample size factor into the power calculation, but so does the assumed standard deviation. Thus, to calculate power, the following are required: alpha, sample size, difference in means under the null hypothesis (usually 0), the difference in means under the alternative hypothesis, and the standard deviation in each group. The researchers expect that the mean 25(OH)D levels will be 55 ng/mL in the low-dose group and 65 ng/mL in the high-dose group after 6 months of supplementation. Under the null hypothesis, the means would be the same; and under the alternative hypothesis, the difference in means would be 10 ng/mL:

$$H_0 : u_2 - u_1 = 0 \text{ ng/mL}$$

$$H_1 : u_2 - u_1 = 10 \text{ ng/mL}$$

To achieve 90% power with a two-sided alpha level of 5%, and assuming that the standard deviation is 14 ng/mL in each group, the research team would need to enroll 42 patients in each group. Figure 2a shows the distributions of the difference in means under the null and the alternatives, assuming a sample size of 42 per group, and a standard deviation (SD) of 14 ng/mL in each group. All else being the same, if the assumed SD were larger, the power would decrease. Having a larger SD in each group adds more variance and thus more imprecision in the estimates. Figure 2b shows the effect of the larger SD on power if the sample size remains 42 per group. Notice that the curves are wider, the overlap is greater, and the area under the alternative distribution curve representing power (i.e., the red shaded portion) is smaller. If the SD is 16 ng/mL in each group instead of 14, the power decreases from 90% to 82%. In the example above, it was assumed that the standard deviation in the two groups is the same (14 ng/mL). Power calculations can also be performed assuming a different standard deviations in each group.

Time-to-Event Outcomes

In many trials, the outcome of interest is a time interval. For example, in many phase III randomized clinical trials in cancer research, survival time is the outcome, that is, the time from enrollment on the trial until death. The challenging aspect of survival time as an outcome is that not all patients have the event of interest (death) when the data are analyzed. The patients who are still alive at the time of data analysis have survival times that are "censored," meaning that we know that they lived for a certain amount of time but we do not know their actual survival time (which will occur in the future). Statisticians have approaches for analyzing time-to-event outcomes, such as survival time. Randomized trials with time-to-event outcomes which have inferences based on the hazard ratio (i.e., the ratio of events in two groups being compared) only require a few elements: the hazard ratio under the null hypothesis (usually assumed to be 1, meaning equal event rates), the hazard ratio under the alternative, and the type I and type II errors. With these quantities, one can solve for the number of events required to achieve the desired power. While the simplicity is convenient, when planning a trial, knowing the number of events needed is not sufficient: clinical trial protocols require that the number of patients enrolled be stated. Using additional information, including the expected accrual rate and the minimum amount of time each patient will be followed for events combined with the required number of events to achieve the desired power, the number of patients required for enrollment can be calculated.

The hypothesis for evaluating a time-to-event outcome could be set up as follows, where the null hypothesis assumes there is no difference in the event rates in the two groups; the alternative in this example assumes that the event rate in group 2 (λ_2) is half as large as the event rate in group 1 (λ_1). If this were a cancer treatment trial with two treatments with survival time as the outcome, the alternative assumes that the rate of death occurring in group 2 is half of that in group 1, meaning the treatment in group 2 doubles the expected survival time:

$$H_0 : \lambda_2/\lambda_1 = 1$$

$$H_1 : \lambda_2/\lambda_1 = 0.5$$

Going back to the characteristics that affect sample size, if the hazard ratio were 0.75 instead of 0.5, the sample size would be required to be larger due to a smaller difference in rates in the two treatments. And, knowing that the power is driven by the number of events, the sample size for a trial with 2 events per month would need to be larger than a trial with 20 events per month to be completed in a similar amount of time. Sample size for trials based on time-to-event outcomes also depends on the accrual rate and the planned length of follow-up. For example, based on the expected accrual rate of ten patients per month, a trial with only 1 year of follow-up (after the last patient has enrolled) will require more patients than a trial with 2 years of follow-up because the latter trial will observe more events prior to stopping the trial.

Single-Treatment Studies

In single-treatment studies, the null hypothesis is based on an "historical control" estimate of a control setting (e.g., the effect under the standard of care). Using our previous example, imagine that instead of performing a trial with two treatments where patients are randomized to the experimental and the control group, information from patients previously treated with the control treatment is used to develop an appropriate null hypothesis regarding what an ineffective response rate would be, but no patients are enrolled in a control condition. In practice, patients are enrolled to the experimental treatment, and at the end of the trial, their response rate (p) is compared to what would have been expected had they been treated using the control treatment. This is written (using our previous terminology) as

$$H_0 : p = 0.10$$

$$H_1 : p = 0.25$$

where p is the response rate and H_0 represents a response rate too low for further consideration and H_1 a response rate that is sufficiently high for further study of the treatment. The power calculation includes the same elements of alpha, beta, null, and alternative hypothesis, but the calculation will have smaller sample sizes than the comparative trial. This is due to lower variance – with only one treatment group included, and a fixed comparator, there is only variance in the experimental condition.

The same trade-offs between type I and II errors, clinical effect size, and sample size are present in single-treatment studies as in randomized trials.

Single-Treatment Trial, Binary Outcome

Single Stage

In the example in section "Single-Treatment Studies," with a null response rate of 0.10 and an alternative response rate of 0.25, the sample size can be calculated using either an approximation (e.g., a normal approximation or chi-square approximation) or an exact test. Because single-treatment studies tend to be smaller than comparative studies, using Fisher's exact test is often preferred (recall that the approximations work best when sample sizes are large). If we assume a type I error (two-sided) of 0.05 and power of 90%, this trial would require 59 patients. If the research team determined that they did not have sufficient resources to enroll 59 patients and could only enroll 50 patients, the trial would have 83% power.

Multistage

As described in section "Interim Analyses and Early Stopping Rules" (Practical Considerations), many trials are designed to have sufficient sample size to maintain power and alpha when interim analyses or early stopping rules are incorporated into the design. One common single-treatment trial design for binary outcomes is the Simon two-stage design which includes two stages, where n_1 patients are enrolled in the first stage and n_2 patients are enrolled in the second stage, and uses a one-sided test (Simon 1989). After n_1 patients are enrolled, the number of responses is compared to a predefined threshold (r_1). If there are r_1 or fewer responses, the trial stops for futility. That is, if there are r_1 or fewer responses at the end of stage 1, it is unlikely that sufficient responses could be seen by the end of stage 2 to reject the null hypothesis, and so no more patients are enrolled. If more than r_1 responses are seen at the end of stage 1, the trial continues, enrolling an additional n_2 patients (for a total of n_1+n_2 patients at the end of stage 2). At the end of stage 2, the total number of responses (from stage 1 and 2 combined) are counted up, and the null hypothesis is rejected if there are sufficient responses.

Technically, there are many designs that can fit the criteria (due to the flexibility induced by allowing the early look). Simon suggested a criterion minimizes the expected sample size of the trial if the null hypothesis is true. He referred to this version of the design as the "optimal" two-stage design.

Because the trial has two "looks" at the data, the type I and II errors will differ from that in a trial with only one look. In this type of trial, early stopping is only allowed for futility, meaning there are two opportunities for a type II error and only one opportunity for a type I error. To ensure that the errors are controlled, the sample size is usually slightly larger than if the trial was performed in a single stage. For example, a single-stage trial with H_0: $p = 0.20$ versus H_1: $p = 0.40$ requires a sample size of 42 for a one-sided alpha of 0.05 to maintain a power of 0.90. Simon's optimal two-stage design requires 54 patients, with 19 patients in stage 1 and stopping early for futility if fewer than 5 patients has responses. Other two-stage designs with alpha of 0.05 and power of 90% could be selected that would allow a sample size closer to 42, but they would not meet the optimality criterion defined above.

Single-Treatment Trial, Continuous Outcome

Single-treatment studies with continuous outcomes include primarily the same information as for two-treatment studies for continuous outcomes. If one were to undertake a trial of high-dose vitamin D supplementation described as a single-treatment trial, the trial would enroll patients into a high-dose vitamin D group (2000 IU). The null hypothesis was an expected mean of 25(OH)D level of

55 ng/mL, which is what the research team assumed would occur in a low-dose (400 IU) setting; the researchers assumed that giving a high dose would lead to a higher mean, a mean of 65 ng/mL. This would be set up as follows:

$$H_0 : u = 55 \text{ ng/mL}$$

$$H_1 : u = 65 \text{ ng/mL}$$

The additional requirements to complete the power calculation would be the assumed standard deviation (14 ng/mL from above) and the alpha and power levels. With alpha of 0.05, and power of 90%, the required sample size was only 17. Note that the sample size in the comparative trial described in section was 84 (42 patients per treatment). As expected the sample size for the single-treatment trial is smaller, due to the lower variance with just one treatment.

Single-Treatment Trial with TTE Outcome

When designing a single-treatment trial with a time-to-event outcome, the standard approaches are (1) to compare the median event time to a presumed median event time in a control setting or (2) to compare the event rate to a presumed event rate in a control setting. The first of these will require a larger sample size, because the median event time tends to be imprecise. In the example below, this is expressed as null hypothesis of a median (m) of 6 months and an alternative hypothesis median of 9 months. Power calculations can be based on a test for differences in medians (Brookmeyer and Crowley 1982).

$$H_0 : m = 6 \text{ months}$$

$$H_1 : m = 9 \text{ months}$$

Comparing event rates is more efficient but will require that assumption that the event rate is constant over time. For example, the example below shows a null hypothesis with an event rate (λ) of 0.30; the alternative hypothesis event rate is 0.20. If the assumption that the event rate is constant over time is untrue, the inferences from the trial could be invalid. Power calculations in this setting can be based on a test of the rate parameter from the exponential distribution.

$$H_0 : \lambda = 0.30$$

$$H_1 : \lambda = 0.20$$

Power Calculations for Non-inferiority Studies

Most trials are designed as superiority studies; that is, the goal is to show that a treatment is better than another treatment setting (which might be an active treatment, a placebo, or no treatment at all). However, some trials have the primary objective of showing that a new treatment is similarly effective to another treatment. For example, the standard-of-care treatment might be reasonably efficacious but have unpleasant side effects. A new treatment may be hypothesized to have similar efficacy to the standard of care but a better side effect profile. In this example, the research team would want to design a trial to show that for the efficacy outcome, the new treatment is non-inferior to the standard of care. Non-inferiority trials require the research team to define a margin of non-inferiority to set up the hypothesis test. That, is how much worse could the new treatment be without being considered significantly worse? As an example, if the standard of care had a response rate of 50%, by setting a non-inferiority margin of 5% would mean that a response rate of 45% for the new treatment would be considered non-inferior.

The hypothesis test is set up in the opposite way from superiority trials. The null hypothesis assumes that the new treatment is worse than the standard of care; the alternative hypothesis assumes that the new treatment is equal to or better than the standard of care (based on the margin of non-inferiority). Power is still the probability that the null hypothesis is rejected if the alternative is true; alpha is still the probability that the null hypothesis is rejected if the null hypothesis is true. For obvious reasons, non-inferiority margins should be rather small. It would be hard to argue that a treatment with a response rate that is 10–20% worse than the standard of care is non-inferior. As a result, non-inferiority trials seek to focus on small differences in treatment and require large sample sizes to demonstrate non-inferiority for levels of power and alpha that are comparable to those in superiority trials.

Approaches for Calculation of Power and Sample Size

Available Software and Websites

Although there are formulas for power and sample size calculations that can be implemented by hand (or with a calculator), clinical trial power calculations are performed using software packages specifically designed for power and sample size estimation (e.g., NQuery, PASS, GPower, EAST), standard all-purpose statistical software (e.g., SAS, Stata, R, or SPSS), or using online websites (e.g., www.crab.org, http://powerandsamplesize.com).

Sample size estimation software packages provide many options and user-friendly interfaces for standard trial designs and some more complex settings, such as ANOVA, clustered designs, and early stopping rules. Many academic institutions and companies involved in trial design have a license for at least one package, and some are free to download (e.g., GPower). Statistical packages like SAS and Stata include standard trial design options for power calculations (e.g., one- and two-sample comparisons of mean and proportions). While R has standard designs available, it also has user-contributed libraries that allow users to perform power calculations for more complex designs (e.g., cluster-randomized trials can be designed using the "`clusterPower`" library.

Simulation Studies for Power Calculations

Not all trials designs will fall into the categories discussed above. For example, for a trial with a longitudinal design where the primary objective includes comparing trajectories (or slopes) based on repeated measures per individual in two or more groups, there may not be a standard software package that will suit the trial design needs. In that case, sample size could be determined based on simulation studies. That is, just as above where assumptions were made regarding effect size, variance, sample size, and alpha, assumptions are made for all the relevant parameters, and trials are simulated under the set of assumptions. For each trial simulated under the parameters consistent with the alternative hypothesis, the trial results are analyzed, and it is determined if the null hypothesis is rejected or accepted (at the predefined alpha level). The proportion of simulated trials for which the null hypothesis is rejected provides an estimate of the power. To get a precise estimate of power, the number of simulated trials has to be reasonably large. If the power is too low for a given sample size, the sample size can be increased, and the simulations can be performed using the larger sample size; this can be repeated until the desired power level is reached.

While simulations allow the research team to investigate trial properties for complex designs, they have the drawback that they usually have quite a few parameters for which the research team needs to make assumptions. However, it is not always possible to have preliminary information to make assumptions. This leads the research team to consider a range of values for some parameters. Additionally, simulations require skill in programming and depth of knowledge of statistics and probability distributions. Simulations can be time-consuming: they may take considerable time to develop and undertake (depending on the number of simulations, the number of parameters, and the range of parameters considered) and to summarize and present in graphical or tabular format.

Power Calculations for Fixed Sample Size Studies

In clinical trials, the sample size is planned prior to embarking on the trial, and so the planning for the sample size incorporates the clinical effect size, alpha, power, and variance. Once the sample size is determined, there may be additional analyses the research team plans to perform to address secondary objectives of the trial. It is unlikely that the sample size would be increased to ensure sufficient power for secondary objectives, but it can be helpful to calculate power for secondary analyses or to report the effect size that is detectable for secondary analyses based on a fixed power and the sample size for the trial.

In some cases, after the trial is completed, the data from the trial may be used for "secondary data analyses," which implies that the data were collected but not intended to be used for these analyses. The researchers may write a proposal for these additional data analyses and the proposal should justify that the objectives of the secondary data analyses can be achieved with the sample size of the dataset. This can be helpful perspective for the research team proposing the analyses as it will determine the effect sizes that are detectable for the predetermined sample size for a given power level. The research team may have an overpowered trial, in which case they may want to use a relatively small alpha level to conclude "significance." If the trial is underpowered (i.e., the sample size is too small to detect clinically relevant effect sizes), the research team may decide that the analysis should not be conducted, or they may decide to perform the analysis, but will be cognizant of the low power and take it into account when interpreting their results, and they may choose to avoid significance testing altogether.

Alternatives to Power

Inferences for some trials are not based on traditional hypothesis tests, and therefore power is not relevant.

Precision

Some trials have goals of estimation. For example, a single-treatment trial of a new agent in a patient population defined by a biomarker could have the primary objective of estimation of median progression-free survival. Instead of testing that median survival is larger than a null value, the sample size can be motivated by the precision with which the median survival is estimated. If the research team wants to estimate the median survival with a 95% confidence interval with a width no greater than 2 months, the research team can use information regarding expected accrual rate, assumptions about possible observed values of median survival, and determine how many patients to enroll to ensure that the width is within 2 months.

Although this is a sensible approach, there are not standard guidelines that allow one to determine what a sufficiently precise confidence interval might be. Additionally, at the end of the trial, the 95% confidence interval still needs to be interpreted, and a decision has to be made regarding whether or not further study of the agent should be pursued in the patient population. The lower limit of the confidence interval in this case could be used to determine if the treatment should be pursued in additional research studies and for calculating effect sizes for future studies.

Sample Size Calculations in Bayesian Settings

The approaches in this chapter have focused primarily on frequentist interpretations of hypothesis testing and frequentist calculations. Bayesian statistics use different concepts for analysis and interpretation of data. Thus, Bayesian trial designs differ in the way that they determine sample sizes and in the concepts that they use that are similar to type I and II errors. Although some quantities can be directly calculated, power and sample size calculations for Bayesian trial designs are calculated using simulations because Bayesian trial designs tend to be adaptive. See Lee and Chu for more details, including advantages to Bayesian trial designs (Lee and Chu 2012).

Practical Considerations

Evaluability of Patients

Clinical trials must state a planned sample size for review and approval by institutional review boards (IRBs) and for other scientific review committees. Technically, studies should not enroll beyond the planned sample size, and doing so can result in punitive actions for not following the trial protocol. But, in the practical implementation of trials, not all patients contribute information to address the primary objective and are deemed "inevaluable" as per a definition in the protocol. For example, a patient may enroll in the trial but drop out of the trial prior to receiving the trial treatment, and thus the patient did not receive treatment and has no information on the outcome of interest. Some trials may have approaches for how this patient may contribute to the analysis, but many trials would deem this patient as inevaluable. In trials in which there are expected to be patients who are inevaluable, the research team should take this into account when planning the sample size. For example, if the sample size calculation requires 60 patients for sufficient power and the team anticipates 10% of patients will be inevaluable, the projected enrollment should be at least 67 ($67 \times (1–0.10) = 60.3$).

Interim Analyses and Early Stopping Rules

The examples provided in previous sections (except for the Simon's two-stage design) have assumed single-stage designs, where the trial enrolls patients and does not evaluate the data until the trial ends. In practice, many trials have early stopping rules or are designed to have interim analyses, which may affect the trial's enrollment.

Early Stopping Rules

Trials with early stopping rules allow trials to stop prior to total planned enrollment if there is early evidence to stop early. Stopping rules can be included for early evidence of futility and/or efficacy. As noted above, futility stopping allows an early look where a type II error could be made. Early stopping for efficacy (i.e., early evidence suggests the alternative hypothesis is true) allows an early look where a type I error could be made. Trials in which both futility and efficacy stopping are included will need to account for these looks at the data and increase the sample size accordingly to ensure that the desired power and alpha can be achieved. If the power calculations do not account for the early looks, the true type I and II error rates will be higher than assumed.

Interim Analyses

In addition to early stopping rules, other analyses can be planned to take place in the midst of a trial. For example, the research team may be required to make assumptions regarding the trial, such as the accrual rate or the event rate, without much preliminary data, and the team designs the trial to adjust the sample size to account for any incorrect assumptions. This does not allow the team free reign to make changes to the trial based on interim results – this type of analysis must be planned carefully in advance with clearly defined plans for how any changes would be made. In addition, these mid-trial analyses are usually planned so that the research team is blinded from knowing efficacy estimates. One type of interim analysis that could be planned is an estimation of "conditional power" where the trial team determines the likelihood of rejecting the null hypothesis based on the evidence in the data collected thus far. If the conditional power is very high, the trial may continue without any revisions to the sample size; if the conditional power is moderate (e.g., between 50% and 80%), the sample size may be increased to bring the power up to a level of 80% or higher; if the conditional power is low, the trial may be discontinued due to futility (i.e., with a low conditional power, a very large sample size increase would be required, suggesting that the detectable effect size would be considered too small to be clinically relevant).

Summary and Conclusions

Power and sample size calculations are an important part of clinical trial planning. There are standard approaches for many traditional designs, including those for continuous, binary, or time-to-event outcomes, and for single-treatment and for randomized trials. For more complex designs, including those with adaptive designs, interim analyses, or early stopping, more sophisticated calculations need to be performed to ensure that type I and type II errors are controlled. While some power calculations can be conducted using standard software or online tools, it is wise to engage a biostatistician to ensure the calculations are performed properly and any nuances of the design have been accounted for.

Key Facts

- Type I and II errors must be controlled when designing trials to ensure that inferences lead research team to correct conclusions with a high probability.
- There are many types of trial designs, and power and sample size calculations can be performed using simple approaches (which are available in software or online) or using complex simulation studies.
- Practical considerations need to be considered in addition to output from formulas for power or sample size.

References

Brookmeyer R, Crowley JJ (1982) A confidence interval for the median survival time. Biometrics 38:29–41

Ellis LM, Bernstein DS, Voest EE, Berlin JD, Sargent D, Cortazar P, Garrett-Mayer E, Herbst RS, Lilenbaum RC, Sima C, Venook AP, Gonen M, Schilsky RL, Meropol NJ, Schnipper LE (2014) American Society of Clinical Oncology perspective: raising the bar for clinical trials by defining clinically meaningful outcomes. J Clin Oncol 32(12):1277–1280

Lee JJ, Chu CT (2012) Bayesian clinical trials in action. Stat Med 31(25):2955–2972

Simon R (1989) Optimal two-stage designs. Control Clin Trials 10:1–10

Sobrero A, Bruzzi P (2009) Incremental advance or seismic shift? The need to raise the bar of efficacy for drug approval. J Clin Oncol 27(35):5868–5873

Controlling Bias in Randomized Clinical Trials

42

Bruce A. Barton

Contents

Abstract

Clinical trials are considered to be the gold standard of research designs at the top of the evidence chain. This reputation is due to the ability to randomly allocate subjects to treatments and to mask the treatment assignment at various levels, including subject, observers taking measurements or administering questionnaires, and investigators who are overseeing the performance of the study. This chapter section deals with the five major causes of bias in clinical trials: (1) selection bias, or the biased assignment of subjects to treatment groups; (2) performance bias, or the collection of data in a way that favors one treatment group over another; (3) detection bias, or the biased detection of study outcomes (including both safety and efficacy) to favor one treatment group over another;

B. A. Barton (✉)
Department of Population and Quantitative Health Sciences, University of Massachusetts Medical School, Worcester, MA, USA
e-mail: Bruce.Barton@umassmed.edu

© Springer Nature Switzerland AG 2022

S. Piantadosi, C. L. Meinert (eds.), *Principles and Practice of Clinical Trials*,
https://doi.org/10.1007/978-3-319-52636-2_214

(4) attrition bias, or differential dropout from the study in one treatment group compared to the other; and (5) reporting and publication bias, or the tendency of investigators to include only the positive results in the main results paper (regardless of what is specified in the study protocol) and the tendency of journals to publish only papers with positive results. While other biases can (and do) occur and are also described here, they tend to have lower impact on the integrity of the study. The definitions of these biases will be presented, along with how to proactively prevent them through study design and procedures.

Keywords

Treatment randomization · Treatment masking · Selection bias · Performance bias · Detection bias · Attrition bias · Reporting bias

Introduction

Clinical trials are generally considered the least biased of any research study design and are widely considered to the gold standard of research designs (Doll 1998). The two major factors credited for the lower risk of bias in clinical trials are the use of random treatment assignment for subjects and masking of the assigned treatment. No matter how it is performed, treatment randomization "levels the playing field" so that the treatment groups are typically similar in terms of baseline patient characteristics, medical history, etc. Assignment to treatment is not influenced by factors of any kind – for example, severity of disease, previous history, gender, age, or location do not affect the probability of randomization for any subject. The treatment masking of the assigned treatment alleviates any bias of the observer to record data in a way that is preferential to one treatment group over the other.

However, clinical trials are not impervious to bias, although the risk is certainly reduced compared to other designs (Lewis and Warlow 2004). Perhaps the best compendium of biases in clinical trials is the *Cochrane Handbook for Systematic Reviews of Interventions* (Higgins et al. 2008), which lists the potential biases in clinical trials: (1) selection bias, (2) performance bias, (3) detection bias, (4) attrition bias, (5) reporting/publication bias, and (6) other sources of bias. The Cochrane Collaboration has developed a tool for assessing the risk of bias, which is recommended for the evaluation of studies to include in each systematic review submitted to the Cochrane Reviews, but is also useful to help investigators reduce, if not eliminate, bias in their studies. In addition, the CONSORT Statement and, in particular, the Elaboration and Extension information can help investigators avoid inadvertent biases in their study design, protocol, and reporting.

The following sections describe the types of problems that can result in each type of bias, how to detect these problems, how serious they are, and how a researcher can design a study that avoids them.

Sources of Bias

Selection Bias

Selection bias refers to how subjects are allocated to treatment groups. There are many examples in the literature of nonrandomized studies yielding positive results for a treatment only to have a subsequent randomized study overturn those results (e.g., Wangensteen et al. 1962; Ruffin et al. 1969). The underlying reason for the positive results in a nonrandomized setting is that the investigators give the treatment to patients preselected to be responsive. Without a randomized control group, it is not possible to estimate the treatment effect. Bias can also arise if patient outcomes are compared to historical or other non-contemporaneous (or nonrandomly chosen) controls. The solution to this source of bias is the randomization of subjects between (or among) treatment/control groups.

In a randomized clinical trial, subjects are randomly allocated to treatment/control groups according to a masked allocation sequence, either static or dynamic. It is important to understand that the randomization must be masked so that the investigators are not able to determine what the next treatment assignment might be. For example, if the "randomization" is based on the last digit of the patient's medical record number, investigators will be able to determine what treatment the current patient will receive – and advise the patient (either directly or indirectly) on whether to enroll in the study based on that knowledge and their own bias related to treatment efficacy. In RCTs, randomization means masked randomization with barriers built into the sequence to prevent determining the next treatment allocation. The section below discusses approaches to do this.

Typically, this is done through a randomization process as part of the allocation; for example, subjects are assigned to treatment groups based on a sequence of random numbers. The complete process is as follows.

Before the study is started, a sequence of random numbers is generated, either from a table of random numbers or from a computer program/web site. That sequence can take a number of forms, ranging from single digits (e.g., 1, 2, 3,. . .) to multiple digits (e.g., 001, 002, 003,. . .) or (especially from computer programs) any decimal sequence between 0.0 and 1.0. Once the full range of the random numbers is known, subjects who receive numbers in the lower half of the sequence of random numbers are assigned to one treatment group, while subjects who receive numbers in the top half are assigned to the other treatment group. Once the treatment assignments have been determined for each random number, the numbers are put back into the original order to achieve a fully randomized list (Lachin 1988).

This simple approach, however, does not assure balance of the numbers of subjects between the treatment groups. It also does not avoid a lengthy string of the same treatment. The usual approach to assure the balance is through a permuted block randomization (Matts and Lachin 1988). In this approach to random allocation, random sequences are generated in groups of numbers, known as "blocks." Each block of, say, four random numbers is sorted by the random numbers in the block with the lowest two numbers assigned to one treatment group and the other two numbers assigned to the other treatment group. The random numbers are then put back into the original sequence, forcing a balance between the numbers of subjects assigned to each treatment group while generating a truly random sequence. The down side to this approach is that, if it becomes known what the block size is, the final treatment assignment in the block is easy to determine. The way to eliminate this potential bias is to randomly set the block size (e.g., for a particular study, the block sizes could be 2, 4, or 6) so that it is not possible to determine the next treatment assignment without knowledge of the block size that is currently being filled. This information is, of course, hidden from the investigators as only the random sequence of treatment assignments is available to the randomization system.

In addition to the allocation bias described above, there is a potential bias related to an imbalance of factors that are highly predictive of outcomes. For example, in studies of diabetes in which HbA1c is the outcome, body mass index (BMI) could be an important predictor of HbA1c. To assure a balance of BMI in the two treatment groups so that a biased outcome is not generated by a BMI imbalance, stratification can be used. Patients' BMI could be classified as "normal" (BMI 18–25) or "elevated" (BMI >25.0). The patients with normal BMI would have a separate randomization to assure an equal distribution of normal BMI patients between the treatment groups, as would the patients with elevated BMI. It should be noted that typically there is a separate randomization within the clinical center in a multicenter clinical trial so that the treatments are balanced within each clinic, eliminating any treatment bias within center.

Typically, a formal stratification using this approach would be limited to three variables because of complexity of maintaining the randomizations across multiple strata. For situations where it is important to balance the randomization for more than three important factors, the alternate strategy is a minimization or dynamic allocation strategy. This strategy keeps track of the treatment allocations for each factor of interest. As patients are randomized using a standard approach, an imbalance may develop with, say, females so that more females are assigned to one treatment group (Treatment A) compared to the other (Treatment B). The usual approach, to preserve an element of randomization, is to reduce the probability of being assigned to Treatment A so that Treatment B has a higher probability of assignment for the next female. This reduction in the probability of assignment to Treatment A is a function of the imbalance, so that the usual probability of assignment to Treatment A of 0.50 is reduced to 0.40 or even 0.25 depending on the decisions during the study design phase related to how much tolerance to imbalance is possible. The adjustment of this probability also implies that an a priori randomization scheme is not possible since the probability of assignment will vary for each new patient depending on the balance across the important factors. For each new patient ready for randomization, this recalculation of probability of assignment to Treatment A (and the associated probability of assignment to Treatment B) must take into account any imbalance for each important factor, so that an overall probability is calculated. Thus, the randomization system must be available at all times with access to the previous randomizations so that these calculations can be made in real time.

In a cluster-randomized study, the randomization is generated at the facility level (e.g., nursing home, ERs, hospitals) so that everyone recruited from that facility receives the same treatment. In this type of study, masking is less of an issue since everyone is getting the same treatment. However, the main problem is that the baseline characteristics of the randomized units may not be similar, as they are when the randomization is at the individual level. For cluster-randomized studies, a recently described approach, the minimal sufficient balance randomization method (Zhao et al. 2011), and other approaches can balance the covariates of the randomization units so that even a small number of clusters (e.g., nursing homes within a city) will be reasonably balanced on important covariates.

Unfortunately, there are few, if any, flexible randomization programs available online or even in the more advanced statistical software packages (e.g., SAS, Stata, SPSS, R). Programs can certainly be written in these languages to implement any of the above techniques, but programming knowledge of each package is required. The implementation of adaptive randomization strategies, in particular, will require specialized programming. While there are a few R-based programs, such as RRApp, to provide more capability, the more advanced techniques still require programming capability.

Cautionary Note

Many database management systems, such as REDCap, have randomization capabilities built into the system. While the primary purpose is to provide convenient randomizations within the one system, a secondary purpose is to allow for real-time verification of eligibility of a patient before he/she is randomized to a study. Under intention-to-treat principles, once a patient is randomized, he/she is in the study without exception. To avoid randomizing ineligible patients, verification of eligibility criteria is essential before the randomization is issued.

It is critical that all randomizations have tracking for patient eligibility and group assignment that cannot be changed after the randomization decision is issued. REDCap offers this capability as do other similar systems. This ability is to verify the randomization that was issued for the subject, which is critical if any dispute over the "intention-to-treat" paradigm develops. In addition, it can be used to routinely check on the performance of the randomization system, especially in terms of verification of eligibility.

Selection bias also includes a bias in the actual performance of the randomization of subjects. This can include randomization under difficult situations, such as transport to emergency departments, in trauma situations, or when the subject is not conscious. In situations where it may not be possible to contact a central randomization facility (e.g., data coordinating center or research pharmacy) to randomize the subject, recent publications have proposed a "step-forward" randomization design (Zhao et al. 2010). Database systems, such as REDCap, have a mobile app which can be programmed to have the next randomization ready, but in a masked format. In the case of REDCap, even if the cell phone/tablet is not in contact with the central REDCap database, the next randomization is available – and the individual can still be checked for eligibility prior to the randomization. Once contact with REDCap is restored, the information is transmitted to the main study database, and the next randomization is downloaded.

If the randomization cannot be done electronically, then an opaque sealed envelope system can be used, but it is much easier to get around the masked treatment assignments and "game" the masking. Various methods are used to maintain the mask of the next randomization in the nonelectronic randomization. For example, the person obtaining the randomization must sign the opaque envelope (along with the date and time) on the seal on the back of the envelope as well as signing the actual card with the treatment assignment. A third party, not otherwise associated with the study, could be in charge of the randomization envelopes and log the date, time, and requestor for each envelop. Once the envelope is opened, that subject is in the study.

Berger et al. (Berger and Christophi 2003) have made the point that allocation concealment (i.e., no ability to predict the next random treatment allocation) is critical to the successful randomization of patients to form equivalent treatment groups. The impact of selection bias is hard to estimate, although a recent review of oral health intervention studies (Saltaji et al. 2018) indicated that studies with inadequate or unknown method of sequence generation/masking had larger effect sizes (diff. in effect size = 0.13 (95% CI: 0.01–0.25)) than studies where the generation/masking of treatment allocation was adequate.

Finally, some studies use a "run-in" period to assess a subject's ability to adhere to the study requirements and to the intervention as well as to detect any early adverse effects (Laursen et al. 2019). There is some concern that a run-in period can create a selection bias because the run-in explicitly tests the ability of subjects to adhere to the intervention, whereas, in studies without a run-in, the ability of people to adhere to the intervention becomes part of the study post-randomization. Because of this selection bias, the results of these studies could be less generalizable than otherwise. However, the counterargument is that, with an intervention that requires that the subject performs a task in some way, medical personnel would not prescribe the intervention without knowing if the subject could (and would) perform the task. In the HIPPRO study, for example, the intervention was the wearing of hip pads to prevent hip fractures in nursing home residents. If the resident was not able (or willing) to wear the pads daily during the run-in period, he/she was not included in the main study. In reality, medical personnel would not ask a nursing home resident to wear hip pads if the resident was not capable of wearing them all day every day. So, in some cases, a run-in period makes sense. In a drug study, however, a run-in period could eliminate people who experience a specific side effect, while, in reality, these people could be prescribed the drug. So the question of whether to include a run-in period should be considered carefully to be sure that generalizability is not compromised. In a systematic review by Laursen et al. (2019) of 470 clinical trials reported in Medline in 2014, 5% (25 studies) had a run-in period of varying design and duration. Of the 25 studies, 23 had incomplete reports of the run-in period in the study results paper. Industry-sponsored studies were more likely to have run-in periods than studies funded by other sources.

Performance Bias

Performance bias refers to the collection of data from subjects in a way that does not accurately reflect subject responses, i.e., the collection of data in a way that is favorable to the data collector's treatment of choice. If the data collection staff are not masked, a number of biases can enter into the data, including exaggeration (or diminishing) of outcomes, failing to record adverse events, failing to administer all data collection forms in a neutral way, and misinterpreting laboratory results. For example, a data collector/interviewer could record "headaches" as an expected and nonserious adverse event for study participants in one treatment group but the same symptoms as unexpected and serious for the other group. To avoid this bias, all clinic staff responsible for any form of data collection must be masked to the treatment assignment. This is inclusive of all data collection staff or anyone who can influence the staff, such as the principal investigator of the study or of the clinical site. This implies that only the person obtaining the randomization would be unmasked – such as pharmacy staff who are packaging or providing the study treatments in a study of medications. In these clinical trials, the clinic staff and even the laboratory staff should be masked to study treatment.

Care must be taken if there are laboratory results that could unmask the study physicians or nurses. For example, in studies of a new treatment in type 2 diabetics with uncontrolled diabetes, HgbA1c or fasting glucose values could unmask the physician reviewing the results. Similarly, in patients with sickle cell disease, patients taking hydroxyurea will have higher fetal hemoglobin levels than those not taking it. In these situations, the laboratory results may need to be first sent to the data center to be masked (especially placebo results) prior to forwarding to the clinic staff, but the true results always need to be recorded in the patient's medical records. In the WARCEF study (Pullicino et al. 2006), in which patients were randomized to aspirin or warfarin (coumadin), the INRs for the warfarin patients were put into the study/clinical records without modification, but the data center generated INRs for the aspirin patients to avoid unmasking those patients. The process of masking laboratory results depends on the condition being studied, but generally involves imputing a random level in one (or both) groups that will not distinguish between the treatments. This will need to be stated explicitly in the protocol and to the IRB along with the explanation of how these results will be handled in the clinical center. It is important to note that the actual results be recorded in a fashion that will not jeopardize patient care but will mask the information for study personnel. Depending on the electronic health record system used at each site, this may need specialized programming to be done effectively.

In studies of behavioral interventions, the same is true, although it may be difficult to maintain masking if there is a difference in the level of "attention" in the intervention group compared to the control group. Many behavioral clinical trials now include an equivalent number of sessions for both groups to avoid a bias created by this additional attention in the intervention group.

Subjects should also be masked to their treatment group (if possible) so that all reporting by the subjects is accurate and not related to the perceived effects of the treatment. This is particularly true in studies where subjective or patient-reported outcomes are used, including occurrence of nonserious adverse events as well as quality of life scales. Because consent forms typically list expected adverse events of the treatments (and these expected AEs are readily available on various drug information web sites), subjects may be more inclined to report symptoms, such as headaches or colds, as treatment-related AEs if they know that they are in the intervention group. It has been reported in the research journals (*The Lancet Oncology* Editorial 2014) and even the lay press (Marcus 2014) that subjects in masked clinical trials have formed groups on social media, such as Facebook, to offer support for others and to compare treatment effects. Participants in these social groups typically compare symptoms and effects and try to determine (based on other information on the internet) which treatment they are on. If subjects do determine what treatment they are on, this can lead to other "downstream" biases, such as detection bias or attrition bias, both discussed below.

All clinic personnel should have a complete understanding of the protocol and protocol-specific procedures. This can be accomplished through webinars and online training sessions. It can also be reinforced through testing of personnel on the protocol – with emphasis on specific elements that are important to the different types of clinic staff. There should also be refresher sessions through the study.

Finally, ongoing monitoring of study performance is critical to identify problems and biases before they critically disrupt the integrity of the study. This involves generating Quality Assurance/Quality Control reports for the study leadership and for the Data and Safety Monitoring Board to review. Included in these reports should be presentations of data quality (e.g., time to submit information after a visit, percent of data that is "clean" on initial entry), measurement quality (e.g., number of measurements within study-defined limits and with normal variability, variability of measurements across staff taking them), laboratory quality (e.g., results from masked duplicate assays, variability of coefficients of variation across time), and quality assurance activities (e.g., retraining, site visit reports). Techniques for these reports should include techniques such as Shewhart Plots (Dunn 2019) to display unusual variability (either excessive or lack of variability) across visits and across clinic staff.

Detection Bias

Detection bias refers to a systematic bias in determining outcomes in subjects by treatment groups (Wirtz et al. 2017; Rundle et al. 2017; Dusingize et al. 2017) . Even in a well-masked study, there are frequently unavoidable indicators of treatment group in a subject that can contribute to a biased determination of an outcome, particularly a subjective outcome, such as pain level, but it can also influence the assessment of a clinical outcome, such as myocardial infarction in cardiology or acute chest syndrome in sickle cell disease or even cause of death. For example, in a study of multiple sclerosis treatments, the initial assessment of stage of disease and progression by study (unmasked) neurologists showed an advantage of the intervention over the standard of care treatment. However, when the same assessment was conducted by masked neurologists, there was no advantage shown by the analysis of the masked results (Noseworthy et al. 1994). In general, masked observers produce smaller treatment effect sizes that are also more reproducible (Hróbjartsson et al. 2012). A recent state-of-the-art review by Kahan et al. (2017) indicated that the best approach to adjudication of events and outcomes in a clinical trial is dependent of the nature of the study and of the event/outcomes that are subject to adjudication.

The approach that can typically minimize or even eliminate detection bias is to engage a group of clinicians, unrelated to the study, to determine the outcome based on prespecified criteria listed in the final study protocol. It is important that these criteria are finalized before any outcome data are reviewed. This Outcomes Adjudication Committee would receive only data, reports, and notes that are de-identified and on which any reference to the study (and any potentially unmasking information) is redacted. The minutes should be taken at Committee meetings and become part of the study documents. Decisions by the committee should be clearly indicated in the Committee meeting minutes and should be entered into the study database by the Committee secretary and verified by the Committee chair or designee. The adjudications could only be changed by the Committee chair through the database audit trail and such actions noted in subsequent Committee meeting minutes.

The independent adjudication could also include a review of unexpected serious adverse events (SAEs) to verify the relatedness of the SAE to the study therapy (i.e., drug, behavior modification, device, or biologics). The same basic approach as for clinical outcomes should be taken with SAEs.

An additional detection bias is the inability to determine if an outcome, especially a soft or subjective outcome, has occurred due to subject recall bias. For example, in studies of sickle cell disease, if a patient is feeling better in general, he/she may forget about the pain episode 2 weeks ago, while a patient who feels miserable may not. Electronic daily pain diaries (especially cell phone apps) have been very useful in capturing transient subject outcomes with corroborative information, such as prescription use, in a number of disease areas, such as sickle cell disease, atrial fibrillation, and diabetes glucose monitoring. A number of these apps are being paired with sensors to help determine if, for example, a sickle cell pain crisis is about to start, if an episode of atrial fibrillation has started or is imminent, or if a subjects' continuous glucose monitor is indicating out-of-control blood sugar levels. With the availability of wearable devices, including those that can run apps, it is practical to design studies that collect daily information on these types of outcomes or adherence information (such as length of Transcendental Meditation or yoga practice sessions) to avoid recall bias.

Attrition Bias

Attrition bias can have two causes. First, some outcomes, although recorded in the database, may be excluded from analysis for a variety of reasons. Some reasons may be technical in nature (e.g., outcome not assessed within prespecified time window or not assessed using protocol specified lab test). Others may be more logistic (e.g., subject did not receive protocol mandated intervention, patient found to be ineligible after randomization). Second, subjects may have dropped out of the study or can no longer be located for follow-up. These subjects may have dropped out of the study for reasons related to treatment (Hewitt et al. 2010), so that it is critical to keep this "missingness" to a minimum and preferably less than 5%. Differential attrition between the two treatment groups may be an indication that side effects (or even treatment effects) are not acceptable to subjects, and, rather than confront clinic staff with that decision, the subjects are walking away quietly. It is important that the Informed Consent Form (ICF) be written in such a way as to allow indirect (at least) searching for subject information, including vital status (through the National Death Index). If the subject has died, the causes of death (through the NDI) can be obtained and would be important to complete the mortality information.

A systematic review (Akl et al. 2012) assessed the reporting, extent, and handling of loss to follow-up and its potential impact of treatment effects in randomized controlled trials published in the five top medical journals. The authors calculated the percentage of trials in which the relative risk would no longer be significant when participant's loss to follow-up varied. In 160 trials, with an average loss to follow-up of 6%, and assuming different event rates in the intervention groups relative to the control groups, between 0% and 33% of trials were no longer significant.

The least biased approach to analysis of a clinical trial in general is the intention-to-treat (ITT) approach. This approach, devised at the time of the Anturane Study controversy (The Anturane Reinfarction Trial Research Group 1978; Temple and Pledger 1980), has three principles: (1) all patients are analyzed in the treatment group to which they were assigned; (2) outcomes for each subject must be recorded; and (3) all randomized subjects should be included in the analysis. The problem is that it is rare that a study has the outcome(s) for all subjects. So, some form of imputation is usually required to satisfy all three of the ITT principles. The rule of thumb is that, if the level of missing outcome data is 5% or less, it will not affect the overall study results and imputation is not critical. If the level of missingness is 10% or more, multiple imputation is a good clinical practice and should be performed. If the level of missingness is 20% or more, imputation can overly influence the results and, in a sense, drive the results. In these situations, other approaches for dealing with the missingness would be necessary. These approaches will depend on the study, but could include checking other sources for information (NDI, Social Security, Medicare, all-payer claims databases, or contacting other family members).

Briefly, multiple imputation is a strategy that generates expected outcomes for patients missing them (Sterne et al. 2009). This is usually done using a model-based approach based on observed data. However, because even model-based imputation can produce the same expected outcome for multiple patients, the end result of a single imputation is likely to yield a smaller standard deviation (and, thus, standard error of the regression coefficients), making it easier to reject the null hypothesis than in reality. The solution is to produce multiple sets of imputed data, each with a random variation of the imputed values designed to restore the full variability of the outcome. The same strategy can be used to generate expected predictors when important predictors are missing. The multiply imputed data sets are then analyzed using an analysis stratified by imputation data set and the results combined to produce a single analytic result.

A second approach to the analysis, sometimes called the "modified intention to treat," excludes subjects who have not received a protocol-specified minimum "dose" of the intervention. The problem with the modified ITT approach is that people who drop out early due to immediate adverse events are excluded from the analysis – the exact problem that ITT was designed to prevent. This approach is used frequently in oncology studies that enroll patients with advanced disease. The rationale is that a number of these patients do not live long enough after randomization to receive the minimum dose – or potentially any dose. Thus, using ITT for efficacy analysis could artificially reduce the success rate in those studies.

A third approach, the "per-protocol" approach, excludes subjects who do not receive the protocol-specified complete dose for the treatment to which they were assigned. It is typical that studies report the ITT as the primary analysis and the per-protocol as the secondary analysis of the primary outcome. Thus, the readers see the most unbiased result as well as the "full dose" result. An additional concept that is sometimes included under the per-protocol approach is to analyze subjects according to the treatment received, not as randomized. The rationale for this is that this is a "cleaner" approach to estimating treatment effect, rather than keeping people in their original groups, regardless of what they received. The ITT analysis tends to minimize the treatment effect, whereas the "as-treated" approach tends to report the observed treatment effect.

The study may also inadvertently cause differential attrition. In a study of growth in children (not a clinical trial, but the lesson is valuable), the blood pressure of the children was measured at one of the visits, and a note was given to the children with elevated blood pressure to take home to their parents. A higher proportion of the children who received the note did not return for future visits compared to those who did not receive the notes. Actions may have unintended consequences and need to be pilot tested for acceptance by subjects.

Attrition bias can lead to nonrandom missingness (as in the example above), so that study results could be compromised, even if the nonrandomness is recognized. If follow-up (and, thus, outcome) data are missing not at random, interpretation of the study is not straightforward and could be curtailed to certain subgroups. In conjunction with the Data and Safety Monitoring Board and QA/QC reports discussed above, analyses of missingness should be included so that the DSMB can identify early any nonrandom missingness and potential causes.

Reporting/Publication Bias

Reporting bias relates to the reporting of significant treatment comparisons and the underreporting of nonsignificant comparisons. As Chan and Altman (2005) says, this could be the most substantial of the biases that can affect clinical trials. The

Catalog of Bias lists several types of selective reporting of outcomes: (1) reporting only those outcomes that are statistically significant, (2) adding new outcomes after reviewing the data that are statistically significant, (3) failing to report the safety data (i.e., adverse events) from the trial, and (4) changing outcomes of interest to include only those that are statistically significant (Catalog of Bias Collaboration 2019). The CONSORT statement and associated checklist (Consolidated Standards of Reporting Trials; http://www.consort-statement.org) is a comprehensive list of items that should be included in the reporting of clinical trials (Schulz et al. 2010; Moher et al. 2010). Most medical journals now subscribe to the CONSORT principles, including the principles that all primary and secondary outcomes should be reported (Item 17a) and all adverse events reported (Item 19). With the enforced use of CONSORT by the ICMJE (International Committee of Medical Journal Editors), which requires that all outcomes and adverse events be reported for a clinical trial, the reporting bias should be minimized (Thomas and Heneghan 2017). This does assume that studies will follow CONSORT and that the journals verify that.

It should also be noted that outcome data must be posted on ClinicalTrials.gov, along with the study protocol and adverse event information. There are strict timelines for posting the outcome results from the study, with financial penalties for failure to comply. This requirement will also tend to diminish this bias in the future. A number of systematic reviews of publications versus protocols filed on ClinicalTrials.gov or other publicly accessible data sources have documented that between 6% and 12% of reported studies have different primary outcomes than specified in the protocol or a different analytic approach (Dwan et al. 2008, 2013, 2014; Zhang et al. 2017; Perlmutter et al. 2017). This is complicated by the possibility that protocols were updated after data were viewed (or even analyzed), and it is not possible to review previous protocol versions, indicating that this may be a substantial underestimate of the problem. So even the manuscript statement "Analyses were conducted according to the protocol" is not necessarily meaningful. There is no clear way to determine if the analyses were conducted using prespecified analytic techniques or if a number of analytic approaches were used until one that produced a significant result was found and the statistical section of the protocol (or the SAP) was changed to reflect the new approach. One indicator of this possibility is if an "esoteric" statistical technique is used without a clear explanation why.

The second aspect of this type of bias, the publishing bias, is the tendency of journals to publish studies with significant results. This is much more difficult for an investigator or research group to counter. This bias can have a wide-reaching impact since meta-analyses use predominately published results, although more are starting to include results posted on ClinicalTrials.gov. Because meta-analyses are frequently used in reports to policy makers regarding health care, this bias can lead to the exaggeration of the efficacy of a new medication or procedure and, potentially, the underestimation of safety issues. Because the sample of patients in a clinical trial does represent a single sample in meta-analytic terms, investigators working on meta-analyses need to be very careful of the publication bias in RCTs. To help counter this bias is not easy, since the journal editors have control over what gets published; investigators involved in negative studies should argue in the article

Discussion section (as well as in the cover letter to the editor) that publication of the negative results is important to keep the literature balanced. Statisticians and epidemiologists who develop meta-analyses for treatments of specific conditions should be careful to search ClinicalTrials.gov for negative, non-published results to enhance the balanced inclusion of studies in the meta-analysis.

Other Sources of Bias

Other sources of bias include statistical programming quality control concerns. The data collected by a clinical trial will be recorded in a database, such as REDCap. The data is typically longitudinal with repeated drug administration, clinical visits, laboratory tests, adverse events, and outcome adjudication results. Assembling these data into an analytic database can be challenging, requiring the merging of multiple data sets into a set of longitudinal records for each patient. That aspect of each study is a high-risk program that must be closely checked through a documented quality control process. The programming to determine the outcomes for each patient are also high-risk programs. All of these programs need to be subjected to multiple layers of quality control to verify the accuracy of the preparation of the data for analysis. The actual analysis programming is less risky because those programs are using the prepared analytic data sets. However, with today's statistical software, a mistake in one line of computer code can reverse the treatment groups for efficacy and for safety outcomes.

Another source of bias occurs in cluster-randomized studies where it is known that recruitment of subjects in the control facility is more difficult than in the intervention facility. It will likely be necessary to allow a longer recruitment period in control facilities to achieve the appropriate sample size. There is also concern that the characteristics of the subjects recruited in control facilities could be different than those in intervention facilities. These characteristics should be monitored during recruitment to verify that the two cluster-randomized treatment groups are similar. The DSMB reports should contain information on patient characteristics in these studies. In addition, the characteristics of the facilities should be compared as well. In the advent of an imbalance in patient characteristics between treatment groups, if discovered early in the study, an adaptive randomization plan could be implemented so that the patient characteristics would balance themselves prior to the end of recruitment.

In studies that are not FDA monitored, a statistical analysis plan (SAP) either does not exist or is vague and not followed very well. FDA typically requires a SAP to be filed before the final analysis can be conducted. The reason is simple – if the analytic techniques are not prespecified, the investigators are able to select the analytic technique that supports their research without concern for what was stated in a SAP. While a preliminary analysis approach was likely included in an NIH application, that can easily be dismissed as preliminary and not even reported. If a reduced version of a SAP is included in the protocol (and, thus, on ▶ ClinicalTrials.gov), it is much harder to ignore it. But few protocols include much more than a cursory explanation of the analysis plan unless there is FDA oversight, in which case the major elements of the SAP are included in the protocol.

Summary

This section describes the major sources of bias in RCTs and possible solutions. In most cases, depending on the nature of the study, other solutions can be found in addition to those described here. There is no "push button" approach to safeguarding a trial from bias – every RCT is different and will require different approaches to controlling and, hopefully, eliminating bias. New sources of bias can arise through the electronic social media. For example, a slight difference in the appearance of a placebo (or the inherent differences in behavioral study treatments/conditions) can give study participants enough information that, combined with a study-related social media group, can unmask a study, resulting in misleading results based on patient-related outcomes. Investigators, therefore, must be constantly watchful for bias to proactively prevent bias from occurring and to retroactively correct existing problems.

Key Facts

1. Biases can still occur in randomized clinical trials, the study design that is considered to be the gold standard.
2. Random treatment group assignment and data collection masked to subjects' treatment group assignment will prevent most biases.
3. Random treatment assignments are always required for an RCT; treatment group masking can be more challenging.
4. Other types of bias, such as reporting and publication bias, are unrelated to randomization and masking. While reporting bias can be avoided by following the CONSORT statement and checklist, publication bias is in the hands of the journal editors.

Cross-References

▶ Adherence Adjusted Estimates in Randomized Clinical Trials
▶ Administration of Study Treatments and Participant Follow-Up
▶ ClinicalTrials.gov
▶ Financial Conflicts of Interest in Clinical Trials
▶ Design and Development of the Study Data System
▶ Fraud in Clinical Trials

► Good Clinical Practice
► Intention to Treat and Alternative Approaches
► Masking of Trial Investigators
► Masking Study Participants
► Missing Data
► Participant Recruitment, Screening, and Enrollment
► Patient-Reported Outcomes
► Principles of Clinical Trials: Bias and Precision Control
► Reporting Biases

References

Akl AE, Briel M, You JJ, Sun X, Johnston BC, Busse JW, Mulla S, Lamontagne F, Bassler D, Vera C, Alshurafa M, Katsios CM, Zhou Q, Cukierman-Yaffe T, Gangji A, Mills EJ, Walter SD, Cook DJ, Schünemann HJ, Altman DG, Guyatt GH (2012) Potential impact on estimated treatment effects of information lost to follow-up in randomized controlled trials (LOST-IT): systematic review. BMJ 344:e2809

Berger VW, Christophi CA (2003) Randomization technique, allocation concealment, masking, and susceptibility of trials to selection bias. J Mod Appl Stat Methods 2(1):80–86

Catalog of Bias Collaboration (2019). Catalog of Bias, November 19. Retrieved from catalogofbias.org

Chan A-W, Altman DG (2005) Identifying outcome reporting bias in randomised trials on PubMed: review of publications and survey of authors. BMJ 330(7494):753

Doll R (1998) Controlled trials: the 1948 watershed. BMJ 317:1217

Dunn K (2019) Shewhart charts, July 17. Retrieved from https://learnche.org/pid/process-monitoring/shewhart-charts

Dusingize JC, Olsen CM, Pandeya NP, Subramaniam P, Thompson BS, Neale RE, Green AC, Whiteman DC, Study QS (2017) Cigarette smoking and the risks of basal cell carcinoma and squamous cell carcinoma. J Invest Dermatol 137(8):1700–1708

Dwan K, Altman DG, Arnaiz JA, Bloom J, Chan AW, Cronin E, Decullier E, Easterbrook PJ, Von Elm E, Gamble C, Ghersi D, Ioannidis JP, Simes J, Williamson PR (2008) Systematic review of the empirical evidence of study publication bias and outcome reporting bias. PLoS One 3(8): e3081

Dwan K, Gamble C, Williamson PR, Kirkham JJ, Reporting Bias Group (2013) Systematic review of the empirical evidence of study publication bias and outcome reporting bias – an updated review. PLoS One 8(7):e66844

Dwan K, Altman DG, Clarke M, Gamble C, Higgins JP, Sterne JA, Williamson PR, Kirkham JJ (2014) Evidence for the selective reporting of analyses and discrepancies in clinical trials: a systematic review of cohort studies of clinical trials. PLoS Med 11(6):e1001666

Editorial (2014) #Trial: clinical research in the age of social media. Lancet Oncol 15(6):539

Hewitt CE, Kumaravel B, Dumville JC, Torgerson DJ, Trial Attrition Study Group (2010) Assessing the impact of attrition in randomized controlled trials. J Clin Epidemiol 63(11): 1264–1270

Higgins JPT, Altman DG, Behalf of the Cochrane Statistical Methods Group and the Cochrane Bias Methods Group (2008) In: JPT H, Green S (eds) Cochrane handbook for systematic reviews of interventions. Wiley, Chichester

Hróbjartsson A, Thomsen AS, Emanuelsson F, Tendal B, Hilden J, Boutron I, Ravaud P, Brorson S (2012) Observer bias in randomized clinical trials with binary outcomes: systematic review of trials with both blinded and unblinded assessors. BMJ 344:e1119

Kahan BC, Feagan B, Jairath V (2017) A comparison of approaches for adjudicating outcomes in clinical trials. Trials 18:266

Lachin J (1988) Properties of simple randomization in clinical trials. Control Clin Trials 9:312–326

Laursen DRT, Paludan-Muller AS, Hrobjartsson A (2019) Randomized clinical trials with run-in periods: frequency, characteristics and reporting. Clin Epidemiol 11:169–184

Lewis SC, Warlow CP (2004) How to spot bias and other potential problems in randomised controlled trials. J Neurol Neurosurg Psychiatry 75:181–187. https://doi.org/10.1136/jnnp.2003.025833

Marcus AD (2014) Researchers FRET as social media lift veil on drug trials: online chatter could unravel carefully built construct of 'blind' clinical trials. Wall Street Journal, July 29

Matts J, Lachin J (1988) Properties of permuted-block randomization in clinical trials. Control Clin Trials 9:327–344

Moher D, Hopewell S, Schulz KF, Montori V, Gøtzsche PC, Devereaux PJ, Elbourne D, Egger M, Altman DG (2010) Explanation and elaboration: updated guidelines for reporting parallel group randomised trials. BMJ 340:c869

Noseworthy JH, Ebers GC, Vandervoort MK, Farquhar RE, Yetisir E, Roberts R (1994) The impact of blinding on the results of a randomized, placebo-controlled multiple sclerosis clinical trial. Neurology 44(1):16–20

Perlmutter AS, Tran VT, Dechartres A, Ravaud P (2017) Statistical controversies in clinical research: comparison of primary outcomes in protocols, public clinical-trial registries and publications: the example of oncology trials. Ann Oncol 28(4):688–695

Pullicino P, Thompson JLP, Barton B, Levin B, Graham S, Freudenberger RS (2006) Warfarin versus aspirin in patients with reduced cardiac ejection fraction (WARCEF): rationale, objectives, and design. J Card Fail 12(1):39–46

Ruffin JM, Grizzle JE, Hightower NC, McHardy G, Shull H, Kirsner JB (1969) A Cooperative Double-Blind Evaluation of Gastric Freezing in the Treatment of Duodenal Ulcer. New England Journal of Medicine 281(1):16–19

Rundle A, Wang Y, Sadasivan S, Chitale DA, Gupta NS, Tang D, Rybicki BA (2017) Larger men have larger prostates: detection bias in epidemiologic studies of obesity and prostate cancer risk. Prostate 77(9):949–954. https://doi.org/10.1002/pros.23350

Saltaji H, Armijo-Olivo S, Cummings GG, Amin M, da Costa BR, Flores-Mir C (2018) Impact of selection bias on treatment effect size estimates in randomized trials of oral health interventions: a meta-epidemiological Study. J Dent Res 97(1):5–13

Schulz KF, Altman DG, Moher D, for the CONSORT Group (2010) CONSORT 2010 statement: updated guidelines for reporting parallel group randomised trials. BMJ c332:340

Sterne JAC, White IR, Carlin JB, Spratt M, Royston P, Kenward MG, Wood AM, Carpenter JR (2009) Multiple imputation for missing data in epidemiological and clinical research: potential and pitfalls. BMJ 338:b2393

Temple R, Pledger G (1980) The FDA's critique of the Anturane Reinfarction trial. NEJM 303(25):1488–1492

The Anturane Reinfarction Trial Research Group (1978) Sulfinpyrazone in the prevention of cardiac death after myocardial infarction. NEJM 298(6):289–295

Thomas ET, Heneghan C (2017) Catalogue of bias collaboration, outcome reporting bias. In: Catalogue of biases. http://www.catalogueofbiases.org//outcomereportingbias

Wangensteen OH (1962) Achieving "Physiological Gastrectomy" by Gastric Freezing. JAMA 180(6):439

Wirtz HS, Calip GS, Buist DSM, Gralow JR, Barlow WE, Gray S, Boudreau DM (2017) Evidence for detection bias by medication use in a cohort study of breast cancer survivors. Am J Epidemiol 185(8):661–672

Zhang S, Liang F, Li W (2017) Comparison between publicly accessible publications, registries, and protocols of phase III trials indicated persistence of selective outcome reporting. J Clin Epidemiol 91:87–94

Zhao W, Ciolino J, Palesch Y (2010) Step-forward randomization in multicenter emergency treatment clinical trials. Acad Emerg Med 17(6):659–665

Zhao W, Hill MD, Palesch Y (2011) Minimal sufficient balance—a new strategy to balance baseline covariates and preserve randomness of treatment allocation. Statistical Methods in Medical Research 24(6):989–1002

Masking of Trial Investigators

43

George Howard and Jenifer H. Voeks

Contents

Abstract

The substantial investment of both time and money to mount a clinical trial would not be made without an underlying belief that the new treatment is likely beneficial. While a lack of definitive evidence can underpin the equipoise of investigators that is necessary to mount a new trial, the success in previous early phase trials (or even animal models) provides a natural foundation for an expected benefit in subsequent phase trials. Both investigators and patients can share this belief, and these expectations of treatment efficacy for new therapies introduce the potential for bias in clinical trials. The benefits, completeness, and reporting of masking in clinical trials are described, as they are approaches for implementing and maintaining the mask.

Keywords

Masking · Blinding · Assessment of outcomes

G. Howard (✉)
Department of Biostatistics, University of Alabama at Birmingham, Birmingham, AL, USA
e-mail: ghoward@uab.edu

J. H. Voeks
Department of Neurology, Medical University of South Carolina, Charleston, SC, USA
e-mail: voeks@musc.edu

© Springer Nature Switzerland AG 2022
S. Piantadosi, C. L. Meinert (eds.), *Principles and Practice of Clinical Trials*,
https://doi.org/10.1007/978-3-319-52636-2_215

Introduction

The substantial investment of both time and money to mount a clinical trial would not be made without an underlying belief that the new treatment is likely beneficial. While a lack of definitive evidence can underpin the equipoise of investigators that is necessary to mount a new trial, the success in previous early phase trials (or even animal models) provides a natural foundation for an expected benefit in subsequent phase trials. Such an underlying belief of efficacy is demonstrated when investigators were asked to guess whether patients were assigned to active versus placebo in a trial treating depression and were more likely to guess assignment to active treatment among patients who had better clinical outcomes (and also among patients with more adverse events) (Chen et al. 2015). Likewise, patients either have a predisposition or are transferred a confidence that active treatment is superior, with patients even in early-phase cancer trials are optimistic that new therapies will be beneficial (Sulmasy et al. 2010; Jansen et al. 2016). These expectations of treatment efficacy for new therapies introduce the potential for bias in clinical trials (see Fig. 1).

Why Mask Randomized Trials

Masking (or blinding) of the treatment assignment stands as one of the pillars to protect the study from potential biases introduced through these expectations. These expectations could consciously or unconsciously influence the messaging by investigators to subjects in the description of expected outcome and adverse events, the

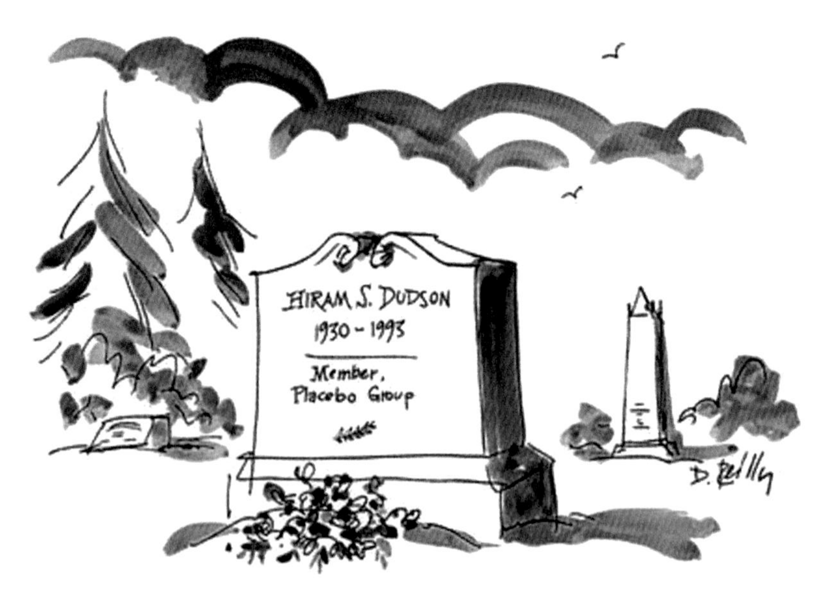

Fig. 1 Cartoon demonstrating expectation of beneficial efficacy of experimental therapies. Reprinted from the New Yorker with permission

Table 1 Potential benefits accruing depending on those individuals successfully masked. (From Schulz and Grimes (2002))

Individual masked	Potential benefit
Participants	Less likely to have biased psychological of physical responses to intervention
	More likely to comply with trial regimens
	Less likely to seek additional adjunct interventions
	Less likely to leave trial without providing outcome data, including lost to follow-up
Trial investigators	Less likely to transfer their inclinations or attitudes to participants
	Less likely to differentially administer co-interventions
	Less likely to differentially adjust dose
	Less likely to differentially withdraw participants
	Less likely to differentially encourage or discourage participants to continue trial
Assessors	Less likely to have biases affect their outcome assessments, especially with subjective outcomes of interest

diligence of the surveillance for outcomes by investigators, and the adjudication of suspected study events. Through masking, the treatment assignment can be obscured to three groups: study participants, study investigators, and those assessing study outcomes. While the language is not precise, "double mask" commonly refers to obscuring treatment assignment to all three groups (hence, sometimes alternatively referred to as "triple masking") (Schulz and Grimes 2002; Bang et al. 2004). While more confusion surround the use of the term "single mask," which can refer to obscuring treatment assignment to any of these three groups, it most frequently refers to obscuring treatment assignment to the participants (Schulz and Grimes 2002; Bang et al. 2004). Schulz and Grimes (2002) offer a list of the benefits to the study in masking each of these groups (see Table 1), with 5 of the 10 advantages accruing to the masking of investigators. A study without masking is commonly referred to as "open label." This chapter focuses on methods for masking of investigators, including both double masking and the single masking of investigators.

Meta-analyses of specific therapies, where some of the component studies were masked and others were not, offer the opportunity to assess the magnitude of potential bias attributable to a failure to mask. These meta-analyses can estimate the difference in treatment effect between masked and unmasked studies, with any larger treatment effect in open-label studies assumed to arise from a bias introduced by the lack of masking. For example, a recent analysis of 64 meta-analyses including 540 trials of oral health treatments estimated the standardized difference in treatment effect between masked and unmasked/inadequately masked trials. Among these trials, 71% provided adequate masking of patients, and 59% provided adequate masking of the outcome assessor. The standardized difference in the treatment effect was 0.12 (95% CI, 0.00 to 0.23) larger in trials where the patient was not masked to the treatment and 0.19 (95% CI, 0.06 to 0.32) for trials where the assessor was not masked. In the same set of analyses, masking of caregivers and principal investigators was not associated with differences in estimated treatment effect between adequately and inadequately masked studies (Saltaji et al. 2018). Similarly among trials in osteoarthritis, there was a substantially larger treatment effect among inadequately masked studies than in adequately masked studies when the magnitude of the overall treatment effect was larger (difference in treatment effect = −0.79; 95% CI, −1.02 to −0.50), but (not surprisingly) little difference in treatment effect between unmasked and masked sites for treatments with smaller overall treatment effects (difference in treatment effect = −0.02; 95% CI, −0.10 to 0.06) (Nuesch et al. 2009). Other meta-analyses using a similar approach also show unmasked studies tend to have a larger treatment effect than those that are masked, and the bias is larger when subjective outcomes are used (Savovic et al. 2012; Page et al. 2016). Hence with this approach, there is strong empirical evidence that the lack of masking can introduce bias to overestimate the magnitude of the treatment effect.

The current (2010) Consolidated Standard for Reporting Trials (CONSORT) statement has two statements for reporting of masking: (1) "if done, who was blinded after assignment to interventions (for example, participants, care provided, those assessing outcomes)" and (2) "if relevant, description of the similarities of interventions" (Schulz et al. 2010). Despite this requirement, numerous authors have noted that the documentation of the methods underpinning masking is commonly poorly reported (Armijo-Olivo et al. 2017; Boutron et al. 2006). In a systematic review of 819 trials published in major medical journals in 2004, only 472 (58%) reported the methods of masking, with the authors speculating that a lack describing the methods of masking is in part a product of an under emphasis of the importance in the CONSORT guidelines (Boutron et al. 2006). However, it also seems that pressure from word-count policies of journals could also be a contributor.

Approaches to assess the completeness masking in trials are largely based on asking patients to report their suspected assignment group or a response they don't know to which group they are assigned. Two approaches have been proposed to quantify the quality of masking and to provide for statistical inference. The approach of James and colleagues is related to the kappa statistic for disagreement and heavily weights the proportion of subjects responding that they do not know to which group they are assigned and provides a single index of the quality of masking across the treatment groups (James et al. 1996). The dependence of this index on the proportion that is unsure of their assignment implies that if this proportion is large ($\approx>$30%), that unmasking in one or both arms may not be detected (Bang et al. 2004). Additionally, that the approach provides a single index pooling results across multiple treatment arms may result in failing to detect unmasking in a single arm (e.g., in the case of a strong treatment effect in the experimental arm, but little effect in the control arm). These shortcomings were overcome by the subsequent proposal for masking indices by Bang that provides an estimate of the quality of masking for specific treatment groups. Under the assumption that those uncertain of their assignment are masked, the Bang can be interpreted as the proportion of unmasked patients in each treatment (Bang et al. 2004).

However, the success in masking is frequently not assessed. Only 40 of 2,467 (1.6%) psychiatric trials (Freed et al. 2014), and only 23 or 408 (5.6%) pain trials (Colagiuri et al. 2019), reported assessing masking with information for meta-analysis of the masking index. Likewise, the reporting of the success of efforts to mask was reported in only 31 of 1,599 (2%) trials described as masked, included in the Cochrane Central Register of Control Trials, and published in 2001 (Hrobjartsson et al. 2007). The guideline for reporting the success of masking included in the 2001 CONSORT guidelines was removed from the 2010 CONSORT guidelines because of a lack of empirical evidence supporting the practice and concerns regarding the validity of assessments (Schulz et al. 2010). Reports that do report the frequency of assessing the success of masking are inconsistent, for example, with the previously mentioned meta-analysis of psychiatric trials showing masking success in both arms (Freed et al. 2014), while the masking was not successful in the pain trials (Colagiuri et al. 2019). Success in masking appears higher in trials with smaller effect sizes (Freed et al. 2014). However, as many as half of masked trials conducted some assessment of the quality of masking without reporting it in the literature (Bello et al. 2017), where 20% or less of the trials with formal assessments of masking reported these results in publications (Hrobjartsson et al. 2007; Bello et al. 2017). Hence, reporting bias and other factors challenge efforts to describe whether masking can be successfully implemented and factors associated with masking success.

Among the mechanisms through which the lack of masking could introduce bias is the possibility that knowledge of the treatment assignment may make affect the vigilance of investigators in their surveillance of potential study outcomes. For example, an unmasked investigator may consciously or unconsciously more aggressively probe potential symptoms for patients in the placebo arm, "ensuring" that the events presumed to be more common are not missed. Conversely, the investigator may have a higher threshold to declare an outcome event in the actively treated arm. But, as outcomes become more objective, there is less judgment in probing for potential events and less leeway for judgment by the investigator assessing outcomes. Hence, with objective outcomes, there is less opportunity for investigators (or subjects) to introduce bias, with little contribution for very objective outcomes such as mortality or outcomes determined through direct measurement (e.g., weight loss, blood pressure, lipid levels, etc.). This possibility that masking is less important with increasing objectivity of the outcome is supported by empirical evidence. For example, in analyzing the difference in the treatment effect between 532 trials with adequate masking versus 272 with inadequate masking, there was no evidence of a difference for all-cause mortality (ratio of odds ratio = 1.04; 95% CI, 0.95 to 1.14), while the difference between masked and unmasked was significantly different (ratio of odds ratio = 0.83; 95% CI, 0.70 to 0.98). When these differences were assessed at the threshold where outcomes were classified as "objective" versus "subjective" outcomes, the ratio of odds ratios were 1.01 (95% CI, 0.92 to 1.10) for objective studies and 0.75 (95% CI, 0.61 to 0.82) for subjective outcomes (Wood et al. 2008). However, while such evidence does support a lower importance of masking with outcomes that are more objective, it is important to remember there are other pathways through which unmasked investigators could introduce bias. For example, in the setting of intensive care units (ICUs), knowledge of the treatment assignment could affect the decision to provide or withhold life support therapy and thereby have an effect on mortality as an outcome (Anthon et al. 2017). However, a systematic review with a published a priori protocol (Anthon et al. 2017) suggests this theoretical possibility provided little support that it is a major concern. The authors considered published systematic reviews and reanalyzed the data clustering the studies included into those with and without masking. The results of this effort showed that for the primary outcome of death (at the longest follow-up time), only 1 of 22 studies showed a larger treatment effect for those unmasked than masked (odds ratio = 0.58; 95% CI, 0.35–0.98 versus odds ratio = 1.00; 95% CI, 0.87–1.16) (Anthon et al. 2018). With 22 assessments (and testing interaction at $\alpha = 0.10$), this is nominally fewer treatments showing heterogeneity of effect than expected. Similar findings were shown for other outcomes including in-hospital and in-ICU mortality (Anthon et al. 2018). Still, even in studies with very objective outcomes, the possibility that alternative pathways could introduce bias should be carefully considered before abandoning masking.

There is a growing literature supporting the position that estimation of treatment effects based on events as reported by site investigators is quite similar to results when information is centrally retrieved and processed by adjudication committees (Ndounga Diakou et al. 2016). However, it is important to recognize that decision to use or not use adjudication committees differs fundamentally from the decision to mask or not mask studies. That is, it is straightforward to maintain a mask within the clinics for pharmacological treatments with active versus placebo treatments, and hence the decision for the use of adjudication becomes a comparison of masked local determination of outcomes versus the masked central adjudication of outcomes. However, for other trials where maintaining a mask within the clinical center is problematic (such as surgical trials), providing adequate masking for the determination of outcomes may require either additional staff in the clinical centers who are masked to treatment allocation (and trust to believe that a "wall" there between the masked and unmasked clinical center staff) or the use of central adjudication committee that can be masked (discussed below).

It does seem intuitive that investigators (and subjects) could be influenced by the knowledge of the treatment allocation, and this intuition is supported by empirical data showing a bias for larger treatment effects in unmasked studies. While a large number of studies are masked, there appears to be substantial room for improvement in the reporting of the methods for implementing the mask, and the methods and benefit for assessing the success of masking remain questionable.

How to Mask Investigators in Randomized Trials

While double mask active versus placebo treatments in pharmacologic trials are frequently the first thought of when discussing masking in clinical trials, the mask of treatment assignment is much more complex for many trials. Different treatments give rise to a spectrum of challenges to the masking of investigators, with perhaps surgical trials giving rise to the largest number of issues. Here, clearly those providing the therapy cannot be masked, nor can patients generally be masked (without the use of sham surgery, i.e., frequently considered unethical (Macklin 1999)), nor can many assessors be masked from the scars associated with procedures. Implementation of masking in lifestyle treatments (e.g., diet, exercise, etc.) is similarly difficult to implement. However, as noted above, the lack of masking can give rise to biased estimates of treatment effect, and as such the effort to provide the most complete masking feasible is central to the good conduct of studies. As such, an array of tools and approaches have been developed to reduce bias. Karanicolas and colleagues have proposed three consideration to consider in the implementation of these approaches: they should successfully conceal the group allocation, they should not impair the ability to successfully assess outcomes, and they must be acceptable to the individuals assessing the outcome (Karanicolas et al. 2008).

Boutron and colleagues' outstanding systematic review of methods for masking studies among 819 trials offered an effective strategy for classifying masking tools and approaches, specifically whether they primarily (1) mask patients and healthcare providers, (2) maintain the mask of patients and healthcare providers, or (3) support the masking of assessor of outcomes (Boutron et al. 2006). We will follow this structure in the review of these methods.

Among approaches to support the masking of patients and healthcare providers, by far, the most common technique is the central preparation of oral/topical active treatments with masked alternative treatments, an approach employed by 193 of 336 (57%) of studies reporting approaches to mask the patient and healthcare provider (Boutron et al. 2006). This approach for masking is nearly ubiquitous in pharmacological clinical trials, and use of a central pharmacy effectively masks the treatment assignment from the investigators. While this approach is common, the effort and cost to identify and contract with a central pharmacy partner for the trial are considerable, and the time line for implementation and production of active and placebo treatment should not be underestimated. In addition, investigators in the central pharmacy have unique experience and insights that are often remarkably useful for the trial; it is critical to identify and involve these scientists as early as possible in the trial planning process. Specifically, while the active drug may be readily available, the creation of a placebo treatment with similar characteristics sometimes requires encapsulation to conceal the active drug, or the addition of flavors to mask the taste. Care and due diligence are still required, as while never published in the reports from the trial, the investigators in the Vitamin Intervention in Stroke Prevention (VISP) trial fortunately had the foresight to bioassay the first batch of active and placebo medications provided by the central pharmacy, finding the placebo to have levels of the treatment medications (folate, B_6, and B_{12}) nearly indistinguishable from the active medication (obviously resolved prior to the onset of the trial). Trials with an active alternative treatments (e.g., a trial of teriparatide versus risedronate for new fractures in postmenopausal women (Kendler et al. 2018)) offer additional challenges, where it could be difficult to produce treatment that appear similar even with encapsulation. Such a situation may call for a placebo to be created for each of the two active treatments, or a "double-dummy" design.

Once masking of treatment assignment is established, efforts need to focus on maintaining that mask during patient follow-up during which several factors work to potentially unmask the treatment assignment. A particular challenge to maintaining the masking of investigators are pharmacological trials that require dose adjustments, where the mask can be maintained by having a centralized office that creates the adjustment orders with the inclusion of sham adjustments for those patients on placebo. The investigators can also be partially or completely unmasked by the availability of results of laboratory or other assessments at the clinical site. This possibility can be reduced by the use of a central laboratory or reading facility with only selected information required for safety being returned to the clinical site. The masking of investigators is also challenged by the occurrence of specific adverse events, and again the use of a central facility to process and report adverse events can reduce this possibility and by systematic treatments to prevent adverse events that are applied equally in both treatment groups. Finally, it is critical for the investigators to avoid "messaging" to the patient about the therapeutic effect ,and the expected side effects have to be carefully considered to maintain the mask.

However, there are treatments where maintaining the mask in the clinical center is quite difficult or even impossible. Examples would include randomization to surgery versus medical management for the management of asymptomatic carotid stenosis (Howard et al. 2017), randomization to Mediterranean diet versus alternative diets (Estruch et al. 2013), or randomization to different treatment algorithms (such as different blood pressure levels (SPRINT Research Group et al. 2015)). In this case, a first-line approach to provide masking is to have independent clinic staff who are not involved in providing treatment be masked to the treatment allocation and assess the trial outcomes; however, such an approach requires faith that the clinic staff will maintain a "wall" between staff who may know each other well. Alternatively, outcomes can be centrally processed by trial staff that are masked to treatment allocation, an approach referred to as a prospective randomized open-blinded end-point (PROBE) design (Hansson et al. 1992). Examples of the approach include the video recording of a neurological examination with centralized scoring of the modified Rankin score that serves as the primary study outcome (Reinink et al. 2018) or the retrieval of medical records for suspected stroke events that can be redacted to mask treatment allocation and adjudicated by clinicians who are masked to treatment allocation (Howard et al. 2017). Even with the use of PROBE designs, investigators must be careful to not let the actions of the unmasked clinic staff introduce bias. For example, the clinic staff could be more sensitive to the detection of potential events in the medically managed group and be more likely to report these events for the central adjudication. This can be partially overcome by the introduction of triggers, such as a 2-point increase in a clinical stroke scale, and requiring records to be provided each time the trigger occurs. This potential bias can also be reduced by setting a very low threshold for suspected events, so that many more records are centrally reviewed with a relatively small proportion being adjudicated as a study outcome. That PROBE approaches could reduce but not eliminate bias is supported by a meta-analysis of oral anticoagulants to reduce stroke risk estimating the treatment difference between trials using a double mask approach (4 trials) versus a PROBE design (9 trials). This analysis observed a nonsignificantly ($p = 0.16$) larger effect for stroke prevention in the PROBE studies (relative risk = 0.76; 95% CI, 0.65–0.89) than for the double mask studies (relative risk = 0.88; 95% CI, 0.78–0.98) and a significantly larger effect ($p = 0.05$) for the prevention of hemorrhagic stroke in the placebo trials (relative risk = 0.33; 95% CI, 0.21–0.50) than the double mask studies (relative risk = 0.55; 95% CI, 0.41–0.73) (Lega et al. 2013). While the use of PROBE methods likely reduces bias in outcome ascertainment, it is not clear that these methods are as widely used as possible. For example, in a review of 171 orthopedic trials, masking of clinical assessors was considered feasible in 89% of studies and masking of radiographic assessors in 83% of trials; however, less than 10% of these trials used masked assessors (Karanicolas et al. 2008).

While simple active/placebo masking is possible for some treatments, many trials will require creativity and determination to implement masking of investigators. Additionally, once masking is in place, efforts need to be directed to maintain the mask.

Conclusions

Masking stands as one of the pillars to reduce or eliminate bias in the conduct of clinical trials. Without masking, intentional or unintentional prejudice can influence the outcome of the trial, and as such ignorance is truly bliss.

References

Anthon CT, Granholm A, Perner A, Laake JH, Moller MH (2017) The effect of blinding on estimates of mortality in randomised clinical trials of intensive care interventions: protocol for a systematic review and meta-analysis. BMJ Open 7(7):e016187

Anthon CT, Granholm A, Perner A, Laake JH, Moller MH (2018) No firm evidence that lack of blinding affects estimates of mortality in randomized clinical trials of intensive care interventions: a systematic review and meta-analysis. J Clin Epidemiol 100:71–81

Armijo-Olivo S, Fuentes J, da Costa BR, Saltaji H, Ha C, Cummings GG (2017) Blinding in physical therapy trials and its association with treatment effects: a meta-epidemiological study. Am J Phys Med Rehabil 96(1):34–44

Bang H, Ni L, Davis CE (2004) Assessment of blinding in clinical trials. Control Clin Trials 25 (2):143–156

Bello S, Moustgaard H, Hrobjartsson A (2017) Unreported formal assessment of unblinding occurred in 4 of 10 randomized clinical trials, unreported loss of blinding in 1 of 10 trials. J Clin Epidemiol 81:42–50

Boutron I, Estellat C, Guittet L et al (2006) Methods of blinding in reports of randomized controlled trials assessing pharmacologic treatments: a systematic review. PLoS Med 3(10):e425

Chen JA, Vijapura S, Papakostas GI et al (2015) Association between physician beliefs regarding assigned treatment and clinical response: re-analysis of data from the Hypericum Depression Trial Study Group. Asian J Psychiatr 13:23–29

Colagiuri B, Sharpe L, Scott A (2019) The blind leading the not-so-blind: a meta-analysis of blinding in pharmacological trials for chronic pain. J Pain 20:489–500

Estruch R, Ros E, Salas-Salvado J et al (2013) Primary prevention of cardiovascular disease with a Mediterranean diet. N Engl J Med 368(14):1279–1290

Freed B, Assall OP, Panagiotakis G et al (2014) Assessing blinding in trials of psychiatric disorders: a meta-analysis based on blinding index. Psychiatry Res 219(2):241–247

Hansson L, Hedner T, Dahlof B (1992) Prospective randomized open blinded end-point (PROBE) study. A novel design for intervention trials. Prospective Randomized Open Blinded End-Point. Blood Press 1(2):113–119

Howard VJ, Meschia JF, Lal BK et al (2017) Carotid revascularization and medical management for asymptomatic carotid stenosis: protocol of the CREST-2 clinical trials. Int J Stroke 12(7):770–778

Hrobjartsson A, Forfang E, Haahr MT, Als-Nielsen B, Brorson S (2007) Blinded trials taken to the test: an analysis of randomized clinical trials that report tests for the success of blinding. Int J Epidemiol 36(3):654–663

James KE, Bloch DA, Lee KK, Kraemer HC, Fuller RK (1996) An index for assessing blindness in a multi-centre clinical trial: disulfiram for alcohol cessation – a VA cooperative study. Stat Med 15(13):1421–1434

Jansen LA, Mahadevan D, Appelbaum PS et al (2016) Dispositional optimism and therapeutic expectations in early-phase oncology trials. Cancer 122(8):1238–1246

Karanicolas PJ, Bhandari M, Taromi B et al (2008) Blinding of outcomes in trials of orthopaedic trauma: an opportunity to enhance the validity of clinical trials. J Bone Joint Surg Am 90(5):1026–1033

Kendler DL, Marin F, Zerbini CAF et al (2018) Effects of teriparatide and risedronate on new fractures in post-menopausal women with severe osteoporosis (VERO): a multicentre, double-blind, double-dummy, randomised controlled trial. Lancet 391(10117):230–240

Lega JC, Mismetti P, Cucherat M et al (2013) Impact of double-blind vs. open study design on the observed treatment effects of new oral anticoagulants in atrial fibrillation: a meta-analysis. J Thromb Haemost 11(7):1240–1250

Macklin R (1999) The ethical problems with sham surgery in clinical research. N Engl J Med 341 (13):992–996

Ndounga Diakou LA, Trinquart L, Hrobjartsson A et al (2016) Comparison of central adjudication of outcomes and onsite outcome assessment on treatment effect estimates. Cochrane Database Syst Rev 3:MR000043

Nuesch E, Reichenbach S, Trelle S et al (2009) The importance of allocation concealment and patient blinding in osteoarthritis trials: a meta-epidemiologic study. Arthritis Rheum 61(12):1633–1641

Page MJ, Higgins JP, Clayton G, Sterne JA, Hrobjartsson A, Savovic J (2016) Empirical evidence of study design biases in randomized trials: systematic review of meta-epidemiological studies. PLoS ONE 11(7):e0159267

Reinink H, de Jonge JC, Bath PM et al (2018) PRECIOUS: PREvention of Complications to Improve OUtcome in elderly patients with acute Stroke. Rationale and design of a randomised, open, phase III, clinical trial with blinded outcome assessment. Eur Stroke J 3(3):291–298

Saltaji H, Armijo-Olivo S, Cummings GG, Amin M, da Costa BR, Flores-Mir C (2018) Influence of blinding on treatment effect size estimate in randomized controlled trials of oral health interventions. BMC Med Res Methodol 18(1):42

Savovic J, Jones H, Altman D et al (2012) Influence of reported study design characteristics on intervention effect estimates from randomised controlled trials: combined analysis of meta-epidemiological studies. Health Technol Assess 16(35):1–82

Schulz KF, Grimes DA (2002) Blinding in randomised trials: hiding who got what. Lancet 359 (9307):696–700

Schulz KF, Altman DG, Moher D (2010) CONSORT 2010 statement: updated guidelines for reporting parallel group randomised trials. J Pharmacol Pharmacother 1(2):100–107

SPRINT Research Group, Wright JT Jr, Williamson JD et al (2015) A Randomized Trial of Intensive versus Standard Blood-Pressure Control. N Engl J Med 373(22):2103–2116

Sulmasy DP, Astrow AB, He MK et al (2010) The culture of faith and hope: patients' justifications for their high estimations of expected therapeutic benefit when enrolling in early phase oncology trials. Cancer 116(15):3702–3711

Wood L, Egger M, Gluud LL et al (2008) Empirical evidence of bias in treatment effect estimates in controlled trials with different interventions and outcomes: meta-epidemiological study. BMJ 336(7644):601–605

Masking Study Participants

44

Lea Drye

Contents

Abstract

Masking or blinding in clinical trials refers to the process of keeping the identity of the assigned treatment hidden from specific groups of individuals such as participants, study staff, or outcome assessors. The purpose of masking is to minimize conscious and unconscious bias in the conduct and interpretation of a trial. Masking participants in clinical trials is a key methodological procedure since patient expectations can introduce bias directly through how a participant reports patient-reported outcomes but also indirectly through his or her willingness to participate in and adhere to study activities.

The complexity of operational aspects of masking participants is often underestimated. Masking is facilitated by placebos, dummies, sham devices, or sham procedures/surgeries. The success of masking depends on how closely the

L. Drye (✉)
Office of Clinical Affairs, Blue Cross Blue Shield Association, Chicago, IL, USA
e-mail: latdrye@gmail.com

© Springer Nature Switzerland AG 2022

S. Piantadosi, C. L. Meinert (eds.), *Principles and Practice of Clinical Trials*,
https://doi.org/10.1007/978-3-319-52636-2_216

placebo or sham matches the active treatment. Creation of a completely identical placebo is generally possible only when active drug and matching placebo are provided by the manufacturer. Masking of participants becomes more complicated if there are more than two experimental treatment groups, an active control, if treatments are taken at different intervals or via different routes, or if sham devices or procedures are required.

Trials in which participants are masked should have procedures in place to unmask. Most unmasking is routine unmasking in which investigators communicate treatment assignment with participants after treatment and follow-up are complete. In addition to this routine unmasking, masked trials should have procedures to immediately unmask at any hour of the day in the event of an emergency.

Keywords

Blind · Mask · Single mask · Double mask · Unmask · Placebo · Sham

Definitions

Mask or blind: Withholding treatment assignment identification from a group or groups of individuals in a clinical trial.

Single mask: Withholding treatment assignment identification from a single group, usually used to refer to withholding treatment assignment from participants.

Double mask: Withholding treatment assignment identification from two groups of individuals, usually used to refer to withholding treatment assignment from both participants and from study staff.

Unmask: Unintentional or intentional revealing of the treatment assignment to groups of individuals who were previously masked.

Introduction

Masking in clinical trials is the process of keeping one or more parties (e.g., participants, study staff, outcome assessors, data analysts) unaware of the identity of the treatment assignment during the conduct of the trial. The purpose of masking is to prevent conscious or subconscious notions and expectations regarding the treatment effects from affecting outcomes. To minimize behavior that can lead to differential effects on outcomes, the preferred design strategy is to mask as many individuals as is practically possible while maintaining safety. Blinding is a term synonymous with masking that is frequently used.

The term single masking is usually used to refer to the masking of study participants, while double masking is usually used to refer to masking of study participants and study staff. Additional levels of masking, such as masking of data analysts or treatment effects monitoring committees (also known as data and safety monitoring boards), may also be used. It is important to note that the terms single, double, and triple masked, which are used to describe the level of masking, are not universally standardized. Readers must evaluate the description of masking in trial publications or study documentation such as the protocol to understand which groups were masked.

Goals of Masking

Masking is a crucial methodologic feature of randomized controlled trials. While randomization minimizes selection bias and confounding in the assignment of treatment, it does not prevent subsequent differential reporting or assessment of outcomes or behaviors that indirectly affect outcomes. Masking should not to be confused with allocation concealment, which is preventing the disclosure of upcoming treatment assignments until enrollment.

The masking of participants is particularly important for patient-reported outcomes such as symptom scales, adverse events, and concomitant medications. However, the participant's knowledge of treatment assignment could affect outcomes in less direct ways through his or her willingness to continue participation in study activities, adherence to assigned treatment, avoidance of other treatments, and risk behaviors. There are no analytical techniques that can "correct" for biased assessment of outcomes.

The effect of masking on outcomes was explored in Hrobjartsson et al. (2014). The authors reported results of a systematic review of 12 randomized clinical trials including 3869 patients in which the trial had one sub-study involving masked participants and another, otherwise identical, sub-study involving unmasked participants. In trials with patient-reported outcomes, the authors reported that effect sizes based on unmasked participants were exaggerated by an average of 0.56 standard deviations compared to masked participants. In addition to the effect on patient-reported outcomes, the average risk of participant attrition in the control groups of RCTs including more than 2 weeks follow-up duration was 7% (4% to 11%) in the unmasked treatment groups versus 4% (2% to 6%) in masked treatment groups, and more participants in the unmasked control groups used co-interventions compared to masked control group.

Alerting Participants That Masking Will Be Used

Study staff should explain to study participants that treatments will be masked and the reasons for masking. Masking should not be attempted if accomplishing it requires lying to participants or deception.

Both the Common Rule and FDA clinical trial regulations require (45 CFR Part 46.116 and 21 CFR 50.25) that descriptions of procedures related to research, such as masking, should be included in the informed consent process. Participants should be informed that they will be kept unaware of their treatment assignments in masked studies as well as whether the study staff or physician will be aware of the treatment assignment.

Operationalizing Masking

Placebos and Shams

Operationally, masking participants is facilitated by placebos and shams. Both serve the same purpose regarding bias control.

Placebo or dummy treatments are inert or inactive substances that are taken or applied as a substitute for the active treatment to prevent the participant from knowing which treatment he or she received. In device trials, both the terms placebo device and sham device are used.

Sham procedures or surgeries refer to something done to study participants to prevent them from knowing which treatment they received. Sham procedures have additional ethical concerns given that they are not inert like placebo treatments. They generally involve potential risks to participants due to sedation and possibly surgical wounds.

Mechanics

The success of masking depends on how closely the placebo or sham matches the active treatment. The brief statements regarding masking in most published reports of clinical trials belie how complicated the task of masking truly is.

Masking participants in drug trials depends on whether pills, tablets, patches, injections, liquid formulations, etc. can be made to match the active treatment with respect to obvious characteristics such as size, shape, and color but also with respect to smell and taste, particularly if the drug is known to have a characteristic feature. In practice, this is generally possible only when active drug and matching placebo are provided by the manufacturer since formulating an identical product to one that is marketed is not legal. In the Alzheimer's Disease Anti-inflammatory Prevention Trial (ADAPT), Bayer and Pfizer supplied investigators with identical placebos matching their marketed products (Martin et al. 2002).

When the manufacturer does not provide matching placebo, overencapsulation is a technique that can be used to produce identical active and placebo capsules for a trial of treatments that are in pill, tablet, or capsule formulation. This process is expensive and may require lab testing to confirm bioavailability. Depending on how large the overencapsulated study drug becomes, it can add additional eligibility criteria for participation, i.e., participants must be able to swallow the capsule to enroll.

Masking of drugs goes beyond creating identical product. The packaging also must be identical. This will require repackaging of drug in some situations which adds cost and time and also may have implications for product stability.

Masking of participants in drug trials becomes even more complicated if there are more than two treatment groups or an active control, or if the treatments are taken at different intervals or via different routes. In these cases, placebos will need to be created so that participants take active and placebo treatments at the appropriate treatment intervals and routes for all treatments. If one treatment requires administration twice as often as another, all participants must take study treatment at the most frequent interval to maintain masking. Similarly, if one treatment is a tablet and another is an injection, participants in both groups must receive both tablets and injections. For example, the Oral Psoriatic Arthritis Trial (OPAL) Broaden phase 3 trial compared tofacitinib to adalimumab for psoriatic arthritis in patients with inadequate response to previous disease-modifying antirheumatic drugs (Mease et al. 2017). Patients were randomized in a 2:2:2:1:1 ratio to receive tofacitinib 5 mg twice daily, tofacitinib 10 mg twice daily, adalimumab 40 mg administered subcutaneously once every 2 weeks, placebo with switch to the 5 mg tofacitinib at 3 months, or placebo with switch to the 10 mg tofacitinib at 3 months. In order to mask the trial, all patients had to take two tablets twice daily and receive biweekly injections. The content of the tablets and injections varied according to treatment group.

Masking of participants in device or surgery trials is difficult but not always impossible. Sham devices are manufactured to appear the same as active devices but are manipulated so that they do not function as required to administer the treatment. The Escitalopram versus Electrical Current Therapy for Treating Depression Clinical Study (ELECT-TDCS) compared transcranial direct-current stimulation with escitalopram in patients with major depressive disorder (Brunoni et al. 2017). Patients received active or placebo escitalopram and active or sham transcranial direct-current stimulation. Sham transcranial direct-current stimulation was accomplished using fully automated devices that were programmed to turn off the current automatically after 30 s. In a sham-controlled trial of 5 cm H2O and 10 cm H2O of continuous positive airway pressure (CPAP) in patients with asthma, "sham" CPAP was delivered via identical devices calibrated by the manufacturer to deliver pressure at less than 1 cm H2O with masked display of pressure level and intake flow rates and noise levels similar to the active devices (Holbrook et al. 2016).

In a sham surgery, an imitation procedure is performed to mimic the active surgery. This might include patients receiving anesthesia, having scopes inserted, having incisions, etc. Therefore, sham surgeries do carry risks that are more difficult to justify ethically and have been used less often than placebos. If patients are not under general anesthesia, then the surgical team may also have to mimic sounds, smells, and dialogue of surgery so that patients cannot distinguish whether or not they underwent the actual surgery. Any imaging to check success of surgery or medication to prevent infection must also be mimicked in patients assigned to sham. While difficult, sham surgeries are not impossible to perform if risks to patients can be minimized. In a trial investigating transplantation of retinal pigment epithelial cells as a treatment for Parkinson's disease, surgeons performed not only skin incision but also burr holes in the skull. In the sham group, the burr holes did not penetrate the dura matter (Gross et al. 2011).

Unmasking

To the extent possible, it is important to maintain participant masking until outcomes assessment is complete. In reality, no masking scheme is perfect. Participants who are determined to figure out their treatment assignment may be able to do so by comparing their treatments to other participants to look for tell-tale subtle differences between the treatments or, in the case of overencapsulated study drug, by opening the capsules to examine the contents.

Most unmasking occurs after treatment and follow-up are complete as a matter of process in closing out a trial. During the trial, there should be few instances where unmasking is required. When participants are experiencing side effects, unmasking is usually not needed as the study drug can simply be stopped. However, all masked trials should have procedures in place to immediately unmask at any hour of the day in emergency situations. This might be accomplished through a study website, 24-h call-in service or through tear-off labels on containers or devices. Situations which require immediate unmasking are:

- The treatment assignment is needed to care for the participant because decisions on how to proceed depend on which treatment the participant has received particularly in an emergency setting.
- Potential allergic reaction.
- Potential overdose of the participant or another person.

Occasionally, a participant will be adamant that he or she be told the treatment assignment during conduct of the trial. In these cases, the study staff have no choice but to unmask the participant.

Conclusion

Masking minimizes conscious and unconscious bias in the conduct and interpretation of a trial and as such is a key methodological procedure. While the importance of participant masking is well understood, the complexity of its implementation is often underestimated. It is rarely possible to create or purchase a completely identical placebo or sham. Masking of participants is difficult if there are more than two treatment groups or an active control, if the treatments are taken at different intervals or via different routes, or if sham procedures are required. Investigators should have procedures in place for routine unmasking of participants after treatment and follow-up are complete as well as procedures to immediately unmask at any hour of the day in the event of an emergency.

Key Facts

- Masking (also called blinding) is used to minimize the likelihood of differential treatment or assessments of outcomes due to conscious or unconscious bias.

Cross-References

▶ Administration of Study Treatments and Participant Follow-Up
▶ Issues for Masked Data Monitoring
▶ Masking of Trial Investigators
▶ Patient-Reported Outcomes

References

Brunoni AR, Moffa AH, Sampaio-Junior B, Borrione L, Moreno ML, Fernandes RA, Veronezi BP, Nogueira BS, Aparicio LVM, Razza LB, Chamorro R, Tort LC, Fraguas R, Lotufo PA, Gattaz WF, Fregni F, Bensenor IM (2017) Trial of electrical direct-current therapy versus Escitalopram for depression. N Engl J Med 376(26):2523–2533

Gross RE, Watts RL, Hauser RA, Bakay RA, Reichmann H, von Kummer R, Ondo WG, Reissig E, Eisner W, Steiner-Schulze H, Siedentop H, Fichte K, Hong W, Cornfeldt M, Beebe K, Sandbrink R (2011) Intrastriatal transplantation of microcarrier-bound human retinal pigment epithelial cells versus sham surgery in patients with advanced Parkinson's disease: a double-blind, randomised, controlled trial. Lancet Neurol 10(6):509–519

Holbrook JT, Sugar EA, Brown RH, Drye LT, Irvin CG, Schwartz AR, Tepper RS, Wise RA, Yasin RZ, Busk MF (2016) Effect of continuous positive airway pressure on airway reactivity in asthma. A randomized, sham-controlled clinical trial. Ann Am Thorac Soc 13(11):1940–1950

Hrobjartsson A, Emanuelsson F, Skou Thomsen AS, Hilden J, Brorson S (2014) Bias due to lack of patient blinding in clinical trials. A systematic review of trials randomizing patients to blind and nonblind sub-studies. Int J Epidemiol 43(4):1272–1283

Martin BK, Meinert CL, Breitner JC (2002) Double placebo design in a prevention trial for Alzheimer's disease. Control Clin Trials 23(1):93–99

Mease P, Hall S, FitzGerald O, van der Heijde D, Merola JF, Avila-Zapata F, Cieslak D, Graham D, Wang C, Menon S, Hendrikx T, Kanik KS (2017) Tofacitinib or Adalimumab versus placebo for psoriatic arthritis. N Engl J Med 377(16):1537–1550

Issues for Masked Data Monitoring

45

O. Dale Williams and Katrina Epnere

Contents

Abstract

The essential, primary purpose of a clinical trial is to provide a fair test for the comparison of treatments, drugs, strategies, etc. A challenge to this fairness is the appropriate utilization, or lack thereof, of masking or blinding. Masking generally refers to restricting knowledge as to the treatment group assignment for the individual or, in the case of a Data and Safety Monitoring Board (DSMB), to the summary of information comparing treatment groups. Fundamentally, masking is important to consider for those situations wherein knowledge of the treatment assignment could alter behavior or otherwise impact inappropriately on trial results. Masking may, however, while protecting against this bias, make it more difficult for the DSMB properly to protect trial participants from undue risk of adverse or serious adverse events. While there are several dimensions to this

O. D. Williams (✉)
Department of Biostatistics, University of North Carolina, Chapel Hill, NC, USA

Department of Medicine, University of Alabama at Birmingham, Birmingham, AL, USA
e-mail: odalewilliams@yahoo.com

K. Epnere
WCG Statistics Collaborative, Washington, DC, USA
e-mail: epnere@gmail.com

© Springer Nature Switzerland AG 2022

S. Piantadosi, C. L. Meinert (eds.), *Principles and Practice of Clinical Trials*,
https://doi.org/10.1007/978-3-319-52636-2_217

overall situation, this chapter addresses the important issue as to whether a trial's DSMB should be fully aware of which treatment group is which as it reviews data summaries for an ongoing trial.

Keywords

Data and safety monitoring board · Data monitoring committee · Masking · Blinding · Open report · Closed report · Interim analysis · Risk/benefit

Introduction

DSMBs, sometimes called Data Monitoring Committees (DMCs) or Safety and Data Monitoring Boards (SDMBs), have been utilized and referenced in the context of clinical trials since the 1960s (Greenberg Report 1967; Gordon et al. 1998; Wittes 1993). From that time to the present, the field of clinical trials methods and applications has grown enormously (► Chap. 37, "Data and Safety Monitoring and Reporting"). This period experienced an enormous expansion of the types of research questions that the field addresses. Some of these require long-term, complex trials, some address treatment regimens with inherent adverse event and serious adverse event issues, and some address those regimens without such issues. Global policies impacting on the conduct of trials should take this diversity into account.

The typical situation providing context for this discussion has to do with how reports prepared for the Board's review are organized and how Board meetings tend to be conducted. For the reports, their presentation schedule is roughly defined at the outset; this schedule is followed unless a critical issue arises that needs attention prior to a scheduled report release or meeting. These reports tend to have three components: an investigator's report to the DSMB, the open report, and the closed report. The investigator's report tends to deal with overall trial progress, responses to Board recommendations, synopsis of the protocol, review of the protocol history and amendments, and emerging results from relevant clinical studies. Typically, the open and closed reports contain a core set of tables and figures that are based on an agreed-upon data analysis plan. The typical open report provides recruitment and compliance information, demographic and baseline characteristic summaries for the combined treatment groups, and other relevant information. The closed report may include some of the same information, adverse event data, and outcome summaries, all by treatment group. "The closed report should allow the DMC to assess the risk/benefit (► Chap. 99, "Safety and Risk Benefit Analyses") of the study treatments as well as the integrity of the data, including completeness and timeliness, used in the interim analyses" (► Chap. 59, "Interim Analysis in Clinical Trials") (Neaton et al. 2018).

The meetings tend to follow this same structure with separate open and closed sections. Access to the open reports and participation in their discussion typically are limited to investigators and others involved in the study under careful confidentiality restrictions. Access to the closed report and participation in the closed session are restricted to Board members and those responsible for preparing the closed reports. For publically funded trials, representatives of the funding agency may attend (Anand et al. 2011; Bierer et.al 2016; DeMets et al. 2004; Wittes et al. 2007).

Main Focus

This chapter focuses on how these treatment groups are identified in the closed reports and during the consequent Board discussions.

Context is a critical issue, elements of which include:

1. No masking – Also sometimes called "open label," generally implies neither the participants enrolled in the trial, the staff conducting the trial, nor the DSMB are masked to treatment assignment. Even for this situation, trial site staff and potential enrolled participants typically – and importantly – are masked with respect to the treatment assignment for participants in line to be randomized.
2. Almost no masking – A special case of the "no masking" situation whereby the process of assessing the trial's primary outcome is done in a masked fashion. That is, the individuals or panels assessing or measuring trial outcomes for individual enrolled participants do so without knowledge as to the participant's treatment group. This is often considered a critically important need for any trial.
3. Single-masked trial – Generally refers to the situation where the participants enrolled in the trial do not know which treatment they are receiving, but the trial site staff and others are aware of treatment assignment (▶ Chap. 44, "Masking Study Participants").
4. Double masked – Generally refers to the situation where neither the enrolled participants nor the trial site staff are aware of the treatment assignments.
5. Triple masked – Generally refers to the double-masked situation plus the masking of the DSMB when reviewing ongoing results by treatment group.
6. Only DSMB unmasked – The critical question herein is whether the DSMB should be masked or should be the only operational entity, except for the staff preparing reports for the DSMB, which should be unmasked.

There is an important difference between the masking issues for a DSMB relative to those for the other components mentioned above. For the others, the frame of reference is possible bias for data items for individual enrolled participants. For the DSMB, the judgment is whether differences between the treatment groups as represented by summary data merit some action. This is, by its very nature, a broader, more important assessment of benefit and risk, often with societal implications (▶ Chaps. 99, "Safety and Risk Benefit Analyses").

In this context, the operative question is whether the Board should be masked as to the identity of the treatment groups and how should this operational decision be made and implemented. Some options are listed below:

1. Masked mandated – The implication is that during the ongoing trial, the Board would review differences between treatment groups with the treatment groups

identified by codes (e.g., group A and B). They would learn the actual identity of said groups only at the end of the trial. This strategy gives considerable weight to the concern that the knowledge of treatment group could bias the interpretation of interim results and lead to perhaps inappropriate action. It gives lesser weight to the concern that the strategy would perhaps impair the Board's ability to address adverse event issues in a timely and appropriate manner.
2. Unmasked mandated – The implication is that the likelihood of the Board not properly being able to assess harm or benefit without knowing the identity of the treatment groups outweighs the concern about possible bias.
3. Something in between – If so, who decides and how will it be structured.

Although Boards typically have purview over additional issues, the two most central issues tend to be:

1. Adverse events, including those considered attributable to a trial treatment regimen and those not so considered
2. Trial outcomes, with a priority focus on the primary, design outcome but also on those outcomes considered secondary or otherwise not primary

Operational implications can be quite different for these two issues: a masking policy for one may well not be appropriate for the other. The adverse event situation typically involves the Board's review of individual events in addition to summaries comparing treatment groups. Further, the review of adverse events may be undertaken on the occurrence of each individual event along with a careful investigation of differences between treatment groups subsequently at a Board's formal meeting. The fundamental issue is risk to the enrolled individuals. A careful assessment of this risk may require that the Board be informed as to treatment assignment.

Outcome comparisons may be made at each of the Board's formal meetings. These comparisons are critical to the purpose of the trial, and any factors that could impact on the fairness of the comparison need careful attention. In this context, some Board members may prefer to be masked and others may not. A special case is the issue of interim analyses. There is often pressure for the Board not to formally review interim analyses dealing with primary outcomes. Further, if the Board also is not able to conduct "informal" looks at such efficacy data, there is an interesting situation with respect to masking. *If there are no such interim analyses or looks, then the Board is inherently totally masked as to the assessment of outcomes prior to the end of the trial* (▶ Chap. 59, "Interim Analysis in Clinical Trials"). In this case, arguments for or against the Board being masked with respect to primary outcomes are moot.

Some Current Guidelines and Opinions

The critical aspects of assessing the pros and cons of masking Board are the expectations and opinions of funding agencies, of governmental agencies, of investigators, and of experts in the field. Highlighted below are excerpts from relevant documents and publications:

1. From the European Medicines Agency (EMA), (European Medicines Agency 2005):

> A Data Monitoring Committee is a group of independent experts external to a study assessing the progress, safety data and, if needed critical efficacy endpoints of a clinical study. In order to do so a DMC may review unblinded study information during the conduct of the study and provide the sponsor with recommendations regarding study modification, continuation or termination. Operating procedures describing how the DMC works and how it communicates with other study participants (e.g. with the data centre or the sponsor) should be in place at the start of the trial. [..] procedures should also describe how the integrity of the study with respect to preventing dissemination of unblinded study information is ensured.

Note that the EMA does not mandate unblinded reports; rather it indicates that the DMC "may review unblinded study information."

2. From the US Food and Drug Administration (FDA) (US DHHS FDA CBER CDER CDRH 2016):

> We recommend that a DMC have access to the actual treatment assignments for each study group. Some have argued that DMCs should be provided only coded assignment information that permits the DMC to compare data between study arms, but does not reveal which group received which intervention, thereby protecting against inadvertent release of unblinded interim data and ensuring a greater objectivity of interim review. This approach, however, could lead to problems in balancing risks against potential benefits in some cases.

Note that this report references possible problems in some cases in "balancing risk against potential benefits" (▶ Chap. 99, "Safety and Risk Benefit Analyses") and thus recommends that the Board be unblinded.

3. From the National Heart, Lung, and Blood Institute (NHLBI) (National Heart, Lung, and Blood Institute National Institutes of Health 2014):

> NHLBI monitoring boards:
>
> - Are convened to protect the interests of research subjects and ensure that they are not exposed to undue risk.
> - Operate without undue influence from any interested party, including study investigators or NHLBI staff.
> - Are encouraged to review interim analysis of study data in an unmasked fashion.

These guidelines reference interim analysis and "encourage" unmasked DSMBs.

4. From Clinical Trials Transformation Initiative (CITI), (Clinical Trials Transformation Initiative 2016):

> DMCs must periodically review the accumulating unmasked safety and efficacy data by treatment group, and advise the trial sponsor on whether to continue, modify, or terminate a trial based on benefit-risk assessment, as specified in the DMC Charter, protocol, and/or

> statistical analysis plan. During conduct of the trial, DMCs should periodically review by treatment group and in an unmasked fashion: primary and secondary outcome measures, deaths, other serious and non-serious adverse events, benefit-risk assessment, consistency of efficacy and safety outcomes across key risk factor sub-groups.

These guidelines require periodic reviews during the conduct of the trial by treatment group in an unmasked fashion.

5. From the US Department of Health and Human Services (DHHS) (Department of Health and Human Services, Office of Inspector General 2013):

> The ability of DSMBs to monitor trial progress and ensure the safety of patients may be compromised without access to unmasked data.

Importantly, the weight of the argument of masked vs unmasked DSMBs in these documents is on the side of the Board being unmasked. Note also that these documents tend not to reference the opinions of those on the firing line, so to speak, namely, the Board members themselves and study investigators.

The DSMB masking issue has also been addressed in the scientific literature. Important examples include the following:

1. Clinical Trials Transformation Initiative (CITI) group conducted a survey and a set of focus groups that consisted of DSMB members, statistical data analysis center representatives, patients and/or patient advocate DSMB members, institutional review board and US Food and Drug Administration representatives, industry, government, and nonprofit sponsors:

> Participants indicated that the primary responsibility of a DMC is to be an independent advisory body representing the interests of trial participants. [..]DMCs should have access to unmasked study data in order to periodically review the accumulating safety and efficacy findings and advise the sponsor on whether to continue, modify, or terminate a trial based on an assessment of risks and benefits. Unmasked interim analyses should be identified in the charter and agreed upon beforehand. Charter [..] should fully address whether the DMC will have access to unmasked data at the subject level and aggregate level. (Calis et al. 2017; Lewis et al. 2016)

2. Chen-Mok et al. described the experiences and challenges in data monitoring for clinical trials within an international tropical disease research network:

> The interim reports discussed during closed sessions were presented using treatment codes (eg, A and B), with any needed unblinding done in an executive session of voting members only. The executive secretary kept sealed envelopes containing treatment decoding information [..] These envelopes were available to members for each study being reviewed at a meeting. DSMB members began to consider the arguments for fully unblinded reviews and began to move toward more easily unblinding reports. However, members did not achieve a clear position regarding automatic unbinding of reports. (Chen-Mok et al. 2006)

3. Holubkov et al. summarized the role of DSMB in the comparative pediatric Critical Illness Stress-Induced Immune Suppression (CRISIS) Prevention Trial:

> It is difficult to conjecture whether the DSMB being unmasked at time of the first interim analysis [..] would have led to different decisions regarding study continuation and timing of subsequent data reviews. Blinded review requires simultaneous consideration of different possible scenarios, and the CRISIS DSMB members were sufficiently comfortable with the two possibilities to maintain masking until the second data review. (Holubkov et al. 2013)

4. Recent publications by Fleming et al. have suggested that:

> . . . DMCs should have full access to unblinded accumulating data on safety and efficacy throughout the clinical trial. Some believe a DMC should receive only safety data or that a DMC that receives efficacy data only by blinded codes (e.g., Group A versus Group B) will be more objective in assessing interim data. The consensus of the expert panel was that such blinding was counterproductive, even potentially dangerous to the safety of the study participants. By having access to unblinded data on all relevant treatment outcomes, the DMC can develop timely insights about safety in the context of a benefit-to-risk assessment, as well as about irregularities in trial conduct or in the generation of the DMC reports. (Fleming et al. 2017)
> (Fleming et al. 2018, DeMets and Ellenberg 2016).

5. In 1998, the New England Journal of Medicine published Meinert's opinion regarding masked DSMB reporting:

> Masked monitoring is thought to increase the objectivity of monitors by making them less prone to bias. What is overlooked is what masking does to degrade the competency of the monitors. The assumption underlying masked monitoring is that recommendations for a change in the study protocol can be made independently of the direction of a treatment difference, but this assumption is false. Usually, more evidence is required to stop a trial because of a benefit than because of harm. Trials are performed to assess safety and efficacy, not to "prove" harm. Therefore, it is unreasonable to make the monitors behave as if they were indifferent to the direction of a treatment difference. (Meinert 1998)

Implications and Suggestions

First and foremost, the distinction between the three options for masking listed above can be described simply as differences as to when unmasking occurs. For *Option 1 Masked Mandated*, the unmasking would occur only at the end of the trial. For *Option 2 Unmasked Mandated*, the unmasking would occur at the outset. For *Option 3 Something in between*, there may be masking at the outset but unmasking later in accordance to decisions made jointly by the funding entity, the Board itself, and others as appropriate.

The guidelines and opinions expressed above appear to be more in the context of clinical research for which adverse events and serious adverse events are important. In this context and in view of the information above, a conclusion is that *Option 1 Masked Mandated* above is neither practical nor tenable for many of these trials.

For those investigative issues for which there is limited concern about risk and some concern about judgment bias, the strategy may be more acceptable. Nevertheless, *Option 3* is likely to be a better alternative than mandating masking at the outset and maintaining it until the trial's end.

For *Option 2*, some language in relevant guidelines and used in discussions seems to assume that the only options are *Option 1* and *Option 2*, that is, the assumption appears to be that masking would be mandated in such a manner that unmasking would occur only at the end of the trial. Nevertheless, there is apparent considerable force behind the recommendation that *Option* 2 be the operative strategy.

There are, however, some concerns with *Option 2 Unmasked Mandated* that deserve consideration. The most compelling is the opinion of members of the Board, the funding entity, and any other entity with an explicit role in the Board's deliberations. This collection necessarily has a clear understanding of the needs of the trial and should be well positioned about issues critical to its success. There certainly have been instances where the masking strategy was discussed at the outset and the decision was for the Board to be masked. In this circumstance there is a clear understanding that the Board can chose to be unmasked at any point for which it seems appropriate to do so. When considering unmasking, the discussions tend to focus, as they should, on assessing the joint issue of adverse events and primary and other outcomes.

An important issue is how the masking strategy utilized is reflected in the reports of analyses summarizing adverse events and outcomes. If *Option* 1 is utilized, the reports would necessarily have the treatment groups coded in some way, say Treatment A and Treatment B. For *Option 2*, this would be unnecessary, and the treatment groups could be clearly indicated. For *Option 3*, it may be necessary to code as per *Option 1* and then unmask this coding scheme when the decision to unmask the Board is made. However, it may well be prudent to use coded labels (Buhr et al. 2018) in the reports in any case as this may help prevent the identification of the treatment groups should the reports be accessed inappropriately. If the Board is operating unmasked, then it would simply need access to the interpretation of the codes.

Key Suggestions

A simple strategy consistent with the apparent purpose of the guidelines and opinions above is listed below. This strategy accommodates the wide variety of trials and questions they address and the opinions of the Board members, funding entity, study leaders, and others as appropriate:

Step 1. At the outset of the functioning of the Board, have a clear discussion of the masking strategy that seems most appropriate for the trial in question. This discussion would necessarily involve the funding entity and others as appropriate.

Step 2. If all agree that an unmasked approach is most appropriate and should be used from the outset, then proceed accordingly. However, it still may be prudent to code the labels for the treatment groups in reports, with the code readily available to the Board, as a strategy to diminish the likelihood of inadvertent knowledge of trial status by someone who otherwise would not have access to this information.

Step 3. If all agree that beginning with a masked approach is preferable, then a prudent strategy would be to reconsider this decision at each subsequent meeting so that the mask can be readily lifted if appropriate.

It should be noted that this strategy is not novel (Buhr et al. 2018). It has been used and is being used for clinical trials both recent and underway. It puts the critical decision as to the most appropriate masking strategy in the hands of those responsible for the Board's operation for a specific study. Thus, it takes into account the specific characteristics of both the study in question and the concerns of the appointed Board.

Cross-References

- Data and Safety Monitoring and Reporting
- Interim Analysis in Clinical Trials
- Masking Study Participants
- Safety and Risk Benefit Analyses

References

Anand SS, Wittes J, Yusuf S (2011) What information should a sponsor of a randomized trial receive during its conduct? Clin Trials 8(6):716–719

Bierer BE, Li R, Seltzer J, Sleeper LA, Frank E, Knirsch C, Aldinger CE, Lavine RJ, Massaro J, Shah A, Barnes M, Snapinn S, Wittes J (2016) Responsibilities of data monitoring committees: consensus recommendations. Ther Innov Regul Sci 50(5):648–659

Buhr KA, Downs M, Rhorer J, Bechhofer R, Wittes J (2018) Reports to independent data monitoring committees: an appeal for clarity, completeness, and comprehensibility. Ther Innov Regul Sci 52(4):459–468

Calis KA, Archdeacon P, Bain RP, Forrest A, Perlmutter J, DeMets DL (2017) Understanding the functions and operations of data monitoring committees: survey and focus group findings. Clin Trials 14(1):59–66

Chen-Mok M, VanRaden MJ, Higgs ES, Dominik R (2006) Experiences and challenges in data monitoring for clinical trials within an international tropical disease research network. Clin Trials 3(5):469–477

DeMets DL, Ellenberg SS (2016) Data monitoring committees—expect the unexpected. N Engl J Med 375(14):1365–1371

DeMets D, Califf R, Dixon D, Ellenberg S, Fleming T, Held P, Packer M (2004) Issues in regulatory guidelines for data monitoring committees. Clin Trials 1(2):162–169

Fleming TR, DeMets DL, Roe MT, Wittes J, Calis KA, Vora AN, Gordon DJ (2017) Data monitoring committees: promoting best practices to address emerging challenges. Clin Trials 14(2):115–123

Fleming TR, Ellenberg SS, DeMets DL (2018) Data monitoring committees: current issues. Clin Trials 15(4):321–328

Gordon VM, Sugarman J, Kass N (1998) Toward a more comprehensive approach to protecting human subjects. IRB: A Review of Human Subjects Research 20(1):1–5

Holubkov R, Casper TC, Dean JM, Anand KJS, Zimmerman J, Meert KL, Nicholson C (2013) The role of the data and safety monitoring board in a clinical trial: the CRISIS study. Pediatr Crit Care Med J Soc Crit Care Med World Fed Pediatr Intensive Crit Care Soc 14(4):374

Lewis RJ, Calis KA, DeMets DL (2016) Enhancing the scientific integrity and safety of clinical trials: recommendations for data monitoring committees. JAMA 316(22):2359–2360

Meinert CL (1998) Masked monitoring in clinical trials—blind stupidity? N Engl J Med 338:1381–1382
Neaton JD, Grund B, Wentworth D (2018) How to construct an optimal interim report: what the data monitoring committee does and doesn't need to know. Clin Trials 15(4):359–365
Wittes J (1993) Behind closed doors: the data monitoring board in randomized clinical trials. Stat Med 12(5–6):419–424
Wittes J, Barrett-Connor E, Braunwald E, Chesney M, Cohen HJ, DeMets D, Walters L (2007) Monitoring the randomized trials of the Women's health initiative: the experience of the data and safety monitoring board. Clin Trials 4(3):218–234
Greenberg Report (1967) Organization, Review, and administration of cooperative studies (Greenberg report): a report from the heart special project committee to the National Advisory Heart Council. Control Clin Trials. 1988 9:137–148

Online Documents

Department of Health and Human Services, Office of Inspector General. (2013) Data and safety monitoring boards in NIH clinical trials: meeting guidance, but facing some issues. https://oig.hhs.gov/oei/reports/oei-12-11-00070.pdf
U.S. Department of Health and Human Services Food and Drug Administration, Center for Biologics Evaluation and Research (CBER)Center for Drug Evaluation, and Research (CDER) Center for Devices and Radiological Health (CDRH) (2016) Guidance for clinical trial sponsors establishment and operation of clinical trial data monitoring committee. https://www.fda.gov/downloads/regulatoryinformation/guidances/ucm127073.pdf
European Medicines Agency Committee for medicinal products for human use (2005) Guideline on data monitoring committee. https://www.ema.europa.eu/documents/scientific-guideline/guideline-data-monitoring-committees_en.pdf
National Heart, Lung, and Blood Institute National Institutes of Health (2014) NHLBI policy for data and safety monitoring of extramural clinical studies. https://www.nhlbi.nih.gov/grants-and-training/policies-and-guidelines/nhlbi-policy-data-and-safety-monitoring-extramural-clinical-studies
Clinical Trials Transformation Initiative (CTTI) (2016) CTTI recommendations: data monitoring committees. https://www.ctti-clinicaltrials.org/files/recommendations/dmc-recommendations.pdf

Variance Control Procedures 46

Heidi L. Weiss, Jianrong Wu, Katrina Epnere, and O. Dale Williams

Contents

Abstract

This chapter covers the concepts of variance and sources of variation for clinical trial data. Common metrics to quantify the extent of variability in relation to the mean are introduced as are clinical trial design techniques and statistical analysis methods to control and reduce this variation. The uses of variance as a data quality assessment tool in large-scale, long-term multicenter clinical trials are highlighted.

H. L. Weiss · J. Wu
Biostatistics and Bioinformatics Shared Resource Facility, Markey Cancer Center, University of Kentucky, Lexington, KY, USA
e-mail: heidi.weiss@uky.edu; Jianrong.Wu@uky.edu

K. Epnere (✉)
WCG Statistics Collaborative, Washington, DC, USA

O. D. Williams
Department of Biostatistics, University of North Carolina, Chapel Hill, NC, USA

Department of Medicine, University of Alabama at Birmingham, Birmingham, AL, USA

© Springer Nature Switzerland AG 2022

S. Piantadosi, C. L. Meinert (eds.), *Principles and Practice of Clinical Trials*,
https://doi.org/10.1007/978-3-319-52636-2_218

Keywords

Clinical trial · Variance · Systematic errors · Measurement errors · Random error · Coefficient of variation · Technical error · Matched design · Crossover design · Repeated measures design · Power · Sample size · Analysis of covariance · Multiple regression analysis · Data quality assessment

Introduction

Variance is one of the first topics presented during any basic statistics course, typically occurring shortly after discussions of the mean and other measures of central tendency. Subsequent presentations tend to portray variance in the context of making judgments about the mean and as the denominator in equations that include the mean or other point estimates in the numerator. This tends to indicate that variance is a necessary evil in the computations required for other measures, but otherwise of limited value. This is certainly not true for experimental research and especially not true for large-scale, long-term multicenter clinical trials.

What Is Variance?

Variance is something that can be measured, so what is this something? One simple and somewhat intuitive way to express this is to consider variance as being a consequence of the distances between all the numbers in a dataset. Thus, the closer together these numbers are, the lower the variance and the further apart they are the higher the variance. Mathematically, the sample variance is the sum of squared deviations of each value from the mean value, divided by the sample size minus one.

$$\text{Sample variance} : s^2 = \frac{\sum_{i=1}^{n} (x_i - \overline{x})^2}{n - 1} \quad \text{and standard deviation} : s = \sqrt{s^2}$$

where x_i is the value of the ith element, $\overline{x}$ is the sample mean and n is the sample size.

Thus, the units for the variance are the square of the units for the numbers used for the calculation. To get back to the units of the initial numbers, the square root of the variance, the standard deviation, is used. The magnitude of the variance, per se, is not very informative. It, however, can be highly informative relative to the mean or other relevant point estimates or to compare the variability of one set of numbers to that of another set. This comparison can serve as a critically important data quality assessment and monitoring tool.

What Are the Main Sources of Variance in a Clinical Trial?

Clinical trials, by definition, are comparisons involving persons. In this context, measurements provide data representing differences, that is, variation, among persons and within persons. The process of making the measurements is expected to provide data that represent the underlying true value at the point in time the measurement was made as well as any deviation from this true value due to the measurement process. Measurement error is typically unavoidable so the critical issue is understanding its magnitude and taking steps to reduce it to more comfortable levels should doing so be warranted.

More broadly, in a parallel two group clinical trial, the variances can be divided into two sources: the variance between the treatment groups and the variances within the treatment groups. In general, the variance between the groups should be a consequence of the treatment effects. The variances within the groups, however, reflect the inherent differences among the individuals within the groups plus the errors that occur in the process of making the data measurements. More specifically, measurement errors occurring during data collection can often be due to data collection instrument or process variability, data transfer or transcription errors, simple calculation errors or carelessness. It is good practice for a clinical trial to maximize the treatment effect and to reduce measurement error by using appropriate methods for the study design, data collection, and data analyses.

Why Does Variance in a Clinical Trial Matter?

Data variation is unavoidable in clinical research and such variation due to systematic or random errors can cause unwanted effects and biases. Systematic error (bias) is associated with study design and execution. When bias occurs, the results or conclusions of a trial may be systematically distorted especially should the biases affect one treatment group more or less than the other. These can be quantified and avoided. On the other hand, variances due to random error occur by chance and add noise to the system, so to speak, and thus reduce the likelihood of finding a significant difference between treatment groups (FDA 2019). Publication by Barraza et al. (2019) discusses these two concepts in more detail. Furthermore, variances have great impact on the sample size estimation and precision of outcome measurements of a trial. Underestimation of the variance could result in lower statistical power to detect treatment differences than would otherwise be the case. It can also reduce the ability to comfortably compare the results of one trial to those of other studies.

When Is Variance Uncomfortably Large?

There are two aspects for assessing the magnitude of variance. One is the variance of a set of numbers in relation to the average for that set. This is often assessed by the use of the coefficient of variation (CV),

$$\text{Coefficient of Variation} : \text{CV} = \frac{s}{\overline{x}} \times 100\%$$

where s is the standard deviation and $\overline{x}$ is the sample mean.

which simply is the standard deviation divided by the average. Generally, if the standard deviation is more than 30% of the average, the data may be too highly variable to be fully useful.

The other aspect is technical error (TE), which can be based on the differences between two independent measures of a variable. For example, a clinical chemistry laboratory may be sent two vials of material for analyses, which represent one sample that has been split. The identity of the two samples would not be known by the laboratory. This process could be repeated for several samples so that a dataset based on the assays of these paired observations can be created. These data can be used to calculate the Technical Error for this measurement process, where

$$\text{Technical Error of Measurment : TE} = \sqrt{\frac{\sum_{i=1}^{n} d_i^2}{2n}}$$

where d_i is the difference between measurements made on a given object on two occasions (or by two workers) and n is the sample size.

Detailed instructions for calculating TE are described by Perini et al. (2005). For this situation, data quality is classified as very good if RTE $<10\%$, good if $10\% \leq \text{RTE} < 20\%$, acceptable if $20\% \leq \text{RTE} < 30\%$, and not acceptable if $\text{RTE} \geq 30\%$. The target for key outcome measures for a clinical trial should be $<10\%$, however, there are no universally acceptable cut-off levels.

How to Control Variance Through Clinical Trial Design and Data Collection and Analysis?

Systematic error and measurement error can be reduced by 1) using appropriate statistical designs, blocking, or stratification, 2) successfully implementing standard data collection procedures for key measures and other data quality enhancements, and 3) using appropriate methods of statistical analysis. Particularly important for minimizing measurement errors is the careful use of high-quality methods for data collection with clear procedures and sound quality assurance and quality control methods for instruments and assays to be used. For example, measurement error can be reduced by clear and detailed specifications on standard procedures for measuring clinical and biological outcomes in the protocol. Further, the impact of measurement error can also be reduced through data analysis by using statistical techniques and methods discussed below.

Control Variance Through Clinical Trial Design

Some of the tools that can be used to control or minimize the impact of larger than perhaps desirable variances are described below. These will be helpful in some, but not all situations.

1. Randomization: The process of randomly allocating trial participants to the different treatment groups has many desirable consequences (Suresh 2011). This process results in participants tending to be spread evenly in the treatment groups in items of age, gender, race, genotype, education status, smoking habit, etc. Hence, the potential for systematic differences between groups is reduced, the within group variances are more likely to be similar and the overall variance for trial measurements is likely less in face of the reduced systematic differences. The potential confounding between prognostic factors and outcome variable is also diminished.
2. Matched or paired design: In a matched or paired design, first create pairs of subjects where the individuals within each pair are as alike each other as the situation permits. Then within a pair randomly assign one subject to treatment and the other to control. The primary outcome can then be the differences within pairs across the full trial (Simon and Chinchilli 2007). This strategy has the potential to reduce importantly the confounding between prognostic factors and outcomes.
3. Cross-over design: A more general paired design is a cross-over design. In the simplest cross-over trial, each subject receives two different treatments A and B. Half the subjects receive A first and then after a washout period are crossed over to B. The remaining subjects who initially receive B first are then crossed over to A. Thus, each person serves as their own control, thus eliminating or at least seriously reducing the impact of among person variability on the outcome assessment (Simon and Chinchilli 2007). The use of cross-over designs is not without its risks, however, as there may be difficulty in implementing a fully effective wash out process. For this reason, this design is somewhat infrequently used.
4. Repeated measurements design: Replication provides an efficient way to increase the precision of studies. For example, if the population variance is σ^2, then the variance of sample mean based on the n observation is σ^2/n . Thus, the precision in measuring the mean can be arbitrarily increased with sufficient replications. Using repeated measurements design, the variance due to within subject differences is diminished, perhaps substantially (Tango 2016).
5. Increasing the sample size: In general, increasing sample size reduces the overall error variance and thus increases the study power (Biau et al. 2008).

Control Variance Through Data Collection

Measurement error cannot be eliminated completely, but it can be reduced tremendously by clear and detailed procedures for measuring clinical and biological outcomes in the protocol. Measurement error occurring during the data collection in laboratories is often due to transcription errors, simple calculation errors, or carelessness. Therefore, training of clinicians, nurses, and laboratory technicians is important.

Biologic and clinical data often are generated with the use of sophisticated instrumentation, assays, computers, or questionnaires. The clinical personnel must not only understand the rationale and newly developed technology but also be able to perform consistently throughout the study according to the procedure specified in the protocol (Chow and Liu 2014). Training on use of electronic case report forms (eCRFs), data specification on types of variables within eCRFs, and use of clinical trial management database systems are important.

Control Variance Through Data Analysis

Several statistical techniques and methods can be used in analysis stage of clinical trial to control the variance.

1. ANCOVA: The analysis of covariance (ANCOVA) is a useful statistical analysis method to improve the precision of a clinical trial. The error comes from extraneous variables that vary randomly within the groups. If such extraneous variables cannot be controlled by the experimenter but can be observed along with outcome variable, then ANCOVA can adjust the outcome variable for the effect of the concomitant variable. If such adjustment is not performed, the concomitant variables could inflate the error variance and make the treatment differences difficult to detect (Wang et al. 2019).
2. Analyzing change from baseline: When the outcomes were measured before the patients were randomized, analyzing change from baseline could reduce the variability among subjects. For example, let X be the outcome variable of a treatment group and the corresponding baseline measurement is B and assume

$$\mathrm{var.}(\mathrm{X}) = \mathrm{var.}(\mathrm{B})\sigma^2, \text{ and}$$

$$\mathrm{corr}(\mathrm{X}, \mathrm{B}) = \mathrm{r}.$$

   The analysis ignoring baseline is based on the outcome X with variance σ^2, whereas the analysis based on change from baseline has variance.

$$\mathrm{var.}(\mathrm{X} - \mathrm{B}) = 2\sigma^2(1 - \mathrm{r}).$$

   Thus, the analysis of the difference X-B (change from baseline) will use a smaller variance if $r > 0.5$. This is because of the typically marked positive correlation between the baseline and outcome levels. If the correlation is less than 0.5, then using change from baseline introduces extra noise into the analysis and is not recommended (Mathews 2006; EMA 2015).
3. Multiple regression analysis: Using regression analysis can separate the covariate variance from the error variance, thus reducing the error variance for the treatment assessment. Typical covariates to consider include different sites/centers, demographic and baseline clinical characteristics associated with the trial outcome that were not controlled for in the trial design (EMA 2015).

Variance As a Data Quality Assessment Tool

Measures of variance can be an important data quality assessment tool. In addition to the CV and TE discussed above, additional approaches also can be utilized. Some examples are included below.

Technician Performance. Especially for large-scale, long-term, multicenter clinical trials, numerous measurements are conducted by a variety of technical staff, often with more than one such person at each clinical center. One example is the measurement of blood pressure (BP) with a cuff and stethoscope – the use of automated devices also has similar issues. For example, suppose there are 12 BP technicians and the calculation of the variances for each of these over a prespecified time interval indicates that the BP measurements for one of the technicians have a much *higher variance* than the others. This situation merits further investigation. The first step would be to prepare the frequency distribution of the measurements for this technician and compare it to those for the other technicians. If the measurements for this technician are simply spread out more across the distribution than the others, it likely means this technician is not as careful as the others or perhaps does not hear adequately well. If the distribution is more similar to those for other technicians except for several outliers, then the source of the outliers needs to be ascertained and corrections made as necessary.

Further, an examination of the results for the same technician over several time periods may identify some periods with variances higher than the others. A look at the frequency distribution of the data for this technician or for the time periods of concern may provide some clues. One possibility is that this technician does not follow the protocol carefully.

Sometimes variances can be too small. For many, but not all issues, larger than desirable variances are the concern. However, there are circumstances whereby the calculated *variance is too small*. One such example, again for BP measurements, is the situation whereby the measures of systolic BP completed by a specific technician had a distribution with reasonable mean and variance. Further, the distribution for diastolic BP also had a distribution with reasonable mean and variance; however, when the distribution of the differences between systolic and diastolic BP were examined, the mean was very near 30 and the variance was near zero. It appears that the technician measured the systolic pressure and then rather than taking the time to complete the measurement process correctly, simply subtracted 30 from the systolic measurement and recorded the result as the diastolic pressure.

Other examples can occur if instruments malfunction and get locked at one value or a restricted range of values. In all these cases, simple examinations of the frequency distributions can often provide insights as to the cause of the issue.

Clinical Center Laboratory Performance For those trials that use a local laboratory at each of the participating clinical centers, it can be informative to simply compare the variances for each assay utilized across the different clinical centers, typically for a specific time interval. Further, comparing the variances within laboratory over different time intervals can also be informative. Examining the frequency distributions for those laboratories or time intervals can often provide clues as to the reasons for the higher variances. Outliers, correct values or not, also can create this situation. This can quickly be examined using frequency distributions. There may well be data groupings other than time intervals for which this type of assessment would be informative.

Conclusion/Key Recommendations

- Variance is used to measure the deviation from (or the spread around) the mean in each dataset and it allows us to compare different data sets.
- Coefficient of Variance and Technical Error can be used to assess the amount of variance in each dataset.
- There are several clinical trial design tools as well as data collection and analysis methods that can be used to control variance. Underestimation of the variance could result in lower statistical power to detect treatment differences and it can also reduce the ability to comfortably compare the results between studies.
- Variance can serve as a very useful data quality assessment tool in clinical trials.

Cross-References

▶ Controlling Bias in Randomized Clinical Trials
▶ Cross-over Trials
▶ Data Capture, Data Management, and Quality Control; Single Versus Multicenter Trials
▶ Power and Sample Size

References

Barraza F, Arancibia M, Madrid E, Papuzinski C (2019) General concepts in biostatistics and clinical epidemiology: random error and systematic error. Medwave 19(7):e7687

Biau DJ, Kernéis S, Porcher R (2008) Statistics in brief: the importance of sample size in the planning and interpretation of medical research. Clin Orthop Relat Res 466(9):2282–2288

Chow SC, Liu JP (2014) Design and analysis of clinical trial, 3rd edn. Wiley, Hoboken, NJ. https://www.wiley.com/en-ug/Design+and+Analysis+of+Clinical+Trials%3A+Concepts+and+Methodologies%2C+3rd+Edition-p-9780470887653

European Medicines Agency (EMA) (2015) Guideline on adjustment for baseline covariates in clinical trials. https://www.ema.europa.eu/en/documents/scientific-guideline/guideline-adjustment-baseline-covariates-clinical-trials_en.pdf. Accessed 23 Mar 2021

Mathews J (2006) Introduction to randomized controlled clinical trials, 2nd edn. Chapter 6, p 78, Chapman & Hall/CRC Texts in Statistical Science. https://www.routledge.com/Introduction-to-Randomized-Controlled-Clinical-Trials/Matthews/p/book/9781584886242

Perini TA, de Oliveira GL, Ornellas J d S, de Oliveira FP (2005) Technical error of measurement in anthropometry. Rev Bras Med Esporte 11(1):81–85. https://doi.org/10.1590/S1517-86922005000100009

Simon LJ, Chinchilli VM (2007) A matched crossover design for clinical trials. Contemp Clin Trials 28(5):638–646. https://doi.org/10.1016/j.cct.2007.02.003

Suresh K (2011) An overview of randomization techniques: an unbiased assessment of outcome in clinical research. J Hum Reprod Sci 4(1):8–11. https://doi.org/10.4103/0974-1208.82352

Tango T (2016) On the repeated measures designs and sample sizes for randomized controlled trials. Biostatistics 17(2):334–349. https://doi.org/10.1093/biostatistics/kxv047

U.S. Department of Health and Human Services Food and Drug Administration Center for Drug Evaluation and Research Center for Biologics Evaluation and Research (2019) Enrichment strategies for clinical trials to support determination of effectiveness of human drugs and biological products guidance for industry. https://www.fda.gov/media/121320/download. Accessed 25 Mar 2021

Wang B, Ogburn E, Rosenblum M (2019) Analysis of Covariance (ANCOVA) in randomized trials: more precision, less conditional bias, and valid confidence intervals, without model assumptions. Biometrics 75:1391–1400

Ascertainment and Classification of Outcomes

47

Wayne Rosamond and David Couper

Contents

W. Rosamond (✉)
Department of Epidemiology, Gillings School of Global Public Health, University of North Carolina, Chapel Hill, NC, USA
e-mail: wayne_rosamond@unc.edu

D. Couper
Department of Biostatistics, Gillings School of Global Public Health, University of North Carolina, Chapel Hill, NC, USA
e-mail: david_couper@unc.edu

© Springer Nature Switzerland AG 2022

S. Piantadosi, C. L. Meinert (eds.), *Principles and Practice of Clinical Trials*,
https://doi.org/10.1007/978-3-319-52636-2_233

Abstract

Successful completion and valid conclusions from a clinical trial rely on having complete and accurate outcome data. Misclassification of outcome events can introduce systematic error and bias as well as reduce the statistical power of the trial. Outcomes of interest in clinical trials vary and can include major clinically recognized events; asymptomatic subclinical measurements; and/or patient-centered reported outcomes. Final classification of study outcomes often involves use of standardized computer algorithms, processing of materials and review with outcome classification committees, and linkage with electronic data sources. Processes for accomplishing the goals of outcome ascertainment and classification can be designed as centralized systems, de-centralized networks of investigators, or a hybrid of these two methods. Challenges to obtaining valid outcomes include ensuring complete follow-up of study participants, use of standardized event definitions, capture of relevant diagnostic information, establishing protocols for review of potential events, training of clinical review teams, linkage to data sources across various platforms, quality control, and administrative oversite of the process. Designers of clinical trials need to consider carefully their approach for event identification, capture of diagnostic data, utilization of standardized diagnostic algorithms and/or clinical review committees, and mechanisms for maintaining data quality.

Keywords

Event ascertainment · Outcome classification · Adjudication, bias

Introduction

In the process of conducting clinical trials and observational studies, there is often a heavy focus on treatment and exposure assessment. Although important, this attention can occur at the cost of less consideration of the complexities of complete identification and valid classification of outcomes. Successful completion and valid conclusions of a clinical trial rely on having complete and accurate outcome data, particularly for the primary outcome. In clinical trials, if missingness or misclassification of outcome events is unrelated to treatment group assignment, this may merely reduce the statistical power of the trial and bias results toward the null. However, if the missingness or misclassification varies across treatment or exposure groups, this introduces systematic error in the results of the trial and may bias findings in either direction. There are many challenges to obtaining valid outcomes in clinical trials. These include ensuring complete follow-up of study participants, use of standardized event definitions, capture of relevant diagnostic information, establishing protocols for review of potential events, training of clinical review teams, linkage to data sources across various platforms, quality control, and administrative oversite of the process. This chapter focuses on methods to obtain information needed for the full assessment of trial outcomes and the process of using that information to determine the outcomes for all participants.

Masking to Treatment Assignment

The best designed clinical trials take particular care to reduce the potential for differential misclassification to occur across treatment groups. Even if participants and the investigators and staff involved in treatment provision cannot be masked, it is desirable that those involved in any aspect of the outcome ascertainment and classification be unaware of the participants' treatment group assignments. Otherwise, classifications may be either consciously or subconsciously influenced by knowledge of the treatment group.

Competing Risks

The definition of outcome or the statistical methods for analyzing them need to account for the potential for the outcome to be missing because of competing risks. For instance, in a trial in the elderly of a method to reduce the risk of decline in cognitive function, some participants may be missing information about change in cognitive function because they die before having a follow-up assessment of cognitive function. There are accepted statistical approaches to address competing risks, such as the Fine and Gray model for competing risks in time-to-event analyses (Fine and Gray 1999). Details of these methods are addressed elsewhere in this monograph.

Types of Outcomes

Outcomes of interest in clinical trials may be considered in three main categories. These categories include (1) major clinically recognized events, (2) asymptomatic subclinical measurements, and (3) patient-centered-reported outcomes. Although most clinical trials have a single primary outcome in just one of these domains, some seek to capture information on all three types of outcomes for investigation as secondary outcomes.

Major Clinically Recognized Events

Events that generally come to the attention of medical care services are often primary outcomes in clinical trials. Examples of major clinically recognized outcomes include acute myocardial infarction, acute decompensated heart failure, stroke, all-cause or cause-specific mortality, exacerbations of chronic obstructive pulmonary disease and asthma, venous thromboembolism, gestational diabetes, diabetes mellitus, major infections, trauma, and injury. Events such as acute myocardial infarction generally have a well-defined time of occurrence. Onset dates of other events such as diabetes or heart failure are less well identified. By definition, clinically recognized outcomes involve contact with medical personnel, though often not with staff involved in the clinical trial. For instance, there is generally no expectation that a participant who has an acute myocardial infarction will be treated in hospitals in connection with investigators in the clinical trial. The ease with which such potential events can be identified depends on the type of health-care system in the country in which the trial is conducted. In a country with a single-payer health-care system, information about hospitalizations is collected centrally, and with the appropriate permissions, it is relatively straightforward to obtain the medical records needed for event classification and adjudication. In the USA, if a trial is done using participants from a managed care consortium such as Kaiser Permanente, the situation is similar to a country with a single-payer health system, except that participants may move to a different health-care system during follow-up. When participants are not all in a single managed care consortium, identification of potential events and obtaining the medical records needed for classification are much more complex.

Asymptomatic Subclinical Measurements

Asymptomatic subclinical assessments can be either primary or secondary outcomes of clinical trials and encompass outcomes, conditions, or stages of conditions that generally do not come to the attention of health-care systems. They require independent assessment through either study specific clinical visits, home visits, or contact of study participants through phone, email, or other means. Examples of asymptomatic subclinical outcomes include results from imaging (e.g., white matter lesions in the brain measured by magnetic resonance imaging (MRI); vessel wall thickness of carotid arteries measured by b-mode ultrasound; microvascular narrowing measured by retinal photography; benign electrocardiographic abnormalities from electrocardiography (ECG); coronary calcium measured by computed tomography (CT) scans); biomarker measurements (e.g., serum lipoproteins, cardiac troponin levels); and standardized questionnaire assessments (e.g., cognitive function tests, assessments of diet and physical activity, activities of daily living, range of motion). Outcomes that involve measurement or administration of questionnaires or tests at an in-person study visit may not require adjudication. For instance, in the blood pressure example, the measured blood pressure is the outcome. Similarly, in the COMBINE trial, a participant's outcome was obtained from the structured drinking assessment (Anton et al. 2006). In such instances, procedures need to be in place to ensure good-quality data, such as appropriate training of study personnel, regular equipment checks, and quality control checks, but there is no adjudication of the outcomes themselves.

Patient-Reported Outcomes (PROs)

Patient-centered or patient-reported outcomes are measures of patients' direct experiences of health conditions and health care (Weldring and Smith 2013). Patient-reported outcomes are directly reported by the patient without interpretation of the patient's response by a clinician or anyone else and pertain to the patient's health, quality of life, or functional status associated with health care or treatment. These outcomes may be measured in absolute terms, such as a patient's rating of the severity of pain, and new onset of nausea following administration of a new drug and may include functional status, health service satisfaction, and quality of life. Outcomes such as hospital readmissions may also be included as patient centered and can be measured using administrative claims database or self-report. In the COMBINE study of treatments for alcohol dependence, the co-primary outcomes of percent days abstinent during the 16-week treatment period and time to relapse to heavy drinking were determined from structured in-person interviews. Such interviews could potentially be conducted by telephone (though this was not done in COMBINE). In the Aging and Cognitive Health Evaluation in Elders (ACHIEVE) trial, the primary outcome is change in global cognitive function, which requires assessment at an in-person interview (Deal et al. 2018). A key secondary outcome includes a diagnosis of dementia. Many patient-reported outcome assessments such as dementia do not require an in-person interview. They can be done using a brief telephone interview with the participant or an informant or using hospital records and death certificates. An example of a randomized pragmatic clinical trial that used patient-reported outcomes as the primary study outcome is the Comprehensive Post-Acute Stroke Services (COMPASS) trial (Duncan et al. 2017). Patient-centered outcomes in COMPASS were collected from telephone surveys administered at 90-day post-hospital discharge. A centralized survey research calling center administered the phone interview. The primary outcome was patient-reported functional status as measured by the 16-item Stroke Impact Scale (SIS-16). The SIS-16 is a self-reported questionnaire that can be completed by the patient or a proxy and was selected because it is an outcome that matters to patients, their caregivers, and stroke experts. Interviewers were masked to treatment group and used standardized scripts and interviewing guidelines. COMPASS utilized reminder letters, additional phone contacts, mailed surveys, and proxy interviews to increase follow-up rates.

Time to Event

Time-to-event ("survival") methods are typically used to analyze outcomes from clinical trials. Participants who do not have the event of interest during the trial are censored in the analysis, either at the time they are lost to follow-up or administratively at a designated date for the end of follow-up, whichever is earlier. Censoring should be at the last time at which the participant was known to be free of the event, even if that was earlier than the administrative censoring date, because absence of information about an event does not automatically imply the participant did not have the event. Other outcomes such as heart failure can be thought of as clinical syndromes with a diffuse event onset time. Occurrence time may be defined as first onset of symptoms, which in the case of heart failure could be progressive over an extended period of time. Some trials may choose to define onset of these types of events as the time the condition requires hospitalization or the time it is diagnosed in the outpatient setting. In the case of heart failure, the actual condition may be been present for some time prior to this defined start date.

Models of Event Ascertainment and Classification

The goal of the event ascertainment and classification component of clinical trials is to completely identify all events and establish valid event classification for each. There are several models to identify and classify events. The best choice to employ depends partially on the type of events targeted by the trail and on the size and duration of the clinical trial. Operational structure and resources of the trial also influence the methods used. Models for accomplishing the goals of event ascertainment and classification can be grouped onto three types including centralized systems, decentralized systems, or a hybrid of these two models.

A centralized model is one that establishes special clinics where study participants return for asymptomatic subclinical outcome assessment through a clinic examination, biomarker measurement, and/or questionnaire evaluation. Clinical outcomes may also be determined at central special clinics but would most likely come to attention of other health-care providers within and outside the sphere of the clinical trial investigators. Even though events may be identified in hospitals and clinics outside of special centralized centers, medical records and diagnostic elements are often sent to centralized reading (e.g., electrocardiograms) and/or abstraction centers that employ specially trained medical record abstractors. Using centralized reading centers or review of diagnostic elements helps reduce variation in clinical practice fashions and increases standardization.

Decentralized outcome assessments are also common. Studies that employ a decentralized system rely on identifying and obtaining medical records from all facilities utilized by participants. These facilities could be anywhere around the world. A considerable effort is required to identify and to obtain complete sets of diagnostic information from the various medical systems. These decentralized systems may also incorporate home visits with participants in comparison with having participants return to one or more central specially created clinical sites. An example of this method in a major observations study is the REGARDS study (Howard et al. 2005). In this study of approximately 30,000 participants, mobile units were sent to the homes of participants to capture information on subclinical and patient-reported conditions. Clinical events were identified through participant self-report. Records for reported hospitalizations were then sought and abstracted centrally.

Outcome Event Identification

Outcome ascertainment systems in clinical trials strive for complete capture of the outcomes of interest. This often involves identification of a wide net of events from which outcomes of interest are further evaluated and classified. The type of approach depends on the type of outcomes (i.e., clinical, subclinical, patient-reported) that are of most interest to the study. Studies often apply highly sensitive selection criteria of potential events in order to ensure complete and comprehensive case ascertainment. Clinical trials use a variety of methods that can include participant self-report of potential events, searches of electronic medical records (EMRs) lists obtained from selected health-care facilities and clinics, utilization of wearable devices by participants (e.g., transdermal patch electrocardiographic (ECG) monitors permit extended noninvasive ambulatory monitoring for atrial fibrillation and other cardiac conditions (Heckbert et al. 2018)), and periodic participant examinations (e.g., sequential ECG evaluations to identify silent myocardial infarction).

An example of using participant self-report to obtain comprehensive ascertainment of outcomes in a large observational cohort studies is the Atherosclerosis Risk in Communities (ARIC) study (The ARIC investigators 1989). Briefly, study participants are contacted by phone twice annually to obtain self-reported hospitalizations for any reason. Medical records of all reported hospitalizations are sought. In addition to identifying potential events from patient self-report, electronic files of hospital discharges are obtained from hospitals in the regions from which the cohort was drawn. These files are searched using participants' information to identify hospitalizations for study participants. Approximately 10% of total study outcomes are identified from searching electronic files of discharges from selected hospitals that were not otherwise identified from participant self-report. The result of this case identification approach is a comprehensive list of hospitalized outcomes from which event classification and validation can proceed. In the Hispanic Community Health Study/Study of Latinos (HCHS/SOL), a similar approach is used but includes participant self-report of all visits to an emergency department not leading to hospitalization (Sorlie et al. 2010).

It is important that clinical trials established clear and detailed description of the outcome of interest. This is key to the rigor and reproducibility of findings in the context of other studies and patient populations. An example of this level of outcome description is the RIVUR (Randomized Intervention for Children with Vesicoureteral Reflux) trial, a double-mask placebo-controlled trial of antimicrobial prophylaxis; the primary outcome to evaluate treatment efficacy was recurrence of F/SUTI (febrile or symptomatic urinary tract infection (UTI) (RIVUR Trial Investigators et al. 2014). Suspected recurrent UTI events were reviewed and adjudicated to determine if they met the RIVUR criteria for a primary outcome. The definition of recurrent F/SUTI required the presence of fever or urinary tract symptoms, pyuria based on urinalysis, and culture-proven infection with a single organism. A UTI was defined as recurrent only if its onset occurred more than 2 weeks from the last day of appropriate treatment for the preceding UTI or following a negative urine culture or it was an infection with a new organism. The study had a UTI Classification Committee (UCC). All reported medical care visits required data collection using standardized study procedures, with data entered into the central data management system (DMS). Those visits where a potential UTI was identified were reviewed and classified by the UCC, using standardized criteria to adjudicate each event according to the study definitions. When an algorithm in the data management system identified a potential outcome, relevant data were sent to two randomly selected members of the UCC. Each of the two UCC members classified the event and entered their responses into the DMS. If the classifications by the two reviewers disagreed, the UCC met in person or by conference call to come to a final decision.

Obtaining Diagnostic Data Elements

Once possible outcome events are identified, clinical trials must have standardized approaches to obtain the relevant diagnostic information needed for event validation and classification. Traditional methods of manual abstraction by trained medical records abstractors have been widely used and are successful at reliable collection of diagnostic elements from medical records. More recent approaches employ natural language processing programs to capture information from EMR text fields on symptom presentation, disease course, and other relevant diagnosis elements (e.g., presence of cardiac chest pain, worsening of difficulty breathing). Electronic medical records can also be an efficient method to capture structured data elements (e.g., laboratory values, test results, medications) needed to validate and classify study outcomes. Although the capture of diagnostic elements from EMR relying solely on computer-based methods has great potential for efficiency, challenges remain in the area of interoperability across EMR platforms and establishing and maintaining acceptable sensitivity and specificity compared to traditional medical record review. Once highly reliable and valid data are obtained (either by electronic or manual approach), these data can then be used in computerized standard event classification algorithms. Hybrid approaches to diagnostic data capture are also used. Structured data elements captured from EMR combined with manual abstraction guided by natural language processing are an example of a hybrid data collection approach. Computer systems can be used to search text fields and locate and underscore location of key diagnostic information that can be confirmed by manual overread by trained study personnel.

Development of Data Capture Instruments

Studies typically develop online computer systems for reviewers to use in event classification. After decisions have been made about the information needed to be captured for event classification, case report forms need to be developed and programmed to be used for data entry by abstractors. These systems usually need to include not only fields for capturing specified data elements but also to allow inclusion of narrative sections of the medical record and uploading of images, such as MRIs and other components in electronic formats, such as ECGs. Once data entry for a participant is complete, an algorithm and/or clinician uses the information to decide the event type. When two clinicians or a clinician and the algorithm have reviewed an event, the system compares the reviews. If there are discrepancies, they are resolved either by mutual agreement or adjudication by an additional reviewer. The system needs to be able to incorporate such resolutions or adjudications and record the final decision as to the nature of the event (see section "Classification of Clinical Events").

Training in Data Capture

Standardized initial training and recurrent recertification of staff involved in outcome data capture are essential to maintain high-quality outcome ascertainment and validation. This is important for obtaining data about clinical events as well as when outcomes are derived from participant self-report using interview questionnaires.

Classification of Clinical Events

Once relevant diagnostic data elements captured for potential study outcomes are available, classification of events can proceed. Methods for determining final classification of study outcomes vary and include use of standardized computer algorithms, processing for review with outcome classification committees, and linkage with electronic data sources (e.g., clinical registries, administrative claims, mortality registries, and death indexes).

Computer diagnostic algorithms for determining final study events exist for many major clinical outcomes. For example, a widely used algorithm for classifying acute myocardial infarction utilized data on cardiac pain symptoms, biomarker evidence, and electrocardiographic evidence (Luepker et al. 2003). The results of this and similar algorithms are a spectrum of certainty of classification such as definite, probable, suspect, or no acute myocardial infarction. Input from additional reading of electrocardiograms can be incorporated to identify subclasses of myocardial infarction, namely, ST segment MI (STEMI) or non-ST segment elevation MI (NSTEMI). While widely used in trials, a limitation of these types of algorithms is that they are not specific enough to classify subcategories of events based on newer universal definitions of myocardial infarction (i.e., acute myocardial infarction subtype 1 through subtype 5 (Thygesen et al. 2018)). Clinical overread of diagnostic information is required to produce valid subtyping of these events.

Other major outcomes such as stroke, heart failure, and respiratory disease are less well suited for reliance on diagnostic algorithms and may require processing for final diagnostic classification with outcome review committees. Outcome review committees are commonly used by clinical trials to determine the final diagnostic classification of study outcomes. Methods used to establish and operate outcome review committees vary across studies. Some studies use a consensus model whereby all eligible cases are reviewed by all or a subset of committee member with one member being assigned as the primary reviewer. Under this model, the primary reviewer summarizes the case for the committee, and the case is discussed among all committee members in a conference or webinar. A consensus diagnosis is the result of this method. Another common model is the independent reviewer model with adjudication of disagreements between original reviews. Under this method, eligible cases are independently reviewed and classified by reviewers on the committee. Disagreement between reviews on the case classification is adjudicated by a third reviewer (often the chair of the committee) to create the final study classification. Each reviewer selects a classification by following reviewer guidelines and case law. The reviewer guidelines and case law should be periodically reviewed by members of the committee and modified as needed in order to be consistent both within the committee and with contemporary clinical guidelines. For clinical trials, it is important that possible reviewers should be masked to treatment arm when completing their classification of cases.

Annual recertification of review committee members is recommended. For annual recertification training, all reviewers independently classify a set of selected cases and then review each response in a group setting, seeking clarification from the established guidelines and making new case law as needed. Retention of reviewers is important to help maintained high levels of quality control in the outcome classification process. Methods to ensure retention of committee members include financial compensation on a per case basis or percent effort and/or involvement of review committee members in the development of publications and other scholarly products from the study. Another important aspect of maintaining high-quality outcome assessment in studies using case review committees is the use of online systems to record reviewers' classification and ongoing quality control reporting. In the setting where two reviewers classify each event, with a third reviewer adjudicating disagreements, quality control reports would typically provide information about how frequently reviewers disagree and, when there is adjudication, how frequently the adjudicator agrees with each of the two initial reviewers. The use of online, web-based data systems is important in managing the work of these committee and to keep outcome classification on preestablished timelines. An online event reviewer data collection system with real-time data checks and helps menus that allow reviewers remote access to view standardized summaries of diagnostic data elements, imaging, physicians' notes, procedure notes, and medication lists while they are completing an event classification review form helpful to ensure high-quality data on outcome classification as well as successful management of a review committee.

Ethics

Clinical trials usually require all participants to provide informed consent at the time of entry into the study. There are some types of trials for which a waiver of consent may be granted, such as a trial of a new method of CPR for treating out-of-hospital cardiac arrest (Aufderheide et al. 2011). If medical records are needed for outcome identification and classification, participants also need to sign an agreement allowing their medical records to be obtained from physicians and hospitals.

Administrative Oversight of Outcome Ascertainment

Administrative staff are usually required to manage the outcome ascertainment process. Although many aspects may be automated, an administrator is often responsible for assigning events to reviewers, based on information about their workload and for following up when reviewers are overdue completing their assigned cases. Experienced reviewers are typically busy clinicians who have to fit reviewing into hectic schedules, so having an administrator keeping track of progress is critical for timely classification of events.

Conclusion

Accurate ascertainment of study outcomes is a critical component of a clinical trial. Outcomes need to be defined unambiguously and procedures put in place to maximize completeness and accuracy of outcome classification.

Key Facts

- Complete and accurate outcome ascertainment and classification are important for making valid conclusions from clinical trials.
- Methods for identifying and classifying outcomes vary depending on the aims of the trial and nature of the outcomes of interest.
- Design of clinical trials needs to consider models for event identification, methods to capture relevant diagnostic data, utilization of standardized diagnostic algorithms and/or clinical review committees, and mechanisms for maintaining data quality.

References

Anton RF, O'Malley SS, Ciraulo DA, Cisler RA, Couper D, Donovan DM, Gastfriend DR, Hosking JD, Johnson BA, LoCastro JS, Longabaugh R, Mason BJ, Mattson ME, Miller WR, Pettinati HM, Randall CL, Swift R, Weiss RD, Williams LD, Zweben A (2006) COMBINE Study Research Group. Combined pharmacotherapies and behavioral interventions for alcohol dependence: the COMBINE study: a randomized controlled trial. JAMA 295(17):2003–2017

Aufderheide TP, Frascone RJ, Wayne MA, Mahoney BD, Swor RA, Domeier RM, Olinger ML, Holcomb RG, Tupper DE, Yannopoulos D, Lurie KG (2011) Standard cardiopulmonary resuscitation versus active compression-decompression cardiopulmonary resuscitation with augmentation of negative intrathoracic pressure for out-of-hospital cardiac arrest: a randomized trial. Lancet 377(9762):301–311

Deal JA, Goman AM, Albert MS, Arnold ML, Burgard S, Chisolm T, Couper D, Glynn NW, Gmelin T, Hayden KM, Mosley T, Pankow JS, Reed N, Sanchez VA, Richey Sharrett A, Thomas SD, Coresh J, Lin FR (2018) Hearing treatment for reducing cognitive decline: design and methods of the Aging and Cognitive Health Evaluation in Elders randomized controlled trial. Alzheimers Dement (N Y) 4:499–507. ClinicalTrials.gov entry NCT03243422

Duncan PW, Bushnell CD, Rosamond WD, Jones Berkeley SB, Gesell SB, D'Agostino RB Jr, Ambrosius WT, Barton-Percival B, Bettger JP, Coleman SW, Cummings DM, Freburger JK, Halladay J, Johnson AM, Kucharska-Newton AM, Lundy-Lamm G, Lutz BJ, Mettam LH, Pastva AM, Sissine ME, Vetter B (2017) The Comprehensive Post Stroke Services (COMPASS) study: design and methods of a cluster randomized pragmatic trial. BMC Neurol 17(1):133

Fine JP, Gray RJ (1999) A proportional hazards model for the subdistribution of a competing risk. J Am Stat Assoc 94:496–509

Heckbert SR, Austin TR, Jensen PN, Floyd JS, Psaty BM, Soliman EZ, Kronmal RA (2018) Yield and consistency of arrhythmia detection with patch electrocardiographic monitoring: the multi-ethnic study of atherosclerosis. J Electrocardiol 51(6):997–1002

Howard V, Cushman M, Pulley L, Gomez C, Go R, Prineas R, Graham A, Moy C, Howard G (2005) The reasons for geographic and racial differences in stroke study: objectives and design. Neuroepidemiology 25:135–143

Luepker RV, Apple FS, Christenson RH, Crow RS, Fortmann SP, Goff D, Goldberg RJ, Hand MM, Jaffe AS, Julian DG, Levy D, Manolio T, Mendis S, Mensah G, Pajak A, Prineas RJ, Reddy KS, Roger VL, Rosamond WD, Shahar E, Sharrett AR, Sorlie P, Tunstall-Pedoe H, AHA Council on Epidemiology and Prevention; AHA Statistics Committee; World Heart Federation Council on Epidemiology and Prevention; European Society of Cardiology Working Group on Epidemiology and Prevention; Centers for Disease Control and Prevention; National Heart, Lung, and Blood Institute (2003) Case definitions for acute coronary heart disease in epidemiology and clinical research studies: a statement from the AHA Council on Epidemiology and Prevention; AHA Statistics Committee; World Heart Federation Council on Epidemiology and Prevention; the European Society of Cardiology Working Group on Epidemiology and Prevention; Centers for Disease Control and Prevention; and the National Heart, Lung, and Blood Institute. Circulation 108(20):2543–2549

RIVUR Trial Investigators, Hoberman A, Greenfield SP, Mattoo TK, Keren R, Mathews R, Pohl HG, Kropp BP, Skoog SJ, Nelson CP, Moxey-Mims M, Chesney RW, Carpenter MA (2014) Antimicrobial prophylaxis for children with vesicoureteral reflux. N Engl J Med 370(25):2367–2376

Sorlie PD, Avilés-Santa LM, Wassertheil-Smoller S, Kaplan RC, Daviglus ML, Giachello AL, Schneiderman N, Raij L, Talavera G, Allison M, Lavange L, Chambless LE, Heiss G (2010) Design and implementation of the Hispanic Community Health Study/Study of Latinos. Ann Epidemiol 20:629–641

The ARIC investigators (1989) The atherosclerosis risk in communities (ARIC) study: design and objectives. Am J Epidemiol 129:687–702

Thygesen K, Alpert JS, Jaffe AS, Chaitman BR, Bax JJ, Morrow DA, White HD, Executive Group on behalf of the Joint European Society of Cardiology (ESC)/American College of Cardiology (ACC)/American Heart Association (AHA)/World Heart Federation (WHF) Task Force for the Universal Definition of Myocardial Infarction (2018) Fourth universal definition of myocardial infarction (2018). J Am Coll Cardiol 72(18):2231–2264

Weldring T, Smith S (2013) Patient-reported outcomes (pROs) and patient-reported outcome measures (pROMs). Health Serv Insights 6:61–68

Bias Control in Randomized Controlled Clinical Trials

48

Diane Uschner and William F. Rosenberger

Contents

Abstract

In clinical trials, randomization is used to allocate patients to treatment groups, because this design technique tends to produce comparability across treatment groups. However, even randomized clinical trials are still susceptible to bias. Bias is a systematic distortion of the treatment effect estimate. This chapter introduces two types of bias that may occur in clinical trials, selection

D. Uschner
Department of Statistics, George Mason University, Fairfax, VA, USA
e-mail: duschner@bsc.gwu.edu

W. F. Rosenberger (✉)
Biostatistics Center, The George Washington University, Rockville, MD, USA
e-mail: wrosenbe@gmu.edu

© Springer Nature Switzerland AG 2022

S. Piantadosi, C. L. Meinert (eds.), *Principles and Practice of Clinical Trials*,
https://doi.org/10.1007/978-3-319-52636-2_219

bias and chronological bias. Selection bias may arise from predictability of the randomization sequence, and different models for predictability are presented. Chronological bias occurs due to unobserved time trends that influence patients' responses, and its effect on the rejection rate of parametric hypothesis tests for the treatment effect will be revealed. It will be seen that different randomization procedures differ in their susceptibility to bias. A method to reduce bias at the design stage of the trial and robust testing strategies to adjust for bias at the analysis stage are presented to help to mitigate the potential for bias in randomized controlled clinical trials.

Keywords

Selection bias · Chronological bias · Restricted randomization · Type I error · Power

Introduction

Clinical trials aim at comparing the efficacy and safety of therapeutic agents across treatment groups. It is crucial that the groups are comparable with respect to the demographic features and other prognostic variables. In practice, it is not possible to create comparability deterministically across the groups, particularly, as some underlying prognostic variables, such as pharmacological properties, may still be unknown.

Randomization tends to balance groups with respect to known and unknown covariates and is therefore commonly regarded as the key component of clinical trials that provides comparability of treatment groups (Armitage 1982). In addition, randomized treatment allocation allows the effective concealment of treatments from patients and investigators. When the treatment assignment is deterministic, the concealment of allocations is inherently difficult. Allocation concealment is often referred to as double-blinding, while a loss of concealment is called unblinding. Double-blinding is important, if possible, to achieve an unbiased assessment of the outcomes of the trial.

Despite the favorable properties of randomization, a randomized clinical trial can still suffer from a lack of comparability among the treatment groups. Biases may arise from different sources. For example, long recruitment times, changes in study personal, or learning curves during surgical procedures may cause time trends that affect the outcomes of patients in the trial. It is intuitively clear that time trends will lead to a bias of the treatment effect, when patients that arrive early in the allocation process are allocated to one group and those that arrive later are allocated to the other group. This bias has been termed chronological bias (Matts and McHugh 1978). Randomizing patients in blocks has been recommended as a means to create more similar groups in the course of the trial (ICH 1998). However, blocking introduces predictability of the upcoming treatment assignments. In particular, the pharmacological effects or the side effects of an intervention may be easily distinguishable from those of a standard or placebo intervention. These effects will cause unblinding of the past treatment allocations and may in turn make future allocations more predictable. Predictability can introduce selection bias (Rosenberger and Lachin 2015), a bias caused by a systematic covariate imbalance of the treatment groups.

Several randomization procedures have been developed in the literature to mitigate the effects of chronological bias and selection bias. Each randomization procedure represents a trade-off between balance and randomness, while greater balance leads to higher predictability, and greater randomness leads to more susceptibility to time trends. The extreme of complete randomness is the toss of the fair coin, also called complete randomization or unrestricted randomization. The other extreme is small blocks of two, where after a random allocation to one group, the next patient will be deterministically allocated to the other group. When the allocation of a patient depends on the treatment assignments of the previous patients, a randomization procedure is called restricted. Section "Restricted Randomization in Clinical Trials" reviews restricted randomization procedures that are used to mitigate bias in randomized trials.

Section "Covariate Imbalances and Predictability" shows how predictability and covariate imbalances can be measured in clinical trials. Chronological bias is the focus of section "Chronological Bias." Section "Planning for Bias at the Design Stage" presents an approach to minimize the susceptibility to bias at the design stage. Section "Robust Hypothesis Tests" introduces hypothesis tests that are robust to bias. The chapter closes with a Summary in section "Summary and Conclusions."

Restricted Randomization in Clinical Trials

Consider a randomized clinical trial with an experimental agent E and a control agent C. Patients enter the trial sequentially and are allocated randomly into one of the two groups. When the groups are expected to be balanced in the end of the trial, the random allocation can be achieved by the toss of a fair coin, and a patient will be allocated to the experimental group when the coin shows head and to the control group when the coin shows tails. Let an even $n \in \mathbb{Z}_{>0}$ be the total sample size of the trial. Then the allocation of patient i for $i \in \{1, \ldots, n\}$ is denoted by

$$t_i = \begin{cases} 1 & \text{if patient } i \text{ is allocated to group } E \\ 0 & \text{if patient } i \text{ is allocated to group } C. \end{cases}$$

The allocation t_i of patient i is the realization of a Bernoulli random variable $T_i \sim$ Bern (0.5). The sequence $\mathbf{T} = (T_1, \ldots, T_n)$ with realization $\mathbf{t} = (t_1, \ldots, t_n)$ is called randomization sequence. The set of all randomization sequences with total sample size n is given by $\Omega_n = \{0, 1\}^n$.

The sample size in group E after the allocation of patient i is denoted by $N_E(i) = \sum_{j=1}^{i} t_i$ and in group C by $N_C(i) = i - N_E(i)$. The imbalance after patient i is defined as the difference in group sizes after the allocation of patient i and is given by

$$D_i = N_E(i) = N_C(i) = \sum_{j=1}^{i} 2 \cdot t_j - i.$$

The imbalance D_i is a random variable that describes a random walk (i, D_i) for $i \in 1, \ldots, N$. Figure 1 shows a realization of the random walk in heavy black and all the possible realizations in light gray.

There is a one-to-one correspondence between the set of randomization sequences and realizations of the random walk. Each random walk corresponds to a randomization sequence, and each randomization sequences describes a unique random walk. Using a fair coin toss, each randomization sequence has the same probability

$$P(\mathbf{T} = \mathrm{t}) = \frac{1}{|\Omega_n|} = \frac{1}{2^n},$$

where $|\Omega_n|$ is the cardinality of the set Ω_n. In other words, for each patient i, the random walk has the same probability to go either up or down. As there are no restrictions to the randomization process, this randomization procedure is usually called unrestricted randomization or complete randomization. In particular, complete randomization only maintains the allocation ratio in expectation but may result in high imbalances in the course of the trial, as well as in the end of the trial. As Fig. 1 shows, complete randomization (CR) allows imbalances as high as n.

Several randomization procedures have been proposed to achieve better balance in the clinical trial. A randomization procedure is a (discrete) probability distribution on the set of randomization sequences. Randomization procedures other than the uniform distribution are called restricted randomization procedures.

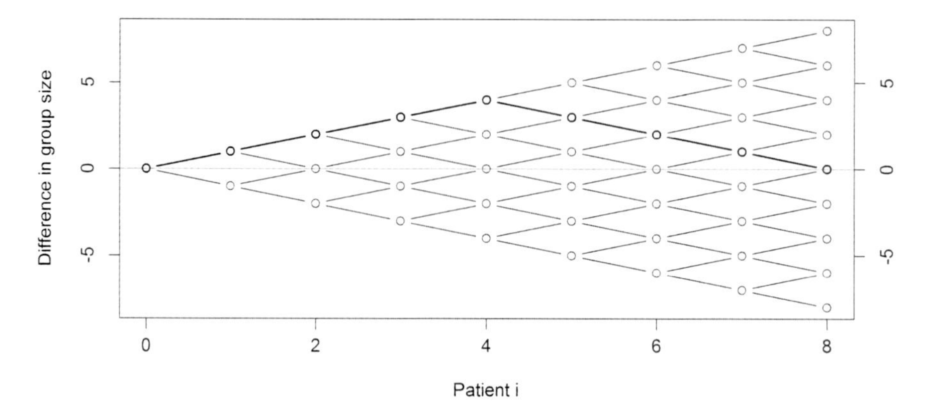

Fig. 1 Random walk of the randomization sequence $\mathbf{t} = (1, 1, 1, 1, 0, 0, 0, 0)$, figure generated using the randomizeR package (Uschner et al. 2018b)

The most commonly used randomization procedures are random allocation rule (RAR) and permuted block randomization (PBR). Random allocation rule forces randomization sequences to be balanced in the end of the trial by giving zero weight to unbalanced sequences and equal probability to balanced sequences. As there are $\binom{n}{n/2}$ sequences, the probability of a sequence $\mathbf{t}$ is

$$P(\mathbf{T}=\mathbf{t}) = \begin{cases} \binom{n}{n/2}^{-1} & \text{if } D_n(t)=0 \\ 0 & \text{otherwise.} \end{cases}$$

Permuted block randomization forces balance not only at the end of a trial but at M points in the trial. The interval between two consecutive balanced points in the trial is called a block. Let every block contain $m = n/M$ patients, where M and m are positive integers, and let $b = m/2$ be the number of patients allocated to E and C in each block. Using PBR, the probability of a sequence is

$$P(\mathbf{T}=\mathbf{t}) = \begin{cases} \binom{2b}{b}^{n/2b} & \text{if } D_{j\cdot k}(t)=0 \text{ for } j=1,\ldots,M \\ 0 & \text{else.} \end{cases}$$

A different way to achieve balance was suggested by Berger et al. (2003). They promote the maximal procedure (MP), a randomization procedure that achieves final balance and does not exceed a maximum tolerated imbalance $b = \max_i |D_i|$. All remaining sequences $\Omega_{n,MP}$ are realized with equal probability.

$$P(\mathbf{T}=\mathbf{t}) = \begin{cases} \frac{1}{|\Omega_{n,MP}|} & \text{if } \max_i |D_i(t)| \leq b \text{ and } D_n=0 \\ 0 & \text{else.} \end{cases}$$

Figure 2 illustrates the set of sequences. The cardinality of the set of sequences of $\Omega_{n,MP}$ depends on n and the imbalance boundary b. There is no closed form, and the generation of the randomization sequences requires an ingenious algorithm proposed by Salama et al. (2008) and implemented in Uschner et al. (2018b).

Another approach that does not force balance in the end of the trial is Efron's biased coin design (EBCD). Here, the probability of the next treatment assignment is based on the current imbalance of the random walk. Let $\frac{1}{2} < p \leq 1$. Then the probability to assign the next patient to group E is given by

$$P(T_{i+1}=1|T_1,\ldots,T_{i-1}) = \begin{cases} p & \text{if } D_i<0 \\ \frac{1}{2} & \text{if } D_i=0 \\ 1-p & \text{if } D_i>0. \end{cases}$$

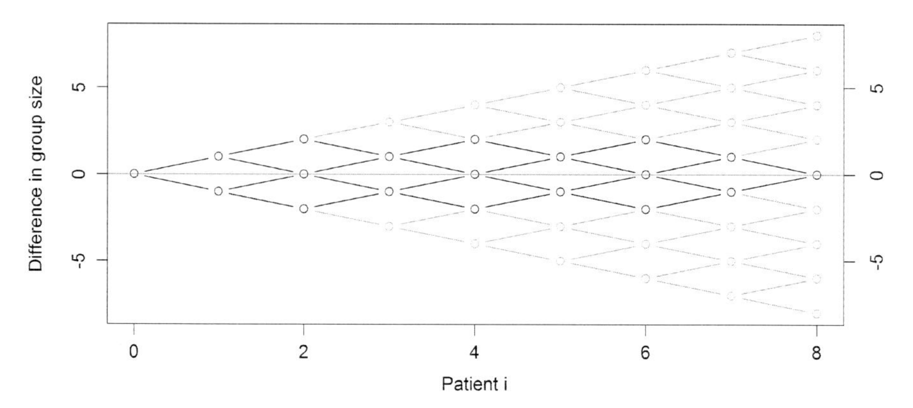

Fig. 2 Set of sequences of the maximal procedure for sample size $n = 8$ with imbalance tolerance $b = 2$, figure generated using the randomizeR package (Uschner et al. 2018b)

The set of all sequences of EBCD is Ω_n, but the probability distribution is different. Sequences with high imbalances have a lower probability. In other words, the probability mass is concentrated about the center of the random walk.

Chen's design and its special case the big stick design (BSD) were developed to avoid the high imbalances still possible in EBCD. Here, an imbalance boundary b is introduced for the random walk, and a deterministic allocation is made to the other treatment group once the random walk attains the imbalance boundary on one side of the random walk. Using Chen's design, the probability to allocate the next patient in group E is

$$P(T_{i+1} = 1|T_1, \ldots, T_{i-1}) = \begin{cases} 1 & \text{if } -b = D_i \\ p & \text{if } -b < D_i < 0 \\ \frac{1}{2} & \text{if } D_i = 0 \\ 1-p & \text{if } 0 < D_i < b \\ 0 & \text{if } D_i = b. \end{cases}$$

The special (and more common) case of the big stick design results if $p = \frac{1}{2}$.

Note that despite the similar set of sequences of the big stick design and the maximal procedure, their probability distributions are very different. Maximal procedure gives equal probability to all sequences. The big stick design, however, introduces deterministic allocations (i.e., allocations with probability one) every time the imbalance boundary is hit. As a consequence, sequences that run along the imbalance boundary have higher probability than those in the middle of the allocation tunnel.

Covariate Imbalances and Predictability

A principal goal of randomization in clinical trials is to produce treatment groups that are comparable with respect to known and unknown prognostic variables. Therefore, randomization is the basis of a meaningful and unbiased comparison of the primary outcome between the treatment groups and allows conclusions about the treatment effect. At the same time, randomization allows the implementation of masking and allocation concealment. A systematic covariate imbalance of the treatment groups is called selection bias. Berger (2005) distinguishes three types of selection bias. First-order selection bias is defined as the bias that results in a non-randomized trial, when the allocation sequence is not generated in advance, and treatments can be assigned based on the patients' and physicians' preferences. The bias that results in a randomized controlled trial that does not use allocation concealment to mask allocations from patients and physicians is called second-order selection bias. Bias that results from predictability of the randomization sequence due to unsuccessful allocation concealment of past treatment assignments in combination with a known target allocation ratio has been termed third-order selection bias (Berger 2005). Third-order selection bias may occur when past treatment assignments are unmasked due to side effects or when the nature of the treatment makes masking of past allocation unfeasible, e.g., in a surgical procedure. While first- and second-order selection bias can be alleviated by a more careful study design, third-order selection bias is harder to mitigate. Intuitively, the more restrictions a randomization procedure induces, the higher the potential for predictability. This section reviews the formal measures of predictability that have been introduced in the literature.

Correct Guesses

The first to propose a measure of selection bias were Blackwell and Hodges (1957). Under the assumption that the investigator knows the target allocation ratio as well as past treatment assignments, they investigate the influence of an investigator who consciously seeks to make one treatment appear better than the other irrespective of the presence of a treatment effect. Assuming that the investigator favors the experimental treatment, he might include a patient with better expected response in the trial when he expects the experimental treatment to be allocated next. Conversely, he would include a patient with worse expected response, when he expects the next treatment assignment to be to the control group. Blackwell and Hodges propose two models for the guess of the investigator. The first model, coined the convergence strategy (CS), assumes that the investigator guesses the treatment that has so far been allocated less. Let $g_{CS}(i, t)$ denote the guess for allocation i using the convergence strategy, and let $R \sim \text{Ber}(0.5)$ be a Bernoulli random variable. Using the convergence strategy, the investigator's guess for the ith allocation is given by

$$g_{\mathrm{CS}}(i,t)=\begin{cases}1 & N_E(i-1,t)<N_C(i-1,t)\\ 0 & N_E(i-1,t)>N_C(i-1,t)\\ R & N_E(i-1,t)=N_C(i-1,t),\end{cases}$$

where a value of 1 corresponds to the experimental treatment, and a value of 0 corresponds to the control treatment. The second model is termed divergence strategy (DS). Here the investigator will guess the treatment which has so far been allocated less frequently. The investigator's guess for the ith allocation is thus given by

$$g_{\mathrm{DS}}(i,t)=\begin{cases}1 & N_E(i-1,t)>N_C(i-1,t)\\ 0 & N_E(i-1,t)<N_C(i-1,t)\\ R & N_E(i-1,t)=N_C(i-1,t).\end{cases}$$

A correct guess is the event that the investigator guesses the treatment that will in fact be allocated next, i.e., $g(i, t) = t_i$ for $g \in \{g_{\mathrm{CS}}, g_{\mathrm{DS}}\}$. The number of correct guesses of a randomization sequence is then defined as

$$G(t)=\sum_{i=1}^{n} I(g(i,t)=t_i).$$

With this notation, the expected number of correct guesses $E(G)$ is given by

$$E(G)=\sum_{t\in\Omega_n} P(T=t)\cdot G(t),$$

where $P(T = t)$ is the sequence probability as induced by the randomization procedure.

It is intuitively clear that the convergence strategy induces a correct guess each step the random walk reduces its imbalance. The divergence strategy induces a correct guess each time the imbalance is increased. In addition, every time the random walk is balanced, a correct guess is made with probability $p = \frac{1}{2}$.

Conditional Allocation Probability

Rosenberger and Lachin (2015) recently proposed a metric that is equivalent to the expected number of correct guesses but does not rely on the guessing model. They propose to investigate the expected difference between the conditional and the unconditional allocation probability. In a clinical trial with target allocation ratio $\frac{1}{2}$, each patient has the probability $\frac{1}{2}$ to be allocated to either of the treatment groups. In other words, for each position $i \in \{1, \ldots, n\}$, the random walk has the same overall probability to go up or down.

Denote the probability to receive the experimental treatment by p, and denote the conditional probability to receive the experimental treatment, given the past treatment assignments by $\phi_i = P(T_i = 1 \mid T_1, \ldots, T_{i-1})$. Then predictability of a sequence t is given by

$$\rho_{\text{PRED}}(t) = \sum_{i=1}^{n} (\phi_i(t) - p)^2.$$

Clearly, if the allocation is completely random, $\rho_{\text{PRED}}(t) = 0$. When each allocation is deterministic (which technically is not a randomized design anymore), $\rho_{\text{PRED}}(t)$ is maximized and takes the value $\rho_{\text{PRED}}(t) = n \cdot (1 - p)^2$. The predictability of a randomization procedure is again given by the weighted mean of the sequence predictability, namely,

$$\rho_{\text{PRED}} = \sum_{t \in \Omega_n} P(T = t) \cdot \rho_{\text{PRED}}(t).$$

It turns out that ρ_{PRED} is mathematically equivalent to the expected number of correct guesses minus the target allocation p, as shown by Rosenberger and Lachin (2015).

Type I Error Probability and Power

Proschan (1994) was the first to propose and investigate the influence of the convergence strategy on the type I error rate of a hypothesis test of the treatment effect. Let the primary outcome Y follow a normal distribution $Y \sim \mathcal{N}(\mu_E \cdot T + \mu_C \cdot (1 - T), \sigma^2)$. If the variance σ is known, the null hypothesis H_0: $\mu_E = \mu_C$ can be tested using a Z-test, and, under the assumption of independent and identically distributed responses, the test statistic $D = \frac{\overline{Y}_E - \overline{Y}_C}{\sqrt{2\sigma}}$ follows a standard normal distribution.

Assume that a higher outcome Y can be regarded as better and that the investigator favors the experimental group, although the null hypothesis is true, i.e., $\mu = \mu_E = \mu_C$. Then the influence of the convergence strategy on the responses can be modeled as follows:

$$E(Y_i) = \begin{cases} \mu + \eta & N_E(i-1,t) > N_C(i-1,t) \\ \mu - \eta & N_E(i-1,t) < N_C(i-1,t) \\ \mu & N_E(i-1,t) = N_C(i-1,t), \end{cases}$$

where $\eta > 0$ denotes the selection effect, the extent of bias introduced by the investigator. It is assumed that $\eta > 0$ to account for the fact that the treatment E is preferred and higher outcomes are regarded as better.

Under this assumption, the responses $Y_1, \ldots, Y_n$ are not identically distributed anymore but are still independent. Proschan gave an asymptotic formula for the type I error probability when random allocation rule is used and investigates the rejection rate in simulations for various values of n and η. It turns out that the rejection probability exceeds the planned significance level even for small values of η.

Kennes et al. (2011) extended the approach of Proschan to permuted block randomization. As expected, the type I error inflation increases with smaller block sizes. Ivanova et al. (2005) adapted the approach for binary outcomes and introduced a guessing threshold to reflect a possibly conservative investigator. The influence of various guessing thresholds was also investigated by Tamm and Hilgers (2014), who further generalized the approach to investigate the influence of predictability on the t test. Rückbeil et al. (2017) investigated the impact of selection bias on time-to-event outcomes.

Langer (2014) gave an exact formula for the rejection rate of the t test conditional on the randomization sequence, when the convergence strategy is used. The approach was published in Hilgers et al. (2017) and implemented in the randomizeR R package in Uschner et al. (2018b). The rejection probability conditional on the randomization sequence $\mathbf{t}$ is given by

$$
\begin{aligned}
r(\mathbf{t}) &= P\left(|S| > t_{n-2}\left(1 - \frac{\alpha}{2}\right)|\mathbf{t}\right) \\
&= F\left(t_{n-2}\left(\frac{\alpha}{2}\right), n-2, \delta, \lambda\right) + F\left(t_{n-2}\left(\frac{\alpha}{2}\right), n-2, -\delta, \lambda\right),
\end{aligned}
$$

where S is the test statistic of the t-test, $t_{n-2}(\gamma)$ is the γ-quantile of the t-distribution with $n - 2$ degrees of freedom, and $F(\cdot, n - 2, \delta, \lambda)$ is the distribution function of the doubly noncentral t-distribution with $n - 2$ degrees of freedom and non-centrality parameters δ, λ that both depend on the randomization sequence $\mathbf{t}$. Figure 3 shows the distribution of the type I error probability for the maximal procedure and the big stick design, both with imbalance tolerance $b = 2$, and for the random allocation rule. All are based on the total sample size $n = 20$ and normally distributed outcomes with group means $\mu_E = \mu_C = 2$ and equal variance $\sigma^2 = 1$.

Notably, all randomization procedures contain sequences with rejection probabilities as high as 100%. These are the alternating sequences. The big stick design has most sequences concentrated around the 5% significance level. The random allocation rule is similar to the big stick design but introduces more variability. The maximal procedure, despite having a similar set of sequences as the big stick design, has a higher probability for sequences that exceed the significance level substantially.

Multi-arm Trials (Generalizations)

The approach to assess susceptibility based on the rejection probability (see section "Type I Error Probability and Power") was generalized to multi-arm trials by

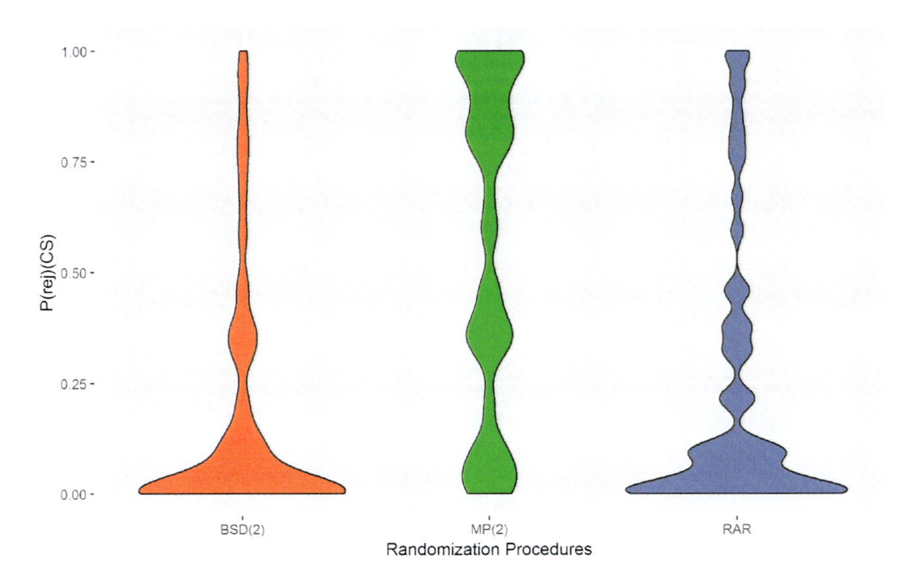

Fig. 3 Distribution of the type I error probability under the convergence strategy with $\eta = 4$ for three randomization procedures, figure generated using the randomizeR package (Uschner et al. 2018b)

Uschner et al. (2018a). They proposed models for selection bias in multi-arm trials that generalize the convergent guessing strategy of Blackwell and Hodges (1957); see section "Correct Guesses." Let $K \geq 2$ denote the number of treatment groups, and assume that a randomization procedure with equal allocation ratio is used for the allocation of patients to the K groups. In the two-arm case, it is assumed that the investigator favors one treatment over the other. In the multi-arm case ($K > 2$), it is assumed that the investigator favors a subset of the K treatment groups and dislikes the rest. Similarly to the two-arm case, it is assumed that the investigator would like to make his favored groups appear better than the disliked groups, despite the null hypothesis H_0: $\mu_1 = \ldots = \mu_K$ being true. Under this assumption, the investigator would thus try to include a patient with better expected response when he guesses that one of his favored groups will be allocated next. Let $\mathcal{F} \subset \{1, \ldots, K\}$ denote the subset of favored treatment groups, and let the complement $\mathcal{F}^C = \{1, \ldots, K\} \setminus \mathcal{F}$ denote the treatment groups that are not favored by the investigator. A reasonable strategy for the investigator would be to guess that one of his favored groups will be allocated next, when *all* of the groups in $\mathcal{F}$ have fewer patients than the remaining groups. Under this assumption, the expected response is given by

$$E(\mathbf{Y}) = \mu + \eta \cdot \mathbf{b},$$

and the components of the bias vector **b** are

$$b_i \begin{cases} 1 & \text{if } \max_{j \in \mathcal{F}} N_j(i-1) < \min_{k \in \mathcal{F}^C} N_k(i-1) \\ -1 & \text{if } \min_{j \in \mathcal{F}} N_j(i-1) > \max_{k \in \mathcal{F}^C} N_k(i-1) \\ 0 & \text{else.} \end{cases}$$

As the responses are no longer identically distributed under the null hypothesis, the F-test of the hypothesis H_0: $\mu_1 = \ldots = \mu_K$, S_F no longer follows a central F-distribution. However, conditional on the realized randomization sequence, S_F follows a doubly noncentral F distribution with degrees of freedom that depends on the bias vector.

Ryeznik and Sverdlov (2018) propose to investigate selection bias in multi-arm groups based on the forcing index (FI) that measures the difference between the conditional allocation probability and the target allocation probability of the randomization procedure. Their approach extends the approach of Rosenberger and Lachin (2015) (see section "Conditional Allocation Probability"). In a trial with K treatment groups, write $T_i = j$ if patient i is allocated to group j, $i = 1, \ldots, n$, $j = 1, \ldots, K$. Then $\phi_{i,j} = P(T_i = j \mid T_1, \ldots, T_{i-1})$ denotes the conditional probability that patient i will be allocated to treatment j, similarly as in section "Conditional Allocation Probability." The Euclidean distance between the vector of conditional allocation probabilities $\phi_i = (\phi_{i,1}, \ldots, \phi_{i,K})$ of patient i and the vector of target allocation probabilities $p = (p_1, \ldots, p_K)$ is defined as the forcing index of patient i,

$$FI_i = \sqrt{\sum_{j=1}^{K} \left(\phi_{i,j} - p_j\right)^2}.$$

The forcing index for the randomization sequence is then given by $FI = \frac{1}{n}\sum_{i=1}^{n} FI_i$. Clearly, the closer the conditional allocation to the target allocation, the more random a randomization sequence can be considered. Therefore, a low forcing index is desirable to reduce predictability.

Chronological Bias

Chronological bias arises when the treatment effect is distorted due to a time trend that affects the patients' responses, i.e., when later observations tend to be systematically higher or lower than previous observations. According to Matts and McHugh (1978), who coined the term chronological bias, clinical trials with a long recruitment phase are particularly prone to suffer from the hidden effects of time. The idea of investigating the effect of an unobserved covariate, such as time, on the estimation of the treatment effect is due to Efron (1971), who termed the resulting systematic distortion of the treatment effect in a linear model accidental bias.

The susceptibility of a randomization procedure to chronological bias may be measured by the degree of balance it yields (Atkinson 2014). In a trial with two treatment arms, a randomization sequence t is said to attain final balance, when the achieved allocation ratio in the end of the trial is equivalent to the target allocation ratio p,

$$N_E(n,t) = n \cdot p.$$

When the target allocation is $p = 0.5$, the maximum difference in group size yields a measure for imbalance throughout the trial,

$$MI = \max_{k=1,\ldots,n} D_k(t),$$

where the difference at time k is given by $D_k(t) = N_E(k, t) - N_C(k, t)$. A generalization of this approach to multiple treatment groups was presented by Ryeznik and Sverdlov (2018).

Impact on Type I Error Probability and Power

A more direct way of measuring the susceptibility of a randomization procedure to chronological bias is by estimating the effects of an unobserved trend on the rejection probability of a parametric test. In a two-arm clinical trial, if the primary outcome Y follows a normal distribution $Y \sim \mathcal{N}(\mu_E \cdot T + \mu_C \cdot (1 - T), \sigma^2)$, we can use a t-test to test the hypothesis H_0: $\mu_E = \mu_C$, assuming that the variance σ^2 is unknown.

In order to assess the effect of a time trend on the type I error rate of the t-test, Tamm and Hilgers (2014) assume that the responses are affected by a trend $\tau(i)$,

$$E(Y_i) = \mu_E \cdot T_i + \mu_C \cdot (1 - T_i) + \tau(i).$$

They propose three different shapes of trend: linear, logarithmic, and stepwise. Under linear time trend, the expected response of the patients increases evenly proportional to a factor θ with every patient included in the trial, until reaching θ after n patients. Linear time trend may occur as a result of gradually relaxing in- or exclusion criteria throughout the trial. The shift of patient i where $i = 1, \ldots, N$ is given by the formula

$$\tau(i) = \frac{i}{n} \cdot \theta.$$

Under logistic time trend, the expected response of the patients increases logistically with every patient included in the study, until reaching θ after n patients. Logistic time trend may occur as a result of a learning curve, i.e., in a surgical trial. Under logistic trend, the shift of patient i where $i = 1, \ldots, N$ is given by the formula

$$\tau(i) = \log\left(\frac{i}{n}\right) \cdot \theta.$$

Under a step trend, the expected response of the patients increases by theta after a given point n_0 in the allocation process. Step trend may occur if a new device is used after the point n_0 or if the medical personal changes at this point. Under a step trend, the shift of patient i where $i = 1, \ldots, N$ is given by the formula

$$\tau(i) = 1_{\{n_0 \leq i \leq n\}} \cdot \theta.$$

Rosenberger and Lachin (2015) present the results of a simulation study in which they investigate the average type I error rate and power of the t-test under a linear time trend for various designs. They find that the mean type I error rate of the designs does not suffer from chronological bias, but power can be deflated substantially. Moreover, more balanced designs lead to better control of power. Tamm and Hilgers (2014) investigate the permuted block design with various block sizes concerning it's susceptibility to chronological bias. They find that strong time trends can lead to a deflation of the type I error rate if large block sizes are used.

It is, however, not necessary to rely on simulation. As in the case of selection bias (see section "Type I Error Probability and Power"), the impact of chronological bias on the rejection probability of the t-test, conditional on the randomization sequence, can be calculated using the doubly noncentral t distribution. Figure 4 shows the exact distribution of the type I error probability under a linear time trend with $\theta = 1$ for the random allocation rule, the maximal procedure, and the big stick design latter two with maximum tolerated imbalance $b = 2$ for sample size $n = 20$.

For all three designs, the most randomization sequences yield a rejection probability that is below the nominal significance level of 5%. The variance of the

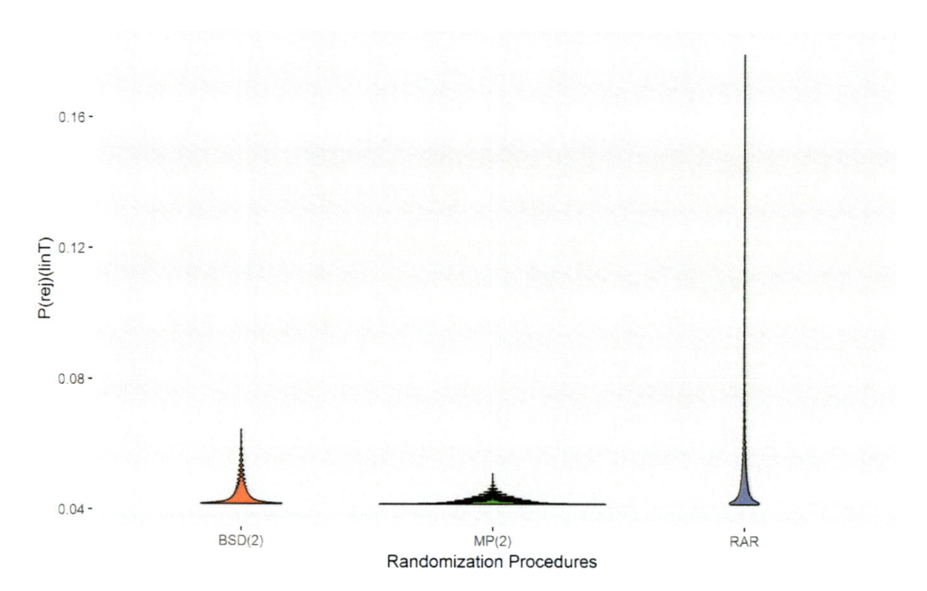

Fig. 4 Distribution of the type I error probability under a linear time trend, figure generated using the randomizeR package (Uschner et al. 2018b)

random allocation rule is higher as for the other designs. The big stick design seems to best attain the significance level.

Planning for Bias at the Design Stage

Hilgers et al. (2017) proposed a framework called ERDO (Evaluation of Randomization procedures for Design Optimization) for the choice of a randomization procedure at the design stage of a clinical trial. Based on the idea that bias that may occur during a trial can be anticipated from previous knowledge of similar trials, their approach consists of assessing a large number of randomization procedures with respect to the anticipated bias and choosing the randomization procedure that has been shown to be susceptible for the design of the new trial. The design is therefore optimal with respect to mitigating the anticipated bias. The assessment is facilitated by the R package randomizeR (Uschner et al. 2018b), which allows the assessment of a large number of restricted randomization procedures, particularly those presented in section "Restricted Randomization in Clinical Trials." In the first step, the objective of choosing an optimal randomization procedure for the study is stated, and prior information as given by previous studies is gathered. Then, the assumptions underlying the study are presented. Information from previous studies is used to estimate the shape of the time trend, its effect size θ, and the selection effect η. Also, the metric of assessment (e.g., mean type I error rate) is stated. Based on these assumptions, a comprehensive evaluation of various randomization procedures will be conducted. Finally, the randomization procedure that best mitigates the biases assumed in the assessment is chosen as the optimal randomization procedure for the study.

Robust Hypothesis Tests

An alternative approach of mitigating the influence of bias in a study is to adjust for bias in the analysis stage of a trial. For the case of normally distributed responses in a trial with two treatment arms and permuted block randomization where the responses are influenced by selection bias, Kennes et al. (2015) proposed to include the selection bias in a linear model in order to estimate the selection bias effect and to get an unbiased estimate of the treatment effect. They further propose asymptotic likelihood ratio test for the treatment effect, adjusted for bias, and for the selection effect. The adjusted test controls the type I error substantially better when the selection effect is medium to large, without losing much power.

Uschner et al. (2018a) employed a similar approach for multi-arm trials, investigating the effects of selection bias on the F-test and comparing several different block sizes. Figure 5 is a reprint of their Fig. 6 and shows the results of a simulation study based on the biasing policy for multi-arm groups that is outlined in section "Multi-arm Trials (Generalizations)." The selection effect η is assumed to be a fraction ρ of Cohen's effect size $f = f_{16,3} = 0.9829$ for 3 treatment arms with 16

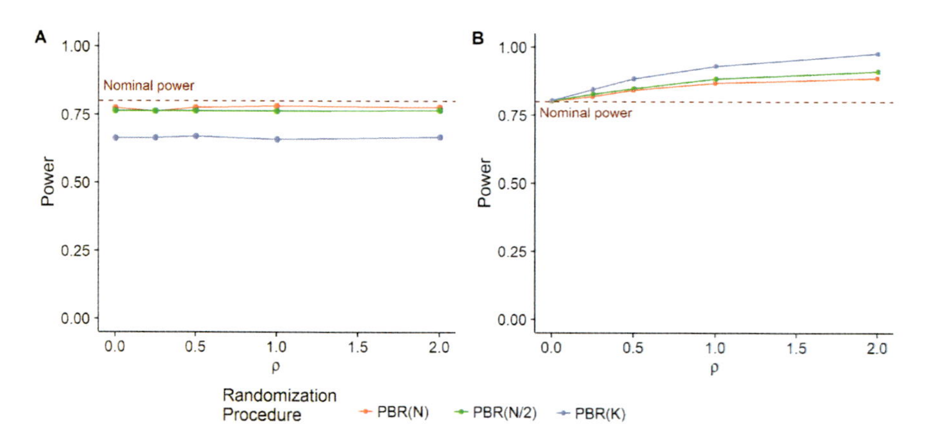

Fig. 5 Power of the F-test. Panel A, adjusted for selection bias; panel B, unadjusted for selection bias. Both panels assume total sample size $n = 48$, $K = 3$ treatment groups, and selection effect $\eta = \rho \cdot f_{16,3}$ with $\rho \in \{0, 0.5, 1, 2\}$. (Originally published in (Uschner et al. 2018a), under Creative Commons Attribution (CC BY 4.0) license)

subjects each. A total number of 10,000 trials was simulated under the assumption $\mu_1 = c \cdot f$, $\mu_2 = c \cdot f$, $\mu_3 = 0$, where c is chosen such that the effect size of the comparison results in 80% power of the F-test $\left(c = 3/\sqrt{2}\right)$, and the estimated power is given by the proportion of trials that led to a rejection of the null hypothesis.

Panel A shows that the power of the adjusted test is close to the nominal power when the block size is large but reduces to about 67% when a small block size is used. The magnitude of the selection effect does not have an impact on the power of the adjusted test. Panel B shows the power of the unadjusted test. As expected, the power increases with increasing selection effect, as a result of an overestimation of the treatment effect. Small block sizes lead to the heaviest inflation, reflecting the higher susceptibility to selection bias.

Randomization Tests

An approach to mitigate the influence of chronological bias is given by randomization tests. They do not rely on parametric assumptions and are thus more robust to deviations and biases. Under the null hypothesis of a randomization test, the patient's responses are independent of the treatment the patient receives. Under this hypothesis, the response vector is fixed, and the treatment assignments are random. A test statistic is then chosen, e.g., the difference in means statistic, and computed for the complete set of randomization sequences (or a Monte Carlo sample thereof), yielding a distribution of the test statistic under the null hypothesis. The p-value is computed as the probability of obtaining a more extreme test statistic than the one that was observed in the trial.

Rosenberger and Lachin (2015) simulated the type I error rate and power for several randomization procedures, using the model

$$Y_i \sim \mathcal{N}(\Delta \cdot T_i + 4 \cdot \tau(i) - 2, 1),$$

where $\Delta \in \{0, 1\}$, and $\tau(i)$ is a linear time trend as in section "Chronological Bias." Their results show that the randomization test maintains the 5% significance level for all randomization procedures. The power is decreased for all randomization procedures except permuted blocks with small block sizes. It results that a smaller degree of balance leads to greater power loss.

The advantages of randomization tests are that they need little effort to compute and can handle heterogeneity in the data that may arise from bias and they do not rely on random sampling from a distribution, such as parametric hypothesis tests. They are therefore the natural choice for hypothesis tests when bias is anticipated in the data.

Summary and Conclusions

Randomization is a design technique that helps to reduce bias in clinical trials. A variety of randomization procedures has been developed in the literature to address different types of bias. At the design stage of a clinical trial, it is crucial to select a randomization procedure that adequately addresses the biases that may potentially occur during the trial. Several restricted randomization procedures are available in the literature to address that need. It has been claimed (Taves 2010) that covariate adaptive allocation, such as minimization, is less susceptible for selection bias. The controversy surrounding this claim and other issues regarding the analysis of covariate adaptive randomization are discussed in Rosenberger and Lachin (2015).

Investigators should take into account information from previous trials to evaluate the potential for bias in a prospective trial, as suggested by Hilgers et al. (2017). When no such information is available, several different scenarios should be anticipated in a sensitivity analysis. For example, clinical trials for rare diseases usually have long recruitment periods in order to identify a larger number of participants that are eligible for participation in the trial. Due to the slow recruitment, changes in study personal or co-medication can be anticipated. Therefore, several different shapes and parameters of time trend should be investigated to assess the potential for chronological bias. A randomization procedure that performs well in all scenarios should consequently be chosen for the design of the trial.

Trials should be assessed for the potential of predictability when the nature of the intervention makes it impossible to blind the investigator or the patient, such as in the case of a surgical intervention. When the investigator knows or can guess the treatment assignment of a patient, there is a potential of predictability of the future allocations. Other examples for potential of predictability are trials where one of the treatments has a side effect that the other treatment has not. Furthermore, when the trial has a single center, or even multiple centers but the randomization is stratified by center, the potential for predictability is high. In any of these cases, the available randomization procedures should be assessed with respect to their potential for selection bias, using a variety of selection bias parameters. Again, a procedure that performs well in all investigated scenarios should be chosen. Lastly, if little is known about the nature of the trial, a combination of chronological and selection bias, as proposed by Hilgers et al. (2017), can be used as a basis for the assessment that will determine the choice of the design. The combination approach will ensure that a trial is protected if both biases occur during the trial.

By choosing a randomization procedure for a particular clinical trial that reflects anticipated bias, the susceptibility to bias can be substantially reduced. While it is recommended to include all available randomization procedures in assessment, randomization procedures that promote balance, such as the permuted block randomization or the big stick design, should particularly be taken into account when chronological bias is anticipated. Procedures that support randomness, such as complete randomization, Efron's biased coin design, or the big stick design with larger imbalance tolerance, are especially recommended when predictability is an issue.

At the analysis stage, when researchers suspect that bias may have affected the results of their trial, they can use testing strategies to detect and adjust for potential bias. The Berger-Exner test (Berger and Exner 1999) can be applied to detect the presence of selection bias with a high accuracy, if all assumptions are met (Mickenautsch et al. 2014). Altman and Royston (1988) recommend to use cumulative sums of the outcomes to detect the presence of time trends. A more general approach to control bias is to use methods that are robust to bias. When a parametric test is used for the treatment effect, it is possible to control for a specific bias by estimating its effect from the data and thus adjusting the treatment effect for the bias. When the focus is not estimation, but testing of the null hypothesis of no treatment effect, randomization tests are recommended to control the effect of bias, particularly chronological bias, on the type I error probability. As randomization tests do not rely on parametric assumptions, their results are robust to biases that arise from heterogeneity in the patient stream, e.g., due to chronological bias.

Key Facts

- The results of a clinical trial can be affected by bias despite randomization.
- The susceptibility to bias varies with the randomization procedure that is employed.
- The susceptibility to bias can be mitigated by chosing suitable randomization procedure at the design stage of a trial.
- Sensitivity analyses are recommended to evaluate the impact of the clinical scenario on the trial results.

Cross-References

▶ Cross-over Trials
▶ Evolution of Clinical Trials Science
▶ Factorial Trials

- ▶ Fraud in Clinical Trials
- ▶ Issues for Masked Data Monitoring
- ▶ Masking Study Participants
- ▶ Multi-arm Multi-stage (MAMS) Platform Randomized Clinical Trials
- ▶ Principles of Clinical Trials: Bias and Precision Control
- ▶ Reporting Biases

References

Altman DG, Royston JP (1988) The hidden effect of time. Stat Med 7(6):629–637. https://doi.org/10.1002/sim.4780070602

Armitage P (1982) The role of randomization in clinical trials. Stat Med 1:345–353

Atkinson AC (2014) Selecting a biased-coin design. Stat Sci 29(1):144–163. https://doi.org/10.1214/13-STS449

Berger VW (2005) Quantifying the magnitude of baseline covariate imbalances resulting from selection bias in randomized clinical trials. Biom J 47(2):119–127. https://doi.org/10.1002/bimj.200410106

Berger VW, Exner DV (1999) Detecting selection bias in randomized clinical trials. Control Clin Trials 20(4):319–327. https://doi.org/10.1016/S0197-2456(99)00014-8

Berger VW, Ivanova A, Deloria Knoll M (2003) Minimizing predictability while retaining balance through the use of less restrictive randomization procedures. Stat Med 22(19):3017–3028. https://doi.org/10.1002/sim.1538

Blackwell D, Hodges JL (1957) Design for the control of selection bias. Ann Math Statist 28(2):449–460. https://doi.org/10.1214/aoms/1177706973

Efron B (1971) Forcing a sequential experiment to be balanced. Biometrika 58(3):403–417

Hilgers RD, Uschner D, Rosenberger WF, Heussen N (2017) ERDO – a framework to select an appropriate randomization procedure for clinical trials. BMC Med Res Methodol 17(1):159. https://doi.org/10.1186/s12874-017-0428-z

ICH (1998) International conference on harmonisation of technical requirements for registration of pharmaceuticals for human use. ICH harmonised tripartite guideline: statistical principles for clinical trials E9

Ivanova A, Barrier RC Jr, Berger VW (2005) Adjusting for observable selection bias in block randomized trials. Stat Med 24(10):1537–1546. https://doi.org/10.1002/sim.2058

Kennes LN, Cramer E, Hilgers RD, Heussen N (2011) The impact of selection bias on test decisions in randomized clinical trials. Stat Med 30(21):2573–2581. https://doi.org/10.1002/sim.4279

Kennes LN, Rosenberger WF, Hilgers RD (2015) Inference for blocked randomization under a selection bias model. Biometrics 71(4):979–984. https://doi.org/10.1111/biom.12334

Langer S (2014) The modified distribution of the t-test statistic under the influence of selection bias based on random allocation rule. Master's thesis, RWTH Aachen University, Germany

Matts JP, McHugh RB (1978) Analysis of accrual randomized clinical trials with balanced groups in strata. J Chronic Dis 31(12):725–740. https://doi.org/10.1016/0021-9681(78)90057-7

Mickenautsch S, Fu B, Gudehithlu S, Berger VW (2014) Accuracy of the Berger-Exner test for detecting third-order selection bias in randomised controlled trials: a simulation-based investigation. BMC Med Res Methodol 14(1):114. https://doi.org/10.1186/1471-2288-14-114

Proschan M (1994) Influence of selection bias on type i error rate under random permuted block designs. Stat Sin 4(1):219–231

Rosenberger W, Lachin J (2015) Randomization in clinical trials: theory and practice. Wiley series in probability and statistics. Wiley, Hoboken

Rückbeil MV, Hilgers RD, Heussen N (2017) Assessing the impact of selection bias on test decisions in trials with a time-to-event outcome. Stat Med 36(17):2656–2668

Ryeznik Y, Sverdlov O (2018) A comparative study of restricted randomization procedures for multi-arm trials with equal or unequal treatment allocation ratios. Stat Med 37(21):3056–3077. https://doi.org/10.1002/sim.7817

Salama I, Ivanova A, Qaqish B (2008) Efficient generation of constrained block allocation sequences. Stat Med 27(9):1421–1428. https://doi.org/10.1002/sim.3014. https://onlinelibrary.wiley.com/doi/abs/10.1002/sim.3014, https://onlinelibrary.wiley.com/doi/pdf/10.1002/sim.3014

Tamm M, Hilgers RD (2014) Chronological bias in randomized clinical trials arising from different types of unobserved time trends. Methods Inf Med 53(6):501–510

Taves DR (2010) The use of minimization in clinical trials. Contemp Clin Trials 31(2):180–184. https://doi.org/10.1016/j.cct.2009.12.005

Uschner D, Hilgers RD, Heussen N (2018a) The impact of selection bias in randomized multi-arm parallel group clinical trials. PLoS One 13(1):1–18. https://doi.org/10.1371/journal.pone.0192065

Uschner D, Schindler D, Hilgers RD, Heussen N (2018b) randomizeR: an R package for the assessment and implementation of randomization in clinical trials. J Stat Softw 85(8):1–22. https://doi.org/10.18637/jss.v085.i08

Part V

Basics of Trial Design

Use of Historical Data in Design

49

Christopher Kim, Victoria Chia, and Michael Kelsh

Contents

Abstract

The goal of clinical research of new disease treatments is to evaluate the potential benefits/risks of a new treatment, which generally requires comparisons to a control group. The control group is selected to characterize what would have happened to a patient if they had not received the new therapy. Although a randomized controlled trial provides the most robust clinical evidence of treatment effects, there may be situations where such a trial is not feasible or ethical, and the use of external or historical controls can provide the needed clinical evidence for granting conditional or accelerated regulatory approvals for novel drugs. Data from previous clinical trials and real-world clinical studies can provide evidence of the outcomes for patients with the disease of interest. However, many methodologic considerations must be considered such as the appropriateness of data sources, the specific data that needs to be collected,

C. Kim · V. Chia (✉) · M. Kelsh
Amgen Inc., Thousand Oaks, CA, USA
e-mail: chrkim@amgen.com; vchia@amgen.com; mkelsh@amgen.com

© Springer Nature Switzerland AG 2022

S. Piantadosi, C. L. Meinert (eds.), *Principles and Practice of Clinical Trials*,
https://doi.org/10.1007/978-3-319-52636-2_69

application of appropriate inclusion/exclusion criteria, accounting for bias, and statistical adjustment for confounding. This chapter reviews the settings in which the use of historical controls or comparators may be appropriate, as well as study designs, limitations to using real-world comparators, and analytic methods to compare real-world data to clinical trial data. When these considerations are appropriately handled, use of historical controls can have immense value by providing further evidence of the efficacy, effectiveness, and safety in the development of novel therapies and increase efficiency of the conduct of clinical trials and regulatory approvals.

Keywords

Real-world comparators · Real-world evidence · Clinical trials · Controls · Historical comparator · Statistical methods · Propensity score

Introduction

The goal of clinical research of new disease treatments is to evaluate the potential benefits/risks of a new treatment, which generally requires comparisons to a control group. The control group is selected to characterize what would have happened to patient if they had not received the new therapy. To minimize bias in this comparison, clinical trial study designs typically involve randomization of eligible patients to treatment and control groups and, where feasible, blinding investigators to patient treatment status. This approach provides the most robust clinical evidence of treatment effects. However, for a variety of reasons and under a number of circumstances, this well-established study design may not be feasible or ethical, and the use of existing "real-world" (RW) data (i.e., external or historical controls) can provide the needed clinical evidence for granting conditional or accelerated regulatory approvals for novel drugs.

Randomized controlled trials (RCTs) may not be feasible because the disease under study is so rare, creating a significant challenge in recruiting a sufficient number of patients or requiring an unreasonably long time period for patient recruitment. Similarly, if a new treatment is targeting a relatively rare "molecular-identified" subgroup of patients, this may require screening a large number of patients to identify the target patient population. In addition, analytical challenges such as patient crossover from the control group to the new treatment group can threaten the study integrity and confound survival analyses. For these feasibility reasons and other ethical considerations (see below), physicians and patients may refuse to participate in RCTs under these circumstances.

The ethical considerations that can impose significant challenges include a lack of equipoise resulting from the early findings of new treatment or the dismal outcomes of the current standard of care (SOC) for many serious life-threatening illnesses. Even if a disease is not life threatening, a study could involve potential invasive/risky monitoring or follow-up procedures, administered to controls who have little to gain in terms of improvement or benefit in their disease status under the current SOC. All of these scenarios could render an RCT as unethical.

Under such circumstances single-arm clinical trials, accompanied with historical controls, can provide the needed comparative data for evaluation of outcomes for patients who did not receive the new treatment. Such studies can be faster and more efficient than RCTs and still generate needed clinical evidence. In some cases, comparative data may be obtained from readily available study group data from completed clinical trial treatment and/or control cohorts, patient cohorts from previous clinical case series, or meta-analyses of previous RCT or observational patient data. However, for more precise comparisons, accounting for important clinical characteristics likely requires individual patient-level data. Use of these data is the focus of the discussion in this chapter.

The broad concept of historical controls has been described previously (Pocock 1976) and has been given various labels such as "nonrandomized control group," "external control," "synthetic control," "natural history comparison," or "historical comparator." Although there are subtle distinctions across these different labels, generally they are used to refer to a comparison group which is not randomized, can be concurrent or historical, and can be derived from a single or multiple sites or data sources. For purposes of discussion in this chapter, we will use the term "historical control" to describe this type of comparison group. These data could be historical or contemporaneous with the new treatment group; with either type of data, similar study design and analytical principles would apply (with the exception of the assessment of trends over time for the historical data). The goal of using historical controls is to provide evidence of the expected patient outcomes in the hypothetical randomized control group in the absence of randomized control study. Additionally, the data could improve the generalizability of the study findings.

Considering the potential ethical and feasibility challenges described above, situations that favor the use of historical controls involve the following:

- A rare disease with a large unmet treatment need.
- Severe or unfavorable outcomes for patients receiving the current SOC.
- The clinical/biological mechanism of the new treatment is well-characterized.
- The natural history of disease is well-understood.
- The new therapy appears to provide significant improvement over current SOC.
- The target patient population is well-defined and can be identified in RW or clinical data sources.
- Disease and outcome classifications are similar between the new treatment group and "real-world" controls, and these measures are collected using objective and repeatable measurements.
- For historical data, disease prognosis and treatment patterns remain relevant for the period under study.

This list is not intended to be exhaustive of all potential scenarios where historical controls may be advantageous or feasible, nor is it a requirement that all of these attributes be present for the use of historical controls in lieu of a randomized control group. Data quality and accessibility are key components to the use of historical controls for evidence generation and regulatory review. Each disease area and specific indication may necessitate one type of data or another.

Controls derived from historical clinical trial data, when "reused" for other studies, are considered observational data (Desai et al. 2013) and, because they involve rigorous data collection and validation procedures, can provide robust historical control data. These data are often limited in how many patients may be eligible to be evaluated as they represent highly selected patient populations. The characteristics of the included patients should be carefully considered for representativeness and comparability to the population being considered. Other data sources include electronic health records, disease registries, insurance administrative claims records, and clinical data abstracted for use as historical controls (USFDA 2018). These data can often provide large numbers of patients but may not have as meticulous collection of data as with other trials. But when the inclusion/exclusion criteria are matched to that of the population being considered, the outcomes can truly reflect what would occur if patient did not receive the investigational intervention. Regardless of the type of data source, historical control data need to include a sufficient number of patients, critical exposure, outcome, and covariate information and systematic and sufficient follow-up to provide reliable comparative information. The potential for bias can be reduced by assuring similar covariate, endpoint, and exposure (e.g., previous treatment information, comorbidity data) definitions, similar SOC across the historical patient cohort, and unbiased patient selection processes. It is also important to fully understand data sources/data systems: how data are recorded, who are the patient populations captured in the data source (e.g., an understanding of patient referral patterns), reasons for missing data, geographic distribution of data, variation in standards of care, and other critical data characteristics or system attributes (Dreyer 2018).

In addition to consideration and evaluation of the quality of historical control data sources, appropriate study design and analytical methods that are aimed at reducing bias and improving comparability/balance between patients receiving new treatment and historical controls are critical aspects in providing an accurate comparison to the new treatment patient group. Study design considerations and analytical strategies to address bias due to confounding generally and, in particular, confounding by indication include descriptive, stratified, weighted analyses, multivariate modeling, propensity score (PS) methods for weighting and matching, and, when appropriate, Bayesian approaches for statistical analysis. Sensitivity analysis should also be proposed to assess impacts of study assumptions. A key to the scientific integrity and successful regulatory evaluation of this process is the upfront specification of these design and analysis strategies. Further details, examples from oncology, and discussion on these topics are provided in this chapter.

In the first section of this chapter, appropriate study design is discussed. Selecting the appropriate data source for the historical control group is critical, and evaluating what data will satisfy the needs is the first key step. Next, defining the study variables between the trial and historical controls is also critical. Without appropriately defined exposures and endpoints, any comparisons will be limited. Finally, appropriate considerations for bias that must be considered are discussed. Randomization typically balances differences between patient populations, but use of historical controls will almost certainly be biased without proper design and analysis. After study design, a number of different analytic options are presented, and examples of comparing single-arm trials to historical controls are discussed.

Study Design

Data Sources

There are three primary methods to conduct a study's data collection, each with its own sets of strengths and limitations: (1) prospective primary data collection, (2) clinical data abstraction from patient charts/clinical databases with a standardized case report form, and (3) databases such as an electronic medical record (EMR) linked to an administrative claims database. The last data option is to use former clinical trial data. The data options that make the most sense will be determined by the disease of interest and what the data will contextualize. The first option is to run a primary prospective data collection. The second option is clinical data abstraction from patient charts or clinical databases with a standardized case report form. Another option is to use existing secondary databases such as comprehensive EMR data, administrative claims data, EMR data linked to administrative claims, disease registry data, or national health screening data. The specific details of each approach are detailed below.

Primary prospective data collection will provide the most in-depth and complete data but will be the most costly and time-consuming effort. This option may be needed if the required data are not regularly collected in clinical practice and cannot be derived from routinely collected measures (e.g., in graft-versus-host disease, measurement of response assessment to therapy by NIH 2014 Consensus Response Criteria Working Group is widely collected and reported in clinical trials but is not integrated into routine clinical care (Lee et al. 2015)). In situations where temporality of the data is particularly important, for example, if standard of care has changed substantially over time, prospective data collection may be the only feasible option. For instance, in 2005, the use of bortezomib was fully approved for the treatment of relapsed or refractory multiple myeloma after compelling data from the phase 3 trial demonstrated bortezomib superiority to dexamethasone in overall survival (Richardson et al. 2005). The introduction of bortezomib changed the SOC of multiple myeloma, and as a result, a reasonable comparison of outcomes for myeloma patients would need to include data after 2005 when bortezomib became a backbone of myeloma therapy. Additionally, some endpoints may have a much more complicated ascertainment than what is routinely conducted under typical clinic care and cannot be derived from existing data. In these circumstances, the only way to collect these assessments is to prospectively design a study that collects such data. This approach will require the most time as sites will need to be enrolled and each patient will need to be screened and provide informed consent.

Retrospective extraction of clinical data using a standardized case report form can provide depth of clinical data with less complexity and time than a prospectively designed study. This option is a good choice if the data needed are commonly collected but not necessarily in a structured field of an electronic medical record (EMR) (e.g., to measure response to therapy for an acute lymphoblastic leukemia patient (Gokbuget et al. 2016a)). The primary benefit of doing a retrospective data collection directly from clinical sites is that most centers will have years of data available. With a specific case report form, a focused effort can extract just the necessary data. In some instances, centers may maintain a database or registry that contains most, if not all, of the data elements needed, which will streamline the data abstraction process. However, many centers do not keep a routine database of clinical data for research purposes. The biggest barrier for these sites will be the process of medical chart abstraction which requires extensive staff support. The process of data abstraction and entry is often a slow and expensive process due to the labor involved. Additionally, many sites and investigators may be less interested in participating in retrospective studies which may not be as novel or impactful as investigational therapies.

Use of databases can be the most time- and cost-efficient method. This option is feasible when the primary endpoints are routinely collected in everyday medical practice in structured EMR or insurance claims diagnosis (e.g., incidence of bleeding events in patients with thrombocytopenia (Li et al. 2018)). The most common types of data used would likely be an EMR linked to an administrative claims database. These data are more likely to be highly generalizable as these data provide a large sampling of centers and providers from a geographic region. Additionally, the sample size provided by these datasets is likely to be far greater than a clinical study. Despite these advantages however, the appropriateness of the databases needs to be considered. For instance, existing electronic databases may lack the specificity and depth of data needed for comparative purposes to clinical trial data. Additionally, because the data are not provided on a protocol or for research purposes, there may be missing elements that were never or rarely collected. Some covariate and endpoint assessments may be less frequently or sporadically measured, as these databases reflect real-world medical practice. Lastly, many types of endpoints cannot be assessed in these types of databases. Understanding the limitations of the data is key to understand if this approach is feasible.

Previous clinical trials can provide robust control data. Clinical trials are considered the gold standard of clinical evidence as they are highly controlled and perform thorough data collection. Many variables may be collected for completeness. Additionally, adherence to medications is often more closely monitored and most potential variables are recorded. This allows investigators to evaluate a wide range of variables during the design and analysis phase. However, clinical trials tend to have highly selected populations, which limits the generalizability and applicability to many populations. Often, most of these data will not mimic the studied population, intervention, or inclusion/exclusion criteria of the population to be compared to, making it difficult to use these data as a source for controls.

Defining Variables

Defining exposure/treatment can vary depending on the type of data collection and study being conducted. In prospective data collection, exposure definition, dates, duration, dose, and any changes due to adverse events can be matched exactly to the trial assessment schedule and definitions. In retrospective data abstraction efforts, it may be straightforward to identify what specific regimen or protocol was anticipated for the patient. However, there may be specific details missing such as the exact dose(s) administered or adjustments for toxicity. Using large databases, treatment regimen typically must be derived using an algorithm which can be prone to errors and assumptions, particularly for multi-agent treatment regimens. For prescriptions that are filled through a pharmacy and not administered in a clinic setting, you only know with certainty that the prescription was picked up but not necessarily whether it was actually taken by the patient. This highlights that in using historical data, assumptions must be made and algorithms developed that need to be validated where possible and/or evaluated in sensitivity analyses (Table 1).

Collection of relevant prognostic covariates is important for assessment of patient population comparability. In a prospective data collection, all baseline covariates can be ascertained with a complete baseline assessment. In a retrospective collection, typically, disease-relevant clinical covariates will be routinely collected. However, a complete assessment as typically done on a trial will not be conducted unless a patient has specific medical conditions necessitating it. In a database, some labs or imaging data may not be routinely available. Claims typically do not contain specific lab values; EMR typically do not contain comorbid conditions captured outside of that specific clinic.

Carefully determined endpoints are critical to study success. In prospective data collection, endpoints can follow assessment schedules and definitions just like in the clinical trial. In retrospective data sources where death is captured, overall survival is

Table 1 Data collection methods suitability for exposure, covariate, and endpoint

Data collection	Exposure	Covariates	Endpoints
Prospective	Collect exact dates, duration, dosing, and changes	Can do a full baseline assessment for all relevant covariates	Set the exact definitions of endpoints and the assessment schedule
Retrospective chart abstraction or clinical database	Identify treatments, but may be missing exact doses and fine details	Demographics and disease-relevant clinical characteristics; some comorbidities	Can be routinely collected in medical practice, but schedule of assessments is less frequent than trial
Claims, registry, or EMR database	Can be inconsistent in details, may require algorithms to identify treatments	Claims can identify demographics and comorbidities; EMR can identify demographics and some clinical characteristics	May lack some endpoints that require lab or imaging results

easiest to evaluate because of limited heterogeneity in endpoint determination (death is death). For composite endpoints such as relapse-free survival, event-free survival, and progression-free survival, ascertainment can vary depending on frequency of assessments, which may be somewhat less frequent and subject to some heterogeneity. However, in administrative or EMR database studies, response to therapy may be difficult to ascertain systematically because of heterogeneity in timing or response assessment is not systematically recorded in real-world medical practice data. Some procedures to ascertain response may not be conducted if there is clear evidence of no treatment response (e.g., if bone marrow aspirate required for response assessment but patient exhibits overt symptoms). Other times, a proxy measure may be sufficient for some endpoints due to similarity in timing of events (e.g., time to next treatment in some scenarios can be similar to progression-free survival). However, these proxies should be validated as a facsimile of the endpoint in question prior to use in a comparative analysis. Lastly, caution should be exercised when assessing safety endpoints from retrospective or databases as they may not be systematically captured except for expected/known toxicities common to the disease/treatments resulting in a visit to the hospital. This may lead to biased ascertainment of adverse events and lead to inappropriate comparisons. Generally, these issues do not apply to prospectively collected data if the assessment schedule is like the trial.

Bias

In 1976, Pocock described the use of historical controls in clinical trials (Pocock 1976), and the acceptability of a historical control group requires that it meet the following conditions:

1. Exposure: such a group must have received a precisely defined standard treatment which must be the same as the treatment for randomized controls.
2. Patient selection: the group must have been part of a recent clinical study which contained the same requirements for patient eligibility.
3. Outcome: the methods of treatment evaluation must be the same.
4. Covariates: the distributions of important patient characteristics in the group should be comparable with those in the new trial.
5. Site selection: the previous study must have been performed in the same organization with largely the same clinical investigators.
6. Confounding: there must be no other indications leading one to expect differing results between the randomized and historical controls.

Only if all these conditions are met can one safely use the historical controls as part of a randomized trial. Although meeting all of these conditions would result in an ideal historical comparator, it is not always feasible. In previous sections, types of data sources, how to define exposures, outcomes, and covariates are discussed. Later, analytic methods to assess and control for confounding will be discussed, and in this section, Pocock's conditions, bias, and how to mitigate bias are discussed. Appropriate control for confounding as described in the analytics section may reduce bias (Greenland and Morgenstern 2001).

Selection Bias

Selection bias may be introduced if the patients selected for the historical comparators are not comparable to the clinical trial-treated subjects (other than treatment exposure) or do not contain the same patient eligibility requirements. Prospective study designs would minimize this bias the most, as investigators are able to define eligibility criteria similarly to that of the clinical trial, with the goal to include patients that would have been able to participate in the clinical trial. For studies using existing data, either from clinical sites or through large existing databases, careful selection of patients restricting inclusion and exclusion criteria is required; however, not all clinical trial eligibility criteria may be found in these types of data sources. Additionally, for existing data sources, selection of patients when the outcome is known can bias the results to produce a favorable evaluation for the drug or device under study. This bias may be mitigated by including all patients who meet the eligibility criteria. If a random sample of patients is selected, then the outcome must be blinded. Random selection can help provide a mix of patients at various lines of therapy. When there are multiple treatments received over time (e.g., different lines of therapy), bias may be introduced when selecting the treatment line for which to assess outcomes. For instance, if subjects in the clinical trial had to have previously failed at least two prior lines of therapy and the majority of subjects only had two prior lines of therapy, bias would be introduced if the majority of patients in the historical comparator had three prior lines of therapy.

In addition to bias resulting from patient selection, for studies using existing data from clinical sites, investigators need to ensure the clinical sites, including type of site (e.g., academic hospitals, large specialty centers), country of site, standard treatments used, and types of patients undergoing treatment at those clinics are comparable to the clinical trial sites and subjects. However, the selected sites do not necessarily have to be performed with the same clinical trial sites and investigators.

Finally, the time period in which the historical comparator is drawn from will need to be carefully assessed for comparators that are nonconcurrent. For instance, if there have been significant changes in medicine or technology over time (e.g., earlier diagnosis of disease, changes in treatment effectiveness, or better supportive care measures), having nonconcurrent comparators can bias the results to favor the drug or device. Thus, it is important to carefully assess changes in the treatment landscape over time when selecting patients for historical comparators.

Information Bias

Appropriate measurement of the exposure, outcomes, and covariates was previously discussed, and appropriate measurement and minimization of missing data can reduce information or measurement bias. When data are collected from multiple existing data sources (e.g., multiple clinical sites), standardization of data collection forms will minimize measurement error. An issue comparative effectiveness observational research is the inappropriate selection of follow-up time. This creates a bias in favor of the treatment group where during a period of follow-up, an event cannot occur due to a delay or wait period for the treatment to be administered. This is known as immortal time bias. Immortal time bias can be appropriately handled by assigning follow-up when events can occur and using a time-varying analysis, not a fixed-time analysis. Finally, the length of follow-up time after the treatment exposure can impact outcomes. For instance, when following patients for death, the longer the follow-up time, the more likely events will accrue. The historical comparator must have a comparable follow-up time as the clinical trial patients.

Analytic Methods

Prior to beginning any comparative analyses, it is important to characterize each patient population by evaluating the important covariates in both populations. The first step is to make sure that the inclusion/exclusion criteria for the historical comparator match as closely as possible to the clinical trial subjects. Once the primary criteria are matched between populations, other baseline clinical characteristics can be described and evaluated for differences. These covariates should be as balanced as possible so the outcomes comparisons can be meaningful and not attributed to one population being sicker/healthier.

As data between studies are collected at different time points and on different schedules, the heterogeneity in endpoints must be accounted for when defining the analysis of time-dependent variables and time-to-event endpoints. These variables will include treatment initiation, treatment response assessment, and overall survival. Alignment on these variables is important so as not to create biased analyses that are invalid and inappropriately favor one group over another as can occur with inappropriate follow-up creating immortal time bias.

Several analytic and design approaches are available to account for information bias. Two analytic methods are the use of simulation-extrapolation or regression calibration to account for measurement error of an exposure/treatment. Depending on how much is known about the type of misspecification in the distribution of the variable, simulation-extrapolation may have less bias if the true measurement distribution is unknown or misspecified compared to regression calibration. Sensitivity analysis with subsets of data to evaluate the consistency of results can also help to identify data/bias issues. During study planning stages, designing data collection and review with multiple checks from data reviewers can also help identify and avoid confirmation biases that are inherent to variables where human judgment is required.

When conducting comparisons between two separate study populations, several different options are available. The simplest method is to conduct a weighted analysis based on a baseline covariate (or a few). This is a straightforward method of adjustment based on levels of a covariate. However, there may be uncontrolled confounding when using such a simple adjustment method as it only adjusts for a few characteristics with simple groupings. But when there are not many prognostic covariates to consider or the populations are relatively well balanced on measured covariates without adjustment, simply weighting may provide adequate and easy-to-interpret comparisons. Another option is to use a multiple regression model. Multiple regression will adjust estimates of an endpoint measure with the assumptions normally associated with fitting multiple covariates in the model. However, many of these assumptions such as linearity or distributions of the covariates may not be met leading to a violation of model assumptions and resulting in biased estimates.

Another method that is more flexible and reduces bias in comparisons is the use of propensity score as adjustment (D'Agostino 1998). Propensity scores estimate the probability of being assigned to a treatment group based on baseline covariates entered in a model. First, the propensity score for each patient is derived using a logistic model with many baseline covariates. It is possible to account for many covariates, including interactions between variables, in deriving the propensity scores. A wide range of variables can be accounted for compared to a traditional multivariate logistic or Cox regression model. The distribution of propensity score for both cohorts should be described and then the adjustment method can be chosen.

Two predominant methods of using propensity scores exist: matching or weighting. When sample size is abundant, matching has some advantages. However, when sample size is a concern, weighting provides a bit more flexibility at the cost of less direct matching. Risk of outcomes associated with treatment exposure can be presented as propensity score-adjusted odds ratios (OR) or hazard ratios (HR) with 95% CIs. Additionally, other covariates may be assessed and adjusted for in the risk models. Propensity score models have been used in comparing phase 2 single-arm trials to historical or real-world studies. Such an example compared blinatumomab to chemotherapy for relapsed/refractory acute lymphoblastic leukemia which will be discussed (Gokbuget et al. 2016b) and alectinib for non-small cell lung cancer compared to real-world clinic outcomes (Davies et al. 2018). When sample size of the assessed studies is small, statistical power can be boosted by including use of a Bayesian prior. This method "borrows" data from a similar statistical analysis (typically the same disease with similar drug) to augment the effect estimates. This may lend additional credibility to study results if the a priori data is a relevant. Additional analytics to consider are outlined well elsewhere (Lim et al. 2018).

Examples of the Use of Historical Comparators to Test Efficacy

Lim et al. describe several examples where drug approvals have used historical comparator data in settings of rare diseases, including oncology and other life-threatening conditions (Lim et al. 2018). One of these examples was for acute lymphoblastic leukemia (ALL) and the use of historical comparators to put the results from the blinatumomab single-arm phase 2 clinical trial into context (Gokbuget et al. 2016b). In this example, historical data were pooled from large study groups and individual clinical sites treating patients with Philadelphia chromosome-negative, B-precursor, relapsed, or refractory ALL with standard of care chemotherapy in Europe and the United States.

Outcomes, such as complete remission and overall survival, in the historical comparator patients were either weighted to the distribution of important clinical prognostic predictors in the blinatumomab trial subjects or were estimated using propensity scores and inverse probability of treatment weighting. Weighted analyses of the historical comparators provided a complete remission (as defined by the study groups) estimate of 24% [95% confidence interval (CI), 20–27%] and a median overall survival of 3.3 months (95% CI, 2.8–3.6 months). In the propensity score model, the predicted complete response was 27% (95% CI, 23–30%) in the historical comparators, with a statistically significant twofold increase in the odds of achieving complete remission in the blinatumomab subjects versus the historical comparators, and a statistically significant hazard ratio for overall survival (0.53, 95% CI, 0.39–0.73) favoring blinatumomab. Several sensitivity analyses were conducted with alternative treatment effect analyses and outlier stabilizations. Yet, the results remained consistent and robust. The authors raised potential issues in residual confounding, temporality of historical data (data included patients as far back as 1990), and heterogeneity in data collection.

Interestingly, the weighted complete remission and overall survival data from the historical comparator was similar to the data in controls from the subsequently completed randomized phase 3 clinical trial of blinatumomab compared to standard of care chemotherapy (Kantarjian et al. 2017). Complete remission in the subjects receiving standard of care chemotherapy was 24.6% (95% CI, 17.6–32.8%), and the median overall survival was 4.0 months (95% CI, 2.9–5.3 months). This example provides a good illustration of the use of historical comparators to put single-arm clinical trial data into context and was reassuringly confirmed to provide data similar to the standard of care arm in the randomized phase 3 clinical trial.

In another example, a comparison of data from two phase 2 trials of alectinib for the treatment of anaplastic lymphoma kinase-positive (ALK) non-small cell lung cancer (NSCLC) were pooled and compared to ALK NSCLC patients treated with ceritinib from the Flatiron electronic health records database and analyzed with IPTW adjustment (Davies et al. 2018). The primary endpoint was overall survival. At baseline, the ceritinib group was older, had less pretreatment, and had less CNS metastases. These covariates were balanced after adjustment with IPTW. The weighted survival of the alectinib group was 24 months (95% CI, 21-NR) and in the ceritinib group was 16 months (95% CI, 16–19) with a hazard ratio of 0.65 (95% CI, 0.48–0.88) favoring the alectinib group. The results were evaluated against a number of sensitivity analyses (i.e., exclusion of outliers, inclusion of additional covariates in model specification, alternative treatment weighting methods), and the results were found to be consistent. The authors pointed out several limitations in the analyses such as residual confounding due to unmeasured covariates, differential follow-up time between the two treatment groups, and inherent differences in the data collection practices between groups. Despite these limitations, these data demonstrated that newer generation of tyrosine kinase inhibitors can reduce the risk of death in ALK NSCLC patients.

Summary and Conclusion

The use of historical controls can serve to provide an alternate form of evidence for understanding treatment effects in nonrandomized studies. In appropriate situations where a randomized trial may be unethical and/or the unmet need is great, historical control may be particularly useful for contextualizing study outcomes in the absence of randomized trials. However, many methodologic considerations must be considered such as the appropriateness of data sources, the specific data that needs to be collected, application of appropriate inclusion/exclusion criteria, accounting for bias, and statistical adjustment for confounding. When these considerations are appropriately handled, use of historical controls can have immense value by providing further evidence of the efficacy, effectiveness, and safety in the development of novel therapies and increase efficiency of the conduct of clinical trials and regulatory approvals.

Key Facts

- External or historical controls can provide the needed clinical evidence for granting conditional or accelerated regulatory approvals for novel drugs.
- Methodologic considerations for the use of external or historical controls must be considered in order to appropriately compare real-world data to clinical trial data.
- When the methodologic considerations are appropriately handled, use of historical controls can have immense value by providing evidence to support the efficacy and safety of novel therapies.

Cross-References

▶ Evolution of Clinical Trials Science

Funding Statement and Declarations of Conflicting Interest CK, VC, and MK are employees and shareholders of Amgen Inc.

References

D'Agostino RB Jr (1998) Propensity score methods for bias reduction in the comparison of a treatment to a non-randomized control group. Stat Med 17:2265–2281

Davies J et al (2018) Comparative effectiveness from a single-arm trial and real-world data: alectinib versus ceritinib. J Comp Eff Res. https://doi.org/10.2217/cer-2018-0032

Desai JR, Bowen EA, Danielson MM, Allam RR, Cantor MN (2013) Creation and implementation of a historical controls database from randomized clinical trials. J Am Med Inform Assoc 20: e162–e168. https://doi.org/10.1136/amiajnl-2012-001257

Dreyer NA (2018) Advancing a framework for regulatory use of real-world evidence: when real is reliable. Ther Innov Regul Sci 52:362–368. https://doi.org/10.1177/2168479018763591

Gokbuget N et al (2016a) International reference analysis of outcomes in adults with B-precursor Ph-negative relapsed/refractory acute lymphoblastic leukemia. Haematologica 101:1524–1533. https://doi.org/10.3324/haematol.2016.144311

Gokbuget N et al (2016b) Blinatumomab vs historical standard therapy of adult relapsed/refractory acute lymphoblastic leukemia. Blood Cancer J 6:e473. https://doi.org/10.1038/bcj.2016.84

Greenland S, Morgenstern H (2001) Confounding in health research. Annu Rev Public Health 22:189–212. https://doi.org/10.1146/annurev.publhealth.22.1.189

Kantarjian H et al (2017) Blinatumomab versus chemotherapy for advanced acute lymphoblastic leukemia. N Engl J Med 376:836–847. https://doi.org/10.1056/NEJMoa1609783

Lee SJ et al (2015) Measuring therapeutic response in chronic graft-versus-host disease. National Institutes of Health consensus development project on criteria for clinical trials in chronic graft-versus-host disease: IV. The 2014 Response Criteria Working Group report. Biol Blood Marrow Transplant 21:984–999. https://doi.org/10.1016/j.bbmt.2015.02.025

Li S, Molony JT, Cetin K, Wasser JS, Altomare I (2018) Rate of bleeding-related episodes in elderly patients with primary immune thrombocytopenia: a retrospective cohort study. Curr Med Res Opin 34:209–216. https://doi.org/10.1080/03007995.2017.1360852

Lim J et al (2018) Minimizing patient burden through the use of historical subject-level data in innovative confirmatory clinical trials: review of methods and opportunities. Ther Innov Regul Sci. https://doi.org/10.1177/2168479018778282

Pocock SJ (1976) The combination of randomized and historical controls in clinical trials. J Chronic Dis 29:175–188

Richardson PG et al (2005) Bortezomib or high-dose dexamethasone for relapsed multiple myeloma. N Engl J Med 352:2487–2498. https://doi.org/10.1056/NEJMoa043445

USFDA USFaDA (2018) Real-world Evidence. https://www.fda.gov/scienceresearch/specialtopics/realworldevidence/default.htm. Accessed 15 Aug 2018

Outcomes in Clinical Trials

50

Justin M. Leach, Inmaculada Aban, and Gary R. Cutter

Contents

Abstract

Selecting outcomes for clinical trials requires a wide range of considerations relating to clinical interpretation, ethics relating to therapy effectiveness and safety, and statistical optimality of measures. Appropriate outcome choice plays a key role in determining the usefulness and/or success of a study and can affect whether a proposed study is view favorably by funding and regulatory agencies. Many regulatory and funding agencies provide guidance on the types of outcomes that are appropriate or acceptable in various contexts, and it is important to understand

J. M. Leach · I. Aban · G. R. Cutter (✉)
Department of Biostatistics, University of Alabama at Birmingham, Birmingham, AL, USA
e-mail: jleach@uab.edu; caban@uab.edu; cutterg@uab.edu

© Springer Nature Switzerland AG 2022

S. Piantadosi, C. L. Meinert (eds.), *Principles and Practice of Clinical Trials*,
https://doi.org/10.1007/978-3-319-52636-2_70

regulatory guidelines, definitions, and expectations when choosing clinical outcomes. This chapter provides an overview of the clinical, practical, and statistical considerations in choosing outcomes, with a focus on the intersection between the considerations themselves and the standards and definitions provided by regulatory and funding agencies. Section "Introduction, Definitions, and General Considerations" introduces basic definitions and broad considerations in clinical trials outcomes. Section "Types of Outcome Measures" discusses clinical distinctions between outcomes, mathematical descriptions of outcomes, and safety considerations. Section "Choosing Outcome Measures" discusses both statistical and practical considerations in outcome choice, introduces approaches for evaluating the quality of selected outcomes, and makes distinctions in reporting outcomes. Section "Multiple Outcomes" examines the intricacies involved in using multiple outcomes, specifically multiple outcomes consisting of different, but possibly related, measures, and longitudinal studies that measure the same outcome for multiple times.

Keywords

Primary outcomes · Secondary outcomes · Biomarker · Multiple measures

Introduction, Definitions, and General Considerations

What Is an Outcome?

All studies consist of taking measurements of varying levels of complexity. While finished studies make included measurements appear obvious and necessary, careful planning is necessary to ensure achievement of study goals. There are two key classes of measurements in studies: outcomes (dependent variables) and predictors (independent variables). In the most basic sense, studies ask whether measured predictors can account for variation in outcomes. In clinical trials the most important predictors are typically therapies, drugs, and outcomes that are measures with clinical significance, e.g., suppose we study the effectiveness of a cigarette smoking cessation method. The (primary) outcome would likely be cigarette cessation (or not); the study then seeks to answer whether the cessation method was associated with higher rates of cigarette smoking cessation. However, decisions regarding outcomes may be more complex than one would naively expect. For smoking cessation, the broad outcome of interest is whether a subject quit smoking, but researchers and regulators may care about how one defines quitting and/or *how long* the cessation lasts. Which measures most adequately capture relevant clinical concerns and are within the practical limits of conducting a trial?

Outcomes in Clinical Trials

The FDA defines a *clinical outcome* as "an outcome that describes or reflects how an individual feels, functions, or survives" (FDA-NIH Biomarker Working GroupB).

Choices regarding outcomes in clinical trials are often further constrained compared to studies in general. Ethical considerations guide the choice of outcomes, and the regulators, i.e., Food and Drug Administration (FDA), EMA, institutional review boards, and/or other relevant funding agencies, ensure that these ethical considerations are considered. Many clinical trials involve therapies that carry significant risks, especially in the case of surgical interventions or drugs. In phase III trials, the FDA requires that the effects of therapies under consideration be clinically meaningful to come to market (Sullivan n.d.). The expectation is that a therapy's benefits will sufficiently outweigh the risks. The FDA gives three reasons for which patients reasonably undertake treatment risks:

1. Increased survival rates
2. Detectable patient benefits
3. Decreased risk of disease development and/or complications

Outcomes inherently vary in importance. A *primary outcome* should be a measure capable of answering the main research question and is expected to directly measure at least one of the above reasons for taking risks. Treatment differences in primary outcomes generally determine whether a therapy is believed to be effective. Researchers often measure a single primary outcome and several *secondary outcomes*. Secondary outcomes may be related to the primary outcomes, but of lower importance or may not be inherently feasible to use as a primary outcome due to duration of the study needed to assess them or the sample size required to defend the study as adequately powered. Outcomes measuring participant safety must ensure that the risk-benefit ratio is sufficiently high. In cigarette cessation trials, perhaps smoking cessation maintained for 6 weeks as the primary outcome and cessation after 6 months and 1 year are secondary outcomes. The longer-duration cessation is actually more important but may make the size and/or duration of the trial not feasible due to expected recidivism or losses to follow-up. Note that therapies not involving drugs typically still require recording adverse events. For example, smoking cessation therapy studies may be concerned about depression or withdrawal symptoms (Motooka et al. 2018). When conducting an exercise study to improve fitness in disabled multiple sclerosis patients, we need to be cognizant of falls and thus measure and record their occurrences.

Where Are We Going?

The focus of this chapter is the mathematical, clinical, and practical considerations necessary to determine appropriate outcomes. Section "Types of Outcome Measures" introduces and discusses biomarkers and direct and surrogate outcomes and defines mathematical descriptions of variables. Section "Choosing Outcome Measures" considers the clinical, practical, and statistical considerations in outcome choice. Finally, Section "Multiple Outcomes" examines the benefits and complications of using multiple outcomes.

Types of Outcome Measures

Clinical Distinctions Between Outcomes

Direct Endpoints

The FDA defines *direct endpoints* as outcomes that directly describe patient well-being; these are categorized as *objective* or *subjective* measures. Objective measures explicitly describe and/or measure clinical outcomes and leave little room for individual interpretation. Some common objective measures are as follows:

1. Patient survival/death.
2. Disease incidence; e.g., did the subject develop hypertension during the study period given they were free of hypertension at the start of the study?
3. Disease progression; e.g., did the subject's neurological function worsen during the study period?
4. Clinical events; e.g., myocardial infarction, stroke, multiple sclerosis relapse.

Subjective measures often depend upon a subject's perception. For health outcomes, this is often in terms of disease symptoms or quality of life (QoL) scores. Subjective endpoints are complicated by their openness to interpretation, either between or within subject's responses or rater's assessments, and whether or which measures adequately capture the quality of interest is often debatable. Ensuring unbiased ascertainment and uniformity of measurement interpretation is difficult when the outcome is, say QoL, global impressions of improvement, etc. compared to objective endpoints such as death or incident stroke. Measure assessment is covered in detail in section "Choosing Outcome Measures."

Note that regulatory agencies prefer direct endpoints as primary outcomes, particularly for new drug approval. There are several issues that arise from using what we will denote as the elusive surrogate measures or biomarkers and how these issues can make their use less than optimal.

Surrogate Endpoints

Surrogate endpoints are substitutes for direct or clinically meaningful endpoints and are typically employed in circumstances where direct endpoints are too costly, are too downstream in time or complexity, or are unethical to obtain. Few true surrogates exist if one uses the definition provided by Prentice (1989). In the Prentice definition, the surrogate is tantamount to the actual outcome of interest (E), but this is often unachievable. While there is some concurrence on the existence of a so-called surrogate, these are often laboratory measures or measurable physical attributes from subjects, such as CD4 counts in HIV trials, although still lacking in meeting the Prentice definition.

Surrogate endpoints may avoid costly or unethical situations, but the researcher must provide strong evidence that the surrogate outcome is predictive of, correlated with, and/or preferably in the therapeutic pathway between the drug or treatment and expected clinically significant benefit. Importantly, while the Prentice criteria argue for complete replacement of the endpoint by the surrogate, the generally accepted goal of a surrogate endpoint is to be sufficiently predictive of the direct endpoint.

In the case of sufficiently severe illness, researchers may obtain "accelerated approval" for surrogate endpoints, but further trials demonstrating the relation between surrogate and direct endpoints are typically required despite initial approval. Surrogate endpoints can be classified into the following stages of validation (Surrogate Endpoint Resources for Drug and Biologic Development n.d.):

1. *Candidate surrogate endpoints* are in the process of proving their worth as predictors of clinical benefits to subjects.
2. *Reasonably likely surrogate endpoints* are "endpoints supported by strong mechanistic and/or epidemiologic rationale such that an effect on the surrogate endpoint is expected to be correlated with an endpoint intended to assess clinical benefit in clinical trials, but without sufficient clinical data to show that it is a validated surrogate endpoint" (FDA-NIH Biomarker Working Group). These are more likely to receive accelerated approval than candidate surrogate endpoints.
3. *Validated surrogate endpoints* "are supported by a clear mechanistic rationale and clinical data providing strong evidence that an effect on the surrogate endpoint predicts a specific clinical benefit" (FDA-NIH Biomarker Working Group). Validated surrogate endpoints are generally accepted by funding agencies as primary outcomes in clinical trials and generally are not required to provide further studies in support of the relationship between the surrogate and direct endpoint.

For validation, regulatory agencies prefer more than one study establishing the relationship between direct and surrogate endpoints. A major drawback to surrogate outcomes is that relationships between surrogate and direct endpoints may not be causal even when the correlation is strong; even if the relationship is (partially) causal, surrogate outcomes may not fully predict the clinically relevant outcome, especially for complicated medical conditions. Two problems thus arise:

1. A drug could have the desired beneficial effect on the surrogate outcome but also have a negative effect on an (possibly unmeasured) aspect of the disease, rendering the drug less effective than anticipated/believed.
2. Drugs designed to treat a medical condition may have varying mechanisms of action, and it does not follow that validated surrogate endpoints are equally valid for drugs with differing mechanisms of action.

These drawbacks can bias the estimate of a benefit-risk ratio, especially in smaller or shorter studies, where there may be insufficient sample size or follow-up time to capture a representative number of adverse events. Pairing underestimation of adverse events with too-optimistic beliefs regarding the therapeutic benefits can result in overselling a mediocre or relatively ineffective therapy.

Surrogates are often used in phase II studies initially before they can be accepted as legitimate for phase III clinical outcomes as surrogate endpoints are not often clinically meaningful in their own right. Phase II trials can use biomarkers or indicators of processes that are not necessarily surrogates.

Biomarkers

Biomarkers are "a defined characteristic that is objectively measured as an indicator of normal biological processes, pathologic processes, or responses to an exposure or intervention, including therapeutic interventions" (FDA-NIH Biomarker Working Group). Biomarkers are often useful as secondary outcomes regarding subject safety or validation that a therapy induces the expected biological response or a primary outcome in phase II proof of concept trials. Most validated surrogate endpoints are in fact biomarkers.

Biomarkers are often chosen as outcomes for the same reasons that surrogates are used: shortened trials, smaller sample sizes, etc. However, biomarkers are often more specific to certain treatments than surrogates. For example, in multiple sclerosis, MRI reveal small areas of inflammation when viewed after injection of a special chemical, gadolinium. Gadolinium-enhanced lesions are used in phase III trials as proof of concept primary outcomes, but they do not clearly predict disability outcomes, which are the goal of disease-modifying therapy, and they are clinically meaningful only through their repeated linkage to successful drug treatment. Sormani et al. have shown that they are acting as surrogates at the study level (Sormani et al. 2009, 2010). These counts of enhancing lesions seem to be biomarkers for inflammation, and their absence following treatment has been taken as a sign of efficacy. However, there are now drugs that virtually eliminate these enhancing lesions, yet progression of disability still occurs, so they are not a good choice for an outcome comparing two effective drugs where both may eliminate enhancing lesions but have differences in their effects on disability.

Biomarkers are also useful not only as outcome variables, but as predictors of outcomes on which to enrich a trial making it easier to see changes in the biomarkers or primary outcomes. Biomarker-responsive trials select individuals who have shown that with certain biomarkers or certain levels of biomarkers, the participants are at increased risk of events or are more responsive to treatment. This seems like a rational approach, but there are several caveats to the uncritical use of this selection. Simon and Maitournam point out that the efficiency of these designs is often not seen unless the proportion of biomarker-positive responders is less than 50% *and* the response in those who are biomarker negative is negligible (Simon and Maitournam 2004). The reasons for this counterintuitive finding are that the cost of screening can overwhelm the dampening of the response by the biomarker-negative individuals making the biomarker selection an added logistic issue while not enhancing the design over simple increases in sample size and stratification. In other situations, the biomarker's behavior needs to be carefully considered. In Alzheimer's trials, it has been argued that more efficient trials could be done if patients were selected based on a protein, tau-beta, found in their spinal cords. This is because patients with these proteins have more rapid declines in their disease as measured by the usual cognitive test outcomes. However, Kennedy et al. (2015) showed that when designing a study based on selection for tau positivity, the gains in sample size reduction due to the greater cognitive declines, which make percent changes easier to detect, were offset by the increased variation in cognitive decline among the biomarker positive subset. This results from assuming that the variance is the same or smaller in the biomarker-positive subset compared to the larger population.

Quantitative and Qualitative Descriptions of Outcomes

Thus far we have definitions of outcomes that relate to *what* we want to measure rather than *how* to quantify the measurement. The biological quantity of interest may be clear, but decisions about how to measure that quantity can affect the viability of a study or the reasonableness of the results. Outcomes are described as either *quantitative* or *qualitative*. In the following sections, we distinguish between these, give several examples, and discuss several common subtypes of outcomes.

Quantitative Outcomes

Quantitative outcomes are measurements that correspond to meaningful numeric scale and can be broken down into *continuous* and *discrete* measurements (or variables). In mathematical terms, continuous variables can take any of the infinite number of values between any two numbers in its support; they are uncountable. On the other hand, discrete variables are countable. A few examples should help clarify the difference.

Systolic blood pressure is a continuous outcome. In theory, blood pressure can take any value between zero and infinity. For example, a subject participating in a hypertension study may have a baseline systolic blood pressure measurement of 133.6224. We may round this number for simplicity, but it is readily interpretable as it stands. In most cases discrete quantitative outcomes consist of positive whole numbers and often represent counts. For example, how many cigarettes did a subject smoke in the last week? The answer is constrained to nonnegative whole numbers: 0, 1, 2, 3, ... While perhaps it is possible to conceive of smoking half a cigarette, the researcher needs to decide a priori whether to record and allow your data collection system to accept fractions or develop clear rules to record discrete values in the same way for all participants.

Categorical Outcomes

Categorical outcomes, or qualitative variables, have neither natural order nor interpretation on a numeric scale and result from dividing study participants into categories. Many drugs are aimed at reducing the risk of negative health outcomes, which are often binary in nature, and common trial aims are reducing the risk of death, stroke, heart attack, or progression in multiple sclerosis. The use of these binary outcomes is not simply convenience or custom, but rather they are much more easily interpreted as clinically meaningful. To say you have reduced blood pressure in a trial by 4.5 mmHg is by conditioning a positive result, but it is not in and of itself immediately clinically meaningful, whereas, if the group that experienced

4.5 mmHg greater change had lower mortality rates, it would be easier to say this is clinically meaningful.

Categories need not be binary in nature. For example, consider a study where it is likely that, in the absence of treatment, patient health is expected to decline over time. A successful drug might slow the decline, stop the decline but not improve patient health, or improve patient health, and so researchers could categorize the subjects as such.

Nominal Versus Ordinal Outcomes

Ordinal outcomes are perhaps best understood as a hybrid of continuous and categorical outcomes. Ordinal outcomes have a natural order, but do not correspond to a consistent, objective numerical scale; moving up/down from one rank to another need not correspond to the same magnitude change and may vary by individual; e.g., categories of worse, the same, or better patient health can be interpreted as an ordinal outcome since there is a natural order. However, it is not immediately clear that the "same" vs. "better" health indicates the same benefit for all patients or is necessarily equal in magnitude to the difference between "worse" and the "same" health. In contrast, nominal outcomes have neither natural ordering nor objective interpretation on a numeric scale. In the context of clinical trials, nominal variables are more likely to be predictors than outcomes; for example, we may have three treatment groups with no natural order, placebo, drug A, and drug B, or they can have an order such as placebo, low dose, and high dose. The former requires certain forms of analyses, while the latter allows us to take advantage of the natural ordering that occurs among the dose groups.

Common Measures

Often outcomes are raw patient measures, e.g., patient blood pressure or incident stroke. However, summary measures are often relevant. Incidence counts the number of new cases of a disease per unit of time and can be divided into cumulative incidence such as that occurring over the course of the entire study or the incidence per unit of time, 30-day mortality following surgery, etc. Incidence can pertain to both chronic issues, e.g., diabetes, and discrete health events, e.g., stroke, myocardial infarction, or adverse reaction to a drug.

Another common summary measure is the proportion: how many patients out of the total sample experienced a medical event or possess some quality of interest? The *incidence proportion* or *cumulative incidence* is the proportion of previously healthy patients who developed a health condition or experienced an adverse heath event. Incidence is also commonly described with an *incidence rate*; that is, per some number of patients, called the radix, often 1000, how many will develop the condition, experience the event, etc.; e.g., supposing 4% of patients developed diabetes during the study, then an incidence rate would say that we expect 40 out of every 1000 (nondiabetic) subjects to develop diabetes. Note that incidence differs from *prevalence*, which is the proportion of all study participants who have the condition. Prevalence can be this simple proportion at some point in time, known as point prevalence or period prevalence, the proportion over some defined period. The period prevalence is often used in studies from administrative databases and counts the number of cases divided by the average population over the period of interest, whereas the point prevalence is the number of cases divided by the population at one specific point in time.

A measure related to incidence is the *time to event*; that is, how long into the study did it take for the incident event to occur? This is often useful for assessing a therapy's effect on survival or health state. For example, a cancer therapy may be considered successful in some cases if patient survival is lengthened; similarly, some therapies may be considered efficacious if they extend the time to a stroke or other adverse health events.

Safety

Measuring/Summarizing Safety

In addition to efficacy outcomes, safety outcomes are also important to consider. We mentioned above that there is a necessary balance between the risks and potential benefits of a therapy. Thus, we need information regarding potential risks, particularly side effects and adverse events. It is possible that a therapy could be highly effective for treating a disease and yet introduce additional negative health consequences that make it a poor option. Safety endpoints can be direct or surrogate endpoints. Some therapies may increase the risk of adverse health outcomes like stroke or heart attack; these direct endpoints can be collected. We often classify events into side effects, adverse effects, and serious adverse effects.

Side Effects: A side effect is an undesired effect that occurs when the medication is administered regardless of the dose. Unlike adverse events, side effects are mostly foreseen by the physician, and the patient is told to be aware of the effects that could happen while on the therapy. Side effects differ from adverse events and later resolve on their own with time.

Adverse Events: An adverse event is any new, undesirable medical occurrence or change (worsening) of an existing condition in a subject that occurs during the study, whether or not considered to be related to the treatment.

Serious Adverse Events: A serious adverse event is defined by regulatory agencies as one that suggests a significant hazard or side effect, regardless of the investigator's or sponsor's opinion on the relationship to investigational product. This includes, but may not be limited to, any event that (at any dose) is *fatal*, is *life threatening* (places the subject at immediate risk of death), requires *hospitalization* or prolongation of existing hospitalization, is a *persistent or significant disability/ incapacity*, or is a *congenital anomaly/birth defect*. Important medical events that may not be immediately life threatening or result in death or hospitalization but may jeopardize the subject or require intervention to prevent one of the outcomes listed above, or result in urgent investigation, may be considered serious. Examples include allergic bronchospasm, convulsions, and blood dyscrasias.

Collecting and monitoring these are the responsibility of the researchers as well as oversight committees such as Data and Safety Monitoring Committees. Collection of these can be complicated, such as when treatments are tested in intensive care units where nearly all actions could be linked to one or the other type of event, to relatively straightforward. Regulators have tried to standardize the recording of these events into System Organ Classes using the Medical Dictionary for Regulatory Activities (MedDRA) coding system. This standardized and validated system allows for mapping of a virtually infinite vocabulary of events into medically meaningful classes of events – infections, cardiovascular, etc. for comparison between groups and among treatments. These aid in the assessment of benefits versus risks by allowing comparisons of the rates of these medical events that occur within specific organs or body functions.

Obstacles to Measuring Safety

It is often the case that direct safety-related endpoints have relatively low incidence rates, especially within the time frame of many clinical trials since many medical conditions manifest after extended exposure; i.e., often weeks, months, or years pass before health conditions manifest. Thus, surrogate endpoints are often necessary, and biomarkers are useful, especially in cases where information on drug toxicity is needed. Using biomarkers to assess toxicity is integral to altering the patient's dose or ceasing treatment before more severe health problems develop (FDA-NIH Biomarker Working Group). Laboratory assessments measure ongoing critical functions, and we often use flags or cut points to identify evolving risks, such three times the upper limit of normal to flag liver function tests or white cell counts to indicate infections. One of the major obstacles to assessing safety is that neither researchers nor regulators can give a specific frequency above which a treatment is considered unsafe. For some events, such as rare fatal events, the threshold may be just a few instances, and for other situations where the participants are extremely sick, high rates of adverse events may be tolerated, such as in cancer trials and treatments.

Choosing Outcome Measures

While some health-related outcomes have obvious metrics, others do not. For instance, if a study is conducted on a drug designed to lower or control blood pressure or cholesterol, then it is straightforward to see that the patient's blood pressure is almost certainly the best primary outcome. However, for many complex medical conditions, arriving at a reasonable metric requires a considerably more twisted, forking path. For example, in multiple sclerosis (MS), the aim is to reduce MS-related disability in patients, but "disability" in such patients is a multidimensional problem consisting of both cognitive and physical dimensions and thus requiring a complex summary metric. Sometimes the choice involves choosing a metric and other times it involves how to use the metric appropriately. For example, smoking cessation therapy studies should record whether patients quit smoking, but at a higher level, we may debate just how long a subject must have quit smoking to be considered a verified nonsmoker, or we may require biological evidence of cessation such as cotinine levels, whereas in MS studies, the debate is more often over which metric most adequately captures patient disability.

Nonstatistical and Practical Considerations

The most important consideration in choosing an outcome measure is to ensure that the outcome measure possesses the ability to capture information that can answer relevant scientific questions of interest, and there can sometimes be a debate about which metrics are most appropriate. In MS studies there has been considerable concern that many commonly used measures of MS-related disability cannot sufficiently capture temporal change nor adequately incorporate or detect patient-perceived quality of life (Cohen et al. 2012).

More practical concerns involve measure interpretability and funding agency approval. Established metrics are more likely to be accepted by funding agencies such as the FDA and NIH, and a considerable amount of work is often necessary to make the case for a new metric. Some of the regulatory preference for established measures is no doubt based in a disposition toward "historical legacy," but we note that there can be good reasons for preferring the status quo in this case (Cohen et al. 2012). Specifically, comparing studies becomes more difficult when different outcome measures are used, complicating interpretation of a body of literature. Therefore, new measures must often bring along detailed and convincing cases for their superiority over established measures. Physicians and other medical professionals must be able to readily interpret trial results in terms of practical implications on their patients, and if an outcome is difficult to practically interpret, it may be resisted even if it possesses other desirable qualities. For example, the Multiple Sclerosis Functional Composite (MSFC) was proposed to answer criticisms of the established and regulator-preferred Expanded Disability Status Scale (EDSS) (Cutter et al. 1999). However, despite its good qualities and improvement on the EDSS in many aspects, the MSFC is resisted by regulators primarily because its mathematical nature, a composite z-score of three functional tests, is a barrier to physician interpretation (Cohen et al. 2001, 2012). Interpretability is closely tied to ensuring that measures are clinically meaningful in addition to possessing desirable metric qualities.

Assessing Outcome Measures

Validity

Validity is the ability of the outcome metric to measure that which it claims to measure. In cases where the outcome is categorical, it is common to assess validity with sensitivity and specificity. Sensitivity is the ability of a metric to accurately determine patients who have the medical condition or experienced the event, and specificity is the ability of a metric to accurately determine which patients do not have the medical condition or did not experience the event. Both sensitivity and specificity should be high for a good metric; for example, consider the extreme case where a metric always interprets the patient as having a medical condition. In such a case, we will identify 100% of the patients with the medical condition (great job!) and 0% of the patients without the medical condition (poor form!). Note that while these concepts are often understood in terms of medical conditions and events, they need not be confined in such a way.

For continuous, and often ordinal, measures, assessing validity is somewhat more complicated. One could impose cutoffs on the continuous measure to categorize the variable, only then using sensitivity or specificity to assess validity. However, this is a rather clumsy approach in many cases; we want continuous outcome measures to capture the continuous value with as little measurement error as possible. This is often more relevant for medical devices. For example, a wrist-worn measure of blood glucose would need to be within +/− of a certain amount of the actual glucose level in the blood to demonstrate validity. Often individuals use regression analyses to demonstrate that a purported measure agrees with a gold standard, but it should be kept in mind that a high correlation by itself does not demonstrate validity. A regression measure should have slope of 1 and an intercept of 0 to indicate validity.

Sensitivity is also used to describe whether an outcome measure can detect change at a reasonable resolution. Consider a metric for disability, on a scale from 1 to 3, where higher scores indicate increased disability. This will be a good metric if generally when a patient's disability increase results in a corresponding increase on the scale, but if the measure is too coarse, then it could be the case, for example, that many patients are having disability increases, but not sufficient to move from a 1 to a 2 on the scale. This measure being insensitive to the worsening at the participant level would lead to high sensitivity (because greater disability would have occurred before the scale recognized it), but poor specificity because being negative does not indicate the participant hasn't progressed. When the metrics pertain to patient well-being or health dimensions of which a patient is conscious, it is expected that when the patient notices a change, the metric will reflect those changes. This is particularly important for determining the effectiveness of therapies in many cases. A measure that is insensitive to change could either mask a therapy's ineffectiveness by incorrectly suggesting that patient conditions are not generally worsening or on the flip side portray an effective therapy as ineffective since it will not detect positive change. Further, because if a participant feels they are worsening, but the measure is insensitive, then this can lead to dropping out of the trial.

Reliability

Reliability is a general assessment of the consistency of a measure's results upon repeated administrations. There are several relevant dimensions to reliability. A measure can be accurate, but not reliable. This occurs because on average the measure is accurate but highly variable. Various types or aspects of reliability are often discussed. Perhaps most prominent is *interrater reliability*. Many trials require raters to assess patients and assign scores or measures describing the patient's condition, and interrater reliability describes the consistency across raters when presented with the same patient or circumstance. A reliable measure will result in (properly trained) raters assigning the same or similar scores to the same patient. When a metric is proposed, interrater reliability is a key consideration and is typically measured using a variant of the intraclass correlation coefficient (ICC), which should be high if the reliability is good (Bartko 1966, Shrout and Fleiss 1979).

Intersubject reliability is also a concern; that is, subjects with similar or the same health conditions should have similar measures. This differs from interrater reliability in that it is possible for raters to be highly consistent within a subject, but inconsistent across subjects, or vice versa. Interrater reliability measures whether properly trained raters assign sufficiently similar scores to the same patient; that is, is the metric such that sufficiently knowledgeable individuals would agree about how to score a specific subject? Intersubject reliability measures whether a metric assigns sufficiently similar scores to sufficiently similar subjects.

Other Concerns

There are several other issues in evaluating outcome measures. *Practice effects* occur when patients' scores on some measure improve over time not due to practice rather than therapy. Studies involving novel outcome measures should verify that either no practice effects are present or that the practice effects taper off; for example, in developing the Multiple Sclerosis Functional Composite (MSFC), practice effects were observed, but these tapered off by the fourth administration (Cohen et al. 2001). Practice effects are problematic in that they can lead to overestimates of a treatment effect because the practice effect improvement is ignored when comparing a post-intervention measure to a baseline measure. In randomized clinical trials, we can assume both groups experience equivalent practice effects and the difference between the two groups is still an unbiased estimate of the treatment effect, but how much actual improvement was achieved is biased unless the practice effects can be eliminated prior to baseline by multiple administrations or adjusted for in the analyses. Practice effects are often complex and require adjustments to the measure or its application; for example, the Paced Auditory Serial Addition Test (PASAT), a measure of information processing speed (IPS) in MS, was shown to have practice effects that increased with the speed of stimulus presentation and was more prominent in relapse-remitting MS compared to chronic-progressive MS (Barker-Collo 2005). Therefore, using PASAT in MS research requires either slower stimulus presentation or some correction accounting for the effects.

Another source of (unwanted) variability in outcome measures, particularly subjective measures, is *response shift*. Response shift occurs when a patient's criteria for a subjective measure change over the course of the study. It is clearly a problem if the meaning of the same recorded outcome is different at different times in a study, and therefore response shift should be considered and addressed when subjective measures and/or patient-reported outcomes are employed (Swartz et al. 2011). This is often the case with long-term chronic conditions such as multiple sclerosis where participants report on their quality of life in the early stages of the disease and when reassessed years later when they have increased disability record the same quality of life scores. Adaptation and other factors are at the root of these response shifts, but outcome measures that are subject to this type of variability can be problematic to use.

Statistical Considerations

In addition to whether a measure is informative to the clinical questions of interest, there are statistical concerns relating to the ability to make comparisons between treatment groups and answer scientific or clinical questions of interest with the data on hand. This section defines the relevant statistical measures and then describes their practical import in outcome choice.

Statistical Definitions

In hypothesis testing, variable selection, etc. there are two kinds of errors to minimize. The first is the *false positive*, formally *Type I error*, which is the probability that we detect a therapy effect, given that one does not exist. False positives are typically controlled by assignment of the *statistical significance threshold*, α, which is generally interpreted as the largest false-positive rate that is acceptable; by convention, $\alpha = 0.05$ is usually adopted.

The second error class is the *false negative*, or *Type II error*, which occurs when we observe no significant therapy effect, when in reality one exists. *Power* is given as one minus the false-negative rate and refers to the *power to detect a difference, given that one exists*. For a given statistical method, the false-positive rate should be as low as possible and the power as high as possible. However, there is a tension in controlling these errors because controlling one in a stronger manner corresponds to a reduction in ability to control the other.

There are several primary reasons that these errors arise in practice (and theory). Sampling variability allows for occasionally drawing samples that are not representative of the population; this problem may be exacerbated if the study cohort is systematically biased in recruitment or changes over time during the recruitment period so that it is doubtful that the sample can be considered as drawn from the population of interest. The second primary reason for errors is sample size. In the absence of compromising systematic recruitment bias, a larger sample size can often increase the chance that we detect a treatment difference if one exists. The fundamental reason for improvement is that sample estimates will better approximate population parameters with less variation about the estimates, on average. Small sample sizes can counterintuitively make it difficult to detect significant effects, overstate the strength of real effects, and more easily find spurious effects. This is because in small samples a relatively small number of outliers can have a large biasing effect, and in general sampling variability is larger for smaller compared to larger samples.

The choice of statistical significance thresholds can also contribute to errors in inference. If the threshold is not sufficiently severe, then we increase the risk of detecting a spurious effect. Correspondingly, a significance threshold that is too severe may prevent detection of treatment differences in all but the most extreme cases. Errors related to the severity of threshold can affect both large and small samples.

Note that caution must be employed with respect to interpreting differences. Statistically significant differences are not necessarily clinically significant or meaningful. It is rare that two populations will be exactly equal in response to a treatment, but small differences between groups, while statistically significant at a large sample size, may not represent a sufficient benefit to the patients.

Common Statistical Issues in Practice

Statistical significance thresholds, power, and clinically meaningful treatment differences are determined a priori. Using these values and some estimate of variance gleaned from similar studies, we can calculate the necessary sample size. In cases with continuous outcomes, the calculations are often relatively straightforward and tend to have few, if any, additional restrictions beyond (usually) normality on the outcome's values. However, the situation is more complicated when the outcomes are no longer continuous (or normal). A common problem is near or complete separability when the outcome is binary, that is, when almost all the patients have one or the other outcome. Model fitting problems will arise when separability applies to the whole study sample but also when (nearly) all patients in one group have one outcome and (nearly) all patients in the other group have the other outcome. This is especially true in retrospective and observational studies which seek to make comparisons among subgroups within the population. For example, in a study presented at the European Association for Cardiothoracic Surgery in 2016, a retrospective study of a vein graft preservation by a buffered solution compared to saline for use during harvesting and bypassing heart vessels attempted to adjust for the two time periods of comparison, the saline period prior to the introduction of the new product and after introduction. However, when the propensity scores were plotted by type of storage solution used, there was almost complete separation of the two populations before and after (Haime 2016). Here nearly all saline patients had a more favorable risk profile as the willingness to perform bypasses was directed toward younger healthier patients and after the buffered solution was adopted, so did the willingness to accept higher-risk patients for bypass.

Another common way such a situation arises is when the study length is too short for a sufficient number of events to arise. This is an issue whether the study is collecting time-to-event outcomes or simply recording incidence at the study terminus. In such cases it is highly relevant to know the required number of events necessary to detect a clinically significant difference. This problem is generalized to cases where there are more than two categories for the outcome, e.g., ordinal or multinomial data. In such cases where the study length cannot be extended to a sufficient length, nonbinary outcomes and/or surrogate outcomes may be necessary alternatives.

Common Simplifications and Their Up- and Downsides

As noted above, due to the ease of interpretation on the clinical meaningfulness of binary events, a common approach to analysis is to categorize continuous measures so long as the cutoffs are clinically relevant and decided before conducting a study. As discussed in the previous section, this simplification can cause analysis and interpretation issues if there are not sufficient numbers of patients in each category. There is also a tendency to reanalyze the data to better understand what has happened and that can lead to arbitrary cutoffs, and without the a priori specification of the outcome, finding a cut point that "works" is certainly changing the chances of a false-positive result.

On the other hand, it is sometimes useful to treat a discrete variable as continuous; the most common instance of this is count data, where counts are generally very large. In some cases, ordinal data may be treated as continuous with reasonable results. Even though analyzing the ordinal data implicitly assumes that each step is the same in meaning, this provides a simple summarization of response rate. Nevertheless, treating these ordinal data as ranks can be shown to have reasonable properties in detecting treatment effects. However, one should use caution when analyzing ordinal data by applying statistical methods designed for continuous outcomes; in particular, models for continuous outcomes perform badly when the number of ranks is small, and/or the distribution of the ordinal variable is skewed or otherwise not approximately normally distributed (Bauer and Sterba 2011; Hedeker 2015).

Reporting Outcomes

There are several main approaches for assessing outcomes: patient-reported outcomes, clinician-reported outcomes, and observer-reported outcomes. We define and discuss each below.

Patient-Reported Outcomes

Patient-reported outcomes (PROs) are outcomes dependent upon a patient's subjective experience or knowledge; PROs do not exclude assessments of health that could be observable to others and may include the patient's perception of observable health outcomes. Common examples include quality of life or pain ratings (FDA-NIH Biomarker Working Group). These outcomes have gained a lot of acceptance since the Patient-Centered Outcomes Research Institute (PCORI) came into existence. The FDA and other regulators routinely ask for such outcomes as they are indicative of the meaningfulness of treatments. Rarely have patient-reported outcomes been used as primary outcomes in phase III trials, except in those instances, such as pain, where the primary outcomes are only available in this manner. Most often they are used to provide adjunctive information on the patient perspective of the treatments or study. Nevertheless, researchers should be cautioned not simply to accept the need for PROs, but rather think carefully about what and when to measure PROs. PROs are subjective assessments and can be influenced by a wide variety of variables that may be unrelated to the actual treatments or interventions under study. Asking a cancer patient about their quality of life during chemotherapy may not lead to the conclusions of benefits of survival because of the timing of the ascertainment. Similarly, a participant in a trial who is severely depressed may be underwhelmed with the benefits of a treatment that doesn't address this depression. In addition, the frame of reference needs to be carefully considered. For example, when assessing quality of life, should one use a tool that is a general measure, such as the Short-Form-36 Health Survey (SF36), or one that is specific to the disease under study?

This depends on the question being asked and should be factored into the design for any and all data to be collected.

PROs, like many outcomes, are subject to biases. If participants know that they are on an active treatment arm versus a placebo, then their reporting of the specific outcome being assessed may be biased. Similarly, participants who know or suspect that they are on a placebo may report they are doing poorly simply because of this knowledge rather than providing accurate assessments as per the goal of the instrument. A general rule is that when one can make blinded assessments, the better. A more detailed discussion of the intricacies involved in PROs is found in Swartz et al., and the FDA provides extensive recommendations and discussion (FDA 2009).

Clinician-Reported Outcomes

Clinician-reported outcomes (CRO) are assessments of patient health by medical or otherwise healthcare-oriented professionals and are characterized by dependence on professional judgment, algorithmic assessment, and/or interpretation. These are typically outcomes requiring medical expertise, but do not encompass outcomes or symptoms that depend upon patient judgment or personal knowledge (FDA-NIH Biomarker Working Group). Common examples are rating scales or clinical events, e.g., Expanded Disability Status Scale, stroke, or biomarker data, e.g., blood pressure.

Observer-Reported Outcomes

Observer-reported outcomes (OROs) are assessments that require neither medial expertise nor patient perception of health. Often OROs are collected from parents, caregivers, or more generally individuals with knowledge of the patient's daily life and often, but not always, are useful for assessing patients who cannot, for reasons of age or impairment, reliably assess their own health (FDA-NIH Biomarker Working Group). For example, in epilepsy studies caregivers often keep seizure diaries to establish the nature and number of seizures a patient experiences.

Multiple Outcomes

Most studies have multiple outcomes (e.g., primary, secondary, and safety outcomes), but it is sometimes desirable or necessary to include multiple primary outcomes. These generally consist of repeatedly measuring the same (or similar) outcomes over time and/or including multiple measures, which can encompass multiple primary outcomes or multiple secondary outcomes. This section describes common situations where multiple outcomes are employed and discusses relevant considerations arising thereof.

Multiple (Possibly Related) Measures

When the efficacy of a clinical therapy is dependent upon more than one dimension, it may be inappropriate to prioritize one dimension or ignore lower-priority dimensions. For example, in a trial of thymectomy, a surgical procedure by which one's thymus is removed, to control myasthenia gravis, a neuromuscular disease, a joint outcome was needed (Wolfe et al. 2016). The treatments were thymectomy plus prednisone versus prednisone alone. The primary outcome was the clinical condition of the participant over 3 years and the amount of prednisone utilized to control the disease. The need for both outcomes was due to the fact that the clinical condition could be made better by using more prednisone, so analyzing the clinical condition as the outcome would not correctly answer the question of how well a participant was doing, nor would use of the amount of prednisone used since using less prednisone could be done at the expense of the clinical condition.

Primary outcomes are generally analyzed first. For a therapy to achieve an efficacy "win," it usually must meet some criteria pertaining to success in the primary endpoints (Huque et al. 2013). This may consist of all, some proportion, or at least one of the primary endpoints achieving significance by specified criteria and is typically conditional on demonstration of acceptable safety outcomes. Primary outcomes that must be all significant in order to demonstrate efficacy are called *coprimary* (FDA 2017). Significance in secondary outcomes tends to be supportive in nature and is generally not considered an efficacy "win" in the absence of significance for the therapy on primary outcome terms. Additionally, tertiary and exploratory outcomes are often reported, but conditional on primary endpoint efficacy. Nevertheless, the regulators often refer to the "totality of the evidence" when evaluating any application for licensing, and there have been treatments approved when showing statistically significant effectiveness on secondary outcomes, but not primary outcomes. This is more often done when there are no or few treatments available for a condition.

Composite Outcomes

Composite outcomes are functions of several outcomes. These can be relatively simple, e.g., the union of several outcomes. Such an approach is common for time-to-event data, e.g., major adverse cardiovascular events (MACE) or to define an event as when a patient experiences one of the following: death, stroke, or heart attack. Composite outcomes can also be more complex in nature. For example, many MS trials are focused on MS-related disability metrics, which tend to be composites of multiple outcomes of interest and which may be related to either physical or cognitive disability; two common options are the Expanded Disability Status Scale (EDSS) and the Multiple Sclerosis Functional Composite (MSFC).

Composite events are often used in time-to-event studies to increase the numbers of outcomes and, thus for the same relative risk reductions, increase the power as the power of a time-to-event trial is directly related to the number of events. When such events are not reasonably correlated however, care must be given not to dominate signal by noise. For example, as noted previously MS impacts patients differently and variably. The EDSS assesses seven functional systems and combines them into a single ordinal number ranging from 0 to 10 in 0.5 increments. For a person who is impacted in only one functional system, the overall EDSS may not be moved even by changes in this one functional system, thereby reducing its sensitivity to change.

In composites, such as z-scores of multiple tests, it is recommended that no more than four or five components be used because most composites are averages or sums of the individual items. This means that any signal can be dominated by noise. Consider five ordinal scales, four of which only vary due to measurement error or variability and only one is in the affected domain. If all five scales were 2 at the baseline and all but one are 2 s later on and the one that changes goes from a 2 to 4, the overall average score would go from 2.0 to 2.4 because of the lack of change in four of the five measures. Many measurements are more variable than that in this example, and thus, understanding or even identifying changes becomes more difficult because of the signal-to-noise problem.

Multiple Comparisons/Testing Considerations

Multiple testing issues arise when individual outcomes are to be evaluated individually, either as components of a composite outcome or without a global test. When efficacy depends on more than one outcome, controlling the false-positive rate becomes more complicated, and there are two general metrics for false-positive control, each of which has multiple approaches to control. The family-wise error rate (FWER) is the probability of one or more false positives in a family of tests; control of the FWER is divided into *weak control*, which controls the FWER under the *complete null hypothesis*, i.e., when no outcomes have a significant treatment effect, and *strong control*, which controls the FWER when any subset of the outcomes has no significant treatment effect. Note that in confirmatory trials, strong control of the FWER is often required (Huque et al. 2013; FDA 2017). Alternatively, the false discovery rate (FDR) is the expected proportion of false rejections in a family. A good heuristic for determining which false-positive rate is appropriate is whether a single false positive would significantly affect the interpretation of the study. FWER is usually appropriate if a false positive would invalidate the study, while in contrast, FDR is often appropriate in the presence of a large number of tests, where a few false positives would not alter the study interpretation.

The utility of controlling complex false-positive rates was once viewed with suspicion, not least because many traditional methods resulted in severe decreases in statistical power, for example (Pocock 1997). However, advances in methodology for control and concern about study reliability have renewed focus on controlling false-positive rates; e.g., Huque et al. (2013) provide an overview of approaches to FWER control, and Benjamini and Cohen (2017) propose a weighted FDR controlling procedure in similar contexts. In addition to improvements in the quality of the procedures for false-positive control, regulatory agencies are also more aware and concerned with false-positive control (FDA 2017). The pharmaceutical industry is under control by regulators, but the academic community has been less well-regulated with regard to these multiple comparison issues. However, the requirement to list trials with ClinicalTrials.gov has made it more concrete that these issues must be decided in advance. Often, such testing approaches are not determined explicitly at the initiation of the protocol, but codified at the time the statistical analysis plan is created, prior to locking the database and in double blind studies, prior to unblinding. These details are often in the statistical analysis plan and, thus, not available on

ClinicalTrials.gov. While the specific corrections are beyond the scope of this chapter, it is useful to contrast traditional approaches to false-positive control with modern extensions.

In many cases traditional methods for controlling FWER or FDR have been adapted to handle multiple testing in a more nuanced manner. Traditionally, one defined a family of tests and then applied a particular method for controlling false positives, but a study may reasonably consist of more than one family of tests; e.g., one may divide primary and secondary outcome analyses into two separate families. Furthermore, families need not be treated as having equal importance, which is the basis for *hierarchical ordered families or a so-called step-down approach*. This approach applies to controlling FWER or FDR when "win" criterion is achieved in the families of primary endpoints which is required before testing secondary (and possibly tertiary) outcomes. The two most common frameworks are α-propagation and gatekeeping. α-Propagation divides the significance level across a series of ordered tests, and when a test is significant, its portion of the α is "propagated" or passed to the next test. Gatekeeping approaches depend on a hierarchy of families. In regular gatekeeping, a second family of tests is only tested if the first family passes some "win" criteria, but some gatekeeping procedures allow for retesting, and many methods incorporate both gatekeeping and α-propagation. A detailed discussion is found in Huque et al. (2013).

Defining power and calculating the required sample size in complex multiplicity situations may not be straightforward (Chen et al. 2011). However, using traditional methods in the absence of updated methodology is likely to result in conservative results, especially since many methods control FWER *at or below* the specified significance value and so are often more conservative than the desired value so that higher sample sizes are required to achieve the desired power. Note that there are no multiplicity issues when considering coprimary endpoints, since each must successfully reject the null hypothesis, but power calculations are nonetheless complicated and require considering the dependency between test statistics; unnecessarily large sample sizes will be required if an existing dependency is ignored (Sozu et al. 2011); for a detailed discussion on power and sample size with coprimary endpoints, see Sozu et al. (2012).

Longitudinal Studies

What Are Longitudinal Studies?

Multiple outcomes also arise when following patients over time, recording measurements for outcomes at several time points throughout the trial. The circumstances for such a situation can be quite varied. In Alzheimer's disease, we are interested in the trajectory or slope of the decline in cognitive function over time or in chronic obstructive pulmonary disease, the rate of lung function decline. In many cases where adverse medical events (e.g., death, stroke, etc.) are recorded, it is of interest to know *when* the event occurred, and follow-up may be conducted at pre-specified times to determine whether or not an event occurred for each (qualifying) patient; in such cases therapies may be distinguished by whether they prolong the time to event instead of, or in addition to, whether they prevent the event entirely. Some events, such as exacerbations (relapses) in MS, can occur repeatedly over time, and thus assessing these for the intensity of their occurrence (often summarized as the annualized relapse rate) is common. Other less extreme examples involve recording patient attributes, e.g., quality of life assessments or biomarkers like blood pressure or cholesterol; these and similar situations assess changes over time and address the existence and/or form of differences between treatment groups.

Benefits

A major benefit of recording patients at multiple time points is that it allows for a better understanding of the trajectory of change in a patient's outcome; for example, nonlinear trends may be discovered and modeled, thereby allowing researchers to seek understanding of the clinical reasons for each part of the curve. For example, longitudinal studies of blood pressure have established that human blood pressure varies according to a predictable nonlinear form (Edwards and Simpson 2014). Such a model may be used to better define and evaluate healthy ranges for patient blood pressure. Second, patient-specific health changes and inference are available when a patient is followed over time. A simple example is given by comparing a cross-sectional study, a rarity in clinical trials, to a pre-post longitudinal study. Whereas in a cross-sectional study, we only have access to observed group differences in raw scores, longitudinal studies provide insight into whether and how a particular patient's metrics have changed over time; generalizing beyond pre-post to many observations allows better modeling for individuals as well as groups. Additionally, unless the repeated measures are perfectly correlated, the power to detect group differences is generally increased when using longitudinal data and may require a smaller sample size to detect a specified treatment difference.

Drawbacks and Complications

The increased use and acceptance of the (generalized) linear mixed model (GLMM) have allowed increased flexibility in modeling dependence and handling missing outcomes compared to traditional methods such as repeated measures ANOVA or MANOVA approaches, which require strong assumptions and trouble including patients with missing observations (Hedeker and Gibbons 2006). While GLMM work by making some assumptions that are rarely testable, there are far more flexible. However, while modeling has been greatly improved in recent decades, longitudinal studies still have drawbacks and complications. An obvious drawback is the corresponding increase in study cost; trials must balance the benefit of additional information with the ability to pay for that information. Power is generally increased in these repeated measures designs, but few studies seem designed based on the balance of the gain per dollar for each measurement.

A perhaps more pressing concern is that while missing data is no longer an impediment to modeling and inference, the reason that missingness occurs is relevant to interpretation of trial results (Carpenter and Kenward 2007). Data *missing completely at random (MCAR)* are associated with neither observed nor unobserved outcomes of interest. Data *missing at random (MAR)* may be associated with observed, but not unobserved, outcomes. Data *missing not at random (MNAR)* are associated with unobserved outcomes. The assumptions of MCAR are often not well-substantiated. In particular, using complete case analyses where participants with missing observations are excluded can bias results (Mallinckrodt et al. 2003; Powney et al. 2014). Likewise, many common imputation methods, such as last observation carried forward, are often not valid approaches; GLMMs are valid when the assumptions of MAR are reasonable and do not require imputation methods to include all subjects but verifying missingness is not MNAR is difficult. In the interest of transparency, studies should report reasons for dropout and prepare detailed and well-justified approaches for handling missing data (Powney et al. 2014). Performing sensitivity analyses is essential, not just to get agreement on what the primary analysis showed, but to provide evidence that the results are not the product of hidden biases.

Summary/Conclusion

It is imperative that researchers think deeply about which outcomes to employ in studies and are aware of the various issues and complications that can arise from those choices. This chapter has introduced outcomes in clinical trials, delineated their different purposes and manifestations, and discussed regulatory and statistical issues in selecting appropriate study outcomes so that researchers have a clear idea of what to consider as they make choices on which outcomes to include in their studies.

Key Facts

- Primary outcomes should be measures capable of answering the main research/clinical question and are often expected to measure rates, scale outcomes, detectable patient benefits, risk of disease development, and/or complications, while secondary outcomes are often related to the primary outcomes but typically of lesser importance and/or may be infeasible due to sample size limitations; both are typically related to assessing the efficacy of a therapy.
- Direct endpoints directly describe patient well-being, and may be objective, i.e., explicitly measure clinical outcomes, or subjective, which often depend on subject self-report.
- Surrogate or biomarker endpoints substitute for direct endpoints and are often employed when direct endpoints are infeasible and/or unethical to measure. Many are biomarkers, which objectively measure biological processes, pathologies, and/or responses to exposures or interventions, whereas surrogate endpoints are tantamount to the outcome of interest itself.
- Safety outcomes measure negative health consequences such as side effects or adverse events and help assess the trade-offs between the benefits and risks of therapies.

- Choosing outcome measures requires both practical and statistical considerations. Practical considerations include the ability to capture the physical phenomenon of interest, interpretability, while statistical considerations include validity, reliability, and the ability to answer the clinical questions.
- Outcome measurements may depend on a patient's subjective experience (patient-reported), require some degree of medical/professional expertise (clinician-reported), or be measurable by some other third party who is neither a medical professional nor the patient (observer-reported).

References

Barker-Collo SL (2005) Within session practice effects on the PASAT in clients with multiple sclerosis. Arch Clin Neuropsychol 20:145–152. https://doi.org/10.1016/j.acn.2004.03.007

Bartko JJ (1966) The intraclass correlation coefficient as a measure of reliability. Psychol Rep 19:3–11

Bauer DJ, Sterba SK (2011) Fitting multilevel models with ordinal outcomes: performance of alternative specifications and methods of estimation. Psychol Methods 16(4):373–390. https://doi.org/10.1037/a0025813

Benjamini Y, Cohen R (2017) Weighted false discovery rate controlling procedures for clinical trials. Biostatistics 18(1):91–104. https://doi.org/10.1093/biostatistics/kxw030

FDA-NIH Biomarker Working Group. BEST (Biomarkers, EndpointS, and other Tools) Resource [Internet]. Silver Spring (MD): Food and Drug Administration (US); 2016-. Available from: https://www.ncbi.nlm.nih.gov/books/NBK326791/ Co-published by National Institutes of Health (US), Bethesda (MD).

Carpenter JR, Kenward MG (2007) Missing data in randomised controlled trials – a practical guide. National Institute for Health Research, Birmingham

Chen J, Luo J, Liu K, Mehrotra DV (2011) On power and sample size computation for multiple testing procedures. Comput Stat Data Anal 55:110–122

Cohen JA, Cutter GR, Jill FS, Goodman AD, Heidenreich FR, Jak AJ, ... Whitaker JN (2001) Use of the multiple sclerosis functional composite as an outcome measure in a phase 3 clinical trial. Arch Neurol 58: 961–967

Cohen JA, Reingold SC, Polman CH, Wolinsky JS (2012) Disability outcome measures in multiple sclerosis clinical trials: current status and future prospects. Lancet Neurol 11:467–476

Cutter GR, Baier ML, Rudick RA, Cookfair DL, Fischer JS, Petkau KS, ... Reingold S (1999) Development of a multiple sclerosis functional composite as a clinical trial outcome measure. Brain 122(5): 871–882. https://doi.org/10.1093/brain/122.5.871

Edwards LJ, Simpson SL (2014) An analysis of 24-hour ambulatory blood pressure monitoring data using orthonormal polynomials in the linear mixed model. Blood Press Monit 19(3):153–163. https://doi.org/10.1097/MBP.0000000000000039

FDA (2009) Guidance for industry patient-reported outcome measures: use in medical product development to support labeling claims. U.S. Department of Health and Human Services Food and Drug Administration. Retrieved from https://www.fda.gov/downloads/drugs/guidances/ucm193282.pdf

FDA (2017) Multiple endpoints in clinical trials: guidance for industry. U.S. Department of Health and Human Services Food and Drug Administration. Retrieved from https://www.fda.gov/downloads/drugs/guidancecomplianceregulatoryinformation/guidances/ucm536750.pdf

Haime M (2016) Somahlution announces study results showing DuraGraft® vascular graft treatment improves long-term outcomes in coronary artery bypass grafting surgery. European Association for cardio-thoracic surgery annual meeting. Barcelona. Retrieved from https://www.somahlution.com/vascular-graft-treatment/

Hedeker D (2015) Methods for multilevel ordinal data in prevention research. Prev Sci 16(7):997–1006. https://doi.org/10.1007/s11121-014-0495-x

Hedeker D, Gibbons RD (2006) Longitudinal data analysis. Wiley, Hoboken

Huque MF, Dmitrienko A, D'Agostino R (2013) Multiplicity issues in clinical trials with multiple objectives. Stat Biopharmaceut Res 5(4):321–337. https://doi.org/10.1080/19466315.2013.807749

Kennedy RE, Cutter GR, Wang G, Schneider LS (2015) Using baseline cognitive severity for enriching Alzheimer's disease clinical trials: how does mini-mental state examination predict rate of change? Alzheimer's Dementia: Transl Res Clin Interven 1:46–52. https://doi.org/10.1016/j.trci.2015.03.001

Mallinckrodt CH, Sanger TM, Dubé S, DeBrota DJ, Molenberghs G, Carrol RJ, . . . Tollefson GD (2003) Assessing and interpreting treatment effects in longitudinal clinical trials with missing data. Biol Psychiatry 53:754–760

Motooka Y, Matsui T, Slaton RM, Umetsu R, Fukuda A, Naganuma M, . . . Nakamura M (2018) Adverse events of smoking cessation treatments (nicotine replacement therapy and non-nicotine prescription medication) and electronic cigarettes in the Food and Drug Administration Adverse Event Reporting System, 2004–2016. SAGE Open Med 6:1–11. https://doi.org/10.1177/2050312118777953

Pocock SJ (1997) Clinical trials with multiple outcomes: a statistical perspective on their design, analysis, and interpretation. Control Clin Trials 18:530–545

Powney M, Williamson P, Kirkham J, Kolamunnage-Dona R (2014) A review of handling missing longitudinal outcome data in clinical trials. Trials 15:237. https://doi.org/10.1186/1745-6215-15-237

Prentice RL (1989) Surrogate endpoints in clinical trials: definition and operational criteria. Stat Med 8(4):431–440. https://doi.org/10.1002/sim.4780080407

Shrout PE, Fleiss JL (1979) Intraclass correlations: uses in assessing rater reliability. Psychol Bull 86(2):420–428

Simon R, Maitournam A (2004) Evaluating the efficiency of targeted designs for randomized clinical trials. Clin Cancer Res 10:6759–6763. https://doi.org/10.1158/1078-0432.CCR-04-0496

Sormani MP, Bonzano L, Luca R, Cutter GR, Mancardi GL, Bruzzi P (2009) Magnetic resonance imaging as a potential surrogate for relapses in multiple sclerosis: a meta-analytic approach. Ann Neurol 65:268–275. https://doi.org/10.1002/ana.21606

Sormani MP, Bonzano L, Luca R, Mancardi GL, Ucceli A, Bruzzi P (2010) Surrogate endpoints for EDSS worsening in multiple sclerosis. A meta-analytic approach. Neurology 75(4):302–309. https://doi.org/10.1212/WNL.0b013e3181ea15aa

Sozu T, Sugimoto T, Hamasaki T (2011) Sample size determination in superiority clinical trials with multiple co-primary correlated endpoints. J Biopharm Stat 21:650–668. https://doi.org/10.1080/10543406.2011.551329

Sozu T, Sugimoto T, Hamasaki T (2012) Sample size determination in clinical trials with multiple co-primary endpoints including mixed continuous and binary variables. Biom J 54(5):716–729. https://doi.org/10.1002/bimj.201100221

Sullivan EJ (n.d.) Clinical trials endpoints. U.S. Food and Drug Administration. Retrieved November 19, 2018, from https://www.fda.gov/downloads/Training/ClinicalInvestigatorTrainingCourse/UCM337268.pdf

Surrogate Endpoint Resources for Drug and Biologic Development (n.d.) U.S. Food and Drug Administration. Retrieved November 19, 2018, from https://www.fda.gov/Drugs/DevelopmentApprovalProcess/DevelopmentResources/ucm606684.htm

Swartz RJ, Schwartz C, Basch E, Cai L, Fairclough DL, Mendoza TR, Rapkin B (2011) The king's foot of patient-reported outcomes: current practice and new developments for the measurements of change. Qual Life Res 20:1159–1167. https://doi.org/10.1007/s11136-011-9863-1

Wolfe GI, Kaminski HJ, Aban IB, Minisman G, Kuo H-C, Marx A, . . . Evoli A (2016) Randomized trial of thymectomy in myasthenia gravis. N Engl J Med 375(6):511–522. https://doi.org/10.1056/NEJMoa1602489

Patient-Reported Outcomes

51

Gillian Gresham and Patricia A. Ganz

Contents

G. Gresham
Samuel Oschin Comprehensive Cancer Institute, Cedars-Sinai Medical Center, Los Angeles, CA, USA
e-mail: gillian.gresham@cshs.org

P. A. Ganz (✉)
Jonsson Comprehensive Cancer Center, University of California at Los Angeles, Los Angeles, CA, USA
e-mail: PGanz@mednet.ucla.edu

© Springer Nature Switzerland AG 2022

S. Piantadosi, C. L. Meinert (eds.), *Principles and Practice of Clinical Trials*,
https://doi.org/10.1007/978-3-319-52636-2_241

Abstract

Patient-reported outcomes (PROs) are defined as any report that comes directly from a patient. Their use as key outcomes in clinical trials has increased significantly, especially during the last decade. PROs encompass a variety of measurements including health-related quality of life (HRQOL), symptoms, functional status, safety, utilities, and satisfaction ratings. Selection of the PRO in a trial will depend on a variety of factors including the trial's objectives, study population, disease or condition, as well as the type of treatment or intervention. PROs can be used to inform clinical care and to support drug approval and labeling claims. This chapter will provide an overview of the different types of PROs with examples and their role in healthcare within the context of clinical trials. Summaries of important regulatory documents including the FDA PRO guidance and recommendations (SPIRIT and CONSORT PRO extensions) will also be provided. Considerations when designing clinical trials are described in the last section, highlighting important issues and topics that are unique to PROs. Many methodologic and analytic features of PROs are similar to those of any outcomes used in clinical trials; thus they require the same methodological rigor with special attention to missing data. This chapter is written with a focus on the use of PROs in interventional trials in the United States, although most information can be applied to any context. Information presented in this chapter is relevant to clinicians, researchers, policy makers, regulatory and funding agencies, as well as patients. When used appropriately, PROs can generate high-quality data about the effects of a particular intervention on a patient's physical, psychological, functional, and symptomatic experience.

Keywords

Patient-reported outcomes (PROs) · Quality of life · Health-related quality of life · Health status · Symptoms · Adverse events · NIH PROMIS

Introduction

During the last two decades, patient-reported outcomes (PROs) have increasingly been used in clinical trials to inform clinical care and to support drug approval and labeling claims. PROs are defined as: "any report of the status of a patient's health condition that comes directly from the patient, without interpretation of the patient's response by a clinician or anyone else" (FDA 2009). A list of key terms related to PROs and their definitions is included in Table 1.

There are several key regulatory and academic events that led to the increased incorporation of PROs in clinical trials. Some of the first research studies to use PROs included the Alameda County Human Population Laboratory Studies, the RAND Health Insurance Experiment, and the Medical Outcome Studies occurring in the 1970s and 1980s (Ganz et al. cited in Kominski 2013). In July 1990, the US

Table 1 List of key terms and definitions related to PROs

Term	Definition
Comparative effectiveness research (CER)	The generation and synthesis of evidence that compares the benefits and harms of alternative methods to prevent, diagnose, treat, and monitor a clinical condition or to improve the delivery of care[a]
Construct validity	Evidence that relationships among items, domains, and concepts conform to a priori hypotheses concerning logical relationships that should exist with other measures or characteristics of patients and patient groups[b]
Content validity	Evidence from qualitative research demonstrating that the instrument measures the concept of interest including evidence that the items and domains of an instrument are appropriate and comprehensive relative to its intended measurement concept, population, and use. Testing other measurement properties will not replace or rectify problems with content validity[b]
Criterion validity	The extent to which the scores of a PRO instrument are related to a known gold standard measure of the same concept. For most PROs, criterion validity cannot be measured because there is no gold standard[b]
Domain	A subconcept represented by a score of an instrument that measures a larger concept comprised of multiple domains. For example, psychological function is the larger concept containing the domains subdivided into items describing emotional function and cognitive function[b]
Health-related quality of life (HRQOL)	A subcomponent of overall quality of life that relates to health and that focuses on the patient's own perception of Well-being and the ability to function as a result of health status or disease experience[a]
Item	An individual question, statement, or task (and its standardized response options) that is evaluated by the patient to address a particular concept[b]
Outcomes of care	Refers to specific indicators of what happens to the patient once care has been rendered[a]
Patient-reported outcome (PRO)	A measurement based on a report that comes directly from the patient (i.e., study subject) about the status of a patient's health condition without amendment or interpretation of the patient's response by a clinician or anyone else. A PRO can be measured by self-report or by interview provided that the interviewer records only the patient's response.[b]
Process of care	Refers to the content of the medical and psychological interactions between patient and provider[a]
Quality-adjusted life years (QALY)	A measure of life expectancy with adjustment for quality of life that integrates mortality and morbidity to express health status in terms of equivalents of well-years of life[a]
Quality of life	A range of human experience, including but not limited to access to the daily necessities of life such as food and shelter, intrapersonal and interpersonal response to life events, and activities associated with professional fulfillment and personal happiness[a]

(continued)

Table 1 (continued)

Term	Definition
Questionnaire	A set of questions or items shown to a respondent to get answers for research purposes. Types of questionnaires include diaries and event logs[b]
Reliability	The ability of a PRO instrument to yield consistent, reproducible estimates of true treatment effect[b]
Sign	Any objective evidence of a disease, health condition, or treatment-related effect. Signs are usually observed and interpreted by the clinician but may be noticed and reported by the patient[b]
Structure of care	Refers to how medical and other services are organized in a particular institution or delivery system[a]
Symptom	Any subjective evidence of a disease, health condition, or treatment-related effect that can be noticed and known only by the patient[b]

[a]Definitions transcribed from Ganz et al. (2014)
[b]Definitions transcribed from US Department of Health and Human Services: Food and Drug Administration (2009)

National Cancer Institute held an all-day workshop to discuss the inclusion of PROs in cancer clinical trials, informing subsequent strategies for their use in federally funded cancer trials (Nayfield et al. 1992). Additional regulatory advancements in the early 2000s include the draft of the EMA Reflection Paper on HRQL (2005) and release of the Food and Drug Administration (FDA) draft guidance in 2006. In 2009, the FDA published final guidance regarding the use of PROs for medical product development to support labeling claims (FDA 2009). The guidance provides information related to the evaluation of a PRO instrument and clinical trial design and protocol considerations. This guidance will be used throughout this chapter to support recommendations for the design of clinical trials that incorporate PROs.

Another key event in the history of PROs in the United States was the establishment of the Patient-Centered Outcomes Research Institute (PCORI) as part of the 2010 Affordable Care Act (Frank et al. 2014). PCORI is an independent nonprofit, nongovernmental organization that funds a wide range of research that incorporates the patient perspective and will improve healthcare delivery and patient outcomes. It is the largest public research funder that focuses on comparative effectiveness research (CER) having funded over $2 billion dollars in research and related projects to date. A unique feature of PCORI includes the active engagement of patients and stakeholders throughout the research and review process (Frank et al. 2014). The PCORI merit review includes five criteria that address the "impact of the condition on the health of individuals and populations, population for the study to improve health care and outcomes, technical merit, patient-centeredness, and patient and stakeholder engagement" (Frank et al. 2014). Additional funding information and details about PCORI can be found at the following web link: https://www.pcori.org/.

The purpose of this chapter is to provide a summary of the role of PROs within the context of clinical trials, describe different types of PROs currently being used, and include PRO-specific considerations to take into account when designing a clinical trial. Additional information regarding outcomes more broadly and the analysis of PROs are provided in ▶ Chaps. 50, "Outcomes in Clinical Trials" and ▶ 92, "Statistical Analysis of Patient-Reported Outcomes in Clinical Trials," respectively.

Role of PROs in Clinical Trials

PROs play different, but equally important roles across each phase of drug development (e.g., Phase I, II, III, IV). The role of the PRO depends largely on the clinical trial endpoint model, defined in the FDA 2009 PRO guidance as "a diagram of the hierarchy of relationships among all endpoints, both PRO and non-PRO, that corresponds to the clinical trial's objectives, design, and data analysis plan" (FDA 2009). The conceptual framework for each endpoint model is illustrated in Figs. 1 and 2 as adapted from the FDA guidance. A PRO may be defined as the primary, secondary, or exploratory endpoint in a clinical trial. If used as a primary endpoint, the methods for sample size determination and power calculations should be included, as described further in ▶ Chap. 92, "Statistical Analysis of Patient-Reported Outcomes in Clinical Trials." Regardless of the type of outcome, the specific PRO hypothesis and objectives should be clearly stated a priori along with details of the instrument's conceptual framework and measurement properties in the protocol.

The use of PROs across all phases of clinical trials, as registered in clinicaltrials.gov between 2000 and 2018, has increased over time as displayed in Fig. 3. Based on a general search of clinicaltrials.gov, we identified approximately 146 trials that included PROs or HRQOL as outcomes in 2000, 693 in 2005, 1056 in 2010, and

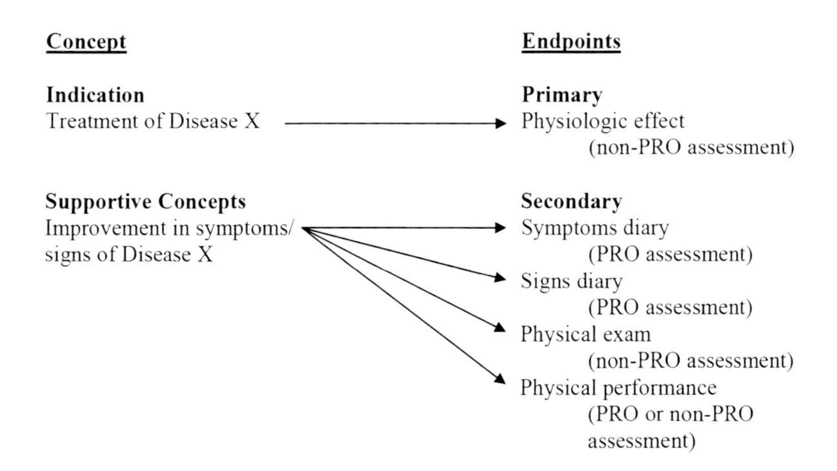

Fig. 1 Endpoint model: Treatment of disease X

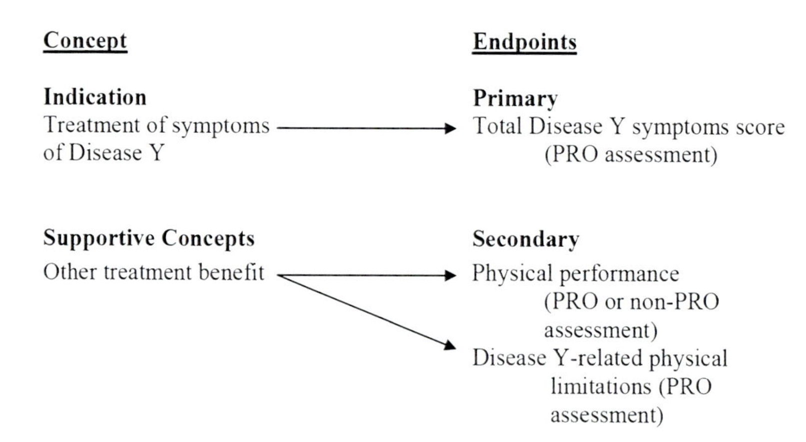

Fig. 2 Endpoint model: Treatment of symptoms associated with disease Y

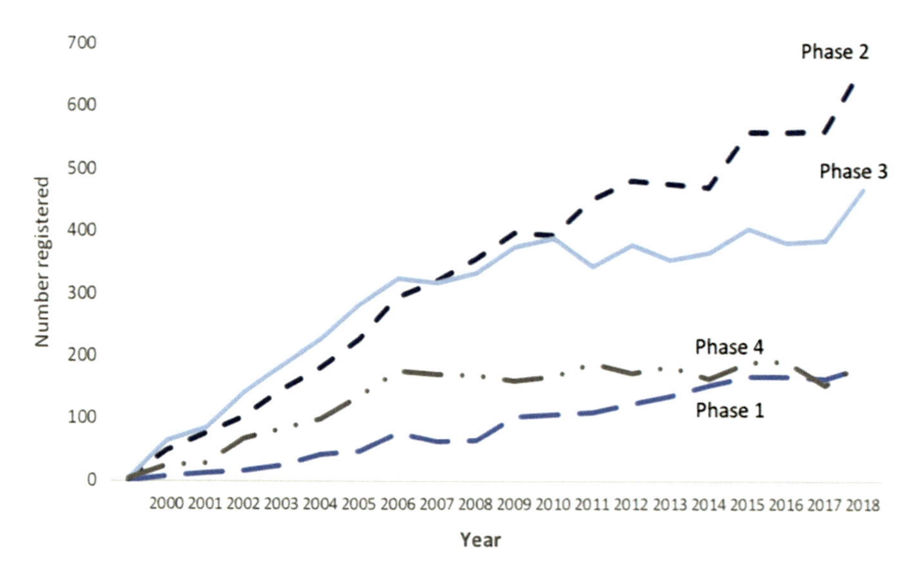

Fig. 3 Number of clinical trials with PROs registered in clinicaltrials.gov by phase

1505 in 2018. The majority of trials registered during this period were phase 2 ($n = 6768$), phase 3 ($n = 5807$) followed by phase 4 (2715), and phase 1 ($n = 1769$).

In early development trials (phase I/II), PROs can provide important information about specific toxicities and symptoms before the treatment progresses to the next phase (Lipscomb et al. 2005; Basch et al. 2016). In the earlier phases of clinical trials, disease-specific measures and PROs may be more useful and clinically relevant to clinicians and patients (Spilker 1996). Because early phase trials enroll selective groups of subjects, PROs should be employed cautiously (Lipscomb et al. 2005). Early phase trials are less likely to support PRO labeling claims but can provide early insight into toxicity and tolerability of new drugs or devices.

PROs are especially informative in situations where a disease may be well-controlled by either of the interventions being compared but the symptom profile and HRQOL are different. Thus, the use of PRO assessments as primary outcomes in middle to late development (Phase II–III) studies is appropriate in this setting and can help inform clinical decisions (Piantadosi 2017). In middle and late development trials, PROs can provide important information regarding the baseline and treatment symptom profiles as well as provide additional data for comparing the tolerability between treatments (Basch et al. 2016). Thus, well-designed phase III trials with PROs may inform policy and support labeling claims. PROs may also play a role in post-marketing (phase IV) studies with regard to the long-term treatment effects and safety surveillance (Basch et al. 2016).

PROs to Support Labeling Claims in the United States

There has been an increasing call for the incorporation of the patient voice into FDA drug approval and labeling claims. This led to the release of PRO-specific FDA guidance for industry (FDA 2009). The 2009 FDA guidance for use of PROs to support labeling claims provides recommendations for areas that should be addressed in PRO documents that are submitted to the FDA for review (FDA 2009). To ensure high-quality PRO data that is used to support the labeling claims, the guidance focuses on the evaluation of the PRO instrument and design considerations. Briefly, these areas include as follows: (I) the PRO instrument being used along with instructions; (II) targeted claims or target product profile related to the trial outcome measures (e.g., disease or condition, intended population, data analysis plan); (III) the endpoint model; (IV) the PRO instrument's conceptual framework; (V) documentation for content validity; (VI) assessment of other measurement properties (e.g., reliability, construct validity); (VII) interpretation of scores; (VIII) language translations (if applicable); (IX) the data collection method; (X) any modifications to the original instrument with justification; (XI) the protocol including PRO-specific content; and (XII) key references. Detail and explanation for each of these topics are included in the Appendix of the final 2009 FDA guidance document and described within the context of clinical trial design in a later section.

While the FDA PRO guidance marks a significant advancement for the field, the use of PROs to support labeling claims and their inclusion in published reports of clinical trials remains low (Basch 2012). In the United States, it has been reported that approximately 20-25% of all drug approvals were supported by PROs between 2006, when the FDA draft guidance was released, and 2015, despite the fact that 50% of drug approval packages included PRO endpoints (Basch 2012; DeMuro et al. 2013). A literature review identified 182 NDAs between 2011 and 2015, for which 16.5% had PRO labeling, defined as any treatment benefit related to PROs that are mentioned in the FDA product label (Gnanasakthy et al. 2017). Authors found that the majority of PRO labeling has been based on primary outcomes in PRO-dependent diseases (e.g., mental, behavioral, and neurodevelopment disorders, diseases of the respiratory system, diseases of the musculoskeletal system, etc.) as compared to non-PRO-dependent diseases (e.g., neoplasms, infection and parasitic diseases, diseases of the circulatory system, etc.) The majority of new drugs approved supported by PRO labeling were in diseases of the nervous system, musculoskeletal system, and genitourinary system. For example, there were 23 new drugs approved in diseases of the nervous system between 2006 and 2015, for which over half ($n = 13$) were approved based on PRO labeling (Gnanasakthy et al. 2017). Treatment approvals included gabapentin enacarbil for restless legs syndrome, where the International Restless Legs Syndrome (IRLS) Rating Scale was used to support labeling, perampanel and eslicarbazepine acetate to treat seizures using patient diaries to record seizures, and tasimelteon or suvorexant to treat sleep disorders using patient-reported sleep latency and time.

Other notable PROs used to support drug approvals included the Pain Visual Analog Scale (VAS) for conditions of the musculoskeletal system (e.g., arthritis), diaries for rescue medication in diseases of the respiratory system, and other diaries and self-reported accounts of gastrointestinal or genitourinary symptoms. Of the 69 new drug approvals in neoplasms between 2006 and 2015, none of them had PRO labeling (Gnanasakthy et al. 2017). A second review identified three treatments that used PRO data to support their FDA approval, including the Brief Pain Inventory-Short Form (BPI-SF) for abiraterone in prostate cancer (2011), the Myelofibrosis Symptom Assessment Form (MFSAF) to support the approval of ruxolitinib for myelofibrosis (2011), and the Visual Symptom Assessment Questionnaire-Anaplastic Lymphoma Kinase (VSAQ-ALK) to support the approval of crizotinib for non-small cell lung cancer (Gnanasakthy et al. 2016). Authors suggest that the low rates of PRO labeling in oncology are due to the fact that the development of cancer drugs mostly relies on survival-related outcomes and tumor growth to assess treatment efficacy (Gnanasakthy et al. 2017; Kluetz and Pazdur 2016). However, the inclusion of PROs in pivotal cancer studies may help increase PRO labeling in future drug approvals and are essential to the development and review of oncology drugs (Basch 2018). Additional recommendations for sponsors and the FDA to increase the success of including PROs in clinical trials and US drug labels have been provided in Basch (2012).

PROs to Support Labeling Claims in Other Countries

While other countries have not issued formal guidelines specific to PROs such as the US 2009 FDA guidance for PROs, recommendations exist for the use of PROs to support the evaluation and approval of drug products. Perspectives of different International regulatory scientists, focusing on the incorporation of PROs into the regulatory decision-making process has been described in a recent paper by Kluetz et al. (2018). In Europe, the European Medicines Agency (EMA) published a reflection paper that provides recommendations on HRQOL evaluation within the context of clinical trials (European Medicines Agency 2005; DeMuro et al. 2013). A review published in 2013 compared PRO label claims granted by the FDA to those granted by the EMA between 2006 and 2010 (DeMuro et al. 2013). The authors found that the EMA granted more PRO labels with 47% of products with at least one EMA-granted PRO label compared to 19% by the FDA. They also observed that the majority of FDA claims focus on symptoms, while the EMA-granted claims are more likely to approve treatments based on higher-order concepts such as HRQOL, patient global ratings, and functioning. Of the 52 PRO label claims granted by both agencies, 14 products were approved by both the FDA and EMA (DeMuro et al. 2013). The UK National Institute for Clinical Excellence (NICE) has also provided guidance for the inclusion of patients and public in treatment evaluations (NICE 2006).

In most parts of Europe, Australia, and Canada, PROs are included as an important component of health technology assessment (HTA). The WHO defines HTA as: "The systematic evaluation of properties, effects, and/or impacts of health technology." HTA was first developed in the United States in the 1970s as a policy tool and later introduced to Europe, Canada, the United Kingdom, and Scandinavia (Banta 2003). HTA is used to support healthcare policy and inform reimbursement and coverage insurers (Banta 2003). Although the United States supports HTA research, also as a component of comparative effectiveness research, no formal HTA agencies exist in the United States. Within the context of clinical trials, survival, QOL, and cost-effectiveness outcomes generated from clinical trials are subsequently used to inform HTA. Thus, it is important that trials are designed to incorporate these important and informative outcomes in order to generate high-quality evidence.

Types of PROs

PROs encompass a variety of measurements including health-related quality of life (HRQOL), symptoms, functional status, safety, utilities, and satisfaction ratings (FDA 2009; Calvert et al. 2013). The following sections describe some key PRO measurements that can be included as outcomes in clinical trials.

There are several instruments that have been developed to target different populations with different purposes. PRO assessments can be categorized into generic and disease-specific instruments based on the concepts they are measuring. Generic measures may be useful when evaluating core domains of function and well-being across various populations and to detect differential effects on more general aspects of health status (Spilker 1996; Lipscomb et al. 2005). While they may allow comparison across interventions, they may not focus adequately on a specific area of interest and may not be as responsive as disease-specific measurements (Spilker 1996). Generic measures may be appropriate when there is a large trade-off between length of life and quality of life, which feeds into the concept of quality-adjusted life years (QALY) and quality-adjusted time without symptoms or toxicity (Q-TWIST), where generic population-based assessments have been used (see discussion of QALYs later).

Utility measures are a second type of generic instrument, which "reflect the preferences of patients for different health states" (Spilker 1996). Their use may be appropriate when it is of interest to assess health states as they relate to death or if investigators want to conduct cost-utility analyses. Because utility measures provide a single summary score of the net change in HRQL, they do not allow for examination of effect on the different aspects of quality of life (Spilker 1996).

Finally, disease-specific measures focus on the distinguishing features of functional status and well-being that are specific to different diseases or conditions (e.g., heart failure, cancer), populations (e.g., frail or elderly), functions (e.g., sleep, sexual function), or problems (e.g., pain) (Spilker 1996). Because they only include the aspects of PROs that are relevant to the patients being studied, they may result in improved responsiveness. Often, several disease-specific measures are used together in a battery to obtain a more comprehensive picture of the impact of treatment interventions (Spilker 1996). For example, a clinical trial that is evaluating the effect of a particular treatment on HRQL may include measures of physical function, pain, sleep, and side effects as they relate to that treatment. Some weaknesses of disease-specific assessments include the fact that they may be limited in terms of populations and interventions, there may be restricted domains of relevance to the specific disease, population, function, or problem, and they do not allow cross-condition comparisons (Spilker 1996).

Health-Related QOL (HRQOL)

HRQOL is a special type of PRO that is widely used in clinical trials (Piantadosi 2017). It is considered an outcome of care that focuses on a "patient's own perception of well-being, and the ability to function as a result of health status or disease experience" (Ganz et al. 2014). The World Health Organization (WHO) defines health as: "A state of complete physical, mental and social well-being and not merely the absence of disease or infirmity," and it has been schematically represented in three levels of QOL that included the overall assessment of well-being, broad domains, and the specific components of each domain (Spilker 1996). Early reviews of the MEDLINE database demonstrated an exponential increase in the number of studies that used QOL evaluation, with only five studies identified in 1973 and 9291 articles in 2010 (Testa and Simonson 1996; Ganz et al. 2014). In 2018, this number is just over 34,000 articles, using "quality of life" as a topic heading with 1532 if restricted to human clinical trials. In a clinicaltrials.gov search of the term "quality of life," a total of 28,886 interventional trials started between 01/01/2000 and 12/31/2018 were identified. It is anticipated that this number will continue to grow as the relevance and value of QOL are increasingly recognized.

HRQOL is measured using instruments (self-administered questionnaires) that contain questions or items that are subsequently organized into scales (Ganz et al. 2014). HRQOL instruments may be general, addressing common components of functioning and well-being, or disease-targeted, which focus on the specific impact of the particular organ dysfunctions that affect HRQOL (Patrick and Deyo 1989 in: Ganz et al. 2014). HRQOL is considered multidimensional, consisting of different domains (physical, psychological, economic, spiritual, social) and specific measurement scales within each domain (Testa and Simonson 1996; Spilker 1996). The overall assessment of well-being or global HRQOL score is often achieved by summing scores across the different domains or may contain a global rating scale for summary. Scores can also be established by each of the broad domains (e.g., physical domain) or of the specific item (e.g., symptoms, functioning, disability).

One of the most common generic HRQOL instruments, emerging from the Medical Outcomes Study (RAND Corporation), is the SF-36. It is composed of 36 items across 8 scales (physical functioning, role-physical, bodily pain, general health, vitality, social functioning, role-emotional, mental health), which can be further grouped into physical health and mental health summary measures. An abbreviated, but equivalent version of the SF-36 was also developed through the MOS and includes 12 items (SF-12) summarized into the mental and physical domains. The SF-36 and SF-12 have been particularly useful in comparing the relative burden of different diseases. They also have potential for evaluating the QOL burden from different treatments (Spilker 1996).

An example of a disease-specific instrument of QOL is the European Organization for Research and Treatment of Cancer (EORTC) QLQ-30 questionnaire (Aaronson et al. 1993). The QLQ-30 is a cancer-specific questionnaire that was developed from an international field study of 305 patients from centers across 13 different countries. The QLQ-C30 is composed of nine multi-item scales, which include functional scales (physical, role, emotional, cognitive, social), symptom scales (fatigue, nausea/vomiting, pain, dyspnea, sleep disturbance, appetite loss, constipation, diarrhea, financial impact), and a global health and QOL scale. The EORTC questionnaire and its many cancer-specific modules have been used throughout the world to evaluate the HRQOL outcomes in cancer treatment trials: (https://www.eortc.org/). Comprehensive inventory of HRQOL instruments is available online at https://eprovide.mapi-trust.org/ with information for over 2000 generic and disease-specific instruments.

Healthcare Utility and Cost-Effectiveness

HRQOL can be used as utility coefficients to weight or adjust for outcomes such as survival or progression-free survival and inform policy and healthcare decisions. For example, quality-adjusted life years (QALY) are a measure of life expectancy that adjusts for QOL (Kominski 2014). QALYs are often used to evaluate programs and assist in decision-making processes where the Institute of Medicine (IOM) Committee on Public Health Strategies to Improve Health recommended that QALYs are used to monitor the health status of all communities (Institute of Medicine 2011). Consequently, there have been an increasing number of studies in which QALYs have appeared in the literature, and advancements in methodologies for measuring and reporting QALYs have been made (Ganz et al. in Kominski 2014). QALYs can also be combined with cost evaluations, where the cost per QALY can be used to show the relative efficiency of different health programs. While QALYs have played an important role in health policy, they are also associated with limitations and obstacles for which the Affordable Care Act states that QALYs cannot be used for resource allocation decisions, and thus studies funded by PCORI do not include these assessments (Ganz et al. in Kominski 2014). However, in the United Kingdom, and other jurisdictions, their assessments play an important role in drug and device approval processes.

Another measure that incorporates quantity and quality of life is the quality-adjusted time without symptoms of disease and toxicity of treatment (Q-TWIST). It is based on the concept of QALYs and represents a utility-based approach to QOL assessment in clinical trials (Spilker 1996). Q-TWIST is calculated by subtracting the number of days with specified disease symptoms or treatment-induced toxicities from the total number of days of survival (Lipscomb et al. 2005). It requires calculation of QOL-oriented clinical health states, for which treatments can then be compared using a weighted sum of the mean duration of each health state with weights being utility-based (Spilker 1996; Lipscomb et al. 2005). Often, the area under the Kaplan-Meier survival curves is partitioned to calculate the average time a patient spends in each clinical health state. An example of where Q-TWIST was informative is in the case of adjuvant chemotherapy with tamoxifen for breast cancer versus tamoxifen alone, where findings demonstrated the additional burden the cytotoxic chemotherapy imposed on patients (Gelber et al. cited in Lipscomb et al. 2005). Another example is in a trial that demonstrated lengthened progression-free survival (0.9 months) with zidovudine in patients with mildly symptomatic HIV infection. However, Q-TWIST showed that patients who were treated with zidovudine did worse (Spilker 1996). Additional details and analysis information related to QALYs and Q-TWIST are described in ▶ Chap. 92, "Statistical Analysis of Patient-Reported Outcomes in Clinical Trials."

PROs Developed by the National Institutes of Health (NIH)

NIH PROMIS®

In 2004, the NIH established the Patient-Reported Outcomes Measurement Information System (PROMIS®) as part of a multicenter cooperative group with the purpose of developing and validating PROs for clinical research and practice (Cella et al. 2010). PROMIS® consists of over 300 self-reported and parent-reported measures of global, physical, mental, and social health. This domain mapping process was built based on the WHO framework of physical, mental, and social health. Qualitative research and item response theory (IRT) analysis from 11 large datasets informed an item library of close to 7000 PRO items to be further reviewed and evaluated in field testing (Cella et al. 2010). PROMIS® measurement tools have been validated in adults and children from the general population and those living with chronic conditions. Additional information and PROMIS® measures are available through the official information and distribution center: HealthMeasures (http://www.healthmeasures.net/index.php).

The adult PROMIS® measures framework is composed of the PROMIS® profile domains and additional domains, which are further categorized into physical, mental, or social health components (HealthMeasures 2019). Physical health measures include fatigue, pain intensity, pain interference, physical function, and sleep disturbance. Mental health profile domains include anxiety depression, and social health includes the ability to participate in social roles and activities. A general global health measure also makes up the self-reported health framework. The complete framework and a list of additional PROMIS® domains can be accessed at http://www.healthmeasures.net/explore-measurement-systems/promis/intro-to-promis.

A framework for pediatric self-reported and proxy-reported health was also developed including the same health measures (physical, mental, social, global health) with slightly different profile and additional domains. For instance, physical health adds mobility and upper extremity function to the list of physical profile domains, while sleep disturbance is not included. Anxiety and depressive symptoms represent profile domains for mental health, while peer relationships are assessed as part of social health.

PROMIS® measures can be administered using computer adaptive testing or on paper through short forms or profiles (HealthMeasures 2019). The PROMIS® self-report measures are intended to be completed by the respondent themselves without the help from others, unless they are unable to answer on their own, in which case a parent or proxy measure may be used. Computer adaptive tests and short forms can be imported into common data platforms and web applications such as REDCap, Epic, OBERD, the Assessment Center (SM), and the Assessment Center Application Programming Interface (API), which can connect any data collection software application with the full library of PROMIS® measures.

PROMIS® items include questions accompanied by Likert-type responses (e.g., not at all, very little, somewhat, quite a lot, cannot do), which are associated with a numerical score (0–5). The sums of the scores can then be converted into standardized T-scores through the HealthMeasures scoring service, automatic scoring in data collection tools, or manually. T-score metrics have a mean of 50 and standard deviation of 10, making it easy to compare to reference populations including the general population and clinical samples (e.g., cancer, pain populations) (Cella et al. 2007). PROMIS® scores can also be converted to similar items from different instruments such as the SF-36. For example, a PROMIS® physical T-score for physical function can be linked to the SF-36 physical function score (www.prosettastone.org). This allows for PRO evaluation and comparisons even when different measures are used.

The use of PROMIS® measures in clinical trials has significantly increased since their development, with over 2000 observational or interventional studies identified in clinicaltrials.gov as of January 2021. The majority of trials that use NIH PROMIS® measures are for pain conditions, musculoskeletal diseases, and mental and psychotic disorders. Their use is also increasing in cancer clinical trials, especially breast cancer, and diseases of the central nervous system.

Patient-Reported Common Terminology Criteria for Adverse Events (PRO-CTCAE)

In 2014, the NCI developed PRO-CTCAE in order to incorporate the patient perspective and improve symptom monitoring in cancer (Basch et al. 2014; Dy et al. 2014; Atkinson et al. 2017; Dueck et al. 2015), reflecting toxicities and adverse events typically measured by clinical trial staff as part of the Common Terminology Criteria for Adverse Events (CTCAE) assessment system. The PRO-CTCAE measurement system includes 78 treatment toxicities that patients can systematically use to document the frequency, severity, and interference of each toxicity (Basch et al. 2014). PRO-CTCAE includes a library of 124 questions that can be selected to include as relevant to the specific trial. Each question includes a measure of the frequency of the AE (e.g., "never," "rarely," "occasionally," "frequently," "almost constantly"), the severity ("none," "mild," "moderate," "severe," "very severe"), or the interference with usual or daily activities ("not at all," "a little bit," "somewhat," "quite a bit," "very much") (Basch et al. 2016). The patient-reported AEs can be systematically collected at baseline, during active treatment, and during follow-up using a pre-populated questionnaire.

An electronic platform for PRO-CTCAE also exists allowing for customized data tailored to a particular treatment schedule and the incorporation of patient reminders and clinician alerts (Dy et al. 2011; Basch et al. 2017b). Studies of both the PRO-CTCAE and electronic PRO-CTCAE symptom collection system have demonstrated feasibility, validity, and reliability of both the PRO-CTCAE and electronic PRO-CTCAE in cancer patients (Dy et al. 2011; Basch et al. 2017a). Their use has also been associated with enhanced care, improved QOL, and survival, possibly as the result of earlier responsiveness to patient symptoms by medical personnel (Basch et al. 2014, 2017; Aaronson et al. 1993).

Design Considerations

The following sections provide summaries of PRO-specific considerations to account for when designing a clinical trial and to include in the clinical trial protocol.

Selection of the Instrument

Selection of the PRO in a trial will depend on a variety of factors including the trial's objectives, study population, disease or condition, as well as the type of treatment or intervention to a certain extent (Piantadosi 2017). When designing a clinical trial, the instrument(s) used should be specified a priori and appropriately selected for the specific population being enrolled in the clinical trial. For instance, additional measurement considerations may need to be accounted for when assessing PROs in pediatric, cognitively impaired, or seriously ill patients (FDA 2009). Investigators should first determine whether an adequate PRO instrument exists to assess and measure the concepts of interest (FDA 2009). In some cases, a new PRO instrument may be developed or modified, with additional steps that would need to be taken to ensure validity and reliability.

Validity and reliability should be supported before using an instrument in a clinical trial. The FDA guidance requires that content validity as well as other validity and reliability to be established as a component of FDA review. The content validity of an instrument, or the extent to which the instrument measures the concept of interest, should be supported by evidence from the literature or preliminary studies and established prior to the evaluation of other measurement properties (FDA 2009). The PRO instrument should also demonstrate reliability, or the ability to yield consistent, reproducible estimates of the true treatment effect (e.g., test-retest reliability), as well as construct validity, the relationships among items, domains, and concepts, and criterion validity, or the extent to which the scores of a PRO instrument are related to a gold standard measure of the same concept, if available (FDA 2009). FDA definitions of validity and reliability are included in Table 1, and a detailed description of how validity and reliability are assessed is described in ► Chap. 50, "Outcomes in Clinical Trials."

The FDA also provides guidance on the review of PRO instrument characteristics including the modes of administration and data collection methods, the frequency and duration of assessments, as well as other considerations specific to the clinical trial design as described in the following sections:

Modes of Administration and Data Collection Methods

There are several different ways that PROs can be administered including self-administration, interview-administered, telephone-administered, surrogate- (or proxy) administered, or a combination of modes (Spilker 1996; Lipscomb et al. 2005; FDA 2009). When selecting the mode of administration and data collection method in a trial, it is important to consider its intended use, the cost, and how missing data can be reduced (Lipscomb et al. 2005). While self-administrated PROs require the minimal amount of resources, they are associated with increased likelihood for missing items, misunderstanding, and lower response rates (Spilker 1996). For both face-to-face and telephone interviews, response rates are maximized, while missing data and errors of misunderstanding are minimized (Spilker 1996). Disadvantages of these methods are that more time and resources are required to train the interviewers and administer the questionnaires. Additionally, for telephone interviews, the format of the instrument is further limited (Spilker 1996). A third option is the use of surrogate responders to complete the assessments. Advantages of using surrogates or proxies are that it is more inclusive of patients who may not be able to complete the questionnaires themselves such as children and those who are cognitively impaired or have language barriers (Spilker 1996). A risk associated with using surrogate responders is that the perceptions of the surrogate may be different from those of the target group and not accurately represent the patient's perspective. For example, proxy reports of more observable domains such as physical or cognitive function domains may be overestimated, while symptoms or signs may be underestimated by proxy respondents (Spilker 1996). Thus, it is important to consider the strengths and weaknesses of each mode of administration and identify the mode that is most relevant and appropriate for each context.

Methods to collect PRO data from either self-administered or interviewer-administered questionnaires include entry on paper by the patient or interviewer or using computer-assisted assessments. While paper-based methods of assessment are the most widely used and may be preferred by some patients, they can result in higher risk of missing items or data due to skipped questions or pages. Alternatively, computer-assisted assessments, such as electronic PROMIS® questionnaires, can include skip patterns, data checks, and forced responses to ensure complete data. The FDA guidance has highlighted specific issues associated with the use of electronic PRO instruments including the entry, maintenance, and transmission of electronic data (FDA 2009). If the electronic PRO instrument is used as the source document, additional requirements must be met including 21 CFR Part 11 compliance and a plan to ensure data security and integrity. As part of the FDA PRO guidance, the FDA will review the clinical trial protocol to determine the steps used to ensure that the patients complete the entries at the specified period using the appropriate administration mode (FDA 2009).

Frequency and Duration of PRO Assessments

The frequency and duration of PRO assessments must correspond to the specific research question and objectives of the particular clinical trial. The frequency of assessments will depend on the natural history of disease, the timing of the therapeutic and diagnostic interventions, and the likelihood of changes in the outcome within the time period (Lipscomb et al. 2005; FDA 2009). Clinical trials with PROs will often require at least one baseline assessment and several PRO assessments over the course of the study period. Assessments should be frequent enough to capture the meaningful change without introducing additional burden to the patients. They should also not be more frequent than the specific period of recall, explained in the next section, as defined in the instrument. For example, if an instrument has a 1-month recall period, assessments should not occur weekly or daily.

The duration of the assessment will also depend on the research question and should cover the period of time that is sufficient to observe changes in the outcome (Lipscomb et al. 2005). Investigators should also consider whether they are interested in specific changes that occur during therapy or the long-term effect of the therapy on that particular outcome. Therefore, the duration of follow-up with a PRO assessment may be the same of other measures of efficacy or may be longer in duration if the study objectives require continued assessment. In the former case, it is important that efforts are made to reduce missing data and loss to follow-up.

Investigators should also take the recall period for the PRO instrument into consideration when designing a trial. This is defined as the period of time patients are asked to consider in responding to a PRO or question and can be momentary or retrospective of varying lengths (FDA 2009). The recall period will depend on the purpose and intended use of the PRO instrument, the concept being measured, and the specific disease and treatment schedule. Items with shorter recall periods are preferred over retrospective as patients are likely to be influenced by their current state during the time of recall (FDA 2009). Thus, the use of PRO instruments with short recall periods administered at regular intervals (e.g., 2, 4, 6 weeks) may enhance the quality of the data and reduce the risk for recall bias but have more chance of missing data.

Other Design Considerations

The FDA PRO guidance also reviews clinical trial design principles unique to PRO endpoints. The first consideration relates to masking (blinding) and randomization of trial participants. In the case of open-label trials, patients may overestimate the treatment benefit in their responses, while those who are not receiving active treatment may underreport any potential improvements (FDA 2009). Authors suggest administering the PRO assessments prior to clinical assessments or procedures to minimize the potential influence on patient perceptions. It is rare that such open-label trials will be adequate to support labeling claims based on PRO instruments. In masked clinical trials, there is still a possibility for inadvertent unblinding if a treatment has obvious effects, such as adverse events. Consequently, similar over- or underreporting of the treatment effect may occur if a patient thinks they are receiving one treatment over the other. To decrease the risk of possible unblinding, the guidance suggests using response options that ask for current status, not giving patients access to previous responses, and using instruments that include many items about the same concept (FDA 2009). Investigators should also take specific host factors into consideration, where randomization may not achieve balance with regard to the specific PROs (psychological and functional outcomes) that participants have at baseline or develop as a result of treatment.

The FDA guidance provides additional recommendations for clinical trial quality control when using PROs in order to ensure standardized assessments and processes. Specifically, the protocol should include information on how both patients and interviewers (if applicable) will be trained for the PRO instrument along with detailed instructions. The protocol should also include instructions regarding the supervision, timing, and order of questionnaire administration as well as the processes and rules for the questionnaire review for completeness; documentation of how and when data are filed, stored, and transmitted to/from a clinical trial site; and plans for confirmation of the instrument's measurement properties using the clinical trial data (FDA 2009).

A third recommendation as it relates to the use of PROs is to provide detailed plans on how investigators will minimize and handle missing data (FDA 2009). Because longitudinally measured PROs are subject to informative missingness, they can introduce bias and interfere with the ability to compare effects across groups. Thus, the protocol should include plans for collecting reasons that patients discontinued treatment or withdrew their participation. Efforts should also be made to continue to collect PRO data, regardless of whether patients discontinued treatment, and a process should be established for how to obtain PRO measurement before or after patient withdrawal to prevent loss to follow-up. Details on statistical methods to account for missing data in the analysis plan are further described in ▶ Chap. 92, "Statistical Analysis of Patient-Reported Outcomes in Clinical Trials," of this book. Despite more stringent guidance on the assessment of PROs in clinical research, there remains a need for a more standardized and coordinated approach to further improve the efficiency for which PROs are collected and to maximize the benefits of PROs in healthcare (Calvert et al. 2019).

Clinical Trial Protocol Development

It is essential that clinical trial protocols incorporating PROs are designed with the same methodological rigor and detail as any other clinical trial protocol. To improve standardization and enhance quality across clinical trial protocols, the SPIRIT (Standard Protocol Items: Recommendations for Interventional Trials) statement was developed, with the most recent version being published in 2013 (Chan et al. 2013) (Appendix 10.7). It consists of 33 recommended items to include in clinical trial protocols organized by protocol section. To address PRO content-specific recommendations, a PRO extension of the SPIRIT statement was developed in 2017. In addition to the 33 checklist items from the SPIRIT statement, the PRO extension includes 11 extensions and 5 elaborations that focus on PRO-specific issues across each protocol section (Calvert et al. 2018). Extensions and elaborations for the PRO-specific elaborations and extensions to the standard SPIRIT checklist are paraphrased in the following section.

As part of the administrative information and introduction components of the trial protocol, PRO elaborations and extensions include *SPIRIT-5a* specifying the individual(s) responsible for the PRO content of the trial; *SPIRIT-6a* describing the PRO-specific research question and rationale for PRO assessment and summarizing PRO findings in relevant studies; and *SPIRIT-7* stating the PRO objectives or hypotheses. PRO extensions related to the methods section of the protocols are:

SPIRIT-10 Specify any PRO-specific eligibility criteria. If PROs are only collected in a subsample, provide rationale and description of methods for obtaining the PRO subsample.

SPIRIT-12 Specify the PRO concepts/domains used to evaluate the intervention and, for each one, the analysis metric and principle time point or period of interest.

SPIRIT-13 Include a schedule of PRO assessments (with rationale for the time points) and specify time windows and whether order of administration will be standardized if using multiple questionnaires.

SPIRIT-14 State the required sample size and how it was determined (if PRO is the primary endpoint). If sample size is not established based on PRO, discuss the power of the principal PRO analyses.

SPIRIT-18a(i) Justify the PRO instrument that will be used and describe domains, number of items, recall period, instrument scaling, and scoring. Provide information about the instrument measurement properties, interpretation guidelines, patient acceptability and burden, as well as the user manual, if available.

SPIRIT-18a(ii) Include the data collection plan that outlines the different modes of administration and the setting.
SPIRIT-18a(iii) Specify whether more than one language version will be used and state whether translated versions have been developed and will be used.
SPIRIT-18a(iv) If trial requires a proxy-reported outcome, state and justify the use of a proxy respondent and cite the evidence of the validity of the proxy assessment, if available.
SPIRIT-18b(i) Specify the PRO data collection and management strategies used to minimize missing data.
SPIRIT-18b(ii) Describe the process of PRO assessment for participants who discontinue or deviate from the assigned intervention.
SPIRIT-20a State PRO analysis methods and include plans for addressing multiplicity and type 1 error.
SPIRIT-20c State how missing data will be described and outline methods for handling missing items or entire assessments.
SPIRIT-22 State whether PRO data will be monitored during the study to inform patient care and how it will be managed in a standardized way.

In summary, the SPIRIT-PRO extension provides important consensus-based guidance on PRO-specific information that should be included in clinical trial protocols. Currently, literature reviews suggest that PRO-specific content in clinical trial protocols is frequently absent or incomplete from clinical trial protocols (Kyte et al. 2014). By following the SPIRIT PRO statement and checklist, researchers can enhance the quality of the design, conduct, and analysis of clinical trials for which PROs are primary, secondary, or exploratory outcomes. By conducting high-quality clinical trials with PRO-specific content, results can contribute to the global PRO evidence base and appropriately inform decision-making, labeling claims, clinical guidelines, and health policy (Calvert et al. 2018).

Reporting PRO Results from Clinical Trials

Standards exist to improve the quality and completeness of reporting PROs from clinical trials (Calvert et al. 2013). The Consolidated Standards of Reporting Trials (CONSORT) statement is intended for use as a tool for authors, reviewers, and consumers and endorsed by major journals and editorial groups. A CONSORT extension was published in 2013 that includes recommendations for RCTs that incorporate PROs in order to facilitate interpretation of PRO results and inform clinical care. CONSORT statement was first published in 1996 to improve clinical trial reporting (Calvert et al. 2013) (Appendix 10.5). Since then, extensions have been developed to address specific trial designs and methods, including the CONSORT PRO extension. The CONSORT PRO extension describes five specific recommendations that have been added to supplement the standard CONSORT guidelines. The specific PRO items include the following: (1) PROs should be identified as primary or secondary outcomes in the abstract; (2) the scientific background and rationale as well as a description of the hypothesis and relevant domains (for multidimensional instruments) should be provided; (3) evidence for the validity and reliability of the instrument should be provided or cited; (4) statistical approaches to handle missing PRO data should be explicitly stated; and (5) PRO-specific limitations and generalizability of results should be discussed (Calvert et al. 2013). The CONSORT PRO extension includes specific examples and explanations for each of these recommendations (Calvert et al. 2013). The complete CONSORT PRO statement and checklist can be accessed online at the following link: http://www.consort-statement.org/extensions

Summary and Conclusion

PROs are important sources of information for the evaluation of clinical trial outcomes. There is an increasing emphasis on the use of PROs to inform healthcare policy and clinical care. Routine collection of PROs has also been shown to improve quality of care, engagement, and survival in some cases (Basch 2010). To ensure high-quality PRO data, guidance and recommendations exist for the design of trials (FDA PRO guidance), protocol development (SPIRIT-PRO), as well as the reporting of PROs (CONSORT). The role of PROs in clinical trials will depend on the study objectives, the disease/condition, and the treatment/intervention. It is important to recognize some of the challenges with using PROs in clinical trials, such as the difficulty validating different PRO measures, missing data, and the reporting biases that inheriently exist in their assessment. Given the added value that PROs provide as well as their potential for improving patient-centered care, PROs should be incorporated into clinical trial design following the available guidelines and recommendations that exist to ensure high-quality PRO data.

Key Facts

- The use of PROs in clinical trials can provide added value about the efficacy and tolerability of an intervention
- PROs are increasingly being used as primary or secondary outcomes to support labeling claims in the United States and inform clinical decision making
- There remains a need to standardize methods and coordinate efforts in the collection, assessment, analysis, and reporting of PROs
- Guidance and recommendations have been established to improve the quality and methodologic rigor of clinical trials that incorporate PROs

References

Aaronson NK, Ahmedzai S, Bergman B, Bullinger M, Cull A, Duez NJ, Filiberti A, Flechtner H, Fleishman SB, de Haes JC et al (1993) The European Organization for Research and Treatment of Cancer QLQ-C30: a quality-of-life instrument for use in international clinical trials in oncology. J Natl Cancer Inst 85(5):365–376

Atkinson TM, Stover AM, Storfer DF, Saracino RM, D'Agostino TA, Pergolizzi D, Matsoukas K, Li Y, Basch E (2017) Patient-reported physical function measures in cancer clinical trials. Epidemiol Rev 39(1):59–70

Banta D (2003) The development of health technology assessment. Health Policy 63(2):121–132

Basch E (2010) The missing voice of patients in drug-safety reporting. New England Journal of Medicine 362(10):865–869

Basch (2012) Beyond the FDA PRO Guidance: Steps toward Integrating Meaningful Patient-Reported Outcomes into Regulatory Trials and US Drug Labels Value in Health 15(3):401–403

Basch E (2018) Patient-reported outcomes: an essential component of oncology drug development and regulatory review. The lancet Oncology 19(5):595–597

Basch E, Reeve BB, Mitchell SA, Clauser SB, Minasian LM, Dueck AC, Mendoza TR, Hay J, Atkinson TM, Abernethy AP, Bruner DW, Cleeland CS, Sloan JA, Chilukuri R, Baumgartner P, Denicoff A, Germain DS, O'Mara AM, Chen A, Kelaghan J, Bennett AV, Sit L, Rogak L, Barz A, Paul DB, Schrag D (2014) Development of the National Cancer Institute's patient-reported outcomes version of the common terminology criteria for adverse events (PRO-CTCAE). J Natl Cancer Inst 106(9):dju244. https://doi.org/10.1093/jnci/dju244. PMID: 25265940; PMCID: PMC4200059

Basch E, Rogak LJ, Dueck AC (2016) Methods for implementing and reporting patient-reported outcome (PRO) measures of symptomatic adverse events in cancer clinical trials. Clin Ther 38 (4):821–830

Basch E, Deal AM, Dueck AC, Scher HI, Kris MG, Hudis C, Schrag D (2017a) Overall survival results of a trial assessing patient-reported outcomes for symptom monitoring during routine cancer treatment overall survival for patient-reported symptom monitoring in routine cancer treatment letters. JAMA 318(2):197–198

Basch E, Dueck AC, Rogak LJ, Minasian LM, Kelly WK, O'Mara AM, Denicoff AM, Seisler D, Atherton PJ, Paskett E, Carey L, Dickler M, Heist RS, Himelstein A, Rugo HS, Sikov WM, Socinski MA, Venook AP, Weckstein DJ, Lake DE, Biggs DD, Freedman RA, Kuzma C, Kirshner JJ, Schrag D (2017b) Feasibility assessment of patient reporting of symptomatic adverse events in multicenter cancer clinical trials patient reporting of symptomatic adverse events in multicenter cancer trials patient reporting of symptomatic adverse events in multicenter cancer trials. JAMA Oncol 3(8):1043–1050

Calvert M, Blazeby J, Altman DG, Revicki DA, Moher D, Brundage MD (2013) Reporting of patient-reported outcomes in randomized trials: the CONSORT PRO extension. JAMA 309 (8):814–822

Calvert M, Kyte D, Mercieca-Bebber R, Slade A, Chan A-W, King MT, a. t. S.-P. Group (2018) Guidelines for inclusion of patient-reported outcomes in clinical trial protocols: the SPIRIT-PRO extension guidelines for inclusion of patient-reported outcomes in clinical trial protocols guidelines for inclusion of patient-reported outcomes in clinical trial protocols. JAMA 319 (5):483–494

Calvert M, Kyte D, Price G, Valderas JM, Hjollund NH (2019) Maximising the impact of patient reported outcome assessment for patients and society. BMJ 24;364

Cella D, Yount S, Rothrock N, Gershon R, Cook K, Reeve B, Ader D, Fries JF, Bruce B, Rose M (2007) The patient-reported outcomes measurement information system (PROMIS): progress of an NIH roadmap cooperative group during its first two years. Med Care 45(5 Suppl 1):S3

Cella D, Riley W, Stone A, Rothrock N, Reeve B, Yount S, Amtmann D, Bode R, Buysse D, Choi S, Cook K, Devellis R, DeWalt D, Fries JF, Gershon R, Hahn EA, Lai JS, Pilkonis P, Revicki D, Rose M, Weinfurt K, Hays R (2010) The patient-reported outcomes measurement information system (PROMIS) developed and tested its first wave of adult self-reported health outcome item banks: 2005–2008. J Clin Epidemiol 63(11):1179–1194

Chan A-W, Tetzlaff JM, Altman DG, Laupacis A, Gøtzsche PC, Krleža-Jerić K, Hróbjartsson A, Mann H, Dickersin K, Berlin JA, Doré CJ, Parulekar WR, Summerskill WSM, Groves T, Schulz KF, Sox HC, Rockhold FW, Rennie D, Moher D (2013) SPIRIT 2013 statement: defining standard protocol items for clinical trials. Ann Intern Med 158(3):200–207

DeMuro C, Clark M, Doward L, Evans E, Mordin M, Gnanasakthy A (2013) Assessment of PRO label claims granted by the FDA as compared to the EMA (2006–2010). Value Health 16 (8):1150–1155

Dueck AC, Mendoza TR, Mitchell SA, Reeve BB, Castro KM, Rogak LJ, Atkinson TM, Bennett AV, Denicoff AM, O'Mara AM, Li Y, Clauser SB, Bryant DM, Bearden JD 3rd, Gillis TA, Harness JK, Siegel RD, Paul DB, Cleeland CS, Schrag D, Sloan JA, Abernethy AP, Bruner DW, Minasian LM, Basch E (2015) National Cancer Institute PRO-CTCAE Study Group. Validity and Reliability of the US National Cancer Institute's Patient-Reported Outcomes Version of the Common Terminology Criteria for Adverse Events (PRO-CTCAE). JAMA Oncol 1(8):1051–1109. https://doi.org/10.1001/jamaoncol.2015.2639. Erratum in: JAMA Oncol. 2016 Jan;2 (1):146. PMID: 26270597; PMCID: PMC4857599

Dy SM, Roy J, Ott GE, McHale M, Kennedy C, Kutner JS, Tien A (2011) Tell us™: a web-based tool for improving communication among patients, families, and providers in hospice and palliative care through systematic data specification, collection, and use. J Pain Symptom Manag 42(4):526–534

Dy SM, Walling AM, Mack JW, Malin JL, Pantoja P, Lorenz KA, Tisnado DM (2014) Evaluating the quality of supportive oncology using patient-reported data. J Oncol Pract 10(4):e223–e230

European Medicines Agency, C. f. M. P. f. H. U (2005) Reflection paper on the regulatory guidance for the use of health related quality of life (HRQL) measures in the evaluation of medicinal products. Retrieved March 3, 2019, from https://www.ema.europa.eu/en/regulatory-guidance-use-health-related-quality-life-hrql-measures-evaluation-medicinal-products

Frank L, Basch E, Selby JV, F. t. P.-C. O. R. Institute (2014) The PCORI perspective on patient-centered outcomes research the PCORI perspective on patient-centered research the PCORI perspective on patient-centered research. JAMA 312(15):1513–1514

Ganz PA, Hays RD, Kaplan RM, Litwin MS (2014) Measuring health-related quality of life and other outcomes. In: Kominski GF (ed) Changing the U.S. health care system: key issues in health services policy and management. Wiley, San Francisco, pp 307–341

Gnanasakthy A, DeMuro C, Clark M, Haydysch E, Ma E, Bonthapally V (2016) Patient-reported outcomes labeling for products approved by the Office of Hematology and Oncology Products of the US Food and Drug Administration (2010–2014). J Clin Oncol 34(16):1928–1934

Gnanasakthy A, Mordin M, Evans E, Doward L, DeMuro C (2017) A review of patient-reported outcome labeling in the United States (2011–2015). Value Health 20(3):420–429

HealthMeasures. PROMIS (2019) Explore measurement systems. Retrieved March 20, 2019 from http://www.healthmeasures.net/explore-measurement-systems/promis/intro-to-promis

Institute of Medicine (2011) Leading health indicators for healthy people 2020: letter report. National Academies Press, Washington, DC. Retrieved 15 March 2019 from http://books.nap.edu/openbook.php?record_id=13088&page=R1

Kluetz PG, Pazdur R (2016) Looking to the future in an unprecedented time for cancer drug development. Semin Oncol 43(1):2–3

Kluetz PG, O'Connor DJ, Soltys K (2018) Incorporating the patient experience into regulatory decision making in the USA, Europe, and Canada. The lancet Oncology 19(5):e267–e274

Kyte D, Duffy H, Fletcher B, Gheorghe A, Mercieca-Bebber R, King M, Draper H, Ives J, Brundage M, Blazeby J, Calvert M (2014) Systematic evaluation of the patient-reported outcome (PRO) content of clinical trial protocols. PLoS One 9(10):e110229

Lipscomb JG, Gotay CC, Snyder C (2005) Outcomes assessment in cancer: measures, methods, and applications. Cambridge University Press, Cambridge

Nayfield SG, Ganz PA, Moinpour CM, Cella DF, Hailey BJ (1992) Report from a National Cancer Institute (USA) workshop on quality of life assessment in cancer clinical trials. Qual Life Res 1 (3):203–210

Piantadosi S (2017) Clinical trials: a methodologic perspective. Wiley, Hoboken

Spilker B (1996) Quality of life and pharmacoeconomics in clinical trials. Lippincott-Raven Publishers, Philadelphia

Testa MA, Simonson DC (1996) Assessment of quality-of-life outcomes. N Engl J Med 334 (13):835–840

US Department of Health and Human Services (USDHHS): Food and Drug Administration. Accessed 1 March 2019; Draft guidance for industry. Patient-reported outcome measures: use in medical product development to support labeling claims. 2006 February.; www.ispor.org/workpaper/FDAPROGuidance2006.pdf

US Department of Health and Human Services (USDHHS): Food and Drug Administration. Accessed 1 March 2019; Guidance for industry. Patient-reported outcome measures: use in medical product development to support labeling claims. 2009 December.; www.fda.gov/downloads/Drugs/GuidanceComplianceRegulatoryInformation/Guidances/UCM193282.pdf

Translational Clinical Trials

52

Steven Piantadosi

Contents

Abstract

Translational research and clinical trials are often discussed especially in academic centers from the perspective that such efforts are difficult or endangered. Yet every new therapeutic must pass through this stage of investigation where promising evidence supports staged development with the goal of product registration. Many clinical investigators instinctively know that relatively small clinical trials can be essential in translation, but this is often contrary to the statistical rigors of later development. This chapter attempts to reconcile these equally valid perspectives.

Keywords

Translational research · Translational clinical trials · Biomarkers · Information · Entropy · Sample size

S. Piantadosi (✉)
Department of Surgery, Division of Surgical Oncology, Brigham and Women's Hospital, Harvard Medical School, Boston, MA, USA
e-mail: spiantadosi@bwh.harvard.edu

© Springer Nature Switzerland AG 2022

S. Piantadosi, C. L. Meinert (eds.), *Principles and Practice of Clinical Trials*,
https://doi.org/10.1007/978-3-319-52636-2_76

Introduction

The terms *basic research*, *clinical research*, and *translational research* require some practical definitions. Basic and clinical investigations are the ends of a spectrum and therefore have always been part of the research landscape by default. Basic implies that the research does not need an immediate application but represents knowledge for its own sake. Clinical is the direct application to care or prevention of illness – literally "at the bedside." Without fanfare, translational research takes place between the two ends of the spectrum, so it too has always been with us but perhaps less obvious.

Historically, academic centers seem to have concentrated on basic and clinical research, while commercial entities focused on translational research. Translational research began to be characterized explicitly mostly in the 1990s and later. Translation is difficult to define universally, but many academic institutions and sponsors try to foster it alongside basic and clinical research at least in the sense that they know it when they see it. A problem with a precise definition is that there is no single anchor for the domain of translation like the laboratory or clinic. In fact, the apparent gap between basic and clinical research often seems to be widening (Butler 2008). There is a National Center for Advancing Translational Sciences (NCATS) as part of the National Institutes of Health. But NCATS does not offer a simple clear definition.

Translational clinical trials are elusive because the label is often applied even when the research has conventional developmental purposes such as dose finding. A search of ClinicalTrials.gov (National Library of Medicine 2019) found only 243 trials with the term "translational" out of over 300,000 entries in the database. The search filters were "recruiting," "enrolling by invitation," "interventional," "early phase 1," "phase 1," and "phase 2." Removing all filters except "interventional" raised the number to 2888. These are imperfect snapshots. For example, a randomized trial came up under the filter "early phase 1." ClinicalTrials.gov does not have an explicit filter for translational trials.

The clinical scope of trials captured was universal as one might expect. Most of the trials were probably not translational in the sense to be developed in this chapter. But many trials have components or sub-studies that have translational objectives. Many other studies in the database used similar descriptors but were not obviously interventional trials. It seems unlikely that less than one in a thousand trials is translational, but this low number points to nonuniformity in the way the concept is used. The characterizations of translational trials in this chapter will push toward common concepts and usage.

Presently there are about 100 medical journals in at least 5 languages with the word "translational" in their title or self-identified as translational. Most of these are online. A wide range of disciplines and diseases are represented among them, including pediatrics, cardiovascular disease, cancer, psychiatry, immunology, and informatics. As one might expect from the minority of clinical trials that are classified as translational, publications in such journals seem to emphasize technological and pre-developmental studies.

This chapter will attempt to define and characterize translational clinical trials as a distinct type apart from the typical developmental classifications such as phase I, II, or III. Major conceptual differences are that unlike developmental trials, translational clinical trials are unlikely to employ clinical outcome measures and may beget laboratory experiments as readily as additional clinical trials. Due to the high uncertainty regarding treatment effects when they are begun, even the relatively weak evidence produced from translational trials is informative for initiating or suspending developmental steps.

Definitions

For this chapter, I will define translational research simply as *converting observations from the laboratory into clinical interventions*. This definition keeps away from the ends of the spectrum in the following sense. Basic science observations must already exist: translational research does not discover them. Clinical interventions are created and await confirmation: translational research does not prove health benefits.

With this simple definition of translational research, a translational clinical trial (TCT) will be seen to be something special. First, although a TCT takes place in the clinic, it relies heavily on laboratory foundations. Second, a TCT will not provide strong evidence for therapeutic efficacy. Third, a TCT must inform the subsequent clinical trials or laboratory experiments that will lead to strong evidence.

For the purposes of this chapter, I will use the following definition of a translational clinical trial (Piantadosi 2005):

> A clinical trial where the primary outcome: 1) is a biological measurement (target) derived from a well-established paradigm of disease, and 2) represents an irrefutable signal regarding the intended therapeutic effect. The design and purposes of the trial are to guide further experiments in the laboratory or clinic, inform treatment modifications, and validate the target, but not necessarily to provide reliable evidence regarding clinical outcomes.

Therapy acts on a signal derived from a disease model but measured in the clinic where it implicates definitive effects (Fig. 1). A TCT should inform the design of subsequent experiments by reducing uncertainty regarding effects on the target. Hence it should be designed to yield useful evidence whether the treatment succeeds or fails. It must contain two explicit definitions for lack of effect: one for each study subject and another for the entire study cohort. A TCT will not carry formal hypothesis tests regarding therapeutic efficacy. One result for such a trial might be that the treatment requires modifications or replacement: translational trials are circular between the laboratory and clinic.

A translational treatment is not fixed. Imagine needing to modify a small molecule or antibody based on an initial human trial. Not only might the treatment itself change, but it is being tracked by a signal derived from the laboratory and measured in people. Clinical outcomes will come only in later more definitive studies.

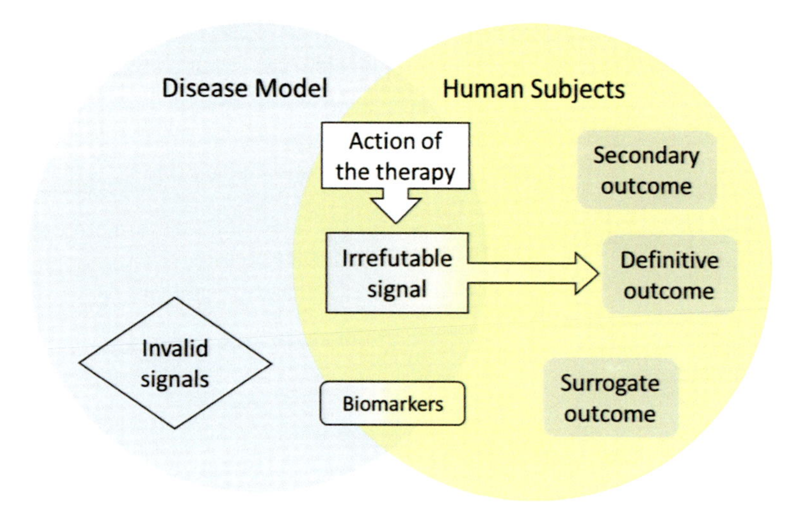

Fig. 1 Translational clinical trial paradigm. The irrefutable signal is derived from understanding of the disease model but it is measured in human subjects. The treatment modifies the signal which then implies alteration in a definitive outcome

Table 1 Additional characteristics of translational trials

The disease model must contain relevant elements of the actual disease process
The target draws support from the disease model to implicate an effect on the definitive outcome
There can be no targets (surrogates) for safety
Can observe high risks but cannot reliably establish safety
Evidence for efficacy can evolve prior to strong evidence regarding safety, reversing the typical sequence
Informs the design of subsequent experiments by reducing uncertainty regarding effects on the target

Therefore, TCTs are pre-developmental. Such studies can sometimes be nested within typical developmental clinical trials. Most often they will be single-cohort studies. Additional requirements and characteristics of a translational trial are listed in Table 1.

Issues in Translational Trials

TCTs may focus on any of several natural questions. The most pointed question is **targeting** – does the therapy hit the biological target and does it appear to produce the intended effect. A small molecule or biologic might target a cellular receptor, enzyme, antibody ligand, or gene, for example. The answer to this question implies quantitative measurement of the relevant product.

Another question in translation might be **signaling** – are there products or effects (signals) downstream from the target that reveal the intended effect after treatment. If we observe and measure the signal, we can reasonably infer that the target was hit. A signal might be a change in activity level or switching of a gene expression, for example.

A TCT could focus on **feasibility** – can we successfully implement and refine an unproven complex method for delivering a therapy. Feasibility is vital when it is a legitimate question but a straw man otherwise. Feasibility is not an appropriate objective when the ability to administer a treatment is neither complex nor questionable. Such questions are sometimes chosen merely to deflect criticism from small or poorly designed studies.

In a feasibility study, two definitions for *infeasible* are essential because it represents a type of failure mentioned above. One definition pertains to each study participant so there is an outcome measure relevant to the primary objective in every subject. A second definition of infeasible refers to the entire study cohort so there will be a prespecified measure of success. That tolerance specification also needs a precision or confidence level. For example, suppose our translational trial addresses delivery feasibility and we have an appropriate list of show-stopping problems that could be encountered. Assume we can continue development only if 85% or more of subjects have no clinically significant delivery problems. The smallest possible study that can satisfy our requirement is 20 subjects, none of whom could have feasibility problems. Then the lower 95% confidence bound on the success rate would exceed 85%.

The potential scope of delivery issues in translation is wide as a few examples will illustrate. A drug might depend on its size, polarity, or solubility for reaching its target. The dose or schedule will determine blood and tissue levels. For oral medications subject behavior, adherence, or diet may also be factors. Individual genetic or epigenetic characteristics can affect drug exposure via metabolism. For gene or cell therapies, properties of the vector, dose or schedule, need for replication, immunological characteristics of the recipient, and individual genetic or epigenetic characteristics may affect delivery. Devices or skill-dependent therapies may depend on procedural technique, function of a device, or the anatomy of the subject or disease. This daunting array of issues indicates that study goals must be set thoughtfully, and off-the-shelf drug development designs may not be appropriate for many feasibility questions.

TCTs may involve **biomarkers** at any of several levels. They are not unique in this regard, but some uses of biomarkers are specific to translational trials. A biomarker is an objective measurement that informs disease status or treatment effects. Surrogate outcomes also track the effects of treatment but also change in proportion to the way a definitive outcome would respond to the treatment. From the perspective of trial design, a biomarker creates a subset in the study population. It predicts whether a treatment works or carries information regarding prognosis. A principal design question for a biomarker is if the study population should be enriched with respect to it. If the biomarker indicates definitively whether treatment will work, the population should be selected accordingly.

In some cases, **companion diagnostics** are at issue in translational trials. A companion diagnostic is the test that reveals the biomarker level or presence. Such a test might be new and could be based on evolving technology. The diagnostic test could therefore be refined alongside the therapeutic. Different companion diagnostic tests, if they exist, could yield different study compositions and potentially different results.

Examples

As a hypothetical example of a TCT, suppose we have a local gene therapy for brain tumors to be delivered using a well-studied (safe) lentiviral vector. The virus delivers the gene product to tumor cells where it stops their growth and kills them. Suppose further that production of the delivery vector is straightforward, injecting the viral particles is feasible, and the correct dose is known from previous studies. The treatment will be administered days prior to routine surgical resection of the tumor so effects can be measured clinically and in the specimens.

An appropriate design for the first human trial in this circumstance will not emphasize a dose question. To rule out adverse events at a 10% threshold requires at least 30 subjects yielding zero such events. Then the upper 95% confidence bound on the adverse event rate would be 0.1. This would be a relatively large early clinical trial. However, we might reliably establish the presence of gene product in resected tumor cells with many fewer subjects. Furthermore, seeing a handful of tumor responses prior to surgery would also be promising evidence of efficacy. Hence a translational trial could reveal more about efficacy than safety.

An example of an actual translational trial is in the ClinicalTrials.gov database at record NCT02427581 which is a breast cancer vaccine trial (Gillanders et al. 2019). Subjects in this trial have not had a complete response after chemotherapy and are at very high risk for disease recurrence. The planned sample size is 15, and the primary outcome measure is grade and frequency of adverse events at 1 year. Secondary outcomes of the trial are immunogenicity measures for the vaccine.

Another translational trial is illustrated by a test of mushroom powder for secondary breast cancer prevention in 24 subjects (Palomares et al. 2011). The trial was formally described as "dose finding" although up to 13 g of white button mushroom was not a difficult tolerance challenge, especially compared to typical cancer therapies. The translational objectives were aromatase inhibition, with response defined as a $\geq$50% decrease in free estradiol. No participants met the predefined response criterion in this trial according to the report.

A final example of a translational clinical trial is a test of valproate for upregulating CD20 levels in patients with chronic lymphocytic leukemia (Scialdone et al. 2017). This trial was planned in four subjects but one dropped out due to a hearing disorder. No upregulation of CD20 mRNA or protein could be detected in vivo in cells from patients on this trial according to the report.

Reducing Uncertainty

Clinicians want translational clinical trials to be small. I have often heard excellent clinical investigators indicate that there would be much to learn from an early test of a new therapeutic idea in a handful of subjects, say 6 or 8, for example. This is consistent with some of the examples just cited. Resource limitations are partly at the root of clinicians' concerns to make TCTs small. But the reasoning is more considered than resources alone. Small experiences can be critical when uncertainty is high. But statisticians tend to disrespect this notion because statistical learning is connected to narrowing confidence or probability intervals around estimands. A handful of observations does not do much by those measures.

Both perspectives are correct. Statisticians are usually interested in definitive evidence in service of decisions. Clinical investigators often seek ways to reduce uncertainty regarding the biological effects of a new therapy as a prerequisite for further clinical trials. In settings of high uncertainty, relatively few observations can reduce uncertainty and lead in the correct direction for further experimentation. Here I will illustrate some hypothetical circumstances of high uncertainty and its reduction using small trials.

Suppose that our therapy can yield a positive, neutral, or negative outcome. Before the trial, assume we are maximally uncertain as to the effect that the treatment will produce. This means that we hypothesize that each outcome is equally likely. We hope our experiment will reveal a dominance of positive outcomes. When the trial is over, we assess the information gained and decide what studies should be performed next. We will temporarily put aside concerns over sample size and focus only on the outcome frequencies produced by such a trial.

Table 2 shows a hypothetical example. Before the trial, each outcome is assumed to have an equal chance of happening. After the trial, suppose half the subjects have a positive result, and 25% have each negative or neutral. Gain in information can be calculated using entropy (Gillanders et al. 2019) and yields a value of 0.6. Alternatively, the relative information from these results can be calculated using the Kullback-Leibler divergence (Kullback and Leibler 1951) and yields a value of 0.05. The Kullback-Leibler divergence is sometimes called relative entropy and can be taken as a measure of surprise. Most of us do not have an intuitive feel for these information values, but both indicate a small gain in information. Depending on the clinical context, this might be a very promising result because half the subjects seemed to benefit from the therapy.

The consequences of assuming too much prior to the experiment can be serious. Consider the hypothetical results in Table 3 where optimism prior to the trial was very strong. The same trial results from Table 2 are measured against that very optimistic initial hypothesis. The information value is −0.52, and the divergence is 0.28 indicating that before and after are quite different. However, we seem to know less after the trial than before because we have "lost" information. In a sense this is true because the initial hypothesis implied too

Table 2 Hypothetical prior (before) and outcome (after) probabilities for a translational clinical trial. Before the trial, maximum uncertainty regarding the treatment effect was assumed

	Outcome probabilities		
Time	Neg	Neutral	Pos
Before	0.33	0.33	0.33
After	0.25	0.25	0.50

Table 3 Hypothetical prior (before) and outcome (after) probabilities for a translational clinical trial. Before the trial, strong assumptions were made regarding the treatment effect. Implications are different compared to Table 2, despite the outcome data being identical

	Outcome probabilities		
Time	Neg	Neutral	Pos
Before	0.05	0.10	0.85
After	0.25	0.25	0.50

Table 4 Hypothetical prior (before) and outcome (after) probabilities for a translational clinical trial. Prior assumptions were strong. Formally there is no gain in information but the results are divergent and carry biological implications

	Outcome probabilities		
Time	Neg	Neutral	Pos
Before	0.10	0.50	0.40
After	0.50	0.40	0.10

much certainty. This might be a very unpromising result if the strong optimism prior to the trial was justified.

As a third example, consider the scenario in Table 4. There the anticipated outcome probabilities are the same as those observed after the trial but rearranged. The information gain is apparently zero. The divergence is 0.5, indicating before and after are substantially different. Such a result would likely prevent development because half the subjects show negative outcomes.

These examples have assumed we have reasonable estimates of the classification or response probabilities when the TCT is complete. In small sample sizes, the calculated information and its variance are biased (Butler 2008). The bias can be substantially reduced in modest sample sizes, meaning that we can then obtain reasonable quantitative estimates of information gain.

These simple examples show that simple prior hypotheses coupled with outcome summaries yield quantifiable information and relative information. It seems appropriate to assume we are uncertain before human data are obtained. The clinical setting and properties of existing treatments must be brought into the assessment of how promising results are.

Sample Size

We can now return to the question of how large such trials need to be. What does it take to get reasonable estimates of information gain? Simulation according to the following algorithm provides an answer. We begin with a fixed sample size and combinatorically enumerate all possible outcomes, calculating entropy and divergence for each. Each outcome has a probability of occurring according to a multinomial distribution that is assumed to represent the truth of nature. From the probabilities we construct the cumulative distribution functions (CDFs) of entropy and divergence. Then by varying the sample size, we can observe its effect on the CDF or expected values of entropy and divergence. The impact of different assumed true multinomial distributions can also be studied.

CDFs for entropy and divergence from such a simulation with varying sample sizes are shown in Figs. 2 and 3. Small sample sizes with coarse estimates of the CDF are biased as one would expect intuitively. This is demonstrated by the rightward shift of the CDFs as sample size increases in Figs. 2 and 3. However, the bias diminishes rapidly with increasing sample size, especially for the KL divergence CDF. Very similar curves result from alternative true multinomial distributions. This indicates that nearly bias-free estimates of information and divergence for a TCT can be obtained using small sample sizes. Large sample sizes will, of course, increase the precision of estimated outcome probabilities, but a picture of (relative) information emerges sooner. For example, returning to Table 1, the simulations suggest that sample sizes in the range of 12–18 subjects give an accurate assessment of the distribution of KL divergence values for all possible outcomes.

There is a sense in which the results regarding sample size seem too good to be true. Small sample sizes relative to conventional standards are useful with respect to acquiring information. We know such sample sizes would be inadequate for most consequential clinical decisions such as comparing treatments. But the usefulness of information measures depends on context. When uncertainty about a treatment effect is high as it is in translation, weaker evidence than it would otherwise take to change

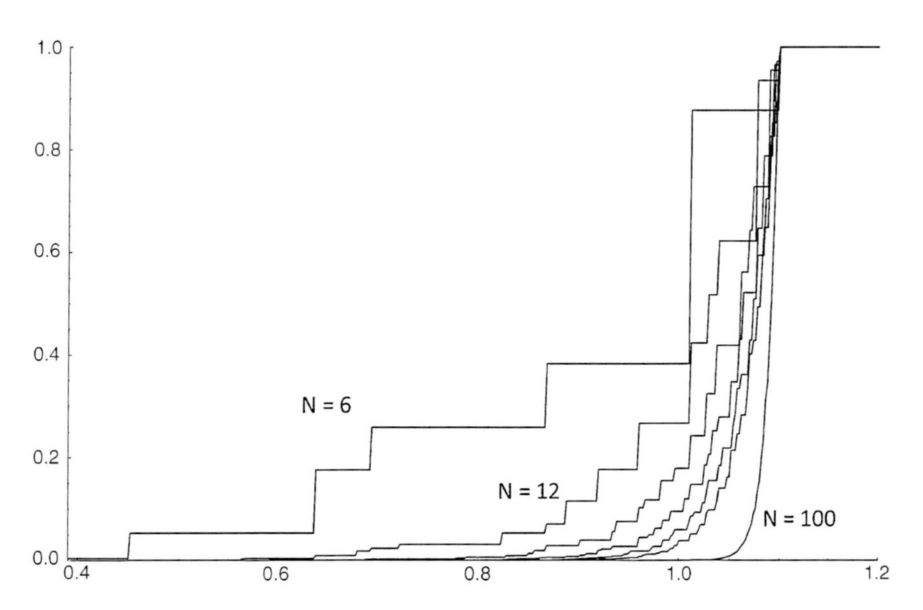

Fig. 2 CDF of entropy as defined in Shannon [1948]. Three outcome categories were used as in Table 1 in the text and the multinomial probabilities were uniform. Curves correspond to sample sizes ranging from 6 to 36. A reference curve for $N = 100$ is shown to indicate how small sample sizes perform relative to it

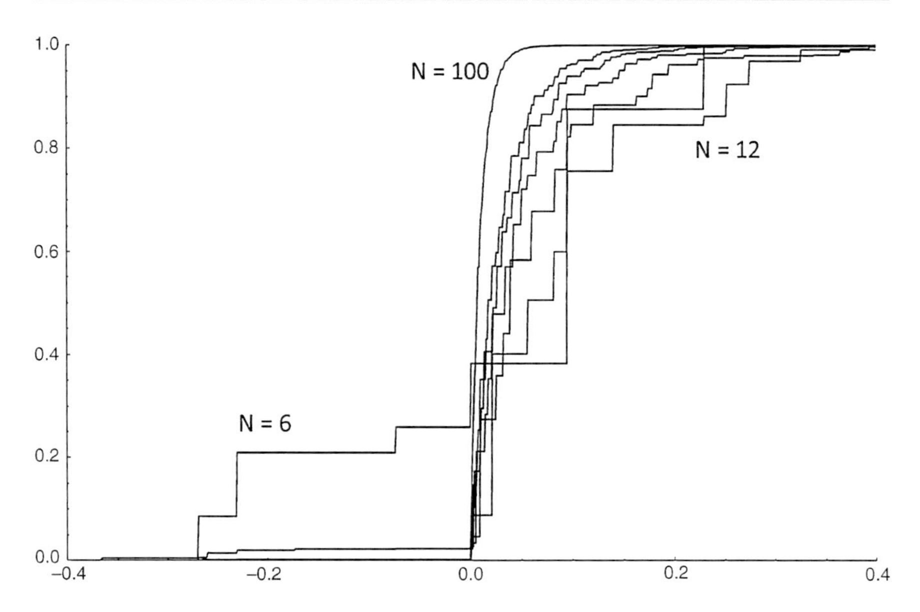

Fig. 3 CDF of Kullback-Leibler divergence. The same conditions as in Fig. 2 apply

medical practice is valuable and can guide subsequent experimental steps. A TCT shares as many characteristics with lab experiments as with definitive clinical trials. The decisions faced after a TCT are treatment effects on the irrefutable signal and what is the best next experiment. Whether or not to accept a treatment for wide use is not an issue. Therefore, lesser evidence is required to guide the next experimental steps.

Safety Versus Efficacy

Another dimension for translational clinical trials is the extent to which they can reassure investigators as to the safety of the intervention in question. Safety is a ubiquitous concern in clinical trials but is more aspirational than real in small studies. There are two strong reasons for this. One is biological: there are no surrogates for safety, so we never have more promising evidence than zero events in the trial cohort. In contrast, efficacy may show promise via the irrefutable signal which is its intended purpose.

A second reason why proof of safety is unattainable in TCTs derives from statistical considerations. Safety is not a measurement but is a clinical judgment based on an informative absence of events. Only sizable experiences are informative. For example, if 10% is the upper tolerance for serious adverse events, data would have to show zero events in 30 subjects for the confidence bound on the event rate to be below the 10% limit. A 5% limit would require 60 event-free subjects. These are realistic tolerances for serious adverse events putting proof of safety out of reach of many TCTs that enroll only a few subjects.

To contrast, far fewer subjects could show evidence of efficacy. For example, a handful of disease responses out of 10 or 12 participants in a TCT could be very promising. Hence, we must be alert to the chance to learn about efficacy before safety in such trials. This is a reverse of the stereotypical sequence.

Summary and Conclusion

The goal of this chapter has been to describe features of translational clinical trials that codify them as a distinct type of study. There are trials that fit this paradigm very well. However, many studies labeled as such have only certain components that are translational. Still others are relatively ordinary developmental trials that carry a translational label probably to make them appear more vital because of the importance of the term.

The key feature of a translational trial is the intersection of a well-characterized laboratory model of disease with the actual human condition. An irrefutable signal is derived and validated from laboratory studies but measured as an outcome in the clinical trial. If it does not reflect favorably on the treatment, investigators must either abandon or redesign the therapy.

Statistical precision is not obtained in the small experiences of many translational trials. But measurable gains in information relative to a state of maximal uncertainty can be obtained. The acceptability of this perspective may be a point of divergence for the instincts of clinician investigators versus statisticians. In any case, translational trials must provide enough information to justify performing more expensive developmental studies or to terminate or not begin development at all. Trialists should be alert to the needs of clinical studies in translation so they are not forced into unserviceable commonplace designs.

Key Facts

Translation is a key step in the evolution of a new therapeutic idea, whether viewed as predevelopment or as part of staged development. It constitutes the bridge between basic science and preclinical investigations and human trials. Relatively small translational trials can reduce the considerable uncertainty regarding therapeutic effects at this stage of development. Such trials rely on biological models as implemented in the laboratory and biological targets and signaling. Simple approaches to quantifying information gained show that small sample sizes can reduce uncertainly enough to guide subsequent clinical trials.

Cross-References

▶ Power and Sample Size

References

Butler D (2008) Translational research: crossing the valley of death. Nature 453(7197):840–842
Gillanders WE et al (2019) Safety and immunogenicity of a personalized synthetic long peptide breast cancer vaccine strategy in patients with persistent triple-negative breast cancer following neoadjuvant chemotherapy. ClinicalTrials.gov identifier: NCT02427581
Kullback S, Leibler RA (1951) On information and sufficiency. Ann Math Stat 22(1):79–86
National Library of Medicine (2019) ClinicalTrials.gov. https://clinicaltrials.gov
Palomares MR et al (2011) A dose-finding clinical trial of mushroom powder in postmenopausal breast cancer survivors for secondary breast cancer prevention. J Clin Oncol 29(15_suppl): 1582–1582
Piantadosi S (2005) Translational clinical trials: an entropy-based approach to sample size. Clin Trials 2:182–192
Scialdone A et al (2017) The HDAC inhibitor valproate induces a bivalent status of the CD20 promoter in CLL patients suggesting distinct epigenetic regulation of CD20 expression in CLL in vivo. Oncotarget 8(23):37409–37422. https://doi.org/10.18632/oncotarget.16964
Shannon CE (1948) A mathematical theory of communication. Bell Syst Tech J 27(3):379–423

Dose-Finding and Dose-Ranging Studies

53

Mark R. Conaway and Gina R. Petroni

Contents

Abstract

There is a growing recognition of the importance of well-designed dose-finding studies in the overall development process. This chapter is an overview of designs for studies that are meant to identifying one or more doses of an agent to be tested in subsequent stages of the drug development process. The chapter also provides

M. R. Conaway (✉)
University of Virginia Health System, Charlottesville, VA, USA
e-mail: mconaway@virginia.edu

G. R. Petroni
Translational Research and Applied Statistics, Public Health Sciences, University of Virginia Health System, Charlottesville, VA, USA
e-mail: gpetroni@virginia.edu

© Springer Nature Switzerland AG 2022

S. Piantadosi, C. L. Meinert (eds.), *Principles and Practice of Clinical Trials*,
https://doi.org/10.1007/978-3-319-52636-2_77

a summary of dose-finding designs that have been developed to meet the challenges of contemporary dose-finding trials, including the use of combinations of agents, more complex outcome measures, and heterogeneous groups of participants.

Keywords

Interval-based methods · Model-based methods · Operating characteristics · Coherence · Combinations of agents · Patient heterogeneity

Introduction

This chapter describes the design of studies that have the goal of identifying one or more doses of an agent to be tested in subsequent stages of the drug development process. Piantadosi (2017) makes a distinction between dose-ranging studies, in which doses are to be explored without a pre-specified objective, and dose-finding, where the objective is to find a dose that meets a pre-specified criterion such as a target rate of toxicities. This chapter provides a description of designs for both dose-ranging and dose-finding studies.

Some early-phase studies are designed as randomized trials (Eussen et al. 2005; Partinen et al. 2006; Schaller et al. 2010; Vidoni et al. 2015), with participants allocated randomly among several pre-specified doses. Design considerations for these trials, such as the choice of outcome measures, sample size, the use of stratification factors, or interim monitoring, are common to randomized clinical trials and are covered in Sections 4 (▶ Bias Control and Precision) and 5 (▶ Basics of Trial Design). The distinguishing feature of the designs described in this chapter is that allocation of participants to study dose is done sequentially; the choice of a dose for a participant is determined by the observed outcomes from participants previously treated in the trial. These trials often involve the first use of an agent or combination of agents, and the sequential allocation is intended to avoid exposing participants to undue risk of adverse events. While there are examples of sequential dose-ranging studies in many fields, including anesthesiology (Sauter et al. 2015) and addiction research (Ezard et al. 2016), these designs are most commonly associated with "phase I" trials in oncology.

Designs Based on Increasing Dose-Toxicity Curves

A primary goal of a dose-finding trial is to learn about the safety and adverse events related to study agent(s) and is often labeled "phase I." Historically, for phase I trials involving cytotoxic agents in oncology, a main objective was to identify the "maximum tolerated dose" (MTD). This remains a main objective even for noncytotoxic agents. The MTD is defined as the highest dose that can be administered to participants with an "acceptable" level of toxicity where toxicity is assessed based upon observed adverse events. The amount of toxicity at a given dose level is considered "acceptable" if the proportion of participants treated at that dose who experience a "dose-limiting toxicity" (DLT) is less than or equal to a target level of toxicity. The definition of a DLT is study specific, depends on the type of agent being studied, and is used to set the study target level. Traditionally, the target level has been in the range of 20–33%. Participants are sequentially assigned to dose levels with the starting dose being the lowest dose. Dose allocations can be done for individual participants or in groups of participants where groups of participants are referred to as cohorts. Each participant is assigned to a single dose level and is observed on a binary outcome measure specifying whether or not the participant experienced a DLT. Many of the methods for these trials were developed for cytotoxic agents, where it is assumed that the dose-toxicity and dose-efficacy relationships are monotonic, in which the probability of a DLT and the potential for clinical benefit, often termed "efficacy," both increase with dose (see Fig. 1).

In this setting, the MTD is to be chosen from a pre-specified set of doses, $d_1 < d_2 < \ldots < d_K$, with the probability that a participant given dose level d_k experiences a DLT denoted by π_k, $k = 1, \ldots, K$. The probability of a DLT is assumed to increase with dose, $\pi_1 < \pi_2 < \ldots < \pi_K$. At any point in the trial, there are n_k participants who have been observed on dose level d_k, and of the participants treated, Y_k have experienced a DLT. The target level of toxicity is denoted by θ.

Although the discussion in this chapter will center on dose-finding and dose-ranging studies in oncology, the designs can be applied more widely to any clinical setting in which both the probability of an adverse event and efficacy can be expected to increase with dose. One example is the study of a new anesthetic. The probability of an adverse event and efficacy, defined in this case as sufficient sedation, both increase with dose. As in the oncology studies, the goal is to find the highest dose that can be administered safely, with the added requirement that the dose yields sufficient sedation to an acceptable proportion of participants.

For these trials the statistical design revolves around two questions: (Ananthakrishnan et al. 2017) How should doses be allocated to participants as the

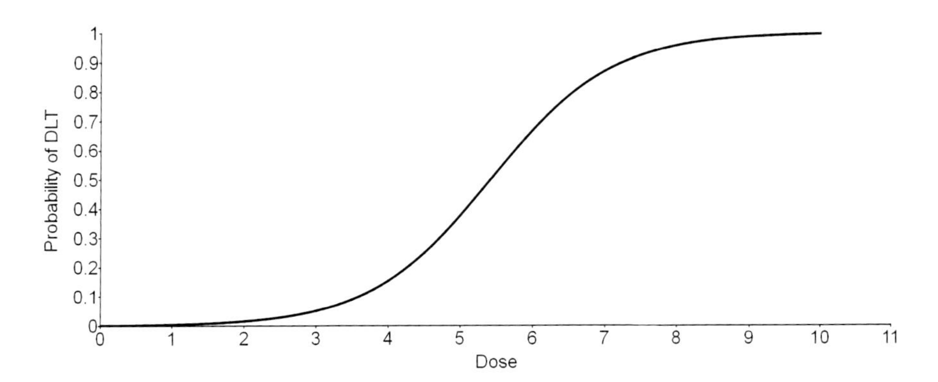

Fig. 1 An example of a monotonic dose-toxicity relationship

trial proceeds? and (Babb et al. 1998) At the end of the trial, what dose should be nominated as the MTD? There are, of course, many other clinical and statistical issues to be made in carrying out a dose-finding or dose-ranging trial, including the pre-specification of dose levels and the definition of a DLT (Senderowicz 2010), but this chapter focuses primarily on the statistical issues of dose allocation and estimation of the MTD at the end of the study.

Methods in this situation are broadly categorized as "rule-based," in which decisions to decrease, increase, or assign the same dose level for a new participant are determined by rules for the observed proportion of toxicities at the current dose, or "model-based," in which a parametric model is fit to all the accumulated data and used to guide dose allocation and the estimation of the MTD (Le Tourneau et al. 2009). In practice, the distinction between rule-based and model-based is not completely clear, as there are methods that use rule-based dose allocation (Storer 1989; Stylianou and Flournoy 2002; Ji et al. 2007) but use a parametric model or isotonic regression at the end of the trial to estimate the MTD. Other methods (Shen and O'Quigley 1996; Wages et al. 2011a) are model-based but start with an initial rule-based stage before using the parametric model. In this chapter, methods are designated as rule-based or model-based depending on how participants are allocated to doses.

Rule-Based Algorithm

The 3+3 Algorithm for Dose-Ranging

The "3+3" algorithm was used originally for finding the MTD for a single cytotoxic agent and applies decision rules based upon outcomes from cohorts of three participants. Rogatko et al. (2007) reviewed phase I clinical trials reported over a 15-year period, from 1991 to 2006, and found that 98% of the trials used some version of the 3+3 algorithm. More recently, Conaway and Petroni (2019b) noted that in 2018, a leading cancer journal published 37 articles that report on dose-finding or dose-ranging studies. Of the 37 studies, 32 (86%) still used the 3+3, even though few of the studies involved finding the MTD. There are a few versions of this algorithm with varying decision rules (Storer 1989; Piantadosi 2017).

Notwithstanding the prevalence of its use in applications, the 3+3 is generally dismissed in the statistical literature for its poor operating characteristics. Lin and Shih (2001) provide an in-depth evaluation of the properties of algorithmic designs in general, including the 3+3. The authors present results for three scenarios, each with five dose levels, and show that if the target toxicity were 25%, the percent of times that the 3+3 correctly selected the true MTD was only 26%, 30%, and 29% in the three scenarios. Given that choosing a dose at random, without even doing a trial, would recommend the correct MTD 20% of the time, the results for the 3+3 design are not impressive. Lin and Shih (2001) also demonstrate that despite the perception that the 3+3 targets the dose with a 1/3 probability of a DLT, the 3+3 algorithm design does not have a target toxicity level. Thus, it remains an applied design that does not target a specific population characteristic but instead describes the outcome from a small sample which provides little information on what proportion of future patients would experience a DLT. Similar results are found in Storer (1989), Reiner et al. (1999), and Iasonos et al. (2008). More general versions of this design, "A+B," have been proposed (Ananthakrishnan et al. 2017). An R Shiny app that can be used to investigate the operating characteristics of A+B designs, including the 3+3, is given by Wheeler et al. (2016).

Biased Coin Designs

Durham et al. (1997) describe a method for sequential dose allocation and estimation of the MTD based on random walks which allocates participants to dose level in cohorts of 1. If the current participant has been treated at dose level d_k and experiences a DLT, the next participant is treated at the next lower dose level d_{k-1}. If the current participant does not experience a DLT, the next participant is treated at the current dose, d_k, with probability $\theta/(1-\theta)$ or at the next higher dose level d_{k+1} with probability $1-[\theta/(1-\theta)]$, where $\theta < 0.5$ is the pre-specified target level of acceptable toxicity. The trial ends when a pre-study specified total of participants have been accrued to the study. Durham, Flournoy, and Rosenberger (1997) and Stylianou and Flournoy (2002) propose several estimators for the MTD at the end of the trial, including estimates based on logistic regression, means based on the number of participants assigned to each dose level, or based on isotonic regression. There are a number of good features to this design. It relies only on the assumption of an increasing dose-toxicity curve, the escalation and de-escalation rules are easy to implement, and both the small sample properties and asymptotic distribution theory for the estimators have been derived (Durham and Flournoy 1994, 1995).

Interval-Based Methods for Dose-Finding

The original interval-based method is the "cumulative cohort design" (CCD) proposed by Ivanova et al. (2007). Given a target toxicity probability, θ, the term "interval-based" derives from basing decision rules for treating the next set of participants at a lower, higher, or the same dose as the current cohort of participants on intervals placed around θ. If the current dose level is d_k and there are Y_k participants experiencing a DLT out of the n_k participants who have been treated at that dose, the decision rules proposed by Ivanova et al. (2007) are:

- If $\widehat{q} \leq \theta - \Delta_L$, "escalate the dose": treat the next group of participants at dose d_{k+1}.
- If $\widehat{q} \geq \theta + \Delta_U$, "de-escalate the dose": treat the next group of participants at dose d_{k-1}.
- If $\theta - \Delta_L \leq \widehat{q} \leq \theta + \Delta_U$, "stay": treat the next group of participants at dose d_k.

where $\widehat{q} = Y_k/n_k$ is the proportion of participants treated at dose d_k who have experienced a DLT. The interval values Δ_L and Δ_H are chosen to allocate, on average, as many participants as possible to the MTD. Ivanova et al. (2007) simplify the design further by taking $\Delta_L = \Delta_H = \Delta$ so that the decision intervals are symmetric around the target θ. They recommend $\Delta = 0.09$ for target toxicity probabilities between 0.10 and 0.25 and $\Delta = 0.10$ for target toxicity probabilities of 0.30 and 0.35. As an example, with a target toxicity probability of 0.20, the cumulative cohort design would indicate escalating to the next higher dose if the observed proportion of toxicities at the current dose is less than or equal to 0.11. If the observed proportion of toxicities is 0.29 or greater, the next cohort of participants would be treated at the next lower dose. The current dose would be allocated if the observed proportion of participants experiencing a DLT is between 0.21 and 0.29. This process of adaptively recommending doses to participants continues until a pre-specified number of participants have been observed.

A number of other interval-based designs have been proposed, including the modified toxicity probability interval (mTPI) method (Ji et al. 2007) and a subsequent modification of this method, the mTPI-2 (Guo et al. 2017). Liu and Yuan (2015) proposed a Bayesian optimal interval design (BOIN). A related method, the "Keyboard design," was proposed by Yan, Mandrekar, and Yuan (2017) and is equivalent to the mTPI-2 design. In this chapter, these methods are categorized as "interval-based" methods, although the authors also use the term "model-assisted" to refer to this class of method. All of these methods share a common goal, to develop designs for dose-finding studies that are simple to implement and have better operating characteristics than the 3+3. The methods differ on the criteria on which the intervals are derived, and the use of a point estimate, such as $\widehat{q}$ in the cumulative cohort design, or the Bayesian posterior probability associated with the intervals indicating de-escalation, escalation, or staying at the current dose.

In addition, these interval-based methods, unlike the cumulative cohort design, implement additional rules on the dose assignment process. A dose, and all higher doses, can be eliminated from consideration if the observed proportion of toxicities at the current dose is too great. The need for such a rule is clear with a simple, if somewhat unrealistic, example. Suppose that four dose levels are under consideration, and the levels were chosen such that the true toxicity probabilities associated with dose levels 1 and 2 are near 0 and dose levels 3 and 4 are near 1. Without these stopping rules, the design would oscillate between recommending dose escalation from dose level 2 to 3 and de-escalation from dose level 3 to 2. Other than the CCD, the other interval-based methods also implement rules that stop the trial if too much toxicity is observed at the lowest dose level.

As a practical matter, these designs differ little in their decision rules. Table 1 shows the decision rules for a target toxicity level of 0.20, for up to ten participants treated at a dose, and the possible number of participants observed to have a DLT. The CCD method was modified to have the same dose elimination rules as BOIN and Keyboard. The values for CCD, BOIN, and Keyboard (mTPI-2) were computed from the "get.boundary" function in R (Lin 2018). In this table, if only a single entry appears, all three methods gave the same recommendation. In the few cases where the recommendations differ, the recommendations from each of the methods are given in the order CCD, BOIN, and Keyboard. There are few points of disagreement among the three methods and the BOIN and Keyboard methods never disagree. The

Table 1 Comparison of dose allocation rules for three interval-based methods

	Number of participants observed on the current dose									
Number of participants with a DLT on the current dose	1	2	3	4	5	6	7	8	9	10
0	E	E	E	E	E	E	E	E	E	E
1	D	D	D	S;D;D	S	S	S;E;E	S;E;E	S;E;E	E
2		D	D	D	D	D	S;D;D	S;D;D	S	S
3			R	R	R	R	D	D	D	D
4				R	R	R	R	R	R	D
5					R	R	R	R	R	R
6						R	R	R	R	R
7							R	R	R	R
8								R	R	R
9									R	R
10										R

E, escalate dose; S, stay at current dose; D, de-escalate; R, de-escalate and remove the dose from consideration

similarity in the dose allocation rules is not surprising; Clertant and O'Quigley (2017, 2019) develop a semiparametric method that can be calibrated to produce identical operating characteristics to all of these individual methods.

Model-Based Methods for Dose-Finding

The most widely recognized model-based method for dose-finding trials is the continual reassessment method (CRM). The original CRM paper proposed a single-stage design; a later version (Shen and O'Quigley 1996) is a two-stage design using a rule-based algorithm in the first stage and maximum likelihood estimation in the second stage. An excellent overview of the theoretical properties and guidelines for the practical application of the method is given in Cheung (2011) and O'Quigley and Iasonos (2012). The CRM assumes a parametric model for the dose-toxicity curve, but it does not require that the model be correct across all the doses under consideration. The model only needs to be increasing in dose and be such that there is a parameter value that enables the function to equal the target value, θ, at the true MTD. The original CRM paper discussed one- and two-parameter models but focused primarily on one-parameter models because the simpler models tended to have better properties in terms of identifying the correct MTD.

The most common implementation of the CRM uses the "empiric" model for π_k; the probability of a DLT at dose level d_k is assumed to be equal to

$$\pi_k = (\varphi_k)^{\exp(a)}$$

where $0 < \varphi_1 < \varphi_2 < \ldots < \varphi_K < 1$ are pre-specified constants, often referred to as the "skeleton" values and "a" is a scalar parameter to be estimated from the data. The parametrization exp(a) ensures that the probability of toxicity is increasing in dose for all values of the parameter a. The original CRM paper (O'Quigley et al. 1990) was a Bayesian method that put a prior distribution on the parameter, a. The paper provided guidance on eliciting a gamma prior for exp(a) but noted that in many cases, the special case of an exponential prior with mean 1 gave satisfactory performance. The skeleton values can be based on the prior, as suggested in the original CRM paper, or by using the method of Lee and Cheung (2009) where the skeleton values are calibrated in a way to give good performance for the CRM across a variety of true dose-toxicity curves.

Once the prior and skeleton values are chosen, the first participant is assigned to the dose level with prior probability closest to the target θ. After that, the CRM allocates participants sequentially, with each participant assigned to the dose level with the model-based estimated probability of toxicity closest to the target. To be specific, suppose that $j-1$ participants have been observed on the trial, with $n_k \geq 0$ participants observed on dose levels k, k = 1, ..., K. Of the n_k participants, Y_k participants experienced a DLT. Using the data accumulated from the $j-1$ participants observed, the updated model-based toxicity probabilities are

$$\widehat{\pi}_k = (\varphi_k)^{\exp\left(\widehat{a}\right)}$$

where $\widehat{a}$ can be the posterior mean computed via numerical integration, an approximation to the posterior mean as in O'Quigley et al. (1990), the posterior mode, or the posterior median (Chu et al. 2009). The next participant is assigned to the dose level k with the estimated toxicity probability closest to the target, where "closest" is according to a pre-specified measure of distance between the estimate and the target. The original paper uses a quadratic distance, but asymmetric distance functions, which give greater loss to deviations above the target than below, could also be used. The updating of "a" and the allocation of participants to the dose with updated toxicity probability closest to the target continues until a pre-specified number of participants have been observed. At the end of the study, the MTD is taken to be the dose that the next participant would have received had the trial not ended.

A two-stage version of the CRM is presented by Shen and O'Quigley (1996). The first stage uses a rule-based design and continues until at least one participant experiences a DLT and one participant does not experience a DLT. Once heterogeneity in responses is observed, the trial proceeds as in the original CRM, except that the estimate of the parameter "a" is based on maximum likelihood. The paper uses a rule-based design using single-participant cohorts: if a participant does not experience a DLT, the next participant is treated at the next higher dose level, but the authors note that any rule-based design could be used in stage I until heterogeneity is observed.

The "escalation with overdose control" (EWOC) method of Babb et al. (1998) is a popular method for dose-finding. As with the previous dose-finding methods, Babb et al. (1998) set a target toxicity probability, θ, and assume that the true MTD, defined as the dose that has a toxicity probability equal to the target, is in a pre-specified interval [X_{min}, X_{max}]. Their method is designed to identify the MTD while providing "overdose control," limiting the proportion of participants exposed to doses above the MTD.

The EWOC design is based on a two-parameter model for the probability of a DLT at dose x in [X_{min}, X_{max}]. One of several possibilities for the dose-toxicity relationship model is the logistic model:

$$logit[P(DLT\ |x)] = \beta_0 + \beta_1 x$$

where β_1 is restricted to be greater than 0 so that the probability of a DLT is increasing in x. Babb et al. (1998) propose a Bayesian method, assuming priors on the pair (β_0, β_1).

The first participant or cohort of participants is assigned dose X_{min}. From there, the study proceeds much like the original CRM. Data from the first j-1 participants is used to update the posterior distribution for (β_0, β_1) and used to guide the dose administered to the jth participant. Unlike the CRM, which allocates the jth participant to the dose that has a toxicity probability estimated to be closest to the target, the EWOC method assigns the dose, x*, such that the posterior probability that the toxicity probability associated with x* exceeds the target is equal to a pre-specified value.

This process of updating the posterior distribution of (β_0, β_1) and allocating participants to doses based on the updated posterior distribution continues until a pre-specified number of participants have been observed. At the end of the trial, the MTD is chosen as the value that minimizes the expected loss with respect to the posterior distribution of the MTD. This loss is taken as an asymmetric loss function, penalizing overdosing more than underdosing.

Babb et al. (1998) showed that EWOC and the Bayesian CRM with a symmetric loss function had similar properties for identifying the MTD and were more efficient than any of the rule-based designs they considered which include the four up-and-down designs of Storer (1989) and two methods based on stochastic approximation. On average, the EWOC method tended to treat more participants on low and possibly sub-therapeutic doses than did the CRM but treated fewer participants at dose levels above the MTD than did CRM. Over all the simulations, the average proportion of participants with DLTs with CRM was almost exactly equal to the target level (33%); this proportion was between 25% and 30% for EWOC. An excellent overview of EWOC and its extensions is given in Tighiouart and Rogatko (2014).

Semiparametric and Order-Restricted Methods for Dose-Finding

These methods do not fall neatly into either the interval-based or model-based classifications. The semiparametric dose-finding method of Clertant and O'Quigley (2017) is more of a class of methods than a specific design. If parametric conditions are added to the class, the result is the CRM design. Using less structure on the class results in the interval-based designs, including the CCD, mTPI-2, and BOIN. Clertant and O'Quigley (2017) present results for a "semiparametric" design that corresponds to CRM with an additional nuisance parameter. This formulation leads to a design that reduces the dependence of the CRM on a single model and produces results similar to those of the CRM.

The methods of Leung and Wang (2001) and Conaway et al. (2004) are based on methods for order-restricted inference. These methods are, in a way, model-based designs but rely only on the assumption that the probability of a DLT increases with dose. The methods do not specify a full parametrized parametric model. Recent work (Wages and Conaway 2018) has shown that the order-restricted methods are competitive in performance to the CRM, the method that generally has the best operating characteristic, as described in the following section, in dose-finding studies over a wide range of scenarios.

Evaluating Methods for Dose-Finding and Dose-Ranging

There are a number of criteria on which the methods can be compared. These include the statistical properties, the ease of implementation and adaptability to changes in the study conduct, and principles for conducting early-stage studies.

Operating Characteristics

Comparisons of the properties of the methods are complicated by the lack of consensus in the criteria on which the methods should be judged and the necessity of focusing on selected true dose-toxicity scenarios. The most common criterion for evaluation is the "percent correct selection" (PCS) (Cheung 2011), the proportion of times that the method correctly selects the true MTD, or how often the method selects a dose within a certain range, such as 5 or 10 percentage points within the target toxicity. Comparisons may be also made on the percent of participants treated at the MTD or at doses close to the MTD or on the basis of the proportion of participants treated at doses above the MTD.

The accuracy index (Cheung 2011) is a useful measure that takes into account the entire distribution of dose recommendations:

$$\text{Accuracy index} = 1 - K\,\frac{\sum_{k=1}^{K}\rho_k\, P(\text{design selects dose } k)}{\sum_{k=1}^{K}\rho_k}$$

where ρ_k is a measure of the deviation of the true toxicity probability, π_k, at dose k from the target toxicity probability θ. Cheung (2011) gives several choices for ρ_k, including an absolute deviation, $\rho_k = |\pi_k - \theta|$. The accuracy index has a maximum value of 1, which occurs when the design always recommends the correct MTD.

With few exceptions, comparisons among the methods are made based on simulations, and historically, these simulations were done using a limited number of true dose-toxicity curves. Even when exact small sample results are available (Durham and Flournoy 1994, 1995; Lin and Shih 2001), these results depend on the true unknown underlying dose-toxicity curve. This can make comparisons difficult, since every method has some scenarios under which it will perform well. A tool for evaluating the properties of designs is given in O'Quigley et al. (2002) and Paoletti et al. (2004). The benchmark cannot be used in practice because it requires knowledge of the true underlying dose-toxicity curve; however, it has been shown to be useful in investigating the efficiency of proposed designs (Wages et al. 2013) in the context of studies with monotone dose-toxicity curves.

It is important, when evaluating a design, to consider the performance across a broad range of scenarios, varying the location of the MTD and the steepness of the dose-toxicity curve. To this end, a number of families of dose-toxicity curves have been proposed. Evaluating methods for specific dose-toxicity curves randomly sampled from the family of curves is intended to test the method across a range of curves that vary in MTD location and steepness. One of the first families of curves was generated by Paoletti et al. (2004); subsequent proposals can be found in Horton et al. (2017), Clertant and O'Quigley (2017), and Conaway and Petroni (2019a).

Ease of Implementation and Adaptability

Rule-based methods have the practical advantage of being simpler to carry out because all of the decision rules can be laid out in a table prior to starting the study. The model-based methods also have some practical advantages over rule-based methods. Model-based methods can enroll participants even if the follow-up period for previously enrolled participants is not yet complete. Model-based methods can accommodate revisions to data errors; on subsequent review, participants thought not to have had DLTs could be found to have had DLTs, or vice versa, participants thought not to have DLTs could be classified upon further review as having had a DLT. Subsequent allocations can proceed based on models fit to the corrected data.

Principles

Cheung (2005) defined the principle of coherence for single-agent dose-finding and dose-ranging studies. By this definition, a method is coherent for dose escalation if the method does not increase the dose following an observed DLT and coherent for dose de-escalation if the method does not decrease the dose following the observation of a non-DLT. This is an important principle in implementing a study, since clinicians can be reluctant to follow an incoherent design, particularly one that is incoherent in dose escalation.

The 3+3, despite its poor operating characteristics, is at least coherent by this definition. The biased coin design (Durham et al. 1997), EWOC (Tighiouart and Rogatko 2014), and the semiparametric CRM (Clertant and O'Quigley 2017) are all coherent. Cheung (2011) shows that the one-stage Bayesian CRM is coherent and that the two-stage CRM is coherent as long as it does not produce an incoherent transition between the rule-based and model-based stages. Clertant and O'Quigley (2017) show that the semiparametric CRM is coherent. In general, the interval-based methods are not coherent by this definition, and in practice, incoherent decisions occur frequently with these designs (Wages et al. 2019 under review).

Interval-based designs defined a separate principle and unfortunately also used the term "coherence" (Liu and Yuan 2015). The principle, defined as "long-term memory coherence," means that a method will not increase the dose for the next participant if the observed proportion of participants at the current dose who have experienced a DLT exceeds the target toxicity rate and the method will not reduce the dose for the next participant if the observed proportion of DLTs at the current dose is less than the target. By construction, the interval-based designs are all "long-term memory coherent."

An example from Wages et al. (2019 under review) serves to illustrate the difference between the original definition of coherence and "long-term memory coherence." Table 2 shows the dose allocations from BOIN and Keyboard for a simulated trial using the settings in Scenario 2 in Table S2 of Zhou et al. (2011). Decisions at participants 9 and 13 represented incoherence in dose de-escalation; in each case, the next participant is treated at a lower dose immediately following a non-DLT. Both of these decisions are "long-term memory coherent." The decision at participant 16 is incoherent in dose escalation. Even though this participant

Table 2 Example of incoherent dose escalations

				Accumulated data on each dose (# DLTs/# participants)				
Participant	Dose assigned	Outcome	Decision	1	2	3	4	5
1	1	Non-DLT	Escalate	0/1	0/0	0/0	0/0	1/1
2	2	Non-DLT	Escalate	0/1	0/1	0/0	0/0	1/1
3	3	Non-DLT	Escalate	0/1	0/1	0/1	0/0	1/1
4	4	Non-DLT	Escalate	0/1	0/1	0/1	0/1	1/1
5	5	DLT	De-escalate	0/1	0/1	0/1	0/1	1/1
6	4	DLT	De-escalate	0/1	0/1	0/1	1/2	1/1
7	3	DLT	De-escalate	0/1	0/1	1/2	1/2	1/1
8	2	Non-DLT	Escalate	0/1	0/2	1/2	1/2	1/1
9[a]	3	Non-DLT	De-escalate	0/1	0/2	1/3	1/2	1/1
10	2	Non-DLT	Escalate	0/1	0/3	1/3	1/2	1/1
11	3	DLT	De-escalate	0/1	0/3	2/4	1/2	1/1
12	2	Non-DLT	Escalate	0/1	0/4	2/4	1/2	1/1
13[a]	3	Non-DLT	De-escalate	0/1	0/4	2/5	1/2	1/1
14	2	Non-DLT	Escalate	0/1	0/5	2/5	1/2	1/1
15	3	DLT	De-escalate	0/1	0/5	3/6	1/2	1/1
16[b]	2	DLT	Escalate	0/1	1/6	3/6	1/2	1/1
17	3	Non-DLT	De-escalate	0/1	1/6	3/7	1/2	1/1

[a]Not coherent in dose de-escalation
[b]Not coherent in dose escalation

experienced a DLT on dose level 2, both BOIN and Keyboard treat the next participant at a higher dose, dose level 3, which has an observed proportion of toxicities greater than the target.

Extensions Beyond Single-Agent Trials with a Binary Toxicity Outcome

Single-agent dose-finding or dose-ranging trials are becoming less frequent, particularly in oncology, giving way to studies that involve combinations of agents or studies that involve heterogeneous groups of participants. Designs that have been developed to meet the challenges of studies of combinations of agents or studies conducted in heterogeneous groups of participants are discussed in this chapter. Other features of contemporary dose-finding or dose-ranging trials include the study of noncytotoxic agents or studies that collect preliminary assessments of efficacy, but space limitations preclude a full discussion of methods in these areas.

Time-to-Event Toxicity Outcomes

The original CRM paper (O'Quigley et al. 1990) noted that the observation of a toxicity does not occur immediately. As a result, there may be new participants ready to enroll in the study before all the prior participants have been observed for a DLT. O'Quigley et al. (1990) suggested treating the new participants at the last allocated dose, or given the uncertainty in the dose allocations, treating participants' one level above or one level below the most recent model-recommended dose.

Cheung and Chappell (2010) proposed an extension to the continual reassessment method known as the "time-to-event CRM" (TITE-CRM). This method allows for a weighted toxicity model, with weights proportional to the time that the participant has been observed. They consider a number of weight functions, but simulation results suggested that a simple linear weight function of the form $w(u) = u/T$, where T is a fixed length of follow-up observation time for each participant, is adequate. If a participant is observed to have a toxicity at time $u < T$, the follow-up time u is set to equal T. If DLT information has been observed for all participants, the method reduces to the continual reassessment method of O'Quigley et al. (1990).

Normolle and Lawrence (2006) discuss the use of the TITE-CRM in radiation oncology studies, where the toxicities tend to occur late in the follow-up period. Polley (2011) observes that in studies with rapid participant accrual and late toxicities, the TITE-CRM can allocate too many participants to overly toxic doses. The paper has a comparison of a modification of the TITE-CRM that was suggested in the original TITE-CRM paper, as well as a modification that incorporates wait times between participant accruals. A version of EWOC with time-to-event endpoints is described in Mauguen et al. (2011) and Tighiouart et al. (2014a).

A modification of the 3+3, called the rolling 6 (Skolnik et al. 2008), is meant to reduce the time to completion of a dose-ranging trial by allowing participants to enter a trial before complete information is available for participants in the prior cohort. Zhao et al. (2011) has shown that this method is less efficient and less accurate than TITE-CRM.

Combinations of Agents

The simplest form of a study with a combination of two agents is depicted below. Each of two agents (A and B) is being studied at two dose levels ("low" and "high"). The probability of a DLT with agent at level "a" and agent B at level "b" is denoted by π_{ab}. The problem of dose-finding or dose-ranging differs from the single-agent case in that the probabilities of toxicity no longer follow a complete order, in which the ordering or any two toxicity parameters are known, but instead follow a "partial order" (Robertson et al. 1988). In a partial order, there are pairs of parameters whose ordering is not known. For example, it is not known whether $\pi_{HL} > \pi_{LH}$ or $\pi_{HL} < \pi_{LH}$. A second distinction from the single-agent case is that in a combination study, there may be more than one "MTD," meaning more than one dose combination with a toxicity probability close to the target.

The initial suggestion for studies of drug combinations was to lay out a specific ordering of the combinations (Korn and Simon 1993; Kramar et al. 1999). While simple to implement, this approach follows only one path through the combinations and could have poor properties in identifying an MTD, particularly if the assumed ordering is incorrect.

As in the single-agent case, methods can broadly be classified as rule-based or model-based methods. The interval-based "Bayesian optimal interval design (BOIN)" has been extended to studies involving combinations (Lin and Yin 2017). Based on the observed proportion of participants experiencing a DLT at the current dose, a decision is made to "escalate," "de-escalate," or "stay" at the current dose. More than one dose combination might be considered an "escalation" or a "de-escalation," and Lin and Yin (2017) propose pre-specifying, for each dose combination, a set of "admissible escalation doses" and "admissible de-escalation doses." A similar idea had been proposed by Conaway et al. (2004), who used the estimation method of Hwang and Peddada (1994) as well as "possible escalation sets" for each dose combination to guide dose combination allocations. Similarly, bivariate isotonic regression was the basis of the method proposed by Wang and Ivanova (2005). This method estimates the probability of a DLT for each combination under the assumption that for a fixed row, the toxicity probabilities increase across columns and for each column, toxicity probabilities increase across each column. In Table 3 for example, it is known that $\pi_{LL} < \pi_{LH}$, $\pi_{HL} < \pi_{HH}$, $\pi_{LL} < \pi_{HL}$ and $\pi_{LH} < \pi_{HH}$.

The majority of methods for dose-finding and dose-ranging for combinations of agents are model-based. Extensions of the CRM were proposed by Wages et al. (2011a, b). These methods consider either a subset or all possible orders of the toxicity probabilities. For example, in Table 3 for the simplest case, there are two possible orders:

Table 3 A study with two agents, each at two dose levels

	Agent B	
Agent A	Low	High
High	π_{HL}	π_{HH}
Low	π_{LL}	π_{LH}

$$\text{Order 1}: \quad \pi_{LL} < \pi_{LH} < \pi_{HL} < \pi_{HH}$$

$$\text{Order 2}: \quad \pi_{LL} < \pi_{HL} < \pi_{LH} < \pi_{HH}$$

The CRM is fit separately within each order. After each participant is observed, the recommendation is based on the order that yields a greater value of the likelihood. In many studies with more than two dose levels for each of the agents, there can be too many possible orderings to specify all of them. In this case, clinical judgment can be used to guide the choice of orders under consideration, or the default set of orders recommended by Wages and Conaway (2013) can be used.

Yin and Yuan (2009) also generalize the single-agent CRM for studies considering combinations of J levels of agent A and K levels of agent B. They pre-specify values $p_1 < p_2 < \ldots < P_K$ for agent A and values $q_1 < q_2 < \ldots < q_J$ for agent B and use a model for the probability of a DLT that depends on the pre-specified values as well as three parameters to be estimated from the data. At the end of the trial, the estimate of the MTD is the dose with the estimated DLT probability closest to the pre-specified target.

Other model-based methods are based on a full mathematical specification of the probabilities of toxicity for each combination. Thall et al. (2003) propose a nonlinear six-parameter model to describe how the probability of toxicity depends on the dose combination.

All of the previous methods are for studies in which a discrete set of combinations have been pre-specified. For dose-finding studies, Shi and Yin (2013) and Tighiouart et al. (2014b) have generalized the EWOC method for combinations. Both of these generalizations use a logistic model for the probability of toxicity that included main effects for the dose level of each combination and a multiplicative interaction term to specify the joint effect of the two agents.

Heterogeneity of Participants

In some dose-finding trials, there are several groups of participants, and the goal is to estimate a MTD within each group. These groups may be defined by the participants' degree of impairment at baseline (Ramanathan et al. 2008; LoRusso et al. 2012) or genetic characteristics (Kim et al. 2013). For example, Ramanathan et al. (2008) enrolled 89 participants with varying solid tumors to develop dosing guidelines for the administration of imatinib in participants with liver dysfunction. Prior to dosing, participants were stratified into "none," "mild," "moderate," or "severe" liver dysfunction at baseline, according to serum total bilirubin and AST. A similar classification is used by LoRusso et al. (2012). Kim et al. (2013) define three groups of participants according to the number of defective alleles, either 0, 1, or 2.

In each of these cases, parallel phase I studies were conducted within each group but did not account for the expectation that the MTD would be lower in the more severely impaired participants at baseline or in the subset of participants with a greater number of defective alleles. In these cases, even with an efficient design, given the sample sizes typically seen in phase I trials, ignoring the orderings among the groups can lead to reversals in the MTD estimates, meaning that the estimated MTDs in the groups can contradict what is known clinically (Horton et al. 2019b). Furthermore, even in cases where the ordering is not known, running parallel studies can be inefficient compared to a design that uses a model to pool information from all participants across all groups in order to estimate the dose-toxicity relationship.

O'Quigley, Shen, and Gamst (1999) and O'Quigley and Paoletti (2003) were the first to investigate the consequences of using parallel trials. More recently, Raphael et al. (2010) discussed the use of parallel trials of heavily pretreated and lightly pretreated participants in dose-finding trials in pediatric participants and recommended that parallel trials only be undertaken when there is a strong rationale for doing so.

To avoid the issues with parallel groups, a number of statistical methods have been proposed for estimating MTDs when there is heterogeneity among participants. All of the methods proposed to date for accounting for participant heterogeneity in dose-finding are either generalizations of model-based methods or order-restricted methods for single-agent trials. O'Quigley, Shen, and Gamst (1999) and O'Quigley and Paoletti (2003) account for participant heterogeneity by adding a covariate to represent participant characteristics. In O'Quigley and Paoletti (2003), the ordering of probabilities of DLTs between the groups is known, and this knowledge is incorporated into the model through the prior distribution.

An alternative to adding a covariate to account for discrete groups in dose-finding studies is to combine model-based methods and order-restricted inference. The first method to do this is Yuan and Chappell (2004), who are estimating the MTD for a single agent in each of G ordered groups. In Yuan and Chappell (2004), the single-agent CRM is applied separately to the data in each group. Using the bivariate isotonic regression estimator (Robertson et al. 1988), the resulting DLT probability estimates are modified so that the estimates increase with increasing dose within each group, and there are no reversals, meaning there are no dose levels where a lower-risk group has greater DLT probability estimates than a higher-risk group. Once the isotonic estimates are computed, dose allocation proceeds as in the single-group CRM, the next participant in group "g" is allocated to the dose with an estimated toxicity probability in group "g" closest to the target θ. Similar ideas are found in Conaway (2017a, b) which propose methods for completely ordered groups, such as the example in Ramanathan (2008), or partially ordered groups, in which some of the orderings between the groups are unknown.

Several methods take advantage of the discrete dose levels often found in dose-finding studies. The "shift model" (O'Quigley 2006), described more fully in

O'Quigley and Iasonos (2014), takes a different approach to generalizing the CRM to two ordered groups. For two groups, the assumption underlying this method is that the MTD in group 2 will be Δ dose levels less than the MTD in group 1, with Δ a nonnegative integer. O'Quigley and Iasonos (2014) restrict Δ to be 0, 1, 2, or 3 levels, but their method applies to any shift in the MTD. Horton et al. (2019a) generalize the shift model to more than two groups and to either completely or partially ordered groups.

Babb and Rogatko (2001) extend the EWOC method to allow for a continuous covariate. In their application (Babb and Rogatko 2001), the covariate was protective, with increasing levels of the covariate associated with a lower probability of a DLT. Data from a previous study of the agent allowed the investigators to set bounds on the permissible doses for a participant with a specific covariate value. With this method, participants can receive individualized doses according to their level of the covariate. Similar methods are found in Tighiouart et al. (2012).

Summary and Conclusion

This chapter has presented a number of designs for dose-finding and dose-ranging studies for a single agent and in which the primary objective of the study is to establish a maximum safe dose. Many of the applications of these designs are in oncology, which is currently undergoing a change in the complexity and objectives of dose-finding and dose-ranging studies. This chapter has also reviewed a number of designs that have been developed recently to meet the challenges of contemporary dose-finding and dose-ranging studies.

Key Facts

1. The dose-finding design must be conducted in a way that addresses the study objectives.
2. Dose-finding studies are an integral part of the overall drug development process.
3. The commonly used "3+3" algorithm has poor operating characteristics.
4. Interval-based dose-finding designs are simple to implement and provide better operating characteristics than the "3+3."
5. In general, model-based dose-finding designs have superior operating characteristics and provide the flexibility needed to handle data revisions and delayed dose-limiting toxicities.

Cross-References

▶ Bayesian Adaptive Designs for Phase I Trials
▶ Dose Finding for Drug Combinations
▶ Implementing the Trial Protocol

▶ Interim Analysis in Clinical Trials
▶ Monte Carlo Simulation for Trial Design Tool
▶ Participant Recruitment, Screening, and Enrollment
▶ Power and Sample Size
▶ Principles of Clinical Trials: Bias and Precision Control

References

Ananthakrishnan R, Green S, Chang M, Doros G, Massaro J, LaValleya M (2017) Systematic comparison of the statistical operating characteristics of various phase I oncology designs. Contemp Clin Trials Commun 5:34–48

Babb J, Rogatko A (2001) Patient specific dosing in a cancer phase I clinical trial. Stat Med 20:2079–2090

Babb J, Rogatko A, Zacks S (1998) Cancer phase I clinical trials: efficient dose escalation with overdose control. Stat Med 17:1103–1120

Cheung YK (2005) Coherence principles in dose-finding studies. Biometrika 92:203–215

Cheung YK (2011) Dose finding by the continual reassessment method. Chapman and Hall/CRC Biostatistics Series, New York

Cheung YK, Chappell R (2010) Sequential designs for phase I clinical trials with late-onset toxicities. Biometrics 56:1177–1182

Chu PL, Lin Y, Shih WJ (2009) Unifying CRM and EWOC designs for phase I cancer clinical trials. J Stat Plann Inference 139:1146–1163

Clertant M, O'Quigley J (2017) Semiparametric dose finding methods. J R Stat Soc Ser B 79 (5):1487–1508

Clertant M, O'Quigley J (2019) Semiparametric dose finding methods: special cases. Appl Stat 68 (2):271–288

Conaway M (2017a) A design for phase I trials in completely or partially ordered groups. Stat Med 36(15):2323–2332

Conaway M (2017b) Isotonic designs for phase I trials in partially ordered groups. Clin Trials 14 (5):491–498

Conaway M, Petroni G (2019a) The impact of early stage design on the drug development process. Clin Cancer Res 25(2):819–827

Conaway M, Petroni G (2019b) The role of early-phase design-response. Clin Cancer Res 25 (10):3191

Conaway M, Dunbar S, Peddada S (2004) Designs for single- or multiple-agent phase I trials. Biometrics 60:661–669

Durham S, Flournoy N (1994) Random walks for quantile estimation. In: Gupta S, Berger J (eds) Statistical decision theory and related topics V. Springer, New York, pp 467–476

Durham S, Flournoy N (1995) Up-and-down designs I: stationary treatment distributions. In: Flournoy N, Rosenberger W (eds) Adaptive designs. Institute of Mathematical Statistics, Hayward, pp 139–157

Durham S, Flournoy N, Rosenberger W (1997) A random walk rule for phase 1 clinical trials. Biometrics 53(2):745–760

Eussen S, de Groot L, Clarke R, Schneede J, Ueland P, Hoefnagels W, van Staveren W (2005) Oral cyanocobalamin supplementation in older people with vitamin B12 deficiency: a dose-finding trial. Arch Intern Med 165:1167–1172

Ezard N, Dunlop A, Clifford B, Bruno R, Carr A, Bissaker A, Lintzeris N (2016) Study protocol: a dose-escalating, phase-2 study of oral lisdexamfetamine in adults with methamphetamine dependence. BMC Psychiatry 16:428

Guo W, Wang S-J, Yang S, Lynna H, Ji Y (2017) A Bayesian interval dose-finding design addressing Ockham's razor: mTPI-2. Contemp Clin Trials 58:23–33
Horton B, Wages N, Conaway M (2017) Performance of toxicity probability interval based designs in contrast to the continual reassessment method. Stat Med 36:291–300
Horton BJ, Wages NA, Conaway MR (2019a) Shift models for dose-finding in partially ordered groups. Clin Trials 16(1):32–40
Horton BJ, O'Quigley J, Conaway M (2019b) Consequences of performing parallel dose finding trials in heterogeneous groups of patients. JNCI Cancer Spectrum. https://doi.org/10.1093/jncics/pkz013. Online ahead of print
Hwang J, Peddada S (1994) Confidence interval estimation subject to order restrictions. Ann Stat 22:67–93
Iasonos A, Wilton AS, Riedel ER, Seshan VE, Spriggs DR (2008) A comprehensive comparison of the continual reassessment method to the standard 3+3 dose escalation scheme in phase I dose-finding studies. Clin Trials 5(5):465–477
Ivanova A, Flournoy N, Chung Y (2007) Cumulative cohort design for dose-finding. J Stat Plann Inference 137:2316–2327
Ji Y, Li Y, Bekele B (2007) Dose-finding in phase I clinical trials based on toxicity probability intervals. Clin Trials 4:235–244
Kim K, Kim H, Sym S, Bae K, Hong Y, Chang H, Lee J, Kang Y, Lee J, Shin J, Kim T (2013) A UGT1A1*28 and *6 genotype-directed phase I dose-escalation trial of irinotecan with fixed-dose capecitabine in Korean patients with metastatic colorectal cancer. Cancer Chemother Pharmacol 71:1609–1617
Korn E, Simon R (1993) Using tolerable-dose diagrams in the design of phase I combination chemotherapy trials. J Clin Oncol 11:794–801
Kramar A, Lebecq A, Candalh E (1999) Continual reassessment methods in phase I trials of the combination of two agents in oncology. Stat Med 18:849–864
Le Tourneau C, Lee J, Siu L (2009) Dose escalation methods in phase I clinical trials. J Natl Cancer Inst 101:708–720
Lee S, Cheung YK (2009) Model calibration in the continual reassessment method. Clin Trials 6:227–238
Leung D, Wang Y-G (2001) Isotonic designs for phase I trials. Clin Trials 22:126–138
Lin R (2018) R codes for interval designs. https://github.com/ruitaolin/IntervalDesign
Lin Y, Shih W (2001) Statistical properties of traditional algorithm-based designs for phase I cancer clinical trials. Biostatistics 2(2):203–215
Lin R, Yin G (2017) Bayesian optimal interval design for dose finding in drug-combination trials. Stat Methods Med Res 26(5):2155–2167
Liu S, Yuan Y (2015) Bayesian optimal interval designs for phase I clinical trials. J R Stat Soc Ser C Appl Stat 32:2505–2511
LoRusso P, Venkatakrishnan K, Ramanathan R, Sarantopoulos J, Mulkerin D, Shibata S, Hamilton A, Dowlati A, Mani S, Rudek M, Takimoto C, Neuwirth R, Esseltine D, Ivy P (2012) Pharmacokinetics and safety of Bortezomib in patients with advanced malignancies and varying degrees of liver dysfunction: phase I NCI Organ Dysfunction Working Group Study NCI-6432. Clin Cancer Res 18(10):1–10
Mauguen A, Le Deleya M, Zohar S (2011) Dose-finding approach for dose escalation with overdose control considering incomplete observations. Stat Med 30:1584–1594
Normolle D, Lawrence T (2006) Designing dose-escalation trials with late-onset toxicities using the time-to-event continual reassessment method. J Clin Oncol 24:4426–4433
O'Quigley J (2006) Phase I and phase I/II dose finding algorithms using continual reassessment method. In: Crowley J, Ankherst D (eds) Handbook of statistics in clinical oncology, 2nd edn. Chapman and Hall/CRC Biostatistics Series, New York
O'Quigley J, Iasonos A (2012) Dose-finding designs based on the continual reassessment method. In: Crowley J, Hoering (eds) Handbook of statistics in clinical oncology, 3rd edn. Chapman and Hall/CRC Biostatistics Series, New York

O'Quigley J, Iasonos A (2014) Bridging solutions in dose-finding problems. J Biopharm Stat 6 (2):185–197
O'Quigley J, Paoletti X (2003) Continual reassessment method for ordered groups. Biometrics 59:430–440
O'Quigley J, Pepe M, Fisher L (1990) Continual reassessment method: a practical design for phase I clinical trials in cancer. Biometrics 46(1):33–48
O'Quigley J, Shen L, Gamst A (1999) Two sample continual reassessment method. J Biopharm Stat 9:17–44
O'Quigley J, Paoletti X, Maccario J (2002) Nonparametric optimal design in dose finding studies. Biostatistics 3(1):51–56
Paoletti X, O'Quigley J, Maccario J (2004) Design efficiency in dose finding studies. Comput Stat Data Anal 45:197–214
Partinen M, Hirvonen K, Jama L, Alakuijala A, Hublin C, Tamminen I, Koester J, Reess J (2006) Efficacy and safety of pramipexole in idiopathic restless legs syndrome: a polysomnographic dose-finding study – the PRELUDE study. Sleep Med 7:407–417
Piantadosi S (2017) Clinical trials: a methodologic perspective, 3rd edn. Wiley, Hoboken
Polley M (2011) Practical modifications to the time-to-event continual reassessment method for phase I cancer trials with fast patient accrual and late-onset toxicities. Stat Med 30:2130–2143
Ramanathan R, Egorin M, Takimoto C, Remick S, Doroshow J, LoRusso P, Mulkerin D, Grem J, Hamilton A, Murgo A, Potter D, Belani C, Hayes M, Peng B, Ivy P (2008) Phase I and pharmacokinetic study of Imatinib Mesylate in patients with advanced malignancies and varying degrees of liver dysfunction: a study by the National Cancer Institute Organ Dysfunction Working Group. J Clin Oncol 26:563–569
Raphael M, le Deley M, Vassal G, Paoletti X (2010) Operating characteristics of two independent sample design in phase I trials in paediatric oncology. Eur J Cancer 46:1392–1398
Reiner E, Paoletti X, O'Quigley J (1999) Operating characteristics of the standard phase I clinical trial design. Comput Stat Data Anal 30(3):303–315
Robertson T, Wright FT, Dykstra R (1988) Order restricted statistical inference. Wiley, New York
Rogatko A, Schoeneck D, Jonas W, Tighiouart M, Khuri F, Porter A (2007) Translation of innovative designs into phase I trials. J Clin Oncol 25(31):4982–4986
Sauter A, Ullensvang K, Niemi G, Lorentzen H, Bendtsen T, Børglum J, Pripp A, Romundstad L (2015) The shamrock lumbar plexus block: a dose-finding study. Eur J Anaesthesiol 32:764–770
Schaller S, Fink H, Ulm K, Blobner M (2010) Sugammadex and neostigmine dose-finding study for reversal of shallow residual neuromuscular block. Anesthesiology 113:1054–1060
Senderowicz A (2010) Information needed to conduct first-in-human oncology trials in the United States: a view from a former FDA medical reviewer. Clin Cancer Res 16(6):1719–1725
Shen L, O'Quigley J (1996) Continual reassessment method: a likelihood approach. Biometrics 52:673–684
Shi Y, Yin G (2013) Escalation with overdose control for phase I drug combination trials. Stat Med 32:4400–4412
Skolnik JM, Barrett JS, Jayaraman B, Patel D, Adamson PC (2008) Shortening the timeline of pediatric phase I trials: the rolling six design. J Clin Oncol 26(2):190–195
Storer B (1989) Design and analysis of phase I clinical trials. Biometrics 45(3):925–937
Stylianou M, Flournoy N (2002) Dose finding using the biased coin up-and-down design and isotonic regression. Biometrics 58(1):171–177
Thall P, Millikan R, Mueller P, Lee S-J (2003) Dose-finding with two agents in phase I oncology trials. Biometrics 59:487–496
Tighiouart M, Rogatko (2014) A dose finding with escalation with overdose control (EWOC) in cancer clinical trials. Stat Sci 25(2):217–226
Tighiouart M, Cook-Wiens G, Rogatko A (2012) Incorporating a patient dichotomous characteristic in cancer phase I clinical trials using escalation with overdose control. J Probab Stat 10:Article ID: 567819

Tighiouart M, Liu Y, Rogatko A (2014a) Escalation with overdose control using time to toxicity for cancer phase I clinical trials. PLoS One 9(3):e93070
Tighiouart M, Piantadosi S, Rogatko A (2014b) Dose finding with drug combinations in cancer phase I clinical trials using conditional escalation with overdose control. Stat Med 33 (22):3815–3829
Vidoni ED, Johnson DK, Morris JK, Van Sciver A, Greer CS, Billinger SA et al (2015) Dose-response of aerobic exercise on cognition: a community-based, pilot randomized controlled trial. PLoS One 10(7):e0131647
Wages NA, Conaway MR (2013) Specifications of a continual reassessment method design for phase I trials of combined drugs. Pharm Stat 12(4):217–224
Wages N, Conaway M (2018) Revisiting isotonic phase I design in the era of model-assisted dose-finding. Clin Trials 15(5):524–529
Wages N, Conaway M, O'Quigley J (2011a) Dose-finding design for multi-drug combinations. Clin Trials 8:380–389
Wages N, Conaway M, O'Quigley J (2011b) Continual reassessment method for partial ordering. Biometrics 67:1555–1563
Wages N, Conaway M, O'Quigley J (2013) Performance of two-stage continual reassessment method relative to an optimal benchmark. Clin Trials 10:862–875
Wages NA, Iasonos A, O'Quigley J, Conaway MR (2019) Coherence principles in interval-based dose-finding. Submitted
Wang K, Ivanova A (2005) Two-dimensional dose finding in discrete dose space. Biometrics 61:217–222
Wheeler G, Sweeting M, Mander A (2016) AplusB: a web application for investigating A+B designs for phase I cancer clinical trials. PLOS. https://doi.org/10.1371/journal.pone.0159026. Published: July 12, 2016
Yan F, Mandrekar S, Ying Y (2017) Keyboard: a novel Bayesian toxicity probability interval design for phase I clinical trials. Clin Cancer Res 23(15):3994–4003
Yin G, Yuan Y (2009) Bayesian dose finding in oncology for drug combinations by copula regression. Appl Stat 58(2):211–224
Yuan Z, Chapell R (2004) Isotonic designs for phase I cancer clinical trials with multiple risk groups. Clin Trials 1(6):499–508
Zhao L, Lee J, Mody R, Braun T (2011) The superiority of the time-to-event continual reassessment method to the rolling six design in pediatric oncology phase I trials. Clin Trials 8(4):361–369

Inferential Frameworks for Clinical Trials 54

James P. Long and J. Jack Lee

Contents

J. P. Long · J. J. Lee (✉)
Department of Biostatistics, University of Texas MD Anderson Cancer Center, Houston, TX, USA
e-mail: jplong@mdanderson.org; jjlee@mdanderson.org

© Springer Nature Switzerland AG 2022

S. Piantadosi, C. L. Meinert (eds.), *Principles and Practice of Clinical Trials*,
https://doi.org/10.1007/978-3-319-52636-2_271

Abstract

Statistical inference is the process of using data to draw conclusions about unknown quantities. Statistical inference plays a large role both in designing clinical trials and in analyzing the resulting data. The two main schools of inference, frequentist and Bayesian, differ in how they estimate and quantify uncertainty in unknown quantities. Typically, Bayesian methods have clearer interpretation at the cost of specifying additional assumptions about the unknown quantities. This chapter reviews the philosophy behind these two frameworks including concepts such as p-values, Type I and Type II errors, confidence intervals, credible intervals, prior distributions, posterior distributions, and Bayes factors. Application of these ideas to various clinical trial designs including 3 + 3, Simon's two-stage, interim safety and efficacy monitoring, basket, umbrella, and platform drug trials is discussed. Recent developments in computing power and statistical software now enable wide access to many novel trial designs with operating characteristics superior to classical methods.

Keywords

Bayes factors · Bayesian · Confidence intervals · Credible intervals · Frequentist · Hypothesis testing · P-value · Prior distribution · Sequential designs · Statistical inference

Introduction

Statistical inference is the process of using data to draw conclusions about unknown quantities. Rigorous frameworks for statistical inference ensure that the conclusions are backed by some form of guarantee. For example, in drug development, one is interested in estimating the response rate of a new agent with certain precision and/or concluding whether the new agent has at least 30% response rate with certain confidence. The two dominant frameworks for statistical inference, Bayesian and Frequentist, both provide these guarantees in the form of probabilistic statements. Inference frameworks play an important role both in designing clinical trials and in analyzing and interpreting the information contained in the collected data.

Consider the popular oncology Phase I 3 + 3 dose escalation design with a set of predefined dose levels (Storer 1989). Starting at the lowest dose level, three patients are enrolled. If none experience a toxicity, the dose is escalated. If one experiences a toxicity, an additional three are enrolled at the same dose level. Among the additional three patients, if none experience a toxicity, the dose is escalated. If one experiences a toxicity, the current dose or one dose lower is defined as the maximum tolerated dose (*MTD*). If two or more patients experience toxicity in three or six patients, the dose exceeds the *MTD*.

Table 1 lists the probability of dose escalation for given toxicity probability p based on Eq. 1.

Table 1 Probability of dose escalation in the 3 + 3 design for given toxicity probability

Toxicity probability	Escalation probability
0.1	0.91
0.2	0.71
0.3	0.49
0.4	0.31
0.5	0.17
0.6	0.08

$$\text{Escalation Probability} = (1-p)^3 + 3p\,(1-p)^5 \tag{1}$$

The table provides assurance that as the probability of toxicity of the current dose increases, the chance of escalation decreases. This table requires simple probability computations to construct.

The 3 + 3 design (and variants; see Le Tourneau et al. (2009), Lin and Shih (2001)) is a rule-based method in which the trial design and interpretation of results are typically not performed within a formal statistical inference framework. This results in several weaknesses:

1. The algorithm does not explicitly produce an estimate of the toxicity rate at the *MTD*. Studies show that the targeted toxicity rate is not the widely believed 33% and depends on extraneous factors such as the number of dose levels used (Lin and Shih 2001). In most typical applications, the targeted toxicity rate resulting from a 3 + 3 design is between 23% and 28%, but it can be much lower or higher (Smith et al. 1996).
2. Depending on the circumstances, investigators can elicit maximum targeted toxicities for drugs (higher for drugs with higher potential efficacy and lower for preventive agents), yet the 3 + 3 algorithm cannot incorporate this information when finding the *MTD*.

A statistical inferential framework is necessary for addressing these issues. Such a framework can provide a formal method for evaluating the clinical trial data, e.g., answering questions about the drug's toxicity profile after the data has been collected and providing an estimate of the probability of toxicity at the reported *MTD*. Equally important, the framework can be used to design a trial with favorable operating characteristics, e.g., ensure that enough, but not too many, patients are enrolled at each of the potential dose levels, that the dose levels and patient allocations are sensible, etc. Computer simulations show that 3 + 3 is deficient as a trial design (O'Quigley et al. 1990; O'Quigley and Chevret 1991). Despite these weaknesses, reviews suggest that over 90% of Phase I oncology drug trials use a 3 + 3 design (Le Tourneau et al. 2009).

The last 250 years have seen extensive methodological development in the frequentist and Bayesian inferential frameworks. Frequentist inference views parameters, unknown quantities of interest, as fixed. Probabilities are considered only with respect to the data given these fixed parameters. Conversely, Bayesian inference views parameters as random following a particular statistical distribution. The data is fixed since it has been collected. Bayesian inference applies probabilistic statements to estimate these unknowns directly given the data. While the frameworks exhibit important differences, the fact that both have been successfully used in nearly every scientific field demonstrates their breadth and versatility. These characteristics are critical for clinical trials which seek answers to a broad range of questions, including evaluation of efficacy, safety monitoring, dose identification, treatment assignment, adaptation to interim events, go/no-go decision on drug development, cost-benefits analysis, etc.

In the context of clinical trials, frequentist inference dominated the design and analysis of clinical trials in the twentieth century. However, in the last 25 years, Bayesian methods have increased in popularity due to a number of factors including advances in computing power, better computational algorithms, deficiencies in frequentist measures of evidence (such as the p-value), and the need for complex, adaptive trial designs (Biswas et al. 2009; Lee and Chu 2012; Tidwell et al. 2019).

This chapter is organized as follows. Section "Inferential Frameworks: Samples, Populations, and Assumptions" contrasts inferential frameworks with rule-based methods for inference and discusses sampling assumptions common to both frequentist and Bayesian frameworks. The two dominant inferential frameworks, frequentist and Bayesian, are reviewed in sections "Frequentist Framework" and "Bayesian Framework," respectively. Popular designs are discussed such as the frequentist Simon's optimal two-stage design (Simon 1989) and the Bayesian design of Thall et al. (1995). In section "Inferential Frameworks: Connections and Synthesis," efforts to connect the frameworks as well as Bayesian-frequentist hybrid designs are reviewed. Section "Inferential Frameworks and Modern Trial Design Challenges" describes recent developments and challenges in trial design. Section "Summary and Conclusion" concludes with a discussion.

Inferential Frameworks: Samples, Populations, and Assumptions

Consider a hypothetical Phase II trial of an experimental cancer drug in which the investigator would like to determine p, the percentage of all patients in some population (e.g., patients with Stage III pancreatic cancer) who would achieve complete or partial response if given the drug. It is costly and unethical (this is an experimental drug) to treat every patient with the new drug, so it is given to a sample of $n = 10$ patients, of whom six achieve responses. One would like to answer questions such as:

1. What is a reasonable best guess (i.e., estimate) for p? Typically, this sample-based estimate of p is denoted by $\widehat{p}$ (read "p hat").
2. Is the new treatment better than standard of care? If standard of care produces a response in 20% of patients, this statement becomes is p greater than 20%?
3. What is a range of plausible values for p?
4. What is the probability that the response rate is greater than 40%?

All of these questions except question #4 can be addressed in the frequentist and Bayesian inferential frameworks. Question #4 can only be answered by the Bayesian framework because it assumes that the unknown response rate is random, while in the frequentist framework, the unknown response rate is considered fixed and does not have a distribution. Note that the unknown, population response rate p is treated separately from the sample-based estimate $\widehat{p}$. This separation of sample and population is critical for formal inferential reasoning and is not typically discussed in the 3 + 3 dose finding algorithm. In 3 + 3, the MTD is defined based on the sample. In fact, 3 + 3 produces a number more akin to $\widehat{MTD}$, an estimate of the true MTD. The 3 + 3 design does not precisely define the true MTD which it is attempting to estimate. However, one could posit the true MTD as the highest of the prespecified doses which will produce a toxicity in no more than 33% of all patients in the population. With this definition, one can now ask questions akin to 2 and 3, such as how likely is $\widehat{MTD}$ to be no higher than MTD? The 3 + 3 design does not offer any answer to this seemingly important question and in fact makes this question difficult to even ask by not conceptually separating the estimate, $\widehat{MTD}$, from what is being estimated, MTD.

Inferential frameworks require the existence of a population on which inferences are to be drawn. Typically, the population of interest in clinical trials is all patients who would receive the treatment if it were to be approved by a regulatory agency. In the case of the experimental cancer drug, this may be all present and future patients in the United States with Stage III pancreatic cancer.

Nearly all clinical trial designs, both Bayesian and frequentist, assume that the sample is collected by randomly selecting patients from the population with each patient being equally likely to be selected. In practice this random sampling is not done for several reasons including that there do not exist easily accessible lists of all patients in the population and that the resulting selection would result in a geographically diverse set of patients who would be difficult to treat. Instead patients are enrolled at one or a small set of usually academic institutions (thus geographically biasing the sample) and must consent to be treated (thus biasing the sample towards individuals with a high desire for new treatments). The resulting sample may differ from the population in terms of socioeconomic status, ethnicity, present health condition, disease severity, etc.

The extent to which deviations in sampling assumptions occur is situation dependent. Phase II clinical trials typically seek to demonstrate treatment efficacy relative to efficacy on historical controls. Observed differences between treatment and control may be the result of treatment efficacy or differences between trial subjects and historical controls, e.g., the trial may systematically select healthier patients than the historical control group. In this setting, standard Bayesian and frequentist methods will both produce biased results. Phase III double-blinded randomized studies are less likely to suffer from selection bias caused by deviations in sampling assumptions. Yet problems can arise regarding generalization of study findings to patient groups not meeting study eligibility criteria. See Jüni et al. (2001) for a discussion of these issues. In addition, journals are more likely to publish studies with positive findings. Hence, readers must be aware that the publication bias may portray a rosier picture than what the truth is.

Frequentist Framework

Frequentist approaches to addressing questions 1, 2, and 3 above are now discussed. There are many variants of these approaches tailored to fit specific types of data (Casella and Berger 2002; Agresti and Franklin 2009). A few of the most common versions are reviewed with an emphasis on correct frequentist interpretation of the resulting quantities.

With regard to question 1, the best guess of p is referred to as a point estimator. Common frequentist methods for point estimation include maximum likelihood estimators (MLEs) and method of moment (MOM) estimators. Often these methods agree with intuition. In the Phase II cancer trial, the most intuitive estimator for p is the percentage of patients in the sample who achieved response. MLE and MOM both require a *likelihood function*, the probability of observing data given a particular value of the unknown parameter. The most natural likelihood for the cancer example with $n = 10$ patients is the binomial distribution with the mathematical form

$$f(x|p) = \binom{10}{x}\left(\frac{p}{100}\right)^{x}\left(1-\frac{p}{100}\right)^{10-x} \tag{2}$$

where x is the number of responses. Figure 1 provides a graphical illustration of the function $\mathrm{f}(x|p = 20\%)$. From the graph, the probability of observing six responses, assuming a population response rate of 20%, is about 0.0055, calculated by mathematically computing $\mathrm{f}(x = 6|p = 20\%)$ in Eq. 2.

With the binomial model, both the MLE and MOM methods suggest using the intuitive estimator of the percentage of patients who achieved response, in this case 60%. Statistical theory for these estimation methods provides theoretical guarantees on its quality. While the percentage of responses in the sample may seem like the

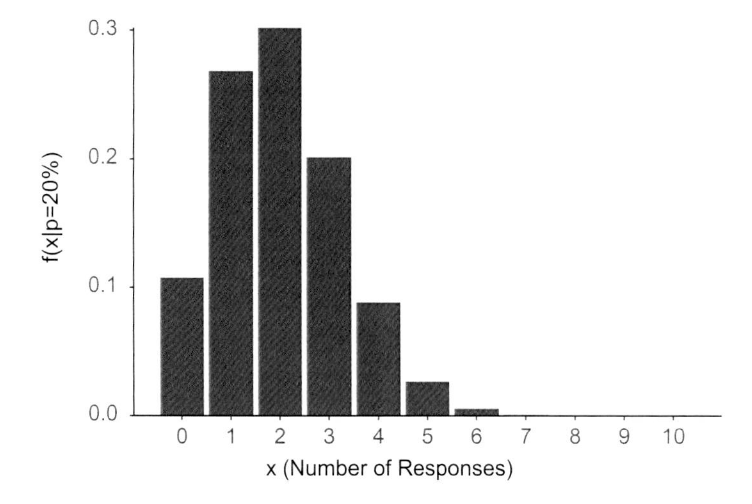

Fig. 1 Binomial probability mass function. This is a graphical illustration of Eq. 1 with p = 20%

only reasonable estimator, the Bayesian inferential approach discussed in the next section typically suggests a different estimate. In this response example, MLE and MOM theory do not produce a particularly surprising result. However, for more complicated statistical models, these methods can be used to derive estimators when intuition fails. For example, suppose dozens of candidate biomarkers (SNPs, protein expression levels, prior treatments, etc.) are measured and some of them are associated with the response status. MLE, in conjunction with a logistic regression statistical model, could be used to identify combinations of biomarkers which predict response.

Hypothesis testing in conjunction with p-values is used to answer 2. Typically, the hypothesis that the experimental treatment does not exceed standard of care ($p = 20\%$) is termed the null hypothesis, while experimental treatment beating standard of care ($p > 20\%$) is termed the alternative hypothesis. These may be written as

$$
\begin{aligned}
H_0 &: p \leq 20\% \\
H_a &: p > 20\%.
\end{aligned}
$$

A decision about whether to accept H_a may be based on the p-value, the probability of observing a result as extreme or more extreme than the one actually obtained, assuming that the null hypothesis is true. Since 6 out of 10 responses were observed, the p-value is the probability of getting 6, 7, 8, 9, or 10 responses assuming the true response rate in the population is 20% which equals about 0.0064. Note that the p-value is not the probability that the null hypothesis is correct, i.e., the probability that p is less than 20% (or equals 20%). While this would seem like the most natural definition, frequentist statistics cannot apply probabilities to the unknown quantity p because p is assumed to be fixed. Many statisticians see the convoluted definition of the p-value as a major disadvantage of frequentist hypothesis testing.

The p-value does have an interpretation in the context of error rates. Consider rejecting the null hypothesis (i.e., concluding that p is greater than 20% and that the experimental drug works) if the p-value is less than some threshold, usually taken to be 0.05. Then the probability of rejecting the null hypothesis when the null hypothesis is actually true, known as a Type I error or the false positive rate, is equal to the threshold.

Another way to understand p-values is to imagine running the trial over and over again with a separate set of n patients. Suppose the experimental drug is not effective. Then if one uses a p-value threshold of 0.05 to reject the null hypothesis, in 5% of the hypothetical trials, one will erroneously conclude that the drug is effective. The mental experiment of rerunning the trial and calculating the p-value is an important component of frequentist reasoning. The distribution of p-values from these hypothetical experiments is known as the sampling distribution.

Confidence intervals are used for addressing 3. Frequentist statisticians use confidence intervals to determine a range of plausible values for an unknown parameter. In the context of the example, with six in ten responses, a 95% confidence interval for p may span 31–83% (Wilson binomial confidence interval. Wilson 1927). Here, again, the natural interpretation is to claim that the probability that p is in the interval 31–83% is 95%. However, the frequentist inferential framework cannot apply probabilities to p, so this statement does not have meaning. Instead, the 95% refers to what would occur if the trial were run again and again, and in each trial, one made a 95% confidence interval. Approximately 95% of these intervals would contain p. However, any individual interval either does or does not contain p. Again, under the frequentist approach, the data is random while the parameter is unknown but fixed.

Figure 2 illustrates this concept. Here 100 hypothetical trials were run each with 10 patients. The true response rate is 40%. For each trial, a 95% confidence interval is produced. The horizontal lines in Fig. 1 show the confidence intervals for each trial. The black lines denote trials in which the resulting confidence interval includes the true response rate, while the red lines denote trials in which the resulting confidence interval does not include the true response rate. For about 95% of trials (in this particular example, 96%), the confidence interval will include the true response rate. However, under the frequentist paradigm, any particular trial confidence interval either does or does not contain the true response rate, so the 95% interpretation can only be applied to the average coverage probability of confidence intervals, not any single interval. The "frequentist" framework studies the property of long-run frequency of an estimator by how often it occurs, hence the name. In both the hypothesis testing and confidence interval estimation, the frequentist approach answers the question of interest indirectly.

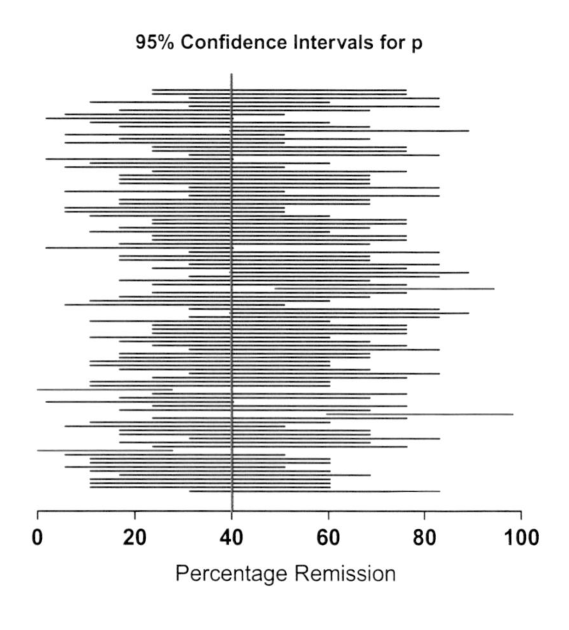

Fig. 2 Illustration of correct interpretation of frequentist confidence interval

Optimizing Trial Design Using Frequentist Statistics

In addition to analyzing the results of a clinical trial, the frequentist inferential framework is used to design trials with favorable operating characteristics. In simple cases, the main design decision is selecting the sample size. For example, the sample size could be chosen such that the width of the resulting confidence interval is no wider than 10%. Alternatively, the sample size could be chosen so that one will successfully reject the null hypothesis with a specified probability assuming some true difference between treatment and control, i.e., power calculations. These design decisions ensure that the trial will accrue enough patients to make conclusions (such as to proceed to a Phase III trial) but not incur excess costs in terms of time, money, and patient exposure to experimental drugs. Note that 3 + 3, as a fixed algorithmic design, cannot be easily modified to achieve any of these objectives.

While a simple trial design may involve determining a single sample size, more complicated designs can often achieve more efficient allocation of resources. For example, Simon's optimal two-stage design for Phase II trials terminates the trial early if the experimental treatment is deemed ineffective based on an interim analysis of the data (Simon 1989). Simon's method chooses two sample sizes n_1 and n_2. After accrual of n_1 patients, the data is examined to determine if the treatment response rate is sufficient to merit further investigation. If yes, additional n_2 patients are enrolled, and the combined sample of $n_1 + n_2$ is analyzed for efficacy. If not, the trial terminates and the treatment is deemed ineffective. The methodology for determining effectiveness follows the frequentist hypothesis testing framework. Simon's optimal two-stage design determines sample sizes n_1 and n_2 which minimize the expected number of patients to be treated when the null hypothesis is true while maintaining Type I and Type II error guarantees. Alternatively, Simon's minimax design finds a design which minimizes the maximum sample size when the null hypothesis is true with specified Type I and Type II error rates.

Limitations and Guidance on Frequentist Statistical Inference

Frequentist statistics is often criticized for the complicated interpretation of its output. The p-value can be used to claim whether or not statistical significance is reached for rejecting the null hypothesis while controlling Type I error. However, it cannot be directly translated into the probability that the null hypothesis is true, a quantity that is likely of greater interest. In order to assign probabilities to the null and alternative hypothesis, one needs prior probabilities on these quantities, a feature of Bayesian statistics.

The p-value threshold of 0.05 is commonly used to denote statistical significance and is often the boundary between publishable and non-publishable results. The 0.05 threshold is quite arbitrary. Statisticians have argued for cutoffs of 0.005 and 0.001 to denote significant and highly significant results (Johnson 2013). The following key points were outlined in a recent statement from the American Statistical Association regarding context, process, and purpose of p-values (Wasserstein and Lazar 2016):

- P-values can indicate how incompatible the data are with a specified statistical model.
- P-values do not measure the probability that the studied hypothesis is true, or the probability that the data were produced by random chance alone.
- Scientific conclusions and business or policy decisions should not be based only on whether a p-value passes a specific threshold.
- Proper inference requires full reporting and transparency.
- A p-value, or statistical significance, does not measure the size of an effect or the importance of a result.
- By itself, a p-value does not provide a good measure of evidence regarding a model or hypothesis.

The frequentist hypothesis testing paradigm does not offer a method to conclude that the null hypothesis is true. The result of the test is generally a p-value and a conclusion that the null was rejected at some Type I error control rate (usually 0.05) or the null hypothesis was not rejected. The conclusion is never that the null hypothesis is true or highly likely to be true. Bayesian hypothesis testing permits reaching these conclusions as will be discussed in Sections "Bayesian Framework" and "Reducing Subjectivity and Calibrating P-Values with Bayes Factors."

In other words, since null hypothesis significance testing (NHST) calculates the p-value assuming that the null hypothesis H_0 is true, the p-value is not the probability that H_0 is true. No specific alternative hypothesis H_1 needs to be specified. No estimation of the treatment effect is given. The inference is based on unobserved data and violates the likelihood principle (Berger and Wolpert 1988).

In a recent special issue of the *American Statistician*, a collection of 43 articles provides further discussion on p-values and statistical inference in general (Wasserstein et al. 2019). There are a few "Do's" and "Don't's" offered in the editorial. For the "Don't's":

- Don't base your conclusions solely on whether an association or effect was found to be "statistically significant" (i.e., the p-value passed some arbitrary threshold such as $p < 0.05$).
- Don't believe that an association or effect exists just because it was statistically significant.
- Don't believe that an association or effect is absent just because it was not statistically significant.
- Don't believe that your p-value gives the probability that chance alone produced the observed association or effect or the probability that your test hypothesis is true.
- Don't conclude anything about scientific or practical importance based on statistical significance (or lack thereof).

For the "Do's":

- Accept Uncertainty
- Be Thoughtful

  - Thoughtfulness in the big picture, context, and prior knowledge
  - Thoughtful alternatives and complements to p-values
  - Thoughtful communication of confidence
- Be Open
  - Openness to transparency and to the role of expert judgment
  - Openness in communication
- Be Modest
  - Being modest requires a reality check, in recognizing there is not a "true statistical model" underlying every problem.
  - Be modest about the role of statistical inference in scientific inference, encouraging others to reproduce your work.

Bayesian Framework

Bayesian statistics applies probabilistic statements directly to unknown quantities. It assumes that the data is fixed and the parameter is random. For example, one may state that given the data collected, the probability that the response rate for the experimental treatment is greater than the response rate for standard of care (20%) is 95%. In mathematics this is

$$P(p > 20\%) = 0.95$$

This statement avoids the opaque interpretation of p-values and can be seen as a benefit of the Bayesian inferential framework (Berger 2003). Bayesian approaches to questions 1, 2, 3, and 4 are now discussed in the context of the response example. More complex analyses are discussed in references (Berry et al. 2010; Gelman et al. 2013).

In order to make probabilistic statements, prior knowledge about the unknown parameters is formalized into a prior distribution. The prior is then combined with the data to produce a posterior distribution. The mathematical machinery for combining the prior with the data is Bayes theorem, from whence the framework gets its name (Bayes 1763). Bayes theorem states that for two events A and B

$$P(A|B) = \frac{P(B|A)P(A)}{P(B)}.$$

The left side of the equation is read "the probability that A is true given that B is true." In the context of the response example, A could be "the population response rate p is greater than 20%" and B could be data such as six out of ten patients responded. The left side of the equation, $P(A|B)$, then reads the probability that the response rate is greater than 20% (in the population) given that six out of ten responses were observed in the sample.

The central concept of Bayesian statistics is information synthesis. Specifically, Bayesian 1-2-3 is that prior plus data becomes posterior. The current posterior can be considered as an updated prior for future data acquisition. The Bayesian method takes a "learn-as-we-go" approach to perform continual learning by synthesizing all available information at hand.

Note that it is a misconception that frequentist statisticians do not use Bayes theorem. Bayes theorem is a mathematical fact, accepted and used by all statisticians. The frequentist framework objects to the representation of unknown quantities using distributions, in particular the prior, not the existence of Bayes theorem.

Figure 3 demonstrates simple Bayesian statistics with the response example. The x-axis represents different possible response rates p for the experimental drug. The blue and red curves and area under the corresponding curves represent prior knowledge about p (prior distribution) and the updated knowledge of p after observing the data (posterior distribution). The word prior refers to prior to data collection. The mathematical form for this prior is a beta distribution. For Fig. 3, left panel,

$$\pi(p) = \frac{1}{B(0.6, 1.4)}\left(\frac{p}{100}\right)^{-0.4}\left(1 - \frac{p}{100}\right)^{0.4}. \tag{3}$$

This prior favors low response percentages with a mean response rate of 0.3 and an effective sample size of 2. The source of prior knowledge can be subjective and is sometimes controversial in Bayesian statistics. However, it is reasonable to formulate the prior distribution based on response rates observed with past experimental drugs.

The prior distribution in Eq. 3 is combined with the likelihood function of Eq. 2 to produce a posterior distribution. The posterior distribution of p after observing six responses out of ten evaluated patients is mathematically computed by

$$\pi(p|x = 6) = \frac{f(x = 6|p)\pi(p)}{\int f(x = 6|p)\pi(p)dp} = \frac{1}{B(6.6, 5.4)}\left(\frac{p}{100}\right)^{5.6}\left(1 - \frac{p}{100}\right)^{4.4}.$$

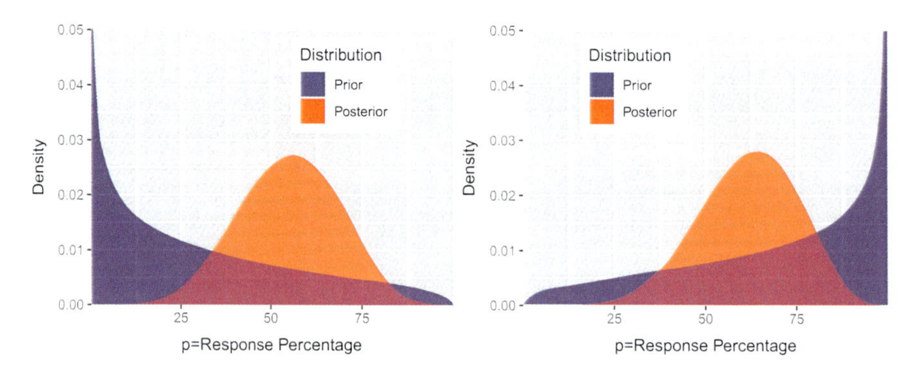

Fig. 3 (Left) Prior and posterior distributions. The prior is Beta(0.6,1.4), while the posterior is Beta (6.6,5.4). (Right) A second example with the same data but a different prior. The prior is Beta (1.4,0.6) and the posterior is Beta(7.4,4.6). The posterior distribution is different than (Left), representing the subjective nature of Bayesian analyses

The first equality is Bayes theorem, while the second equality involves algebraic manipulations. Notice the probabilities have shifted considerably after observing the data of six responses out of ten patients. While the prior states that the probability p is greater than 20% is only 53%, the posterior assigns greater than 99% chance to this event.

The posterior distribution in red is used to answer questions 1, 2, 3, and 4. The most common Bayesian point estimator is the posterior mean or the average value of p as indicated by the posterior distribution. With six out of ten responses, the posterior mean is 55%. This is different than the sample percentage of response of 60%. The reason for this difference is that the prior distribution (in blue) favored low percentages and is still exerting an effect on the point estimate even after collecting the data. As the amount of data increases, the prior will have less and less effect. The posterior mean estimator will become closer to the percentage of responses in the sample. For example, with 60 responses out of 100 patients, the posterior mean (using the blue prior) is 59%. Since the typical frequentist estimator is 60%, the sample proportion, this example illustrates that as the sample size increases, Bayesian and frequentist methods become more in agreement. This is common in many other settings.

For addressing question 2, one can use the posterior distribution which shows there is a 99.6% chance that the experimental treatment exceeds standard of care (20% response). This is determined by calculating the percentage of the red posterior area which is greater than 20% on the x-axis. This efficacy result would likely form the basis for proceeding to a Phase III trial. For example, one could decide to proceed to a Phase III trial if there is at least a 95% chance that the experimental treatment exceeds standard of care. In practice, such decisions usually involve a number of factors including toxicity analysis. In section "Multiple Outcomes and Utility Functions" statistical methodology for formal incorporation of multiple objectives (e.g., efficacy and safety) in decisions is discussed.

For addressing question 3, the red posterior distribution indicates there is a 95% chance that the response rate is between 28% and 81%. This is known as a 95% credible interval, the Bayesian equivalent of a confidence interval. These endpoints, 28% and 81%, are the 2.5 and 97.5 percentiles of the red curve (i.e., the area of the red region to the left of 28% is 0.025, and the area of the red region to the left of 81% is 0.975).

For addressing question 4, the tail probability of the response rate greater than 40% can be calculated by summing up or integrating the area under the curve from the response rate of 0.4 to 1.0, which is 85%.

The frequentist testing paradigm treats the null and alternative hypotheses asymmetrically, and there is no clear way to conclude the null is true or make a statement about confidence in the null hypothesis. In contrast Bayesian hypothesis tests treat the null and alternative symmetrically. A posterior probability for each hypothesis may be reported (sum of probabilities of null and alternative will of necessity equal 1). In section "Reducing Subjectivity and Calibrating P-Values with Bayes Factors," we will discuss Bayesian hypothesis testing using Bayes factor.

Sequential Design

In many data analysis applications, the sample size is fixed and the data is analyzed only after collection. However, in clinical trials patients accrue sequentially, offering the opportunity for stopping based on interim analysis of safety and efficacy results. The Bayesian framework is particularly simple because the reason for stopping formally has no impact on the subsequent data analysis (Berger and Wolpert 1988). A caveat to this message is that data-dependent stopping rules can increase sensitivity to prior distribution assumptions. For example, Bayesian credible intervals constructed using conservative priors can have anti-conservative coverage probability (lower than the specified amount) when data-dependent stopping rules are used (Rosenbaum and Rubin 1984). Frequentist measures of evidence, such as p-values, explicitly require incorporating the reason for stopping. This can be implemented a priori, such as in Simon's optimal two-stage design, in which interim stopping is accounted for in the hypothesis test decision with the specified Type I and Type II error rates.

Thall et al. (1995) is a popular Bayesian sequential design for Phase II clinical trials. The design is used for monitoring multiple outcomes, such as safety and efficacy. Data can be monitored patient by patient, but typically interim analyses are conducted in cohort sizes of five or ten to reduce logistical burden. At each interim analysis, such as five patients with toxicity and efficacy data available, the method produces a probability distribution for the parameters, similar to Fig. 3. Prior to the trial, tolerable safety and efficacy boundaries are established. For example, stop if the probability of efficacy being greater than 20% is less than 5% or the probability of toxicity greater than 25% is greater than 95%. Thus, the trial is stopped whenever one becomes confident in efficacy less than 20% or toxicity greater than 25%. From these probabilistic thresholds, one can determine stopping boundaries (number of toxicities or treatment failures which will terminate the trial) at various interim analysis points. In this way the trial design produces simple rules for continuing or terminating the trial, much like a 3 + 3 design, but with probabilistic guarantees about the decisions. In addition to stopping boundaries, operating characteristics of the trial such as the probability of stopping early given some efficacy and toxicity levels can be tabulated prior to trial initiation.

Bayesian Computation

Although Bayes theorem was published more than 250 years ago, its use was limited to conjugate models in which the posterior distribution has the same parametric form as the prior distribution (such as the beta-binomial example discussed in the previous section). In these cases, analytic solutions are available for computing the posterior distribution. Bayesian computation beyond conjugate cases can be demanding. Since the late 1980s, a combination of faster computers and better algorithms (e.g., Gibbs sampling, Metropolis-Hastings sampling, and general Markov Chain Monte Carlo (MCMC)) has made Bayesian computation for clinical trial data sets feasible and even routine. Software tools such as BUGS, JAGS, STAN, and SAS PROC MCMC allow easy implementation of a wide spectrum of Bayesian models (Spiegelhalter et al. 1996; Plummer 2003; Chen 2009; Carpenter et al. 2017).

Prior Distributions and Schools of Bayesian Thought

The posterior distribution is computed using Bayes theorem and is dependent upon both the prior distribution and the data. Different prior distributions can produce different conclusions from the data. For example, in Fig. 3 (right), the prior belief about effectiveness has been changed (relative to Fig. 3 (left)) to a Beta(1.4,0.6) in order to favor high response rates. Using the same data as before, six out of ten observed responses, the posterior is now the red curve in the right plot. Notice that the two posterior distributions differ even though the data collected are the same. This will result in different numerical summaries of the posterior and possibly even different decisions about whether to proceed to the next clinical trial phase. For example, with the Fig. 3 (left) posterior, the probability the response rate is greater than 40% is about 85%, while for the Fig. 3 (right) posterior, it is about 94%.

Within Bayesian statistics, there are different views about how to construct prior distributions. Spiegelhalter et al. (2004) identified four schools of Bayesian thinking which may represent a continuity from frequentist to fully Bayesian methods:

1. Empirical: Prior distributions are constructed from data, usually in the context of a hierarchical model which has multiple levels of parameters (see diagnostic testing example below for a definition and example of a hierarchical model). While empirical Bayesian analyses use Bayes theorem, the resulting inferences typically reported are frequentist (e.g., confidence intervals rather than credible intervals, MLEs rather than posterior means). Many statisticians who consider themselves frequentists use empirical Bayes methods.
2. Reference (or Objectivist): A set of default, or reference, prior distributions are used which do not attempt to incorporate subjective knowledge about the parameters. Default priors may be chosen to have favorable mathematical properties (Jeffreys 1946). Reference Bayesians may employ *improper* priors or non-informative/vague priors which do not correspond to prior belief because they are not probability densities such as Uniform $(0, \infty)$ or a normal distribution prior with infinite variance.
3. Proper (or Subjectivist): The prior is chosen to reflect subject matter knowledge about the parameter. Different practitioners will have different beliefs about the parameter, resulting in different informative priors and different inferences.
4. Decision Theoretic: Utility functions, which assign numeric values to different outcomes, are combined with posterior distributions, which reflect uncertainty about the state of nature, to make decisions. The particular choice of utility function adds an additional level of subjectivity to the analysis, for example, in the trade-off of toxicity versus efficacy or cost versus benefit.

An example from diagnostic testing may help illustrate the differences, similarities, and continuity in these schools of thought. Suppose a test for lung cancer has 95% sensitivity and 90% specificity. For a particular individual, let the parameter θ equal 1 if the person has cancer and 0 if not. Let Y equal 1 if the test is positive for the individual and 0 if negative. What is the probability that this person has cancer given she tests positive, i.e., $P(\theta = 1 | Y = 1)$? The following steps illustrate a dynamic back-and-forth among the various schools of statistical thinking on how to address this question:

(i) Since this question involves computing probabilities of parameters, it can naturally be addressed in a Bayesian framework once a prior for θ has been chosen. Supposing this individual was selected randomly from a population, the appropriate prior (the probability the individual has the disease prior to administering the test) is the disease prevalence in the population, termed p. Mathematically $P(\theta = 1) = p$. The post-test probability is then computed using Bayes formula

$$P(\theta = 1|Y = 1) = \frac{P(Y = 1|\theta = 1)P(\theta = 1)}{P(Y = 1|\theta = 1)P(\theta = 1) + P(Y = 1|\theta = 0)P(\theta = 0)}$$
$$= \frac{0.95p}{0.95p + 0.1(1 - p)}$$

For example, with $p = 0.1$, the post-test probability is 0.51. This could be viewed as a subjective Bayesian analysis in which the prior was chosen based on the practitioner's belief about disease prevalence.

(ii) A frequentist statistician may object to this analysis as subjective. Where does the disease prevalence number originate? The frequentist statistician may engage in a literature search and find that 100 individuals from the population were given a gold standard lung cancer test (always provides correct result), and X had cancer. The frequentist computes a (binomial) MLE estimate of $\widehat{p} = X/_n$, the sample proportion who have the disease. The posttest probability estimate is

$$\widehat{P}(\theta = 1|Y = 1) = \frac{0.95\widehat{p}}{0.95\widehat{p} + 0.1(1 - \widehat{p})}$$

This could be viewed as a simple empirical Bayes model or as a frequentist application of the invariance property of MLEs (Theorem 7.2.10 from Casella and Berger (2002)). This is a hierarchical model because there are two levels of parameters, a parameter describing the population (p in this case) and a parameter describing an individual (θ in this case). Empirical Bayesians consider individual level parameters random, but population-level parameters fixed. If $\widehat{p} = 0.1$, then the empirical Bayesian estimate will match the subjectivist Bayesian from (i).

(iii) Now that the frequentist (or empirical Bayesian) has included X formally in the analysis, a Bayesian would seek an analysis that uses both Y and X. While the frequentist treated the population-level parameter p as fixed, the Bayesian will put a prior on this quantity. This distribution represents belief about the population prevalence prior to observing the gold standard data X. A subjectivist Bayesian will incorporate beliefs into this prior, e.g., most diseases are not common, so the prior on p will favor disease prevalences less than 0.5. In contrast, the two objective Bayesian priors for this model are Beta(1/2,1/2) (Jeffreys prior) and Beta(1,1) (suggested by Laplace); see Mossman and Berger (2001).

(iv) While the empirical, reference, and proper Bayesian will all report $\widehat{P}(\theta = 1|Y = 1)$, a decision theoretic Bayesian will go a step further and seek to use the data X and Y (along with the prior distributions) to make some choice of action. For example, given that an individual tests positive, should she undergo an additional invasive test which has some potential side effects? This decision requires balancing many factors, including the risks associated with having undetected disease and side effects of the invasive test, along with the measure $\widehat{P}(\theta = 1|Y = 1)$. The consideration of all these factors is typically formalized in a utility function.

Mossman and Berger (2001) discuss this problem in the more complex case where the sensitivity and specificity must be estimated from data and confidence bounds (rather than simply point estimates) for $\widehat{P}(\theta = 1|Y = 1)$ are desired. They find the objectivist Bayesian method has desirable properties relative to frequentist/empirical Bayesian analyses.

The schools of thought above involve considerable overlap. Some statisticians advocate using multiple approaches within the same problem. For example, calibrated Bayes recommends using Bayesian (either reference or proper) analysis for fitting statistical models while using frequentist methods to test the quality of the model itself (Little 2006).

Guidance on Bayesian Inference

Several important elements for applying Bayesian methods are listed below.

1. Define the primary endpoint(s) under the Bayesian probability model.
2. Determine prior information.
   (a) Historical data of similar studies.
   (b) Elicit expert opinion.
   (c) Non-informative or objective prior.
3. Extensive simulations.
   (a) Calibrate design parameters to reach desirable operating characteristics such as accuracy for making correct decisions, study accrual and duration, early stopping probabilities, etc.
   (b) Maintain the desirable frequentist properties such as controlling Type I and Type II errors.
4. Sensitivity analysis.

An important principle of the Bayesian analysis is that one should not manipulate the prior in order to obtain desirable results post data collection. After setting the prior, sensitivity analysis can be applied to study its influence. For example, the two posteriors in Fig. 3 are based on two priors (with different parameters a and b) and can help illustrate to what extent posterior conclusions are influenced by the prior.

Inferential Frameworks: Connections and Synthesis

Rule-based, frequentist, and Bayesian trial designs all exist and are in use because each approach has strengths: rule-based methods are simple to follow, frequentist methods avoid prior selection, and Bayesian methods are flexible. The strengths of each approach have motivated trial design and statistical methodology which incorporate ideas from multiple frameworks.

Reducing Subjectivity and Calibrating P-Values with Bayes Factors

In the response example above, the prior belief about p (blue curve in Fig. 3 left) implied a prior belief about whether the response rate of the experimental treatment exceeded that of the standard of care (20%). In particular, prior to collecting any data, one assumed a 53% chance that the experimental treatment had response rate greater than 20% (the area under the blue curve to the right of 20%) and hence a 47% chance that the experimental treatment was worse than standard of care (the area under the blue curve to the left of 20%). The act of assigning prior probabilities to the null and alternative hypothesis may be seen as especially subjective.

One Bayesian remedy for this problem is to construct prior distributions for the null hypothesis and alternative hypothesis separately. One may then calculate the probability of the data given the null hypothesis is true and the probability of the data given the alternative hypothesis is true. The ratio of these two quantities is known as the Bayes factor. Letting D denote data, H_0 denote the null hypothesis, and H_1 denote the alternative hypothesis, the Bayes factor links the posterior odds with the prior odds:

$$\underbrace{\frac{P(H_0|D)}{P(H_1|D)}}_{\text{posterior odds}} = \underbrace{\frac{P(D|H_0)}{P(D|H_1)}}_{\text{Bayes factor}} \times \underbrace{\frac{P(H_0)}{P(H_1)}}_{\text{prior odds}} \tag{4}$$

Table 2 (adapted from Goodman (1999) Table 1) relates the Bayes factor, the prior probability of the null hypothesis, and the posterior probability of the null hypothesis. For example, with a Bayes factor of 1/5 and a prior probability on the null hypothesis of 90%, the posterior probability of the null is 64%. This is determined by noting that a 90% prior on the null is equivalent to a 9:1 odds, so the posterior odds is $\frac{1}{5} \times \frac{9}{1} = \frac{9}{5}$. The posterior odds is then converted to a posterior probability with

$\frac{\frac{9}{5}}{\frac{9}{5}+1} \approx 0.64$. Reporting the Bayes factor (BF) does not require specifying the prior odds (i.e., the Bayes factor does not depend on the prior probability of the null hypothesis) and is thus is perceived as testing a hypothesis "objectively" (Berger 1985) and removes "an unnecessary element of subjectivity" (Johnson and Cook 2009).

In Fig. 3 (left), the Bayes factor can be computed as a way to remove the influence of the initially specified prior probability of the null $P(H_0)= 0.47$ and only consider the conditional priors $P(p|\ H_0)$ and $P(p|\ H_1)$ when making a decision about the veracity of the null hypothesis. The Bayes factor can be determined for Fig. 3 (left) by noting that $P(H_0|\ D) = P(p < 0.2|\ \text{data}) = 0.0041$ and thus $P(H_1|\ D) = P(p > 0.2|\ \text{data}) = 0.9959$ resulting in posterior odds of 0.0042. The prior distribution Beta(0.6,1.4) implies $P(H_0)= 0.47$ and $P(H_1)= 0.53$ with prior odds $= 0.87$. Thus, the Bayes factor is the ratio of posterior odds divided by prior odds which is 0.0048 in favor of the alternative hypothesis that the response rate is greater than 0.2.

A user of the Bayes factor can specify his own prior probability and then compute the posterior probability of the alternative or consider several possible prior probabilities (as in Table 2). For example, a Bayes factor of 1/100 is considered strong–very strong evidence for the alternative hypothesis because even assuming a 90% prior probability on the null, the posterior probability on the null is 8%.

Bayes factors can also be used to calibrate p-values in an attempt to find more objective cutoffs than 0.05. Johnson (2013) developed connections between Bayes factors and p-values based on Bayesian uniformly most power tests. He argued that the p-value thresholds of 0.005 and 0.001 should be used to denote significant and highly significant results in clinical trials, rather than the typical 0.05.

A simple version of this idea can be seen with the Gaussian null hypothesis testing problem. Suppose the common scenario of testing a simple null hypothesis (population mean equals some constant) and that under the null and alternative hypotheses, the frequentist test statistic has a normal distribution (Z score). Then

Table 2 Bayes factors, prior probabilities, and posterior probabilities

		Change in probability of null (i.e., $P(H_0)$ to $P(H_0\|D)$)	
Strength of evidence	Bayes factor	From (%)	To (%)
Weak	1/5	90	64
		50	17
		25	6
Moderate	1/10	90	47
		50	9
		25	3
Moderate–strong	1/20	90	31
		50	5
		25	2
Strong–very strong	1/100	90	8
		50	1
		25	0.3

Table 3 P-values, Bayes factors, and posterior probabilities

		Change in probability of null (i.e., $P(H_0)$ to $P(H_0 \mid D)$)	
P-value (Z score)	Minimum Bayes factor	From (%)	To (%)
0.1 (1.64)	0.26 (1/3.8)	75	44
		50	21
		17	5
0.05 (1.96)	0.15 (1/6.8)	75	31
		50	13
		26	5
0.03 (2.17)	0.095 (1/11)	75	22
		50	9
		33	5
0.01 (2.58)	0.036 (1/28)	75	10
		50	3.5
		60	5
0.001 (3.28)	0.005 (1/216)	75	1
		50	0.5
		92	5

for a given Z-score (equivalently p-value), one can derive a minimum Bayes factor and hence a maximum level of support for the alternative hypothesis. Table 3 (adapted from Goodman (1999) Table 2) displays these relations. The common p-value threshold of 0.05 implies a minimum Bayes factor of 0.15. If one assigns a 50% chance that the null hypothesis is true a priori, then the posterior on the null is 13%. Thus a p-value of 0.05 could be considered moderate, but certainly not definitive evidence of the alterative.

For more on Bayes factors, see Johnson and Cook (2009) for a Phase II single-arm trial design and Goodman (1999) and Kass and Raftery (1995) for general reviews (https://biostatistics.mdanderson.org/softwaredownload/ hosts software for implementing clinical trial designs with Bayes factors.).

Model-Based and Model-Assisted Phase I Designs Constructed Using Inferential Frameworks

The Continual Reassessment Method (CRM) is a Bayesian Phase I trial design meant to address some of the deficiencies in 3 + 3 (O'Quigley et al. 1990). CRM assumes a dose-toxicity relationship curve and, using a Bayesian framework, updates estimates of the curve with each new patient. The next patient is given the dose with estimated toxicity probability closest to the targeted toxicity probability. CRM can estimate the maximum tolerated dose (*MTD*) at any desired target toxicity probability, e.g., at 15%, 30%, or 40%, etc. depending on the respective clinical trial setting. It can escalate and de-escalate dose levels an arbitrary number of times and produce an estimate of the toxicity probability at each dose level, features absent in traditional 3 + 3 designs.

The traditional 3 + 3 remains popular likely due to its simplicity. While the rule-based 3 + 3 dose levels can be assigned by any clinical trialist, CRM requires evaluating the posterior distribution at each cohort, a task that requires computer software and a statistician.

To address this concern, new trial designs have attempted to merge the good operating characteristics of CRM with the simplicity of rule-based methods such as 3 + 3. These represent one sort of hybrid trial. A particular example of this new approach is the Phase I Bayesian Optimal Interval Design (BOIN) (Liu and Yuan 2015). In BOIN, users specify a toxicity interval. The design seeks a dose with toxicity in the interval. BOIN escalates or de-escalates doses based on the results of a Bayesian hypothesis test of whether the current dose toxicity is in the acceptable toxicity interval. Similar to CRM, the method can result in an arbitrary number of escalations and de-escalations. However, unlike CRM, these decisions are made only based on the toxicities observed at the current dose, not other doses. This feature results in simple interval boundaries for the escalation decision which can be pre-computed at the design level. Thus the trial runs without consultation to computer software, much like the 3 + 3 design. Figure 4 displays a decision flowchart for a BOIN trial design with a targeted toxicity probability of 0.3. Dose escalation, de-escalation, and retention decisions are entirely based on comparing the DLT rate at the current dose to fixed thresholds provided in the diagram. BOIN designs (including these operational flowcharts) can be created using freely available web applications (http://trialdesign.org).

Model-Based and Model-Assisted Phase II Designs

The Phase II sequential monitoring design of Thall et al. (1995) (TSE) proposes early stopping for safety and efficacy based on posterior probabilities. A disadvantage of this procedure is that, unlike Simon's two-stage design (Simon 1989), the method does not provide a recommendation about proceeding to a Phase III trial. TSE suggest performing a separate analysis on the final data using either a frequentist or Bayesian framework. A challenge of using frequentist methods in this setting is that standard frequentist hypothesis tests will not control Type I or Type II error at the specified level due to the previous sequential monitoring. Control of these errors is considered desirable by regulatory agencies because they are not based on prior distributions and are thus seen as more objective than traditional Bayesian hypothesis testing.

Recent Bayesian designs calibrate parameters to obtain desirable frequentist properties, such as Type I and Type II error control, while simultaneously making interim decisions in a straightforward Bayesian probabilistic manner. Two such Phase II designs are the predictive probability design (Lee and Liu 2008) and the Bayesian Optimal Phase II design (BOP2) (Zhou et al. 2017).

The predictive probability design adds early stopping for efficacy based on the probability that the trial will achieve its objective, given all current information.

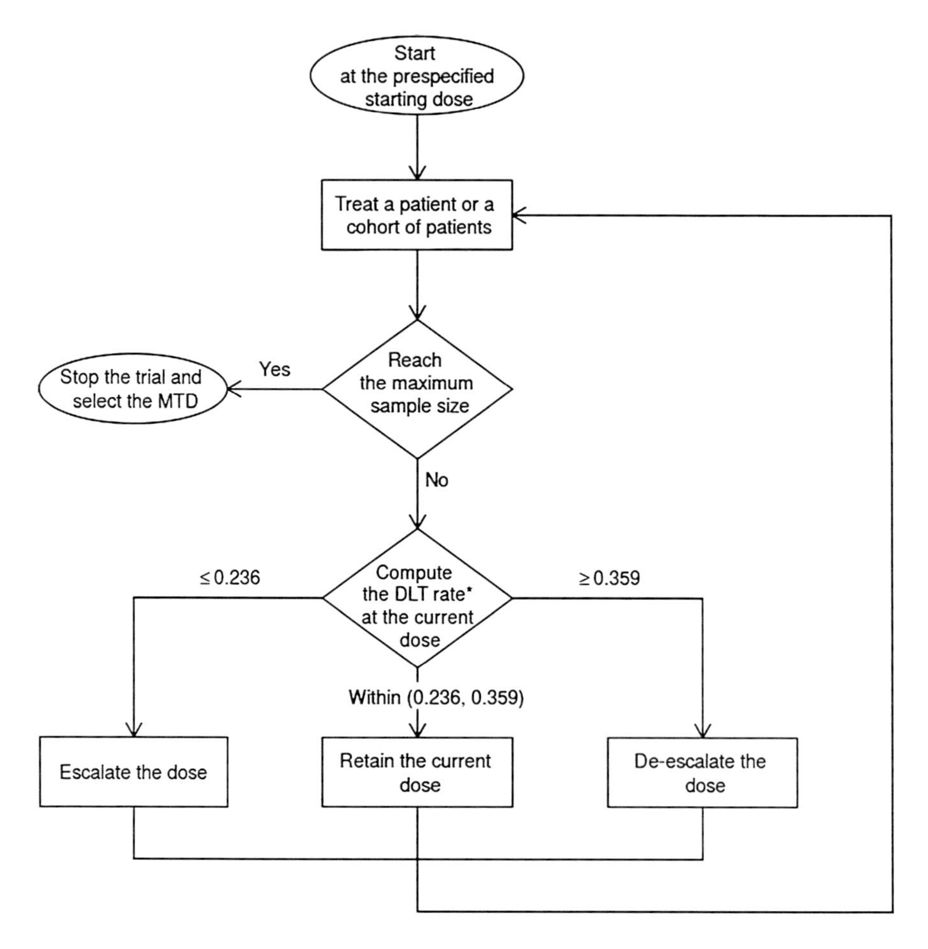

Fig. 4 BOIN flowchart with a targeted probability of toxicity of 0.3. BOIN retains the operational simplicity of 3 + 3 but with better statistical properties

The null hypothesis is that the true experimental efficacy rate p is no better than standard of care efficacy rate p_0 (i.e., $H_0 : p \leq p_0$). The targeted efficacy for the experimental treatment is p_1. At final sample size of N, the null hypotheses will be rejected, and the treatment determined more effective than standard of care, if $P(p > p_0 \mid \text{data on } N \text{ patients}) > \theta_T$. Rather than waiting until all N patient responses have been observed, the trial computes the probability of attaining this result in cohorts of arbitrary size. The trial is terminated early if the probability falls below θ_L (treatment determined ineffective early) or above θ_U (treatment determined effective early). Similar to Simon's two-stage design, the predictive probability design optimizes over N, θ_U, θ_L, and θ_T to obtain specified Type I and Type II error rates and minimum sample size. By controlling Type I and Type II error, the design ensures good frequentist properties while making decisions based on straightforward posterior probabilities.

The BOP2 design operates in a similar manner to Thall et al. (1995) (TSE) but tunes the posterior probability cutoffs at each interim cohort in order to control Type I error at some predefined threshold while maximizing power (i.e., minimizing Type II error). The posterior probability cutoffs become more stringent as the trial progresses, requiring more evidence of treatment efficacy. Like TSE, BOP2 can monitor multiple endpoints, such as safety and efficacy.

To illustrate BOP2, consider a hypothetical Phase II single-arm study with a maximum of 50 patients. Each patient will be evaluated for a binary treatment response and a binary toxicity response. BOP2 requires a user-specified null hypothesis probability of efficacy, toxicity, and efficacy AND toxicity. These probabilities could be determined from historical controls and are here assumed P(Eff) = 0.2, P (Tox) = 0.4, and P(Eff & Tox) = 0.08. BOP2 then constructs a vague prior distribution belonging to the Dirichlet class with these historical control probabilities as the prior parameter means.

The power is computed at a user input value under the alternative hypothesis, here specified as P(Eff) = 0.4, P(Tox) = 0.2, and P(Eff & Tox) = 0.08. A Type I error rate, here 0.05, is chosen as well as interim monitoring at 10, 20, 30, and 40 patients. BOP2 then seeks probability stopping thresholds to maximize power. These probability thresholds are converted into stopping criteria in terms of number of toxicities and number of responses at each interim cohort. The stopping boundaries are listed in Table 4. This design obtains a power of 0.95 to reject the null hypothesis and conclude that the treatment is more efficacious and less toxic than the null hypothesis.

One can also assume particular efficacy and toxicity values and calculate the probability of stopping, the probability of claiming the treatment is acceptable, and the expected sample size. These are known as the operating characteristics for the trial and are contained in Table 5. Higher efficacy and lower toxicity probabilities lead to lower chance of early stopping and higher chance of claiming acceptable. At the null value of Pr(Eff) = 0.2 and Pr(Tox) = 0.4 (second row), the probability of claiming acceptable is 3.57%, below the specified 5% threshold. At the alternative value of Pr(Eff) = 0.4 and Pr(Tox) = 0.2, the power of the test is 95.36%.

The dynamic performance of the BOP2 design can be visualized with animations. A still image from one such animation is contained in Fig. 5. Patients are monitored in cohorts of size 10 up to a maximum of 50. At each interim cohort, a Go/No Go decision is made based on the number of responses (left plot) and toxicities (right

Table 4 Stopping rules for a BOP2 trial design with the null hypothesis of P (Eff) = 0.2, P(Tox) = 0.4, and P(Eff & Tox) = 0.08, 5% Type I error

Cohort size	STOP IF # responses < =	OR # toxicities > =
10	0	6
20	3	10
30	5	13
40	8	16
50	12	18

Table 5 Operating characteristics for a BOP2 trial design with the null hypothesis of P(Eff) = 0.2, P(Tox) = 0.4, and P(Eff & Tox) = 0.08, 5% Type I error, and the alternative hypothesis of P (Eff) = 0.4, P(Tox) = 0.2, and P(Eff & Tox) = 0.08, 95% power

Pr (Eff)	Pr (Tox)	Pr(Eff & Tox)	Early stopping (%)	Claim acceptable (%)	Sample size
0.2	0.2	0.04	66.63	15.9	32.6
0.2	0.4	0.08	87.17	3.57	25.3
0.2	0.6	0.12	99.93	0	13.9
0.4	0.2	0.08	3.59	95.36	48.9
0.4	0.4	0.16	61.85	20.89	34.3
0.4	0.6	0.24	99.73	0.03	14.9

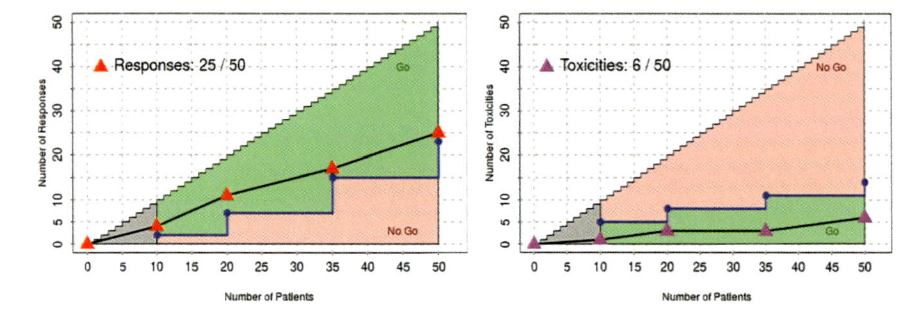

Fig. 5 Visualization of a BOP2 study

plot). This study did not stop early because the number of responses and toxicities stayed within the green regions.

Inferential Frameworks and Modern Trial Design Challenges

The flexibility of the Bayesian and frequentist inferential frameworks enables adaptation and development of new statistical methodology to address challenges and opportunities in modern medicine. Here two recent directions for trial design are reviewed with an emphasis on how the inferential frameworks are impacting design decisions.

Precision Medicine, Master Protocols, Umbrella Trials, Basket Trials, Platform Trials, and Adaptive Randomization

The advent of widely available genetic tests enables selective targeting of drugs to specific patient subpopulations. For example, cancer patients may be screened for dozens of genetic mutations and then given a treatment which produces optimal results for their genetic profile. Whereas traditional clinical trials focused on answering a single question (is this drug effective for a given patient population), newer trial designs seek to find optimal matches between patient profiles and particular drugs.

Master protocols coordinate several closely linked investigations into a single trial, enabling efficient use of resources (Mandrekar et al. 2015; Redman and Allegra 2015; Renfro and Sargent 2016; Woodcock and LaVange 2017). For example, umbrella trials select patients from a certain disease site (e.g., lung cancer), perform genetic testing on patients, and assign them to multiple treatments according to the matched drug targets. Basket trials take patients from multiple disease sites but with a certain mutation (e.g., BRAF mutation) and assign them to the corresponding target therapy (e.g., BRAF inhibitors) (Redig and Jänne 2015; Simon et al. 2016; Hobbs and Landin 2018). Platform trials provide efficient screening of multiple treatments in a certain disease in which a steady flow of patients is available (Berry et al. 2015; Hobbs et al. 2018). A common control group such as the standard of care can be incorporated as the reference groups. New treatments can be added to the platform and evaluated. If a treatment is promising, it can "graduate" and, if a treatment is not promising, it can be dropped from the platform. The trial can run perpetually to efficiently screen for effective treatments (Simon 2017).

Accrual of sufficient sample sizes can be challenging because of the number of disease and treatment combinations. For example, the Biomarker-integrated Approaches of Targeted Therapy for Lung Cancer Elimination (BATTLE) trial is an umbrella trial for non-small cell lung cancer tested 4 treatments and 4 genetic marker strata for a total of 16 possible marker-treatment combinations applying a Bayesian hierarchical model with 8-week disease control rate as the primary endpoint (Zhou et al. 2008; Kim et al. 2011; Liu and Lee 2015; Simon 2017). Prespecifying a fixed sample size for each combination would result in a large overall sample size due to the large number of combinations. Instead the trial used Bayesian adaptive randomization in which the most promising combinations continued accruing patients while combinations with disappointing response rates were suspended. With adaptive randomization designs, suspended combinations may be reopened if initially promising combinations begin to show poor performance. This accrual strategy optimizes use of limited resources and has the potential to speed up drug development (Berry 2015).

The I-SPYII Phase II platform trial for women with locally advanced breast cancer (Barker et al. 2009) is testing standard neoadjuvant chemotherapy against five new chemotherapy drugs, each being added to the standard regimen. Each drug is tested in a minimum of 20 and maximum of 120 patients. Patients are randomized based on hormone receptor status, HER2 status, and MammaPrint score. As the trial progresses, biomarker-drug combinations with more favorable outcomes (pathological complete response after resection) are assigned more patients so that they can accumulate more data. These promising arms then proceed to separate Phase III trials. The GBM-Agile for glioblastoma multiforme includes many of the inferential elements of I-SPY2 while adding a transition from Phase II to III as part of the trial for the promising arms (Alexander et al. 2018). NCI-Match trial and a BRAF trial are examples of basket trials (Hyman et al. 2015; Mullard 2015). Platform trials are currently underway for several cancer types (Herbst et al. 2015; Alexander and Cloughesy 2018).

Multiple Outcomes and Utility Functions

Clinical trials typically collect data on several outcomes, such as safety and efficacy, thus offering several metrics on which to compare treatments. This can make decisions about identifying the "best" treatment difficult, as one drug may be more effective but also more toxic. A simple and common solution is to define a maximum toxicity threshold and then select as superior the treatment with acceptable toxicity and highest efficacy. Alternatively a new drug may undergo a noninferiority trial for efficacy and then be deemed superior based on safety (Mauri and D'Agostino Sr 2017).

Decision theory offers a more nuanced alternative. In decision theory, a utility function determined a priori by the clinician is used to summarize potentially complex treatment effects as a single number. Murray et al. (2016) discuss utility functions in the context of cancer patients where treatment efficacy may be recorded as complete response, partial response, stable disease, and progressive disease (four categories) while nonfatal toxicities may be recorded as none, minor, and major (three categories). Each patient has one of 13 possible responses to treatment (four possible efficacies x three toxicity levels + death). The clinician then defines a desirability, or utility, of each of these possible 13 responses. Murray et al. (2016) recommend assigning a utility score of 100 to the best possible response (complete response with no toxicity) and 0 to the worst outcome (death). The utility is then computed for each patient enrolled in the trial. The distribution of utilities in treatment and control groups can be compared using either frequentist or Bayesian methods. Hypothesis testing can be used to determine if the experimental treatment convincingly delivers better average utility than standard of care.

The AWARD-5 trial used a utility function to find the optimal dose of dulaglutide for treating type 2 diabetes patients (Skrivanek et al. 2014). The trial combined four safety and efficacy measures (glycosylated hemoglobin A1c versus sitagliptin, weight, pulse, and diastolic blood pressure) into a clinical utility index (CUI) with larger values indicating more favorable profile. The trial computed posterior distributions for CUI at various dose levels and recommended a dose based on these distributions.

Summary and Conclusion

Inferential frameworks enable clinicians to conduct clinical trials and draw principled conclusions from the resulting data. Four essential aspects of inferential frameworks are:

1. *Assumptions relating to the data collection of the sample from the population*: Both frequentist and Bayesian methods will produce valid results when the sample is selected in an unbiased manner. Random sampling of patients,

treatment randomization, and objective evaluation of treatment outcomes blinded to the treatment assignment are critical for obtaining valid inferences.

2. *Separation of the concepts of parameter estimate* ($\widehat{p}$) *from the true unknown parameter in the population (p)*: Both Bayesian and frequentist statistics separate sample-based estimates from true population-based quantities. The particular estimated values produced by Bayesian and frequentist statistical methods are often different.
3. *Frequentist framework assumes that the parameter is fixed and data are random. Conversely, Bayesian framework assumes that the parameter is random and data are fixed.*
4. *Quantification of uncertainty in how close the estimate* $\widehat{p}$ *is to the true unknown population value* p: Here Bayesian and frequentist methods differ. Bayesian statistics uses the posterior distribution of the parameter to quantify uncertainty, while frequentist statistics uses sampling distributions. Bayesian measures of uncertainty typically have a more straightforward interpretation, at the cost of having to specify a prior distribution.

While constructing new trial designs involves complex statistical considerations, software for implementing existing designs is increasingly available via web applications and free downloads. The website http://trialdesign.org hosts web applications for implementing over 30 trial designs, both frequentist and Bayesian, including classical methods such as Simon's optimal two-stage and newer Bayesian adaptive methods for basket and platform trials. This software is freely available to the scientific research community and requires only an Internet browser to use.

In the past, Bayesian and frequentist schools were combative. They countered each other's points and had heated debate and argument fiercely. At the present time, the two schools of inference are competitive. There is abundant literature comparing the pros and cons of each approach. In the future, they will be more cooperative. Bayesian and frequentist's approaches offer complementary views, and both approaches can learn from each other. Convergence of Bayesian and frequentist's methods was inconceivable in the past but inevitable in the future.

Cross-References

▸ Adaptive Phase II Trials
▸ Bias Control in Randomized Controlled Clinical Trials
▸ Confident Statistical Inference with Multiple Outcomes, Subgroups, and Other Issues of Multiplicity
▸ Dose Finding for Drug Combinations
▸ Essential Statistical Tests
▸ Power and Sample Size
▸ Statistical Analysis of Patient-Reported Outcomes in Clinical Trials

References

Agresti A, Franklin CA (2009) Statistics: the art and science of learning from data. Prentice Hall, Upper Saddle River
Alexander BM, Cloughesy TF (2018) Platform trials arrive on time for glioblastoma. Oxford University Press US
Alexander BM et al (2018) Adaptive global innovative learning environment for glioblastoma: GBM AGILE. Clin Cancer Res 24(4):737–743
Barker A et al (2009) I-SPY 2: an adaptive breast cancer trial design in the setting of neoadjuvant chemotherapy. Clin Pharmacol Ther 86(1):97–100
Bayes T (1763) LII. An essay towards solving a problem in the doctrine of chances. By the late Rev. Mr. Bayes, FRS communicated by Mr. Price, in a letter to John Canton, AMFR S. Philos Trans R Soc Lond 53:370–418
Berger JO (1985) Statistical decision theory and Bayesian analysis. Springer Science & Business Media
Berger JO (2003) Could fisher, Jeffreys and Neyman have agreed on testing? Stat Sci 18(1):1–32
Berger JO, Wolpert RL (1988) The likelihood principle. IMS
Berry DA (2015) The brave New World of clinical cancer research: adaptive biomarker-driven trials integrating clinical practice with clinical research. Mol Oncol 9(5):951–959
Berry SM et al (2010) Bayesian adaptive methods for clinical trials. CRC press
Berry SM et al (2015) The platform trial: an efficient strategy for evaluating multiple treatments. JAMA 313(16):1619–1620
Biswas S et al (2009) Bayesian clinical trials at the University of Texas MD Anderson cancer center. Clin Trials 6(3):205–216
Carpenter B et al (2017) Stan: a probabilistic programming language. J Stat Softw 76(1)
Casella G, Berger RL (2002) Statistical inference. Duxbury Pacific Grove, Belmont
Chen F (2009) Bayesian modeling using the MCMC procedure. Proceedings of the SAS Global Forum 2008 Conference. SAS Institute Inc., Cary
Gelman A et al (2013) Bayesian data analysis. Chapman and Hall/CRC
Goodman SN (1999) Toward evidence-based medical statistics. 2: the Bayes factor. Ann Intern Med 130(12):1005–1013
Herbst RS et al (2015) Lung Master Protocol (Lung-MAP) – a biomarker-driven protocol for accelerating development of therapies for squamous cell lung cancer: SWOG S1400. Clin Cancer Res 21(7):1514–1524
Hobbs BP, Landin R (2018) Bayesian basket trial design with exchangeability monitoring. Stat Med 37(25):3557–3572
Hobbs BP et al (2018) Controlled multi-arm platform design using predictive probability. Stat Methods Med Res 27(1):65–78
Hyman DM et al (2015) Vemurafenib in multiple nonmelanoma cancers with BRAF V600 mutations. N Engl J Med 373(8):726–736
Jeffreys H (1946) An invariant form for the prior probability in estimation problems. Proc R Soc Lond A Math Phys Sci 186(1007):453–461
Johnson VE (2013) Revised standards for statistical evidence. Proc Natl Acad Sci 110(48):19313–19317
Johnson VE, Cook JD (2009) Bayesian design of single-arm phase II clinical trials with continuous monitoring. Clin Trials 6(3):217–226
Jüni P et al (2001) Assessing the quality of controlled clinical trials. BMJ 323(7303):42–46
Kass RE, Raftery AE (1995) Bayes factors. J Am Stat Assoc 90(430):773–795
Kim ES et al (2011) The BATTLE trial: personalizing therapy for lung cancer. Cancer Discov 1 (1):44–53
Le Tourneau C et al (2009) Dose escalation methods in phase I cancer clinical trials. J Natl Cancer Inst 101(10):708–720
Lee JJ, Chu CT (2012) Bayesian clinical trials in action. Stat Med 31(25):2955–2972

Lee JJ, Liu DD (2008) A predictive probability design for phase II cancer clinical trials. Clin Trials 5(2):93–106
Lin Y, Shih WJ (2001) Statistical properties of the traditional algorithm-based designs for phase I cancer clinical trials. Biostatistics 2(2):203–215
Little RJ (2006) Calibrated Bayes: a Bayes/frequentist roadmap. Am Stat 60(3):213–223
Liu S, Lee JJ (2015) An overview of the design and conduct of the BATTLE trials. Chin Clin Oncol 4(3)
Liu S, Yuan Y (2015) Bayesian optimal interval designs for phase I clinical trials. J R Stat Soc Ser C Appl Stat 64(3):507–523
Mandrekar SJ et al (2015) Improving clinical trial efficiency: thinking outside the box. American Society of Clinical Oncology educational book. American Society of Clinical Oncology. Annual Meeting
Mauri L, D'Agostino RB Sr (2017) Challenges in the design and interpretation of noninferiority trials. N Engl J Med 377(14):1357–1367
Mossman D, Berger JO (2001) Intervals for posttest probabilities: a comparison of 5 methods. Med Decis Mak 21(6):498–507
Mullard A (2015) NCI-MATCH trial pushes cancer umbrella trial paradigm. Nature Publishing Group
Murray TA et al (2016) Utility-based designs for randomized comparative trials with categorical outcomes. Stat Med 35(24):4285–4305
O'Quigley J, Chevret S (1991) Methods for dose finding studies in cancer clinical trials: a review and results of a Monte Carlo study. Stat Med 10(11):1647–1664
O'Quigley J et al (1990) Continual reassessment method: a practical design for phase 1 clinical trials in cancer. Biometrics:33–48
Plummer M (2003) JAGS: a program for analysis of Bayesian graphical models using Gibbs sampling. In: Proceedings of the 3rd international workshop on distributed statistical computing. Austria, Vienna
Redig AJ, Jänne PA (2015) Basket trials and the evolution of clinical trial design in an era of genomic medicine. J Clin Oncol 33(9):975–977
Redman MW, Allegra CJ (2015) The master protocol concept. Seminars in oncology. Elsevier
Renfro L, Sargent D (2016) Statistical controversies in clinical research: basket trials, umbrella trials, and other master protocols: a review and examples. Ann Oncol 28(1):34–43
Rosenbaum PR, Rubin DB (1984) Sensitivity of Bayes inference with data-dependent stopping rules. Am Stat 38(2):106–109
Simon R (1989) Optimal two-stage designs for phase II clinical trials. Control Clin Trials 10 (1):1–10
Simon R (2017) Critical review of umbrella, basket, and platform designs for oncology clinical trials. Clin Pharmacol Ther 102(6):934–941
Simon R et al (2016) The Bayesian basket design for genomic variant-driven phase II trials. Seminars in oncology. Elsevier
Skrivanek Z et al (2014) Dose-finding results in an adaptive, seamless, randomized trial of once-weekly dulaglutide combined with metformin in type 2 diabetes patients (AWARD-5). Diabetes Obes Metab 16(8):748–756
Smith TL et al (1996) Design and results of phase I cancer clinical trials: three-year experience at MD Anderson Cancer Center. J Clin Oncol 14(1):287–295
Spiegelhalter DJ et al (1996) BUGS: bayesian inference using Gibbs sampling. Version 0.5, (version ii). http://www.mrc-bsu.cam.ac.uk/bugs. 19
Spiegelhalter DJ et al (2004) Bayesian approaches to clinical trials and health-care evaluation. Wiley
Storer BE (1989) Design and analysis of phase I clinical trials. Biometrics 45(3):925–937
Thall PF et al (1995) Bayesian sequential monitoring designs for single-arm clinical trials with multiple outcomes. Stat Med 14(4):357–379
Tidwell RSS et al (2019) Bayesian clinical trials at The University of Texas MD Anderson Cancer Center: an update. Clin Trials:1740774519871471

Wasserstein RL, Lazar NA (2016) The ASA's statement on p-values: context, process, and purpose. Am Stat 70(2):129–133

Wasserstein RL et al (2019) Moving to a world beyond "p< 0.05". Taylor & Francis

Wilson EB (1927) Probable inference, the law of succession, and statistical inference. J Am Stat Assoc 22(158):209–212

Woodcock J, LaVange LM (2017) Master protocols to study multiple therapies, multiple diseases, or both. N Engl J Med 377(1):62–70

Zhou X et al (2008) Bayesian adaptive design for targeted therapy development in lung cancer – a step toward personalized medicine. Clin Trials 5(3):181–193

Zhou H et al (2017) BOP2: bayesian optimal design for phase II clinical trials with simple and complex endpoints. Stat Med 36(21):3302–3314

Dose Finding for Drug Combinations

55

Mourad Tighiouart

Contents

Abstract

We present early phase cancer clinical trial designs for drug combinations focusing on continuous dose levels. For phase I trials, the goal is to estimate the maximum tolerated dose (MTD) curve in the two-dimensional Cartesian plane. Parametric models are used to describe the relationship between the doses of the two agents and the probability of dose limiting toxicity (DLT). Trial design proceeds using cohorts of two patients receiving doses according to univariate escalation with overdose control (EWOC) or continual reassessment method (CRM). The maximum tolerated dose curve is estimated as a function of

M. Tighiouart (✉)
Cedars-Sinai Medical Center, Los Angeles, CA, USA
e-mail: mourad.tighiouart@cshs.org

© Springer Nature Switzerland AG 2022

S. Piantadosi, C. L. Meinert (eds.), *Principles and Practice of Clinical Trials*,
https://doi.org/10.1007/978-3-319-52636-2_80

Bayes estimates of the model parameters. In the case where some DLTs can be attributed to one agent but not the other, we describe how these parametric designs can be extended to account for an unknown fraction of attributable DLTs. For treatments where efficacy is resolved after few cycles of therapy, it is standard practice to perform single or randomized phase II trials using the MTD(s) obtained from a phase I trial. In our setting, we show how the MTD curve is carried out into a phase II trial where patients are allocated to doses likely to have high probability of treatment efficacy using a Bayesian adaptive design. The methodology is illustrated with an application to an early phase trial of cisplatin and cabazitaxel in advanced stage prostate cancer patients with visceral metastasis. Finally, we describe how these methods are adapted to the case of a pre-specified set of discrete dose combinations.

Keywords

Dose fiinding · Drug combinations · MTD · DLT · EWOC · CRM · Adaptive designs · Attributable toxicity · Efficacy · Cubic splines

Introduction

Early phase cancer clinical trials are small studies aimed at identifying tolerable doses with promising signal for efficacy. These trials use drug combinations of cytotoxic, biologic, immunotherapy, and/or radiotherapy agents to better target different signaling pathways simultaneously and reduce potential tumor resistance to chemo- or targeted therapy. However, most of these trials are designed to estimate the maximum tolerated dose (MTD) of a single agent for fixed dose levels of the other agents. This approach may provide a single safe dose for the combination, but it may be suboptimal in terms of therapeutic effects. Statistical designs that allow more than one drug to vary during the trial have been studied extensively in the last decade (see, e.g., Thall et al. 2003; Wang and Ivanova 2005; Yin and Yuan 2009a, b; Braun and Wang 2010; Wages et al. 2011; Shi and Yin 2013; Tighiouart et al. 2014b, 2016, 2017b; Riviere et al. 2014; Mander and Sweeting 2015). Some of these designs are aimed at identifying a single MTD, whereas others can recommend more than one MTD combination and even an infinite number of MTDs Tighiouart et al. (2014b, 2016, 2017b). Most of these methods use a parametric model for the dose-toxicity relationship

$$P(T = 1|\text{dose} = \boldsymbol{x}) = F(\boldsymbol{x}, \boldsymbol{\xi}), \tag{1}$$

where $\boldsymbol{x} = (x_1, \ldots, x_k)$ is the dose combination of k drugs, F is a known link function, T is the indicator of dose limiting toxicity (DLT), and $\boldsymbol{\xi} \in \mathbb{R}^d$ is an unknown parameter. Let S be the set of all dose combinations available in the trial. The MTD is defined as the set C of dose combinations $\boldsymbol{x}$ such that the probability of DLT for a patient given dose combination $\boldsymbol{x}$ equals to a target probability of DLT θ:

$$C = \{\boldsymbol{x} \in S : F(\boldsymbol{x}, \boldsymbol{\xi}) = \theta\}. \tag{2}$$

An alternative definition of the MTD is the set of dose combinations $\boldsymbol{x}$ that satisfy $|F(\boldsymbol{x}, \boldsymbol{\xi}) - \theta| \leq \delta$ since the set C in (2) may be empty. This can happen, for example, when S is finite and the MTD is not part of the dose combinations available in the trial. The threshold parameter δ is referred to as $100 \times \delta -$ point window in Braun and Wang (2010) and is pre-specified by the clinician. In general, the above methods proceed by treating successive cohorts of patients with dose escalation starting from the lowest dose combination and the model parameters and estimated probabilities of toxicities are sequentially updated. Dose allocation to the next cohort of patients is carried out by minimizing the risk of exceeding the target probability of DLT θ according to some loss function. In section "Dose Finding to Estimate the Maximum Tolerated Dose Curve" of this chapter, we present a drug combination design based on escalation with overdose control (EWOC) (Babb et al. 1998; Tighiouart et al. 2005, 2012a, b, 2014a, 2017a; Tighiouart and Rogatko 2010, 2012; Chen et al. 2012a; Wheeler et al. 2017; Diniz et al. 2019). We will focus on drug combination of two agents with continuous dose levels, and the goal of the trial is to estimate the MTD curve. The design proceeds by treating consecutive cohorts of two patients receiving different dose combinations determined using univariate EWOC. In section "Attributable Toxicity," we extend model (1) to account for an unknown fraction of attributable DLTs. This may arise when combining drugs with different mechanisms of action such as Taxotere and metformin. The design is similar to the one in section "Dose Finding to Estimate the Maximum Tolerated Dose Curve" except that the estimated doses for the next cohort of patients use the continual reassessment method criteria (CRM) (O'Quigley et al. 1990; Faries 1994; Goodman et al. 1995; O'Quigley and Shen 1996; Piantadosi et al. 1998).

In section "Phase I/II Dose Finding" of this chapter, we show how the estimated MTD curve from a phase I trial can be used in a phase II study with the goal of determining a dose combination along the MTD curve with maximum probability of efficacy. This setting corresponds to a phase I/II cancer clinical trial design where the MTD is first determined in a phase I trial and then is used in a phase II trial to evaluate treatment efficacy. Such situations occur when response evaluation takes few cycles of therapy or the phase I and II patient populations are different. In the case where both toxicity and efficacy are resolved within one or two cycles of therapy, sequential designs that update the probabilities of DLT and efficacy are used instead, and the goal is to determine a tolerable dose combination with maximum probability of treatment response. Finally, we show how the methods described in sections "Dose Finding to Estimate the Maximum Tolerated Dose Curve" and "Attributable Toxicity" can be adapted to the setting of a discrete set of dose combinations in section "Discrete Dose Combinations." Properties of these designs are evaluated by presenting operating characteristics derived under a large number of practical scenarios. For phase I trials, summary statistics of safety and precision of the estimate of the MTD curve are calculated. For the phase II trial, Bayesian power and type I error probabilities are provided under scenarios favoring the alternative and null hypotheses, respectively.

Dose Finding to Estimate the Maximum Tolerated Dose Curve

Model

Consider the dose-toxicity model of the form

$$P(T = 1|x, y) = F(\eta_0 + \eta_1 x + \eta_2 y + \eta_3 xy), \tag{3}$$

where T is the indicator of DLT, $T = 1$ if a patient given the dose combination (x, y) exhibits DLT within one cycle of therapy, and $T = 0$ otherwise, $x \in [X_{min}, X_{max}]$ is the dose level of agent A_1, $y \in [Y_{min}, Y_{max}]$ is the dose level of agent A_2, and F is a known cumulative distribution function. Here, X_{min}, X_{max} and Y_{min}, Y_{max} are the lower and upper bounds of the continuous dose levels of agents A_1 and A_2, respectively. Suppose that the doses of agents A_1 and A_2 are standardized to be in the interval [0, 1] using the transformations $h_1(x) = (x - X_{min})/(X_{max} - X_{min})$, $h_2(y) = (y - Y_{min})/(Y_{max} - Y_{min})$, and the interaction parameter $\eta_3 > 0$.

We will assume that that the probability of DLT increases with the dose of any one of the agents when the other one is held constant. A necessary and sufficient condition for this property to hold is to assume $\eta_1, \eta_2 > 0$. The MTD is defined as any dose combination (x^*, y^*) such that

$$\text{Prob}(T = 1|x^*, y^*) = \theta. \tag{4}$$

The target probability of DLT θ is set relatively high when the DLT is a reversible or nonfatal condition and low when it is life threatening. We reparameterize model (3) in terms of parameters clinicians can easily interpret. One way is to use ρ_{10}, the probability of DLT when the levels of drugs A_1 and A_2 are 1 and 0, respectively; ρ_{01}, the probability of DLT when the levels of drugs A_1 and A_2 are 0 and 1, respectively; and ρ_{00}, the probability of DLT when the levels of drugs A_1 and A_2 are both 0. It can be shown that

$$\begin{cases} \eta_0 = F^{-1}(\rho_{00}) \\ \eta_1 = F^{-1}(\rho_{10}) - F^{-1}(\rho_{00}) \\ \eta_2 = F^{-1}(\rho_{01}) - F^{-1}(\rho_{00}) \end{cases} \tag{5}$$

Using (3), the definition of the MTD in (4), and reparameterization (5), we obtain the MTD curve C as a function of the model parameters ρ_{00}, ρ_{01}, ρ_{10}, and η_3 and target probability of DLT θ as

$$C = \left\{ (x^*, y^*) : y^* = \frac{\left(F^{-1}(\theta) - F^{-1}(\rho_{00})\right) - \left(F^{-1}(\rho_{10}) - F^{-1}(\rho_{00})\right)x^*}{\left(F^{-1}(\rho_{01}) - F^{-1}(\rho_{00})\right) + \eta_3 x^*} \right\}. \tag{6}$$

This reparameterization allows the MTD curve to lie anywhere within the dose range $[X_{min}, X_{max}] \times [Y_{min}, Y_{max}]$. If there is strong a priori belief that $\Gamma_{A1|A2=0}$, the MTD of drug A_1 when the level of drug A_2 is equal to Y_{min} is in the interval [X_{min},

$X_{max}]$ and $\Gamma_{A2\,|A1\,=0}$, the MTD of drug A_2 when the level of drug A_1 is equal to X_{min} is in the interval $[Y_{min}, Y_{max}]$, then the reparameterization ρ_{00}, $\Gamma_{A1\,|A2\,=0}$, $\Gamma_{A2\,|A1\,=0}$, η_3 is more convenient (see Tighiouart et al. 2014b for more details on this reparameterization).

A prior distribution on the model parameters is placed as follows. ρ_{01}, ρ_{10}, and η_3 are independent a priori with $\rho_{01} \sim \text{beta}(a_1, b_1)$, $\rho_{10} \sim \text{beta}(a_2, b_2)$, and conditional on (ρ_{01}, ρ_{10}), $\rho_{00}/\min(\rho_{01}, \rho_{10}) \sim \text{beta}(a_3, b_3)$. The prior distribution on the interaction parameter η_3 is a gamma with mean a/b and variance a/b^2. If $Dk = \{(x_i, y_i, T_i)\}$ is the data after enrolling k patients to the trial, the posterior distribution of the model parameters is

$$\pi(\rho_{00},\rho_{01},\rho_{10},\eta_3) \propto \prod_{i=1}^{k} \left(G(\rho_{00},\rho_{01},\rho_{10},\eta_3;x_i,y_i)\right)^{T_i}\left(1 - G(\rho_{00},\rho_{01},\rho_{10},\eta_3;x_i,y_i)\right)^{1-T_i}$$
$$\times \pi(\rho_{01})\pi(\rho_{10})\pi(\rho_{00}|\rho_{01},\rho_{10})\pi(\eta_3),$$

where

$$G(\rho_{00},\rho_{01},\rho_{10},\eta_3;x_i,y_i) = F\left(F^{-1}(\rho_{00}) + \left(F^{-1}(\rho_{10}) - F^{-1}(\rho_{00})\right)x_i + \left(F^{-1}(\rho_{01}) - F^{-1}(\rho_{00})\right)y_i + \eta_3 x_i y_i\right). \quad (7)$$

Features of the posterior distribution are estimated using WinBUGS (Lunn et al. 2000) and JAGS (Plummer 2003).

Trial Design

Dose escalation/de-escalation proceeds by treating cohorts of two patients simultaneously. It is based on the escalation with overdose control (EWOC) principle where at each stage of the trial, the posterior probability of overdosing a future patient is bounded by a feasibility bound α (see, e.g., Babb et al. 1998; Tighiouart et al. 2005; Tighiouart and Rogatko 2010, 2012). For a given cohort, one subject receives a new dose of agent A_1 for a given dose of agent A_2 that was previously assigned, and the other patient receives a new dose of agent A_2 for a given dose of agent A_1 that was previously assigned. Specifically,

(i) The first two patients receive the same dose combination $(x_1, y_1) = (x_2, y_2) = (0, 0)$ and let $D_2 = \{(x_1, y_1, T_1), (x_2, y_2, T_2)\}$.
(ii) In the second cohort, patients 3 and 4 receive doses (x_3, y_3) and (x_4, y_4), respectively, where $y_3 = y_1$, $x_4 = x_2$, x_3 is the α-th percentile of $\pi\left(\Gamma_{A_1|A_2=y_1}|D_2\right)$, and y_4 is the α-th percentile of $\pi\left(\Gamma_{A_2|A_1=x_2}|D_2\right)$. Here, $\pi\left(\Gamma_{A_1|A_2=y_1}|D_2\right)$ is the posterior distribution of the MTD of drug A_1 given that the level of drug A_2 is y_1, given the data D_2.
(iii) In the i-th cohort of two patients, if i is even, then patient $(2i - 1)$ receives dose (x_{2i-1}, y_{2i-3}), and patient $2i$ receives dose (x_{2i-2}, y_{2i}), where $x_{2i-1} =$

$\Pi^{-1}_{\Gamma_{A_1|A_2=y_{2i-3}}}(\alpha|D_{2i-2})$ and $y_{2i} = \Pi^{-1}_{\Gamma_{A_2|A_1=x_{2i-2}}}(\alpha|D_{2i-2})$. If i is odd, then patient $(2i-1)$ receives dose (x_{2i-3}, y_{2i-1}), and patient $2i$ receives dose (x_{2i}, y_{2i-2}), where $y_{2i-1} = \Pi^{-1}_{\Gamma_{A_2|A_1=x_{2i-3}}}(\alpha|D_{2i-2})$ and $x_{2i} = \Pi^{-1}_{\Gamma_{A_1|A_2=y_{2i-2}}}(\alpha|D_{2i-2})$. Here, $\Pi^{-1}_{\Gamma_{A_1|A_2=y}}(\alpha|D)$ denotes the inverse cdf of the posterior distribution $\pi(\Gamma_{A_1|A_2=y}|D)$.

(iv) Repeat step (iii) until N patients are enrolled to the trial subject to the following stopping rule.

Stopping Rule

Enrollment to the trial is suspended for safety if $P\ (P\ (T = 1|(x, y) = (0, 0)) > \theta + \xi_1|\text{data}) > \xi_2$, i.e., if the posterior probability that the probability of DLT at the minimum available dose combination in the trial exceeds the target probability of DLT is high. The design parameters ξ_1 and ξ_2 are chosen to achieve desirable model operating characteristics.

At the end of the trial, we estimate the MTD curve using (6) as

$$C_{\text{est}} = \left\{ (x^*, y^*) : y^* = \frac{\left(F^{-1}(\theta) - F^{-1}(\widehat{\rho}_{00})\right) - \left(F^{-1}(\widehat{\rho}_{10}) - F^{-1}(\widehat{\rho}_{00})\right)x^*}{\left(F^{-1}(\widehat{\rho}_{01}) - F^{-1}(\widehat{\rho}_{00})\right) + \widehat{\eta}_3 x^*} \right\}, \quad (8)$$

where $\widehat{\rho}_{00}, \widehat{\rho}_{01}, \widehat{\rho}_{10}$,and $\widehat{\eta}$ are the posterior medians given the data D_N.

Operating Characteristics

The performance of this design is evaluated for a prospective trial by assessing the safety of the trial and efficiency of the estimated MTD curve under various plausible scenarios elicited by the clinician in collaboration with the statistician.

Safety

For trial safety, the percent of DLTs across all patients and all simulated trials is reported in addition to the percent of trials with an excessive DLT rate, for example, greater than $\theta + 0.1$. The latter is an estimate of the probability that a prospective trial will result in a high rate of DLTs for a given scenario.

Efficiency

Uncertainty about the estimated MTD curve is evaluated by the pointwise average bias and percent selection. For $i = 1, \ldots, m$, let C_i be the estimated MTD curve and C_{true} be the true MTD curve, where m is the number of simulated trials. For every point $(x, y) \in C_{\text{true}}$, let

$$d^{(i)}_{(x,y)} = \text{sign}(y' - y) \times \min_{\{(x^*,y^*):(x^*,y^*) \in C_i\}} \left((x - x^*)^2 + (y - y^*)^2 \right)^{1/2}, \quad (9)$$

where y' is such that $(x, y') \in C_i$. This is the minimum relative distance of the point (x, y) on the true MTD curve to the estimated MTD curve C_i. Let

$$d_{(x,y)} = \frac{1}{m} \sum_{i=1}^{m} d_{(x,y)}^{(i)}. \tag{10}$$

Equation (10) can be interpreted as the pointwise average bias in estimating the MTD.

Let $\Delta(x, y)$ be the Euclidean distance between the minimum dose combination (0, 0) and the point (x, y) on the true MTD curve and $0 < p < 1$. Let

$$P_{(x,y)} = \frac{1}{m} \sum_{i=1}^{m} I\left(|d_{(x,y)}^{(i)}| \leq p\Delta(x,y)\right). \tag{11}$$

This is the pointwise percent of trials for which the minimum distance of the point (x, y) on the true MTD curve to the estimated MTD curve C_i is no more than $(100 \times p)\%$ of the true MTD. This statistic is equivalent to drawing a circle with center (x, y) on the true MTD curve and radius $p\Delta(x, y)$ and calculating the percent of trials with MTD curve estimate C_i falling inside the circle. This will give us the percent of trials with MTD recommendation within $(100 \times p)\%$ of the true MTD for a given tolerance p. This is interpreted as the pointwise percent selection for a given tolerance p.

Application to the CisCab Trial

The algorithm described in section "Trial Design" was used to design the first part of a phase I/II trial of the combination cisplatin and cabazitaxel in patients with prostate cancer with visceral metastasis. A recently published phase I trial of this combination by Lockhart et al. (2014) identified the MTD of cabazitaxel/cisplatin as 15/75 mg/m^2. This trial used a "3 + 3" design exploring three pre-specified dose levels 15/75, 20/75, and 25/75. In part 1 of the trial, nine patients were evaluated for safety, and no DLT was observed at 15/75 mg/m^2. In part 2 of the study, 15 patients were treated at 15/75 mg/m^2, and 2 DLTs were observed. Based on these results and other preliminary efficacy data, it was hypothesized that there exists a series of active dose combinations which are tolerable and active in prostate cancer. Cabazitaxel dose levels will be selected in the interval [10, 25], and cisplatin dose levels were selected in the interval [50, 100] administered intravenously. The plan is to enroll $N = 30$ patients and estimate the MTD curve. The target probability of DLT is $\theta = 0.33$, and a logistic link function for $F(\cdot)$ in (3) was used. DLT is resolved within one cycle (3 weeks) of treatment. Although the algorithm dictates that the first two patients receive dose combination 10/50 mg/m^2, the clinician Dr. Posadas preferred to start with 15 mg/m^2 cabazitaxel and 75 mg/m^2 cisplatin since this combination was tolerable based on the results of the published phase I trial and a number of patients he treated at this combination. The prior distributions were calibrated so that the prior mean probability of DLT at the dose combination 15/75 mg/m^2 equals the target probability of DLT. Specifically, informative priors were used for the model parameters ρ_{01}, $\rho_{10} \sim$ beta (1.4, 5.6), and conditional on ρ_{01}, ρ_{10}, $\rho_{00}/\min(\rho_{01}, \rho_{10}) \sim$ beta(0.8, 7.2) and a vague prior for η_3 with mean 20, and variance 540 was used so that $E(P\ (DLT\ |(15; 75))) \approx 0.33$ a priori. Operating characteristics were derived by simulating $m = 2000$ trial replicates under various scenarios for the true MTD curve. Figure 1 shows the true and estimated MTD curve obtained using (6) with the parameters ρ_{00}, ρ_{01}, ρ_{10}, and η_3 replaced by their posterior median averaged across all 2000 simulated trials. Scenario A shown on the left panel of Fig. 1 is a case where the true MTD curve passes through a point very close to the dose combination (15, 75) identified as the MTD from the previous trial. Scenario B shown on the right panel is a case where the MTD curve is way above this dose combination. In each case, the estimated MTD curves are very close to the true MTD curves. This is also evidenced by the pointwise bias and percent selection (graphs included in the supplement). The trial was also safe since the percent of trials with DLT rate above $\theta + 0.1$ were 3.5% for the scenario on the left and 5.0% for the scenario on the right.

Figures 2 and 3 show the pointwise average bias and percent selection for tolerances $p = 0.05, 0.1$ under scenarios A and B. In both cases, the absolute average bias is less than 0.05, which corresponds to 5% of the standardized dose range of either agent. We conclude that the pointwise average bias is practically negligible. The pointwise percent selection when $p = 0.05$ varies between 40% and 90% under scenario A for most doses and between 60% and 75% under scenario B. These are reasonable percent selections comparable to dose combination phase I trials. Other scenarios were included in the clinical protocol.

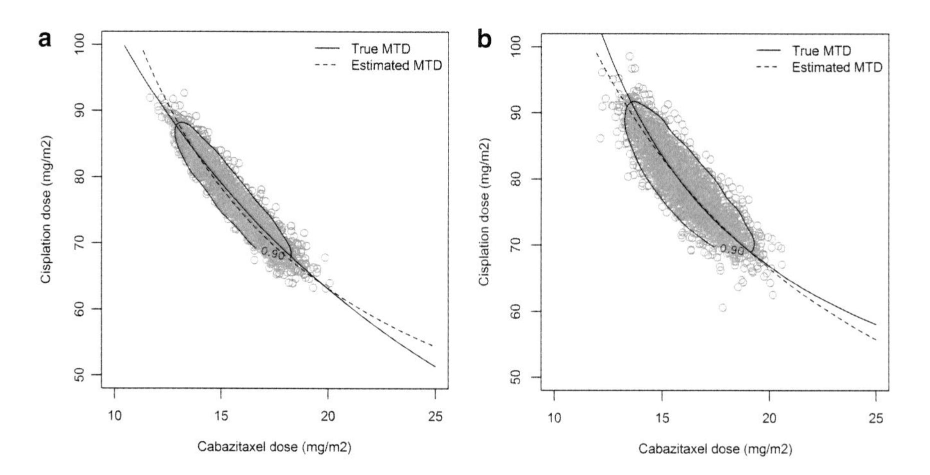

Fig. 1 True and estimated MTD curve under two different scenarios for the MTD curve. The gray diamonds represent the last dose combination from each simulated trial along with a 90% confidence region

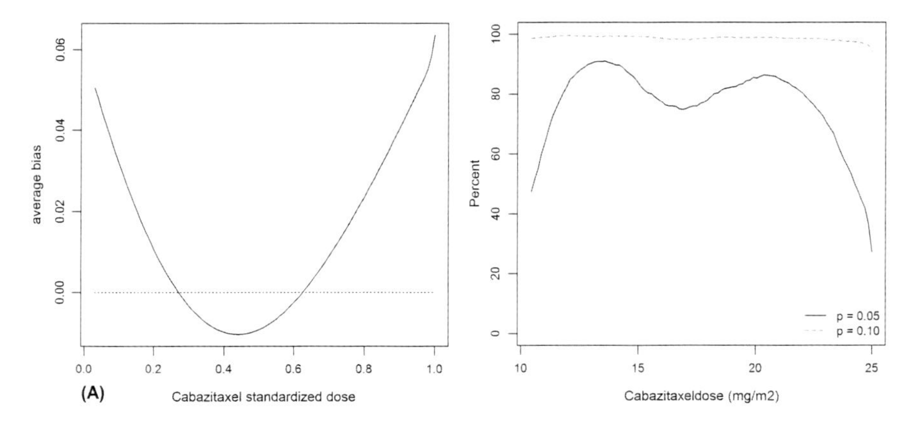

Fig. 2 Pointwise average bias (left) and percent selection (right) under scenario A

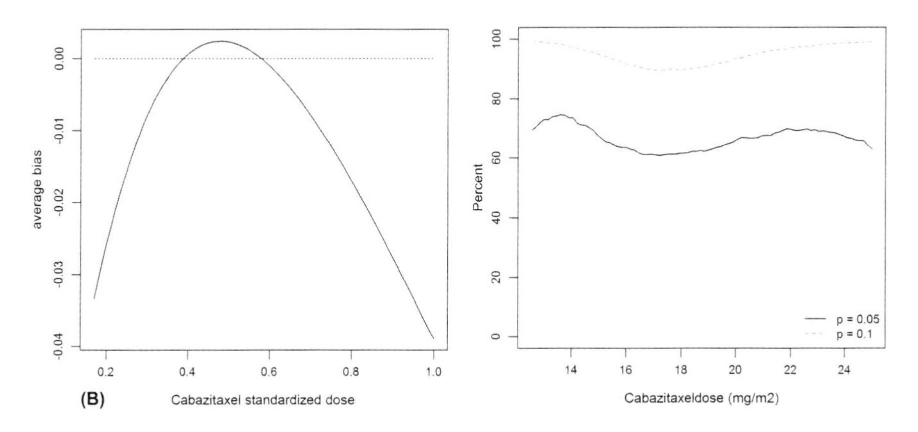

Fig. 3 Pointwise average bias (left) and percent selection (right) under scenario B

Attributable Toxicity

In section "Dose Finding to Estimate the Maximum Tolerated Dose Curve" and Eq. (3), a DLT event is assumed to be caused by drug A_1 or drug A_2, or both. In some applications, some DLTs can be attributed to one agent but not the other. For example, in a drug combination trial of Taxotere, a known cytotoxic agent, and metformin, a diabetes drug, in advanced or metastatic breast cancer patients, the clinician expects that some DLTs can be attributable to either agent or both. For example, a grade 3 or 4 neutropenia can only be attributable to Taxotere and not metformin. In this section, we present a dose combination trial design that accounts for an unknown fraction of attributable DLTs.

Dose-Toxicity Model

Let $F_\alpha(\cdot)$ and $F_\beta(\cdot)$ be parametric models for the probability of DLT of drugs A_1 and A_2, respectively. We specify the joint dose-toxicity relationship using the Gumbel copula model (see Murtaugh and Fisher 1990) as

$$\pi^{(\delta_1,\delta_2)} = \text{Prob}(\delta_1,\delta_2|x,y) = F_\alpha^{\delta_1}(x)\left[1-F_\alpha(x)\right]^{1-\delta_1}\times$$
$$F_\beta^{\delta_2}(y)\left[1-F_\beta(y)\right]^{1-\delta_2} + (-1)^{(\delta_1+\delta_2)}F_\alpha(x)\left[1-F_\alpha(x)\right]F_\beta(y)\left[1-F_\beta(y)\right]\frac{e^{-\gamma}-1}{e^{-\gamma}+1}, \tag{12}$$

where x and y are the standardized dose levels of drugs A_1 and A_2, respectively, δ_1 and δ_2 are the binary indicators of DLT attributed to drugs A_1 and A_2, respectively, and γ is the interaction coefficient. Similar to section "Dose Finding to Estimate the Maximum Tolerated Dose Curve," we assume that the probability of DLT $\pi = 1 - \pi^{(0,0)}$ increases with the dose of any one of the agents when the other one is held constant. A sufficient condition for this property to hold is to assume that $F_\alpha(\cdot)$ and $F_\beta(\cdot)$ are increasing functions with $\alpha > 0$ and $\beta > 0$. We take $F_\alpha(x) = x^\alpha$ and $F_\beta(y) = y^\beta$. Using (12), if the DLT is attributed exclusively to drug D_1, then

$$\pi^{(\delta_1=1,\delta_2=0)} = x^\alpha\left(1-y^\beta\right) - x^\alpha(1-x^\alpha)y^\beta\left(1-y^\beta\right)\frac{e^{-\gamma}-1}{e^{-\gamma}+1}. \tag{13}$$

If the DLT is attributed exclusively to drug D_2, then

$$\pi^{(\delta_1=0,\delta_2=1)} = y^\beta(1-x^\alpha) - x^\alpha(1-x^\alpha)y^\beta\left(1-y^\beta\right)\frac{e^{-\gamma}-1}{e^{-\gamma}+1}. \tag{14}$$

If the DLT is attributed to both drugs D_1 and D_2, then

$$\pi^{(\delta_1=1,\delta_2=1)} = x^\alpha y^\beta + x^\alpha(1-x^\alpha)y^\beta\left(1-y^\beta\right)\frac{e^{-\gamma}-1}{e^{-\gamma}+1}. \tag{15}$$

Equation (13) represents the probability that A_1 causes a DLT and drug A_2 does not cause a DLT. This can happen, for example, when a type of DLT of Taxotere, such as grade 4 neutropenia, is observed. However, this type of DLT can never be observed with metformin. This can also happen when the clinician attributes a grade 4 diarrhea to Taxotere but not to metformin in the case of a low dose level of this later even though both drugs have this common type of side effect. The fact that dose level y is present in Eq. (13) is a result of the joint modeling of the two marginals and accounts for the probability that drug A_2 does not cause a DLT. This later case is, of course, based on the clinician's judgment. Equations (14) and (15) can be interpreted similarly. The probability of DLT is

$$\pi = \text{Prob}(\text{DLT}|x,y) = \pi^{(\delta_1=1,\delta_2=0)} + \pi^{(\delta_1=0,\delta_2=1)} + \pi^{(\delta_1=1,\delta_2=1)} =$$
$$x^\alpha + y^\beta - x^\alpha y^\beta - x^\alpha(1-x^\alpha)y^\beta\left(1-y^\beta\right)\frac{e^{-\gamma}-1}{e^{-\gamma}+1}. \tag{16}$$

The MTD is any dose combination (x^*, y^*) such that Prob(DLT$|x^*, y^*) = \theta$. It follows that the MTD set $C(\alpha, \beta, \gamma)$ is

$$C(\alpha,\beta,\gamma) = \left\{ (x^*,y^*) : y^* = \left[\frac{-(1-x^{*\alpha}-\boldsymbol{\kappa}) \pm \sqrt{(1-x^{*\alpha}-\boldsymbol{\kappa})^2 - 4\boldsymbol{\kappa}(x^{*\alpha}-\theta)}}{2\boldsymbol{\kappa}} \right]^{\frac{1}{\beta}} \right\}, \tag{17}$$

where

$$\boldsymbol{\kappa} = x^{*\alpha}(1-x^{*\alpha})\frac{e^{-\gamma}-1}{e^{-\gamma}+1}.$$

Let T be the indicator of DLT, $T = 1$ if a patient treated at dose combination (x, y) experiences DLT within one cycle of therapy that is due to either drug or both, and $T = 0$ otherwise. Among patients treated with dose combination (x, y) who exhibit DLT suppose that an unknown fraction η of these patients has a DLT with known attribution, i.e., the clinician knows if the DLT is caused by drug A_1 only, or drug A_2 only, or both drugs A_1 and A_2. Let A be the indicator of DLT attribution when $T = 1$. It follows that for each patient treated with dose combination (x, y), there are five possible toxicity outcomes: $\{T=0\}$, $\{T=1, A=0\}$, $\{T=1, A=1, \delta_1=1, \delta_2=0\}$, $\{T=1, A=1, \delta_1=0, \delta_2=1\}$, and $\{T=1, A=1, \delta_1=1, \delta_2=1\}$. Using Eqs. (13), (14), (15), and (16) and Fig. 4, the likelihood function is

$$L(\alpha,\beta,\gamma,\eta|\text{data}) = \prod_{i=1}^{n} \left[\left(\eta\pi_i^{(\delta_{1_i},\delta_{2_i})} \right)^{A_i} (\pi_i(1-\eta))^{1-A_i} \right]^{T_i} (1-\pi_i)^{1-T_i}, \tag{18}$$

and the posterior distribution of the model parameters is

$$\pi(\alpha,\beta,\gamma,\eta|\text{data}) \propto L(\alpha,\beta,\gamma,\eta|\text{data}) \times \pi(\alpha,\beta,\gamma,\eta). \tag{19}$$

Features of the posterior distribution are estimated using JAGS (Plummer 2003).

Dose Allocation Algorithm

Dose escalation is similar to section "Dose Finding to Estimate the Maximum Tolerated Dose Curve" except that univariate continual reassessment method (CRM) (O'Quigley et al. 1990) is carried out to estimate the next dose instead of EWOC. In a cohort with two patients, the first one would receive a new dose of agent A_1 given the dose y of agent A_2 that was previously assigned. The new dose of agent A_1 is defined as $x_{\text{new}} = \text{argmin}_u \mid \widehat{\text{Prob}}(\text{DLT}|u, y) - \theta \mid$, where y is fixed and $\widehat{\text{Prob}}(\text{DLT}|u, y)$ is computed using Eq. (16) with α, β, γ replaced by their posterior medians. The other patient would receive a new dose of agent A_2 given the dose of agent A_1 that was previously assigned. Specifically, the design proceeds as follows:

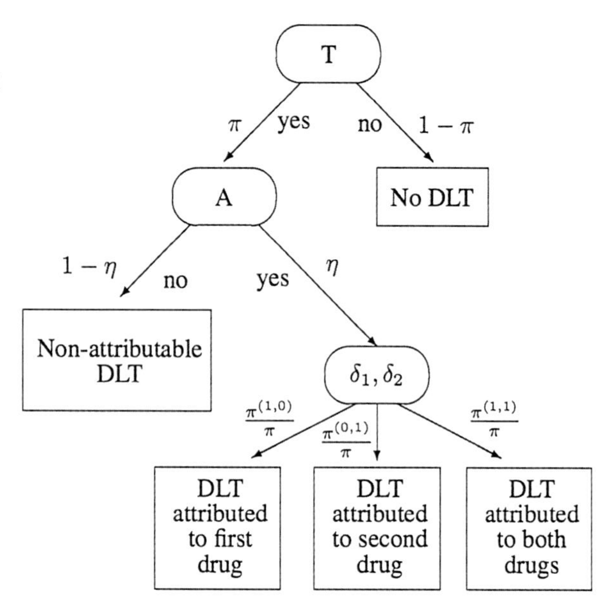

Fig. 4 A chance tree illustrating the five possible outcomes we can find in a trial

(i) The first two patients receive the same dose combination ($X_{\min}$, $Y_{\min}$).

(ii) In the i-th cohort of two patients,

- If i is even, patient $(2i - 1)$ receives dose combination (x_{2i-1}, y_{2i-1}), where $x_{2i-1} = \underset{u}{\operatorname{argmin}}\left|\widehat{\text{Prob}}(\text{DLT}|u, y_{2i-3}) - \theta\right|$, and $y_{2i-1} = y_{2i-3}$. For ethical reason, if a DLT was observed in the previous cohort of two patients and was attributable to drug A_1, then x_{2i-1} is further restricted to be no more than x_{2i-3}. Patient $2i$ receives dose combination (x_{2i}, y_{2i}), where $y_{2i} = \underset{v}{\operatorname{argmin}}\left|\widehat{\text{Prob}}(\text{DLT}|x_{2i-2}, v) - \theta\right|$, and $x_{2i} = x_{2i-2}$. If a DLT was observed in the previous cohort of two patients and was attributable to drug A_2, then y_{2i} is further restricted to be no more than y_{2i-2}.
- If i is odd, patient $(2i-1)$ receives doses (x_{2i-1}, y_{2i-1}), where $y_{2i-1} = \underset{v}{\operatorname{argmin}}\left|\widehat{\text{Prob}}(\text{DLT}|x_{2i-3}, v) - \theta\right|$, and $x_{2i-1} = x_{2i-3}$. If a DLT was observed in the previous cohort of two patients and was attributable to drug A_2, then y_{2i-1} is further restricted to be no more than y_{2i-3}. Patient $2i$ receives doses (x_{2i}, y_{2i}), where $x_{2i} = \underset{u}{\operatorname{argmin}}\left|\widehat{\text{Prob}}(\text{DLT}|u, y_{2i-2}) - \theta\right|$, and $y_{2i} = y_{2i-2}$. If a DLT was observed in the previous cohort of two patients and was attributable to drug A_1, then x_{2i} is further restricted to be no more than x_{2i-2}.

(iii) Repeat step 2 until the maximum sample size is reached subject to a safety stopping rule as described in section "Trial Design."

Here, we used univariate CRM instead of EWOC to estimate the next dose for computational efficiency. A comparison of the two methods in drug combination setting can be found in Diniz et al. (2017).

Simulation Studies

Dose levels of drugs A_1 and A_2 are standardized to be in the interval [0.05, 0.30], and we consider three scenarios for the true MTD curve shown by the black dashed curves in Fig. 5. We evaluate the effect of toxicity attribution in these three scenarios using four different values for η: 0, 0.1, 0.25, and 0.4. These values are reasonable because higher values of η in practice are very rare. Data are randomly generated as follows. For a given dose combination (x, y), a binary indicator of DLT T is generated from a Bernoulli distribution with probability of success computed using Eq. (16). If $\{T = 1\}$, we generate the attribution outcome A using a Bernoulli distribution with probability of success η. If $\{T = 1, A = 1\}$, we attribute the DLT to drug A_1, A_2, or to both with equal probabilities. We assume that the model parameters α, β, γ, and η are independent a priori. We assign vague prior distributions to α, β, and γ as in Yin and Yuan (2009a), where $\alpha \sim$ Uniform(0.2, 2), $\beta \sim$ Uniform(0.2, 2), and $\gamma \sim$ Gamma (0.1, 0.1). The prior distribution for the fraction of attributable toxicities η is set to be Uniform(0, 1). Using these prior distributions, the true parameter values for each scenario are as follows: in scenario 1, $\alpha = \beta = 0.9$ and $\gamma = 1$; in scenario 2, $\alpha = \beta = 1.1$ and $\gamma = 1$; and last, in scenario 3, $\alpha = \beta = 1.3$ and $\gamma = 1$. For each scenario, $m = 1000$ trials will be simulated. The target risk of toxicity is fixed at $\theta = 0.3$, the sample size is $n = 40$, and the values for ξ_1 and ξ_2 will be 0.05 and 0.8, respectively. Figure 5 shows the estimated MTD curves for each scenario as a function of η. In general, increasing the value of η until 0.4 corresponds to estimated MTD curves closer to the true MTD curve.

Table 1 shows the average percent of toxicities as well as the percent of trials with toxicity rates greater than $\theta + 0.05$ and $\theta + 0.1$ for scenarios 1–3. In general, we

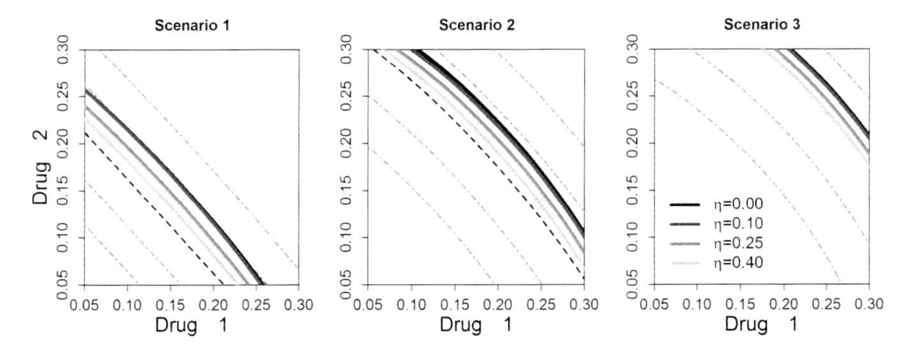

Fig. 5 Estimated MTD curves for $m = 1000$ simulated trials. The black dashed curve represents the true MTD curve, the gray dashed lines represent the contours at $\theta \pm 0.05$ and $\theta \pm 0.10$, and the solid curves represent the estimated MTD curves for each value of η

Table 1 Operating characteristics summarizing trial safety in $m = 1000$ simulated trials

		Average % of toxicities	% of trials with toxicity rate > $\theta + 0.05$	% of trials with toxicity rate > $\theta + 0.10$
Scenario 1	$\eta = 0.00$	33.62	25.90	4.10
	$\eta = 0.10$	32.67	22.60	4.80
	$\eta = 0.25$	31.55	17.60	2.70
	$\eta = 0.40$	30.70	13.30	2.00
Scenario 2	$\eta = 0.00$	30.64	9.40	0.90
	$\eta = 0.10$	29.69	7.30	0.40
	$\eta = 0.25$	28.76	5.00	0.20
	$\eta = 0.40$	28.04	4.10	0.30
Scenario 3	$\eta = 0.00$	27.47	2.00	0.00
	$\eta = 0.10$	26.80	1.80	0.00
	$\eta = 0.25$	25.99	1.30	0.00
	$\eta = 0.40$	25.37	0.70	0.00

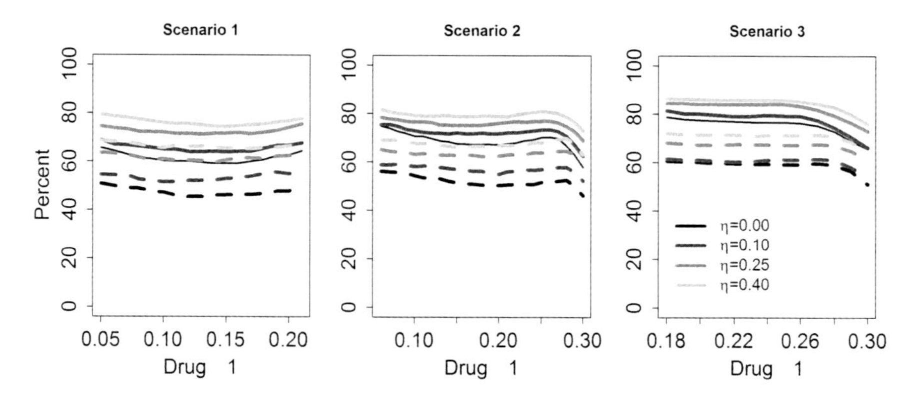

Fig. 6 Pointwise percent of MTD recommendation for $m = 1000$ simulated trials. Solid lines represent the pointwise percent of MTD recommendation when $p = 0.2$, and dashed lines represent the pointwise percent of MTD recommendation when $p = 0.1$

observe that increasing the fraction of toxicity attributions η reduces the average percent of toxicities and percent of trials with toxicity rates greater than $\theta + 0.05$ and $\theta + 0.10$. These results show that the design is safe in the sense that the probability that a prospective trial will result in an excessive rate of toxicity (greater than $\theta + 0.10$) is less than 5%. Figure 6 shows the pointwise percent of MTD recommendation of the three proposed scenarios for each value of η. In general, increasing the value of η increases the pointwise percent of MTD recommendation, reaching up to 80% of correct recommendation when $p = 0.2$ and up to 70% of correct recommendation when $p = 0.1$. Based on these simulation results, we conclude that in continuous dose setting, the approach of partial toxicity attribution generates safe trial designs and efficient estimation of the MTD. Further details about the approach and computer codes can be found in Jimenez et al. (2019).

Phase I/II Dose Finding

In this section, we describe a phase I/II design with the objective of determining a tolerable dose level that maximizes treatment efficacy. For treatments where efficacy is ascertained in a relatively short period of time such as one or two cycles of therapy, sequential designs for updating the joint probability of toxicity and efficacy and estimating the optimal dose have been studied extensively in the literature (for single agent trials, see, e.g., Murtaugh and Fisher (1990), Thall and Russell (1998), Braun (2002), Ivanova (2003), Thall and Cook (2004), Chen et al. (2015), and Sato et al. (2016), and for dose combination trials Yuan and Yin (2011), Wages and Conaway (2014), Cai et al. (2014), Riviere et al. (2015), and Clertant and Tighiouart (2017)). For treatments where response evaluation takes few cycles of therapy, it is standard practice to perform a two-stage design where a maximum tolerable dose (MTD) of a new drug or combinations of drugs is first determined, and then this recommended phase II dose is studied in stage II and evaluated for treatment efficacy, possibly using a different population of cancer patients from stage I (see Rogatko et al. 2008; Le Tourneau et al. 2009; Chen et al. 2012b for a review of such a paradigm). For drug combination phase I trials, more than one MTD can be recommended at the conclusion of the trial and choosing a single MTD combination for efficacy study may result in a failed phase II trial since other MTDs may present higher treatment efficacy. Hence, adaptive or parallel phase II trials may be more suitable for searching an optimal dose combination that is well tolerable with desired level of efficacy.

Stage I

Stage I proceeds as in section "Dose Finding to Estimate the Maximum Tolerated Dose Curve." Let C_{est} be the estimated MTD curve obtained at the end of the phase I trial, and suppose it is defined for $x \in [X_1, X_2]$ and $y \in [Y_1, Y_2]$. Here, $[X_1, X_2] \subset [X_{min}, X_{max}]$ and $[Y_1, Y_2] \subset [Y_{min}, Y_{max}]$. Let E be the indicator of treatment response such as tumor shrinkage, $E = 1$ if we have a positive response after a pre-defined number of treatment cycles and $E = 0$ otherwise. Let p_0 be the probability of efficacy of the standard of care treatment. We propose to carry out a phase II study to identify dose combinations $(x, y) \in C_{est}$ such that $P(E = 1|(x, y)) > p_0$.

Stage II

For every dose combination $(x, y) \in C_{est}$, let x be the unique vertical projection of (x, y) on the interval $[X_1, X_2]$. Next, denote by $z \in [0, 1]$ the standardized dose of $x \in [X_1, X_2]$ using the transformation $z = h_3(x) = (x - X_1)/(X_2 - X_1)$. In the sequel, we will refer to z as dose combination since there is a one-to-one transformation mapping $z \in [0, 1]$ to $(x, y) \in C_{est}$, $x \in [X_1, X_2]$, $y \in [Y_1, Y_2]$. We model the probability of treatment response given dose combination z in C_{est} as

$$P(E = 1|z, \boldsymbol{\psi}) = F(\ f(z; \boldsymbol{\psi})), \tag{20}$$

where F is a known link function, $f\,(z;\, \boldsymbol{\psi})$ is an unknown function, and $\boldsymbol{\psi}$ is an unknown parameter. A flexible way to model the probability of efficacy along the MTD curve is the cubic spline function

$$f(z; \boldsymbol{\psi}) = \beta_0 + \beta_1 z + \beta_2 z^2 + \sum_{j=3}^{k} \beta_j (z - \boldsymbol{\kappa}_j)_+^3, \tag{21}$$

where $\boldsymbol{\psi} = (\boldsymbol{\beta}, \boldsymbol{\kappa}), \boldsymbol{\beta} = (\beta_0, \ldots, \beta_k), \boldsymbol{\kappa} = (\boldsymbol{\kappa}_3, \ldots, \boldsymbol{\kappa}_{;k})$ with $\boldsymbol{\kappa}_3 = 0$. Let $D_m = \{(z_i, E_i),\ i = 1, \ldots, m\}$ be the data after enrolling m patients in the trial, where E_i is the response of the i-th patient treated with dose combination z_i, and let $\pi(\boldsymbol{\psi})$ be a prior density on the parameter $\boldsymbol{\psi}$. The posterior distribution is

$$\pi(\boldsymbol{\psi}|D_m) \propto \prod_{i=1}^{m} [F(\ f(z_i; \boldsymbol{\psi}))]^{E_i} [1 - F(\ f(z_i; \boldsymbol{\psi}))]^{1-E_i} \pi(\boldsymbol{\psi}). \tag{22}$$

Let p_z be the probability of treatment efficacy at dose combination z and denote by p_0 the probability of efficacy of a poor treatment or treatment not worthy of further investigation. An adaptive design is used to conduct a phase II trial in order to test the hypothesis.

H_0: $p_z \leq p_0$ for all z versus H_1: $p_z > p_0$ for some z.

Trial Design

(i) Randomly assign n_1 patients to dose combinations $z_1, \ldots, z_{n_1}$ equally spaced along the MTD curve C_{est} so that each combination is assigned to one and only one patient.
(ii) Obtain a Bayes estimate $\widehat{\boldsymbol{\psi}}$ of $\boldsymbol{\psi}$ given the data D_{n_1} using (22).
(iii) Generate n_2 dose combinations from the standardized density $F\,(f\,(z;\, \widehat{\boldsymbol{\psi}}))$, and assign them to the next cohort of n_2 patients.
(iv) Repeat steps (ii) and (iii) until a total of n patients have been enrolled to the trial subject to pre-specified stopping rules.

This algorithm can be viewed as an extension of a Bayesian adaptive design to select a superior arm among a finite number of arms Berry et al. (2011) to selecting a superior arm from an infinite number of arms.

Decision rule. At the end of the trial, we accept the alternative hypothesis if

$$\text{Max}_z[P(F(\ f(z; \boldsymbol{\psi})) > p_0|D_n)] > \delta_u, \tag{23}$$

where δ_u is a design parameter.

Stopping rules. For ethical considerations and to avoid exposing patients to subtherapeutic doses, we stop the trial for futility after j patients are evaluable for efficacy if there is strong evidence that none of the dose combinations are promising, i.e., $\text{Max}_z\ [P\,(F\,(f\,(z;\boldsymbol{\psi})) > p_0|D_j)] < \delta_0$ where δ_0 is a small pre-specified threshold. In cases where the investigator is interested in stopping the trial early for superiority, the trial can be terminated after j patients are evaluable for efficacy if $\text{Max}_z\ [P\,(F\,(f\,(z;\ \boldsymbol{\psi})) > p_0|D_j)] > \delta_1$ where $\delta_1 \geq \delta_u$ is a pre-specified threshold and the corresponding dose combination $z^* = \text{argmax}_u\{P\,(F\,(f\,(u;\boldsymbol{\psi})) > p_0|D_j)\}$ is selected for future randomized phase II or III studies.

CisCab Trial (Continued)

In section "Application to the CisCab Trial," we described the phase I part of the CisCab trial where 30 patients are enrolled and the MTD curve estimated. In stage II, $n = 30$ patients will be enrolled to identify dose combinations along the MTD curve with maximum clinical benefit rate. Clinical benefit is defined as either a complete response, partial response, or stable disease within three cycles of treatment. The probability of a poor clinical benefit is $p_0 = 0.15$, and we expect that a tolerable dose combination achieves a clinical benefit rate of $p = 0.4$. We present simulations based on six scenarios that include three situations favoring the alternative hypothesis and three instances supporting the null hypothesis. A logistic link function $F\,(u) = (1 + \exp(u))^{-1}$ is used in (20), and $f\,(z;\ \boldsymbol{\psi})$ is modeled as a cubic spline function with two knots in (0, 1). This is a very flexible class of efficacy curves and accommodates cases of constant probability of efficacy along the MTD curve, high probability of efficacy around the middle of the MTD curve, and high probability of efficacy at one or both edges of the MTD curve. Vague priors are placed on the model parameters by assuming that $\beta \sim \mathcal{N}(\mathbf{0}, \sigma^2 I_6)$ with $\sigma^2 = 10^4$ and $(\boldsymbol{\kappa}_4,\ \boldsymbol{\kappa}_5) \sim \text{Unif}\{(u,\ v)\colon 0 \leq u < v \leq 1\}$. It can be shown that the induced prior mean and variance of the probability of treatment response are $E_{\text{prior}}(F\,(f\,(z;\ \boldsymbol{\psi}))) \approx 0.5$ and $Var_{\text{prior}}(F\,(f\,(z;\ \boldsymbol{\psi}))) \approx 0.25$ for all dose combinations $z \in [0,\ 1]$. The initial number of patients enrolled to the trial was set to $n_1 = 10$, and $n_2 = 5$ was used in the adaptive randomization phase of the design. The design parameter for the decision rule in (23) was taken as $\delta_u = 0.8$. In each scenario, we simulated $M = 2000$ trial replicates. The true probability of response curves under scenarios (a,b,c) is shown in blue in Fig. 7. The black horizontal lines correspond to the probability of a poor treatment response $p_0 = 0.15$, and the green horizontal lines represent the target probability of response $p = 0.4$. Scenario (a) is a case where the probability of efficacy is maximized near the middle of the estimated MTD curve with dose combinations in the interval (0.03, 0.76) having probability of efficacy greater than $p_0 = 0.15$. The target probability of response is achieved at a single dose combination $z = 0.42$. Scenario (b) is a case where higher doses of cisplatin and lower doses of cabazitaxel achieve higher efficacy. Specifically, standardized dose combinations in the interval (0.00, 0.49) have probability of efficacy greater or equal to $p_0 = 0.15$. Scenario (c) is an unusual situation where the probability of efficacy is maximized at the edges of the MTD curve. In this case, dose combinations in the interval $(0.00, 0.41) \cup (0.90, 1.00)$ have probability of efficacy greater or equal to $p_0 = 0.15$. Corresponding to these scenarios are situations (d–f) favoring the null hypothesis shown in Fig. 7d, e, f. The true probability of response curves shown in blue has been shifted downward so

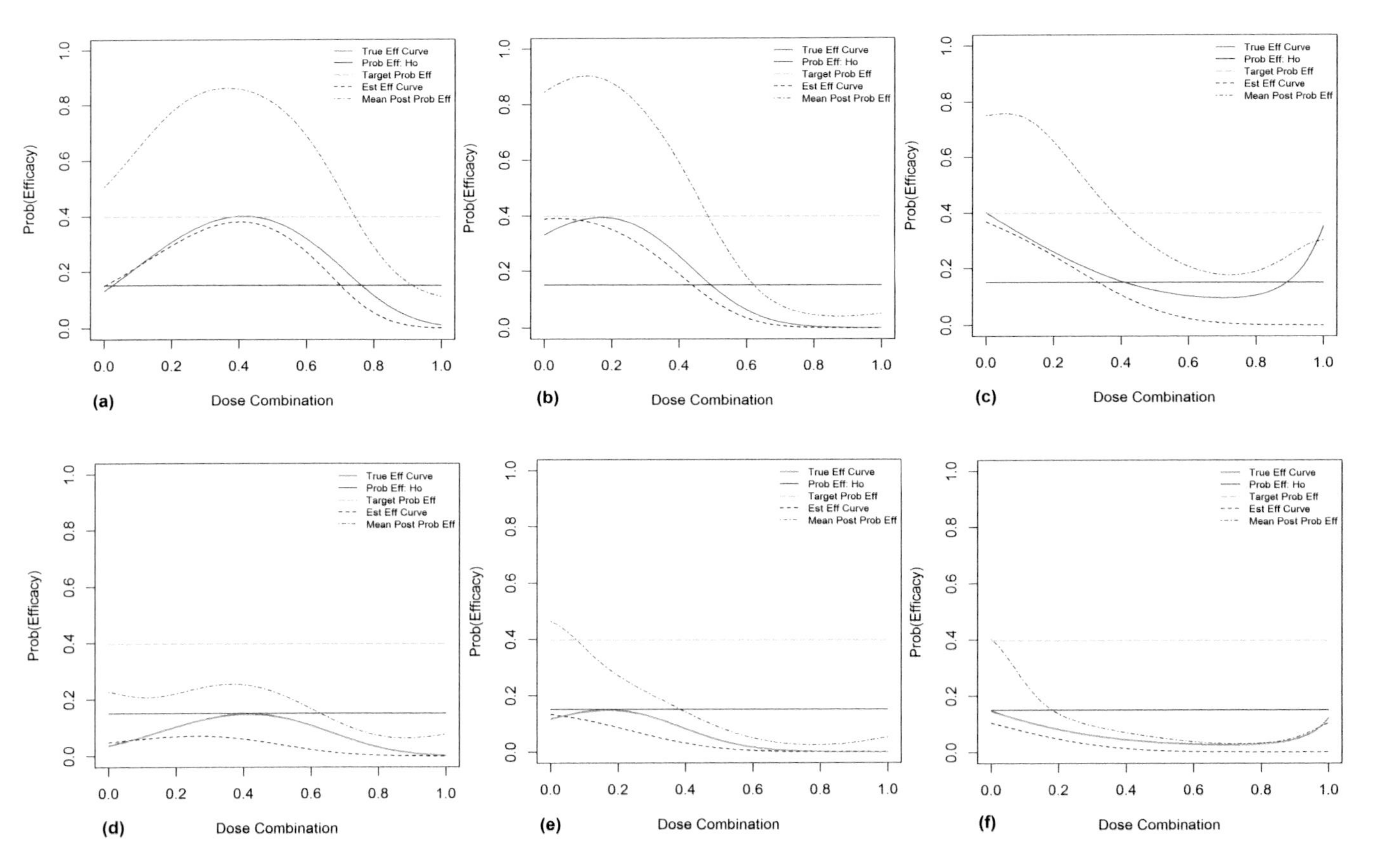

Fig. 7 True and estimated efficacy curve under six scenarios favoring the null and alternative hypotheses

that the probability of response equals to p_0 at one dose combination only for scenarios (d), (e), and (f).

Operating Characteristics

For each scenario favoring the alternative hypothesis, we estimate the Bayesian power as

$$\text{Power} \approx \frac{1}{M}\sum_{i=1}^{M} I[\text{Max}_z\{P(F(f(z;\boldsymbol{\psi}_i)) > p_0|D_{n,i})\} > \delta_u], \tag{24}$$

where $P(F(f(z;\boldsymbol{\psi}_i)) > p_0|D_{n,i})$ is estimated using an MCMC sample of $\boldsymbol{\psi}_i$,

$$P(F(f(z;\boldsymbol{\psi}_i)) > p_0|D_{n,i}) \approx \frac{1}{L}\sum_{j=1} I\left[F\left(f\left(z;\boldsymbol{\psi}_{i,j}\right)\right)L > p_0\right], \tag{25}$$

where $\boldsymbol{\psi}_{i,j}$, $j = 1, \ldots, L$ is an MCMC sample from the i-th trial. For scenarios favoring the null hypothesis, (24) is the estimated Bayesian type I error probability. The optimal or target dose from the i-th trial is

$$z_i^* = \text{argmax}_v\{P(F(f(v;\boldsymbol{\psi}_i)) > p_0|D_{n,i})\}. \tag{26}$$

We also report the estimated efficacy curve by replacing $\boldsymbol{\psi}$ in (20) by the average posterior medians across all simulated trials

$$F(f(z;\overline{\boldsymbol{\psi}})), \tag{27}$$

where $\overline{\boldsymbol{\psi}} = (\overline{\beta}, \boldsymbol{\kappa}), \overline{\beta}_l = M^{-1}\sum_{i=1}^{M}\widehat{\beta}_{i,l}, l = 0, \ldots, 5, \overline{\boldsymbol{\kappa}}_k = M^{-1}\sum_{i=1}^{M}\widehat{\boldsymbol{\kappa}}_{i,k}, l = 4, 5$, and $\widehat{\beta}_{i,l}, \widehat{\boldsymbol{\kappa}}_{i,k}$ are the posterior medians from the i-th trial. Finally, we also report the mean posterior probability of declaring the treatment as efficacious for all dose combination z as

$$\frac{1}{M}\sum_{i=1}^{M} P(F(f(z;\boldsymbol{\psi}_i)) > p_0|D_{n,i}). \tag{28}$$

The estimated efficacy curves shown in black dashed lines in Fig. 7 computed using Eq. 27 are fairly close to the true probability of efficacy curve in all scenarios except for scenario (c) near the lower edge of the MTD curve. The mean posterior probability of efficacy curve shown in red dashed line computed using Eq. 28 is 80% or more at dose combinations where the true probability of efficacy is maximized for scenarios (a, b) and close to 80% for scenario (c). Similar conclusions can be drawn for scenarios favoring the null hypothesis where the maximum of the mean posterior probability of efficacy is less than 50%. Figure 8 is the estimated density of the target dose z^* defined in Eq. 26 under scenarios favoring the alternative hypothesis (a–c), and the shaded region corresponds to dose combinations with corresponding true

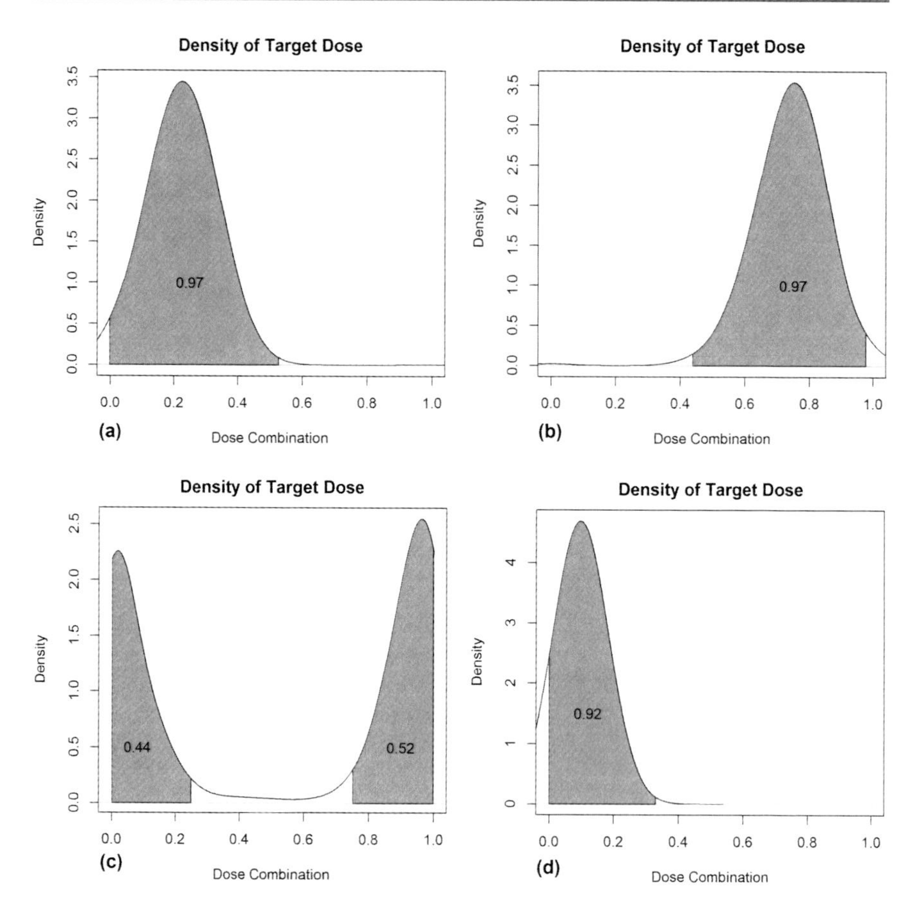

Fig. 8 Estimated density of the target dose combination under three scenarios favoring the alternative hypothesis

Table 2 Bayesian power, type I error, and coverage probabilities

Scenarios	Power	Scenarios	Prob(Type I error)	Coverage prob.
(a)	0.896	(d)	0.100	0.964
(b)	0.921	(e)	0.190	0.897
(c)	0.810	(f)	0.143	0.937

probability of efficacy greater than $p_0 = 0.15$. The mode of these densities is close to the target doses. Moreover, the estimated probabilities of selecting a dose with true probability of efficacy greater than $p_0 = 0.15$ vary between 0.90 and 0.96 across the three scenarios. The Bayesian power for scenarios (a–c) and type I error probability for scenarios (d–f) estimated using Eq. 24 using a threshold $\delta_u = 0.8$ are reported in Table 2. Power varies between 0.81 and 0.92, and the type I error probability varies between 0.10 and 0.19. The coverage probability in the last column of Table 2 is the estimated probabilities of selecting a dose with true probability of efficacy greater than $p_0 = 0.15$. We conclude that the design has good operating characteristic in identifying tolerable dose combinations with maximum benefit rate. We refer the reader to Tighiouart (2019) for sensitivity analysis regarding n_1, n_2, δ_u, and other values of p_0 and effect size.

Discrete Dose Combinations

In sections "Dose Finding to Estimate the Maximum Tolerated Dose Curve," "Attributable Toxicity," and "Phase I/II Dose Finding," the methodologies for estimating the MTD curve and tolerable dose combination with maximum probability of efficacy were described for continuous dose levels of the two agents. These methods can be adapted to the case of pre-specified discrete dose levels as follows. Let $(x_1, \ldots, x_r)$ and $(y_1, \ldots, y_s)$ be the doses of agents A_1 and A_2, respectively. Following the notation of section "Dose Finding to Estimate the Maximum Tolerated Dose Curve," $X_{\min} = x_1$, $X_{\max} = x_r$, $Y_{\min} = y_1$, and $Y_{\max} = y_s$ and the doses are standardized to be in the interval [0, 1]. Dose escalation proceeds using the algorithms described in sections "Trial Design" and "Dose Allocation Algorithm" where the recommended continuous doses in steps (ii) and (iii) of the algorithms are rounded to the nearest discrete dose levels. At the end of the trial, a discrete set Γ satisfying conditions (a) and (b) below is selected as the set of MTDs. Let $d((x_j, y_k), C_{\text{est}})$ be the Euclidean distance between dose combination (x_j, y_k) and the estimated MTD curve C_{est}.

(a) Let $\Gamma_{A_1} = \bigcup_{t=1}^{s} \left\{ (x, y_t) : x = \underset{x_j}{\operatorname{argmin}}\ d\left((x_j, y_t), C_{\text{est}}\right) \right\}$,

$$\Gamma_{A_2} = \bigcup_{t=1}^{r} \left\{ (x_t, y) : y = \underset{y_j}{\operatorname{argmin}}\ d\left(\left(x_t, y_j\right), C_{\text{est}}\right) \right\}, \text{and } \Gamma_0 = \Gamma_{A_1} \cap \Gamma_{A_2}.$$

(b) Let $\Gamma = \Gamma_0 \backslash \{(x*, y*) : P(|\ P(DLT|\ (x*, y*)) - \theta| > \delta_1 |\ D_n) > \delta_2\}$.

The set Γ_0 in (a) consists of dose combinations closest to the MTD curve obtained by first minimizing the Euclidean distances across the levels of drug A_1 and then across the levels of drug A_2. Doses in Γ_0 that are either likely to be too toxic or subtherapeutic are excluded in (b). The design parameter δ_1 is selected after consultation with a clinician. The parameter δ_2 is selected after exploring a large number of practical scenarios when designing a trial. In our experience with the sample sizes and scenarios used in Wang and Ivanova (2005), we found that $\delta_2 = 0.3, 0.35$ result in good design operating characteristics.

Illustration

We consider five scenarios studied in Wang and Ivanova (2005) and shown in Table 3. The sample size for the first four scenarios is $n = 54$ and $n = 60$ for the

Table 3 Dose limiting toxicity scenarios with θ = 0.2

Dose level	1	2	3	4	5	6
Scenario 1						
3	0.08	0.13	**0.2**	0.29	0.40	0.53
2	0.05	0.08	0.13	**0.2**	0.29	0.40
1	0.03	0.05	0.08	0.13	**0.2**	0.20
Scenario 2						
3	0.05	0.08	0.11	0.15	**0.21**	0.29
2	0.04	0.06	0.09	0.13	**0.18**	0.25
1	0.04	0.05	0.08	0.11	15	**0.21**
Scenario 3						
3	**0.20**	0.30	0.41	0.53	0.65	0.70
2	0.10	**0.20**	0.25	0.32	0.41	0.50
1	0.03	0.05	0.13	**0.20**	0.27	0.35
Scenario 4						
3	**0.20**	0.40	0.47	0.56	0.65	0.76
2	0.08	0.13	**0.20**	0.32	0.41	0.50
1	0.03	0.05	0.08	0.13	0.17	**0.20**
Scenario 5						
4	**0.20**	0.29	0.40	0.53		
3	0.13	**0.20**	0.29	0.40		
2	0.08	0.13	**0.20**	0.29		
1	0.05	0.08	0.13	**0.20**		

last scenario. The target probability of DLT is $\theta = 0.2$, and the prior distributions for ρ_{00}, ρ_{01}, ρ_{10}, and η_3 are described in section "Dose Finding to Estimate the Maximum Tolerated Dose Curve" with hyperparameters $a_i = b_i = 1$, $i = 1, \ldots, 3$. A tight gamma(1,1) prior was put on the interaction parameter η_3 since the model in Wang and Ivanova (2005) has two parameters with no interaction coefficient. We assess the performance of the method by simulating $m = 2000$ trials and calculating the accuracy index introduced in Cheung (2011).

$$AI_n = 1 - K \times \frac{\sum_{k=1}^{K} \Delta_k \times p_{n,k}}{\sum_{k=1}^{K} \Delta_k}, \tag{29}$$

where n is the trial sample size, K is the number of discrete doses available in the trial, $p_{n,k}$ is the probability of selecting dose k in a trial with n patients, and Δ_k is a distance measure between the true probability of DLT p_k at dose k and the target probability of DLT θ. It can be shown that $AI_n < 1$ and higher values of AI_n are desirable. We also report a measure of percent selection defined as follows. For a given scenario, let $\Gamma_\delta = \{(x_i, y_j): |P(DLT|(x_i, y_j)) - \theta| < \delta\}$ be the set of true MTDs where the threshold parameter δ is fixed by the clinician. Let Γ_i the set of estimated MTDs at the end of the i-th trial as described in section "Discrete Dose Combinations," $i = 1, \ldots, m$. The percent of MTDs selection is

$$\%\text{Selection} = \frac{1}{m}\sum_{i=1}^{m} I(\Gamma_i \subset \Gamma_\delta). \tag{30}$$

This statistic is an estimate of the probability that for a given scenario, a prospective trial will recommend a set of dose combinations that are all MTDs. Other measures of percent selection when recommending more than one MTD can be found in Diniz et al. (2017). Table 4 gives the summary statistics of the accuracy index using the square discrepancy (sq) $\Delta_k = (p_k - \theta)^2$, absolute discrepancy (abs) $\Delta_k = |p_k - \theta|$, and overdose error (od) $\Delta_k = \alpha^\star(\theta - p_k)^+ + (1 - \alpha^\star)(p_k - \theta)^+$ with $\alpha^\star = 0.25$, the percent selection with $\delta = 0.1$, and safety of the trial for the proposed approach (conditional EWOC) and the two-dimensional design of Wang and Ivanova (2005). Conditional EWOC performs well relative to the two-dimensional design under scenarios 1, 3, and 5 according to the three measures of discrepancies. Scenario 2 is more complex due to the location of the true MTDs, and this is reflected by the negative values of the accuracy index across the three measures of discrepancies for the two approaches. The two-dimensional design performs better than conditional EWOC under scenario 4 according to two of the three discrepancy measures. When the accuracy index AI_n is averaged across the five scenarios, conditional EWOC performs better than the two-dimensional design for each discrepancy measure. The percent selection is higher using conditional EWOC under scenarios 1, 3, and 4 and higher on the average across all five scenarios relative to the two-dimensional design. The last three columns of Table 4 show that the trial is safe using both approaches under these five scenarios. Other simulation results using informative priors matching the priors used in Wang and Ivanova (2005) lead to similar conclusions and much higher percent selection under scenarios 1, 3, 4, and 5. Further details can be found in Tighiouart et al. (2017b).

Summary and Conclusion

Model-based designs for drug combinations in early phase cancer clinical trials have been studied extensively in the last decade. For phase I trials, these methods are designed to estimate one or more MTDs for use in future phase II trials. It is important to note that designs that recommend more than one MTD for efficacy studies should be used as this may decrease the likelihood of a failed phase II trial. In this chapter, we focused on dose finding using two drugs with continuous dose levels. For a phase I trial design, consecutive cohorts of two patients were treated simultaneously with different dose combinations to better explore the space of doses. The method was studied extensively in Tighiouart et al. (2014b, 2016, 2017b) and Diniz et al. (2017) via extensive simulations and was shown to be safe in general with high percent of MTD recommendation. We also showed how this was applied to design the first part of the CisCab trial using a relatively small sample size and calibrate prior distributions of the model parameters. In practice, active involvement of the clinician is required at the design stage of the trial to facilitate prior calibration and to specify scenarios with various locations of the true MTD set of doses.

Table 4 Operating characteristics for the two designs

	Accuracy index			% Selection	Mean % DLTs	% Trials: DLT rate > θ + 0.05	% Trials: DLT rate > θ + 0.10
	sq	abs	od				
Scenario 1							
Cond. EWOC	0.37	−0.13	0.07	75.2	15.05	0.30	0.00
Two-dim	0.17	−0.45	−0.08	58.8	16.56	0.65	0.00
Scenario 2							
Cond. EWOC	−0.34	−0.63	−0.62	53.6	12.54	0.00	0.00
Two-dim	−0.13	−0.72	−0.82	81.6	13.37	0.08	0.00
Scenario 3							
Cond. EWOC	0.80	0.40	0.46	92.65	19.08	6.30	0.00
Two-dim	0.70	0.20	0.43	68.58	20.08	6.90	0.10
Scenario 4							
Cond. EWOC	0.57	0.10	0.20	45.95	17.10	2.30	0.00
Two-dim	0.62	0.05	0.36	39.93	19.35	3.55	0.00
Scenario 5							
Cond. EWOC	0.54	−0.01	0.23	78.55	16.34	0.01	0.00
Two-dim	0.27	−0.5	−0.12	87.40	17.72	0.88	0.00
Average							
Cond. EWOC	0.39	−0.05	0.07	69.19	16.02	1.78	0.00
Two-dim	0.33	−0.28	−0.05	67.26	17.42	2.41	0.02

It is well known that optimal treatment protocols use drug combinations that have nonoverlapping toxicities. However, cancer drugs with nonoverlapping toxicities of any grade are rare. In this chapter, we described situations where the clinician is able to attribute the DLT to one or more drugs in an unknown fraction of patients by extending the previous statistical models. This is practically useful when the two drugs do not have many overlapping toxicities (see, e.g., Miles et al. (2002)) for some examples of drug combination trials with these characteristics. We showed by simulations that as the fraction of attributable toxicities increases, the rate of DLT decreases, and there is a gain in the precision of the estimated MTD curve. In cases where we expect a high percent of overlapping DLTs, designs that do not distinguish between drug attribution listed in the introduction and described in section "Dose Finding to Estimate the Maximum Tolerated Dose Curve" may be more appropriate. It is also important to note that the method relies on clinical judgment regarding DLT attribution.

In the second part of the chapter, we showed how the estimated MTD curve from a phase I trial is carried to a phase II trial for efficacy study using Bayesian adaptive randomization. This design can be viewed as an extension of the Bayesian adaptive design comparing a finite number of arms (Berry et al. (2011)) to comparing an infinite number of arms. In particular, if the dose levels of the two agents are discrete, then methods such as the ones described in Thall et al. (2003), Wang and Ivanova (2005), and Wages (2016) can be used to identify a set of MTDs in stage I, and the trial in stage II can be done using adaptive randomization to select the most efficacious dose. Unlike phase I/II designs that use toxicity and efficacy data simultaneously and require a short period of time to resolve efficacy status, the use of a two-stage design is sometimes necessary in practice if it takes few cycles of therapy to resolve treatment efficacy or if the populations of patients in phases I and II are different. In fact, for the CisCab trial described in section "Phase I/II Dose Finding," efficacy is resolved after three cycles (9 weeks) of treatment, and patients in stage I must have metastatic, castration-resistant prostate cancer, whereas patients in stage II must have visceral metastasis. The uncertainty of the estimated MTD curve in stage I is not taken into account in stage II of the design in the sense that the MTD curve is not updated as a result of observing DLTs in stage II. This is a limitation of this approach since patients in stage II may come from a different population and may have different treatment susceptibility relative to patients in stage I. This problem is also inherent to single agent two-stage designs where the MTD from the phase I trial is used in phase II studies and safety is monitored continuously during this phase. Due to the small sample size, methods to estimate the MTD curves for each subpopulation in the phase I trial (Diniz et al. 2018) may not be appropriate. An alternative design would account for first, second, and third cycle DLT in addition to efficacy outcome at each cycle. In addition, the nature of DLT (reversible vs. nonreversible) should be taken into account since patients with a reversible DLT are usually treated for that side effect and kept in the trial with dose reduction in subsequent cycles. For the CisCab trial, a separate stopping rule using Bayesian continuous monitoring for excessive toxicity is included in the clinical protocol.

Cross-References

- ▶ Adaptive Phase II Trials
- ▶ Bayesian Adaptive Designs for Phase I Trials
- ▶ Dose-Finding and Dose-Ranging Studies
- ▶ Inferential Frameworks for Clinical Trials
- ▶ Interim Analysis in Clinical Trials

Acknowledgments This work is supported in part by the National Institute of Health Grant Number R01 CA188480-01A1 and the National Center for Research Resources, Grant UL1RR033176, and is now at the National Center for Advancing Translational Sciences, Grant UL1TR000124, P01 CA098912, and U01 CA232859-01.

References

Babb J, Rogatko A, Zacks S (1998) Cancer phase I clinical trials: efficient dose escalation with overdose control. Stat Med 17:1103–1120
Berry SM, Carlin BP, Lee JJ, Muller P (2011) Bayesian adaptive methods for clinical trials. Chapman & Hall, Boca Raton
Braun TM (2002) The bivariate continual reassessment method: extending the CRM to phase I trials of two competing outcomes. Control Clin Trials 23:240–256
Braun TM, Wang SF (2010) A hierarchical Bayesian design for phase I trials of novel combinations of cancer therapeutic agents. Biometrics 66:805–812
Cai C, Yuan Y, Ji Y (2014) A Bayesian dose finding design for oncology clinical trials of combinational biological agents. Appl Stat 63:159–173
Chen Z, Tighiouart M, Kowalski J (2012a) Dose escalation with overdose control using a quasi-continuous toxicity score in cancer phase I clinical trials. Contemp Clin Trials 33:949–958
Chen Z, Zhao Y, Cui Y, Kowalski J (2012b) Methodology and application of adaptive and sequential approaches in contemporary clinical trials. J Probability Stat 2012:20
Chen Z, Yuan Y, Li Z, Kutner M, Owonikoko T, Curran WJ, Khuri F, Kowalski J (2015) Dose escalation with over-dose and under-dose controls in phase I/II clinical trials. Contemp Clin Trials 43:133–141
Cheung YK (2011) Dose-finding by the continual reassessment method, 1st edn. Chapman & Hall, Boca Raton
Clertant M, Tighiouart M (2017) Design of phase I/II drug combination cancer trials using conditional continual reassessment method and adaptive randomization. In: JSM Proceedings, Biopharmaceutical Section. Alexandria, VA: American Statistical Association 1332–1349
Diniz MA, Quanlin-Li, Tighiouart M (2017) Dose Finding for Drug Combination in Early Cancer Phase I Trials Using Conditional Continual Reassessment Method. J Biom Biostat 8: 381. https://doi.org/10.4172/2155-6180.1000381
Diniz MA, Kim S, Tighiouart M (2018) A Bayesian adaptive design in cancer phase I trials using dose combinations in the presence of a baseline covariate. J Probab Stat 2018:11
Diniz MA, Tighiouart M, Rogatko A (2019) Comparison between continuous and discrete doses for model based designs in cancer dose finding. PLoS One 14:e0210139
Faries D (1994) Practical modifications of the continual reassessment method for phase I cancer clinical trials. J Biopharm Stat 4:147–164
Goodman S, Zahurak M, Piantadosi S (1995) Some practical improvements in the continual reassessment method for phase I studies. Stat Med 14:1149–1161
Ivanova A (2003) A new dose-finding design for bivariate outcomes. Biometrics 59:1001–1007

Jimenez JL, Tighiouart M, Gasparini M (2019) Cancer phase I trial design using drug combinations when a fraction of dose limiting toxicities is attributable to one or more agents. Biom J 61 (2):319–332

Le Tourneau C, Lee JJ, Siu LL (2009) Dose escalation methods in phase I cancer clinical trials. J Natl Cancer Inst 101:708–720

Lockhart AC, Sundaram S, Sarantopoulos J, Mita MM, Wang-Gillam A, Moseley JL, Barber SL, Lane AR, Wack C, Kassalow L, Dedieu JF, Mita A (2014) Phase I dose-escalation study of cabazitaxel administered in combination with cisplatin in patients with advanced solid tumors. Investig New Drugs 32:1236–1245

Lunn DJ, Thomas A, Best N, Spiegelhalter D (2000) WinBUGS – a Bayesian modelling framework: concepts, structure, and extensibility. Stat Comput 10:325–337

Mander A, Sweeting M (2015) A product of independent beta probabilities dose escalation design for dual-agent phase I trials. Stat Med 34:1261–1276

Miles D, Von Minckwitz GJ, Seidman AD (2002) Combination versus sequential single-agent therapy in metastatic breast cancer. Oncologist 7:13–19

Murtaugh PA, Fisher LD (1990) Bivariate binary models of efficacy and toxicity in dose-ranging trials. Commun Stat Theory Methods 19:2003–2020

O'Quigley J, Shen LZ (1996) Continual reassessment method: a likelihood approach. Biometrics 52:673–684

O'Quigley J, Pepe M, Fisher L (1990) Continual reassessment method: a practical design for phase I clinical trials in cancer. Biometrics 46:33–48

Piantadosi S, Fisher JD, Grossman S (1998) Practical implementation of a modified continual reassessment method for dose-finding trials. Cancer Chemother Pharmacol 41:429–436

Plummer M (2003) JAGS: a program for analysis of Bayesian graphical models using Gibbs sampling. 3rd International Workshop on Distributed Statistical Computing (DSC 2003); Vienna, Austria. 124

Riviere M, Yuan Y, Dubois F, Zohar S (2014) A bayesian dose-finding design for drug combination clinical trials based on the logistic model. Pharm Stat 13:247–257

Riviere MK, Yuan Y, Dubois F, Zohar S (2015) A Bayesian dose-finding design for clinical trials combining a cytotoxic agent with a molecularly targeted agent. J R Stat Soc Ser C 64:215–229

Rogatko A, Gosh P, Vidakovic B, Tighiouart M (2008) Patient-specific dose adjustment in the cancer clinical trial setting. Pharm Med 22:345–350

Sato H, Hirakawa A, Hamada C (2016) An adaptive dose-finding method using a change-point model for molecularly targeted agents in phase I trials. Stat Med 35:4093–4109

Shi Y, Yin G (2013) Escalation with overdose control for phase I drug-combination trials. Stat Med 32:4400–4412

Thall PF, Cook JD (2004) Dose-finding based on efficacy toxicity trade-offs. Biometrics 60:684–693

Thall PF, Russell KE (1998) A strategy for dose-finding and safety monitoring based on efficacy and adverse outcomes in phase I/II clinical trials. Biometrics 54:251–264

Thall PF, Millikan RE, Mueller P, Lee SJ (2003) Dose-finding with two agents in phase I oncology trials. Biometrics 59:487–496

Tighiouart M (2019) Two-stage design for phase I/II cancer clinical trials using continuous-dose combinations of cytotoxic agents. J R Stat Soc Ser C 68(1):235–250

Tighiouart M, Rogatko A (2010) Dose finding with escalation with overdose control (EWOC) in cancer clinical trials. Stat Sci 25:217–226

Tighiouart M, Rogatko A (2012) Number of patients per cohort and sample size considerations using dose escalation with overdose control. J Probab Stat 2012:16

Tighiouart M, Rogatko A, Babb JS (2005) Flexible Bayesian methods for cancer phase I clinical trials. Dose escalation with overdose control. Stat Med 24:2183–2196

Tighiouart M, Cook-Wiens G, Rogatko A (2012a) Escalation with overdose control using ordinal toxicity grades for cancer phase I clinical trials. J Probab Stat 2012:18. https://doi.org/10.1155/2012/317634

Tighiouart M, Cook-Wiens G, Rogatko A (2012b) Incorporating a patient dichotomous characteristic in cancer phase I clinical trials using escalation with overdose control. J Probab Stat 2012:10

Tighiouart M, Liu Y, Rogatko A (2014a) Escalation with overdose control using time to toxicity for cancer phase I clinical trials. PLoS One 9:e93070

Tighiouart M, Piantadosi S, Rogatko A (2014b) Dose finding with drug combinations in cancer phase I clinical trials using conditional escalation with overdose control. Stat Med 33:3815–3829

Tighiouart M, Li Q, Piantadosi S, Rogatko A (2016) A Bayesian adaptive design for combination of three drugs in cancer phase I clinical trials. Am J Biostat 6:1–11

Tighiouart M, Cook-Wiens G, Rogatko A (2017a) A Bayesian adaptive design for cancer phase I trials using a flexible range of doses. J Biopharm Stat 31:1–13

Tighiouart M, Li Q, Rogatko A (2017b) A Bayesian adaptive design for estimating the maximum tolerated dose curve using drug combinations in cancer phase I clinical trials. Stat Med 36:280–290

Wages NA (2016) Identifying a maximum tolerated contour in two-dimensional dose finding. Stat Med 36:242–253

Wages NA, Conaway MR (2014) Phase I/II adaptive design for drug combination oncology trials. Stat Med 33:1990–2003

Wages NA, Conaway MR, O'Quigley J (2011) Continual reassessment method for partial ordering. Biometrics 67:1555–1563

Wang K, Ivanova A (2005) Two-dimensional dose finding in discrete dose space. Biometrics 61:217–222

Wheeler GM, Sweeting MJ, Mander AP (2017) Toxicity-dependent feasibility bounds for the escalation with overdose control approach in phase I cancer trials. Stat Med 36:2499–2513

Yin GS, Yuan Y (2009a) A latent contingency table approach to dose finding for combinations of two agents. Biometrics 65:866–875

Yin GS, Yuan Y (2009b) Bayesian dose finding by jointly modelling toxicity and efficacy as time-to-event outcomes. J R Stat Soc Ser C Appl Stat 58:719–736

Yuan Y, Yin G (2011) Bayesian phase I/II adaptively randomized oncology trials with combined drugs. Ann Appl Stat 5:924–942

Middle Development Trials

56

Emine O. Bayman

Contents

Abstract

Phase I trials are the first application of the new treatment on humans. The main goal of the phase I trial is to establish the safety of the new treatment and determine the maximum tolerable dose for use in subsequent phase II clinical trial. When moved from phase I to phase II trial, the focus shifts from toxicity (safety) to efficacy. In phase II trials, the aim is to decide whether the new treatment is sufficiently promising relative to the standard therapy so that the new treatment can be included in a large-scale phase III clinical trial.

E. O. Bayman (✉)
University of Iowa, Iowa City, IA, USA
e-mail: emine-bayman@uiowa.edu

© Springer Nature Switzerland AG 2022

S. Piantadosi, C. L. Meinert (eds.), *Principles and Practice of Clinical Trials*,
https://doi.org/10.1007/978-3-319-52636-2_81

In this chapter, first frequentist one-arm two-stage phase II clinical trials will be introduced. Then, a brief background for Bayesian trials will be provided. Finally, one-arm Bayesian design using predictive probability approach will be explained. Calculations or software to implement the examples will also be provided when available.

Keywords

Phase II · Clinical trial · Bayesian · Predictive probability · Two-stage design

Introduction

After one or more successful phase I trials have been completed, phase II trials may be initiated. Phase II clinical trials are aimed to decide whether a new treatment is sufficiently promising, relative to the standard therapy, to include in large-scale randomized clinical trials. Phase II trials provide a bridge between small phase I trials, where maximum tolerated dose is determined, and large-scale randomized phase III trials. Compared to phase I trials, phase II trials run on larger groups of patients, generally 40 to 200 patients. Compared to phase III trials, phase II trials tend to use surrogate markers as earlier endpoints (tumor shrinkage within first few weeks instead of survival at 5 years) to shorten the study duration. Generally, sample size is not large enough to have sufficient power. The design provides decision boundaries, a probability distribution for the sample size at termination, and operating characteristics under fixed-response probabilities with the new treatment.

There are three basic requirements for any clinical trial: (1) the trial should examine an important research question; (2) the trial should use rigorous methodology to answer the question of interest; and (3) the trial must be based on ethical considerations and assure that risks to subjects are minimized. Because of the small sample size, meeting these requirements in early-phase clinical trials can be more challenging compared to phase III trials. Therefore, the importance of study planning is magnified in these settings.

Single-Arm Versus Two-Arm Phase II Trials

Phase II studies could be single arm, where only the treatment of interest is tested, or two-arm with a concurrent control group. One-arm designs are used more frequently to expedite the phase II clinical trials and will be presented here.

The main goal of phase II studies is to provide assessment of efficacy of the treatment of interest. Accordingly, the goal is to determine if new treatment is sufficiently promising to justify inclusion in large-scale randomized trials. Otherwise, ineffective treatments should be screened out. In addition, the safety profile of the treatment of interest is further characterized in phase II trial. Generally a binary primary endpoint of favorable/unfavorable outcome (efficacy/no efficacy) is used in phase II designs. If the probability of efficacy is higher than a predetermined threshold at the end of the phase II trial, then the treatment of interest will be tested in a larger phase III clinical trial (Yuan et al. 2016).

Frequentist Two-Stage Designs

Most commonly used frequentist two-stage designs are Gehan's design (Gehan 1961), Simon's optimal design, and minimax design (Simon 1989). The optimal design minimizes the expected sample size under the null hypothesis, and sample size. The user needs to specify the fixed target response rate for the new therapy (p_1) and the existing treatment (p_0) along with the type I (α) and type II error (β) rates to obtain the sample sizes and stopping boundaries for each stage for two-stage designs. In this setting, type I error rate can be interpreted as the probability of finding the treatment of interest as efficacious and recommending for further study when it is not in fact efficacious. Similarly, type II error is the probability of finding the treatment of interest as not efficacious and not recommending for further study when it is in fact efficacious. Therefore, in phase II trials, it is more important to control type II error rate than the type I error rate so that efficacious treatments are not missed. Type I and II error rates are larger and around 10% in phase II trials.

Because of the small sample size, when available, exact methods are preferred (Jung 2013). More complex phase II designs with more than one interim monitoring also exist (Yuan et al. 2016).

At the end of the first stage, frequentist two-stage designs allow early termination of the trial for futility, if the interim data indicate that the new treatment is not effective (Lee and Liu 2008). Both Simon and minimax designs can be implemented online for pre-specified inputs using the NIH Biometric Research Program website: https://linus.nci.nih.gov/brb/samplesize/otsd.html.

Example 1 Let the current favorable response rate with the standard therapy be 30% ($p_0 = 0.3$). New treatment is expected to increase the favorable response rate to 50% ($p_1 = 0.5$). The outcome will be recorded as favorable versus unfavorable for each patient. Both type I and type II error rates will be kept below 10%. Null and alternative hypothesis for this study can be written as follows: $H_0: p \leq 0.3$; $H_1: p \geq 0.5$.

The stopping boundaries for each of the two stages can be calculated for both optimum and minimax designs from the website provided above.

For the optimum design, 22 (n_1) patients should be enrolled in the first stage. If there are 7 (r_1) or less favorable outcomes, out of 22 patients, the trial should be stopped early due to futility, and the new treatment should be declared as ineffective. If there are more than 7 favorable outcomes, 24 more patients should be enrolled in the second stage so that the overall sample size of the study is 46 (n). If there are 17 (r) or less favorable outcomes, out of 46 patients, the new treatment will be declared as ineffective. If there are more than 17 favorable outcomes, null hypothesis will be rejected and the new treatment will be declared as effective (Fig. 1).

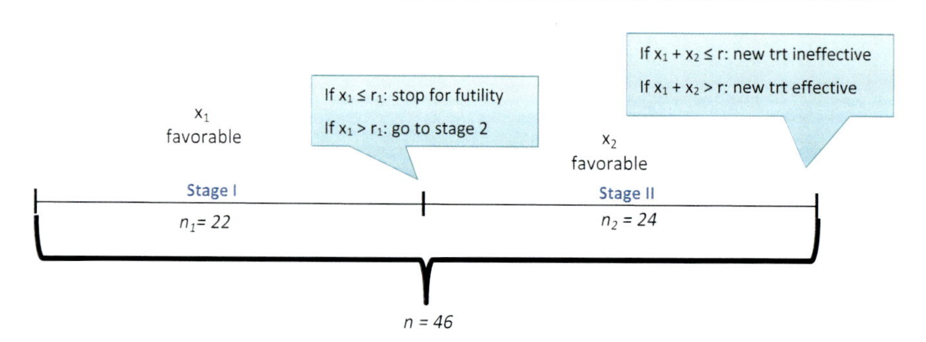

Fig. 1 Frequentist two-stage design example

The probability of early termination under the null hypothesis, PET(p_0), is the probability of observing 0 to 7 favorable outcomes out of the first 22 subjects where the probability of favorable outcomes is 0.3. Let x_1 be the number of favorable outcomes out of the first n_1 patients in the first stage. The probability of early termination can be calculated in R with the following codes: PET(p_0) = Pr $(x_1 \leq r_1 \mid H_0)$ = sum(dbinom((0:7), 22, 0.3)) = 0.67.

The expected sample size of the study under the null hypothesis is the combination of early termination at the end of the first stage or not terminating and enrolling all 46 patients. Therefore, it can be written as E(N|p) = [n1 × PET(p_0)] + [n × (1 − PET(p_0))] = [22 × 0.67] + [46 × (1–0.67)] = 29.9.

A good two-stage frequentist design would have type I and type II error rates lower than the initial constraints (0.1 for each in our example), high probability of early termination, and small expected sample size under the null hypothesis (Lee and Liu 2008).

Oncology Example: Ray-Coquard et al. investigated antitumor activity of sorafenib in patients with metastatic or advanced angiosarcomas in a phase II clinical trial (Ray-Coquard et al. 2012). The primary endpoint was the progression-free rate (PFR) at 9 months after the initiation of sorafenib. Only part of the study including superficial angiosarcoma patients will be considered here. Simon's two-stage minimax design was used. Based on the previous study using paclitaxel in angiosarcoma patients, the 9-month PFR rate was assumed 12.7% ($p_0 = 0.127$). It was assumed that sorafenib will increase the 9-month PFR rate to 31.7% ($p_1 = 0.317$). Type I and type II error rates were selected as 10% and 5%.

Stopping boundaries according to minimax designs are as follows. Enroll 26 patients in the first stage. If there are 3 or less patients with 9-month PFR, out of 26 patients, the trial should be stopped early due to futility, and the sorafenib should be declared as ineffective. If there are more than 3 patients with disease-free PFR, 17 more patients should be enrolled in the second stage. If there are 8 or less favorable outcomes, out of 43, sorafenib will be declared as ineffective to reduce PFR at 9 months.

In this study, there was only 1 patient with PFR at 9 months out of the 26 patients enrolled in the first stage. Therefore, no more patients were enrolled in stage 2 and the study was stopped early for futility. It was concluded that sorafenib is ineffective on PFR at 9 months (Ray-Coquard et al. 2012).

Pitfalls with Conventional Frequentist Designs

Multistage designs have better statistical properties than single-stage designs because they allow users to incorporate the interim data in decision-making (Lee and Liu 2008). The two-stage design also has limitations. In the extreme case scenario, consider the Example 1 presented above: $p_0 = 0.3$, $p_1 = 0.5$, $n_1 = 22$, $r_1 = 7$, $n = 46$, and $r = 17$. Let's assume 8 favorable outcomes were observed at the first stage of the study, and 24 more patients should be enrolled in the second stage. To be able to show the efficacy at the end of the second stage, nine more patients should have favorable outcome ($r = 17$). If the number of favorable outcomes out of the next 16 patients is 0, it is impossible to observe 9 more favorable outcomes for the next 8 patients to declare efficacy at the end of the second stage of the study (Fig. 2). However, investigators cannot stop the study at this point under this design. In other words, eight more patients should be enrolled in this study even if their results will be very likely to be unfavorable and the overall results of the study will not change. Therefore, more flexible designs that allow users to incorporate interim data at multiple stages of the study are needed.

Bayesian Methods

Due to incorporating prior information and more frequent monitoring, Bayesian designs may require a smaller sample size and therefore may take shorter time to conduct compared to frequentist designs. The opportunity of arriving at the same decision with a smaller sample size makes Bayesian designs more appealing than frequentist designs, especially for phase I and phase II clinical trials where preliminary data is limited. Bayesian methods are being increasingly used in the design and analysis of clinical trials (Biswas et al. 2009). As with the frequentist design, the

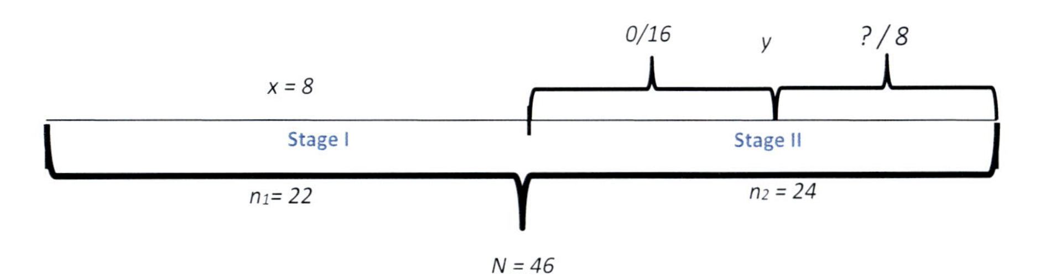

Fig. 2 Frequentist two-stage design with an extreme case

statistical analysis plan should be predefined in Bayesian designs. Similarly, the prior information should be identified in advance and justified.

A study design can be a stand-alone Bayesian design or a hybrid approach with Bayesian and frequentist approaches for different outcomes. The FDA Guidance for the Use of Bayesian Statistics in Medical Device Clinical Trials requires the frequentist properties of Bayesian procedures to be investigated (FDA 2010).

To implement most of the commonly used frequentist designs for phase II trials, the clinician must specify a single value of the patient's favorable outcome rate, p_0, to the standard therapy. In many cases there is uncertainty regarding p_0. In contrast to frequentist design, the parameter of interest, p_0, is considered as a random variable with a prior distribution with density $\pi(p_0)$ in Bayesian designs. Both in planning the phase II trial and interpreting its results, a more realistic approach should explicitly account for the clinician's uncertainty regarding p_0.

The design and conduct of phase II clinical trials would benefit from statistical methods that can incorporate external information into the design process. With the Bayesian design, the prior information and uncertainty can be quantified into a probability distribution. This prior information can be updated and easily implemented in a sequential design strategy.

Bayesian inference requires a joint distribution of the unknown parameters p and the data y. This is usually specified through a prior distribution $\pi(p)$ over the parameter space θ and a likelihood, the conditional distribution of y, the data, given p the parameters. Bayesian inference about p is through the posterior distribution, the conditional distribution of p given y.

As data accumulate, the prior distribution is updated, and the posterior distribution from the previous step becomes the prior distribution. Therefore, there is a continuous learning as data accumulates with the Bayesian approach:

$$P(p|y) \propto L(y\,|p)\pi(p). \tag{1}$$

How to Construct Prior Distributions

If there is a historical data available for the standard therapy, they may be incorporated formally into the trial design and subsequent statistical inferences. If there is no such data that exists, clinical experience and a clinician's current belief regarding the efficacy of the standard therapy may be represented by a probability distribution on p_0. This prior probability distribution can be elicited from subjective opinions of the experts in the field (Chaloner and Rhame 2001) or the subjective opinion of the investigator. In this case the Bayesian approach becomes even more appropriate.

Noninformative Prior Distributions

When the prior distribution and the posterior distribution are from the same family, this is called conjugacy. For example, the beta prior distribution is a conjugate family for the binomial likelihood (Gelman et al. 2004), and the normal distribution with a known variance is a conjugate to itself (Chen and Peace 2011). When the prior distribution of p is not conjugate, the posterior distribution should be calculated numerically. It is often mathematically convenient to use conjugate family of distributions so that the posterior distribution follows a known parametric form. Most real applied problems cannot be solved by conjugate prior distributions.

If there is some information about the distribution, parameters of the prior distribution can be derived. For example, binomial endpoint is commonly used in phase II clinical trials in terms of favorable versus unfavorable outcomes. In such case, because of the conjugacy, using beta prior distribution would make calculations easier (Gelman et al. 2004). Let's assume from the historical data that the median and the upper confidence bound are known for the favorable outcome rates. Using these two values, a search algorithm can be used to find the parameters of the prior distribution for the favorable outcome rate. It is advised to use a larger standard error to add some uncertainty to the prior distribution (Lynch 2007). When conducting Bayesian analyses, it is recommended to use different prior distributions as a sensitivity analysis to assess the robustness of the results (Gelman et al. 2004).

Another approach is to make statistical inferences from a posterior distribution based on simulation (Chen and Peace 2011). Modern computational methods can be used to calculate posterior distributions. For example, WinBUGS is a popular software specifically developed for Bayesian analyses which can also be used to easily implement Markov chain Monte Carlo methods to generate a random sample from any posterior distribution. A large class of prior distributions can be specified in WinBUGS. R packages such as R2WinBUGS (Sturtz 2005) allow users to use WinBUGS within R which are relatively easy framework for many analyses. Additionally, there are stand-alone R packages, such as MCMCpack (Martin et al. 2011), that can be used for Bayesian analyses. The MCMCpack can be used for an extensive list of statistical models such as hierarchical longitudinal models and multinomial logit model (Chen and Peace 2011).

Bayesian inferences are made based on the posterior distribution. It should also be noted that there is no p-value in the Bayesian analysis. Instead, the 95% (or 1 – type I error rate) credible interval of the posterior distribution can be used to evaluate the strength of evidence of the results.

Beta-Binomial Example

Assume p is the favorable outcome rate of the new treatment, and the interest is to test the following hypothesis in a one-arm phase II clinical trial: H_0: $p \leq p_0$; H_1: $p > p_1$.

Let $Y_1, Y_2, \ldots, Y_n$ denote patient responses to the new treatment with each $Y_i = 1$ or 0 as success or failure, respectively. $X_n = Y_1 + Y_2 + \ldots + Y_n$ denotes the total number of favorable outcomes out of the n subjects treated. X_n follows a binomial distribution with parameters n and p. Because of the conjugacy of the beta prior distribution for the binomial likelihood, it is common to use a beta prior distribution for the favorable response rate, p. Let the prior distribution for p follow a beta distribution with parameters a and b:

$$\pi(p) = \frac{\Gamma(a+b)}{\Gamma(a)\,\Gamma(b)} p^{a-1}(1-p)^{b-1}$$

The mean of this beta distribution is $a/(a + b)$.

The posterior distribution of the favorable response rate, given X_n, follows another beta distribution:

$$\begin{aligned} p(p|X_n) &\propto L(X_n|p)\pi(p) \\ &\propto p^{X_n}(1-p)^{n-X_n} p^{a-1}(1-p)^{b-1} \\ &\propto p^{X_n+a-1}(1-p)^{n-X_n+b-1} \\ \mathrm{p} \mid \mathrm{X_n} &\sim \text{Beta}\,(a+X_n, b+n-X_n). \end{aligned} \tag{2}$$

The mean of this posterior distribution is $(a + X_n) / (a + b + n)$. Therefore, the prior distribution can be interpreted as contributing $a + b$ patients where a patients are with favorable outcomes and b patients with unfavorable outcomes. It is recommended to keep the worth of the prior distribution, $a + b$, relatively small, compared to the size of the actual patients, n (Geller 2004). Some authors recommended choosing a equal to the mean probability of favorable outcome and b as 1- a, 2- a, or 3- a depending on how much weight investigators are planning to put on prior distribution (Zohar et al. 2008). In other words, if the expected favorable outcome rate is 40%, a can be selected as 0.4, and b can be 0.6, 1.6, or 2.6.

Bayesian Phase II Clinical Trials

Efficacy, safety, and cost of the proposed therapy are assessed at phase II trials (Stallard 1998). The data can be assessed only at two stages in traditional frequentist phase II clinical trials. In contrast, Bayesian methods allow users to examine the interim data by updating the posterior probability of parameters and make relevant predictions and decisions at multiple stages. At each stage, the posterior distribution can be used to draw inferences concerning the parameter of interest. Accordingly, at each stage, there are three possible actions (Lee and Liu 2008):

I: Stop the study because of futility and declare that the new drug is not promising.
II: Stop the study because of efficacy and declare that the new drug is promising.
III: Continue with phase II study until the next inspection or the maximum sample size is reached.

Predictive Probability Approach

Bayesian decision in phase II clinical trials is based on the predictive probabilities (PP). The approach introduced by Lee and Liu for single-arm designs will be presented here (Lee and Liu 2008). The PP is obtained by calculating the probability of rejecting the null hypothesis (concluding efficacy) should the trial be conducted to the maximum planned sample size (N_{max}), based on the current data from the patients already enrolled in the study (Lee and Liu 2008). Then, depending on the strength of this probability, the decision to continue or stop (go/no go) is made.

Assume the response is binary and the data is monitored continuously. The goal is to provide simple and practical guidelines to decide whether the new treatment is promising relative to the standard therapy while accounting for the uncertainty regarding the response rates in each group. The trial continues until the new treatment is shown with high posterior predictive probability to be either promising, not promising, or until the N_{max} is reached.

First, the posterior probability of target response rate being greater than the pre-specified alternative response probability should be calculated. If this posterior probability is greater than a pre-specified threshold (θ_T), the design can declare efficacy. Therefore, if Pr ($p > p_0 \mid X_1, X_2) > \theta_T$, the new treatment will be deemed efficacious and the study will proceed to phase III clinical trial.

The steps for the Bayesian PP approach are as follows. First, the prior distribution for the favorable outcome rate is pre-specified. Second, the group of n patients is enrolled, and favorable (X) versus unfavorable ($n-X$) outcome is observed from each of these n patients. At this point in time (marked as red in Fig. 3), the posterior distribution for the favorable outcome rate is obtained based on the prior information and the data. As shown in Equation 2, the posterior distribution based on n patients where X patients had favorable would be Beta ($a + X$, $b + n-X$). This posterior distribution would be used as prior distribution for the calculations for the not observed future m patients.

Let Y be the number of favorable outcomes among the potential $m = N_{max}-n$ future patients. The distribution of Y future responses can be derived as

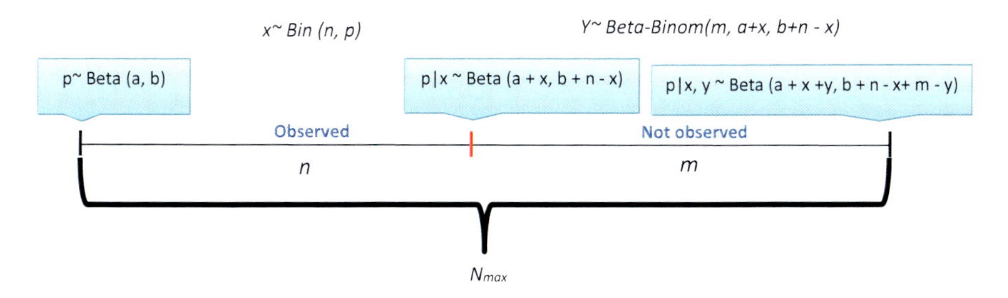

Fig. 3 Bayesian design with the PP approach

$$
\begin{aligned}
P(\tilde{y}|y) &= \int_0^1 p(\tilde{y}\,|p)p(p|y)dp \\
&= \int_0^1 \binom{m}{y} p^y (1-p)^{m-y} \frac{\Gamma(a+b+n)}{\Gamma(a+x)\Gamma(b+n-x)} p^{a+x-1}(1-p)^{b+n-x-1}dp \\
&= \frac{m!}{y!(m-y)!}\frac{\Gamma(a+b+n)}{\Gamma(a+x)\Gamma(b+n-x)}\int_0^1 p^{y+a+x-1}(1-p)^{b+n-x+m-y-1}dp \\
&= \frac{\Gamma(m+1)}{\Gamma(y+1)\Gamma(m-y+1)}\frac{\Gamma(a+b+n)}{\Gamma(a+x)\Gamma(b+n-x)}\frac{\Gamma(y+x+a)\Gamma(b+n-x+m-y)}{\Gamma(a+b+n+m)}
\end{aligned}
$$

and follows a beta-binomial distribution ($m,\ a+x,\ b+n-x$).

For the future m potential patients, the number of favorable outcomess, Y, will be between 0 and m. The probabilities of observing each possible value of $Y = i,\ i = 0, 1, \ldots, m$ favorable outcomes can be calculated from this beta-binomial distribution. In addition, when $Y = i$ favorable outcomes out of the m patients are observed, the posterior distribution of the favorable outcome rate will follow another beta distribution: $P|X = x,\ Y = i \sim Beta\ (a + x + y,\ b + n - x + m-y)$. From this beta distribution, the probability of $p>p_0$ can be calculated and will be called B_i:

$$B_i = \text{Prob}(\,P > p_0 \mid \text{x}, \text{Y} = \text{i})$$

Then, this B_i value will be compared to the threshold value, θ_T. If B_i is greater than θ_T, for that realization of Y = i, it is expected that the new treatment will be efficacious at the end of the trial. The predictive probability is the weighted average of the positive trial ($B_i>\theta_T$) and the trial continuing until N_{max} patients are enrolled (Lee and Liu 2008). The predictive probability approach looks at the strength of evidence for concluding efficacy at the end of the trial, based on the current evidence in terms of the prior information and the data. The decisions to stop the study early due to efficacy/futility or continue because the current data are not conclusive will depend on this PP. If the PP is high, it is expected that the new treatment will be efficacious at the end of the study, given the current data. On the other hand, low PP indicates that the new treatment may not have sufficient activity by the end of the study. To prevent any ambiguity, lower (Q_L) and upper (Q_U) stopping thresholds should be pre-specified:

$$
\begin{aligned}
\text{PP} &= \sum_{i=0}^{m} \Pr(Y = i|x) x\, I_{\left(\Pr\left(p>p_0|x,\, Y=i\right)>\theta_T\right)} \\
&= \sum_{i=0}^{m} \Pr(Y = i\,|x) I_{(B_i>\theta_T)}
\end{aligned}
$$

The decision of early stopping or continuing the trial will be based on the following thresholds.

If PP<θ_L: with the given current information, it is unlikely that the response rate will be larger than the p_0 at the end of the trial. Stop for futility and reject H_1.

If PP>θ_U: the current data suggest that, if the same trend continues, it is highly likely that the treatment will be efficacious at the end of the trial. Stop for efficacy and reject H_0.

If θ_L<PP<θ_U: continue to the next stage until reaching N_{max} patients.

Both lower (θ_L) and the upper (θ_U) stopping thresholds set between 0 and 1. It is advised to stop early if the drug is not promising. Therefore, θ_L is chosen to be closer to 0. In contrast, if the drug is promising, it is better not to stop the trial early. Therefore, θ_U is chosen as close to 1.

Example 2 Assume an investigator wants to design a study with a binary favorable/unfavorable outcome. Suppose she does not want to enroll more than 30 (N_{max}) subjects into this trial. To date, she has enrolled 16 (n) subjects and observed favorable outcomes from 12 (x) of the 16 subjects. Assume Y is the number of positive outcomes for the 14 future subjects. What is the probability of favorable outcome rate being greater than 65% at the end of the trial?

The following vague beta prior distribution for the favorable outcome rate can be used: Beta(0.65, 0.35). Note that, as explained above, the mean of this beta distribution is 0.65 (0.65 / (0.65 + 0.35)), and the worth of the prior distribution is only 1 (0.65 + 0.35).

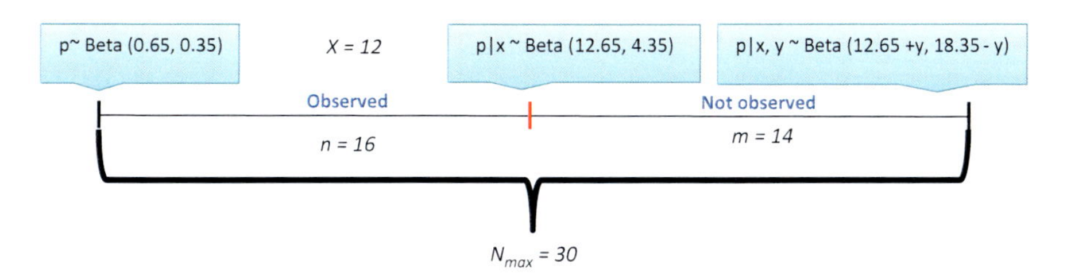

A table showing each possible number of favorable outcomes for the future 14 patients can be created (Table 1).

Note that, for example, to calculate the Prob(Y = 11 | X = 12) in column 2, the beta-binomial distribution should be used, beta-binomial(i = 11, m = 14, 12.65, 4.35). dbetabinom.ab function in VGAM package in R can be used to calculate this probability: dbetabinom.ab(11, 14, shape1 = 12.65, shape2 = 4.35). Similarly, to calculate the probability of p>0.65 given x = 12 and i = 11 presented in column 3, beta distribution should be used: Beta(23.65, 12.35). In R, 1−pbeta(0.65, 23.65, 7.35) function can be used. The last column is an indicator function showing whether B_i is greater than the threshold of $\theta_T = 0.9$.

For values of Y between 0 and 10, B_i is less than 0.9. In other words, if 0 to 10 favorable outcomes are observed, out of the future 14 patients, the null hypothesis will be failed to be rejected, and it will be concluded that the new treatment is not

Table 1 Calculation of Bi and PP

Y = i	Prob(Y = i |x)	B_i = Prob(p>0.65 | x, Y = i)	I (Bi>0.9)
0	0.0000	0.0031	0
1	0.0001	0.0088	0
2	0.0004	0.0223	0
3	0.0017	0.0504	0
4	0.0051	0.1015	0
5	0.0128	0.1832	0
6	0.0275	0.2981	0
7	0.0516	0.4393	0
8	0.0856	0.5909	0
9	0.1261	0.7319	0
10	0.1635	0.8450	0
11	**0.1832**	**0.9225**	**1**
12	**0.1706**	**0.9672**	**1**
13	**0.1209**	**0.9885**	**1**
14	**0.0509**	**0.9968**	**1**

$N_{max} = 30$, $n = 16$, $x = 12$, $m = 14$, $a = 0.65$, $b = 0.35$, $\theta_T = 0.9$, $\theta_L = 0.1$, and $\theta_U = 0.95$

effective. On the other hand, if number of favorable outcomes out of the future 14 patients is 11 or more, new treatment will be deemed effective.

Finally, the PP for this table can be calculated as 0.1832 + 0.1706 + 0.1209 + 0.0509 = 0.5256. This PP value is $>\theta_L = 0.1$. Therefore, the trial cannot be stopped for futility. It is less than $\theta_U = 0.95$. Thus, it cannot be stopped for efficacy. According to this PP value, based on the interim data, the study should continue because the evidence is insufficient to draw a definitive conclusion in either stopping early for futility or efficacy yet.

This predictive probability value can be calculated using the R package "ph2bayes" with the following R code:

```
predprob(12, n = 16, nmax = 30, alpha_e = 0.65, beta_e = 0.35,
p_s = 0.65, theta_t = 0.9).
```

Oncology Example with the PP Approach

For example, for the oncology example presented earlier, the 9-month PFR rate was assumed 12.7% ($p_0 = 0.127$) for the standard therapy group. It was expected that sorafenib will increase the 9-month PFR rate to 31.7% ($p_1 = 0.317$). Same example can also be handled with the Bayesian PP approach. Let both type I and type II error rates to be 10%. In addition to the existing frequentist assumptions, let's assume the data will start to be monitored after data from the first 14 ($N_{min} = 14$) patients are observed and $N_{max} = 43$. Let the response rate to follow a beta prior distribution with parameters 0.127 and 0.873 (1–0.127). Note that this distribution has a prior mean of 0.127 (0.127/(0.127 + 0.873)) and worth only one patient (0.127 + 0.873).

The corresponding rejection regions for this study would be 0/14, 1/24, 2/29, 3/33, 4/37, 5/39, 6/41, 7/42, and 8/43. The trial will stop for futility, the first time the number of favorable outcomes falls into the rejection region. In the actual study, Ray-Coquard et al. observed 1 patient with PFR at 9 months, out of the 26 enrolled patients (Ray-Coquard et al. 2012). Consistent with the frequentist design, Bayesian design would also recommend stopping at this point. Indeed, with the PP approach, the study would have been stopped after 14 patients if there was no favorable outcome or after only 24, instead of 26, patients if there was only 1 patient with favorable outcome.

Rejection regions can be calculated using the following R code in "ph2bye" package:

```
DT.design(type = "PredP", a=0.127, b=0.873, nmin=14, nmax=43,
p0=0.127, p1=0.317, theta0 = 0.001, theta1 = 0.9, theta_t = 0.85).
```

In addition, following Lee and Liu's (Lee and Liu 2008) approach, M.D. Anderson Cancer Center group developed a software (https://biostatistics.mdanderson.org/SoftwareDownload/) to implement further calculations to determine stopping regions for futility and search for N_{max}, θ_L, $\theta_{T,}$ and θ_U. Similarly, to be able to use the software, users should specify the minimum (N_{min}) and maximum sample sizes (N_{max}), response rates of the standard therapy (p_0) and the new treatment (p_1) groups, type I and type II error rates, and the parameters of the beta prior distribution for the success in the standard therapy group (Berry et al. 2011). It is recommended to start monitoring the data after the first ten patients ($N_{min} = 10$) have been treated and outcomes were observed. The software can be used for different N_{max} values and be searched for θ_L and θ_U space to generate designs satisfying both type I and type II error rate criteria (Berry et al. 2011).

Frequentist Two-Stage Design Versus Bayesian PP Approach

In contrast to looking at the data only at the end of the first and second stages with the frequentist two-stage design, the Bayesian PP approach allows users to assess the data continuously after outcomes from at least ten patients were observed. In other words, for the extreme case presented in Fig. 2, the frequentist design would not be stopped even if no favorable outcome is observed for the first 16 patients in the second stage of the study. Bayesian design would allow users to stop the study much earlier, in fact, after the first six unfavorable outcomes in the second stage of the study for futility. The Bayesian PP approach allows more frequent monitoring; therefore it is more flexible than the frequentist two-stage design. The Bayesian PP design enables users to stop at any time if the accumulating evidence does not support the new treatment's efficacy over the standard therapy.

Bayesian Phase I–II Trials

It is more common to focus to the outcome of toxicity only in phase I trials and for the outcome of efficacy in phase II trials. However, it is also possible and may be more efficient to include a bivariate binary outcome of efficacy and toxicity in a single phase I–II clinical trial. Readers can learn more about Bayesian phase I–II trials on Yuan, Nguyen, and Thall (Yuan et al. 2016).

Summary and Conclusion

The main goal of phase II studies is to provide assessment of efficacy of the treatment of interest. Frequentist two-stage designs are common and easy to implement. However, data is assessed only at the end of two stages. Bayesian approach allows synthesis of external information into the design and allows updating the evidence based on the accumulated data, more frequent monitoring, and calculating predictive probabilities based on the current information (Biswas et al. 2009). Accordingly, Bayesian designs are more flexible compared to frequentist two-stage designs and allow for continuous decision of stopping the study for futility and efficacy or enrolling more patients. With the availability of computer programs utilizing Bayesian predictive probability approach, Bayesian designs are now easier to implement and being used increasingly (Biswas et al. 2009).

Key Facts

- With the Bayesian design, it is possible to incorporate external information and update evidence based on the accumulated data.
- Bayesian designs using predictive probability approach are more flexible than frequentist two-stage designs and allow continuous monitoring.

Cross-References

▶ Dose-Finding and Dose-Ranging Studies
▶ Randomized Selection Designs

References

Berry SM, Carlin BP, Lee JJ, Muller P (2011) Bayesian adaptive methods for clinical trials. Chapman & Hall/CRC Biostatistics Series, vol 38. CRC Press, Boca Raton

Biswas S, Liu DD, Lee JJ, Berry DA (2009) Bayesian clinical trials at the University of Texas M. D. Anderson Cancer Center. Clin Trials (London, England) 6:205–216. https://doi.org/10.1177/1740774509104992

Chaloner K, Rhame FS (2001) Quantifying and documenting prior beliefs in clinical trials. Stat Med 20:581–600. https://doi.org/10.1002/sim.694
Chen DG, Peace KE (2011) Clinical trial data analysis using R. CRC, Boca Raton, pp 1–357
Gehan EA (1961) The determination of the number of patients required in a preliminary and a follow-up trial of a new chemotherapeutic agent. J Chronic Dis 13:346–353
Geller NL (2004) Advances in clinical trial biostatistics. Biostatistics 13:1–52
Gelman A, Carlin JB, Stern HS, Rubin D (2004) Bayesian data analysis. Chapman & Hall/CRC texts in statistical science, Boca Rotan, Florida, 3rd edn
FDA (2010) Guidance for the use of bayesian statistics in medical device clinical trials. U.S. Department of Health and Human Services Food and Drug Administration Center for Devices and Radiological Health Division of Biostatistics Office of Surveillance and Biometrics . http://www.fda.gov/downloads/MedicalDevices/DeviceRegulationandGuidance/GuidanceDocuments/ucm071121.pdf
Jung S-H (2013) Randomized phase II cancer clinical trials. Chapman & Hall/CRC Biostatistics Series. CRC Press/Taylor & Francis Group, Boca Raton
Lee JJ, Liu DD (2008) A predictive probability design for phase II cancer clinical trials. Clin Trials (London, England) 5:93–106. https://doi.org/10.1177/1740774508089279
Lynch SM (2007) Introduction to applied Bayesian statistics and estimation for social scientists. Statistics for social and behavioral sciences. Springer, New York
Martin AD, Quinn KM, Park JH (2011) MCMCpack: Markov Chain Monte Carlo in R. J Stat Softw 42
Ray-Coquard I et al (2012) Sorafenib for patients with advanced angiosarcoma: a phase II Trial from the French Sarcoma Group (GSF/GETO). Oncologist 17:260–266. https://doi.org/10.1634/theoncologist.2011-0237
Simon R (1989) Optimal two-stage designs for phase II clinical trials. Control Clin Trials 10:1–10
Stallard N (1998) Sample size determination for phase II clinical trials based on Bayesian decision theory. Biometrics 54:279–294
Sturtz SL, Ligges U, Gelman A (2005) R2WinBUGS: a package for running WinBUGS from R. J Stat Softw 12:1–16. https://doi.org/10.18637/jss.v012.i03
Yuan Y, Nguyen HQ, Thall PF (2016) Bayesian designs for phase I-II clinical trials. Chapman & Hall/CRC Biostatistics Series. CRC Press, Taylor & Francis Group, Boca Raton
Zohar S, Teramukai S, Zhou Y (2008) Bayesian design and conduct of phase II single-arm clinical trials with binary outcomes: a tutorial. Contemp Clin Trials 29:608–616. https://doi.org/10.1016/j.cct.2007.11.005

Randomized Selection Designs

57

Shing M. Lee, Bruce Levin, and Cheng-Shiun Leu

Contents

Abstract

The general goal of a randomized selection design is *to select* one or more treatments from several competing candidates to which patients are randomly assigned, in such a way that selected treatment(s) are likely to be better than those not selected. For example, if one treatment is clearly superior to all the others, we may demand that the procedure select that treatment with high probability. The experimental treatments could be different doses of a drug or intensities of a behavioral intervention, different treatment schedules, modalities, or strategies, or

S. M. Lee (✉) · B. Levin · C.-S. Leu
Department of Biostatistics, Mailman School of Public Health, Columbia University, New York, NY, USA
e-mail: sml2114@cumc.columbia.edu; Bruce.Levin@columbia.edu; cl94@cumc.columbia.edu

© Springer Nature Switzerland AG 2022

S. Piantadosi, C. L. Meinert (eds.), *Principles and Practice of Clinical Trials*,
https://doi.org/10.1007/978-3-319-52636-2_82

different combinations of treatments. The hallmark feature of a selection design is its ability to achieve its stated goals with surprisingly fewer participants compared with traditional "phase III" trials, precisely because it eschews the formal hypothesis test paradigm with its tight control over type 1 error rates. These designs can be used in clinical research to screen for treatments that are worthy of further evaluation in a subsequent confirmatory clinical trial and to discard unpromising treatments. Thus, they are ideal for middle development settings where we are interested in selecting promising treatments under circumstances typically limited by smaller sample sizes. In this chapter, we discuss the randomized selection designs of Simon, Wittes, and Ellenberg, Steinberg and Venzon, and the Levin-Robbins-Leu family of sequential subset selection procedures. The first two designs select a single treatment, while the latter allows for sequential elimination of inferior treatments, sequential recruitment of superior treatments, and may be used to select treatments with fixed or variable subset sizes.

Keywords

Selection paradigm · Correct selection · Subset selection · Acceptable set · Phase 2 designs · Selection trials

Introduction

The goal of a randomized selection design is to select a truly *best* treatment (given a suitable definition of "best"), or more generally to select a *subset* of $b \geq 1$ treatments, ideally containing the b truly best treatments, using methods that have certain desirable operating characteristics. For example, assuming that one treatment is truly better than all the rest to a prespecified degree, we may wish to select that best treatment with a prespecified *high probability of correct selection*. Furthermore, we may wish to select a treatment or a subset of treatments that are reasonably "acceptable" (suitably defined) with prespecified high probability under any and all circumstances, irrespective of the true efficacy differences among treatments. When selecting treatments, the size of the subset b is typically fixed in advance – most often being $b = 1$ – but we may also wish to select varying numbers of "best" treatments in a data-dependent manner. Alternatively, we may wish to select a subset of treatments of varying size that achieves a prespecified high probability of containing the one truly best treatment. We may even wish to produce a reliable *ranking* of the c candidate treatments. These treatments can be different treatment schedules, doses, or strategies, and may include the standard of care. The statistical theory of ranking and selection, with its strong ties to multiple decision theory, provides an overarching framework for all such selection goals.

It may be helpful here to introduce a taxonomy of randomized selection designs. We shall say that such a trial is a *pure* selection trial if its *primary purpose is to select* (or identify or rank) treatments with goals as stated above *with no further intention of making statements of statistical significance*. Indeed, there is no concern about the type 1 error rate because one simply cannot commit a type 1 error when one doesn't declare efficacy differences statistically significant at the 0.05 level! To the contrary, in pure selection designs we are singularly *uninterested* in the null hypothesis of no difference between treatments. What we care about is making correct selections (or, more generally, *acceptable* selections – see below) with high probability when there are clinically meaningful and worthwhile differences even if we cannot "prove" that they are so. But if there are no meaningful or worthwhile efficacy differences among any of the candidates, then we are generally indifferent to which treatment (or treatments) is (or are) selected, other things being equal such as side effects, tolerability, or costs. This is the so-called *indifference zone* approach of Robert Bechhofer (1954). We will have more to say about this approach in section "Considerations for Designing Randomized Selection Trials."

At this point the reader might be wondering how could one dare to conduct a clinical experiment without some sort of tight control over type 1 error? It seems an unfortunate tendency in some quarters reflexively to identify "clinical research" as synonymous with "testing a null hypotheses at the 0.05 level of significance." There are good reasons regulatory agencies or journal editors insist on such a definition. However, not every important question can or should be addressed this way. For example, when kids in the schoolyard are choosing up sides for a baseball game, the team captains are surely not interested in testing the null hypothesis that all the kids have the same talent, controlling the type 1 error rate. To the contrary, the captains want to *select* the kids best able to help their teams based on observations of their performance. Similarly for choosing a winning horse at the race track or a profitable portfolio for investment. As a further example, during the Ebola outbreak of 2014 in West Africa, some argued (cogently, we believe) that the regulatory dictum – "we *must* use a control group to test the hypothesis of no efficacy while controlling the type 1 error rate, end of debate" – was misguided in the sense that the regulatory mandate was perhaps not the most pressing or important question to settle at that very moment. Rather, a pure randomized selection design of active treatments could have been implemented rapidly to *select* the best candidate treatment option or options, followed by careful rollout and watchful observation to see if patients stopped dying. Best available supportive care, which in West Africa was no better than no treatment at all given the resource poor environment, would not have been required. It would seem the selection goal was urgent and important enough to set aside the agnostic need to control the risk of a type 1 error. Even if the optimal standard of care were available in West Africa and had some efficacy, more rapid results might have been reached by including it in a pure randomized selection design than to insist on its use to demonstrate another treatment's significant improvement over it. See Caplan et al. (2015a, b) for further discussion.

We continue the taxonomy of randomized selection trials in the following sections. In section "Considerations for Designing Randomized Selection Trials" some important considerations for the design of selection trials are introduced. In section "Designs," we discuss some specific pure selection designs that have been proposed in the literature. In section "Other Designs," we briefly mention some other designs such as when selection procedures are used as a preliminary step for a randomized controlled trial or when they are used to formally test whether better-than-placebo treatments exist and if so, to select them. For simplicity in this chapter we shall focus exclusively on the case of binary outcomes as the clinical endpoint of interest, such as tumor response, and we shall use "response" or "success" synonymously. A selection design for time to event outcomes is briefly mentioned in section "Other Designs." In section "Applications of Randomized Selection Designs," we present two examples of actual selection trials to illustrate some practical implementation considerations, one using the prescreening selection approach and the other using an adaptive Levin-Robbins-Leu procedure, both discussed in section "Considerations for Designing Randomized Selection Trials." We conclude with a brief discussion in section "Discussion and Conclusion."

Considerations for Designing Randomized Selection Trials

Approaches to the Subset Selection Problem

A key operating characteristic of any randomized selection trial is its *probability of correct selection* or *PCS*, which is the probability of selecting truly best treatments. Most often one specifies a fixed target number $b \geq 1$ of best treatments in advance and then uses a procedure that selects b treatments. This is called a *fixed subset size* procedure. The *PCS* is then the probability that the selected subset is in fact the b truly best treatments. Fixed subset size procedures use the *indifference zone approach* of Bechhofer (1954) which requires that whatever procedure is used, it shall achieve a minimum pre-specified *PCS*, say P^*, if and when the best treatments' true success probabilities are sufficiently better than the remaining c–b treatments' success probabilities. We say in such cases that the c success probabilities (or parameters) fall in the *preference zone*. For the case of binary outcomes considered in this chapter, by "sufficiently better" we shall mean that the odds on success for the bth best treatment exceeds the odds on success of the next best treatment by a prespecified multiplicative factor, namely, the design *odds ratio* of $\theta > 1$. The choice of θ will depend on the context, but it generally signifies a clinically meaningful and worthwhile degree of relative treatment efficacy. The complement of the preference zone in the parameter space is the *indifference zone*, so-called because presumably one will be indifferent to the fact that the *PCS* may not exceed P^* when the parameters are not sufficiently distinct. Clearly if there are no differences between response probabilities, we are indifferent to which treatments are selected (other factors such as side effects, costs, etc., being equal). At the opposite extreme, though, one should stop being indifferent to the shortfall of the *PCS* below P^* as the separation between the bth best and next-best treatment approaches θ. This often helps to guide the choice of the design odds ratio.

The main drawback of the indifference-zone approach is that in practice one doesn't know whether the population parameters fall in the preference or the indifference zone. This was the principal motivation for Shanti S. Gupta's *subset selection* approach (Gupta 1956, 1965), which selects a *subset* of treatments using a fixed, prespecified sample size, the goal of which is to capture the *one* best treatment in the subset with a prespecified high probability, no matter what the true response probabilities are. To guarantee that, the size of the subset necessarily has to vary randomly according to the observed data. For example, if there are only small differences between success probabilities, all c treatments might have to be "selected." Clearly, the only role played by selection of *subsets* of size one or greater in the Gupta approach is to assure capture of the *best* treatment among those selected with high probability. More generally, to assure capture of b best populations with high probability, subsets of size *b or greater* would have to be selected, with size varying according to the observed data.

We shall not pursue the Gupta subset selection approach any further, referring the reader instead to the book by Bechhofer et al. (1995), because in the sequel we shall mean something very different by the term "subset selection." Henceforth, by *subset selection* we shall mean any procedure whose goal is explicitly *to select subsets of b best treatments,* when b is fixed in advance. In section "Random Subset Size Selection with LRL Procedures" we also briefly consider subset selection procedures that identify subsets of random size, but still the goal will be to select *best subsets* of treatments, albeit of varying size. Such subset selection procedures are called *random subset size* procedures.

Acceptable Subset Selection

The most familiar goal for a pure randomized selection trial in the indifference zone approach is to correctly identify the best treatment with high probability if a minimal clinically meaningful and worthwhile difference exists between the best and the second-best treatment. However, if the success probabilities for the several best treatments are close to one another, assuring a high probability of correct selection is neither meaningful nor possible. When several treatments are close to best in efficacy, we may be indifferent as to which is selected, but we should still want a high probability of selecting one of those near-best treatments if not technically *the* best. This leads to the general notion of *acceptable subset selection* which offers another resolution to the dilemma posed by ignorance of the true parameter values and which, unlike Gupta's approach, stays within the indifference zone approach. We specify these ideas in some more detail next.

Precisely because we generally don't know whether the treatment response probabilities fall in the preference or indifference zone, we will want to know whether or not a procedure will select, if not best subsets, then "acceptable" subsets, with a prespecified high probability *irrespective of the true population parameters.* We shall refer to such a property as *acceptable subset selection,* where the phrase, "with pre-specified probability irrespective of the true population parameters" should be understood. The following notions were introduced by Bechhofer et al. (1968, p. 337, hereinafter BKS) and elaborated upon by Leu and Levin (2008b).

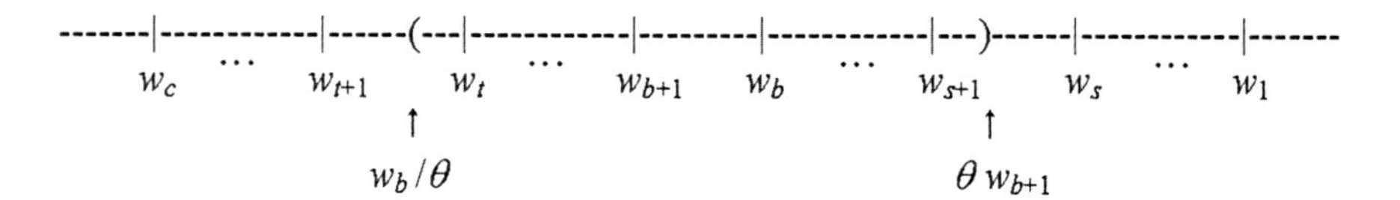

Fig. 1

For any given success odds vector $\boldsymbol{w} = (w_1, \ldots, w_c)$, where $w_j = p_j / (1-p_j)$ and design odds ratio $\theta \geq 1$, we define certain integers s and t given by functions of $\boldsymbol{w}$ and θ, say $s = s(w,\theta)$ and $t = t(w,\theta)$, such that

$$w_{s+1} < w_{b+1}\theta \leq w_s$$

and

$$w_{t+1} \leq w_b/\theta < w_t$$

as illustrated in the following diagram (Fig 1).

These inequalities define an open interval of odds containing w_b and w_{b+1} such that $w_1,\ldots,w_s$ are at least as great as the upper endpoint of the interval, which is given by θ times w_{b+1}, and such that $w_{t+1},\ldots,w_c$ are no greater than the lower endpoint of the interval, which is given by θ^{-1} times w_b. BKS reasoned that with the above configuration of true success odds, in order to be deemed "acceptable" any selection of b treatments ought to contain the s best treatments and ought to exclude the c–t worst treatments, while it would be acceptable to select the remaining b–s treatments in any manner from among the $(s+1)^{st}$ to t^{th} best. In general, then, a θ-*acceptable subset* is any subset of treatments in which the $s = s(\boldsymbol{w},\theta)$ best treatments are selected and all selected treatments are among the $t = t(\boldsymbol{w},\theta)$ best treatments. In other words, a θ-acceptable subset must include all treatments better than the upper endpoint of the defined interval around w_b and w_{b+1} and exclude all treatments worse than its lower endpoint. It is easy to see that if $\boldsymbol{w}$ is in the preference zone, then $s = t = b$ and the only θ-acceptable subset is the correct subset, $(b) = (1,\ldots,b)$. At the other extreme, if the treatments all have equal success odds, $s = 0$ and $t = c$, meaning any b-tuple would be θ-acceptable, in which case we are completely indifferent as to which treatments are selected (other things like cost, side-effects, etc., being equal). The neighborhood around w_b and w_{b+1} creates different regions of the parameter space with a gradation from maximal preference of which treatments to select to maximal indifference.

Fixed Versus Random Subset Sizes

When planning a pure randomized selection trial, it is of course important to decide on how many treatments to select, and if a fixed number of treatments, b, is decided upon, there should be a cogent reason for doing so. For example, there may be several good candidate treatments but the research budget allows for selecting two but not more. Or, we want to screen for three promising candidates in a search process, neither more nor less. Even though most frequently selection procedures aim to identify a single best candidate, that design specification should still be justified.

Often, however, it will not be clear to investigators how best to specify a desired subset size prior to the experiment. For practical reasons we may wish to constrain the size of the selected subset prior to the experiment. For example, budgetary constraints may force us to select *at most* a given number of treatments, but we may be content to select fewer than that number. Or, evidence from pilot work may suggest that at least another given number of promising treatments may exist among the c candidates, in which case we may wish to identify *at least* that number of good treatments. Such practical needs of clinical research call for *random subset size* selection procedures. Random subset size selection procedures should have the acceptable subset selection property.

Designs

The Simon et al. (1985) (hereinafter "SWE") design is a classical fixed sample size selection procedure to select a best treatment, such as discussed in Gibbons et al. (1977). We also discuss an adaptation of the SWE design following a collection of parallel, single-arm, Simon two-stage designs used for prescreening the candidate treatments. The prescreening allows incorporating historical control information to help assure that the selected treatments are better than the current standard of care (Liu et al. 2006). Another extension of the SWE design by Steinberg and Venzon (2002) allows for interim stopping and early termination by requiring a prespecified difference between treatment arms in order to select the most promising treatment at interim looks. The aforementioned designs select one treatment given a fixed sample size. Finally, we discuss the Levin-Robbins-Leu (LRL) family of sequential subset selection procedures, which aim to select subsets of one or more treatments. Extensions allow the size of the selected subset to vary, possibly with prespecified constraints on the (random) size of the selected subsets for practical purposes. Both the fixed- and random-subset size LRL procedures offer acceptable subset selection with high probability, irrespective of true treatment efficacies, while allowing sequentially adaptive elimination and recruitment of treatments.

The Simon et al. (1985) Fixed Sample Size Procedure (SWE)

Suppose we are interested in identifying the one best treatment ($b = 1$), i.e., the treatment with highest success probability, from the c candidates. The SWE procedure draws a fixed sample of size n for each of the c treatment arms, then selects the treatment with the largest observed number of responses, or equivalently largest proportion of responses. If there are ties among the largest, select one randomly as the best (or, more realistically, select one on practical grounds such as side effects, cost, etc.). Simon et al. (1985) provide formulas to calculate the probability of correct selection (*PCS*) under the *least favorable configuration,* that is, the probability of correctly identifying the best treatment if a clinically meaningful difference of Δ exists between the response probability of the best treatment (say $p + \Delta$) and the response probabilities of the remaining c–1 treatments (each assumed equal to p). This configuration is called "least favorable" because any set of response probabilities wherein the best differs from the others by Δ *or more* will have a *PCS* no smaller than that for the least favorable configuration. For given c, p, and Δ, the sample size n per arm may then be determined using the formulas by trial and error to achieve the prespecified level of *PCS.* Table 3 of the SWE paper provides explicit sample sizes per arm in the special case of an absolute difference in response rates of $\Delta = 0.15$ for p ranging from 0.2 to 0.8 in increments of 0.1 with $c = 2$, 3, or 4 treatments that achieve a 90% *PCS* under the least favorable configuration. Alternatively, tables provided in Gibbons et al. (1977) may be used.

Prescreening Using Simon's Two-Stage Design

Liu et al. (2006) describe an adaptation of the SWE procedure following prescreening of several candidate treatments using Simon's two-stage design (Simon 1989). Patients are randomized to the c candidate treatments of interest and parallel single-arm phase II trials are conducted using Simon's two-stage design to screen out nonpromising treatments. We then apply the SWE selection rule among the c' treatments that passed the prescreening step. Note that the sample size for this adaptation is based on the sample size calculation for the original Simon two-stage trials and may not be adequate to guarantee a high probability of correct selection. Of course, the number of treatments that will pass the prescreening step is not known in advance and this complicates the calculation of the overall probability of correct selection. One feature is clear though, which is that the overall *PCS* for the Liu et al. proposal must be smaller than the probability of declaring a treatment promising in the Simon two-stage design under the design alternative. This is because not only must the best treatment pass the Simon prescreening, but in case other less efficacious treatments do too, the best must have more responses than the competitors. We illustrate this feature in the example given in Applications of Randomized Selection Designs.

The Steinberg and Venzon (2002) Design (SV)

The design by Steinberg and Venzon (2002) is an extension of the SWE approach. It differs by allowing an interim look at the data to perform an early selection and terminate the trial. The maximum sample size for the design is calculated using the same method as the SWE procedure. In addition, let d be a prespecified integer such that if the difference in the number of successes between the apparently best and second-best treatment arm is at least d at the interim look, the procedure stops, whereupon the leading treatment is selected as the best. Otherwise, the trial continues to complete its planned accrual. If there is no early stopping, the SWE selection rule is applied. Steinberg and Venzon describe how to determine d to limit the probability of making an incorrect selection in a two-arm trial. They also provide a table with values of d that limit the probability of making an incorrect selection to 0.5%, 1%, 5%, or 10%, assuming a difference of 0.10 or 0.15 in the probability of response between the two treatment arms. These authors also propose their interim stopping rule for use in the context of parallel Simon two-stage screening trials, in effect allowing for early stopping in the design discussed in section "Prescreening Using Simon's Two-Stage Design." Early stopping takes place if the best response tally exceeds the Steinberg and Venzon criterion d among the subset of treatments that have passed the first stage of screening. If the criterion is not met, enrollment continues to complete the second stage with the passing subset and a final selection takes place as in section "Prescreening Using Simon's Two-Stage Design."

The Levin-Robbins-Leu Family of Sequential Subset Selection Procedures

The Levin-Robbins-Leu (LRL) family of sequential subset selection procedures are experimental designs that aim to identify the best treatment, or more generally, the best subset of $b \geq 1$ treatments among $c > b$ candidates. The procedures allow for two adaptive features, namely, sequential *elimination* of apparently inferior treatments as soon as the current weight of evidence indicates that such treatments are not among the b best treatments; and/or sequential *recruitment* of apparently superior treatments as soon as the current weight of evidence indicates that such treatments are among the b best treatments. Four members comprise the LRL family of subset selection procedures: the nonadaptive member with neither the elimination nor recruitment feature; elimination but no recruitment; recruitment but no elimination; and both elimination and recruitment features. Here we shall present only the nonadaptive LRL procedure, which we shall denote by procedure $\mathcal{N}$ and the adaptive procedure featuring both elimination and recruitment, which we shall denote by procedure $\mathcal{E}/\mathcal{R}$. The LRL family of procedures is discussed fully in Leu and Levin (2008a, b, 2017) and Levin and Leu (2013, 2016).

LRL Procedure $\mathcal{N}$

The sampling proceeds vector-at-a-time, meaning that patients are assigned randomly to each of the c treatments in blocks of size c. If desired, the blocking on c patients can also incorporate matching on prognostic factors. Let $r_j^{(n)}$ denote the number of responses in treatment j after n rounds of c-tuplets have been randomized for $j = 1, \ldots, c$. We call the $r_j^{(n)}$ "response tallies." In addition, let $r_1^{[n]} \geq r_2^{[n]} \geq \cdots \geq r_c^{[n]}$ denote the *ordered* response tallies, where the subscripts refer to ordering the number of responses from the greatest ($j = 1$) to the least ($j = c$). Now let d be a positive integer chosen in advance. Procedure $\mathcal{N}$ stops the first time that the difference between the bth largest and $(b + 1)^{st}$ largest response tally equals d, i.e., after $N_{\mathcal{N}} = N_{\mathcal{N}}(b, c, d) = \inf\left\{n \geq 1 : r_b^{[n]} - r_{b+1}^{[n]} = d\right\}$ rounds of c-tuples of patients have had their endpoints observed. At stopping time $N_{\mathcal{N}}$, select the unique set of treatments with the b largest response tallies as the b best.

LRL Procedure $\mathcal{E}/\mathcal{R}$

As above, choose positive integer d in advance. Begin randomizing patients vector-at-a-time, but now *eliminate* the apparently inferior arm or arms as soon as their response tallies fall d heads behind the arm or arms with the currently held b^{th} largest tally. Similarly, *recruit* the apparently superior arm or arms as soon as their response tallies pull d heads ahead of the arm or arms with the currently held $(b + 1)^{st}$ largest tally. By "eliminate" we mean that an arm is withdrawn from the competition with no further patients allocated to it and is classified as outside the set of b best treatments. By "recruit" we mean that an arm is withdrawn from the competition with no further patients allocated to it and is selected to be among the set of b best treatments. Note that there is no claim that the first-recruited arm is equal to the best arm, merely that it qualifies as among the b best. Similarly, there is no claim that the first-eliminated arm is equal to the worst arm, merely that it does not qualify as among the b best.

To specify procedure $\mathcal{E}/\mathcal{R}$ a bit more precisely, let $N_{\mathcal{E}/\mathcal{R}}$ denote *the time of first elimination and/or recruitment* in a c-treatment experiment with treatment labels in the set $C = \{1,\ldots,c\}$. In what follows the subset C will change composition as treatments are eliminated or recruited, resulting in a sequence of subsets $C \supset C' \supset C'' \supset \cdots$ of treatment labels still in competition and we shall let the sequence $c > c' > c'' > \cdots$ denote the size of the corresponding subsets. Then $N_{\mathcal{E}/\mathcal{R}}$ is defined as

$$\begin{aligned} N_{\mathcal{E}/\mathcal{R}} &= N_{\mathcal{E}/\mathcal{R}}(b, C, d) \\ &= \inf\left\{n \geq 1 : r_b^{[n]} - r_c^{[n]} = d\right\} \wedge \inf\left\{n \geq 1 : r_1^{[n]} - r_{b+1}^{[n]} = d\right\} \end{aligned}$$

At round $n = N_{\mathcal{E}/\mathcal{R}}$, we eliminate all treatments i with $r_i^{(n)} = r_c^{[n]}$ if $r_b^{[n]} = r_c^{[n]} = d$ and/or we recruit all treatments i with $r_i^{(n)} = r_1^{[n]}$ if $r_1^{[n]} - r_{b+1}^{[n]} = d$. If fewer than b arms are recruited and/or fewer than c–b arms are eliminated, the procedure continues, starting from the current tallies of the remaining subset of treatments, say $C' \subset C$, and iterates with time of next elimination and/or recruitment $N_{\mathcal{E}/\mathcal{R}}(b', C', d)$, wherein $c' = |C'|$ replaces c and b' is b minus the total number of coins recruited by time $N_{\mathcal{E}/\mathcal{R}}(b, C, d)$. Continuing in this way, we stop whenever there is a recruitment of however many treatments are required to fill out the subset of size b and, simultaneously, an elimination of the other currently remaining treatments, at which point a total of b arms will have been recruited and c–b arms eliminated. Upon stopping we declare the subset of recruited treatments as the b best. The procedure always identifies a well-defined subset of b treatments with no ties.

A Lower Bound Formula for the *PCS* of LRL Procedures

Let $\boldsymbol{w} = (w_1, \ldots, w_c)$ denote the vector of true odds on response with $w_j = p_j/(1 - p_j)$ for $j = 1, \ldots, c$. Because the procedures are symmetric with respect to permutations of the labels of the treatments, we may assume without loss of generality that $w_1 \geq w_2 \geq \cdots \geq w_c$ even though no such assumption is required in practice. Leu and Levin (2008b) proved that the following *lower-bound formula* holds for the *PCS* when using procedure $\mathcal{N}$. For any true success odds vector $\boldsymbol{w}$, the *PCS*, which we denote as $P_{\boldsymbol{w}}[cs]$ to reflect its dependence on the parameters, is bounded from below by

$$P_{\boldsymbol{w}}[cs] \geq \frac{(w_1 \cdots w_b)^d}{\sum_{(b)} w_{(b)}^d}.$$

The sum in the denominator is over all possible b-tuples which we denote generically as $(b) = (i_1, \ldots i_b)$ with integers $1 \leq i_1 < \cdots < i_b \leq c$, and where the summands use the convenient notation $w_{(b)}^d = w_{i_1}^d \cdots w_{i_b}^d$. The above lower bound allows us to choose d in designing selection experiments as follows. It is easy to see that the right-hand side of the above inequality is minimized for any $\boldsymbol{w}$ in the preference zone,

Pref$(b, c, \theta) = \{\boldsymbol{w} : w_b/w_{b+1} \geq \theta\}$ at $\boldsymbol{w}^* = w \cdot (\theta, \ldots, \theta, 1, \ldots 1)$ for any positive constant w. Then

$$P_{\boldsymbol{w}}\{correct\ selection\} \geq \theta^{db} \Big/ \sum_{i=0}^{b \wedge (c-b)} \binom{b}{i} \binom{c-b}{i} \theta^{d(b-i)}.$$

It follows that we can choose a value of d depending only on b, c, θ, and P^*, say $d = d(b, c, \theta, P^*)$, such that the right-hand side of the inequality is at least P^* for any given P^* satisfying $\binom{c}{b}^{-1} < P^* < 1$. We exclude the trivial case $P^* = \binom{c}{b}^{-1}$ since no formal procedure is needed to achieve that lax goal.

Levin and Leu (2013) demonstrate that the lower bound formula holds in fact for each *adaptive* member of the LRL family of sequential subset selection procedures for any number of treatments $c \leq 7$ and numerical evidence strongly supports the conjecture that the inequality holds in complete generality as it does for the non-adaptive procedure $\mathcal{N}$.

Acceptable Subset Selection for LRL Procedures

An analogous lower bound formula holds for the probability of selecting θ-acceptable subsets with LRL procedure $\mathcal{N}$. One simply replaces the term $(w_1 \cdots w_b)^d$ in the numerator of the lower bound for *PCS* with a sum of analogous terms corresponding to each type of θ-acceptable subset. Numerical evidence further suggests that this more general lower bound formula holds for *each* adaptive member of the LRL family. Using the lower bound formula, Leu and Levin (2008b) proved a key result, namely, that for any $1 \leq b < c$, any given design odds ratio $\theta > 1$, and any given probability P^* with $\binom{c}{b}^{-1} < P* < 1$ the LRL procedure $\mathcal{N}$ selects θ-acceptable subsets with probability at least P^* *for any and all true success probabilities.* Thus we can say that the LRL family of subset selection procedures has the *acceptable subset selection* property mentioned in section "Acceptable Subset Selection." See Leu and Levin (2008b) and Levin and Leu (2016) for further details.

Other operating characteristics for LRL subset selection procedures such as the expected number of rounds (number of vectors), $E_{\mathbf{w}}[N_{\mathcal{N}}(r, b, c)]$, expected total number of tosses (sample size), expected number of failures, etc., are typically obtained via simulation.

Random Subset Size Selection with LRL Procedures

An extension of the LRL family of subset selection procedures provides for random subset size selection. Briefly, one simultaneously monitors the accumulating response tallies with *each* of the fixed subset size reference criteria d, say d_b, in LRL procedure $\mathcal{N}$ for $b = 1,\ldots,c-1$. (The various d_b criteria need not be equal.) The first time any stopping criterion is met – that is, the first time $r_b^{[n]} - r_{b+1}^{[n]} \geq d_b$ for some b – we select the subset of b treatments with the largest response tallies. If two or more criteria are simultaneously met, we select the subset with the smallest size. Because the first separation between tallies to meet its corresponding criterion is not predetermined, the resulting selected subset has a random size. Constraints may be imposed on the size of the final selected subset as follows. At the time the first d_b criterion is met, if the size of the subset that would be selected exceeds an upper constraint, sampling continues only among treatments in that subset, i.e., the other treatments are eliminated, and monitoring continues for the next separation in response tallies among that subset, and so on, until the final selected subset size meets the upper constraint. On the other hand, if the size of subset at the first criterion separation is smaller than a lower constraint, the subset is "recruited" and sampling resumes with the remaining treatments monitoring for additional best treatments, and so on, until all constraints are met. Thus subsets of random size can still be selected with the adaptive features of elimination and recruitment. Leu and Levin (2017) provide further details and they show that the LRL family of procedures extended to random subset sizes continues to provide for acceptable subset selection.

Other Designs

Often times randomized selection designs appear as a preliminary stage in larger studies, such as in adaptive phase III RCTs with a preliminary selection stage. A distinguishing feature of such studies is the simultaneous use of the data from the preliminary selection stage *together with* the subsequent efficacy data from the larger trial (as opposed to using a pure selection design first, followed by a completely independent subsequent phase III trial, such as contemplated above). We refer to such applications as a *preliminary selection design* in the sense that the primary purpose of such trials is that of the confirmatory phase III study, i.e., to test a null hypothesis of no efficacy (even with the preferred treatment in the selection stage) with traditional control of the type 1 error rate, whereas the early-stage selection feature is of secondary interest, used for the sake of seamless efficiency leading into the larger study. Because such preliminary selection typically introduces some degree of *selection bias* in the final evaluation of all the data, special statistical adjustments must be made to account for that bias. For example, if the null hypothesis were true, one would be capitalizing purely on chance by selecting the treatment with the apparently best performance, thereby introducing a selection bias when comparing that treatment to a placebo control. We shall not discuss preliminary selection designs further here except to note some examples of such methods: see Stallard and Todd (2003), Stallard and Friede (2008), Levy et al. (2006), Kaufmann et al. (2009), Levin et al. (2011), and the various methods used in adaptive trial design (see, e.g., Coffey et al. 2012, and references cited therein).

A sequential selection design featuring a response-adaptive randomized play-the-winner rule with sequential elimination of inferior treatments was studied by Coad and Ivanova (2005). They show a desirable savings in total sample size compared with fixed sample size procedures together with a palpable increase in the proportion of patients allocated to the superior treatment. They demonstrate the practical benefits of their procedure using a three-treatment lung cancer study and argue that these benefits extend also to dose-finding studies. The same authors also studied the selection bias involved in the maximum likelihood estimators of the success probabilities after the trial stops, using a key identity between the bias and the expected reciprocal stopping time; see Coad and Ivanova (2001).

A novel design called the *comparative selection design* was introduced by Leu et al. (2011) which combines features of a pure selection design with a hypothesis test. One supposes there are one or more active candidate treatments and one or more placebo or other control arms (such as an attention control group or best available standard of care). The primary goal is to *test* the null hypothesis that there does not exist a *better-than-placebo* (BTP) subset of active treatments against the alternative that there does exist a BTP subset of active treatments; *and,* if the null hypothesis is rejected in favor of the alternative, to *select* one such BTP subset of active treatments. The type 1 error rate may be controlled at conventional levels of statistical significance and the probability of *correctly* selecting a BTP subset of active treatments can be made arbitrarily high given a sufficiently wide separation between the efficacy of the BTP active treatments and that of the placebo or other control arms. We refer the reader to Leu et al. (2011) for further details of the comparative selection design.

While we have focused exclusively on randomized selection designs with binary outcomes in this chapter, a selection design has also been proposed for time-to-event outcomes. We refer the reader to Liu et al. (1993) for further details and to Herbst et al. (2010) for an application of the design to evaluate concurrent chemotherapy with Cetuximab versus chemotherapy followed by Cetuximab in patients with lung cancer.

Applications of Randomized Selection Designs

Though randomized selection designs have much to offer, they have seldom been applied in practice. Here we provide two examples of trials using such designs.

The first example is a recently published paper by Lustberg et al. (2010). The study evaluated two schedules of the combination of mitomycin and irinotecan in patients with esophageal and gastroesophageal adenocarcinoma with the goal of selecting the most promising schedule. Patients were randomized (1:1) to either 6 mg/m^2 mitomycin C on day 1 and 125 mg/m^2 irinotecan on days 2 and 9 or 3 mg/m^2 mitomycin C on days 1 and 8 and 125 mg/m^2 irinotecan on days 2 and 9. The Simon two-stage design was used to prescreen the treatments with the primary outcome being response to treatment. Each treatment arm was designed to detect a 20% difference with an alpha of 0.10 and a beta of 0.10 assuming response rates of $\leq$30% under the null and $\geq$ 50% under the alternative hypothesis. This required enrolling 28 patients in the first stage of the Simon two-stage design. If 8 or more responded then an additional 11 patients would be enrolled for a total of 39 patients per arm. Treatment(s) with 16 or more responders would be considered worthy of further evaluation and the SWE procedure would be used to select the most promising one.

Prescreening with Simon's two-stage design followed by an application of the SWE procedure can be considered as an overall selection procedure. Though the probability of passing the screening step with Simon's two-stage procedure is 0.900 in the example at the design alternative of a 50% response rate, the overall *PCS* is only 0.888 for $c = 2$ treatments assuming the inferior treatment has a response rate of 30%. This is because there is a non-negligible chance the inferior treatment will pass the Simon prescreen (with probability 0.094) followed by a small chance that its response tally will actually exceed (or equal) that of the better treatment, leading to an incorrect selection (or a 50% chance of an incorrect selection in the case of a tie). As the response rate of the inferior treatment approaches that of the superior treatment, the *PCS* decreases. For example, with a 35% response rate, the overall *PCS* is 0.855 and with a 40% response rate, the overall *PCS* falls to 0.780.

In the conduct of the actual study, only 6 mg/m^2 mitomycin C on day 1 and 125 mg/m^2 irinotecan on days 2 and 9 passed the screening and was considered worthy for further evaluation. Thus, selection of the most promising treatment was not needed.

The second example is a randomized selection trial the present authors designed using the Levin-Robbins-Leu selection procedures. This study is currently enrolling patients at Columbia University Irving Medical Center to evaluate three types of garments (gloves and socks) for the prevention of taxane-induced peripheral neuropathy, with the goal of selecting the most promising intervention and evaluating it in a large randomized controlled clinical trial. Breast-cancer patients are being randomized in triplets to cryotherapy (cold garments), compression therapy (tight-fitting garments), or placebo (loose garments) with stratification for the chemotherapy schedule. Previous smaller studies have shown that both cryotherapy and compression may be efficacious at preventing taxane-induced peripheral neuropathy.

A “response” is defined as a change from baseline to 12 weeks of less than 5 points in the FACT NTX, a patient self-reported scale of neuropathy symptoms. Though the selection could have been conducted without the placebo arm, it was included in the trial because the investigators were interested in obtaining preliminary effect size estimates for future studies with this unmasked, self-reported endpoint.

The trial uses LRL procedure $\mathcal{E}/\mathcal{R}$ with $c = 3$ and $b = 1$. In this case the trial will stop the first time two intervention arms have been eliminated and the leading arm is recruited. The criterion for elimination of an intervention is defined as a difference of 4 between the currently greatest and smallest response tallies. If and when one arm is eliminated, patients are randomized in pairs to the remaining interventions. If at any time two arms should happen to be tied with 4 fewer responses than the intervention currently in the lead, then both trailing interventions are eliminated at that time. Once the second elimination criterion is reached, the remaining intervention with the largest response tally is selected as the preferred intervention. The trial design modifies the original LRL procedure in two ways. First, sequential monitoring will begin only once 45 patients in 15 triplets have been enrolled. This minimum enrollment requirement will provide unbiased estimates of response proportions for the three arms uncomplicated by selection effects. Second, the trial will be stopped if the second elimination does not occur at or before 100 outcomes have been observed, thus converting the “open” LRL procedure to a “closed” procedure by truncation. If the trial stops by truncation, the intervention with the largest response tally among the remaining competitors is selected. If there are ties for the largest tally at time of truncation, one intervention is selected according to other considerations (safety, ease of compliance, etc.).

The elimination criterion of a lead of 4 between largest and smallest response tallies and the maximum sample size of 100 patients were chosen to achieve a *PCS* of at least 80% for any true success probabilities lying in the *preference zone* characterized by an odds ratio of 2.0 or greater between the true response probabilities of the best two interventions. Based on published studies evaluating the interventions of interest, we assumed a success rate of 79%. Moreover, experience suggests a 40% response rate for the control arm is plausible. Five scenarios were evaluated based on these rates. The first scenario corresponds to response probabilities in the *least favorable configuration* in the preference zone with an odds ratio of 2.0 (79%, 65%, and 65)%. The second scenario corresponds to the abovementioned design alternative based on the observed rates from previously conducted studies (79%, 65% and 40%). The third and fourth scenarios describe the operating characteristics of the selection procedure inside the indifference zone, assuming smaller differences in the response rates for the two interventions. The third scenario assumes that both interventions are superior to the placebo with a smaller difference between them (such that the odds ratio between the best and second-best intervention is less than 2.0); the response rates are 0.75, 0.65, 0.40. The fourth scenario assumes that both interventions are superior to the placebo with no difference between them (an odds ratio of 1.0); the response rates are 0.65, 0.65, 0.40. The fifth scenario illustrates a case where there is no true difference in the rates for all three arms, that is all interventions have a response rate of 0.65.

Table 1 Operating characteristics of the selection procedure for peripheral neuropathy prevention

	Scenario 1	Scenario 2	Scenario 3	Scenario 4	Scenario 5
	(0.79, 0.65, 0.65)	**(0.79, 0.65, 0.40)**	**(0.75, 0.65, 0.40)**	**(0.65, 0.65, 0.40)**	**(0.65, 0.65, 0.65)**
$P[cs]$	0.838	0.912	0.831	0.498	0.336
$P[as]$	0.838	0.912	0.999	0.997	1.00
$P[N = 45]$	0.134	0.272	0.214	0.153	0.075
$P[trunc]$	0.303	0.163	0.231	0.324	0.489
$P[N < 60]$	0.322	0.514	0.435	0.343	0.201
$P[N < 80]$	0.534	0.719	0.638	0.537	0.362
Mean N	75.2	65.7	69.8	74.8	83.1
Med N	76	59	65	75	99

$P[cs]$ is the probability of correct selection overall
$P[as]$ is the probability of an acceptable selection overall
$P[N = 45]$ is the probability of reaching a decision after exactly 45 patients have been randomized
P[trunc] is the probability that the trial will be truncated before the second elimination time
$P[N < 60]$ is the probability that the total number of patients will be less than 60 at stopping
$P[N < 80]$ is the probability that the total number of patients will be less than 80 at stopping
Mean N is the mean of the distribution of the (random) total number of patients
Median N is the median of the distribution of the total number of patients

The operating characteristics of the design shown in Table 1 below were evaluated by simulation studies using 100,000 replications per scenario. The characteristics evaluated were the *PCS*, the probability of an acceptable selection, the probability of stopping at the first look with $N = 45$ patients, the probability of truncation at $N = 100$ patients, the probability of the trial concluding with a sample size below 60 or below 80 (to assess accrual feasibility), and the mean and median sample size.

At the end of the trial the sample proportion of patients with a change in FACT NTX < 5 from baseline to week 12 will be reported for each arm. Additionally, the likelihood of the response tallies for the intervention selected together with the first runner-up will be calculated. This likelihood is given by

$$L\left(p_i, p_j \middle| r_i^{(n)}, r_j^{(n)}\right) = p_i^{r_i^{(n)}} (1 - p_i)^{n - r_i^{(n)}} p_j^{r_j^{(n)}} (1 - p_j)^{n - r_j^{(n)}},$$

where $r_i^{(n)}$ and $r_j^{(n)}$ are the observed tallies for the selected and first runner-up intervention and where p_i and p_j are the respective true response probabilities. The likelihood of the observed response tallies will also be calculated under the assumption that we erred in our selection and that the true probabilities are those for the two interventions *transposed,* namely, $L\left(p_j, p_i \middle| r_i^{(n)}, r_j^{(n)}\right)$. The *likelihood ratio,* or *LR,* is the ratio of these two likelihoods. It can be shown that LR equals the true odds ratio raised to the fourth power,

$$LR = \frac{L\left(p_i, p_j | r_i^{(n)}, r_j^{(n)}\right)}{L\left(p_j, p_i | r_i^{(n)}, r_j^{(n)}\right)} = \left\{\frac{p_i/(1-p_i)}{p_j/(1-p_j)}\right\}^4,$$

in the case where the trial ends meeting the selection criterion. In the case of truncation, the exponent 4 is replaced by $r_i^{(n)} - r_j^{(n)}$. LR will be evaluated at the adjusted sample proportions of p_i and p_j, namely, $\left(r_i^{(n)} + 0.5\right)/(n+1)$ and $\left(r_j^{(n)} + 0.5\right)/(n+1)$, respectively.

The likelihood ratio is an important measure of the weight of evidence in favor of a correct selection after the trial concludes (see, e.g., Royall 1997 and 2000). For example, it indicates strong evidence of correct selection if $LR > 10$ or only weak evidence if it is near 1, and if the *placebo* arm should actually be the selected intervention arm, there would presumably be either weak or even strong evidence *against* either active intervention being the best. Thus the LR will play a crucial role in deciding whether or not to mount a subsequent phase III trial.

Discussion and Conclusion

We began this chapter with the somewhat provocative assertion that not every clinical research problem can – nor should – be addressed with a study design that tests a null hypothesis of no treatment differences while controlling the type 1 error rate to conventional levels such as 0.01, 0.05, or 0.10. Selection problems, addressed by randomized selection trials, are prime examples. While a pure selection design can always be viewed as a multiple decision procedure that tests the null hypothesis of no difference which rejects that hypothesis when one selects the best performing treatment, this view misses the point, which is that when the goal is to select a best treatment, one really doesn't care about the null hypothesis. Indeed, the reason pure selection designs can achieve good PCS (a.k.a. "power" in the hypothesis test context) with smaller sample sizes than conventional phase III designs is exactly because selection trials control the type 1 error rate only at level $\alpha = 1/c$ (or $\binom{c}{b}^{-1}$ for selecting subsets of size b). Pure selection trials are precisely the right tool for the job when a choice between competing alternatives must be made with no negative consequences if the treatments are all of equal efficacy.

Some authors have raised concerns with the use of randomized selection designs in clinical research apart from the hypothesis testing issue; see, e.g., Rubinstein et al. (2009), echoed by Green et al. (2016). Referring to the original SWE design, Rubinstein et al. (2009, p.1886) write,

> The weakness in the original design is that it does not assure that the (sometimes nominally) superior experimental regimen is superior to standard therapy. It was occasionally argued that an ineffective experimental regimen could act as a control arm for the other regimen, but the design was not constructed to be used in this way, since, as designed, one of the two experimental regimens would always be chosen to go forward, even if neither was superior to standard treatment.

To address this concern the authors suggest prescreeing the candidates with Simon's two-stage design, citing Liu et al. (2006). The concern presumes, of course, that standard therapy is not one of the treatments considered for selection. Apart from potential problems with the rate of accrual, there is no intrinsic reason why standard treatment cannot be included among those to be studied in a selection trial, and this option should be carefully considered in the planning stages of the trial. The concern largely evaporates when standard treatments are included.

Whether or not standard treatment is included among the candidates, the stated concern does raise an important question: If one is to give up on statements of statistical significance in the selection paradigm, what then can be said about the quality of the selected treatment(s) based on the accumulated data, a question that will inevitably be asked once the trial ends? We believe that an assessment of the *weight of evidence* using likelihood ratio methodology is perhaps the most appropriate answer, such as was illustrated in the peripheral neuropathy selection trial discussed in section "Applications of Randomized Selection Designs." This approach is not only reasonable insofar as it addresses the right question – How strong is the evidence in favor of having selected the truly best treatment? – it also accords with the current trend away from too-heavy reliance on null hypothesis significance testing and p-values. Weight-of-evidence considerations are especially germane if standard treatment is included among the candidate treatments, but even if not, likelihood ratios against historical control parameters can be quite illuminating.

Such weight-of-evidence considerations complement the more traditional frequentist response to the concern that (a) one has *high confidence* P^* that the selected treatments are acceptable because we use a procedure that has such an operating characteristic (though acknowledging that that does not pertain to any *particular* trial result); and (b) a descriptive review of the maximum likelihood estimates of the treatment response probabilities, possibly together with an estimate of the selection bias adhering thereto following the methods of Coad and Ivanova (2001), can be revealing.

Nevertheless, we suspect some researchers will be unable to overcome the reflex to test some hypothesis, in which case the preliminary selection design or the comparative selection trial mentioned in section "Other Designs" may hold appeal. With the former design, a confirmatory phase III trial ultimately assesses the efficacy of the selected treatment against a control treatment. With the latter design, given several active treatments and possibly several control treatments, it seems quite natural to test whether there is a better-than-placebo active treatment (or a subset of them) and even more reasonable to then wish to correctly identify it (or them) with a high probability of correct (or acceptable) selection.

Finally, in this chapter we have focused on the LRL family of sequential subset selection procedures because we believe its flexibility, adaptive features, and acceptable subset selection property make it an attractive option for randomized selection trials.

References

Bechhofer RE (1954) A single-sample multiple decision procedure for ranking means of normal populations with known variances. Ann Math Stat 25:16–39

Bechhofer RE, Kiefer J, Sobel M (1968) Sequential identication and ranking procedures. University of Chicago Press, Chicago

Bechhofer RE, Santner TJ, Goldsman DM (1995) *Design and analysis of* experiments for statistical selection, screening, and multiple comparisons. Wiley, New York

Caplan A, Plunkett C, Levin B (2015a) Selecting the right tool for the job (invited paper). Am J Bioeth 15(4):4–10. (with open peer commentaries, pp. 33-50)

Caplan A, Plunkett C, Levin B (2015b) The perfect must not overwhelm the good: response to open peer commentaries on "selecting the right tool for the job". Am J Bioeth 15(4):W8–W10

Coad DS, Ivanova A (2001) Bias calculations for adaptive urn designs. Seq Anal 20:91–116

Coad DS, Ivanova A (2005) Sequential urn designs with elimination for comparing $K \geq 3$ treatments. Stat Med 24:1995–2009

Coffey CS, Levin B, Clark C, Timmerman C, Wittes J, Gilbert P, Harris S (2012) Overview, hurdles, and future work in adaptive designs: perspectives from an NIH-funded workshop. Clin Trials 9 (6):671–680

Gibbons JD, Olkin I, Sobel M (1977) Selecting and ordering populations: a new statistical methodology. Wiley, New York

Green S, Benedetti J, Smith A, Crowley J (2016) Clinical trials in oncology, 3rd edn. Chapman and Hall/CRC Press, Boca Raton

Gupta SS (1956) On a decision rule for a problem in ranking means, *mimeograph series 150, Institute of Statistics*. University of North Carolina, Chapel Hill

Gupta SS (1965) On some multiple decision (selection and ranking) rules. Technometrics 7:225–245

Herbst RS, Kelly K, Chansky K, Mack PC, Franklin WA, Hirsch FR, Atkins JN, Dakhil SR, Albain KS, Kim ES, Redman M, Crowley JJ, Gandara DR (2010) Phase II selection design trial of concurrent chemotherapy and cetuximab versus chemotherapy followed by cetuximab in advanced-stage non-small-cell lung cancer: Southwest Oncology Group study S0342. J Clin Oncol 28(31):4747–4754

Kaufmann P, Thompson JLP, Levy G, Buchsbaum R, Shefner J, Krivickas LS, Katz J, Rollins Y, Barohn RJ, Jackson CE, Tiryaki E, Lomen-Hoerth C, Armon C, Tandan R, Rudnicki SA, Rezania K, Sufit R, Pestronk A, Novella SP, Heiman-Patterson T, Kasarskis EJ, Pioro EP, Montes J, Arbing R, Vecchio D, Barsdorf A, Mitsumoto H, Levin B, for the QALS Study Group (2009) Phase II trial of CoQ10 for ALS finds insufficient evidence to justify phase III. Ann Neurol 66:235–244

Leu C-S, Levin B (2008a) A generalization of the Levin-Robbins procedure for binomial subset selection and recruitment problems. Stat Sin 18:203–218

Leu C-S, Levin B (2008b) On a conjecture of Bechhofer, Kiefer, and Sobel for the Levin-Robbins-Leu binomial subset selection procedures. Seq Anal 27:106–125

Leu C-S, Levin B (2017) Adaptive sequential selection procedures with random subset sizes. Seq Anal 36(3):384–396

Leu C-S, Cheung Y-K, Levin B (2011) Chapter 15, Subset selection in comparative selection trials. In Bhattacharjee M, Dhar SK, Subramanian S (eds) Recent advances in biostatistics: false discovery, survival analysis, and other topics. Series in biostatistics 4:271–288. World Scientific

Levin B, Leu C-S (2013) On an inequality that implies the lower bound formula for the probability of correct selection in the Levin-Robbins-Leu family of sequential binomial subset selection procedures. Seq Anal 32(4):404–427

Levin B, Leu C-S (2016) On lattice event probabilities for Levin-Robbins-Leu subset selection procedures. Seq Anal 35(3):370–386

Levin B, Thompson JLP, Chakraborty B, Levy G, MacArthur RB, Haley EC (2011) Statistical aspects of the TNK-S2B trial of Tenecteplase versus Alteplase in acute ischemic stroke: an efficient, dose-adaptive, seamless phase II/III design. Clin Trials 8:398–407

Levy G, Kaufmann P, Buchsbaum R, Montes J, Barsdorf A, Arbing R, Battista V, Zhou X, Mitsumoto H, Levin B, Thompson JLP (2006) A two-stage design for a phase II clinical trial of coenzyme Q10 in ALS. Neurology 66:660–663

Liu PY, Moon J, LeBlanc M (2006) Phase II selection designs. In: Crowly J, Ankerst DP (eds) Handbook of statistics in clinical oncology, 2nd edn. Chapman and Hall/CRC, Boca Raton, pp 155–164

Liu PY, Dahlberg S, Crowley J (1993) Selection designs for pilot studies based on survival. Biometrics 49:391–398

Lustberg MB, Bekaii-Saab T, Young D et al (2010) Phase II randomized study of two regimens of sequentially administered mitomycin C and irinotecan in patients with unresectable esophageal and gastroesophageal adenocarcinoma. J Thorac Oncol 5:713–718

Royall R (1997) Statistical evidence: a likelihood paradigm. Chapman and Hall, London

Royall R (2000) On the probability of observing misleading statistical evidence. J Am Statist Assoc 95(451):760–768

Rubinstein L, Crowley J, Ivy P, LeBlanc M, Sargent D (2009) Randomized phase II designs. Clin Cancer Res 15(6):1883–1890

Simon R (1989) Optimal two-stage designs for phase II clinical trials. Control Clin Trials 10:1–10

Simon R, Wittes RE, Ellenberg SE (1985) Randomized phase II clinical trials. Cancer Treat Rep 69:1375–1381

Stallard N, Friede T (2008) A group-sequential design for clinical trials with treatment selection. Stat Med 27(29):6209–6227

Stallard N, Todd S (2003) Sequential designs for phase III clinical trials incorporating treatment selection. Stat Med 22(5):689–703

Steinberg SE, Venzon DJ (2002) Early selection in a randomized phase II clinical trial. Stat Med 21:1711–1726

Futility Designs

58

Sharon D. Yeatts and Yuko Y. Palesch

Contents

Abstract

Limited resources require that interventions be evaluated for an efficacy signal in Phase II prior to initiation of large and costly confirmatory Phase III clinical trials. The standard concurrently controlled superiority design is not well-suited for this evaluation. Because the Phase II superiority design is often underpowered to detect clinically meaningful improvements, investigators are left to make subjective decisions in the face of a nonsignificant test result. The futility design reframes the statistical hypothesis in order to discard interventions which do not demonstrate sufficient promise. The alternative hypothesis is that the effect is less

S. D. Yeatts (✉) · Y. Y. Palesch
Data Coordination Unit, Department of Public Health Sciences, Medical University of South Carolina, Charleston, SC, USA
e-mail: yeatts@musc.edu; paleschy@musc.edu

© Springer Nature Switzerland AG 2022

S. Piantadosi, C. L. Meinert (eds.), *Principles and Practice of Clinical Trials*,
https://doi.org/10.1007/978-3-319-52636-2_83

than some minimally worthwhile threshold. In this way, the trial can be appropriately powered to evaluate whether the intervention is worth pursuing in Phase III and thus provides a clear "no go" signal. We briefly describe the superiority design in order to compare and contrast with the futility design. We then describe both the single-arm and concurrently controlled futility designs and present case studies of each. Lastly, we discuss some key considerations related to sample size calculation and interim analysis.

Keywords

Phase II · Futility design · Single-arm futility design · Concurrently controlled futility design · Calibration control

Introduction

Each phase of clinical testing has its own objectives, and the optimal trial design should be tailored to the research question at hand. Phase I trials are typically designed to identify the dose (or range of doses) which has desired properties, usually related to safety, and there is a growing body of statistical literature describing various dose-finding/dose-ranging designs, such as the continuous reassessment method (Garrett-Mayer 2006). In Phase II, the selected doses are evaluated for an efficacy signal, in addition to further assessment of safety. Those with sufficient promise then proceed to a confirmatory evaluation of efficacy in Phase III, for which the randomized controlled clinical trial is generally regarded to be the gold standard.

Sacks et al. (2014) conducted a retrospective evaluation of marketing applications submitted to the US Food and Drug Administration for new molecular entities and found that only 50% were approved on first submission. Similarly, Hwang et al. (2016) found that 54% of 640 novel therapeutics entering confirmatory testing between 1998 and 2008 failed and the failure was related to efficacy in 57% of these. This success rate appears to differ by therapeutic area, and the data is conflicting. Hwang et al. (2016) report a failure rate of nearly 70% in cancer, whereas Sacks et al. (2014) report a first round approval rate of 72% in oncology. Djulbegovic et al. (2008) evaluated 624 Phase III clinical trials completed by the National Cancer Institute cooperative groups between 1955 and 2000 and found that only 30% of randomized comparisons were statistically significant and 29% were inconclusive (defined as "equal chance that standard treatment better than experimental or vice versa"). Among trials evaluating treatments for acute ischemic stroke, Kidwell et al. (2001) reported that 23% were considered positive by the reporting authors, but only 3% yielded a positive response on a prespecified primary endpoint at the typical level of significance of 0.05. Chen and Wang (2016) reviewed 430 drugs considered for the treatment of stroke between 1995 and 2015 and found that 70% were discontinued.

Given the disappointing performance of candidate treatments in Phase III clinical trials, there is a need to better screen therapies prior to the implementation of expensive Phase III clinical trials (Brown et al. 2011; Sacks et al. 2014; Levin 2015). Clinical trial conduct requires extensive resources financially (for research personnel efforts and infrastructure support) and in terms of patients with the condition of interest. The available resources are clearly limited, and properly vetting interventions in Phase II allows the finite resources available to be targeted toward confirming efficacy in those with most promise.

The standard concurrently controlled Phase II trial design is often powered to detect very large effect sizes in order to keep the sample size feasible, and hence, it can be criticized as an underpowered Phase III trial (Levin 2015). Failure to find significance may be the result of inadequate power at effect sizes which are still clinically meaningful. The trial results, then, do not provide a clear "go/no go" signal as to whether the intervention should move forward for confirmatory efficacy testing. Consequently, even when the outcome analysis fails to achieve statistical significance, the standard Phase II design assumes that the intervention will move forward.

Rather than evaluating whether an intervention has sufficient promise, the futility design seeks to discard an intervention which clearly lacks sufficient promise. The statistical implication of this distinction is impactful – the futility design can be appropriately powered to declare futility (and hence provide a clear "no go" signal) when an intervention has little or no effect.

Background

The methodologic basis for the futility design stems from the field of cancer clinical trials. To eliminate ineffective therapies from future development, a single-arm clinical trial would be conducted in order to compare the resulting outcome to some minimally acceptable level (Herson 1979).

In recent years, the futility design has received increased attention, particularly in the field of neurology, as a mechanism to weed out interventions which are not sufficiently promising. The IMS I Investigators (2004) adapted the futility design to the acute ischemic stroke treatment with the single-arm futility trial evaluating the effect of intravenous plus intra-arterial tPA. In 2005, Palesch et al. applied this methodology to six past Phase III trials in ischemic stroke and found that the futility design could have prevented three such trials for which the treatment was ultimately determined to be ineffective. The NINDS NET-PD Investigators used the single-arm futility design to test whether creatine or minocycline (2006), as well as Co-Q10 or GPI-1485 (2007), warranted definitive confirmatory testing for Parkinson disease. Kaufmann et al. (2009) conducted a concurrently controlled, adaptive, two-stage selection and futility design to evaluate the promise of coenzyme Q10 in amyotrophic lateral sclerosis (ALS).

As we have stated previously, the traditional concurrently controlled Phase II clinical trial, designed to evaluate the efficacy signal in a test for superiority, can be criticized as an underpowered Phase III trial. We first briefly review the superiority setting in order to demonstrate this point. We then introduce the single-arm futility design and discuss its advantages and disadvantages. Finally, we describe the concurrently controlled futility design.

Superiority Setting

Consider a two-arm concurrently controlled clinical trial designed to evaluate whether there is a difference between the experimental arm and the control arm in the proportion of subjects with good outcome. Let π represent the true proportion of subjects with good outcome, such that π_{tx} is the good outcome proportion associated with the intervention and π_{ctrl} is the good outcome proportion associated with the control. The null hypothesis states that the treatment effect, defined as the absolute difference in the proportions of subjects with good outcome, is zero, and the alternative hypothesis states that the treatment effect is not zero:

$$H_0 : \pi_{tx} - \pi_{ctrl} = 0$$
$$H_A : \pi_{tx} - \pi_{ctrl} \neq 0$$

A Type I error is the rejection of a true null hypothesis, which here means that the treatment arms are declared different when in fact they are not. The commonly used term "false positive" reflects both the statistical framework and the conclusion about the intervention; the investigators declare a positive finding (a difference between the treatments) when none exists. In the superiority setting, the level of significance, which reflects our willingness to make this error, is typically set at 0.05. The scientific community may be more or less willing to tolerate this error, depending on its consequences. The type, safety profile, and cost of the intervention or other considerations may factor into the general willingness to accept the conclusion that a treatment is efficacious when it is not.

A Type II error is the failure to reject a false null hypothesis, which here means that the statistical test fails to conclude a difference when in fact one exists. Again, the commonly used term "false negative" reflects both the statistical framework and the conclusion about the intervention. The investigators consider the trial to be negative (are unable to declare a difference between the treatments) despite a nonzero treatment effect. The willingness to accept such an error is typically set at 0.2 or less; in other words, the statistical power of the trial is set to 0.8 or greater. Again, the scientific community may be more or less willing to tolerate this error, depending on the same factors as for the Type I error.

In order to justify the criticism of a Phase II superiority design as an underpowered Phase III trial, consider a hypothetical Phase II trial intended to evaluate the efficacy signal associated with a new treatment for intracerebral hemorrhage. As the binomial proportion has maximum variance at 0.5, we assume this to be the control proportion to represent the worst case scenario. A concurrently controlled superiority trial of 300 subjects, 150 in each arm, has 81% power to detect an improvement of 16 percentage points. In stroke, recent confirmatory trials have been designed to detect a minimum clinically relevant difference of 10 percentage points; the design has only

42% power to detect this difference. As a result, there is a high likelihood of a statistically nonsignificant finding, even when a clinically relevant treatment effect exists. One can tweak the design in various ways to improve the power. For example, increasing the level of significance (the alpha level) and testing against a one-sided alternative hypothesis will both improve the power for a given sample size. However, even at a one-sided 0.10 level of significance, this design would have only 68% power to detect a 10% absolute improvement over control. As the statistical test is very likely to be not significant, leading to a failure to reject the null hypothesis of no difference between the groups, it is not clear how the efficacy signal can be reliably evaluated in this way.

Single-Arm Futility Design

In the single-arm futility design, all subjects enrolled are treated with the intervention, in order to compare the outcome against a prespecified reference value. The design is intended to establish whether the outcome on the intervention represents less than some minimally clinically relevant improvement over the prespecified reference value, which would lead us to declare the intervention futile. The alternative hypothesis, then, represents futility, and conversely, the null hypothesis assumes that the intervention is not futile. Let π_{tx} represent the true proportion of subjects with good outcome on the intervention, and let π_0 represent this clinically relevant improvement over the reference; we now refer to this improvement as the futility threshold. The statistical hypotheses are written as shown:

$$H_0 : \pi_{tx} \geq \pi_0$$
$$H_A : \pi_{tx} < \pi_0$$

A Type I error is still the rejection of a true null hypothesis; in the context of futility, this means that the treatment response is declared to be less than the threshold when in fact it is not. The commonly used term "false positive" here reflects the statistical framework but does not well describe our conclusions about the intervention; the investigators declare a negative finding (the intervention is futile) when it is not. The prespecified level of significance should take into account both the consequences of this error and the phase of the study. The consequence, here, is that a useful intervention may be unnecessarily discarded. We want to minimize the chance of abandoning effective therapies, certainly, but the community may be more willing to tolerate a Type I error in the futility context than in the superiority context, where the result of such an error is that patients are unnecessarily exposed to an ineffective therapy. In addition, the sample size associated with Phase II trials is expected to be relatively small, at least in comparison to the confirmatory setting. Balancing these needs, a 0.10 level of significance has been suggested (Tilley et al. 2006). Note that the alternative hypothesis is necessarily one-sided, as we wish to discard only interventions for which the response is less than the threshold, and the level of significance should be allocated as such.

A Type II error is still the failure to reject a false null hypothesis; in the context of futility, this means that the statistical test fails to conclude that the treatment is futile despite a treatment response which is less than the threshold. Again, the commonly used term "false negative" reflects the statistical framework but not our conclusions about the intervention; although the response is less than the specified threshold, the intervention is not declared futile. The consequence is that an ineffective therapy will be moved forward for a definitive efficacy evaluation. As our objective is to discard ineffective therapies, we want to limit the chance of this error; however, because additional testing is required before declaring the intervention efficacious, our tolerance for the Type II error can be greater than that for the Type I error.

There is a great efficiency to this single-arm approach in terms of sample size savings. Let us re-envision the previously described concurrently controlled superiority design as a single-arm futility design. Assume, as before, that the literature suggests a good outcome proportion of 0.5 associated with the control; further assume that 10 percentage points can be assumed to be the minimum worthwhile improvement required to warrant further investigation. The statistical hypothesis, then, is written as shown:

$$\begin{aligned} H_0 &: \pi_{tx} \geq 0.6 \\ H_A &: \pi_{tx} < 0.6 \end{aligned}.$$

Calculating the sample size in order to achieve 80% power for declaring futility when there is no improvement associated with the intervention (i.e., when $\pi_{tx} = 0.5$ under the alternative hypothesis), we find that a total sample size of 110 subjects is required to evaluate futility using a one-sided 0.10 level of significance. This is in stark contrast to the superiority approach, which was underpowered to detect clinically relevant improvements in good outcome with a sample size of 300 subjects.

The advantages to this single-arm approach are self-evident. All subjects will receive the intervention of interest, which may increase a potential participant's willingness to enroll. Perhaps more importantly, the trial can be appropriately powered at what might be considered a typical Phase II sample size. Comparison of the outcome proportion against a fixed value yields very real savings in terms of the sample size. This fixed value can be derived from the literature available on outcomes associated with the control intervention, often referred to as historical control data. Decision-making based on the use of such historical control data is also considered to be the primary drawback of the single-arm approach.

Chalmers et al. (1972) summarized the arguments against randomization, both practical and ethical, but ultimately concluded that randomization is necessary to evaluate efficacy and toxicity, even in the early stages of evaluation. Without a concurrent control, one cannot be sure that the historical response would apply to the enrolled population. Estey and Thall (2003) describe this problem as "treatment-trial" confounding. Clinical management, imaging availability, or outcome ascertainment may have changed over time, thus altering outcomes. Subtle differences in eligibility criteria may result in slightly different populations across trials; such differences in baseline characteristics, whether known or unknown, may impact outcomes. When historical data are used for comparison, the observed effect reflects a combination of these trial-specific effects and the true treatment effect, and the specific contribution of each to the observed effect cannot be determined (Estey and Thall 2003). It has also been suggested that outcome is altered simply because of participation in a trial, a phenomenon sometimes referred to as the Hawthorne effect and sometimes referred to as the placebo effect. Because of these limitations, a concurrently controlled design may be preferred.

Pocock (1976) argues that, if it exists, "acceptable" historical control data should not be ignored and presents a case for formally incorporating both randomized and historical controls and describes the associated statistical inference. His definition of acceptability is based on six conditions related to consistency and comparability of the treatment, eligibility criteria, evaluation, baseline characteristics, investigators, and trial conduct. The historical control data typically available would not meet most of the six conditions.

To address concern over the applicability of the specified reference value in a single-arm design, Herson and Carter (1986) proposed the use of a calibration control, a small group of randomized concurrent controls. The calibration control arm is not directly compared to the intervention arm but used to evaluate the relevance of the historical control data in the current study. The utility of the calibration control arm is demonstrated by the NINDS NET-PD Investigators in the case study below.

Case Study: Creatine and Minocycline in Early Parkinson Disease

A brief summary of a randomized, double-blind, futility trial of creatine and minocycline in early Parkinson disease is provided here. The interested reader is referred to NINDS NET-PD Investigators (2006) for a detailed description of the rationale, methods, and findings. Participants were randomly allocated to either (1) active creatine and placebo minocycline, (2) placebo creatine and active minocycline, or (3) placebo creatine and placebo minocycline. The analysis plan specified that each of the active arms would be evaluated using a single-arm futility design, based on historical control data derived from the Deprenyl and Tocopherol Antioxidant Therapy of Parkinsonism (DATATOP) Trial (The Parkinson Study Group 1989). The placebo arm was included as a calibration control – to confirm the historical control assumptions on which the design was based, not for a direct comparison against the active arms. The primary outcome was the change in the Unified Parkinson's Disease Rating Scale (UPDRS), where an increase represents worsening. The futility threshold was defined as 30% less progression on the UPDRS than the increase (10.65, 95% CI 9.63–11.67) observed in DATATOP (NINDS NET-PD Investigators 2006). As shown, the alternative hypothesis describes futility as a mean (μ) increase (worsening) of more than 7.46 points:

$$H_0 : \mu \leq 7.46$$
$$H_A : \mu > 7.46$$

The single-arm futility analysis was conducted as planned, and there was not sufficient evidence to declare either creatine or minocycline futile. However, the mean change observed in the calibration control arm (8.39) was less than anticipated based on the historical control data (10.65), and as a result, the futility threshold was not consistent with 30% less progression than control. However, the investigators had planned for this possibility during the design phase. A series of prespecified sensitivity analyses were undertaken using the calibration control data to update the historical control response in various ways, and the conclusions were not substantively altered. This example demonstrates the potential concern over evaluating futility using historical control data and highlights the potential utility of a concurrent control, whether for calibration, as described above, or for direct comparison, as introduced below.

Concurrently Controlled Futility Design

In the concurrently controlled futility design, subjects are randomly allocated to either an intervention or a control arm, in order to compare the effect of the intervention against some minimum clinically relevant improvement. Let π_{tx} and π_{ctrl} represent the true proportion of subjects with good outcome on the intervention and control, respectively, and let δ represent the futility threshold, defined as a minimum clinically relevant improvement in outcome. As above, the alternative hypothesis represents futility, and the null hypothesis assumes that the intervention is not futile.

$$H_0 : \pi_{tx} - \pi_{ctrl} \geq \delta$$
$$H_A : \pi_{tx} - \pi_{ctrl} < \delta$$

Again, comparing these hypotheses to those in the standard two-arm superiority design, where the alternative hypothesis is that the two arms differ ($H_A : \pi_{tx} - \pi_{tx} \neq 0$), allows us to evaluate the interpretation of the corresponding statistical errors, their implications, and our willingness to tolerate them. These are as described above in the case of the single-arm futility design.

For comparison purposes, let us revisit, again, the previously described concurrently controlled superiority design as a concurrently controlled futility design. Assume, as before, that experience suggests a good outcome proportion of 0.5 associated with the control; further assume that 10 percentage points can be assumed to be the minimum worthwhile improvement required to warrant further investigation. The statistical hypothesis, then, is written as shown:

$$H_0 : \pi_{tx} - \pi_{ctrl} \geq 0.10$$
$$H_A : \pi_{tx} - \pi_{ctrl} < 0.10$$

Calculating the sample size in order to achieve 80% power for declaring futility when there is no improvement associated with the intervention (i.e., when $\pi_{tx} - \pi_{ctrl} = 0$ under the alternative hypothesis), we find that a total sample size of 451 subjects is required to evaluate futility using a one-sided 0.10 level of significance. Although larger than one might expect for a Phase II trial, this sample size would yield only 57% power to detect an absolute 10% improvement in the two-tailed superiority design and is a dramatic increase over the 110 subjects required for the single-arm futility design. However, the inclusion of a concurrent control group for direct comparison with the intervention avoids the pitfalls associated with the use of historical control data to derive the futility threshold and allows for concurrent estimation of the treatment effect.

Case Study: Deferoxamine in Intracerebral Hemorrhage

A brief summary of the Intracerebral Hemorrhage Deferoxamine (i-DEF) trial is provided here; the interested reader is referred to Selim et al. (2019) for a detailed description of the rationale, methods, and findings. This multicenter, randomized, double-blind, placebo-controlled trial was designed to evaluate whether deferoxamine is futile for the purpose of improving good outcome, defined via modified Rankin Scale score 0–2. A weighted average derived from the available literature suggests a good outcome rate in the control arm of 28%. Recently conducted Phase III trials in this patient population have targeted a minimum clinically important difference of 10%. Noting that effect size estimates in confirmatory trials tend to be smaller than the earlier phase counterparts (potentially due to greater heterogeneity with a larger number of participating clinical sites in Phase III), it was decided that a treatment effect less than 12% in favor of deferoxamine would be considered futile, resulting in the following statistical hypotheses:

$$H_0 : \pi_{tx} - \pi_{ctrl} \geq 0.12$$
$$H_A : \pi_{tx} - \pi_{ctrl} < 0.12$$

In order to evaluate futility with 80% power when the two treatments have the same proportion, using a one-sided 0.10 level of significance, 253 subjects are required. The sample size was inflated to account for loss to follow-up, consent withdrawal, etc., resulting in a maximum sample size of 294 subjects. At the conclusion of the trial, the observed good outcome rate in the control arm was slightly higher than anticipated (34%, vs. the anticipated 28%). The power of the trial to declare futility is affected by the discrepancy between the observed control outcome and the assumed control outcome, particularly in binary outcome studies.

However, the futility threshold is not dependent on the assumed control response, and the statistical test for futility is based on the observed response in both groups. Therefore, the concurrent control approach allows the design to compensate, to some extent, for the drawbacks of the single-arm approach, albeit with a larger sample size.

Analysis

Standard statistical testing procedures can be appropriately modified to reflect the key components of the futility design: the one-sided nature of the alternative hypothesis and the nonzero null value. The futility hypothesis can be analyzed via statistical hypothesis test, with the corresponding one-sided p-value used to support the conclusion. It is important to note, however, that the p-value is often used to describe the level of evidence supporting a difference between two treatments, which would not be a correct interpretation in the futility design. As a result, it may be preferable to conduct the futility evaluation using a one-sided confidence boundary on the treatment effect. This would serve to both provide a consistent reminder of the futility threshold and prevent confusion in interpretation.

Sample Size Considerations

Recall the sample size calculation for comparing two independent proportions in a superiority design. Let $z_{1-\alpha/2}$ and $z_{1-\beta}$ represent the corresponding quantiles from the standard normal distribution. Assume the true control response to be π_{ctrl}, and let π_{tx} be derived from the minimum clinically important improvement (ε) over the assumed control response, such that $\pi_{tx} - \pi_{ctrl} = \varepsilon$. The sample size required to achieve power $(1 - \beta)$, using a two-sided α level of significance, and assuming equal allocation to the treatment arms, is defined according the formula below:

$$n = 2\left(\frac{\left(z_{1-\alpha/2} + z_{1-\beta}\right)^2}{\varepsilon^2}\right)\left(\pi_{ctrl}(1 - \pi_{ctrl}) + \pi_{tx}(1 - \pi_{tx})\right)$$

The sample size calculation for the futility design follows the same algebraic formulation but reflects the key components of the futility design:

1. The level of significance is one-sided, as suggested by the trial objectives.
2. Because the superiority setting generally tests against a null value of 0, a placeholder for the null value is often omitted from the formula. The futility hypothesis, however, tests against a nonzero null value, the futility threshold δ, which must be reflected in the calculation.

Using the same notation as above, and letting δ represent the futility threshold, the sample size required to achieve power $(1-\beta)$ for evaluating the futility hypothesis is defined as shown below:

$$n = 2\left(\frac{\left(z_{1-\alpha}+z_{1-\beta}\right)^2}{\left(\varepsilon-\delta\right)^2}\right)\left(\pi_{ctrl}\left(1-\pi_{ctrl}\right)+\pi_{tx}\left(1-\pi_{tx}\right)\right)$$

Another distinguishing feature of the futility calculation is the effect size for which the trial is powered. In the superiority setting, a trial is designed to achieve adequate power to declare superiority under the assumption that some minimum clinically relevant difference ε exists. In the futility setting, however, a trial is designed to achieve adequate power to declare futility under the assumption that any potential improvement in outcomes is less than an effect which is minimally worthwhile from a clinical perspective. A scenario where there is no improvement associated with treatment, for instance, would be considered truly futile, and so one might assume $\varepsilon = 0$ for the power calculation. One might instead wish to target a scenario where there is a small but clinically uninteresting improvement in outcomes. In either case, the trial would have more than adequate power to declare futility if the treatment decreases good outcomes.

The formulas provided here assume equal allocation to each treatment arm but are easily modified to allow for an unequal allocation ratio.

We previously mentioned that the design parameters of the superiority design could be revised in order to improve operating characteristics. Considering instead a one-sided superiority hypothesis (i.e., $H_A: \pi_{tx} - \pi_{ctrl} > 0$), a total sample size of 451 subjects yields 81% power to detect a 10% absolute improvement under a one-sided 0.10 level of significance. Given that the one-sided superiority design and the futility design have approximately equivalent operating characteristics under consistent assumptions, Levin (2012) argues that the futility approach is more consistent with Phase II objectives and the possible conclusions are more concrete. As described in the table below, the form of the statistical hypothesis has a very real implication for the resulting inference. You may recall from introductory statistics that there are only two plausible hypotheses, and we retain our belief in the null hypothesis, unless the data overwhelmingly contradict it, leading us to believe in the alternative hypothesis. In the one-sided superiority setting, a nonsignificant test result leads to a statement that "there is insufficient evidence to conclude that the intervention is better" and therefore requires that we accept as plausible that the intervention does not have a positive effect. In the futility setting, however, a nonsignificant test result leads to a statement that "there is insufficient evidence to conclude that the treatment effect is less than δ" and allows us to accept as plausible that the effect of the intervention is at least minimally worthwhile. In either case, the confidence interval may be used to evaluate which effect sizes remain plausible based on the available data, but in the futility setting, the decision-making process does not rely on such post hoc evaluations of the resulting confidence interval.

	Superiority setting	Futility setting
Statistical hypotheses	$H_0: \pi_{tx} - \pi_{ctrl} \leq 0$ $H_A: \pi_{tx} - \pi_{ctrl} > 0$	$H_0: \pi_{tx} - \pi_{ctrl} \geq \delta$ $H_A: \pi_{tx} - \pi_{ctrl} < \delta$
Significance evaluated via	p-value $< \alpha$	$(1 - \alpha) * 100\%$ one-sided confidence bound
Non-significant result means that	There is insufficient evidence to conclude that the intervention is better	There is insufficient evidence to conclude that the intervention is futile
Implications for future study	Unclear, given the potential for criticism as an underpowered Phase III trial	Confirmatory efficacy evaluation is warranted to definitively evaluate treatment efficacy

Interim Analysis

Interim analysis for statistical futility is somewhat common in today's funding climate. An interim analysis for statistical futility allows the trial to terminate early if it becomes overwhelmingly clear that the trial cannot accomplish its stated objective. Understandably, the funding agency may want to cut their losses if, during the course of the study, it becomes clear that the null hypothesis is very unlikely to be rejected at the conclusion of the trial (i.e., it is statistically futile to continue). Group sequential monitoring approaches, such as alpha- and beta-spending functions, can be applied to the futility design as well. However, such interim analysis for statistical futility is inherently different than the futility design we have described, and as before, it is important to note that the consequences of such interim analysis depend on the formulation of the statistical hypotheses.

In the superiority setting, an interim analysis for statistical futility allows the trial to terminate if it becomes clear that the trial will not demonstrate a difference between the treatment arms. From both a logistical standpoint and an ethnical one, termination of a superiority trial in the face of statistical futility may be of interest. One would not want to continue randomizing participants to an experimental intervention for which there is little chance of showing a benefit. In the context of the futility design, however, an interim analysis for statistical futility allows the trial to terminate if it becomes clear that the trial will not demonstrate that the intervention is futile. Early termination in this scenario is likely not in the best interest of either the scientific community or the funding agency, as continued enrollment would allow a more precise estimate of both the control response and the treatment effect, as well as a more detailed evaluation of the safety profile of the intervention. For this reason, the remainder of our interim analysis discussion is focused on interim analysis for efficacy.

In the context of the futility design, interim analysis for evidence of "efficacy" would allow the trial to terminate if it became overwhelmingly clear that the intervention is futile. It may be worth terminating the trial early in that case, but the operating characteristics of such an analysis should be evaluated during the study design phase. The usual alpha- and beta-spending functions applicable to superiority designs are also applicable in the context of futility designs, but the function which is considered optimal for superiority may not be so for futility. The O'Brien-Fleming spending function (1979) spends alpha more conservatively than its Pocock counterpart (1977), which means that it is more difficult to terminate under O'Brien-Fleming. This may be desirable in the context of the superiority design, where the consequence of such termination is to declare the intervention efficacious, thereby making it available as a treatment option to the target population. In the context of the futility design, however, one might wish to be more liberal in terms of early stopping, given that the consequence of such termination is to declare that the intervention is not sufficiently promising to warrant further study.

Consider a concurrently controlled futility design, sized at 451 subjects in order to achieve 80% power to declare futility against a 10% absolute improvement, with a prespecified interim analysis to be conducted after 50% of subjects have completed the primary follow-up period. The O'Brien-Fleming boundary would call for termination only if the estimated treatment effect were greater than 3.6 percentage points in the wrong direction (in favor of the control arm); under the alternative hypothesis of no difference between the arms, the trial would have a 30% likelihood of terminating early to declare the intervention futile. The Pocock boundary, on the other hand, would call for termination if the estimated treatment effects were greater than 0.2 percentage points in the wrong direction; under the alternative hypothesis of no difference, the trial would have a 49% likelihood of terminating early to declare the intervention futile.

When considering interim analysis, investigators should be aware that treatment effect estimates can be unstable with small sample sizes and tend to stabilize over time as outcomes accrue. Decision-making in the interim, when the effect estimates may yet be unstable, could lead to termination on a random high or low. Bassler et al. (2010) conducted a systematic review and meta-analysis and concluded that trials which are terminated early for benefit yield biased estimates of treatment effect. Early termination yields a smaller than anticipated sample size and a correspondingly imprecise estimate of the treatment effect. In the superiority design, a precise estimate of the treatment effect is desirable, especially when the intervention is shown to be efficacious. One could argue, however, that concern over the imprecision of the effect estimate can be overcome if there is truly overwhelming evidence of benefit. In the futility design, a precise estimate of the treatment effect may not be as important in the face of a futility declaration.

Protocol Adherence

The occurrence of protocol violations (treatment crossovers, failure to administer intervention correctly, inclusion of ineligible subjects, etc.) tends to dilute the treatment effect. In the superiority design, the result is a movement of the estimate away from the alternative of superiority and toward the null hypothesis; the sample size is often increased in order to compensate for the corresponding reduction in power. In the futility design, the result of this dilution is a movement of the estimate toward the alternative hypothesis. The sample size cannot be increased to compensate for the resulting increase in the Type I error probability. While it is always important to encourage strict adherence to the protocol, investigators should be aware that protocol nonadherence can make a futility declaration more likely.

Sequential Futility Designs

One can easily envision the futility design as a second stage in a sequential early phase trial, following either a dose-finding or dose-selection stage. Levy et al. (2006) developed a two-stage selection and futility design to sequentially select the dose of Coenzyme Q10 and subsequently to evaluate the futility of the selected dose, in ALS. The trial design is briefly described here; the interested reader is referred to Levy et al. (2006) for details. The first (selection) stage was designed and conducted according to statistical selection theory, with the sample size determined in order to yield a high probability that the superior dose would be selected. Subjects were randomly allocated to one of three treatment arms (one of two active doses or a concurrent placebo), and at the conclusion of this stage, the preferred active dose was selected. The second stage was designed and conducted according to the futility design. Subjects were randomly allocated to one of two treatment arms (the active dose selected in the first stage or a concurrent placebo). At the conclusion of the second stage, the futility analysis compared the active dose selected in the first to the concurrent placebo, using the subjects randomized to those arms in both stage 1 and stage 2. Levy et al. (2006) note that a bias is introduced into the final futility evaluation because the best dose was selected in the first stage and that same data are used in the second stage analysis, and their methodology includes an appropriate bias correction.

Summary and Conclusion

The futility design can be used to provide a clear “no go” signal for evaluating whether an intervention shows sufficient promise to warrant confirmatory testing. The single-arm futility design yields dramatic sample size savings, but the need to derive a fixed reference value can be difficult. This drawback can be overcome using either a calibration control or a concurrent control, to directly compare against the intervention. The statistical hypotheses, as stated in the futility design, are more in keeping with the Phase II objective than the hypotheses of the superiority design. Because the alternative hypothesis is used to describe futility, a statistically significant finding indicates that the intervention does not warrant confirmatory efficacy testing, whereas a nonsignificant finding suggests that the intervention should be moved forward for further evaluation.

Key Facts

The phase II trial is often used to evaluate whether an intervention has sufficient efficacy signal to warrant confirmatory testing. The typical design, a superiority design powered to detect large effect sizes, can be criticized as an underpowered Phase III trial. The futility design reverses the statistical hypotheses, in order to weed out interventions which do not warrant further testing. The design provides a clear "no go" signal as to whether an intervention should be moved to Phase III efficacy evaluation.

Cross-References

▶ Middle Development Trials
▶ Randomized Selection Designs
▶ Use of Historical Data in Design

References

Bassler D, Briel M, Montori VM, Lane M, Glasziou P, Zhou Q, Heels-Ansdell D, Walter SD, Guyatt GH, The STOPIT-2 Study Group (2010) Stopping randomized trials early for benefit and estimation of treatment effects: systematic review and meta-regression analysis. J Am Med Assoc 303:1180–1187

Brown SR, Gregory WM, Twelves CJ, Buyse M, Collinson F, Parmar M, Seymour MT, Brown JM (2011) Designing phase II trials in cancer: a systematic review and guidance. Br J Cancer 105:194–199

Chalmers TC, Block JB, Lee S (1972) Controlled studies in clinical cancer research. NEJM 287:75–78

Chen X, Wang K (2016) The fate of medications evaluated for ischemic stroke pharmacotherapy over the period 1995–2015. Acta Pharm Sin B 6:522–530

Djulbegovic B, Kumar A, Soares HP, Hozo I, Bepler G, Clarke M, Bennett CL (2008) Treatment success in cancer: new cancer treatment successes identified in phase 3 randomized controlled trials conducted by the National Cancer Institute-Sponsored Cooperative Oncology Groups, 1955–2006. Arch Intern Med 168(6):632–642

Estey EH, Thall PF (2003) New designs for phase 2 clinical trials. Blood 102:442–448

Garrett-Mayer E (2006) The continual reassessment method for dose-finding studies: a tutorial. Clin Trials 3:57–71

Herson J (1979) Predictive probability early termination plans for phase II clinical trials. Biometrics 35:775–783

Herson J, Carter SK (1986) Calibrated phase II clinical trials in oncology. Stat Med 5:441–447

Hwang TJ, Carpenter D, Lauffenburger JC, Wang B, Franklin JM, Kesselheim AS (2016) Failure of investigational drugs in late-stage clinical development and publication of trial results. JAMA Intern Med 176:1826–1833

IMS Investigators (2004) Combined intravenous and intra-arterial recanalization for acute ischemic stroke: the Interventional Management of Stroke Study. Stroke 35:904–911

Kauffman P, Thompson JL, Levy G, Buchsbaum R, Shefner J, Krivickas LS, Katz J, Rollins Y, Barohn RJ, Jackson CE, Tiryaki E, Lomen-Hoerth C, Armon C, Tandan R, Rudnicki SA, Rezania K, Sufit R, Pestronk A, Novella SP, Heiman-Patterson T, Kasarskis EJ, Pioro EP, Montes J, Arbing R, Vecchio D, Barsdorf A, Mitsumoto H, Levin B, QALS Study Group (2009)

Phase II trial of CoQ10 for ALS finds insufficient evidence to justify phase III. Ann Neurol 66:235–244

Kidwell CS, Liebeskind DS, Starkman S, Saver JL (2001) Trends in acute ischemic stroke trials through the 20th century. Stroke 32:1349–1359

Levin B (2012) Chapter 8: Selection and futility designs. In: Ravina B, Cummings J, McDermott MP, Poole M (eds) Clinical trials in neurology. Cambridge University Press, Cambridge

Levin B (2015) The futility study – progress over the last decade. Contemp Clin Trials 45:69–75

Levy G, Kaufmann P, Buchsbaum R, Montes J, Barsdorf A, Arbing R, Battista V, Zhou X, Mitsumoto H, Levin B, Thompson JLP (2006) A two-stage design for a phase II clinical trial of coenzyme Q10 in ALS. Neurology 66:660–663

NINDS NET-PD Investigators (2006) A randomized, double-blind, futility clinical trial of creatine and minocycline in early Parkinson disease. Neurology 66:664–671

NINDS NET-PD Investigators (2007) A randomized clinical trial of coenzyme Q10 and GPI-1485 in early Parkinson disease. Neurology 68:20–28

O'Brien PC, Fleming TR (1979) A multiple testing procedure for clinical trials. Biometrics 35:549–556

Palesch YY, Tilley BC, Sackett DL, Johnston KC, Woolson R (2005) Applying a phase II futility study design to therapeutic stroke trials. Stroke 36:2410–2414

Parkinson Study Group (1989) Effect of deprenyl on the progression of disability in early Parkinson's disease. N Engl J Med 321:1364–1371

Pocock SJ (1976) The combination of randomized and historical controls in clinical trials. J Chronic Dis 29:175–188

Pocock SJ (1977) Group sequential methods in the design and analysis of clinical trials. Biometrika 64:191–199

Sacks LV, Shamsuddin HH, Yasinskaya YL, Bouri K, Lanthier ML, Sherman RE (2014) Scientific and regulatory reasons for delay and denial of FDA approval of initial applications for new drugs, 2000–2012. JAMA 311:378–384

Selim M, Foster LD, Moy CS, Xi G, Hill MD, Morgenstern LB, Greenberg SM, James ML, Singh V, Clark WM, Norton C, Palesch Y, Yeatts SD, on behalf of the iDEF Investigators (2019) Deferoxamine mesylate in patients with intracerebral haemorrhage (i-DEF): a multicenter, placebo-controlled, randomized, double-blind phase 2 trial. Lancet Neurol 18(5):428–438

Tilley BC, Palesch YY, Kieburtz K, Ravina B, Huang P, Elm JJ, Shannon K, Wooten GF, Tanner CM, Goetz GC, on behalf of the NET-PD Investigators (2006) Optimizing the ongoing search for new treatments for Parkinson disease: using futility designs. Neurology 66:628–633

Interim Analysis in Clinical Trials

59

John A. Kairalla, Rachel Zahigian, and Samuel S. Wu

Contents

Abstract

Modern randomized controlled trials often involve multiple periods of data collection separated by interim analyses, where the accumulated data is analyzed and findings are used to make adjustments to the ongoing trial. Various endpoints can be used to influence these decisions, including primary or surrogate outcome data, safety data, administrative data, and/or new external information. Example uses of interim analyses include deciding if there is evidence that a trial should be stopped early for safety, efficacy, or futility or if the treatment allocation ratios

J. A. Kairalla (✉) · S. S. Wu
University of Florida, Gainesville, FL, USA
e-mail: johnkair@ufl.edu; sw45@ufl.edu

R. Zahigian
Vertex Pharmaceuticals, Boston, MA, USA
e-mail: rachel_zahigian@vrtx.com

© Springer Nature Switzerland AG 2022

S. Piantadosi, C. L. Meinert (eds.), *Principles and Practice of Clinical Trials*,
https://doi.org/10.1007/978-3-319-52636-2_84

should be modified to optimize trial efficiency and better align the risk-benefit ratio. Additionally, a decision could be made to lengthen or shorten a trial based on observed information. To avoid unwanted bias, studies known as adaptive design clinical trials pre-specify these decision rules in the study protocol. Extensive simulation studies are often required during study planning and protocol development in order to characterize operating characteristics and validate testing procedures and parameter estimation. Over time, researchers have gained a better understanding of the strengths and limitations of employing interim analyses in their clinical studies. In particular, with proper planning and conduct, adaptive designs incorporating interim analyses can provide great benefits in flexibility and efficiency. However, an increase in infrastructure for development and planning is needed to successfully implement adaptive designs and interim analyses and allow their potential advantages to be achieved in clinical research.

Keywords

Adaptive design · Early stopping · Flexible design · Futility · Interim analysis · Interim monitoring · Group sequential · Safety monitoring · Nuisance parameter · Sample size

Introduction

This chapter describes the concept of interim analysis (IA, also generally referred to as interim monitoring) in clinical trials and how they are used to enhance and optimize the conduct of clinical studies. A specific focus is placed on the use of interim analyses in a class of clinical trials known as adaptive designs (ADs). The chapter begins with an overview including definitions, a brief history, and motivations. It then describes the type of data used in IAs to inform decision-making and various possible applications. Possible study adjustments based on IA data include sample size re-estimation (SSR), early stopping, safety monitoring, and treatment arm modification. Following descriptions of planning considerations, oversight, and results reporting, various examples are summarized. Discussion topics include highlighting the emergence of Bayesian methodology in clinical trials with IAs and describing some logistical barriers that must be addressed in order for clinical research to benefit from interim decision-making.

Background and Motivation

Evidence of efficacy and safety of new interventions is usually provided through the conduct and analysis of randomized controlled trials (RCTs). Traditionally, RCTs are largely inflexible: many design components such as meaningful treatment effects, outcome variability, patient population, and primary endpoint are specified and fixed before trial enrollment begins. The trial is then sized and conducted with statistical power (such as 80%) and an allowable type I error rate (such as 5% for 2-sided tests) in mind for the given set of study assumptions, with analysis conducted once all of the information has been collected. However, if study assumptions are incorrectly specified, the trial may produce inaccurate or ambiguous results, with significant time and resources largely wasted. Additionally, ignoring accruing safety information during study conduct could lead to important ethical concerns. For these reasons, various forms of IAs are included in many modern trial plans. The US Food and Drug Administration (FDA) defines an IA as "any examination of data obtained from subjects in a trial while that trial is ongoing... [including] ...baseline data, safety outcome data, pharmacokinetic, pharmacodynamic or other biomarker data, or efficacy outcome data" (FDA 2018). The idea of IAs was described in the 1967 Greenberg Report (Heart Special Project Committee 1988), which highlighted the potential benefits to stopping a trial early for efficacy or futility. The Greenberg Report also illustrated the necessity of an independent Data Monitoring Committee (DMC, also known as Data Safety and Monitoring Board or similar) to evaluate interim data and provide recommendations. In a trial with IAs, the information that is collected partway through a trial is used to inform a trial's future in some manner. This added flexibility can be very appealing to researchers, stakeholders and sponsors of the trial, regulatory agencies, and study participants. Accumulating data can inform about efficacy, event rates, variability, accrual rates, protocol violations, dropout rates, and other useful study elements. Using this information, various study decisions can be made, including closing a study for safety, efficacy, or futility, updating intervention allocation ratios, altering treatment dosing and regimens, changing primary endpoints, re-estimating the sample size, or altering the study population of interest.

A well-known fact of repeated testing of hypotheses is a potentially inflated overall type I error rate: each time the data is evaluated, there is an additional chance of making a false-positive conclusion (Armitage et al. 1969). In 1977, Pocock proposed repeated significance testing with equally sized groups of sequentially evaluated subjects using a fixed, but reduced nominal significance level to control the overall type I error rate (Pocock 1977). This began the development and implementation of a popular class of study designs called group sequential methods (GSMs).

An alternative approach comes from the idea of partitioning a trial into distinct stages separated by IAs. Each stage is analyzed separately, and the data is combined using a pre-specified combination function (Bauer and Kohne 1994). This method can be implemented for both ADs and *flexible designs*, which allow for planned or unplanned study modifications between stages, including early stopping, trial extensions, and many other stagewise modifications, without type I error rate inflation (Proschan and Hunsberger 1995).

Adaptive designs (ADs) are an important class of RCTs that incorporate IAs in which accumulating data is used to inform how the study should proceed using only pre-specified modification rules (FDA 2018). A beneficial property of this rules-based approach is that study operating characteristics (e.g., power, type I error rate, expected sample size) can be exhaustively explored under various scenarios before trial implementation by undertaking sensitivity analyses based either on known theory or simulation studies (Kairalla et al. 2012). An implementation of ADs that has experienced much attention and methodological development over the last 30 years is sample size re-estimation (SSR). Most SSR procedures aim to stabilize the study power by updating study planning assumptions using observed data, such as using an interim estimate of the treatment effect (Cui et al. 1999), or modifying the sample size based on an updated *nuisance parameter*: a planning parameter, such as variance, that is not of primary concern but that affects the statistical properties of a study (Wittes and Brittain 1990). SSR procedures may or may not include early stopping features in addition to repowering a trial. Methodological development for ADs as a broad category is significant, and implementation frequency is increasing. Years of statistical development and discussion followed before regulatory guidance documents were released in Europe and the United States (EMA 2007; FDA 2018).

When correctly implemented, IAs can lead to improvements in resource and statistical efficiency since there is potentially a higher chance of correctly detecting a treatment effect if one exists or stopping a trial early to save resources if a conclusion is clear. There are also ethical benefits for early stopping and safety monitoring using IAs. These advantages motivate the remainder of this chapter as they highlight the potential benefits to consider when planning a clinical trial using IAs.

Types of Data Used in Interim Analysis

Non-comparative versus Comparative Data: IAs in RCTs use various types of information to make decisions and inform a trial's conduct. This information can be either non-comparative or comparative: non-comparative information does not reveal treatment assignment in any manner, whereas decisions made using accumulating comparative information involve knowledge of actual or masked (e.g., A vs. B) treatment assignments. While investigator's knowledge of non-comparative information (e.g., accrual rates, pooled variance, or event rates) poses less of a concern to trial integrity, it is also more limited in IA possibilities. Of note, a particular IA can use non-comparative information regardless of whether or not the trial team is masked to treatment assignment (FDA 2018).

Administrative: Various administrative items can be used to inform the decisions made in IAs. These usually consist of non-comparative study elements such as accrual rates or overall event rates. A study team (together with a DMC) could make decisions at interim when faced with administrative data. For example, if the accrual or event rates are lower than expected, the desired statistical power for a given effect size will not be reached in an allotted time frame. In order to increase recruitment, the DMC could suggest relaxing eligibility criteria, closing the trial early, or extending the accrual period.

Nuisance Parameters: In the initial design phase, assumptions must be made about nuisance parameters to properly size a trial. However, at IA periods, one can evaluate the accumulated data and use it to modify initial assumptions. The most common nuisance parameters are estimates of variance in continuous outcome settings and estimates of control group event rates in binary outcome settings. While most methods use comparative information by taking advantage of group assignment (such as using residual variance), non-comparative information can also be used to incorporate nuisance parameter updates (Gould and Shih 1992).

Safety:
If an intervention is not proven to be relatively safe, it will not be approved by the FDA or other regulatory bodies regardless of its efficacy for a given endpoint. Early phase clinical trials have safety endpoints, such as dose-limiting toxicities, as primary outcomes. Confirmatory trials also include safety and adverse event monitoring, with both explicit rules and ad hoc safety considerations taken into account at IAs and at final evaluations.

Study and Surrogate Endpoints: Generally, the main study endpoint in a late-phase RCT is intervention efficacy. Decisions made at IAs often involve comparative outcome data among the different treatment arms. In this case, a decision to terminate a trial is reflected directly in the trial's efficacy outcome, e.g., a study could be stopped if there is significant evidence that a new treatment is superior to standard therapy. A surrogate endpoint is a response variable that is assumed to correlate directly to the primary endpoint. With scientific rationale and research justification, it may be possible to use this surrogate outcome as a short-term substitute for the primary outcome of interest at IAs to reduce study timelines. For example, the minimal residual disease is a quantifiable value of residual blood cancer that is correlated with relapse risk; it has been considered as a possible surrogate for event-free survival, which would require waiting until enough patients have relapses or other events to conduct an IA.

External Information: Information gathered outside of an enrolling trial (e.g., from a similar trial) may alter knowledge of expected study outcomes or safety information. Rather than permanently stopping the ongoing trial, changes can be made at interim periods. Unplanned IAs may result, often with study amendments justifying the changes and resulting statistical properties. In order to maintain validity, it is important that internal comparative data are not considered when making such trial modifications. Some designs (e.g., flexible designs) can handle this naturally by analyzing the sequential cohorts separately.

Applications of Interim Analysis

IAs can be ad hoc in nature (typically requiring an amendment to make study modifications), can use flexible design methodology in a manner not anticipated during study design, or can be incorporated into formal, pre-planned ADs. They are useful in both early phase exploratory studies and late-phase confirmatory studies. While the most traditional application of IAs is study outcome monitoring (including early stopping rules for efficacy and futility), they can also inform valuable safety monitoring and monitoring of administrative data, such as patient enrollment rates. Some general areas for application of IAs are described here.

Flexible Designs: Flexible designs are characterized by having multiple stages and IAs that can be both planned and unplanned. Although flexible design methods have advantages and proponents, according to FDA guidance, unplanned modifications create difficulty with statistical properties and trial interpretations and should be limited to pressing issues such as unexpected toxicity in a particular treatment arm or in response to unexpected outside information (FDA 2018). While statistical approaches to incorporating changes and controlling type I error for flexible designs exist (Proschan and Hunsberger 1995), there are other potential statistical and scientific issues associated with unplanned design changes, including reduced interpretability, inefficiency, and potential violation of principles of statistical inference (Burman and Sonesson 2006).

Adaptive Designs: Brannath et al. state that "Many designs have been suggested which incorporate adaptivity, however, are in no means flexible, since the rule of how the interim data determine the design of the second part of the trial is assumed to be completely specified in advance" (Brannath et al. 2007). ADs are a subset of flexible designs characterized by formal or binding procedures with resulting decisions pre-specified in the study protocol. By adhering to a specified plan, uncertain sources of bias can be avoided. Extensive planning can be undertaken to enumerate and describe study operating characteristics before the study plan is implemented. Elements of the study that should be pre-defined in the study protocol include the number and timing of the planned IAs, the types of adaptations and/or possible stopping scenarios, and the statistical inference methods that will be used to prevent erroneous conclusions (FDA 2018). Of note, although GSMs have a somewhat unique developmental history, they do allow a study to stop early for efficacy or futility according to pre-defined rules, falling under the general definition of ADs. Thus, they are the most widely used and well-known form of AD.

Phases of Study: ADs have gained considerable acceptance in early "learning stage" trial settings, where various information about the characteristics of a drug can be gathered, with less focus on tight control of false-positive probabilities. An AD in an exploratory setting may gather valuable information regarding treatment dosing, safety, pharmacodynamics, and patient response that can be used in future confirmatory studies. For example, investigators can use ADs in exploratory settings to determine the maximum tolerated dose, or the highest dose that is deemed to be safe enough for further research (Garrett-Mayer 2006). In late learning stage designs, ADs have been used in dose-ranging studies to find efficacious doses to pass on to confirmatory phase trials (e.g., see the ASTIN study (Krams et al. 2003)). Using IAs in the exploratory phase can efficiently push promising treatments down the development pipeline in a setting where type I errors are less important, since confirmatory trials are still required.

Adaptive methodology can be applied to confirmatory trials in order to evaluate the safety and efficacy of a particular intervention. Generally, confirmatory trials are held to a higher standard with regard to statistical rigor, and thorough justifications and simulations must be conducted (FDA 2018). Adaptive enrichment designs, sample size re-estimation, and adaptive seamless designs are applications of IAs in a confirmatory setting that will be discussed.

Safety Monitoring: Accumulating data can inform investigators about potential safety concerns of a particular intervention or dose. Adaptations at IAs are often planned with both efficacy and safety in mind. For example, exploratory dose-finding trials have adaptations planned on safety and toxicity. Additionally, in confirmatory trials, interventions will not gain regulatory approval unless they have been shown to have an acceptable risk-benefit ratio. It is necessary in the planning phase to consider the minimum amount of data required in order to obtain sufficient safety information; this must be accounted for when planning GSMs (and other IA plans) that may stop early for efficacy (FDA 2018).

Futility Monitoring: Futility stopping in a RCT is an appealing option that can improve overall clinical research efficiency by stopping a trial when there is statistical evidence that a trial is unlikely to show efficacy if allowed to continue. Futility rules can be binding or nonbinding; as futility stopping does not increase the type I error rate, both can be appropriate so long as they are accounted for transparently in the statistical analysis (FDA 2018). In non-binding cases, results can be summarized and presented with recommendations to the DMC, which makes decisions regarding trial alterations or continuations. One class of futility monitoring rules is based on repeatedly testing the alternative hypothesis at a fixed significance level (such at 0.005) and stopping for futility if the alternative hypothesis is rejected at any point (Anderson and High 2011; Fleming et al. 1984). An alternative approach is stochastic curtailment based on conditional power arguments (Lachin 2005). Here, evidence to stop for futility is based on a low probability of correctly detecting a statistically significant result at the end of the study, given the current data.

Methods of Interim Analysis

Once interim data is collected, it is used to inform trial modifications that can better achieve study goals. Methodological results and analytic descriptions of IAs in RCTs are extensive and will not be comprehensively reviewed here. Additionally, complicated and novel designs are frequently proposed that do not neatly fall into one of the below categories. However, some key design classes are highlighted to summarize the various approaches to using interim data in RCTs.

Non-comparative Designs

IAs using non-comparative data do not include information about masked or unmasked treatment assignment. Trial adaptations in this scenario are based on aggregate data across treatment assignments, and pooled analysis is typically used. These methods are appealing from a regulatory standpoint because decisions made based on non-comparative data have negligible effect on type I error rates. One area of application is in updating nuisance parameter values in SSR designs.

To account for the fact that the pooled variance estimate is not independent of the treatment effect, adjustments are made based on the planned treatment effect (Friede and Kieser 2011; Gould and Shih 1992). Another application of non-comparative ADs is in looking at outcome data (such as event rates) for a particular biomarker group in order to assess and optimize an enrichment strategy (FDA 2018).

Comparative Designs

Adaptations that are made based on comparative data, or data that uses information about treatment assignment, can affect the overall type I error rate more drastically than adaptations based on non-comparative data and thus must be justified and accounted for in statistical methods (FDA 2018). There are many described ADs using comparative data, with some broad classes summarized here.

Group Sequential Methods: GSM clinical trials involve several prospectively planned IAs on sequentially enrolled groups of subjects and involve a decision about whether a trial should stop early based on observed interim treatment outcomes. At an IA, a trial can be stopped for efficacy or futility, and the type I error inflation inherent to repeated uncorrected significance testing is controlled through developed stopping bounds. As mentioned in the "Background and Motivation" section, the first proposed bounds involved a fixed, but adjusted nominal significance level at all testing points (Pocock 1977). Other notable GSM stopping bounds include the popular O'Brien-Fleming bounds that start conservative and become more liberal as a study accrues more information (O'Brien and Fleming 1979) and the more flexible GSMs that utilize α-spending functions to allow for flexible number and timing of analyses (Lan and DeMets 1983). GSMs have ethical and efficiency advantages by reducing expected sample size versus fixed sample designs, as well as versus other forms of IAs such as adaptive combination tests and SSRs (Jennison and Turnbull 2006; Tsiatis and Mehta 2003). However, several issues must be considered during planning and before the decision is made to stop early. For one, when using flexible bounds such as those described by Lan and DeMets (1983), the decision to perform an analysis should be specified by calendar time or fractions of available information rather than influenced by observed trends. Additionally, efficacy stopping should be rule-based and involve transparent reporting that includes the stopping bounds considered at each IA. Finally, it is important to consider how much additional precision, as well as secondary outcome and safety information, is lost by stopping a trial early. To account for this, one approach is to allow the first IA only after a minimum fraction of the planned sample has been evaluated.

Adaptive Combination Tests: In RCTs with IAs, outcomes for independent cohorts of participants can be evaluated across time, with standardized test statistics calculated separately in each cohort. By combining these test statistics in a predetermined way, type I error rate can be controlled regardless of whether or not the trial is following pre-defined adaptation rules (Bauer and Kohne 1994; Proschan and Hunsberger 1995). P-values or independent test statistics from different stages can be combined using techniques such as Fisher's p-value combination criterion or the weighted inverse normal method. In general, results at IAs are inspected, and if there is evidence of significance or futility, the trial may stop early. Otherwise, the study continues to enroll an additional cohort of patients using a possibly modified scenario designed to control the overall type I error rate. The advantage of this approach lies in the flexibility that allows for a variety of planned and unplanned adaptations in addition to early stopping.

Sample Size Re-estimation: When calculating a sample size in the initial design phase, information is required about the desired statistical power and significance threshold, and assumptions must be made regarding the treatment effect and nuisance parameters. To protect a study from incomplete knowledge during planning, the assumptions can be re-evaluated, and the sample size can be re-estimated at IAs in order to ensure that the desired statistical power is achieved. These early phases that inform later stages are often referred to as *internal pilots* when based on inspection of nuisance parameters, such as variance (Wittes and Brittain 1990). In a more controversial application, the SSR can also involve inspection of the treatment effect; if the treatment effect is less than the desired a priori planning value but is still deemed important or promising, the sample size can be increased (Cui et al. 1999; Mehta and Pocock 2011). Some concerns with estimating based on treatment effect include decreased interpretability, lost efficiency, and the risk of not clinically meaningful differences (Proschan 2009). Properly planned GSMs have been shown to have efficiency advantages versus planned and unplanned SSRs (Jennison and Turnbull 2006; Tsiatis and Mehta 2003); however, the rigid maximum sample size limits GSMs in certain situations. Tsiatis proposes updating the maximum sample size at each IA in an adaptive GSM (Tsiatis 2006). Mehta and Pocock showed that the adaptive approach is still beneficial in that the initial sample size commitment is small and additional resources are only asked for if needed (Mehta and Pocock 2011).

Adaptive Randomization: For various reasons, it may be beneficial to modify the allocation ratio in which new study participants are randomized to each treatment arm. As one example, randomization may be *covariate-adaptive*, with allocation ratios changing based on the observed covariate allocations to better achieve covariate balance between treatment groups beyond that achieved by simple randomization. Alternatively, randomization may be *response-adaptive*, where observed treatment outcomes from the data are used to inform how the trial should proceed. In a parallel group setting, this can fulfill an ethical desire to increase the chance of giving patients a superior treatment. By noting that dropping or adding arms is equivalent to adjusting its allocation ratio to zero or nonzero values, response-adaptive randomization strategies can also be used in dose-ranging trials, where the trial initially evaluates several different doses and selects a dose based on comparative data, such as dose-limiting toxicities in early phase studies. *Adaptive platform trials* are a specific example of allocation ratio modifications, where prospectively planned adaptations are used to compare multiple treatment arms to one common control arm, with arms added and removed at IAs. However, these studies have many complexities that could limit their practical benefit (FDA 2018).

Enrichment Designs: A particular treatment may be more effective in a group of people who have a particular biomarker or genetic characteristic. For example, a drug to reduce coronary heart disease may show better results in patients with high baseline blood pressure. Targeting a population with known risk factors is known as *enrichment*. When targeted risk factors are not known at study design, *adaptive enrichment* provides a mechanism for a trial to determine promising subgroup(s) of patients to continue on the trial while minimizing efforts toward non-promising groups. Statistical power for chosen subgroups is increased, and improved precision of undiluted effect sizes can be achieved. Correctly implemented adaptive enrichment studies have the capacity to preserve the overall type I error rate while combining the data across multiple stages (Bhatt and Mehta 2016). However, drawbacks include increased complexity, lack of generalizability of results to subsets not included, and potentially biased treatment effect estimates.

Endpoint Modification: An adaptive endpoint selection design could be considered when there is a high degree of uncertainty about treatment effect sizes on multiple patient outcomes in the design phase. Statistical methods have been developed to avoid multiple testing problems (Hommel 2001). However, changing the primary endpoint may reduce interpretability and complicate the regulatory process (FDA 2018; Proschan 2009). Investigators may also attempt to change their primary hypothesis from one of superiority to non-inferiority in cases where two active treatments are being compared. If this is the case, a non-inferiority margin must be pre-specified before enrollment in order to avoid type I error inflation (Hung et al. 2006).

Adaptive Seamless Designs: Adaptive seamless designs, which combine research phases into a single protocol, allow efficiency gains by reducing the time it would normally take to move between the phases as well as by using information from the early phase in final analysis. Most research focus has been placed on adaptive phase II/III designs (Stallard and Todd 2010); however, early development adaptive seamless designs exist as well. Consider a phase I/IIa design with the first stage focusing on dose-finding and the second stage focusing on safety and efficacy confirmation. The first stage can incorporate multiple doses; at the IA, the arm with the best risk-benefit ratio is chosen for the second stage. Since participants from both stages are used to inform the primary aim (which could introduce bias), adaptive seamless designs can be relatively complex, and caution must be weighed against the potential increased efficiency and reduced study timeline.

Planning Considerations

Limitations: Although ADs with IAs provide many advantages, there are limitations that must be considered. For example, terminating a trial early is appealing to sponsors because it saves money and resources and can result in effective treatments being available more quickly. However, evidence collected from a smaller trial is not as precise or reliable; a larger trial allows for more information to be collected on subgroups as well as secondary endpoints and important safety data.

Studies with ADs, and IAs more generally, are not a cure for inadequate planning; in fact, they generally require much more up-front planning than fixed sample studies. This planning process will likely be lengthier and involve more complicated logistical considerations, offsetting some of the time advantages. The added efficiency and flexibility must justify the increase in study complexity and the accompanying difficulties in interpretability. Derived analytic methods and numeric justifications (e.g., simulations) must be used in ADs to avoid bias and type I error inflation, which may be compromised if unplanned IAs arise. Rigidity of an AD implementation plan is a difficultly in practice for complicated RCTs involving hundreds or thousands of subjects across many sites. Any deviations must be documented and subsequent study properties ascertained as well as possible given the actual procedures followed.

Additionally, timing should be considered when contemplating the usefulness of IAs in RCTs. Designs work best when there is a predictable accrual rate and outcomes are known relatively quickly. If there is a fast accrual and outcomes are not known until years of follow-up are completed, then any advantages of efficiency in the study design will be mitigated by the fact that full enrollment is complete before IA results are known. It is important that the design fits the setting and expected outcome time frames, and the usefulness and feasibility of an IA plan must be carefully considered when comparing potential trial designs in the planning stage (Bhatt and Mehta 2016).

Estimation Bias: Much focus when discussing statistical methods for IAs is on hypotheses testing and control of type I error rate. However, any publication or results reporting when a trial is complete would include information about the observed treatment effect, a figure which will be widely cited for a high-profile study. Biased treatment effects from naïve estimates are a concern for any IA plan, especially those involving early stopping. Large fluctuations of early-stage estimated treatment effects could induce stopping, leading to bias and possible overestimation (Bassler et al. 2010). This is also true for estimation of secondary endpoints that are not involved directly in stopping rules but are correlated with the primary endpoint (FDA 2018). Methods can be incorporated prospectively into a trial plan to adjust for potential estimation bias for some designs, but this is an area of research not as well understood or developed as control of type I error rates (Shimura 2019). The extent of potential bias should be explored methodologically or via simulations, with bias corrections considered and estimates and confidence intervals presented with interpretational caution (FDA 2018; Kimani et al. 2015).

Information Sharing and Operational Bias: Comparative results at IAs during trial conduct should be carefully guarded. However, even revealing study decisions based on comparative interim data to those involved with the conduct or management of a trial can lead to substantial bias and unpredictable trial complications. For example, if a statistical plan is known in detail, and a study design changes in a transparent manner such as increasing the sample size to a particular number, then it may be possible for investigators to speculate, infer, or back-calculate treatment effect results. Among other issues, this could compromise study integrity by affecting enrollment and retention for patients currently enrolled and cause hesitancy with sponsors to further support the trial. To limit this bias, the DMC (or other tasked body who evaluates the interim data) should include statistical expertise and a clear understanding of the specified design being implemented by a team independent from those directly involved with the conduct of the trial (Bhatt and Mehta 2016; FDA 2018). Data coordinating centers are useful in creating separation between those directly conducting a trial on a day-to-day level and those responsible for analyzing and reporting IA findings to the DMC. Additionally, a study could consider reporting the details of AD algorithms somewhere other than a public study protocol, such as in a DMC charter.

Role of Simulations: Often, ADs, despite their pre-specified analysis plan, involve complicated components, with hard-to-discern operating characteristics under possible true conditions, such as treatment effects, event rates, and nuisance parameters. In order to justify the validity and advantages of a design, extensive simulation studies can be conducted. Simulations studies use clinical knowledge, programming, and computing technology to create a virtual clinical trial framework that incorporates all IA rules, including SSR, early stopping, and treatment allocation changes. Simulations can provide information about expected study duration and can quantitate power, expected sample sizes, and potential biases. By conducting a sensitivity analysis, researchers can justify their design and explore optimization of study components such as critical value thresholds and sample sizes (FDA 2018; Pallmann et al. 2018).

Generalizability: After adaptation, the results of a trial may not be generalizable to the original study population. For example, in a trial using enrichment strategies, demographics may change over the course of the study based on selected biomarker groups, and study results may be restricted to a particular subgroup. Additionally, a flexible design with resulting study changes at IA such as sample size, participant entry criteria, and primary study endpoint may lead to stagewise study results that are not similar enough for a broad interpretation of a resulting hypothesis test. Careful consideration is necessary when interpreting study conclusions for trials with IAs (Pallmann et al. 2018).

Oversight and Maintaining Integrity

Protocol: Before conducting a RCT, a study protocol must be developed which outlines the study design and intentions of investigators. Since RCTs involving IAs are generally more complicated than fixed sample or historically well-understood designs such as GSMs, detailed study planning results and study operating characteristics (including simulation results) are reported in a study protocol. This includes rationale and information about the chosen study design, a description of potential IAs and their timing, and appropriate statistical methods. The protocol should outline how statistical validity will be maintained and how bias will be minimized throughout the trial. The FDA, other regulatory body, DMC, and/or study sponsors will review the study protocol and provide suggestions before it is approved and the trial begins enrollment. Depending on study adaptations being considered, there may be agreement for certain details (such as exact SSR procedures) to be excluded from the publicly available protocol and documented separately (e.g., in a DMC charter).

Data Monitoring Committee:
DMCs are comprised of some combination of statisticians, epidemiologists, pharmacists, ethicists, patient advocates, and others who are responsible for overseeing IAs in RCTs (Ellenberg et al. 2003). To maintain trial integrity, it is important that the DMC is both intellectually and financially independent from those conducting and sponsoring the trial. The DMC should ideally be involved in protocol development and approval to insure the entire team is on the same page and that the committee understands the design and their responsibilities. At IAs, the DMC considers participant recruitment and compliance to treatment, intervention safety, quality of study conduct, proper measurement of response, and the primary and secondary outcome results. It is recommended that the DMC is unblinded when they conduct or review IAs and their recommendations should follow the previously agreed upon protocol whenever possible. Interim data should be reviewed for intervention efficacy and safety signals, recruitment rates, and subgroup indications. Open reports containing pooled, aggregate information (such as enrollment rates and serious adverse events) can be shared more broadly, and confidential closed reports with specific efficacy information are generated separately for closed DMC review. The DMC should then pass recommendations to a blinded trial steering committee, whose role is to oversee the trial conduct (Pallmann et al. 2018).

Interactions with the FDA: In addition to reviewing protocol information and study design properties, the FDA often reviews marketing applications that highlight the results of a completed RCT. These can include new drug applications (NDAs) or biologic license applications (BLAs). In an AD setting, the FDA's primary concerns of safety and efficacy are coupled with complicated design components that may not be readily understood without further communication. As a result, applications with ADs are often reviewed with greater scrutiny than nonadaptive designs. As described previously, simulations and other justifications are required to rationalize the advantages of a complicated analysis plan with the chosen study parameters. It is also important that the FDA is able to see that the overall type I error rate is controlled despite repeated IAs. Unless patient safety is at risk, results from IAs in ongoing trials are generally not shared with the FDA until the conclusion of the trial (FDA 2018).

Reporting: In the United States, most RCTs that involve human volunteers are required to be registered through the National Library of Medicine at ClinicalTrials.gov in order to provide transparency and give the public, patients, caregivers, and clinical researchers access to trial information. ClinialTrials.gov is a database that summarizes publicly available information and results for registered domestic and international clinical trials. Additionally, a clinical trial should meet the minimum reporting standards outlined in the CONSORT guideline, last updated in 2010 (Moher et al. 2010). This guideline helps investigators worldwide provide complete, transparent reporting with regard to trial design, participant recruitment, statistical methods, and results. The guideline specifically mentions the necessity of reporting IAs (item 7b), regardless of whether or not pre-specified rules are used in decision-making. It is required for investigators to report how many interim looks the DMC completed along with their purpose and the statistical methods implemented.

Applications and Examples

Group Sequential Trials: Consider the Beta-Blocker Heart Attack Trial (Beta-Blocker Heart Attack Study Group 1981), a large, multicenter, double-blind RCT consisting of patients with recent myocardial infarction. The primary aim was to compare mortality in patients taking the active medication, propranolol, versus a placebo. After the independent DMC determined a clear treatment benefit, the trial was terminated 9 months early. The interim data revealed 7% mortality in the propranolol group (135 deaths), compared to 9.5% mortality in the placebo group (183 deaths). In making their recommendation, the DMC ensured no potential confounding existed due to baseline demographics, study compliance, and unanticipated side effects. They were able to conclude that the outcome was unlikely to change if the study continued and, for ethical reasons, it was appropriate to disseminate the trial information as quickly as possible. The study is notable as one of the first major trials to incorporate relatively new GSM monitoring. The rules, based on O'Brien-Fleming-type stopping bounds, were not originally part of the trial design but were incorporated early in the trial implementation. Other examples of pre-specified GSM trials that stopped early include the Herceptin Adjuvant Trial, designed to test the effect of trastuzumab after adjuvant chemotherapy in those diagnosed with HER2-positive breast cancer, and the EXAMINE trial, which studied the use of alogliptin in patients who were considered to be high risk for cardiovascular disease (Piccart-Gebhart et al. 2005; White et al. 2013). Finally, a GSM design combined with information-based SSR was utilized in a multinational study of vitamin D and chronic kidney disease, termed the PRIMO study. The protocol allowed for interim nuisance parameter estimates to modify uncertain design assumptions, and the interim treatment effect was used to influence efficacy-based decision rules. Ultimately, it was found at IA that no SSR was necessary to achieve at least 85% statistical power (Pritchett et al. 2011).

Changing Hypotheses: The EXAMINE trial had an additional adaptive feature in which the hypothesis to be tested could vary from superiority to non-inferiority. The protocol would have allowed the trial to proceed for additional 100 primary events if, at interim, the probability of detecting superiority, assuming it existed, was above 20%. The IA found that the conditional power was less than 20%, and the study was terminated early, declaring non-inferiority (Bhatt and Mehta 2016; White et al. 2013).

Potential Uncertainty and Bias: Consider the recently completed TOTAL trial which studied thrombectomy as adjuvant to traditional percutaneous coronary intervention (PCI) for ST-segment elevation myocardial infarction (STEMI). At an IA ($n = 2{,}791$), the combined intervention group had an observed lower death rate than those with only PCI (with $p = 0.025$) along with no significant evidence of a difference in stroke occurrence; one could deduce from this information that the combined intervention is advantageous. However, the trial continued to completion ($n = 10{,}064$) and found no significant group-wise difference in death rates ($p = 0.48$). Additionally, 1.2% of the combined intervention group experienced stroke at the end of 1 year, compared to only 0.7% of the PCI only group ($p = 0.015$), highlighting an adverse event that was not evident at interim. Due to the results of this study, thrombus aspiration is no longer recommended in the guidelines to reduce mortality in those with STEMI. If the TOTAL trial had shown an increased early signal and stopped at the IA, the benefits associated with the combined intervention could have been overestimated, and the dangerous association of thrombectomy with stroke may not have been initially exposed (Jolly et al. 2018).

Exploratory Response-Adaptive Design: Consider an adaptive double-blind phase II RCT for patients with bipolar depression testing two interventions using a 2x2 factorial trial design (Savitz et al. 2018). This trial examined the anti-inflammatory effects of the antibiotic minocycline and low-dose aspirin, which is known to quicken the response to SSRIs. After half of the patients were evaluated, an IA was conducted for futility testing. This analysis determined that two of the four intervention groups were diverging and provided the only opportunity for a powered result. Thus, enrollment was adjusted with the remaining participants randomized only to the double intervention group and the double placebo group (while maintaining blinding). Additionally, two of the three primary outcomes were reduced to exploratory outcomes due to evidence of insufficient power. This trial proceeded without pre-specified rules, and the protocol was amended to adjust the design going forward; the trial still maintained some integrity through the blinded nature of the analysis, transparency of design decisions, and the preliminary nature of its findings.

Adaptive Seamless Design: A large phase IIb/III trial was recently conducted to efficiently move a potentially more effective nine-valent human papillomavirus vaccine through clinical development (Chen et al. 2015). In the first phase, 1,240 women were equally randomized to three doses of the new vaccine or to active control (four-valent) vaccine. After an IA examined safety data and immunogenicity (used as a short-term biomarker endpoint), one experimental dose was selected, and subjects who received that dose or the control continued follow-up and contributed to the final analysis. Additional 13,400 women were enrolled in the second phase and randomized to the two continuing arms. By not considering the primary endpoint efficacy of viral infections at the IA, claiming small correlation between immunogenicity and infection rates, and using a conservative analysis technique in the confirmatory stage, the investigators justified the seamless design without complex statistical correction. Despite documented challenges, the study met its efficacy goals while shortening the clinical development time frame for the new vaccine formulation.

Allocation Ratio Modifications: In a two-stage AD RCT examining HIV prevention methods in Malawi, pregnant women attending an antenatal care clinic were instructed to encourage their male partners to participate in HIV testing (Choko et al. 2019). In the first stage, participants were randomized to six groups including standard of care (clinic invitation letter) and five other arms defined by HIV self-testing coupled with different incentives. At the IA, enrollment was discontinued in groups not showing improvement over the standard of care (p-value >0.2); in stage 2, randomized enrollment continued equally for the remaining groups. Results showed that secondary distribution of HIV self-testing increased the number of males being tested for HIV, and with incentives, men were more likely to access care and prevention services.

Sample Size Re-estimation: The CHAMPION PHOENIX trial, which evaluated the effects of cangrelor on ischemic complications of percutaneous coronary intervention, incorporated SSR to adjust the trial if observed relative risks differed from the assumed rates (Leonardi et al. 2012). The IA was performed after 70% of patients had completed a short follow-up. The sample size was to be increased if the DMC found the interim results to be in a "promising zone" (as opposed to being clearly favorable or unfavorable) (Bhatt and Mehta 2016). Ultimately, the sample size was not increased since the results were "favorable" at IA. Another example, the CARISA trial was a double-blind, three-group parallel trial to determine whether ranolazine improves treadmill exercise duration of patients with severe chronic angina (Chaitman et al. 2004). An IA based on an updated standard deviation using aggregate data was scheduled after half of the patients were followed for 12 weeks. This "internal pilot-" based SSR allowed the study to maintain stable statistical power despite incorrect initial assumptions.

Enrichment Designs: In a two-stage adaptive enrichment study to test rizatriptan for the treatment of acute migraines in people aged 6–17, the first stage randomized participants at a 20:1 ratio of placebo to intervention (Ho et al. 2012). To enrich the sample by excluding false responders, any patients who noted a quick improvement in migraine symptoms after the first stage were dropped. Of the remaining non-responders, those who took the active treatment in stage 1 were allocated to placebo in stage 2, whereas those assigned to the placebo in stage 1 were randomized equally to rizatriptan and placebo in stage 2. Ultimately, efficacy of rizatriptan was shown, and the drug is now approved by the FDA for acute migraine treatment in this age group.

Discussion

Two discussion points are worth further consideration: the development and potential of ADs using Bayesian methodology and the evolving need for infrastructure in the implementation of RCTs incorporating novel and complicated IAs.

Bayesian Methods: Statistical methods using the Bayesian framework combine prior information with new information to update posterior distributions of interest. While the use of Bayesian methods in early phase ADs has been accepted for years (Garrett-Mayer 2006), interest in their potential use in confirmatory ADs has ramped up considerably over the last decade (Berry et al. 2010; Brakenhoff et al. 2018). To those in the field, the "learn as you go" nature of ADs seems like a natural fit for Bayesian reasoning. For example, to address the uncertainty associated with estimating nuisance parameters in the design phase, Brakenhoff proposed a Bayesian solution combining prior knowledge with data collected at IA (Brakenhoff et al. 2018). Bayesian methods can be useful for predictive modeling, for dose escalation studies, and when statisticians want to explicitly incorporate results from previous or external trials. Computationally intensive simulations are critical to validating adaptive Bayesian designs and ensuring that statistical operating characteristics are being maintained (FDA 2018). An example comes from a phase II enrichment oncology trial using a hierarchical Bayesian design to examine the benefits of a treatment in the whole study population and subpopulations defined by histologic subtype. The hierarchical component borrows treatment effect information from one group and uses it to influence estimation of the treatment effect for another group, making it more likely to correctly conclude efficacy or futility (Berry et al. 2013). Additionally, the trial allows for early stopping for efficacy or futility based on continuously updated posterior estimates of treatment efficacy.

Infrastructure: Although adaptive and flexible designs with IAs have gained significant popularity in private industry, there are barriers preventing their widespread use in publicly funded research. In order to apply for a grant, extensive simulation studies must have already been conducted in order to verify the validity of the study design in a particular setting. Therefore, sufficient infrastructure and resources must be available before the grant is awarded so that the necessary time can be spent on up-front planning. These issues were discussed among representatives from government, academia, and industry at the Scientific Advances in Adaptive Clinical Trial Designs Workshop in November of 2009 (Coffey et al. 2012). Ultimately, the creation of networks across clinical research helps the infrastructure issue by pooling resources and expertise, increasing the feasibility of complicated trial approval. Examples of these networks include the federal Clinical and Translational Science Award program and the Network for Excellence in Neuroscience Clinical Trials (NeuroNEXT). With sufficient resources and infrastructure, adaptive clinical trial designs with IAs can continue to attain their potential and improve trial efficiency.

Summary and Conclusions

IAs in clinical trials are powerful tools that, when properly employed, greatly benefit clinical efficiency, ethics, and chance of a successful trial. Pre-specified ADs in particular (including GSMs) have the advantage of known possible decisions and enumerated study operating characteristics being available for scrutiny before a trial begins. Flexible designs incorporating unplanned analyses while controlling type I error rate can also be useful when unanticipated situations occur during trial conduct. As design understanding and ease of implementation catch up to methodological development, advanced IA designs will benefit health research and patient outcomes in the decades ahead.

Key Facts

- In randomized controlled trials, interim analyses occur periodically during data accumulation to consider adjustments to the ongoing trial.
- These analyses can allow for greater study flexibility and efficiency by updating design considerations with actual information collected during the trial.
- Adaptive designs are a special class of randomized controlled trials with pre-specification of modification rules, which improve a priori understanding of study operating characteristics.
- Through continued methodological and computational advancements, increased investment in trial infrastructure, and careful planning and implementation, successful interim analyses have increasingly become commonplace in clinical research.

Cross-References

▶ Adaptive Phase II Trials
▶ Bayesian Adaptive Designs for Phase I Trials
▶ Biomarker-Driven Adaptive Phase III Clinical Trials
▶ Data and Safety Monitoring and Reporting
▶ Futility Designs

References

Anderson J, High R (2011) Alternatives to the standard Fleming, Harrington, and O'Brien futility boundary. Clin Trials 8(3):270–276. https://doi.org/10.1177/1740774511401636

Armitage P, McPherson C et al (1969) Repeated significance tests on accumulating data. J R Stat Soc Ser A 132(2):235–244. https://doi.org/10.2307/2343787

Bassler D, Briel M et al (2010) Stopping randomized trials early for benefit and estimation of treatment effects: systematic review and meta-regression analysis. JAMA 303(12):1180–1187. https://doi.org/10.1001/jama.2010.310

Bauer P, Kohne K (1994) Evaluation of experiments with adaptive interim analyses. Biometrics 50 (4):1029–1041. https://doi.org/10.2307/2533441

Berry S, Carlin B et al (2010) Bayesian adaptive methods for clinical trials. CRC Press, Boca Raton

Berry S, Broglio K et al (2013) Bayesian hierarchical modeling of patient subpopulations: efficient designs of Phase II oncology clinical trials. Clin Trials 10(5):720–734. https://doi.org/10.1177/1740774513497539

Beta-Blocker Heart Attack Study Group (1981) The beta-blocker heart attack trial. JAMA 246 (18):2073–2074

Bhatt D, Mehta C (2016) Adaptive designs for clinical trials. N Engl J Med 375(1):65–74. https://doi.org/10.1056/NEJMra1510061

Brakenhoff T, Roes K et al (2018) Bayesian sample size re-estimation using power priors. Stat Methods Med Res. https://doi.org/10.1177/0962280218772315

Brannath W, Koenig F et al (2007) Multiplicity and flexibility in clinical trials. Pharm Stat J Appl Stat Pharm Ind 6(3):205–216. https://doi.org/10.1002/pst.302

Burman C, Sonesson C (2006) Are flexible designs sound? Biometrics 62(3):664–669. https://doi.org/10.1111/j.1541-0420.2006.00626.x
Chaitman B, Pepine C et al (2004) Effects of ranolazine with atenolol, amlodipine, or diltiazem on exercise tolerance and angina frequency in patients with severe chronic angina: a randomized controlled trial. JAMA 291(3):309–316. https://doi.org/10.1001/jama.291.3.309
Chen Y, Gesser R et al (2015) A seamless phase IIb/III adaptive outcome trial: design rationale and implementation challenges. Clin Trials 12(1):84–90. https://doi.org/10.1177/1740774514552110
Choko A, Corbett E et al (2019) HIV self-testing alone or with additional interventions, including financial incentives, and linkage to care or prevention among male partners of antenatal care clinic attendees in Malawi: an adaptive multi-arm, multi-stage cluster randomized trial. PLoS Med 16(1). https://doi.org/10.1371/journal.pmed.1002719
Coffey C, Levin B et al (2012) Overview, hurdles, and future work in adaptive designs: perspectives from a National Institutes of Health-funded workshop. Clin Trials 9(6):671–680. https://doi.org/10.1177/1740774512461859
Cui L, Hung H et al (1999) Modification of sample size in group sequential clinical trials. Biometrics 55(3):853–857. https://doi.org/10.1111/j.0006-341X.1999.00853.x
Ellenberg S, Fleming T et al (eds) (2003) Data monitoring committees in clinical trials: a practical perspective. Wiley, Chichester
European Medicines Agency (2007) Reflection paper on methodological issues in confirmatory clinical trials planned with an adaptive design. Retrieved from http://www.ema.europa.eu
Fleming T, Harrington D et al (1984) Designs for group sequential tests. Control Clin Trials 5(4):349–361. https://doi.org/10.1016/S0197-2456(84)80014-8
Food and Drug Administration (2018) Adaptive designs for clinical trials of drugs and biologics: guidance for industry. Retrieved from https://www.fda.gov
Friede T, Kieser M (2011) Blinded sample size recalculation for clinical trials with normal data and baseline adjusted analysis. Pharm Stat 10(1):8–13. https://doi.org/10.1002/pst.398
Garrett-Mayer E (2006) The continual reassessment method for dose-finding studies: a tutorial. Clin Trials 3(1):57–71. https://doi.org/10.1191/1740774506cn134oa
Gould A, Shih W (1992) Sample size re-estimation without unblinding for normally distributed outcomes with unknown variance. Commun Stat Theory Methods 21(10):2833–2853. https://doi.org/10.1080/03610929208830947
Heart Special Project Committee (1988) Organization, review and administration of cooperative studies (Greenberg report): a report from the Heart Special Project Committee to the National Advisory Council, May 1967. Control Clin Trials 9:137–148
Ho T, Pearlman E et al (2012) Efficacy and tolerability of rizatriptan in pediatric migraineurs: results from a randomized, double-blind, placebo-controlled trial using a novel adaptive enrichment design. Cephalalgia 32(10):750–765. https://doi.org/10.1177/0333102412451358
Hommel G (2001) Adaptive modifications of hypotheses after an interim analysis. Biom J 43(5):581–589. https://doi.org/10.1002/1521-4036(200109)43:5<581::AID-BIMJ581>3.0.CO;2-J
Hung H, O'Neill R et al (2006) A regulatory view on adaptive/flexible clinical trial design. Biometr J 48(4):565–573. https://doi.org/10.1002/bimj.200610229
Jennison C, Turnbull B (2006) Efficient group sequential designs when there are several effect sizes under consideration. Stat Med 25(6):917–932. https://doi.org/10.1002/sim.2251
Jolly S, Gao P et al (2018) Risks of overinterpreting interim data: lessons from the TOTAL trial (thrombectomy with PCI versus PCI alone in patients with STEMI). Circulation 137(2):206–209. https://doi.org/10.1161/CIRCULATIONAHA.117.030656
Kairalla J, Coffey C et al (2012) Adaptive trial designs: a review of barriers and opportunities. Trials 13(1):145. https://doi.org/10.1186/1745-6215-13-145
Kimani P, Todd S et al (2015) Estimation after subpopulation selection in adaptive seamless trials. Stat Med 34(18):2581–2601. https://doi.org/10.1002/sim.6506
Krams M, Lees K et al (2003) Acute stroke therapy by inhibition of neutrophils (ASTIN). Stroke 34(11):2543–2548. https://doi.org/10.1161/01.STR.0000092527.33910.89

Lachin J (2005) A review of methods for futility stopping based on conditional power. Stat Med 24 (18):2747–2764. https://doi.org/10.1002/sim.2151

Lan K, DeMets D (1983) Discrete sequential boundaries for clinical trials. Biometrika 70:659–663. https://doi.org/10.1093/biomet/70.3.659

Leonardi S, Mahaffey K et al (2012) Rationale and design of the Cangrelor versus standard therapy to achieve optimal Management of Platelet Inhibition PHOENIX trial. Am Heart J 163 (5):768–776. https://doi.org/10.1016/j.ahj.2012.02.018

Mehta C, Pocock S (2011) Adaptive increase in sample size when interim results are promising: a practical guide with examples. Stat Med 30(28):3267–3284. https://doi.org/10.1002/sim.4102

Moher D, Hopewell S et al (2010) CONSORT 2010 explanation and elaboration: updated guidelines for reporting parallel group randomised trials. J Clin Epidemiol 63(8):e1–e37. Retrieved from www.consort-statement.org

O'Brien P, Fleming T (1979) A multiple testing procedure for clinical trials. Biometrics 35 (3):549–556. https://doi.org/10.2307/2530245

Pallmann P, Bedding A et al (2018) Adaptive designs in clinical trials: why use them, and how to run and report them. BMC Med 16(1):29. https://doi.org/10.1186/s12916-018-1017-7

Piccart-Gebhart M, Procter M et al (2005) Trastuzumab after adjuvant chemotherapy in HER2-positive breast cancer. N Engl J Med 353(16):1659–1672. https://doi.org/10.1056/NEJMoa052306

Pocock S (1977) Group sequential methods in the design and analysis of clinical trials. Biometrika 64(2):191–199. https://doi.org/10.1093/biomet/64.2.191

Pritchett Y, Jemiai Y et al (2011) The use of group sequential, information-based sample size re-estimation in the design of the PRIMO study of chronic kidney disease. Clin Trials 8 (2):165–174. https://doi.org/10.1177/1740774511399128

Proschan M (2009) Sample size re-estimation in clinical trials. Biometr J 51(2):348–357. https://doi.org/10.1002/bimj.200800266

Proschan M, Hunsberger S (1995) Designed extension of studies based on conditional power. Biometrics 51(4):1315–1324. https://doi.org/10.1016/0197-2456(95)91243-6

Savitz J, Teague T et al (2018) Treatment of bipolar depression with minocycline and/or aspirin: an adaptive, 2× 2 double-blind, randomized, placebo-controlled, phase IIA clinical trial. Transl Psychiatry 8(1):27. https://doi.org/10.1038/s41398-017-0073-7

Shimura M (2019) Reducing overestimation of the treatment effect by interim analysis when designing clinical trials. J Clin Pharm Ther 44(2):243–248. https://doi.org/10.1111/jcpt.12777

Stallard N, Todd S (2010) Seamless phase II/III designs. Stat Methods Med Res 20(6):626–634. https://doi.org/10.1177/0962280210379035

Tsiatis A (2006) Information-based monitoring of clinical trials. Stat Med 25(19):3236–3244. https://doi.org/10.1002/sim.2625

Tsiatis A, Mehta C (2003) On the inefficiency of the adaptive design for monitoring clinical trials. Biometrika 90(2):367–378. https://doi.org/10.1093/biomet/90.2.367

White W, Cannon C et al (2013) Alogliptin after acute coronary syndrome in patients with type 2 diabetes. N Engl J Med 369(14):1327–1335. https://doi.org/10.1056/NEJMoa1305889

Wittes J, Brittain E (1990) The role of internal pilot studies in increasing the efficacy of clinical trials. Stat Med 9(1–2):65–72. https://doi.org/10.1002/sim.4780090113

Part VI

Advanced Topics in Trial Design

Bayesian Adaptive Designs for Phase I Trials

Michael J. Sweeting, Adrian P. Mander, and Graham M. Wheeler

Contents

M. J. Sweeting (✉)
Department of Health Sciences, University of Leicester, Leicester, UK

Department of Public Health and Primary Care, University of Cambridge, Cambridge, UK
e-mail: michael.sweeting@le.ac.uk; mjs212@medschl.cam.ac.uk

A. P. Mander
Centre for Trials Research, Cardiff University, Cardiff, UK
e-mail: ManderA@cardiff.ac.uk

G. M. Wheeler
Imperial Clinical Trials Unit, Imperial College London, London, UK

Cancer Research UK & UCL Cancer Trials Centre, University College London, London, UK
e-mail: graham.wheeler@imperial.ac.uk

© Springer Nature Switzerland AG 2022

S. Piantadosi, C. L. Meinert (eds.), *Principles and Practice of Clinical Trials*,
https://doi.org/10.1007/978-3-319-52636-2_92

Abstract

Phase I trials mark the first experimentation of a new drug or combination of drugs in a human population. The primary aim of a cancer phase I trial is to seek a safe dose or range of doses suitable for phase II experimentation. Bayesian adaptive designs have long been proposed to allow safe dose escalation and dose finding within phase I trials. There are now a vast number of designs proposed for use in phase I trials though widespread application of these designs is still limited. More recent designs have focused on the incorporation of multiple sources of information into dose-finding algorithms to improve trial safety and efficiency. This chapter reviews some of the papers that extend the simple dose-escalation trial design with a binary toxicity outcome. Specifically, the chapter focuses on five key topics: (1) overdose control, (2) use of partial outcome follow-up, (3) grading of toxicity outcomes, (4) incorporation of both toxicity and efficacy information, and (5) dual-agent or dose-scheduling designs. Each extension is illustrated with an example from a real-life trial with reference to freely available software. These extensions open the way to a broader class of phase I trials being conducted, leading to safer and more efficient trials.

Keywords

Dose finding · Dose escalation · Phase I trial design · Toxicity · CRM

Introduction

Phase I trials mark the first experimentation of a new drug in a human population. A primary objective is to identify tolerable doses while ensuring the trial is safe, acknowledging the necessary balance of risk versus benefit for participants. In oncology phase I trials, cytotoxic anticancer drugs may have severe toxicity at high doses, yet at low doses little efficacy is expected from the drug. A goal of such trials is therefore to minimize the number of patients allocated to ineffective or excessively toxic doses, and efficient trial designs are required to achieve this and to meet ethical considerations (Jaki et al. 2013).

Phase I trials are conducted as dose-escalation studies, where the dose of the drug under consideration can be adapted as new patients are sequentially recruited into the trial, using dose and outcome data from previously enrolled patients. Designs are often inherently Bayesian in nature since decisions about dose escalation must be made early in the trial when few or no results are available, and thus prior beliefs of the dose-toxicity relationship (and corresponding uncertainty) are often needed. The key quantity in most phase I dose-escalation trials is the maximum tolerated dose (MTD). This is often defined as the dose that has a probability of dose-limiting toxicity (DLT) that is equal to a prespecified target toxicity limit (TTL), which is commonly chosen in cancer trials to be between 20% and 33% (Le Tourneau et al. 2009). A DLT is defined as a drug-induced toxic effect or severe adverse event that is considered unacceptable due to its severity or irreversibility, thus preventing an increase in the dose of the treatment. This definition of the MTD assumes that there is an underlying continuous dose-toxicity relationship, and is central to most model-based phase I designs. An alternative set of designs, called rule-based designs, define the MTD based on the observed proportion of patients in the trial that experience a DLT at a dose level. These designs are not considered in this chapter.

It has been over 30 years since the seminal publication of the continual reassessment method (CRM) (O'Quigley et al. 1990), which was proposed as a model-based adaptive design for dose-escalation phase I trials. The CRM in its simplest form is a one-parameter dose-toxicity model that uses previous dose and DLT outcomes to assign new patients to dose levels as they enter the trial and aims to estimate the MTD. The CRM, and most designs for phase I trials, is based on the assumption of monotonicity, whereby the probability of observing a DLT increases with dose. Since the key interest is in estimating the MTD, a model with a single parameter is sufficient for local estimation of dose response (i.e., if focus is on a single point estimate) (O'Quigley et al. 1990). However, phase I trials may require more complex designs that consider other features, such as limiting the chance of severe overdosing, using partial data from patients who are still under follow-up for DLTs, using toxicity outcomes based on graded responses rather than a dichotomous outcome (DLT or no DLT), considering both toxicity and efficacy outcomes, and designing trials where two drugs are to be administered and their dose levels adapted in combination.

The focus of this chapter is to provide a broad overview of some of the more advanced issues in model-based (Bayesian) adaptive designs for phase I trials and key considerations that have led to these designs being proposed. The chapter is not intended to be all-encompassing, but should provide the reader with a flavor of some of the methodological developments in the area that extend the CRM approach, and to highlight practical considerations for researchers wishing to apply these methods. Examples from real-life trials are given throughout the chapter, along with recommendations of freely available software available to apply the methods. For a more in-depth discussion of the CRM and some of its earlier extensions, readers should refer to the ► chapter 53, "Dose-Finding and Dose-Ranging Studies" by Conaway and Petroni in section ► "Basics of Trial Design" of this book. While this chapter covers some recent designs for dual-agent phase I trials, a more comprehensive discussion of designs for drug combination dose finding is given in section ► "Basics of Trial Design" of this book by Tighiouart.

Escalation with Overdose Control (EWOC)

The CRM was the first model-based adaptive design for phase I dose escalation studies and has been implemented in both Bayesian and frequentist frameworks (O'Quigley et al. 1990; O'Quigley and Shen 1996). The design makes use of the dose and toxicity data accumulating as the trial progresses to make dose selection decisions, giving it a significant advantage over traditional rule-based designs such as the 3 + 3 method (Iasonos et al. 2008; Le Tourneau et al. 2009). Nevertheless, a number of modifications have been proposed since the original design to counter safety concerns about possible overdosing. These include rules that sometimes override model recommendations including always starting at the lowest dose, avoiding dose-skipping when escalating, and treating more than one patient at each dose level (Faries 1994; Korn et al. 1994; Goodman et al. 1995; Piantadosi et al. 1998).

An alternative approach to control overdosing is to modify the CRM dose-finding algorithm. After each patient, the CRM estimates the posterior distribution of the MTD and uses the middle of the distribution (e.g., the mean or median) to recommend the dose to administer to the next patient. However, at least early on in the trial, the posterior mean or median MTD estimate may fluctuate wildly leading to some patients receiving doses high above the true MTD. Overdosing can also occur if the prespecified model is incorrect (Le Tourneau et al. 2009). To overcome this problem Babb et al. (1998) developed the Escalation With Overdose Control (EWOC) design, which modifies the CRM so that it recommends the α quantile of the MTD distribution to the next patient, where $\alpha < 0.5$. The quantile, α, is known as the feasibility bound and governs the predicted chance of overdosing in the trial. For each successive patient the predicted probability of overdosing is α, whereas for the CRM using the median of the MTD distribution the predicted probability is 0.5. Low values of α will result in more cautious escalation; the trade-off for this cautious escalation is that the dose sequence allocated through the trial will generally take longer to converge to the true MTD. In notation, let $F_n(x) = P(MTD \leq x|\mathcal{D}_n)$ denote the probability that the MTD is less than or equal to dose x given the data collected from the previous n patients, namely the doses allocated $x_1, \ldots, x_n$, and the corresponding n DLT outcome indicator variables, $y_1, \ldots, y_n$. The EWOC design selects the dose x_{n+1} for patient $n + 1$ such that

$$F_n(x_{n+1}) = \alpha.$$

The EWOC model has an attractive decision-theoretic loss function interpretation. Given the feasibility bound α, the EWOC model minimizes the risk of toxicity based on the asymmetric loss-function

$$L(x,\gamma) = \begin{cases} \alpha(\gamma - x) & \text{if } x \leq \gamma \\ (1-\alpha)(x-\gamma) & \text{if } x > \gamma \end{cases}$$

where γ is the true MTD. Hence a higher penalty is given to overdosing, and this implies that treating a patient δ units above the MTD is $(1 - \alpha)/\alpha$ times worse than treating them δ units below the MTD.

In practice, with a discrete set of dose levels $d_1, \ldots, d_K$, the EWOC design selects the dose that is within a certain tolerance, T_1, of the EWOC target dose $x^*_{n+1} = F_n^{-1}(\alpha)$ and where the predicted probability of the MTD being less than the dose is within a certain tolerance, T_2, of the feasibility bound. For patient $n + 1$ the next recommended dose is therefore

$$\max\left\{d_1, \ldots, d_K : d_i - x^*_{n+1} \leq T_1 \text{ and } F_n(d_i) - \alpha \leq T_2\right\}.$$

A dose-toxicity model, often used with the EWOC method, is the two-parameter logistic model, where

$$\pi(x) = p(DLT|dose = x) = \text{logit}^{-1}(\beta_0 + \beta_1 x)$$

and x is the dose, either on the original dose scale or standardized. For example, given a reference dose x_R and using $\log(x/x_R)$ as a standardized dose, the intercept β_0 has the interpretation of being the log-odds of toxicity at the reference dose (see, e.g., Neuenschwander et al. 2008). By placing a bivariate normal prior distribution on the parameters β_0 and $\log(\beta_1)$ we ensure a monotonically increasing dose-toxicity relationship since β_1 (the slope) is forced to be positive. An alternative parameterization originally proposed in the EWOC formulation (Babb et al. 1998) is to define $\rho_0 = \pi(x_{min}) = p(DLT|dose = x_{min})$ as the probability of a DLT at the lowest dose, x_{min}, and γ as the MTD. Then it can be shown that

$$\text{logit}(\rho_0) = \beta_0 + \beta_1 x_{min}$$

and

$$\text{logit}(\theta) = \beta_0 + \beta_1 \gamma,$$

where θ is the TTL. The rationale for the re-parameterization is that it may be easier to specify prior distributions for γ and ρ_0, which then can be translated to priors for β_0 and β_1 (using MCMC for example). In a phase I trial of 5-fluorouracil (5-FU) Babb et al. (1998) propose independent Uniform (x_{min}, x_{max}) and $(0, \theta)$ distributions for γ and ρ_0, respectively, which forces the MTD to exist in the prespecified dose range. In further investigations by Tighiouart et al. (2005) a joint prior for γ and ρ_0 with negative correlation structure was found to perform well and which generally resulted in a safer trial. An issue with this parameterization and choice of priors is that the MTD has prior (and hence posterior) probability of 1 of lying between x_{min} and x_{max}. One solution proposed by Tighiouart et al. (2018) is to reparametrize the EWOC model in terms of ρ_0 and ρ_1, the probabilities of DLT at the minimum and maximum doses, respectively.

Example 1: Dose-Escalation Cancer Trial

Neuenschwander et al. (2008) describe a dose-escalation cancer trial designed to characterize the safety, tolerability, and pharmacokinetic profile of a drug. Fifteen doses were prespecified as doses that could be experimented on during the trial: 1, 2.5, 5, 10, 15, 20, 25, 30, 40, 50, 75, 100, 150, 200, and 250 mg. The trial initially recruited five cohorts of individuals of sizes 3, 4, 5, 4, and 2 to doses 1, 2.5, 5, 10, and 25 mg, respectively, with no DLTs experienced in the first four dose levels and 2 (out of 2) DLTs seen at dose 25 mg. The target toxicity was 30% and the original CRM model recommended continued escalation (to dose 40 mg) for cohort 6, using a one-parameter power model and a recommendation rule based on the point estimates for the probability of DLT at each dose. This unexpected recommendation led to further critical re-evaluation of the CRM approach.

An alternative two-parameter model with standardized dose $\log(x/250)$ and a non-informative bivariate lognormal prior on the untransformed parameters was used (see prior B in Neuenschwander et al. (2008)). Figure 1 shows the posterior distribution of the MTD from this model after the first five cohorts had been

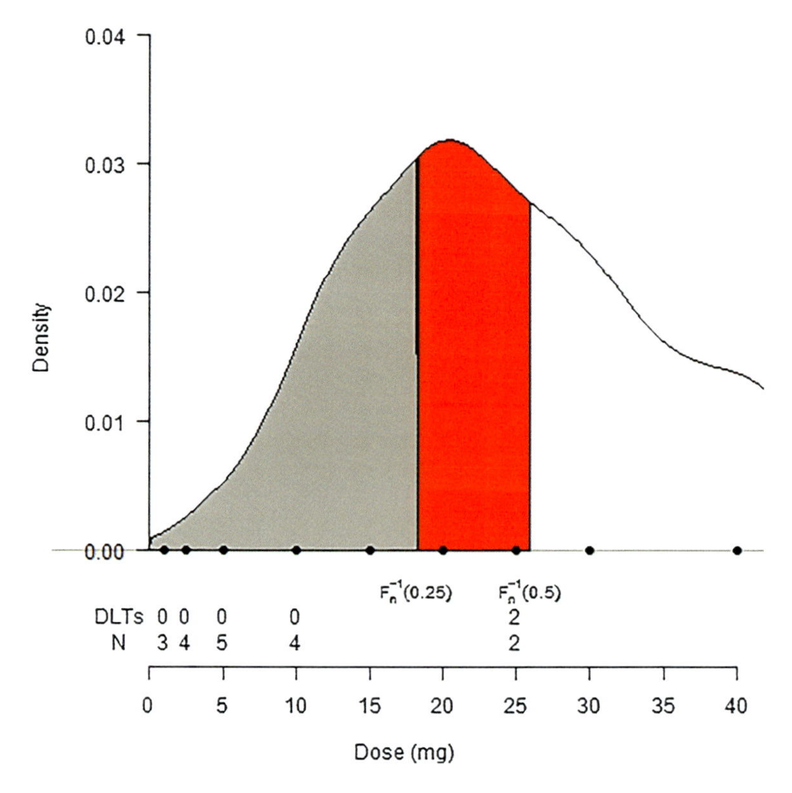

Fig. 1 Posterior distribution of the maximum tolerated dose (MTD) from Example 1 after five cohorts of patients have been recruited, and the $\alpha = 0.25$ and 0.5 quantiles, $F_n^{-1}(0.25)$ and $F_n^{-1}(0.5)$

recruited, where the dose axis is truncated to doses 40 mg. The potential doses that can be tested within the trial are shown as points on the x-axis. At a feasibility bound of $\alpha = 0.25$, the inverse cumulative distribution function of the MTD, denoted $F_n^{-1}(0.25)$ on the figure, is 18.2 mg. To choose from the discrete dose levels, suppose we set strict thresholds such that the next dose is not more than 1 mg above $F_n^{-1}(0.25)$ and the probability that the MTD is below the next dose is not more than $\alpha + 0.05 = 0.30$. That is we set $T_1 = 1$ and $T_2 = 0.05$. Dose 20 mg does not satisfy the first criteria and therefore the recommended next dose would be 15 mg, which does satisfy both constraints. This contrasts to a recommended next dose of 25 mg if the median of the distribution, $F_n^{-1}(0.5)$, is used, which would correspond to the sixth cohort receiving the same dose as the fifth cohort.

Varying the Feasibility Bound

Different proposals have been made for choosing the final dose recommended for phase II study at the end of an EWOC trial (Babb et al. 1998; Berry et al. 2010). One potentially undesirable feature from choosing a central estimate from the posterior MTD distribution (e.g., mean, median, or mode) is that the estimate may be larger than any dose experimented on in the trial. It may also be undesirable to choose a dose that would be given if a new patient were recruited into the trial, based on the feasibility bound, since the final recommended dose is then acknowledged to have posterior probability of $(1 - \alpha)$ being less than the MTD. An alternative approach originally proposed by Babb and Rogatko (2001) and later by Chu et al. (2009) is to vary the feasibility bound as the trial progresses; specifically increasing the bound until it reaches 0.5, at which point the EWOC method would behave like a CRM (with decisions based on the posterior median). The rationale is that early on in the trial there is a lot of uncertainty as to the value of the MTD and hence there is more chance of administering doses that are much greater than the MTD. While, once a number of patients have been recruited, the magnitude of overdosing will be less and hence the feasibility bound can be raised. This *hybrid* approach should therefore converge quicker to the MTD than the traditional EWOC method while also ensuring that the recommended phase II dose coincides with the central estimate from the MTD distribution.

Toxicity-Dependent Feasibility Bounds

Increasing the feasibility bound during the trial is often done using a step-wise procedure. However, it is possible that the approach can lead to *incoherence*; that is despite the most recent patient experiencing a DLT, the recommendation may be to treat the next patient at a higher dose (Wheeler et al. 2017). While both the unmodified CRM and EWOC approaches have been shown to be coherent (the latter for $n \geq 2$) (Cheung 2005; Tighiouart and Rogatko 2010), coherence violations may occur using the EWOC approach with an increasing feasibility bound (Wheeler 2018). To overcome this issue, Wheeler et al. (2017) introduced a toxicity-dependent feasibility bound that guarantees coherence and where the feasibility bound increases as a function of the number of non-DLT responses observed.

Software

EWOC-type designs can be fitted using a number of software packages. The bcrm package in R allows the user to fit EWOC-type designs by specifying the quantile of the MTD distribution that should be used for dose-escalation decisions (Sweeting et al. 2013). The package allows users to conduct a trial interactively or to investigate operating characteristics via simulation. However, the package only allows specification of prior distributions on the regression parameters of the two-parameter logistic model. Alternatively, the ewoc package, also in R (Diniz 2018), is specifically designed for EWOC designs, allowing the user to explicitly set priors for (the probability of DLT at the minimum dose), and γ (the MTD). Users are limited, however, to independent Beta prior distributions for ρ_0 and γ, or priors can be placed on ρ_0 and ρ_1, as proposed by Tighiouart et al. (2018). Finally, a Graphic User Interface application by Dinart et al. (2020) is available to download, allowing users to run and simulate EWOC trials with minimal programming experience (https://github.com/ddinart/GUIP1).

Time-to-Event Endpoints

Many designs for dose-escalation studies require that for a patient's DLT outcome to be included in dose-escalation decision making, a patient must be observed until the end of the DLT observation period, or until a DLT occurs, whichever time point is first. In practice, patients may be recruited to trials whilst other patients are receiving treatment. Therefore, complete outcomes will not be available for all patients, even though a decision on dose allocation for the next patients is required. To accommodate these situations, partial DLT observations may be used to estimate DLT risks at each dose level, conditional on the absence of a DLT up to the current time. This also offers the benefit of reducing the overall trial duration.

Cheung and Chappell (2000) proposed an adaptation to the CRM design to accommodate partial DLT outcomes, known as the Time-to-Event CRM (TITE-CRM). Under the TITE-CRM, the likelihood for the single model parameter a is weighted according to the proportion of each patient's DLT window for which a DLT has not been observed. That is, for patients 1, . . ., n, let x_i and $y_{i,t}$ be the dose given and current DLT outcome at time t for patient i, and let Δ_n be the set of all data for patients 1, . . ., n. The likelihood for parameter a is defined as

$$L(a|\mathcal{D}_n, t) = \prod_{i=1}^{n} \{\pi(x_i; a)\}^{y_{i,t}} \{1 - w_{i,t}\pi(x_i; a)\}^{1-y_{i,t}},$$

where $w_{i,t} = 0$ if a DLT has been observed by time t (i.e., $y_{i,t} = 1$) and $w_{i,t} = (t - t_{i,0})/T$ if $y_{i,t} = 0$ and $t \leq T + t_{i,0}$, where $t_{i,0}$ is the time at which patient i started treatment and T is the length of the DLT observation window. As t increases, the contribution of patient i to the likelihood, in the absence of a DLT, gets bigger. The rest of the trial design process is similar to that of the CRM.

Extensions to the TITE-CRM have also been proposed. Braun et al. (2003) extended the TITE-CRM to adapt the length of schedule (which they refer to as dose) both between and within patients, in order to identify the Maximum Tolerated Cumulative Dose (cumulative, as the schedule may change when a patient is on treatment, and it is the total length of administration that is of interest to the investigators). Braun (2006) also generalized the TITE-CRM approach to borrow information on the timing of toxicity across patients. Furthermore, Mauguen et al. (2011) and Tighiouart et al. (2014) have combined the TITE approach with the EWOC trial design, thus allowing for overdose control methods to be used in dose escalation studies with partial observations over a patient's DLT window.

A similar approach was employed by Ivanova et al. (2016) in their Rapid Enrollment Design (RED); rather than using the weighting structure of Cheung and Chappell (2000), they proposed that a patient who has been followed up for proportion t/T of their DLT window without a DLT being observed has experienced $1 - t/T$ of a *temporary* DLT. As t increases, the weighting ascribed to the patient's DLT risk goes down, and this in turn updates the likelihood. The subtle difference between these two approaches is as follows: in the TITE-CRM, a patient who has completed 70% of their DLT window without having a DLT is included as 0 DLTs out of 0.7 patients; in the RED, the same patient would be included as 0.3 DLTs out of one patient. TITE endpoints have also been included in the design of combination therapy dose-escalation studies (Wages et al. 2013; Wheeler et al. 2019).

Example 2: Dose Escalation of Cisplatin in Pancreatic Cancer

Muler et al. (2004) report the results of a phase I trial with the objective of identifying the MTD of cisplatin when given with fixed doses of gemcitabine and radiotherapy in patients with pancreatic cancer. The investigators planned to investigate four dose levels (20, 30, 40, and 50 mg/m^2), with 30 mg/m^2 as the starting dose and the target toxicity level chosen as 20%. Dose-escalation decisions were recommended using the TITE-CRM design, which used a one-parameter logistic model, with an exponential prior distribution on the model parameter. DLT was defined as either Grade 4 thrombocytopenia, Grade 4 neutropenia lasting more than 7 days, or any other adverse event of at least grade 3, and the DLT observation window was 9 weeks from start of treatment. Prior to the study starting, the skeleton DLT probabilities at each dose were chosen to be 10%, 15%, 20%, and 25%, respectively.

Figure 2 shows the entry and follow-up times for the 18 patients who were considered evaluable for toxicity. Patients 1 through 4 were allocated to the starting

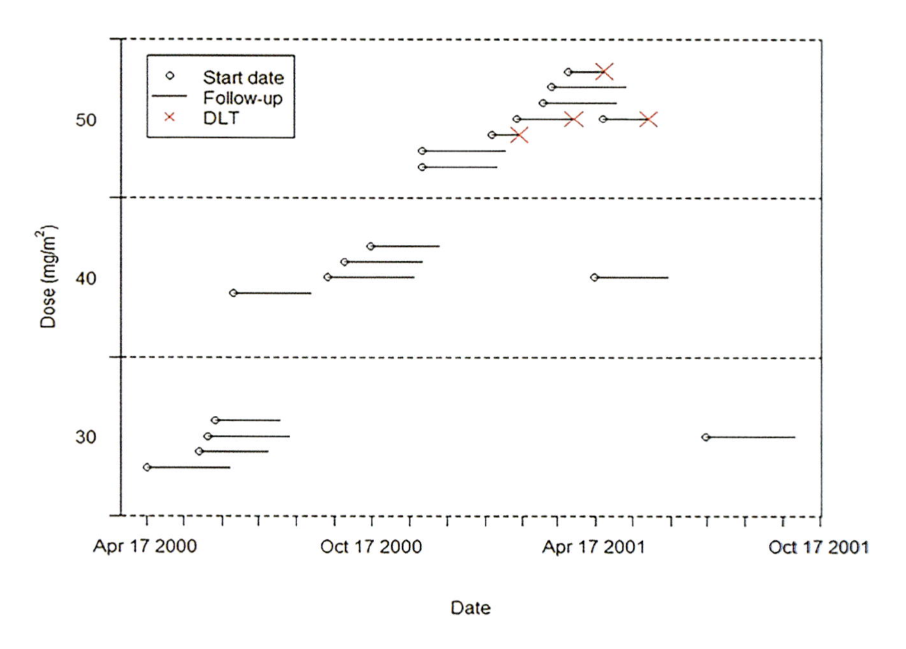

Fig. 2 Trial conduct for Muler et al. (2004)

dose to observe enough time without DLTs before patient 5 was allocated to 40 mg^2 (on June 26, 2000). Patient 9 was allocated to 50 mg/m^2 on November 27, 2000. Patients 11 and 12 experienced DLTs during follow-up at 50 mg/m^2 leading to patient 16 receiving the lower dose of 40 mg/m^2 and patient 18 receiving 30 mg/m^2 following a further DLT in patient 17. At the end of the trial, the 40 mg/m^2 dose had an expected posterior DLT probability of 0.204 (95% credible interval 0.064–0.427).

Software

The R software package dfcrm can be used to design a TITE-CRM trial.

Toxicity Grading

Much of the literature in dose-finding trial designs focuses on the binary DLT outcome in order to identify the MTD. Toxicities are usually graded using the Common Terminology Criteria for Adverse Events (CTCAE) published by the US National Cancer Institute (http://evs.nci.nih.gov/ftp1/CTCAE/About.html) and in turn the dose-limiting toxicities will be tailored to the trial in question. Toxicities are grouped under different System Organ Classes, and each toxicity (e.g. "nausea," "dermatitis," "neutrophil count decreased") is graded from 0 (no toxicity) to

5 (death). A DLT is usually defined as any grade 3+ toxicity whereas a non-DLT is toxicity within grades 0–2. The simplification of the outcome is to help with dose-escalation decision making but it is well known that this results in a reduction in the information used and hence estimation of the MTD may be less efficient. Using graded toxicities in dose-escalation designs can potentially give trialists more information about the speed in which dose escalation should occur; for example, if grade 2 toxicities are being observed in patients, then trialists may wish to slow escalation since this may be indicative of more severe toxicities at nearby higher doses (Van Meter et al. 2012). There has been an increase in the number of papers that handle toxicity gradings directly. The model-based methods for handling toxicity grades fall into two broad categories: those that use ordinal toxicity gradings directly and those that use a score-based (continuous) outcome.

Ordinal Toxicity Gradings

A number of phase I designs have been proposed in the literature that incorporate ordinal toxicity outcomes. Approaches have used either a proportional odds (PO) model (Van Meter et al. 2011; Tighiouart et al. 2012), a continuation ratio (CR) model (Van Meter et al. 2012), or a multinomial extension of the CRM power model (Iasonos et al. 2011) to account for the ordinal toxicity outcome. The PO model relies on the assumption that the odds of a more severe toxicity grade relative to any less severe toxicity is constant among all possible toxicity grades (Van Meter et al. 2012). That is the odds that the toxicity grade is ≥ 2 versus <2 is the same as the odds that the toxicity is ≥ 3 versus <3, etc. Meanwhile, the CR method models the probability that the toxicity is at level g given it is greater than or equal to g but relies on its own assumption of homogeneity of grade-specific dose effects (Cole and Ananth 2001). However, with these assumptions, the models can focus on estimating just one quantile of interest, namely the dose that gives the target probability of observing grades of toxicity that define a DLT. Information from non-DLT grades are used to refine the estimation of the relationship between dose and the common odds ratio. To avoid assumptions imposed by the PO or CR methods, a nonparametric approach has been proposed using a multidimensional isotonic regression estimator (Paul et al. 2004). This allows nonparametric estimation of quantiles for each toxicity grade subject to order constraints and based on a corresponding set of prespecified probabilities for each grade.

Toxicity Score Approach

There are several other approaches of note that collapse the ordinal toxicities into a single equivalent toxicity score (between 0 and 1) such as a beta regression model (Potthoff and George 2009) or a quasi-Bernoulli likelihood approach (Yuan et al. 2007; Ezzalfani et al. 2013). The latter uses a standard CRM model but requires a clinically meaningful toxicity score to be assigned to each grade of toxicity.

Another approach uses an ordinal probit regression with a latent variable, for each toxicity type under consideration (Bekele and Thall 2004; Lee et al. 2010). The probability that the toxicity is at a given level (grade) $g = 0, \ldots, G$ is then modeled using the probit model and $G - 1$ cutoff parameters. Bekele and Thall (2004) used a multivariate ordinal probit regression approach that allowed multiple toxicity types (myelosuppression, dermatitis, liver toxicity, nausea/vomiting, and fatigue), each graded, to be modeled simultaneously with correlation. The authors then quantified the severity of each toxicity type and grade by eliciting numerical weights. For each dose under consideration the posterior expected probability of each toxicity type and grade was multiplied by its associated severity weight and the sum of these across types and grades gave the overall *total toxicity burden* (TTB) for that dose. Dose escalation then proceeded by assigning the next patient the dose with TTB closest to a prespecified target TTB (elicited through a set of scenario analyses with the oncologists).

Software

The R package ordcrm allows the user to fit both the ordinal PO and CR CRM models.

Dual Endpoints

The focus for most dose-escalation designs is purely on toxicity, and the common assumption is that as dose increases, so does both the risk of toxicity and the efficacy of the drug. However, it may be more prudent to model the dose-efficacy relationship as well as dose-toxicity. Efficacy may even plateau after a certain dosage, and therefore, increasing a dose with no increase in efficacy but a potential increase in toxicity would be unwise. Therefore, many approaches have been proposed in order to jointly model dose-efficacy and dose-toxicity outcomes.

The EffTox Design

Thall and Cook (2004) proposed what has come to be known as the EffTox Design, a Bayesian approach that models the efficacy and toxicity risks per dose, and uses the trade-off between toxicity and efficacy to select dose levels for new patients. Specifically, logistic functions are assumed for the dose-toxicity and dose-efficacy curves, that is,

$$\text{logit}(\pi_T(x; \beta_T)) = \beta_{T,0} + \beta_{T,1}x$$

and

$$\text{logit}(\pi_E(x; \beta_E)) = \beta_{E,0} + \beta_{E,1}x + \beta_{E,2}x^2.$$

The dose-efficacy relationship includes the quadratic term $\beta_{E,2}x^2$ to permit a turning point in the curve. Both π_T and π_E are combined using the Gumbel copula model so that the probability of each toxicity-efficacy outcome result (a, b), where a and b take value 0 if toxicity or efficacy does not occur, and 1 if they do respectively, is given as

$$\pi_{a,b} = \pi_T^a(1-\pi_T)^{1-a} + \pi_E^b(1-\pi_E)^{1-b} + (-1)^{a+b}\pi_T(1-\pi_T)\pi_E(1-\pi_E)\frac{e^\phi - 1}{e^\phi + 1}$$

which for patients $1, \ldots, n$, gives the likelihood

$$L(\beta_E, \beta_T, \phi|\mathcal{D}_n) = \prod_{i=1}^{n} \pi_{a,b}(x_i)^{\mathbb{I}[a=a_i, b=b_i]}.$$

As per Thall and Cook (2006) and Brock et al. (2017), prior beliefs on the efficacy and toxicity at each dose must be elicited from the clinicians, along with the prior Effective Sample Size (ESS). It is then possible to transform these prior beliefs and ESS onto the model parameters $\{\beta_{T,0}, \beta_{T,1}, \beta_{E,0}, \beta_{E,1}, \beta_{E,2}, \phi\}$ using specialist software (EffTox Software, MD Anderson, https://biostatistics.mdanderson.org/softwaredownload/SingleSoftware.aspx?Software_Id=2; or the R package trialr). Thall et al. (2014) show how different prior effective sample sizes affect the operating characteristics of the EffTox design, including the probability of selecting each dose as the optimum dose and the probability of terminating the trial early.

The key step under the EffTox approach is to define a utility function that reflects the trade-offs between efficacy and toxicity that the trial team are willing to accept. To do this, three target trade-offs are specified: $\pi_1^* = (\pi_{T,1}^*, 1)$, where $\pi_{T,1}^*$ is the maximum toxicity level at which efficacy is guaranteed; $\pi_2^* = (0, \pi_{E,2}^*)$, where $\pi_{E,2}^*$ is the minimum efficacy level at which toxicity is guaranteed to not occur; $\pi_3^* = (\pi_{T,3}^*, \pi_{E,3}^*)$, an intermediate target between the two marginal targets π_1^* and π_2^* that, with a contour fitted through all three target trade-offs, will provide a suitably steep contour to encourage escalation to doses that are estimated to have substantially higher efficacy probabilities with only a limited increase in toxicity risk (Yuan et al. 2017; Brock et al. 2017). Thall et al. (2014) use L^p norms to model the utility contours, specifically

$$u(\pi_T, \pi_E) = 1 - \left[\left(\frac{1-\pi_E}{1-\pi_{E,2}^*}\right)^p + \left(\frac{\pi_T}{\pi_{T,1}^*}\right)^p\right]^{1/p},$$

where p determines the extent of the curvature of the contours. The utility function u allows us to evaluate the desirability/utility of a dose level based on its estimated probability of toxicity and efficacy. The value of p is obtained by solving $u(\pi_T, \pi_E) = 0$, which denotes the *neutral contour*. We may then recommend a dose level for the next patient that maximizes this utility, subject to any other constraints one may wish to use in the trial. For example, if we have target minimum efficacy π_E^* and target maximum toxicity π_T^*, then for selected cutoffs p_E and p_T, only doses that satisfy the following constraints are available for recommendation:

$$Pr\left(\pi_E(x) \geq \pi_E^*\right) > p_E$$

and

$$Pr\left(\pi_T(x) \leq \pi_T^*\right) > p_T.$$

Example 3: The Matchpoint Trial

Brock et al. (2017) described how they designed the Matchpoint trial, a dose-finding study of Ponatinib plus chemotherapy in patients with chronic myeloid leukemia in blastic transformation phase, using the Efftox design. The aim of the study was to identify the dose of Ponatinib that produced a minimum efficacy response rate of 45%, with an acceptable toxicity level of at most 40%. Four doses were considered: 15 mg every second day, 15 mg daily, 30 mg daily, and 45 mg daily. Clinicians specified prior toxicity and efficacy probabilities as shown in Table 1, and with the help of the trial team, chose cutoffs for admissible doses to be $p_E = 0.03$ and $p_T = 0.05$. The low thresholds permitted that even weak beliefs of the efficacy and toxicity probabilities would still allow doses to be admissible.

For their three target trade-off points, the team chose three points in the toxicity-efficacy space that they felt had equal utility, and solved simultaneous equations to identify what π_1^*, π_2^*, and π_3^* would be. This resulted in $\pi_1^* = (0, 0.40)$ and $\pi_2^* = (0.70, 1)$, giving $p = 2.07$. The resultant utility curves for different utility/desirability levels are shown in Fig. 3; the neutral contour is shown in blue, and yields an interior target point of $\pi_3^* = (0.4, 0.5)$. Any other point lying on this curve could be selected as an interior target point. A trial-and-error approach was used to select the ESS based on the operating characteristics from simulation studies, similar to the approach of Thall et al. (2014). For the Matchpoint trial, the investigators set the ESS as 1.3 to obtain prior distributions on their model parameters.

The Matchpoint trial is currently ongoing, so results are not available. However, Brock et al. (2017) provided results of simulation studies to assess their trial design across six scenarios with different dose-efficacy and dose-toxicity relationships. Figure 4 shows the probability of selecting each dose (or not recommending a

Table 1 Dose levels and prior probabilities for the Matchpoint trial

	1	2	3	4
Dose level Ponatinib dose	15 mg every other day	15 mg daily	30 mg daily	45 mg daily
Prior Pr(Eff)	0.20	0.30	0.50	0.60
Prior Pr(Tox)	0.025	0.05	0.10	0.25

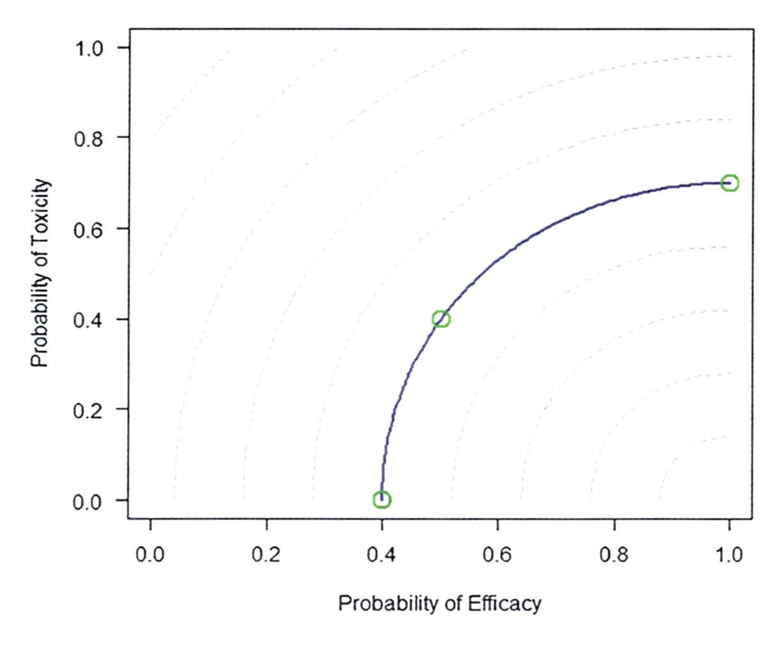

Fig. 3 Utility contours elicited for the Matchpoint trial. Green circles show the three trade-off points used to fit contours. Blue line shows the neutral contour fitted through trade-off points

dose due to safety) across the six scenarios for their proposed design, along with the true toxicity and efficacy probabilities in each scenario.

Other Approaches for Joint Modeling of Efficacy and Toxicity

Additional Bayesian approaches for joint modeling efficacy and toxicity outcomes have been proposed in the literature. Thall and Russell (1998) describe a proportional odds approach to dose-escalation where there are three measurable outcomes concerning adverse events and the onset of Graft versus Host Disease (GvHD): no severe toxicities and no GvHD (outcome 1), no severe toxicities and only moderate GvHD (outcome 2), and either severe toxicity or severe GvHD (outcome 3). The aim is to find the dose that has an expected probability of outcome 2 of at least 50%, but with the expected probability of outcome 3 being no greater than 10%. A parsimonious modeling approach is used, whereby $\gamma_j(x) = \mathbb{P}\,(\text{Outcome} \geq j)$, and

$$\gamma_0(x) = 1$$
$$\gamma_1(x) = \frac{\exp\,(\mu + \alpha + \beta x)}{1 + \exp\,(\mu + \alpha + \beta x)}$$
$$\gamma_2(x) = \frac{\exp\,(\mu + \beta x)}{1 + \exp\,(\mu + \beta x)}.$$

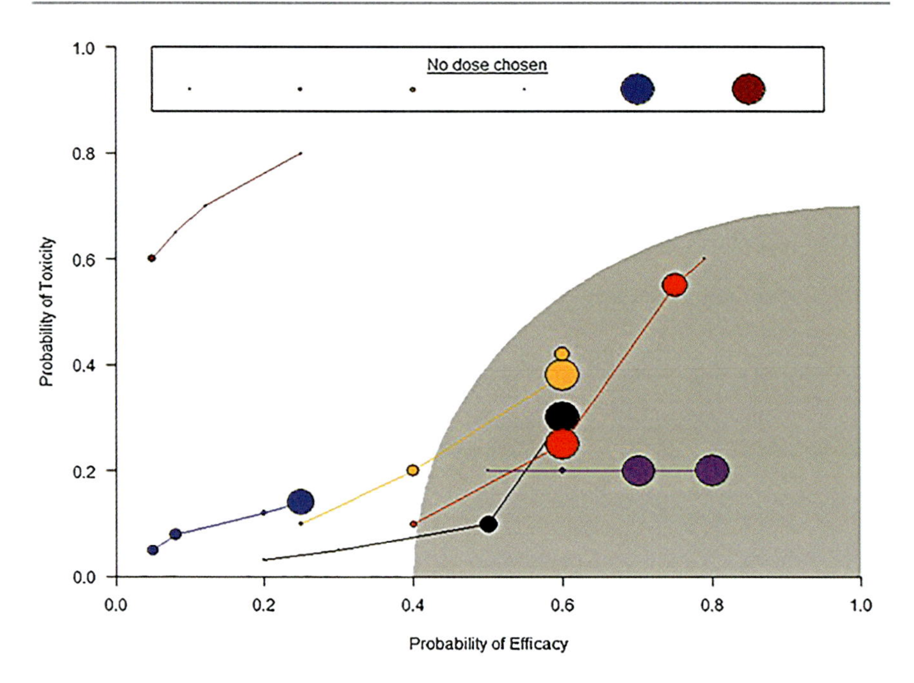

Fig. 4 Simulation results for the EffTox design proposed for the Matchpoint Trial. Gray shaded area shows the set of points that are more desirable than the elicited neutral contour. Areas of points are proportional to the probability of choosing that point as the MTD. Scenario orderings for No dose chosen results are 1 (black), 2 (red), 3 (orange), 4 (purple), 5 (blue), and 6 (brown)

Model parameters are updated by standard Bayesian methods and then the dose with the highest probability for outcome 2 (i.e., moderate GvHD and no severe toxicity) is chosen, subject to the constraint that $\gamma_2(x) \leq 0.10$. A related approach by Braun (2002) extended the CRM to jointly model the probabilities of severe toxicity and disease progression.

Zhang et al. (2006) proposed a continuation-ratio approach for jointly modeling efficacy and toxicity. Specifically, given dose, three probabilities are of interest: $\psi_0(x)$, the probability of no efficacy and no DLT; $\psi_1(x)$, the probability of efficacy and no DLT; $\psi_2(x)$, the probability of DLT, regardless of efficacy status. These probabilities are then modeled to allow toxicity to increase monotonically with dose, but for $\psi_1(x)$ to be non-monotonic with dose:

$$\log\left\{\frac{\psi_1(x)}{\psi_0(x)}\right\} = \alpha_1 + \beta_1 x$$

and

$$\log\left\{\frac{\psi_2(x)}{1-\psi_2(x)}\right\} = \alpha_2 + \beta_2 x.$$

Then, with constraints on the model parameters, specifically $\alpha_1 > \alpha_2$ and β_1, $\beta_2 > 0$, the above equations can be solved to give expressions directly on $\psi_0(x)$, $\psi_1(x)$, and $\psi_2(x)$. Given a target toxicity level θ, the dose-finding algorithm is based on two decision functions:

$$\delta_1(x) = I[\psi_2(x) < \theta]$$

and

$$\delta_2(x) = \psi_1(x) - \lambda\psi_2(x)$$

where λ is the weight for the toxicity risk of dose x relative to its efficacy. The dose x^* for the next patient is that which satisfies $\delta_1(x^*) = 1$ and $\delta_2(x^*) = \max_{x \in \Xi} \{\delta_2(x)\}$, where Ξ is the dose range (or set of doses) under consideration. Other approaches using the continuation ratio model have been published since, including those for combination therapy trials (Mandrekar et al. 2007, 2010).

Dragalin and Fedorov (2006) proposed using optimal design theory for dose-finding studies with joint endpoint data. For a joint probability model $p_{y,z}(x)$, where x is the dose, y is the binary efficacy outcome, and z is the binary toxicity outcome, the authors suggest either a Gumbel-type bivariate logistic regression, such as that used in the EffTox design, or Cox bivariate binary model. In both cases, an analytical expression for the Fisher Information Matrix (FIM) is obtained. A common choice of optimization is the D-optimality criterion, which chooses the dose for the next individual patient that maximizes the determinant of the FIM. An optimal design allows the trial to obtain as much information as possible about the joint probability model. However, the optimal dose may not always be a safe dose. Therefore the range of doses from which the optimal dose is chosen can be restricted to doses within the therapeutic range (above the posterior estimate of the minimum effective dose and below the posterior estimate of the MTD). Other constraints for defining admissible doses are also explored by Dragalin and Fedorov (2006).

The use of D-optimality and an admissible dose range aims to blend together two goals in drug development: doing what is best for the population (by learning as much as possible about the dose-efficacy and dose-toxicity relationships) and doing what is best for the patient (by giving them the dose that has a controlled toxicity risk but some efficacy benefit). Optimal design-theoretic approaches for dose-finding studies have also been proposed by others (Pronzato 2010; Padmanabhan et al. 2010a; Padmanabhan et al. 2010b; Dragalin et al. 2008).

Dual-Agent and Dose-Schedule-Finding Studies

After exploring different endpoints and joint modeling of efficacy and toxicity outcomes for single-agent dose-escalation designs, a natural progression for research and application of such designs was into trials where two or more treatment-related quantities were to be adapted. Since many treatment plans are formed from combinations of drugs, or even different treatment modalities, dose-finding studies may wish to vary the dosage/level of multiple treatments to find one or more maximum tolerated dose combination, or optimal biological dose combinations. Furthermore, even with a single-agent study with one treatment being adapted, it may be of interest to explore different dose administration schedules (e.g., 200 mg daily for two weeks versus 100 mg daily for three weeks) to identify a maximum tolerated dose-schedule combination. As treatments for patients become more complex, so too must trial designs.

Harrington et al. (2013) conducted an extensive review of available trial designs for dual-agent dose-escalation designs, many of which may be also applied to dose-schedule finding trials. This review discusses both rule- and model-based approaches and, though few in number, found several case studies of their implementation in practice. From this and more recent reviews (see Wages et al. 2016; Hirakawa et al. 2018; Riviere et al. 2014), we discuss several designs to illustrate the different trial designs.

Extensions to the CRM

Studies of dual-agent combinations are complicated by the lack of a well-defined ordering with respect to increasing toxicity (and also efficacy if monotonic); that is, the relationship between dose combinations and toxicity risk is only partially ordered. While we may safely assume that, holding all else constant, an increase in one treatment will maintain or increase the risk of toxicity, and that this property also holds when both treatments are increased, we cannot be sure what the relationship is when one treatment is increased and the other is decreased. Figure 5 shows an example dose toxicity grid with six combinations. The grid is partially ordered, in that we know, for example, that d_5 is not as toxic as d_6, but is at least as toxic than both d_1 and d_3; however, we do not know whether d_5 is more or less toxic than d_2 or d_4.

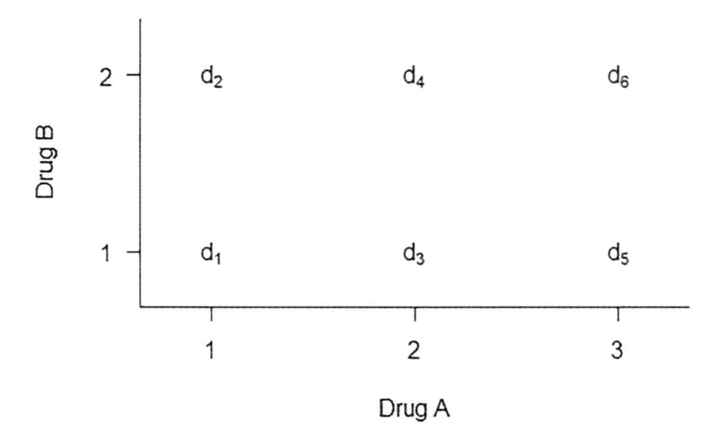

Fig. 5 Dose-toxicity grid and partial ordering

There exist five possible simple orders:

$$1 \to 2 \to 3 \to 4 \to 5 \to 6$$
$$1 \to 2 \to 3 \to 5 \to 4 \to 6$$
$$1 \to 3 \to 2 \to 4 \to 5 \to 6$$
$$1 \to 3 \to 2 \to 5 \to 4 \to 6$$
$$1 \to 3 \to 5 \to 2 \to 4 \to 6.$$

It is the investigators job to identify one or more maximum tolerated dose combinations while accounting for potential uncertainty in the true dose-toxicity relationship given the partial ordering.

Wages et al. (2011a, b) proposed an extension to the standard CRM design, the Partially Ordered CRM (POCRM), which accounts for the partial ordering structure in a dual-agent dose-escalation study setting and conveniently allows for a single-agent dose-escalation approach to be used in a multi-agent setting. For a study of K dose combinations, and under the partial order structure present for the K dose combinations, let us assume there are M possible simple orders. Let $\pi_m(d_k)$ be the probability of DLT at dose combination $k = 1, \ldots, K$ under the assumption that the true dose-toxicity order is that specified by order $m = 1, \ldots, M$. The dose-toxicity function π may be a one-parameter power or logistic as is often used for the CRM. For each possible order m, we may obtain the likelihood for the data and, given some prior belief on how likely order m is to be the true simple ordering for the dose-toxicity relationship, generate a posterior probability that order m is indeed the true simple order. That is, letting $f(m)$ be the prior belief that order m is the true simple order, and $L_m(\Delta_n)$ the likelihood of the model parameters given current trial data Δ_n under simple order m, the posterior probability that order m is the true simple order is

$$\psi(m) = \frac{L_m(\mathcal{D}_n)f(m)}{\sum_{l=1}^{M} L_l(\mathcal{D}_n)f(l)}.$$

We may then choose order $m^* = \arg\max_{m=1,\ldots,M} \psi(m)$ to be the best guess of the true simple order, and apply the CRM for single-agent phase I trials to the dose combinations under this specified ordering. Alternatively, we may randomly select an ordering by using the $\psi(m)$ as selection probabilities; this may be beneficial if two or more orderings have the same or very similar posterior weightings. An extension of this approach including efficacy outcomes has also been proposed (Wages and Conaway 2014).

Dose Toxicity Surface Models

Other approaches model the entire dose-toxicity surface. Gasparini (2013) describes several models for dose-toxicity surfaces, which include logistic-type and copula-type models employed by Thall et al. (2003), Wang and Ivanova (2005), Yin and

Yuan (2009a), and Yin and Yuan (2009b). Further to these, extensions of the EWOC designs for the combination therapy setting have also been proposed for dual-agent phase I dose-escalation studies (Jimenez et al. 2018; Tighiouart et al. 2017; Diniz et al. 2017; Tighiouart 2018); we do not cover these here as they are discussed in other areas of this book.

Example 4: Nilotinib plus Imatinib in Stromal Tumors

Bailey et al. (2009) used an extension of the logistic model to conduct a dose-escalation study of nilotinib plus imatinib in adult patient with imatinib-resistant gastrointestinal stromal tumors. Five doses of nilotinib $\{100, 200, 400, 600, 800\}$mg and two doses of imatinib $\{600, 800\}$mg were considered, though patients could also be given nilotinib alone (so imatinib dose of 0 mg). For each dose level, the probability that the posterior DLT risk is either an underdose (i.e., $\mathbb{P}(\pi(x) \in [0, 0.20))$), in the target range (i.e., $\mathbb{P}(\pi(x) \in [0.20, 0.35))$), an excessive toxicity (i.e, $\mathbb{P}(\pi(x) \in [0.35, 0.60))$), or an unacceptable toxicity (i.e., $\mathbb{P}(\pi(x) \in [0.6, 1])$) are computed. These probability masses are used for dose-escalation decisions.

The model in this trial was a four-parameter logistic-type model. For dose a of nilotinib and dose b of imatinib, the probability of DLT at dose combination (a, b) is.

$$\text{logit}(\pi(a,b)) = \log(\alpha) + \beta\log\left(\left(\frac{a}{a_R}\right)\right) + \gamma_1\mathbb{I}[b \geq 600] + \gamma_2\mathbb{I}[b \geq 800],$$

where a_R is a reference dose level for nilotinib, and $\mathbb{I}[\cdot]$ denotes the indicator function, taking value 1 if true and 0 otherwise. Using suitable priors on $\{\alpha, \beta, \gamma_1, \gamma_2\}$, the trial proceeds like most others in this chapter; after dose and DLT status data are collected, Bayesian methods are used to update the posterior DLT risks per dose, and also to calculate the four aforementioned interval probabilities. Then, the dose for the next patient is that which has the largest probability of being in the target range (i.e., $x_{n+1} = \text{argmax}_{x \in \chi}\, \mathbb{P}(\pi(x) \in [0.20, 0.35))$), subject to the constraint that $\mathbb{P}(\pi(x) \in [0.35, 1]) \leq 0.25$. In addition to this, it was possible for patients to be dosed at combinations that had a smaller target interval probability than $\pi(x_{n+1})$ based on additional clinical data, or if x_{n+1} was a combination where one of the drugs was increased by more than 100% of the current highest level.

To begin, seven patients were recruited to (800, 0) and one had a DLT. Based on the posterior interval probabilities and dose escalation rules, three patients were treated at (200, 800), none of whom had DLTs; during this time an additional two patients received (800, 0) and neither experienced DLTs. Figure 6 shows the trial progress and allocation of patients to different dose combinations throughout the trial, with Bayesian inference and evaluation of the model performed in five stages.

During the course of this trial, several key changes were made. Firstly, severe skin rash was added to the definition of DLT, which meant among the five patients who received the (800,800) combination, four were classes as having experienced DLTs;

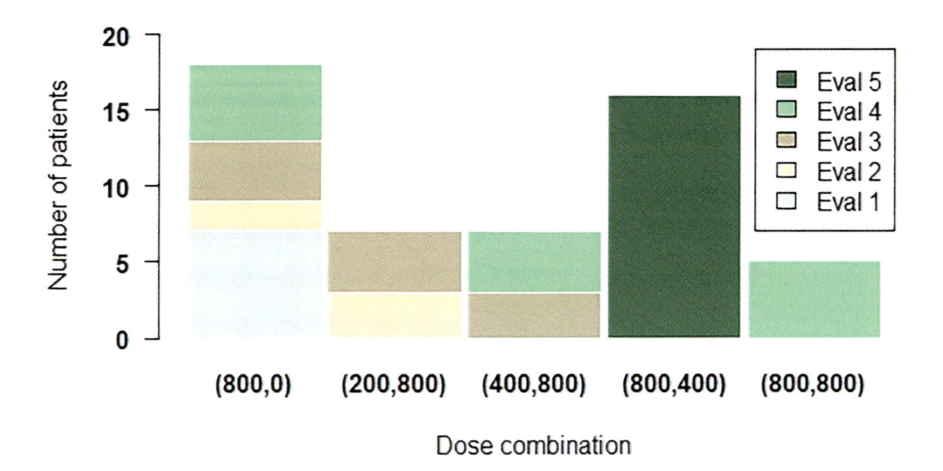

Fig. 6 Trial progress of nilotinib plus imatinib study. Evaluations (Eval) denote when a decision was made to open up a new dose combination to recruitment based on estimates of target interval and overdose interval probabilities

this would previously have been only one patient under the old DLT definition. Secondly, the investigators agreed to open up a 400 mg dose of imatinib after observing the four DLTs at (800,800). This meant that a) the dose-toxicity model had to be modified to include an additional parameter, so the model became

$$\begin{aligned}\text{logit}(\pi(a,b)) = {} & \log(\alpha) + \beta \log\left(\left(\frac{a}{a_R}\right)\right) + \gamma_0 \mathbb{I}[b \geq 400] + \gamma_1 \mathbb{I}[b \geq 600] \\ & + \gamma_2 \mathbb{I}[b \geq 800],\end{aligned}$$

and b) the prior distributions for γ_1 and γ_2 needed to be modified. Once this was completed, posterior estimates for DLT probabilities and dosing interval probabilities were recalculated. A further 16 patients were recruited to the new (800,400) combination, and three of these patients experienced DLT. At the end of the study, the (800,400) dose, which had the largest probability mass in the target range of [0.20, 0.35) and satisfied the aforementioned overdose constraint, was selected as the maximum tolerated dose combination. Figure 7 shows the posterior probability mass for target or overdosing at each dose combination.

Bayesian Model-Free Approaches

Choosing a model for the above designs requires careful consideration, and appropriate priors need to be chosen. Furthermore, for a true dose-toxicity surface with a very asymmetric shape (i.e., increasing one drug adds little to DLT risk, but increasing the other drug adds a lot), it may be difficult to obtain reliable estimates

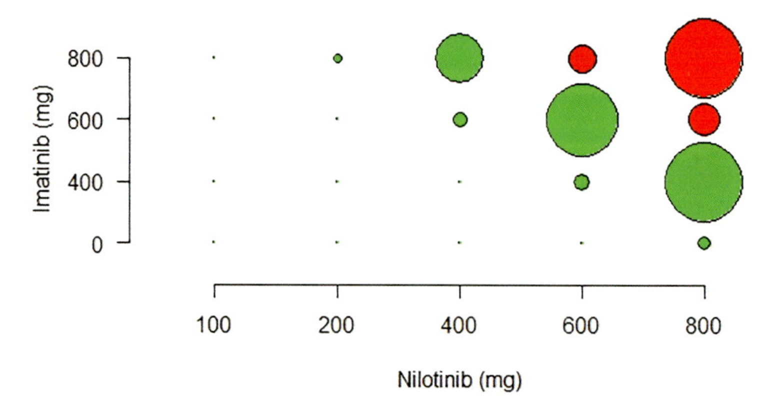

Fig. 7 Summary of posterior probabilities of target (green circles) and overdosing (red circles) per dose combination. Area of circles proportional to probability. Combinations with red circles have $\mathbb{P}(\pi(x) \in [0.35, 1]) > 0.25$, so target probability not shown. Combinations with green circles all have $\mathbb{P}(\pi(x) \in [0.35, 1]) \leq 0.25$

of DLT risks under some models. In light of this, Bayesian approaches have been proposed where a model for the dose-toxicity surface is not required.

Lin and Yin (2017) proposed a Bayesian Optimal Interval (BOIN) design for combination trials, whereby the dose for the next patient is either increased, decreased, or maintained if the expected probability of DLT at the current dose falls within some predefined intervals. Let θ be the target toxicity level, π_{jk} be the DLT risk at dose combination (j, k), and Δ_L and Δ_U be the lower and upper limits for the target DLT interval. If $\widehat{\pi}_{jk}$, equal to the number of DLTs at combination (j, k) divided by the number of patients at (j, k), is less than $\theta - \Delta_L$, then the next patient receives either combination $(j, k + 1)$ or $(j + 1, k)$, whichever combination maximizes $\mathbb{P}(\pi_{jk} \in (\theta - \Delta_L, \theta + \Delta_U)|\Delta_n)$. If $\widehat{\pi}_{jk}$ is greater than $\theta + \Delta_U$, then the next patient receives either combination $(j, k - 1)$ or $(j - 1, k)$, whichever combination maximizes $\mathbb{P}(\pi_{jk} \in (\theta - \Delta_L, \theta + \Delta_U)|\Delta_n)$. Otherwise, the next patient receives the current dose.

Mander and Sweeting (2015) proposed the Product of Independent beta Probabilities dose Escalation design (PIPE), which focused on identifying the Maximum Tolerated Contour (MTC) that divides safe and unsafe doses. A working model is first set up whereby each combination is given an independent beta prior distribution, that is, for combination (j, k), $\pi_{jk} \sim \text{Beta}(a_{jk}, b_{jk})$. With these independent priors and trial data Δ_n, the posterior distribution for each combination is also a beta distribution and it is easy to calculate the probability that the combination is less that the TTL, $p_{jk} = \mathbb{P}(\pi_{jk} \leq \theta | a_{jk}, b_{jk}, \Delta_n)$. The PIPE design then considers each possible contour that can divide a dose-toxicity surface into safe and unsafe combinations and that satisfies the assumption of monotonicity. Using the working model, the probability of each contour being the MTC can then be calculated. For contour

C_m, let $C_m[j, k] = 1$ if combination (j, k) is above the contour (i.e., unsafe), and $C_m[j, k] = 0$ if it is below (i.e., safe). Then

$$\mathbb{P}(\mathrm{MTC} = C_m | \mathcal{D}_n) = \prod_{j=1}^{J} \prod_{k=1}^{K} p_{jk}^{1-C_m[j,k]} \left(1 - p_{jk}\right)^{C_m[j,k]}.$$

The contour that maximizes the above expression is selected as the MTC, and dose-escalation decisions may be made with the MTC as a guide. Software to implement the PIPE designs is available in the R package pipe.design.

Dose-Schedule Finding Designs

Most of the methods for dual-agent phase I trials may be applied directly to dose-schedule finding studies, simply by treating the different administration schedules as another treatment that is varied. However, there are other approaches that consider the subtleties of dose-schedule finding studies. Braun et al. (2007) used time-to-toxicity outcomes to adaptively select dose-schedule combinations where schedules of lower frequency/intensity are nested within more intense ones, with a motivating example of using 5-azacitidine to treat patients with acute myeloid leukemia. Meanwhile, O'Quigley and Conaway (2011) extended the CRM approach so that the skeleton values varied according to which schedule patients were to be treated with.

Summary and Conclusion

This chapter provides an overview and summary of advanced statistical methodology proposed for extending Bayesian adaptive model-based phase I trial designs. A key factor common to many of these methods is the incorporation of data into dose-finding algorithms that is in addition to binary DLT outcomes. This can be in the form of using a more granular classification of toxicity based on CTC criteria, using information on the timing of outcomes for patients during follow-up to allow continual enrollment, use of both toxicity and efficacy outcomes, and the use of dual-agent or dose-schedule finding algorithms. As more complex trials are developed such methodology opens the way to the design of more safe and efficient phase I trials, both in terms of time savings and sample size.

There is a large literature of Phase I trial designs and this chapter is not intended to be all-encompassing. Instead, a wide variety of designs are introduced, which provide a flavor of some of the methodological developments in the area. There are a number of excellent review articles that allow further in-depth exploration of the literature, including O'Quigley and Conaway (2011), Harrington et al. (2013), O'Quigley et al. (2017), Zhou (2009), Wages et al. (2016), and Thall (2010).

References

Babb JS, Rogatko A (2001) Patient specific dosing in a cancer phase I clinical trial. Stat Med 20(14):2079–2090

Babb J, Rogatko A, Zacks S (1998) Cancer phase I clinical trials: efficient dose escalation with overdose control. Stat Med 17(10):1103–1120

Bailey S, Neuenschwander B, Laird G, Branson M (2009) A Bayesian case study in oncology phase I combination dose-finding using logistic regression with covariates. J Biopharm Stat 19(3): 469–484

Bekele BN, Thall PF (2004) Dose-finding based on multiple toxicities in a soft tissue sarcoma trial. J Am Stat Assoc 99(465):26–35

Berry SM, Carlin BP, Jack Lee J, Muller P (2010) Bayesian adaptive methods for clinical trials. Boca Raton, FL: Chapman and Hall/CRC Press

Braun TM (2002) The bivariate continual reassessment method. Extending the CRM to phase I trials of two competing outcomes. Control Clin Trials 23(3):240–256

Braun TM (2006) Generalizing the TITE-CRM to adapt for early- and late-onset toxicities. Stat Med 25(12):2071–2083

Braun TM, Levine JE, Ferrara JLM (2003) Determining a maximum tolerated cumulative dose: dose reassignment within the TITE-CRM. Control Clin Trials 24(6):669–681

Braun TM, Thall PF, Nguyen H, de Lima M (2007) Simultaneously optimizing dose and schedule of a new cytotoxic agent. Clin Trials 4(2):113–124

Brock K, Billingham L, Copland M, Siddique S, Sirovica M, Yap C (2017) Implementing the EffTox dose-finding design in the matchpoint trial. BMC Med Res Methodol 17(1)

Cheung YK (2005) Coherence principles in dose-finding studies. Biometrika 92(4):863–873

Cheung YK, Chappell R (2000) Sequential designs for phase I clinical trials with late-onset toxicities. Biometrics 56(4):1177–1182

Chu P-L, Lin Y, Shih WJ (2009) Unifying CRM and EWOC designs for phase I cancer clinical trials. J Stat Plan Inference 139(3):1146–1163

Cole SR, Ananth CV (2001) Regression models for unconstrained, partially or fully constrained continuation odds ratios. Int J Epidemiol 30(6):1379–1382

Dinart D, Fraisse J, Tosi D, Mauguen A, Touraine C, Gourgou S, Le Deley MC, Bellera C, Mollevi C (2020) GUIP1: a R package for dose escalation strategies in phase I cancer clinical trials. BMC Med Inform Decis Mak 20(134). https://doi.org/10.1186/s12911-020-01149-3

Diniz MA (2018) ewoc: Escalation with overdose control. R package version 0.2.0

Diniz MA, Quanlin-Li, Tighiouart M (2017) Dose finding for drug combination in early cancer phase I trials using conditional continual reassessment method. J Biom Biostat 8(6)

Dragalin V, Fedorov V (2006) Adaptive designs for dose-finding based on efficacy–toxicity response. J Stat Plan Inference 136(6):1800–1823

Dragalin V, Fedorov V, Wu Y (2008) Adaptive designs for selecting drug combinations based on efficacy–toxicity response. J Stat Plan Inference 138(2):352–373

Ezzalfani M, Zohar S, Qin R, Mandrekar SJ, Deley M-CL (2013) Dose-finding designs using a novel quasi-continuous endpoint for multiple toxicities. Stat Med 32(16):2728–2746

Faries D (1994) Practical modifications of the continual reassessment method for phase I cancer clinical trials. J Biopharm Stat 4(2):147–164

Gasparini M (2013) General classes of multiple binary regression models in dose finding problems for combination therapies. J R Stat Soc: Ser C: Appl Stat 62(1):115–133

Goodman SN, Zahurak ML, Piantadosi S (1995) Some practical improvements in the continual reassessment method for phase I studies. Stat Med 14(11):1149–1161

Harrington JA, Wheeler GM, Sweeting MJ, Mander AP, Jodrell DI (2013) Adaptive designs for dual-agent phase I dose-escalation studies. Nat Rev Clin Oncol 10(5):277–288

Hirakawa A, Sato H, Daimon T, Matsui S (2018) Dose finding for a combination of two agents. In: Modern Dose-Finding Designs for Cancer Phase I Trials: Drug Combinations and Molecularly Targeted Agents, pp 9–40. Tokyo: Springer

Iasonos A, Wilton AS, Riedel ER, Seshan VE, Spriggs DR (2008) A comprehensive comparison of the continual reassessment method to the standard 3 + 3 dose escalation scheme in phase I dose-finding studies. Clin Trials 5(5):465–477
Iasonos A, Zohar S, O'Quigley J (2011) Incorporating lower grade toxicity information into dose finding designs. Clin Trials J Soc Clin Trials 8(4):370–379
Ivanova A, Wang Y, Foster MC (2016) The rapid enrollment design for phase I clinical trials. Stat Med 35(15):2516–2524
Jaki T, Clive S, Weir CJ (2013) Principles of dose finding studies in cancer: a comparison of trial designs. Cancer Chemother Pharmacol 71(5):1107–1114
Jimenez JL, Tighiouart M, Gasparini M (2018) Cancer phase I trial design using drug combinations when a fraction of dose limiting toxicities is attributable to one or more agents. Biom J 61 (2):319–332
Korn EL, Midthune D, Chen TT, Rubinstein LV, Christian MC, Simon RM (1994) A comparison of two phase I trial designs. Stat Med 13(18):1799–1806
Le Tourneau C, Jack Lee J, Siu LL (2009) Dose escalation methods in phase I cancer clinical trials. JNCI J Nat Cancer Inst 101(10):708–720
Lee SM, Cheng B, Cheung YK (2010) Continual reassessment method with multiple toxicity constraints. Biostatistics 12(2):386–398
Lin R, Yin G (2017) Bayesian optimal interval design for dose finding in drug-combination trials. Stat Methods Med Res 26(5):2155–2167
Mander AP, Sweeting MJ (2015) A product of independent beta probabilities dose escalation design for dual-agent phase I trials. Stat Med 34(8):1261–1276
Mandrekar SJ, Cui Y, Sargent DJ (2007) An adaptive phase I design for identifying a biologically optimal dose for dual agent drug combinations. Stat Med 26(11):2317–2330
Mandrekar SJ, Qin R, Sargent DJ (2010) Model-based phase I designs incorporating toxicity and efficacy for single and dual agent drug combinations: methods and challenges. Stat Med 29(10): 1077–1083
Mauguen A, Le Deley MC, Zohar S (2011) Dose-finding approach for dose escalation with overdose control considering incomplete observations. Stat Med 30(13):1584–1594
Muler JH, McGinn CJ, Normolle D, Lawrence T, Brown D, Hejna G, Zalupski MM (2004) Phase I trial using a time-to-event continual reassessment strategy for dose escalation of cisplatin combined with gemcitabine and radiation therapy in pancreatic cancer. J Clin Oncol 22(2): 238–243
Neuenschwander B, Branson M, Gsponer T (2008) Critical aspects of the Bayesian approach to phase I cancer trials. Stat Med 27(13):2420–2439
O'Quigley J, Conaway M (2011) Extended model-based designs for more complex dose-finding studies. Stat Med 30(17):2062–2069
O'Quigley J, Shen LZ (1996) Continual reassessment method: a likelihood approach. Biometrics 52(2):673
O'Quigley J, Pepe M, Fisher L (1990) Continual reassessment method: a practical design for phase 1 clinical trials in cancer. Biometrics 46(1):33
O'Quigley J, Iasonos A, Bornkamp B (2017) Handbook of methods for designing, monitoring, and analyzing dose-finding trials. Boca Raton, FL: Chapman and Hall Press/CRC
Padmanabhan SK, Krishna Padmanabhan S, Dragalin V (2010a) Adaptive dc-optimal designs for dose finding based on a continuous efficacy endpoint. Biom J 52(6):836–852
Padmanabhan SK, Krishna Padmanabhan S, Hsuan F, Dragalin V (2010b) Adaptive PenalizedD-optimal designs for dose finding based on continuous efficacy and toxicity. Stat Biopharm Res 2(2):182–198
Paul RK, Rosenberger WF, Flournoy N (2004) Quantile estimation following non-parametric phase I clinical trials with ordinal response. Stat Med 23(16):2483–2495
Piantadosi S, Fisher JD, Grossman S (1998) Practical implementation of a modified continual reassessment method for dose-finding trials. Cancer Chemother Pharmacol 41(6):429–436
Potthoff RF, George SL (2009) Flexible phase I clinical trials: allowing for nonbinary toxicity response and removal of other common limitations. Stat Biopharm Res 1(3):213–228

Pronzato L (2010) Penalized optimal designs for dose-finding. J Stat Plan Inference 140(1): 283–296
Riviere MK, Le Tourneau C, Paoletti X, Dubois F, Zohar S (2014) Designs of drug-combination phase I trials in oncology: a systematic review of the literature. Ann Oncol 26(4):669–674
Sweeting M, Mander A, Sabin T (2013) Bcrm: Bayesian continual reassessment method designs for phase I dose-finding trials. J Stat Softw 54(13)
Thall PF (2010) Bayesian models and decision algorithms for complex early phase clinical trials. Stat Sci 25(2):227–244
Thall PF, Cook JD (2004) Dose-finding based on efficacy-toxicity trade-offs. Biometrics 60(3): 684–693
Thall PF, Cook JD (2006) Using both efficacy and toxicity for dose-finding. In: Statistical methods for dose-finding experiments, pp 275–285. New York: Wiley
Thall PF, Russell KE (1998) A strategy for dose-finding and safety monitoring based on efficacy and adverse outcomes in phase I/II clinical trials. Biometrics 54(1):251–264
Thall PF, Millikan RE, Mueller P, Lee S-J (2003) Dose-finding with two agents in phase I oncology trials. Biometrics 59(3):487–496
Thall PF, Herrick RC, Nguyen HQ, Venier JJ, Norris JC (2014) Effective sample size for computing prior hyperparameters in Bayesian phase I-II dose-finding. Clin Trials 11(6):657–666
Tighiouart M (2018) Two-stage design for phase I-II cancer clinical trials using continuous dose combinations of cytotoxic agents. J R Stat Soc: Ser C: Appl Stat 68(1):235–250
Tighiouart M, Rogatko A (2010) Dose finding with escalation with over-dose control (EWOC) in cancer clinical trials. Stat Sci 25(2):217–226
Tighiouart M, Rogatko A, Babb JS (2005) Flexible Bayesian methods for cancer phase I clinical trials. Dose escalation with overdose control. Stat Med 24(14):2183–2196
Tighiouart M, Cook-Wiens G, Rogatko A (2012) Escalation with over-dose control using ordinal toxicity grades for cancer phase I clinical trials. J Probab Stat 2012:1–18
Tighiouart M, Liu Y, Rogatko A (2014) Escalation with overdose control using time to toxicity for cancer phase I clinical trials. PLoS One 9(3):e93070
Tighiouart M, Li Q, Rogatko A (2017) A Bayesian adaptive design for estimating the maximum tolerated dose curve using drug combinations in cancer phase I clinical trials. Stat Med 36(2): 280–290
Tighiouart M, Cook-Wiens G, Rogatko A (2018) A Bayesian adaptive design for cancer phase I trials using a flexible range of doses. J Biopharm Stat 28(3):562–574
Van Meter EM, Garrett-Mayer E, Bandyopadhyay D (2011) Proportional odds model for dose-finding clinical trial designs with ordinal toxicity grading. Stat Med 30(17):2070–2080
Van Meter EM, Garrett-Mayer E, Bandyopadhyay D (2012) Dose-finding clinical trial design for ordinal toxicity grades using the continuation ratio model: an extension of the continual reassessment method. Clin Trials 9(3):303–313
Wages NA, Conaway MR (2014) Phase I/II adaptive design for drug combination oncology trials. Stat Med 33(12):1990–2003
Wages NA, Conaway MR, O'Quigley J (2011a) Continual reassessment method for partial ordering. Biometrics 67(4):1555–1563
Wages NA, Conaway MR, O'Quigley J (2011b) Dose-finding design for multi-drug combinations. Clin Trials 8(4):380–389
Wages NA, Conaway MR, O'Quigley J (2013) Using the time-to-event continual reassessment method in the presence of partial orders. Stat Med 32(1):131–141
Wages NA, Ivanova A, Marchenko O (2016) Practical designs for phase I combination studies in oncology. J Biopharm Stat 26(1):150–166
Wang K, Ivanova A (2005) Two-dimensional dose finding in discrete dose space. Biometrics 61(1): 217–222
Wheeler GM (2018) Incoherent dose-escalation in phase I trials using the escalation with overdose control approach. Stat Pap (Berl) 59(2):801–811

Wheeler GM, Sweeting MJ, Mander AP (2017) Toxicity-dependent feasibility bounds for the escalation with overdose control approach in phase I cancer trials. Stat Med 36(16):2499–2513

Wheeler GM, Sweeting MJ, Mander AP (2019) A Bayesian model-free approach to combination therapy phase I trials using censored time-to-toxicity data. J R Stat Soc: Ser C: Appl Stat 68(2):309–329

Yin G, Yuan Y (2009a) Bayesian dose finding in oncology for drug combinations by copula regression. J R Stat Soc: Ser C: Appl Stat 58(2):211–224

Yin G, Yuan Y (2009b) A latent contingency table approach to dose finding for combinations of two agents. Biometrics 65(3):866–875

Yuan Z, Chappell R, Bailey H (2007) The continual reassessment method for multiple toxicity grades: a Bayesian quasi-likelihood approach. Biometrics 63(1):173–179

Yuan, Y., Nguyen, H. Q., and Thall, P. F. (2017). Bayesian designs for phase I–II clinical trials. Boca Raton, FL: Chapman and Hall Press/CRC

Zhang W, Sargent DJ, Mandrekar S (2006) An adaptive dose-finding design incorporating both toxicity and efficacy. Stat Med 25(14):2365–2383

Zhou Y (2009) Adaptive designs for phase I dose-finding studies. Fundam Clin Pharmacol 24 (2):129–138

Adaptive Phase II Trials

61

Boris Freidlin and Edward L. Korn

Contents

Abstract

Phase II trials are designed to obtain preliminary efficacy information about a new therapy in order to assess whether the new therapy should be tested in definitive (phase III) trials. Adaptive trial designs allow the design of a trial to be changed during its conduct, possibly using accruing outcome data. Adaptations to phase II trials considered in this chapter include formal interim monitoring, phase II/III trial designs, adaptations related to biomarker subgroups, sample size reassessment, outcome-adaptive randomization, and adaptive pooling of outcome results across patient subgroups. Adaptive phase II trials allow for the possibility of trials reaching their conclusions earlier, with more patients being treated with therapies that have activity for them.

B. Freidlin (✉) · E. L. Korn
Biometric Research Program, Division of Cancer Treatment and Diagnosis, National Cancer Institute, Bethesda, MD, USA
e-mail: freidlinb@ctep.nci.nih.gov; korne@ctep.nci.nih.gov

© This is a U.S. Government work and not under copyright protection in the U.S.; foreign copyright protection may apply 2022

S. Piantadosi, C. L. Meinert (eds.), *Principles and Practice of Clinical Trials*,
https://doi.org/10.1007/978-3-319-52636-2_276

Keywords

Biomarkers · Futility monitoring · Interim monitoring · Outcome-adaptive randomization · Phase II/III · Sample size reassessment

Introduction

Phase II trials are designed to obtain preliminary efficacy information on a new therapy to decide whether development should be pursued with definitive (phase III) trials. Phase II trials are smaller than phase III trials because they relax the error-rate requirements and can use shorter-term endpoints that are more sensitive to biologic activity (regardless of whether they directly measure clinical benefit). For example, oncology phase II trials often use a tumor response (shrinkage) endpoint (rather than, say, overall survival). For evaluating a new agent, a single-arm trial with 32 patients would allow one to distinguish a 20% response rate (interesting activity) from a 5% response rate (uninteresting activity), with both false-positive and false-negative error rates under 10% (Simon 1989). For evaluating addition of a new agent to the standard therapy, a trial that randomly assigns 120 patients to receive either the standard treatment or the standard treatment plus the new agent will have 90% power at a one-sided 0.10 significance level to detect an increase in response rate from 10% to 30% (Green et al. 2016). For randomized phase II trials, one can also use other endpoints for which it would not be as easy to interpret efficacy in a single-arm trial, e.g., progression-free survival.

Adaptive trial designs allow the course of the trial to be changed during its conduct using accruing outcome data. Adaptive features of phase II trial designs considered in this chapter are interim monitoring, phase II/III trial designs, adaptations related to biomarkers, sample size reassessment, outcome-adaptive randomization, and adaptive pooling of outcome results.

Interim Monitoring

The most fundamental adaptive element of a clinical trial is formal interim monitoring, which allows a trial to stop early when its scientific objectives have been met: If it becomes clear in an ongoing phase II trial that the experimental treatment is not going to be worth pursuing, then the trial should be stopped (futility monitoring). This minimizes patient exposure to inactive toxic treatments and conserves resources (Freidlin and Korn 2009). For example, in a single-arm trial targeting a response rate of 20% versus 5%, a Simon optimal two-stage design (Simon 1989) first accrues and evaluates 12 patients. The trial only continues (to a total of 37 patients) if there is at least one response seen in these 12 patients. For a randomized phase II trial, the simple Wieand futility monitoring rule (Wieand et al. 1994) stops the trial half-way through if the experimental arm is doing worse than the standard treatment arm by any amount. For example, in a 120-patient randomized trial to detect an improvement in response rates from 10% to 30%, the trial would stop when the first 60 patients have been evaluated if the observed response rate was lower in the experimental arm than the control arm. With a time-to-event endpoint, Wieand futility monitoring is performed when one-half of the required number of events for the final analysis is observed. Unlike phase III trials, phase II trials generally do not include the possibility of stopping (and discontinuing enrollment) early for positive results (efficacy stopping), e.g., superiority of the experimental treatment over the standard treatment in a randomized phase II trial. This is because it is useful to get more experience with the treatment to inform phase III design (and patients are meanwhile not being given an ineffective experimental therapy). However, it could be useful for phase II trials to allow for the possibility of early reporting of positive results as the trial continues to completion, especially if the trial is relatively large or expected to take a long time to complete (e.g., due to the rarity of the disease). For example, using a version of the Fleming approach (Fleming 1982) to the single-arm two-stage design above, one can report the first-stage (12 patients) results for efficacy with three or more responses as well as stopping the trial for futility with zero responses. For randomized studies, it often would not be acceptable to continue randomization once a positive result is reported. However, in studies with time-to-event endpoints, where the outcome data requires non-trivial follow-up to mature, it might still be useful to conduct an efficacy analysis for potential early reporting once all patients have been enrolled and are off the randomized treatments.

Multi-arm randomized phase II trials with multiple experimental arms being compared to a standard treatment arm are efficient designs as compared to performing separate randomized phase II trials for each experimental treatment (because of the shared standard-treatment arm) (Freidlin et al. 2008). Futility monitoring for each experimental arm/control arm comparison may increase the efficiency further, allowing individual experimental arms to be closed early (increasing the accrual rate on the remaining open arms). An example of such a trial is SWOG 1500 (Pal et al. 2017), which has three experimental arms and a standard treatment arm for metastatic papillary renal carcinoma. The trial design included Wieand futility monitoring rules, and two of the experimental arms stopped early for futility.

There is also the possibility of having a multi-arm trial with a "master protocol" that accommodates adding new experimental treatment arms when they become available for phase II testing. An example of such a trial is ISPY-2 (Barker et al. 2009), which is testing neoadjuvant experimental treatments for women with locally advanced breast cancer. In addition to being less efficient than having all treatments available for testing at the same time (because results from patients on an experimental arm can only be compared to results from patients on the standard-treatment arm who were randomized contemporaneously), trials with master protocols present major logistical challenges to execute (Cecchini et al. 2019).

Phase II/III Trial Designs

A phase II/III design is a phase II trial with an adaptation to possibly extend it to a phase III trial if the phase II results look sufficiently promising (Bretz et al. 2006; Korn et al. 2012). The advantage of phase II/III design over a separate phase II trial followed by a phase III trial (if the phase II trial is positive) is that the patient outcomes from the phase II portion can be used in the phase III analysis. In addition, a phase II/III trial, which requires a single protocol, reduces the development time in that two protocols do not need to be written and receive separate regulatory approvals. The disadvantage to using a phase II/III trial is that one is committing early to the treatment that will be evaluated in a phase III trial (Korn et al. 2012; Cuffe et al. 2014); in a setting where many new treatments are being developed, it may be better to perform a stand-alone phase II trial and then make decision based on what new treatments are available for testing in phase III.

If a phase II/III trial is appropriate, then one first specifies the phase III design parameters: type 1 error (e.g., one-sided 0.025) and sufficient power (e.g., 90%) to detect a clinically meaningful improvement in the phase III endpoint (e.g., improving median overall survival from 12 months to 16 months). The phase III design parameters determine the phase III sample size (e.g., 500 patients randomized), or, for time-to-event endpoints, the number of required events for the final analysis (e.g., 400 deaths). The phase II portion of the trial is then embedded in the phase III trial by evaluating an appropriately selected phase II endpoint on an initial set of randomized patients, typically using a similar design that one would have used for a stand-alone phase II trial (e.g., targeting a 30% versus 10% improvement in response rate in the first 120 randomized patients using the design described in the Introduction). If this phase II analysis rejects the null hypothesis that the response rates are equal at the 0.10 level, then the accrual is continued to the full 500 patients for the phase III analysis. Note that phase II/III designs can have multiple experimental arms with some or all of them dropped at the phase II stage.

For example, SWOG S1117 (Sekeres et al. 2017) is a phase II/III trial that randomly assigned high-risk myelodysplastic syndrome and chronic myelomonocytic leukemia patients to azacitidine (the standard treatment), azacitidine+lenalidomide, or azacitidine+vorinostat arms. The phase II portion of the trial was designed to enroll 240 patients (80 per arm). For each of the combination versus azacitidine comparisons, this provided 81% power at a one-sided 0.05 significance level to detect an increase from 35% to 55% in response rates. If at least one of the combination arms was shown to be promising, the trial would proceed to the phase III portion. The phase III portion was designed to include a total of 452 patients randomly assigned to either azacitidine or the best combination arm (including the phase II stage patients) to provide 80% power to detect an overall survival hazard ratio of 1.4 at a one-sided significance level of 0.025. The study was stopped after the phase II stage because both combination arms failed to pass the phase II decision rule.

Operationally, short-term phase II endpoints like response are easier to employ in the phase II/III framework since they allow a quick evaluation as to whether to continue to the phase III stage of the trial. However, in many clinical settings, a time-to-event endpoint (e.g., progression-free survival) is considered to be a more reliable phase II measure of clinical activity (than response) for deciding whether to proceed to the phase III trial. This leads to another key decision in the trial design: Should one continue to accrue while waiting for the data from the phase II patients to mature, or should one suspend accrual during this time? The advantage of suspending accrual is that no additional patients will have been unnecessarily accrued in the event the phase II analysis suggests not proceeding to phase III. In particular, in some settings, all or practically all the phase III patients will be accrued before the data on the phase II patients are mature enough to make a decision, negating any efficiency in using a phase II/III design. The disadvantage of suspending accrual is that it will take longer to get the phase III results (assuming the phase II analysis is positive), especially if it takes time to ramp up accrual after the suspension. In addition, with a long suspension, one can question the generalizability of the trial results because the patient population may have changed over time. However, a changing patient population can be of theoretical concern for any long trial (whether or not there is an accrual suspension), so this is not a reason to avoid an accrual suspension in a phase II/III trial (Freidlin et al. 2018).

An example of a phase II/III design with accrual suspension is given by RTOG-1216 (Zhang et al. 2019) that compared radiation+docetaxel and radiation +docetaxel+cetuximab arms to a standard radiation+cisplatin arm in advanced head and neck cancer. The phase II design was based on randomly assigning 180 patents between the 3 arms (60 patients per arm), targeting for each of the two experimental versus control comparisons a progression-free survival hazard ratio of 0.6 (with 80% power at a one-sided 0.15 significance level). The phase II analysis for each experimental versus control comparison was scheduled when a total of 56 progression-free survival events were observed for the two arms. If at least one of the experimental arms was significantly positive, the study would proceed to the phase III portion with a total of 460 patients randomized between the best experimental arm and the control arm, targeting an overall survival hazard ratio of 0.67. The study was designed to suspend accrual after the 180-patient phase II portion finished accrual until the phase II analyses were performed requiring 56 events for each of the two experimental versus control comparisons. The protocol projected that the phase II analysis would take place approximately 1.3 years after completion of phase II accrual (but it actually took slightly over 2 years for the phase II data to mature).

An example of a phase II/III trial without an accrual suspension is given by GOG0182-ICON5 for advanced-stage ovarian cancer (Bookman et al. 2009). This trial had four experimental arms that were compared to a standard treatment arm. The phase II endpoint was progression-free survival, and the phase III endpoint was overall survival. The trial accrued 4312 patients rapidly before the phase II analyses determined no difference between the experimental arms and the standard treatment arm (there was also no difference in overall survival). If an accrual suspension of 15 months had been used, the total sample size would have been 1740 (Korn et al. 2012).

Adaptations Related to Biomarkers

Biomarkers can be used to identify patients for whom an experimental treatment is likely to be effective. For example, in metastatic colorectal cancer, it has been well established that the benefit of anti-EGFR monoclonal antibodies (e.g., cetaximab and panitumumab) is restricted to patients with KRAS wild-type tumors (Vale et al. 2012). In the context of phase II trials, it is not known whether the experimental treatment will be effective in either the biomarker-positive or biomarker-negative subgroups, but it is thought that it will be at least as effective in the biomarker-positive subgroup as in the biomarker-negative subgroup. In this case, a biomarker-stratified trial design, in which patients in the two subgroups are separately randomized and analyzed, can be used (Freidlin et al. 2010). It is important to perform interim monitoring separately in these subgroups, which allows for the possibility of adaptively stopping accrual of biomarker-negative patients if it appears that the experimental treatment is not working for them. One should also consider stopping the whole trial (and not just accrual to the biomarker-positive patients) if the biomarker-positive subgroup crosses a futility interim monitoring boundary.

In addition to interim monitoring, a trial may be adaptively modified to increase the number of patients with a specific characteristic, e.g., a specific histology or a specific biomarker value. An example of this type of adaptation is given by the design of the arms of the NCI-Pediatric MATCH trial (Allen et al. 2017). The generic design for each arm (subprotocol) of this trial is the following: Twenty patients with the specific tumor mutation are treated with the agent targeted for this mutation (regardless of cancer histology). The analysis for this primary cohort uses a decision rule of the agent/mutation being considered worthy of further study if at least 3 tumor responses are seen in these 20 patients. Three possible adaptations included in the design are the following. (1) If there are three or more responses in patients with the same histology (after the primary cohort is enrolled), then up to ten patients (in total) can be enrolled with the same histology (who have the mutation). (2) If at any time there are three or more responses in the primary cohort but with less than three responses in the same histology, then a cohort of 10 patients without the mutation (regardless of cancer histology) will be enrolled. (3) If at any time there are three or more responses in the primary cohort with the same histology, then a cohort of ten patients without the mutation but with the same histology will be enrolled. The purpose of these adaptive cohorts is to obtain more information about in which patient subsets the agent is likely to be effective, while minimizing the exposure of patient subsets where the agent is likely not to be effective.

With a biomarker that putatively identifies patients for whom the experimental therapy is better than the standard therapy, the aims of a randomized phase II trial can be expanded from "Does the therapy warrant further testing?" to "Does the therapy warrant further testing only in the biomarker-positive subgroup, in both the biomarker-positive and biomarker-negative subgroups (Freidlin et al. 2010), in the whole population regardless of biomarker status, or not at all?" This allows one to adapt the plan for a future phase III trial. This can be done informally by examining experimental arm versus standard arm comparisons in the biomarker-positive and biomarker-negative subgroups from a completed trial. However, this post hoc approach may not work because of insufficient sample sizes in one or both subgroups. A formal approach to this problem has been proposed (Freidlin et al. 2012), which requires a larger sample size than a single randomized phase II trial, but less total sample size than performing separate randomized phase II trials in the biomarker-positive and biomarker-negative subgroups.

Sample Size Reassessment

Sample size reassessment is a potential adaptation to the sample size of a trial based on promising interim results from the trial. Although mostly used for phase III trials, it has been recommended and used for phase II trials (Wang et al. 2012; Campbell et al. 2014; Meretoja et al. 2014). In the phase II setting, a particular implementation (Chen et al. 2004) initially starts with a plan to enroll a fixed number of patients to target a potentially optimistic treatment effect with 90% power at a one-sided significance level of 10%. When the information from the first-half of the trial becomes available, the design examines the (one-sided) p-value. If this p-value is less than 0.18 but greater than 0.06, then the sample size is increased up to twice the original sample size using a formula that depends on this p-value, with p-values closer to 0.18 leading to larger increases. The idea is that one can gain power to reject the null hypothesis when the interim results appear promising by increasing the sample size.

Sample size reassessment is controversial (Burman and Sonesson 2006; Emerson et al. 2011; Freidlin and Korn 2017; Mehta 2017). The issue is whether sample size reassessment is a reasonable approach to ensuring an adequately powered trial. A simple numerical example illustrates the issues: Consider a randomized phase II trial targeting a response rate of 45% for the experimental therapy versus 20% for the standard treatment arm. With a standard design (maximum of 92 randomized patients with Wieand futility monitoring after 46 patients), the trial would have 90% power for a one-sided significance level of 10% (Green et al. 2016). With the same level and power and using sample size reassessment, the initial sample size can be set to 84, with a possible increase to 168 (based on the interim results after 42 patients have been evaluated, including Wieand futility monitoring at that time). Theoretically, if a sponsor of a trial initially had resources only for an 84-patient trial but not a 96-patient trial, then sample size reassessment would allow the sponsor to obtain additional resources to increase the sample size based on promising interim results. However, as is shown in Table 1, the sample size reassessment design is inferior to the standard design as, on average, it would require more patients (in some cases nontrivially increasing the sample size and duration of the trial). Note that in addition to the efficiency issues, sample size reassessment designs raise some integrity concerns when used with time-to-event outcomes (Freidlin and Korn 2017)

Table 1 Comparison of standard design with sample size reassessment design for comparing response rates of 45% versus 20% (90% power at 0.1 significance level)

Sample size	Standard design (with Wieand futility monitoring)	Sample size reassessment (with Wieand futility monitoring)
Minimum	46	42
Maximum	92	168
Average under null hypothesis	72	73
Average under the alternative hypothesis	91	95

Outcome-Adaptive Randomization

Outcome-adaptive randomization is a technique where the proportion of patients randomized to the different treatment arms changes during the trial based on the accruing outcome data (Lee and Chu 2012). The changes are made so that a higher proportion of patients are randomized to the arm(s) that appear to be doing better. Although this technique is superficially appealing, there are a number of caveats. First, any time trends in the prognosis of patients accruing to the trial can potentially bias (confound) the treatment results and lead to inflated type 1 error (Byar et al. 1976; Korn and Freidlin 2011a). Therefore, this method is not recommended for definitive phase III trials. Second, the operating characteristics of the method are poor for trials with one experimental arm and one control treatment arm (Korn and Freidlin 2011a; Thall et al. 2015), so the technique is also not recommended for two-armed phase II randomized trials. Comparisons of outcome-adaptive randomization with standard fixed randomization (with appropriate futility interim monitoring) are more nuanced in multi-arm trials with multiple experimental agents: Simulations demonstrate similar results, with the outcome-adaptive randomization yielding a slightly higher proportion of patients with good outcomes but also a slightly longer trial with a larger number of patients with bad outcomes (Korn and Freidlin 2011b). Finally, whether using outcome-adaptive randomization is more or less ethical than using fixed randomization has been debated (Hey and Kimmelman 2015).

An example of a multi-arm randomized phase II that used outcome-adaptive randomization is the BATTLE-2 trial (Papadimitrakopoulou et al. 2016). In this trial, patients with advanced non-small cell lung cancer were randomized among four treatment arms (a control arm and three experimental arms), with the outcome being disease control at 8 weeks (complete or partial tumor response or non-progressing disease at 8 weeks). Equal randomization was used for the first 70 patients, and then outcome-adaptive randomization was used for the next 130 patients (adjusted for two biomarkers). For the 186 evaluable patients, the 8-week disease control rates (DCR) were 32% (6/19) for the control arm, and 50% (18/36), 53% (37/70), and 46% (28/61) for the three experimental arms. One can calculate that if one had used equal randomization throughout, then a trial with 120 evaluable patients would have achieved the same statistical power as the 186 evaluable-patient outcome-adaptive randomization trial for the pairwise comparisons between the experimental arms and standard treatment arms (Korn and Freidlin 2017). The equal randomization trial would be expected to have an overall DCR of 45% (54/120), less than the observed rate of 48% (89/186) with the outcome-adaptive randomization, a slight plus for outcome-adaptive randomization. However, equal randomization would have resulted in a shorter trial, with fewer patients, and with fewer patients having a bad outcome (66 versus 97) (Korn and Freidlin 2017).

Note that the outcome-adaptive randomization should not be confused with statistical techniques designed to balance the distribution of baseline covariates between the study arms (Pocock and Simon 1975). Unlike outcome-adaptive randomization that uses study outcome to change the probability of treatment assignment, these methods use prespecified baseline characteristics of the accruing patents to modify the randomization and are not controversial.

Adaptive Pooling of Outcome Results

To account for potential heterogeneity in the activity of an experimental treatment in different patient subgroups, phase II trials often consider the activity separately for the different subgroups. For example, when evaluating an agent targeting a particular molecular target, patients with tumors expressing the target may be separated into histology-based subgroups. It may be reasonable to expect some degree of similarity in the level of activity between the subgroups (although this is not assured). In this case it could be attractive to borrow (pool) activity information across subgroups, especially when the subgroups are small. To address this issue, a variety of adaptive pooling ("adaptive information borrowing") methods that allow the estimate of activity in a given subgroup to be influenced by the outcomes in other subgroups have been proposed. For example, in a trial that is designed to evaluate response rates in different histologic subgroups, the response rate for a specific histology could be estimated as a weighted average of the observed response rate for that histology and the overall response rate across all histologies. The amount of borrowing (pooling) across subgroups is determined by the weights, with weighting the overall rate more representing more borrowing. Most of the adaptive approaches for choosing weights use Bayesian hierarchical modeling (Thall et al. 2003). In this approach the weights are determined by the spread of the observed histology-specific rates: The more narrow the spread, the more weight is given to the overall response rate in estimating the individual histology response. That is, when the observed rates are close to each other, the estimates of the histology-specific means are taken to be close to the observed overall mean. On the other hand, when the observed rates are far apart, the estimated rate for each histology is taken to be close to the corresponding histology-specific mean.

Attractive as it sounds, however, borrowing comes at a price (i.e., just like in life there is no free lunch): In most practical settings, adaptive pooling without proper adjustment can result in nontrivially inflated rates of incorrectly declaring an agent effective in subgroups where it does not work and incorrectly declaring an agent ineffective in subgroups where it does work (Freidlin and Korn 2013). Vigorous methodologic research in refining adaptive pooling designs is continuing (Chu and Yuan 2018; Cunanan et al. 2019). It may not be possible to have a design that allows the use of observed data to guide the pooling across subgroups without inflating the design error rates (Kopp-Schneider et al. 2019).

Summary

Careful application of adaptive features like interim monitoring or biomarker-driven adaptations can dramatically improve the efficiency of phase II trials. This could accelerate development of new therapies, protect patients from exposure to potentially toxic ineffective therapies, and conserve resources. On the other hand, outcome-adaptive randomization has been long known to have suboptimal statistical properties. Less understood methodologies like sample size reassessment and adaptive pooling should be considered carefully, as they provide questionable benefit (if any). Moreover, these more complex statistical methods may pose major transparency and reproducibility challenges. Therefore, their use requires clear justification, and their reporting requires clear description of the study design and conduct.

Key Facts

Application of certain adaptive features like interim monitoring or biomarker-driven adaptations can improve efficiency of phase II trials. Outcome-adaptive randomization has not been shown to improve design performance relative to the properly designed/monitored fixed-randomization trials. Less understood methodologies like sample size reassessment and adaptive pooling increase design complexity without providing tangible benefit.

Cross-References

▶ Biomarker-Guided Trials
▶ Futility Designs
▶ Interim Analysis in Clinical Trials
▶ Multi-arm Multi-stage (MAMS) Platform Randomized Clinical Trials

References

Allen CE, Laetsch TW, Mody R, Irwin MS, Lim MS, Adamson PC, Seibel NL, Parsons DW, Cho YJ, Janeway K, on behalf of the Pediatric MATCH Target and Agent Prioritization Committee (2017) Target and Agent Prioritization for the Children's Oncology Group – National Cancer Institute Pediatric MATCH Trial. J Natl Cancer Inst 109:djw274

Barker AD, Sigman CC, Kelloff GJ, Hylton NM, Berry DA, Esserman LJ (2009) I-SPY 2: an adaptive breast cancer trial design in the setting of neoadjuvant chemotherapy. Clin Pharmacol Ther 86:97–100

Bookman MA, Brady MF, McGuire WP, Harper PG, Alberts DS, Friedlander M, Colombo N, Fowler JM, Argenta PA, De Geest K, Mutch DG, Burger RA, Swart AM, Trimble EL, Accario-Winslow C, Roth LM (2009) Evaluation of new platinum-based treatment regimens in advanced-stage ovarian cancer: a phase III trial of the Gynecologic Cancer Inter Group. J Clin Oncol 27:1419–1425

Bretz F, Schmidli H, König F, Racine A, Maurer W (2006) Confirmatory seamless phase II/III clinical trials with hypothesis selection at interim: general concepts. Biom J 48:623–634

Burman CF, Sonesson C (2006) Are flexible designs sound? Biometrics 62:664–669

Byar DP, Simon RM, Friedewald WT, Schlesselman JJ, DeMets DL, Ellenberg JH, Gail MH, Ware JH (1976) Randomized clinical trials – perspectives on some recent ideas. N Engl J Med 295:74–80

Campbell BC, Mitchell PJ, Yan B, Parsons MW, Christensen S, Churilov L, Dowling RJ, Dewey H, Brooks M, Miteff F, Levi C, Krause M, Harrington TJ, Faulder KC, Steinfort BS, Kleinig T, Scroop R, Chryssidis S, Barber A, Hope A, Moriarty M, McGuinness B, Wong AA, Coulthard A, Wijeratne T, Lee A, Jannes J, Leyden J, Phan TG, Chong W, Holt ME, Chandra RV, Bladin CF, Badve M, Rice H, de Villiers L, Ma H, Desmond PM, Donnan GA, Davis SM, EXTEND-IA Investigators (2014) A multicenter, randomized, controlled study to investigate EXtending the time for Thrombolysis in Emergency Neurological Deficits with Intra-Arterial therapy (EXTEND-IA). Int J Stroke 9:126–132

Cecchini M, Rubin EH, Blumenthal GM, Ayalew K, Burris HA, Russell-Einhorn M, Dillon H, Lyerly HK, Reaman GH, Boerner S, LoRusso PM (2019) Challenges with novel clinical trial designs: master protocols. Clin Cancer Res 25:2049–2057

Chen YH, DeMets DL, Lan KK (2004) Increasing the sample size when the unblinded interim result is promising. Stat Med 23:1023–1038

Chu Y, Yuan Y (2018) Bayesian basket trial design using a calibrated Bayesian hierarchical model. Clin Trials 15:149–158

Cuffe RL, Lawrence D, Stone A, Vandemeulebroecke M (2014) When is a seamless study desirable? Case studies from different pharmaceutical sponsors. Pharm Stat 13:229–237

Cunanan KM, Iasonos A, Shen R, Gönen M (2019) Variance prior specification for a basket trial design using Bayesian hierarchical modeling. Clin Trials 16:142–153

Emerson SS, Levin GP, Emerson SC (2011) Comments on 'Adaptive increase in sample size when interim results are promising: a practical guide with examples'. Stat Med 30:3285–3301

Fleming TR (1982) One-sample multiple testing procedure for phase II clinical trials. Biometrics 38:143–151

Freidlin B, Korn EL (2009) Monitoring for lack of benefit: a critical component of a randomized clinical trial. J Clin Oncol 27:629–633

Freidlin B, Korn EL (2013) Borrowing information across subgroups: is it useful? Clin Cancer Res 19:1326–1334

Freidlin B, Korn EL (2017) Sample size adjustment designs with time-to-event outcomes: a caution. Clinical Trials 14:597–604

Freidlin B, Korn EL, Gray R, Martin A (2008) Multi-arm clinical trials of new agents: some design considerations. Clin Cancer Res 14:4368–4371

Freidlin B, McShane LM, Korn EL (2010) Randomized clinical trials with biomarkers: design issues. J Natl Cancer Inst 102:152–160

Freidlin B, McShane LM, Polley MY, Korn EL (2012) Randomized phase II trials designs with biomarkers. J Clin Oncol 30:1–6

Freidlin B, Korn EL, Abrams JS (2018) Bias, operational bias, and generalizability in phase II/III trials. J Clin Oncol 36:1902–1904

Green S, Benedetti J, Smith A, Crowley J (2016) Clinical trials in oncology, 3rd edn. CRC Press, New York

Hey SP, Kimmelman J (2015) Are outcome-adaptive allocation trials ethical? (and Commentary). Clin Trials 12:102–127

Kopp-Schneider A, Calderazzo S, Wiesenfarth M (2019) Power gains by using external information in clinical trials are typically not possible when requiring strict type I error control. Biom J. https://doi.org/10.1002/bimj.201800395

Korn EL, Freidlin B (2011a) Outcome-adaptive randomization: is it useful? J Clin Oncol 29:771–776

Korn EL, Freidlin B (2011b) Reply to Y. Yuan et al. J Clin Oncol 29:e393

Korn EL, Freidlin B (2017) Adaptive Clinical Trials: advantages and disadvantages of various adaptive design elements. J Natl Cancer Inst 109:dlx013

Korn EL, Freidlin B, Abrams JS, Halabi S (2012) Design issues in randomized phase II/III trials. J Clin Oncol 30:667–671

Lee JJ, Chu CT (2012) Bayesian clinical trials in action. Stat Med 31:2955–2971

Mehta C (2017) Commentary on Freidlin and Korn. Clinical Trials 14:605–608

Meretoja A, Churilov L, Campbell BC, Aviv RI, Yassi N, Barras C, Mitchell P, Yan B, Nandurkar H, Bladin C, Wijeratne T, Spratt NJ, Jannes J, Sturm J, Rupasinghe J, Zavala J, Lee A, Kleinig T, Markus R, Delcourt C, Mahant N, Parsons MW, Levi C, Anderson CS, Donnan GA, Davis SM (2014) The spot sign and tranexamic acid on preventing ICH growth – Australasia Trial (STOP-AUST): protocol of a phase II randomized, placebo-controlled, double-blind, multicenter trial. Int J Stroke 9:519–524

Pal SK, Tangen CM, Thompson IM, Shuch BM, Haas NB, George DJ, Stein MN, Wright JJ, Plets M, Lara P (2017) A randomized, phase II efficacy assessment of multiple MET kinase inhibitors in metastatic papillary renal carcinoma (PRCC): SWOG S1500. J Clin Oncol 35(15_suppl): TPS4599

Papadimitrakopoulou V, Lee JJ, Wistuba II, Tsao AS, Fossella FV, Kalhor N, Gupta S, Byers LA, Izzo JG, Gettinger SN, Goldberg SB, Tang X, Miller VA, Skoulidis F, Gibbons DL, Shen L, Wei C, Diao L, Peng SA, Wang J, Tam AL, Coombes KR, Koo JS, Mauro DJ, Rubin EH, Heymach JV, Hong WK, Herbst RS (2016) The BATTLE-2 study: a biomarker-integrated targeted therapy study in previously treated patients with advanced non-small-cell lung cancer. J Clin Oncol 334:3638–3647

Pocock SJ, Simon R (1975) Sequential treatment assignment with balancing for prognostic factors in the controlled clinical trial. Biometrics 31:103–115

Sekeres MA, Othus M, List AF, Odenike O, Stone RM, Gore SD, Litzow MR, Buckstein R, Fang M, Roulston D, Bloomfield CD, Moseley A, Nazha A, Zhang Y, Velasco MR, Gaur R, Atallah E, Attar EC, Cook EK, Cull AH, Rauh MJ, Appelbaum FR, Erba HP (2017) Randomized Phase II Study of azacitidine alone or in combination with lenalidomide or with vorinostat in higher-risk myelodysplastic syndromes and chronic myelomonocytic leukemia: North American Intergroup Study SWOG S1117. J Clin Oncol 35:2745–2753

Simon R (1989) Optimal two-stage designs for phase II clinical trials. Control Clin Trials 10:1–10

Thall PF, Wathen JK, Bekele BN, Champlin RE, Baker LH, Benjamin RS (2003) Hierarchical Bayesian approaches to phase II trials in diseases with multiple subtypes. Stat Med 22:763–780

Thall P, Fox P, Wathen J (2015) Statistical controversies in clinical research: scientific and ethical problems with adaptive randomization in comparative clinical trials. Ann Oncol 26:1621–1628

Vale CL, Tierney JF, Fisher D, Adams RA, Kaplan R, Maughan TS, Parmar MK, Meade AM (2012) Does anti-EGFR therapy improve outcome in advanced colorectal cancer? A systematic review and meta-analysis. Cancer Treat Rev 38:618–625

Wang S-J, Hung HMJ, Robert O'NR (2012) Paradigms for adaptive statistical information designs: practical experiences and strategies. Stat Med 31:3011–3023

Wieand S, Schroeder G, O'Fallon JR (1994) Stopping when the experimental regimen does not appear to help. Stat Med 13:1453–1458

Zhang QE, Wu Q, Harari PM, Rosenthal DI (2019) Randomized phase II/III confirmatory treatment selection design with a change of survival end points: statistical design of Radiation Therapy Oncology Group 1216. Head Neck 41:37–45

Biomarker-Guided Trials

62

L. C. Brown, A. L. Jorgensen, M. Antoniou, and J. Wason

Contents

L. C. Brown (✉)
MRC Clinical Trials Unit, UCL Institute of Clinical Trials and Methodology, London, UK
e-mail: l.brown@ucl.ac.uk

A. L. Jorgensen
Department of Health Data Science, University of Liverpool, Liverpool, UK
e-mail: aljorgen@liverpool.ac.uk

M. Antoniou
F. Hoffmann-La Roche Ltd, Basel, Switzerland

J. Wason
Population Health Sciences Institute, Newcastle University, Newcastle upon Tyne, UK

MRC Biostatistics Unit, University of Cambridge, Cambridge, UK
e-mail: james.wason@newcastle.ac.uk

© Springer Nature Switzerland AG 2022

S. Piantadosi, C. L. Meinert (eds.), *Principles and Practice of Clinical Trials*,
https://doi.org/10.1007/978-3-319-52636-2_168

Abstract

This chapter describes the field of precision or stratified medicine and the role that clinical trials play in the development and validation of markers, particularly biomarkers, to inform management of patients. We begin by defining various types of biomarker and describe the life cycle of a biomarker in terms of discovery, analytical validation, clinical validation, and clinical utility. We provide a detailed overview of the many types of biomarker-guided trial designs that have been described in the literature and then summarize the analytical methods that are often used for biomarker-guided trials. Much of the research process for biomarker-guided trials does not differ markedly from that used for non-biomarker-guided trials but particular attention must be given to selecting the most appropriate trial design given the research question being investigated and we hope that this chapter helps with decisions on trial design and analysis in the biomarker-guided setting.

Keywords

Biomarker · Stratified · Precision · Personalized · Validation · Prognostic · Predictive · Subgroup · Interaction

Introduction

We begin this chapter with a definition of what is meant by a biomarker-guided trial. The field of stratified medicine (also known as precision or personalized medicine) is dedicated to the identification of patient attributes that can be measured and used to make decisions on the management of their condition. These patient attributes are often called biomarker and they can include anything from complex laboratory tests to simple stratifiers such as gender, age, or stage of disease. Identifying these biomarkers and proving that they are clinically useful is not straightforward: many issues that are challenging in non-biomarker-guided trials tend to be heightened in a biomarker-guided trial setting. This is, in part, because the evidence on which a biomarker performs is based on the comparative evidence between subgroups of patients which by definition will have smaller sample sizes than the non-stratified trial. Furthermore, there can be considerable heterogeneity between patients in terms of their baseline characteristics as well as their responses to treatments.

When undertaking a biomarker-guided clinical trial, many of the design considerations are similar to those for non-biomarker-guided trials but there are particular issues that require attention. This chapter will describe the various different types of biomarkers that can be used in clinical trials as well as the development and validation process that is required before they can be recommended for routine use in clinical practice. A large part of the chapter will be dedicated to describing the different trial designs that have been developed and the advantages and disadvantages of each to help decide which designs might be the most appropriate given the research question. From a statistical perspective, sample size considerations and analytical methods for biomarker trials are important and these are also summarized or referred to in the literature.

Types of Biomarker

There are various different types of biomarkers that are used for different clinical applications. A comprehensive and detailed description of the different types of biomarkers is provided in the FDA-NIH Working Group, Biomarkers, Endpoints and Other Tools (BEST) guidelines (FDA-NIH Working Group 2018) where eight distinct biomarkers have been defined. These are summarized in Table 1.

Biomarkers can be measured using binary, categorical, ordinal, or continuous data, and appropriate statistical methods are required to ensure they are analyzed correctly (both for getting robust results from biomarker assays and analyzing how the biomarker data is associated with the prognosis or treatment effect in a trial). For the purposes of this chapter, the most commonly used biomarkers in clinical trials are prognostic and predictive biomarkers and most of the chapters will be dedicated to these types. Some biomarkers demonstrate both prognostic and predictive qualities so when designing a biomarker-guided trial, it is important to be aware of any existing data that describe the discriminatory performance of the biomarker in question, whether it be prognostic, predictive, or both.

Prognostic Biomarkers

Prognostic biomarkers stratify patients on the basis of the prognosis of the disease in the absence of the new treatment being tested, and thus, they relate to the natural history of the disease. Prognostic biomarkers can be important in biomarker-guided trials as it is usually necessary to understand the behavior of the disease under control conditions. If this is unclear, then it is possible that changes in the course of the disease might be incorrectly attributed to the treatment being tested. Furthermore, if a biomarker is prognostic, then the

Table 1 Summary of types of biomarkers*

Type of biomarker	Description
Diagnostic	A biomarker used to detect or confirm presence of a disease or condition of interest or to identify individuals with a subtype of the disease.
Monitoring	A biomarker measured serially for assessing status of a disease or medical condition or for evidence of exposure to (or effect of) a medical product or an environmental agent.
Pharmacodynamic/ response	A biomarker used to show that a biological response has occurred in an individual who has been exposed to a medical product or an environmental agent.
Predictive	A biomarker used to identify individuals who are more likely than similar individuals without the biomarker to experience a favorable or unfavorable effect from exposure to a medical product or an environmental agent.
Prognostic	A biomarker used to identify likelihood of a clinical event, disease recurrence or progression in patients who have the disease or medical condition of interest.
Surrogate	A biomarker supported by strong mechanistic and/or epidemiologic rationale such that an effect on the surrogate biomarker endpoint is expected to be correlated with an effect on the endpoint intended to assess clinical benefit.
Safety	A biomarker measured before or after an exposure to a medical product or an environmental agent to indicate the likelihood, presence, or extent of toxicity as an adverse effect.
Susceptibility/risk	A biomarker that indicates the potential for developing a disease or medical condition in an individual who does not currently have clinically apparent disease or the medical condition.

[a]*Summarized from the FDA-NIH Working Group, Biomarkers, Endpoints and Other Tools (BEST) guidelines, updated May 2018 (1)*

event rate in the control arm will differ between strata and this may influence the sample size needed for each subgroup. Prognostic biomarkers can potentially also be useful for enriching trials or informing a treatment strategy that avoids toxic treatment in patients that have, for example, a very good or very poor prognosis (Friedlin 2014).

Predictive Biomarkers

Predictive biomarkers (also known as treatment-selection biomarkers) stratify patients on the basis of their expected response (or not) to a particular treatment. For these types of biomarkers, it can be particularly challenging to prove utility as evidence of interaction is often required. In this situation, the target difference is a difference in treatment effects between stratified groups rather than a difference in the overall effect between randomized groups. Often, attaining adequate statistical power for a test of interaction can lead to a potentially unfeasible sample size and tests for interaction are often underpowered in biomarker-guided trials. Thus, the importance of validation of predictive biomarkers in other datasets is particularly important and validation will be discussed later.

The Life Course of a Biomarker

The development and testing of a biomarker ideally follow a typical life course (see Fig. 1). However, this life course is often iterative rather than sequential and a return to earlier stages in the development is often required as more data become available, biomarkers are refined and/or new possibly better biomarkers emerge.

Discovery and Analytical Validity

Biomarkers can be discovered either retrospectively or prospectively. Retrospectively, they can emerge from either preplanned or post-hoc subgroup analyses of previous trials, but they can also be developed prospectively as part of the hypothesis-driven design of a molecule that is specifically intended to work in a biomarker-defined subgroup (targeted therapy). It is important to note that retrospective discovery of biomarkers can be influenced by selection bias in terms of availability of data or tissue on which to retrospectively test the biomarker so caution should be taken in this regard and prospective testing is usually preferable. Regardless of the mode of discovery, biomarkers that are to be used in a clinical trial need to demonstrate analytical validity which means that the test should be reliable (low risk of test failure), accurate (classify the patient into the correct biomarker group), and repeatable (in terms of both inter- and intra-reproducibility). High biomarker test failure rates can make the delivery of a biomarker-guided trial infeasible, and misclassification errors can lead to the dilution of treatment effects (see later section) and thus mask the potential of truly effective treatments. Therefore, establishing analytical validity is an important step in the life course of a biomarker and the extent to which the biomarker is analytically validated will depend on the stage of development of the treatment being tested. For example, during an early phase clinical trial, the development of the analytical validity of the biomarker may still be in progress but it should be validated to a minimum standard before integrating it into the next phases of clinical trial assessment. Furthermore, the analytical validity of the test is required to determine the prevalence of the

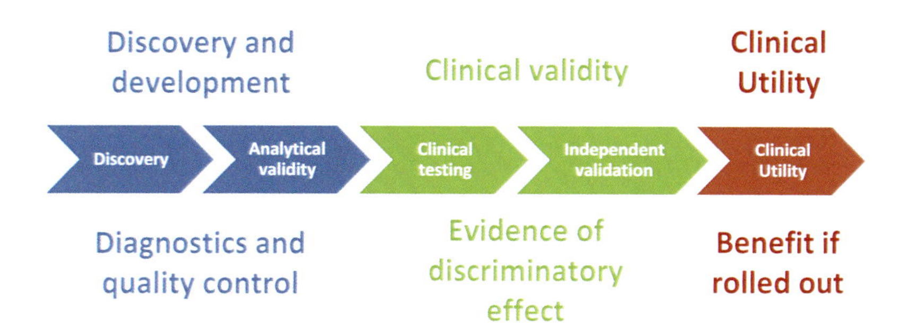

Fig. 1 The life course of a biomarker from discovery to clinical testing and utility

biomarker, and this is an important consideration for the design and sample size calculations for the subsequent trial.

Clinical Validity

If a retrospective subgroup analysis from a clinical trial demonstrates evidence that a particular biomarker might be an important stratifier for patient management, then this finding needs to be validated in an independent dataset, ideally another randomized clinical trial testing the treatment of interest. This is often a challenging aspect of biomarker development as, unless the original trial has built a validation stage into its design, it requires the completion of at least two randomized trials that have not only tested the treatment but also have adequate tissue or data to be able to stratify the patients into the biomarker positive and negative groups. For this reason, clinical validation sometimes occurs in non-randomized, observational datasets or in treated cohorts of patients who are then compared against an appropriately selected historical control group. The use of randomized data should be regarded as the ideal for clinical validation but this is not always possible. The absence of an unbiased control group can lead to type 1 (false positive) and type 2 (false negative) errors. Another important consideration when biomarkers are measured as continuous variables is ensuring reliable estimation of the optimal threshold for classifying patients into the biomarker positive or negative groups on the basis of their benefit (or lack of) with the treatment. Some trial designs such as the adaptive signature design (described later) aim to develop and validate the biomarker cutpoint within the same trial but this can be methodologically challenging.

Clinical Utility

Once a biomarker has passed through all the stages of analytical and clinical validation, it may be necessary to test the utility of the biomarker-guided treatment approach against one that does not use the biomarker to make clinical decisions. These are typically large and expensive trials as they are attempting to measure the real-world effectiveness of biomarker-guided management including reliability, feasibility, and acceptability for patients. If the biomarker testing is complex and expensive, then it may be important to confirm that use of a biomarker-guided approach does indeed lead to better outcomes for patients at a reasonable cost. As a result, cost-effectiveness outcomes can become important in these clinical utility trials.

Biomarker-Guided Trial Designs

Similar to non-biomarker-guided trials, there are two broad categories of biomarker-guided trials: nonadaptive and adaptive. Nonadaptive designs do not allow modifications of important aspects of the trial after its commencement, such as refining biomarker subgroups, adding or dropping treatment arms, sample size, etc. Rather, these factors are defined at the outset and remain fixed for the trial duration. This can be problematic when there is uncertainty surrounding assumptions made at the design stage. There is generally more potential for uncertainty when designing a biomarker-guided trial. For example, new biomarkers or targeted treatments may come to light once the trial is underway; the predictive ability of a potentially promising biomarker may be lower than expected; and there may be uncertainty regarding biomarker prevalence at the outset. Hence an adaptive design, which allows adaptations based on accumulating data, can be an attractive alternative due to its flexibility. However, while offering more flexibility, adaptive designs are more complex and can raise both practical and methodological challenges which need careful consideration.

A summary of the various adaptive and nonadaptive biomarker-guided trial designs is provided below. More in-depth discussion of the various design options, together with an overview of their methodology, guidance on sample size calculations, other statistical considerations, and their advantages and disadvantages in various situations, is provided in two review articles by Antoniou et al. (Antoniou et al. 2016, 2017) and as part of the Delta guidelines for sample size calculations (Cook et al. 2018). Further guidance is also provided in an online tool available at www.bigted.org.

Nonadaptive Biomarker-Guided Trial Designs

Single-Arm Designs Including All Patients

Such designs include the whole study population to which the same experimental treatment is prescribed, without taking into consideration biomarker status. All patients are prescribed the experimental treatment, with no comparison to a control treatment (see Fig. 2). These trial designs can be useful for initial identification and/or validation of a biomarker since they can allow for association to be tested

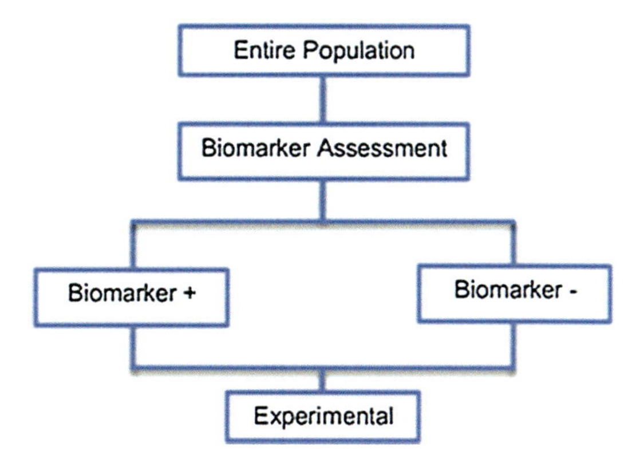

Fig. 2 Schematic for single-arm biomarker exploration design

between biomarker status and efficacy or safety of the experimental treatment. Their aim is not to estimate the treatment effect, nor the clinical utility of a biomarker in a definitive way, but to identify whether the biomarker is sufficiently promising to proceed to a more definitive biomarker-guided randomized controlled trial.

Enrichment Designs

Enrichment designs involve entering and, if appropriate, randomizing only in patients who are positive for a particular biomarker, and comparing the experimental treatment with the standard treatment only in this particular biomarker-positive subgroup. Biomarker-negative patients are excluded from the study at the start but they are sometimes included later if sufficient evidence emerges of a treatment effect in the biomarker-positive group. If this does occur, then consequently, assessing efficacy of the experimental treatment is limited to the biomarker-positive subgroup (see Fig. 3).

These trials are useful for testing treatment efficacy in a specific biomarker-defined subgroup where there is mechanistic evidence to suggest that efficacy is likely to be limited to those within that biomarker-positive subgroup, but this still requires prospective validation. In this situation, these trials can result in cost savings with biomarker-negative patients not randomized unnecessarily. Further, any treatment effect is not inappropriately diluted due to inclusion of biomarker-negative patients, particularly in the case where biomarker-positive prevalence is low. However, these designs are recommended only when both the cut-off for determination of biomarker status and the analytical validity of the biomarker have been well established. They are also only suitable where assessing biomarker status can be done with a rapid turnaround time, to avoid delaying treatment.

Enrichment designs are particularly useful where it would not be appropriate to randomize the biomarker-negative population into different treatment arms, for

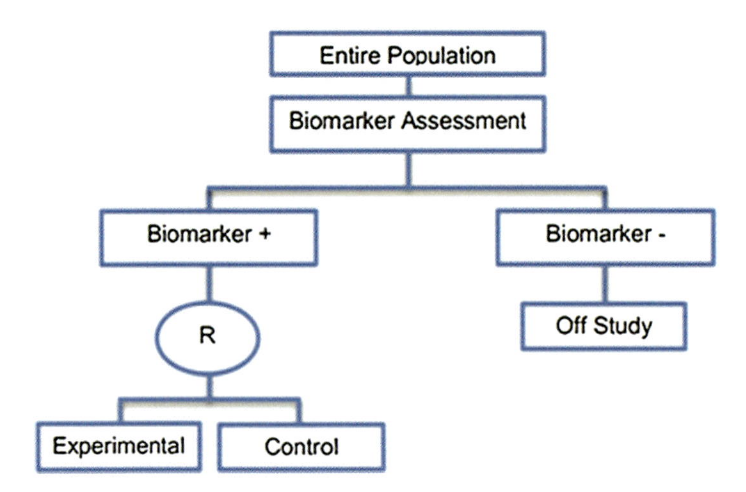

Fig. 3 Schematic for enrichment designs. "R" refers to randomization of patients

example, where there is prior evidence that the experimental treatment is not beneficial for them or is likely to cause them harm. However, when it remains unclear whether or not biomarker-negative individuals will benefit from the novel treatment, the enrichment design is not appropriate and alternative designs, which also assess effectiveness in the biomarker-negative individuals, should be considered.

Marker-Stratified Designs

In marker-stratified design trials, individuals are first stratified into biomarker-positive and biomarker-negative subgroups, then randomized within each of these subgroups to either the experimental or control treatment. Consequently, there are four treatment groups. This allows an assessment of treatment effect not only in the study population overall but also in the biomarker-defined subgroups separately. The design is useful when there is sufficient evidence that the experimental treatment is more effective in the biomarker-positive subgroup than in the biomarker-negative subgroup but insufficient data demonstrating that the experimental treatment is of no benefit to biomarker-negative individuals. However, the design may well be unfeasible when the prevalence of one of the biomarker subgroups is low resulting in chance imbalances between randomized groups for that subgroup (Fig. 4).

Hybrid Designs

In hybrid design trials, the entire population is firstly screened for biomarker status and all individuals enter the trial. However, only biomarker-positive patients are randomly assigned either to the experimental or control treatment, while all

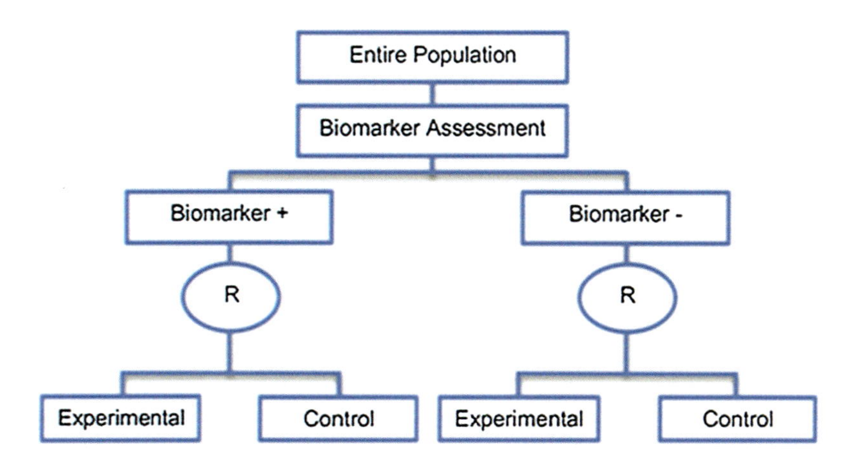

Fig. 4 Schematic for marker-stratified designs. "R" refers to randomization of patients

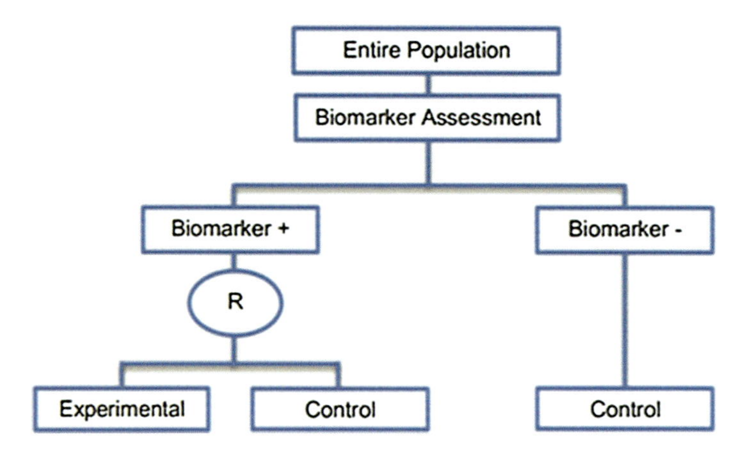

Fig. 5 Schematic for hybrid design. "R" refers to randomization of patients

biomarker-negative patients receive the control treatment. The difference compared to enrichment designs is that biomarker-negative patients are not excluded (see Fig. 5). Such designs are recommended when there is compelling prior evidence showing detrimental effect of the experimental treatment for a specific biomarker-defined subgroup (i.e., biomarker-negative subgroup) or some indication of its possible excessive toxicity in that subgroup, thus making it unethical to randomize patients to the experimental treatment. The strength of the hybrid design is that as well as allowing evaluation of the treatment in the biomarker-positive group, its feasibility as a prognostic biomarker can also be tested.

Biomarker-Strategy Design with Biomarker Assessment in the Control Arm

In this trial design, the entire study population is tested for its biomarker status. Next, patients irrespective of their biomarker status are randomized either to the biomarker-based strategy arm or to the non-biomarker-based strategy arm. In the biomarker-based strategy arm, biomarker-positive patients receive the experimental treatment, whereas biomarker-negative patients receive the control treatment. Patients who are randomized to the non-biomarker-based strategy arm receive the control treatment irrespective of biomarker status (see Fig. 6).

This approach is useful when the aim is to test the hypothesis that a treatment approach taking biomarker status into account is superior to that of the standard of care – that is, the clinical utility of the biomarker. Further, the biomarker-based strategy arm does not necessarily need to be limited to one experimental treatment – in principle, a marker-based strategy involving many biomarkers and many possible treatments could be tested. This type of design can inform researchers whether the biomarker is prognostic, since both biomarker positive and negative patients are exposed to the control treatment. However, it cannot definitively answer the question

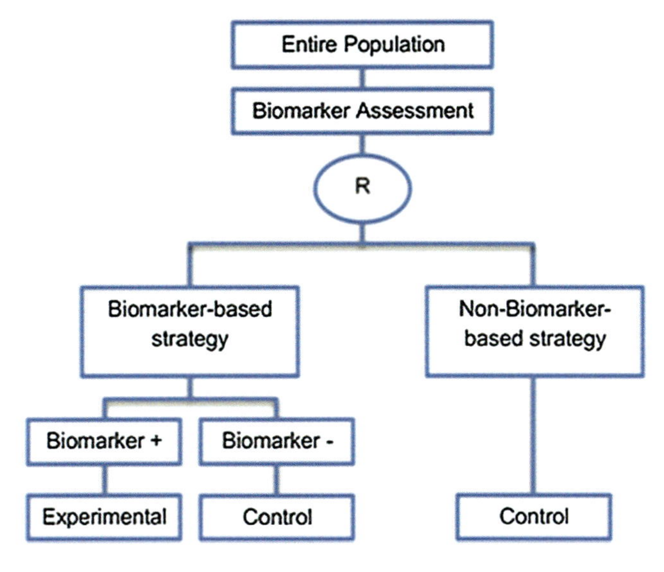

Fig. 6 Schematic for biomarker-strategy design with biomarker assessment in the control arm. "R" refers to randomization of patients

of whether the biomarker is predictive since only biomarker-positive patients are exposed to the experimental treatment.

Furthermore, these designs do not allow for a direct comparison between experimental and control treatment directly as they are designed to compare but the biomarker-strategy and not the treatments.

Biomarker-Strategy Design Without Biomarker Assessment in the Control Arm

Here, patients are again randomized between testing strategies (i.e., biomarker-based strategy and non-biomarker-based strategy) but the design differs in terms of timing of biomarker evaluation. More precisely, first, patients are randomized to either the biomarker-based strategy or to the non-biomarker-based strategy, and biomarkers are evaluated only in patients who are assigned to the biomarker-based strategy arm. Patients found to be biomarker-positive are then given the experimental treatment with biomarker-negative patients given the control treatment. Again, those randomized to the non-biomarker-based strategy receive the control treatment (see Fig. 7).

This design is useful in situations where it is either not feasible or ethical to test the biomarker in the entire population due to several logistical (e.g., specimens not submitted), technical (e.g., assay failure), or clinical reasons (e.g., tumor inaccessible); thus, biomarker status is obtained only in patients who are randomized to the biomarker-based strategy arm. However, biomarker-positive and biomarker-

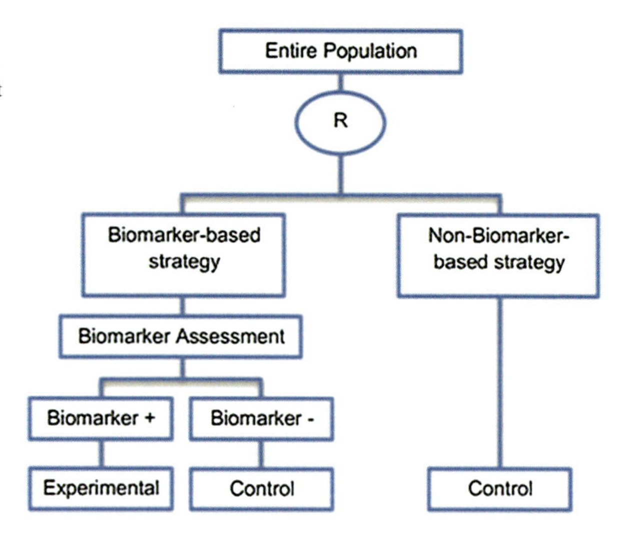

Fig. 7 Schematic for biomarker-strategy design without biomarker assessment in the control arm. "R" refers to randomization of patients

negative subgroups might be more imbalanced as compared to the first type of biomarker-strategy design since randomization is performed before evaluation of biomarker status. This can happen especially when the number of patients is very small.

Biomarker-Strategy Design with Treatment Randomization in the Control Arm

In this design, there is a second randomization between experimental and control treatment in the non-biomarker-guided strategy arm. While the two previously described biomarker-strategy designs can address the question of whether a biomarker-based strategy is more effective than standard treatment, the biomarker-strategy design with treatment randomization in the control arm allows a test of whether the biomarker-based strategy is better not only than the standard treatment but also than the experimental treatment in the overall, unselected population (see Fig. 8).

Patients are first randomly assigned to either the biomarker-based strategy arm or to the non-biomarker-based strategy arm. Next, patients who are allocated to the non-biomarker-based strategy arm are further randomized either to the experimental or to the standard treatment arm, irrespective of biomarker status. The ratio for randomizing in the non-biomarker-based strategy arm should be informed by the prevalence of the biomarker in the population as a whole, to ensure balance between the study arms. Patients randomized to the biomarker-based strategy arm and who are biomarker-positive are given the experimental treatment with biomarker-negative patients given the control treatment.

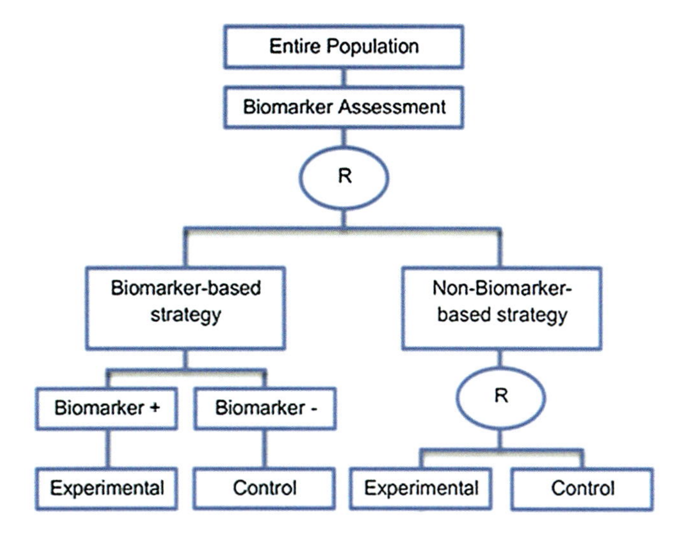

Fig. 8 Schematic for biomarker-strategy design with treatment randomization in the control arm. "R" refers to randomization of patients

The clinical utility of the biomarker is evaluated by comparing treatment effect between the biomarker-based strategy arm and non-biomarker-based strategy arm. It is also possible to test whether the experimental treatment is more effective in the entire population or in a biomarker-defined subgroup only, since both biomarker subgroups are exposed to both treatments.

One benefit of this design as compared to the two previously discussed biomarker-strategy designs is that it allows investigation of not only whether the biomarker is prognostic but also whether it is a predictive treatment effect modifier. A further strength is that it allows clarification of whether a result indicating an advantage in favor of the biomarker-based strategy is due to a true effect of the biomarker itself or due to a treatment effect irrespective of biomarker status.

Reverse Marker-Based Strategy Design

Here, patients are randomized either to the biomarker-based strategy arm or the reverse biomarker-based strategy arm. As in the previous three biomarker-strategy designs, patients who are allocated to the biomarker-strategy arm receive the experimental treatment if they are biomarker-positive whereas biomarker-negative patients receive the control treatment. By contrast, patients who are randomly assigned to the reverse biomarker-based strategy arm receive the control treatment if they are biomarker-positive, whereas biomarker-negative patients receive the experimental treatment (see Fig. 9).

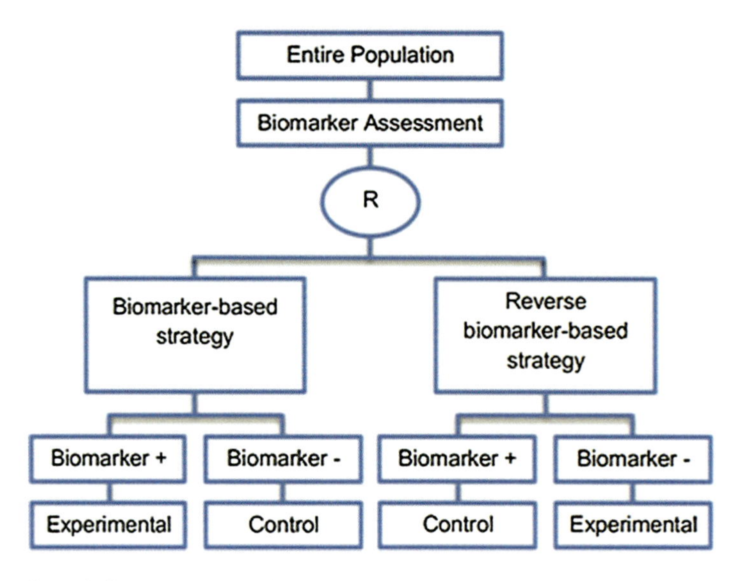

Fig. 9 Schematic for reverse marker-based strategy design. "R" refers to randomization of patients

This design is recommended in cases where prior evidence indicates that both experimental and control treatment are effective in treating patients, but the optimal strategy has not yet been identified. The design enables the evaluation of an interaction between the biomarker and different treatments. Additionally, it allows estimation of the effect size of the experimental treatment compared to control treatment for each biomarker-defined subgroup separately. Also, there is no chance that the same treatment will be allocated to biomarker-positive patients in both arms or to biomarker-negative patients in both arms. This is a problem in the other types of biomarker-based strategy designs where there will be patients with the same biomarker status having the same treatment in both trial arms.

It is important to note that all biomarker-strategy designs will need a larger sample size as compared to the marker-stratified designs.

A Randomized Phase II Trial Design with Biomarker

This is a biomarker-guided phase II clinical trial design which, when completed, recommends which type of phase III trial design should be used. The trial starts with biomarker assessment, with all patients randomized to either an experimental or control treatment. An interim analysis is then undertaken in the biomarker-positive subgroup. If the experimental treatment is found superior to control at a prespecified level of significance, treatment effect is subsequently estimated in the biomarker-negative subgroup. Based on the estimated treatment effect in the biomarker-negative subgroup, and in particular its confidence interval, a recommendation is

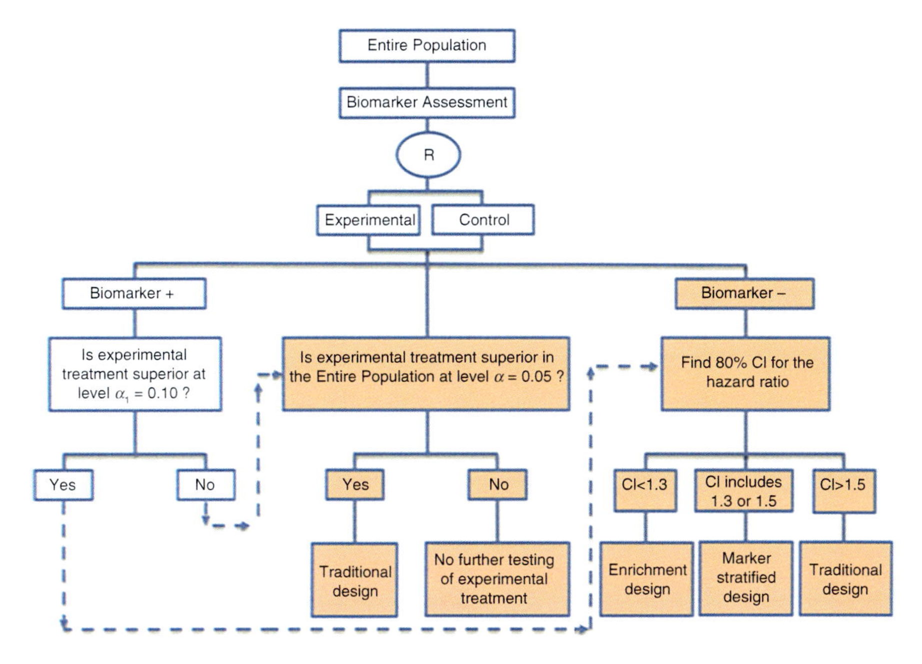

Fig. 10 Schematic for a randomized phase II trial design with biomarkers. "R" refers to randomization of patients. CI refers to the confidence interval. Uncolored boxes refer to the first stage of the trial and colored boxes refer to the second stage of the trial. Different stages refer to the analysis and not to the trial design

given on the type of phase III trial design to be used (enrichment, marker stratified or traditional with no biomarker). If in the interim analysis, however, the treatment effect is not found to be significant in the biomarker-positive subgroup, the experimental treatment is compared to control in the entire study population. If the overall treatment effect is found significant at a prespecified level of significance, a traditional design with no biomarker assessment is recommended for phase III. Otherwise, it is recommended that no phase III trial is undertaken for the experimental treatment (see Fig. 10).

Adaptive Designs

Adaptive Signature Design

The adaptive signature design was proposed for settings where a biomarker signature, defined as a set of biomarkers the combined status of which is used to stratify patients into subgroups, is not known at the outset, and allows the development and evaluation of a biomarker signature within the trial. Generally, this approach is useful when there is no available biomarker at the start of the trial or when there

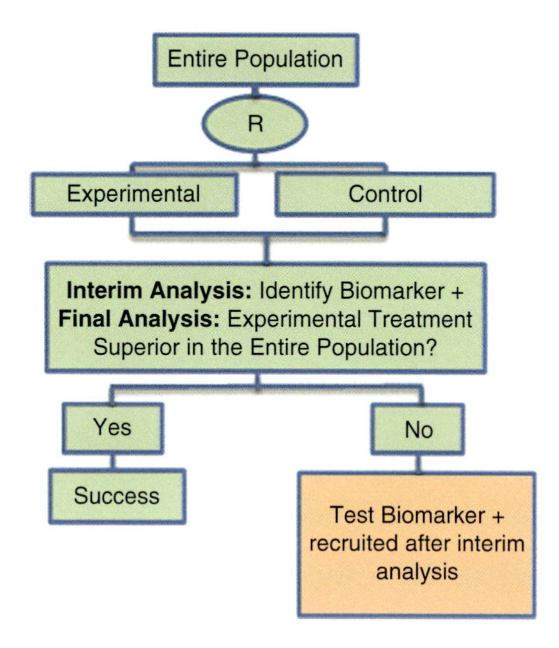

Fig. 11 Schematic for adaptive signature design. "R" refers to randomization of patients

are a great number of candidate biomarkers which could be combined to identify a biomarker-defined subgroup (see Fig. 11).

The design begins with a comparison between the experimental and standard treatment in the entire study population at a prespecified level of significance. If treatment effect is statistically significant, the treatment is considered beneficial, and the trial is closed. If the comparison in the overall population is not promising, then the entire population is divided into two samples in order to develop a biomarker signature in one sample and validate it in another. This is in order to identify a biomarker signature that best identifies subjects for which the experimental treatment is better than the standard treatment (the so-called "biomarker-positive" group). The trial then continues, but recruiting only biomarker-positive patients, as determined by the biomarker signature. Hence, this approach (i) identifies patients who benefit from the experimental treatment during the initial stage of the study (at the interim analysis); (ii) assesses the global treatment effect of the entire randomized study population through a powered test, and (iii) assesses the treatment effect for the biomarker-positive subgroup within patients randomized in the remainder of the trial, the so-called "validation test."

Outcome-Based Adaptive Randomization Design

This design can be useful when the biomarkers are either putative or unknown at the beginning of a phase II trial, and also when there are multiple targeted treatments and biomarkers to be considered. It aims to test simultaneously both biomarkers and

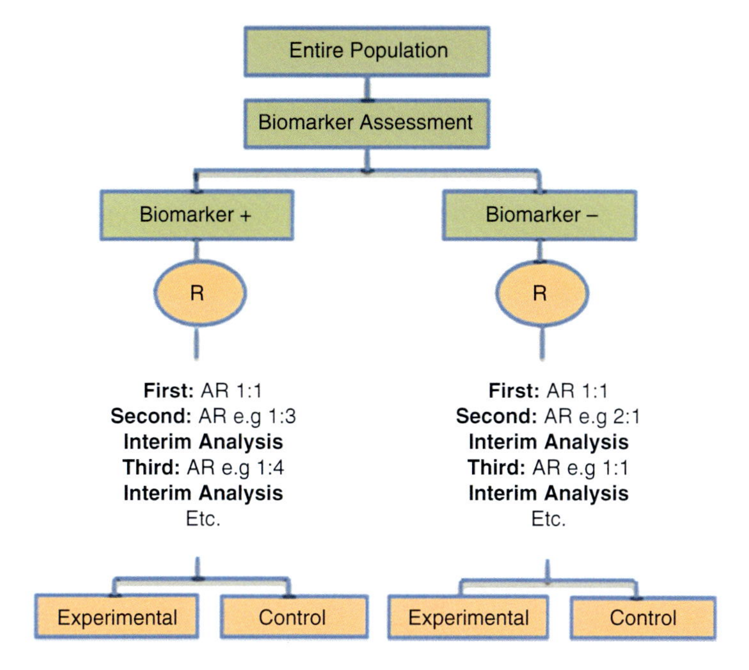

Fig. 12 Schematic for outcome-based adaptive randomization design. "R" refers to randomization of patients

treatments while providing more patients with effective therapies according to their biomarker profiles (see Fig. 12).

The trial begins with the assessment of patients' biomarker status. Within each biomarker subgroup, patients are then randomized equally to one or more experimental arms or control arm. The design permits the modification of the allocation ratio to different treatment arms over time so that the arm(s) which seem(s) to have the best response rate is composed of the higher proportion of randomized patients. This modification in allocation ratio is informed by accumulated patients' data about how well the biomarker performs at each interim analysis stage. For example, when data accrued so far suggests that a particular treatment is superior to others, the ratio will be modified to ensure a higher number of patients are allocated accordingly.

Adaptive Threshold Enrichment Design

This design is based on the former knowledge that a specific biomarker-defined subgroup (biomarker-positive subgroup) is believed to benefit more from a novel treatment as compared to the remainder of the study population (biomarker-negative subgroup). The trial is conducted as follows: (i) accrue and randomize only biomarker-positive patients to experimental or control treatment; (ii) conduct an interim analysis in order to compare the experimental treatment with control

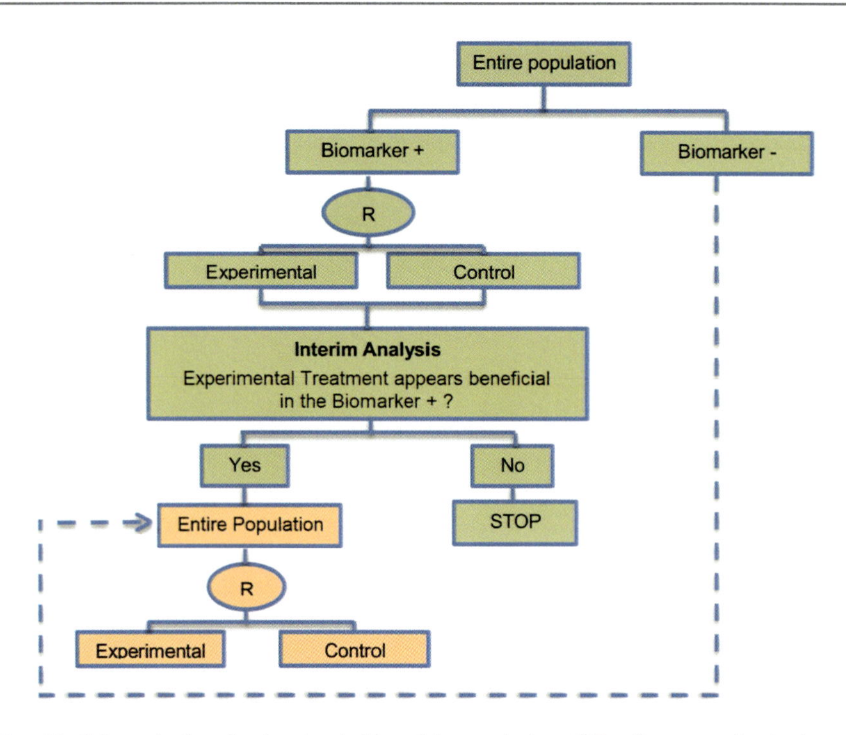

Fig. 13 Schematic for adaptive threshold enrichment design. "R" refers to randomization of patients

treatment within the biomarker-positive subgroup; and (iii) if the interim result is negative, then the accrual stops due to futility in the biomarker-positive subgroup and the trial is closed without showing a treatment benefit; if the result is "promising" for the specific biomarker-positive subgroup, then the study continues with this specific biomarker-positive subgroup and accrual also begins for biomarker-negative patients. Thus, the trial continues with patients randomized from the entire population. A "promising" result in the biomarker-positive subgroup at the interim stage is claimed when the estimated treatment effect is above a particular prespecified threshold (see Fig. 13).

Adaptive Patient Enrichment Design

This design adaptively modifies accrual to two predefined biomarker-defined subgroups based on an interim analysis for futility. The trial is conducted as follows: (i) accrue both biomarker-positive and biomarker-negative patients, and randomize the two subgroups respectively to experimental or control treatment; (ii) perform an interim analysis to evaluate treatment effect in the biomarker-negative subgroup; (iii) if the interim result in that subgroup is "not promising," defined as the observed efficacy for the control group being greater than that for the experimental group and the difference being insufficient to pass the a futility

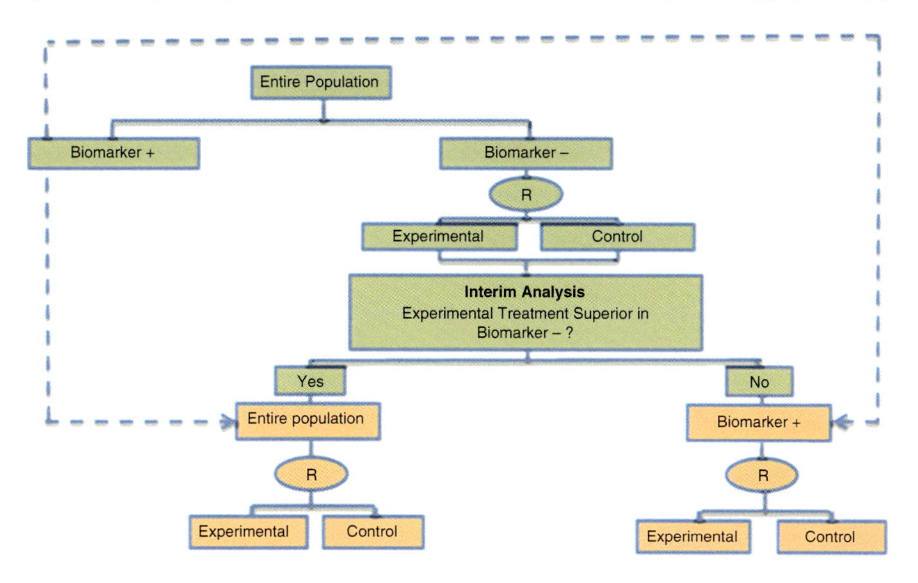

Fig. 14 Schematic for adaptive patient enrichment design. "R" refers to randomization of patients

boundary, then accrual of biomarker-negative patients stops; but the strategy continues with accruing additional biomarker-positive patients in order to substitute the unaccrued biomarker-negative patients until the prespecified total target sample size is achieved; (iv) contrarily, if the interim results are promising in the biomarker-negative patients, the accrual of both biomarker-negative and biomarker-positive patients continues until the total target sample size is achieved (see Fig. 14).

Adaptive Parallel Simon Two-Stage Design

This design allows the efficacy of a novel treatment, which possibly differs in the biomarker-positive subgroup compared to the biomarker-negative subgroup, to be tested. It requires a predefined biomarker with well-established prevalence (see Fig. 15). The design begins with a first stage, which entails two parallel phase II studies, one in the biomarker-positive and the other in the biomarker-negative subgroup. Next, if activity is not observed in either biomarker subgroup during the first stage, the trial stops; if activity of the experimental treatment is observed during the first stage of the study for both the biomarker-positive and biomarker-negative subgroups, additional patients from the general patient population are enrolled into the second stage; if results of the first stage suggest that activity is limited to biomarker-positive patients, the second stage continues with the recruitment of additional biomarker-positive patients only. This design may augment the efficiency of a trial as it allows for early understanding that a particular experimental treatment is beneficial in a specific biomarker defined subgroup.

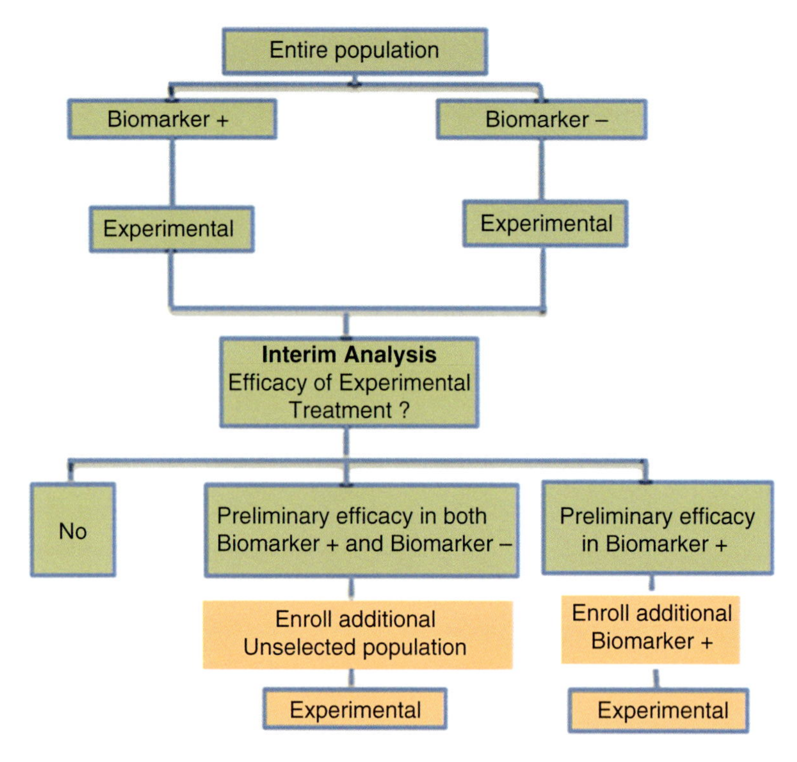

Fig. 15 Schematic for adaptive parallel Simon two-stage design. "R" refers to randomization of patients

Multi-arm Multi-stage Designs (MAMS)

This design as originally proposed was not for biomarker-guided trials but rather was aimed at testing multiple experimental treatments against a control treatment in the same trial. However, it is also useful in a biomarker-guided context since it allows patients to be allocated to a trial of a particular experimental treatment, based on their biomarker status.

The first stage of a MAMS trial (the phase II stage) involves biomarker stratification into one of a number of separate comparisons with each comparing an experimental treatment with a control treatment. The comparison within which a patient is included depends on their biomarker status, for example, patients positive for biomarker 1 may be randomized in comparison 1 to either control or experimental treatment 1 while patients positive for biomarker 2 may be randomized into comparison 2 to either control or experimental treatment 2. At the end of this first stage, an interim analysis is undertaken within each comparison, comparing each experimental treatment with the control treatment. Depending on the outcome of the interim analysis, accrual of patients in a comparison either continues to the second stage of the trial or the accrual of additional patients stops within that comparison (see Fig. 16).

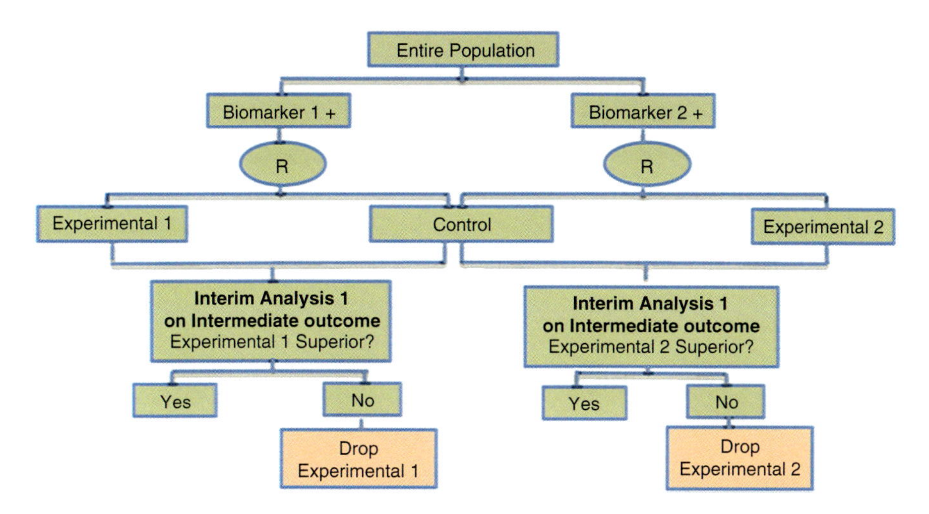

Fig. 16 Schematic for multi-arm, multi-stage (MAMS) design. "R" refers to randomization of patients

This design has the ability to simultaneously compare multiple experimental treatments with a control treatment, therefore achieving results in less time as compared with separate phase II trials to assess each novel treatment individually. Depending on how long the actual endpoint takes to observe, the actual or an intermediate endpoint can be used at the interim analysis stage. Generally, MAMS designs are useful when (i) there are multiple promising treatments in phase II/III studies; (ii) there is no strong belief that a treatment will be more beneficial compared to another therapy; (iii) availability of adequate funds; (iv) there is an adequate number of patients to be enrolled; and (v) there is an intermediate outcome measure that is likely to be on the causal pathway to the primary outcome measure.

Benefits of this design are that the overall trial is unlikely to stop for futility as multiple experimental treatments are tested and hence, it is unlikely that all experimental arms will be ineffective and dropped. Further, the regulatory and administrative burden is reduced as compared to running several separate trials, while unpromising experimental arms can be dropped in a quick and reliable way. Design benefits of this approach have been reported and implemented in trials such as the UK FOCUS4 trial in colorectal cancer and the US Lung Map trial in lung cancer (Kaplan et al. 2013; Lung-Map: Master Protocol for Lung Cancer 2021).

Operational Considerations for Biomarker-Guided Trials

For many biomarkers, measurement can be relatively easy but for some of the more complex laboratory driven and imaging biomarkers, quality assurance is necessary to demonstrate that the biomarker test is reliable and repeatable, particularly between laboratories and between any investigators who are responsible for making judgments on whether the patient is classified as biomarker positive or negative. Much of this relates to the important work completed during the analytical validation stage of the biomarker life course (see Fig. 1), but it is important that quality assurance is performed at the start and during the course of any biomarker-guided clinical trial.

From a regulatory and a patient perspective, there are also important approvals that need to be in place to ensure the appropriate handling and archiving of both patient tissue and clinical data collected from patients. These approvals will vary internationally but all will need to comply with the ICH Guidelines on Good Clinical Practice (ICH GCP guidelines n.d.). The appropriate handling of patient tissue along with the necessary legal requirements for anonymization of patient data is not to be underestimated in these types of trials and adequate resource must be available to ensure that data are secure and test results are turned around in a timely fashion so that patients can be entered into the trial without delays.

Analysis of Biomarker-Guided Trials

There are a number of sources of statistical uncertainty when analyzing biomarker-guided trials (see Fig. 17). Furthermore, as described in the previous section, there are a large number of designs available that utilize biomarkers. In many cases, the primary analysis of biomarker-guided trials aims to demonstrate the performance of the biomarker in terms of decision-making for patient management and this will typically be analyzed using a sensitivity and specificity approach, where area-under-the-curve (AUC) from receiver operator characteristics (ROC) curves will be used. In other cases, it will involve tests of interaction between the biomarker and the treatment. Often both of these aspects are of interest.

The most appropriate statistical analysis is highly dependent on the design used, in particular what is the hypothesis being tested. Ideally any subgroup analyses should be prespecified before data are inspected and analyzed and inclusion in a signed and dated statistical analysis plan is advised to document that the subgroup was prespecified.

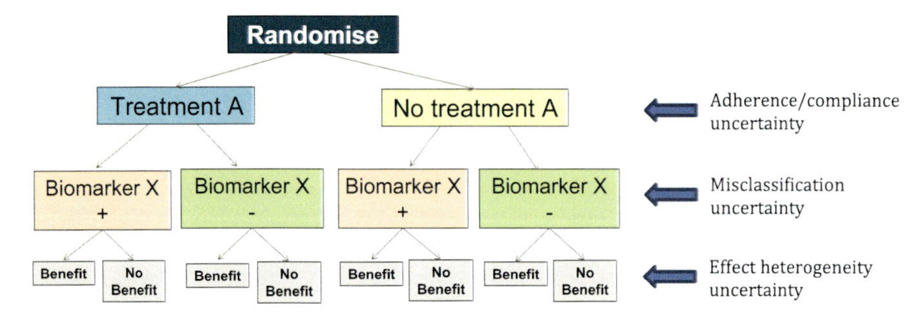

Fig. 17 Sources of statistical uncertainty when exploring the role of a biomarker in a stratified trial

In subsequent subsections, we cover some more specific considerations for the statistical analysis of common types of biomarker-guided trial.

Analysis of Biomarker-Strategy Designs

A biomarker-strategy design tests the hypothesis that using the biomarker to guide treatment will result in superior outcomes to not using it. As discussed above, biomarker-strategy designs can take various forms. The experimental arm may allocate between a number of treatments depending on the results of the biomarker test or may just choose between treatment or nontreatment. The control arm may allocate all patients to one standard treatment or may randomize patients between treatments.

In all cases, the primary analysis of a biomarker strategy will compare outcomes between the experimental and control arm. Thus, methods of analysis will be similar to traditional two-arm RCTs. As biomarker-strategy trials are often assessing the effectiveness of implementing the strategy in routine practice, the primary analysis should generally be by intention to treat, with patients analyzed within their randomized groups. It is likely that some patients in the experimental arm may not follow the specified treatment strategy due to practical issues. In this case, a per-protocol analysis could be useful to determine whether an idealized version of the biomarker strategy, where there were no errors or delays in assessing the biomarker and no deviations from the recommended treatment occur, has a larger advantage. This may be useful in determining if further refinements of the biomarker test could be useful. If a per-protocol analysis is required, then it is important to prespecify the definition of per-protocol clearly in the statistical analysis plan.

One issue with analysis of biomarker strategy designs is that there may be heterogeneity of outcome within each arm which may violate assumptions made by the analysis. If, for example, different types of patients are allocated to different treatments within each arm, then the assumptions of some statistical tests that data from within each arm is similarly distributed will not be true. Analyses that adjust or stratify by the biomarker status may be more appropriate, but still would assume that the mean treatment effect (i.e., the difference in effect of being on the experimental arm compared with the control arm) is the same for different types of patients on some scale. It is important to be clear about the assumptions of the analysis and to ensure the results are robust to them.

Analysis of Marker-Stratified Designs

The gold standard design for testing whether a biomarker is predictive is the marker stratified design. The statistical analysis will generally focus on: (1) the interaction effect between biomarker and treatment on outcome and (2) the marginal effect of the treatment. The primary analysis should be the question that the study was powered to test.

Estimating and testing the interaction effect can be performed by fitting a suitable regression model. This model should include parameters for: (1) the marginal effect of treatment arm; (2) marginal effect of biomarker status; and (3) interaction between treatment arm and biomarker status. For instance, with a normally distributed outcome, the suitable linear model will be:

$$Y_i = \alpha + \beta T_i + \gamma B_i + \delta T_i B_i + \epsilon_i$$

where Yi is the outcome for individual i, T_i is the treatment allocation (1 if experimental, 0 if control), Bi is the biomarker status (e.g., 1 if positive, 0 if negative), and ϵ_i is a normally distributed error term. The parameters in the model, α, β, γ, δ, represent (respectively) the intercept, the marginal effect of treatment, the marginal effect of biomarker, and the interaction between biomarker and treatment. By fitting this model and finding the maximum likelihood estimates $\widehat{\alpha}, \widehat{\beta}, \widehat{\gamma}, \widehat{\delta}$, we can estimate the effect of the treatment in the negative biomarker group ($\widehat{\beta}$), the effect of the treatment in the positive biomarker group ($\widehat{\beta}+\widehat{\delta}$), and the interaction effect ($\widehat{\delta}$). The standard errors of these quantities can be extracted from the model and used to form confidence intervals and Wald tests for testing the null hypothesis of the true parameter (or sum of parameters) being 0.

One consideration that influences interaction and subgroup testing is the presence of measurement error on the biomarker (see section on analytical validity of the biomarker). In epidemiological studies, measurement error can cause bias issues as well as loss of precision when conducting interaction tests (Carroll et al. 2006). This persists in randomized trials, meaning that the estimated interaction effect is likely to be attenuated (i.e., biased towards 0) in the presence of measurement error (Aiken and West 1991). However, as the measurement error of the baseline biomarker status is independent of arm assignment, there is no inflation in the type I error for the interaction test (Pennello 2013). More advanced analysis methods can be used to correct for bias caused by measurement error. It is possible when analyzing a biomarker-guided trial that some high-quality information is available from previous studies assessing the biomarker that could be incorporated into the analysis. For example, if information about the sensitivity and specificity of the biomarker is available, this could be used within a Bayesian framework to correct the measurement error.

Summary and Conclusions

Biomarker-guided trial designs have developed considerably over the last 15 years. The trial design features described in this chapter provide a summary of what is available and the selection of particular design features will depend upon the research question being investigated. We have aimed to provide a high-level summary of issues to consider but other designs will no doubt emerge in the coming years. We would recommend further reading of the extensive literature in this field (Renfro et al. 2016; Freidlin and Korn 2010; Buyse et al. 2011; Mandrekar and Sargent 2009; Freidlin 2010; Stallard 2014; Tajik et al. 2013; Simon 2010; Gosho et al. 2012; European

Medicines Agency 2015; Eng 2014; Baker 2014; Freidlin et al. 2012; Freidlin and Simon 2005; Wang et al. 2009; Karuri and Simon 2012; Jones and Holmgren 2007; McShane et al. 2009; Parmar et al. 2008; Wason and Trippa 2014).

Acknowledgments This work is based on research arising from UK's Medical Research Council (MRC) grants MC_UU_00004/09, MC_UU_12023/29, and MC_UU_12023/20.

References

Aiken LS, West SG (1991) Multiple regression: testing and interpreting interactions. Sage, Newbury Park

Antoniou M, Jorgensen AL, Kolamunnage-Dona R (2016) Biomarker-guided adaptive trial designs in phase II and phase III: a methodological review. PLoS One 11(2):e0149803. https://doi.org/10.1371/journal.pone.0149803

Antoniou M, Kolamunnage-Dona R, Jorgensen AL (2017) Biomarker-guided non-adaptive trial designs in phase II and phase III: a methodological review. J Pers Med 7(1). https://doi.org/10.3390/jpm7010001

Baker SG (2014) Biomarker evaluation in randomized trials: addressing different research questions. Stat Med 33:4139–4140

Buyse M, Sargent G, de Matheson G (2011) Integrating biomarkers in clinical trials. Expert Rev Mol Diagn 11:171–182

Carroll RJ, Ruppert D, Stefanski LA, Crainiceanu CM (2006) Measurement error in nonlinear models: a modern perspective, 2nd edn. Chapman Hall/CRC, Boca Raton

Cook JA et al (2018) DELTA^2 guidance on choosing the target difference and undertaking and reporting the sample size calculation for a randomised controlled trial. BMJ 363. https://doi.org/10.1136/bmj.k3750

Eng KH (2014) Randomized reverse marker strategy design for prospective biomarker validation. Stat Med 33:3089–3099

European Medicines Agency. Reflection Paper on Methodological Issues Associated with Pharmacogenomic Biomarkers in Relation to Clinical Development and Patient Selection. Available online: http://www.ema.europa.eu/docs/en_GB/document_library/Scientific_guideline/2011/07/WC500108672.pdf (Accessed on 10 Oct 2015)

FDA-NIH Working Group, Biomarkers, Endpoints and Other Tools (BEST) guidelines, updated May 2018

Freidlin K (2010) Biomarker-adaptive clinical trial designs. Pharmacogenomics 11(12):1679–1682

Freidlin MS, Korn (2010) Randomized clinical trials with biomarkers: design issues. J Natl Cancer Inst 102:152–160

Freidlin B, Simon R (2005) Adaptive signature design: an adaptive clinical trial design for generating and prospectively testing a gene expression signature for sensitive patients. Clin Cancer Res 11(21):7872–7878

Freidlin B, McShane LM, Polley M-YC, Korn EL (2012) Randomized phase II trial designs with biomarkers. J Clin Oncol 30:3304–3309

Friedlin K (2014) Biomarker enrichment strategies: matching trial design to biomarker credentials. Nat Rev Clin Oncol 11:81–90

Gosho M, Nagashima K, Sato Y (2012) Study designs and statistical analyses for biomarker research. Sensors 12:8966–8986

ICH GCP guidelines.: https://www.ich.org/products/guidelines/efficacy/efficacy-single/article/integrated-addendum-good-clinical-practice.html

Jones CL, Holmgren E (2007) An adaptive Simon two-stage Design for Phase 2 studies of targeted therapies. Contemp Clin Trials 28(5):654–661

Kaplan RK, Maughan TM, Crook AC, Fisher DF, Wilson RW, Brown LC, Parmar MP (2013) Evaluating many treatments and biomarkers in oncology: a new design. J Clin Oncol 31(36): 4562–4568
Karuri SW, Simon R (2012) A two-stage Bayesian design for co-development of new drugs and companion diagnostics. Stat Med 31(10):901–914
Lung-Map: Master Protocol for Lung Cancer.: https://www.cancer.gov/types/lung/research/lung-map. (Accessed 16 Jan 2021)
Mandrekar SJ, Sargent DJ (2009) Clinical trial designs for predictive biomarker validation: theoretical considerations and practical challenges. J Clin Oncol 27(24):4027–4034
McShane LM, Hunsberger S, Adjei AA (2009) Effective incorporation of biomarkers into phase II trials. Clin Cancer Res 15(6):1898–1905
Parmar MKB, Barthel FMS, Sydes M, Langley R, Kaplan R, Eisenhauer E et al (2008) Speeding up the evaluation of new agents in cancer. J Natl Cancer Inst 100(17):1204–1214
Pennello G (2013) Analytical and clinical evaluation of biomarkers assays: when are biomarkers ready for prime time? Clin Trials 10:666–676. [300,301]
Renfro M, Ming-Wen S, Mandrekar (2016) Clinical trial designs incorporating predictive biomarkers. Cancer Treat Rev 43:74–82
Simon R (2010) Clinical trial designs for evaluating the medical utility of prognostic and predictive biomarkers in oncology. Pers Med 7:33–47
Stallard H (2014) Parsons, Friede adaptive designs for confirmatory clinical trials with subgroup selection. J Biopharm Stat 24:168–187
Tajik P, Zwinderman AH, Mol BW, Bossuyt PM (2013) Trial designs for personalizing cancer care: a systematic review and classification. Clin Cancer Res 19:4578–4588
Wang S-J, Hung HMJ, O'Neill RT (2009) Adaptive patient enrichment designs in therapeutic trials. *Biom J Biometrische Zeitschrift* 51(2):358–374
Wason JMS, Trippa L (2014) A comparison of Bayesian adaptive randomization and multi-stage designs for multi-arm clinical trials. Stat Med 33(13):2206–2221

Diagnostic Trials

63

Madhu Mazumdar, Xiaobo Zhong, and Bart Ferket

Contents

M. Mazumdar (✉)
Director of Institute for Healthcare Delivery Science, Mount Sinai Health System, NY, USA
e-mail: madhu.mazumdar@mountsinai.org

X. Zhong · B. Ferket
Ichan School of Medicine at Mount Sinai, New York, NY, USA
e-mail: Xiaobo.Zhong@mountsinai.org; bart.ferket@mountsinai.org

© Springer Nature Switzerland AG 2022

S. Piantadosi, C. L. Meinert (eds.), *Principles and Practice of Clinical Trials*,
https://doi.org/10.1007/978-3-319-52636-2_281

Abstract

The term *diagnostic trial* is generally used in two different ways. A *diagnostic trial type I* describes studies that evaluate accuracy of diagnostic tests in detecting disease or its severity. Primary endpoints for these studies are generally test accuracy outcomes measured in terms of sensitivity, specificity, positive predictive value, negative predictive value, and area under the receiver operating characteristics curves. Although establishing an accurate diagnosis or excluding disease is a critical first step to manage a health problem, medical decision-makers generally rely on a larger evidence base of empirical data that includes how tests impact patient health outcomes, such as morbidity, mortality, functional status, and quality of life. Therefore, the *diagnostic trial type II* evaluates the value of test results to guide or determine treatment decisions within a broader management strategy. Typically, differences in diagnostic accuracy result in differences in delivery of treatment, and ultimately affect disease prognosis and patient outcomes. As such, in the *diagnostic trial type II*, the downstream consequences of tests followed by treatment decisions are evaluated together in a joint construct. These *diagnostic randomized clinical trials* or *test-treatment trials* are considered the gold standard of proof for the *clinical effectiveness or clinical utility* of diagnostic tests. In this chapter, we define the variety of accuracy measures used for assessing diagnostic tests, summarize guidance on sample size calculation, and bring attention to the importance of more accurate reporting of study results.

Keywords

Diagnostic trial type I · Diagnostic trial type II · Test-treatment trial · Sensitivity · Specificity · Positive predictive value · Negative predictive value · Area under the receiver operating characteristics curves

Introduction

Diagnostic tests (such as genetic or imaging tests) are health interventions used to determine the existence or severity of a disease (Sun et al. 2013; Huang et al. 2017). The development and introduction process of diagnostic tests is equivalent to the development of other health technologies such as therapeutic drugs, and similarly the purpose of *diagnostic trials* can be categorized according to different research development phases: varying from exploratory to evaluation of clinical impact (Pepe 2003). The field of diagnostic trials has grown tremendously in the last 40 years (Zhou et al. 2009).

The term *diagnostic trial* is generally used in two distinct ways in the literature. The first, here labeled as *diagnostic trial type I*, is used for studies covering earlier development phases that merely evaluate the accuracy of diagnostic tests in detecting disease or severity of disease (Colli et al. 2014). Primary endpoints for these studies are generally test accuracy measured in terms of sensitivity, specificity, positive predictive value, negative predictive value, and area under the receiver operating characteristics curves. These terms will be explained in more detail below in the section "Definitions of Accuracy." The goal of *type I diagnostic trials* in the early, exploratory phase is to investigate whether the diagnostic test seems promising in distinguishing disease from non-disease and meets criteria for minimally acceptable diagnostic accuracy. The study design used in such early phase is typically the *retrospective case-control study*. This chapter predominantly focuses on *type I diagnostic trials* in later development phases which aim to confirm and refine diagnostic accuracy and compare tests (Colli et al. 2014; Gluud and Gluud 2005; Begg and Greenes 1983; Sackett and Haynes 2002).

Although establishing an accurate diagnosis is a critical first step in the management of a health problem, medical decision-making generally relies on whether there is net health benefit to patients in terms of improvements in morbidity, mortality, functional status, and quality of life. Yet, differences in diagnostic accuracy generally also lead to differences in delivery of treatment, and medical tests thus ultimately affect disease prognosis and patient outcomes. As such, in the final development phase of new medical tests, the downstream consequences of tests followed by treatment decisions should be ideally evaluated together. Here, we explain the role of a late-phase *diagnostic trial type II*. The study design for these *type II diagnostic trials* is equivalent to phase III clinical trials for therapeutic interventions and the purpose is to evaluate test results within the broader management strategy. Such *diagnostic randomized clinical trials* or *test-treatment trials* are considered the gold standard of proof for *clinical effectiveness or clinical utility* of diagnostic tests. In this chapter, we define the variety of accuracy measures used for diagnostic test assessment, summarize guidance on the sample size calculation for various designs, and bring attention to the importance of more accurate reporting of study designs and results.

Diagnostic Trial Type I: Evaluating Diagnostic Accuracy

Assessment of Diagnostic Accuracy of Single Test

Establishing an accurate diagnosis is a critical first step in the management of a health problem; *type I diagnostic trials* or diagnostic accuracy studies attempt to answer this question. To design a *type I diagnostic trial*, investigators must recruit subjects with and without the index disease and obtain valid and precise information about the true disease status. Multiple terms have been used to describe assessment of the true disease status, such as "gold standard," "standard of reference," and "reference standard." In this chapter, we use the term "gold standard."

When using a *case-control* design, study subjects are enrolled in the trial based on their disease status and test results are assessed retrospectively. The alternative is to assess both test results and disease status after enrollment within a *cohort study*. Both study designs, the case-control and the cohort design are subject to a variety of biases. The two most frequently encountered forms of bias are spectrum bias (in case-control studies) and verification bias (in cohort studies) Spectrum bias in case-control studies occurs when subjects with more severe disease than generally observed are selected as cases and healthier subjects are selected as controls. In order to avoid an overestimation of diagnostic accuracy that results from such an induced difference in case-mix between the study and target population, both cases and controls should be randomly selected. Verification bias in cohort studies occurs when the likelihood of obtaining true disease status depends on the results of the diagnostic test. For example, invasive or expensive gold standard tests are oftentimes solely or more frequently performed in subjects with positive test results. The problem of verification bias in *type I diagnostic trials* is equivalent to missing outcome data in cohort studies looking at exposure-outcome relationships. As such, statistical inference about diagnostic accuracy would still be possible but oftentimes requires the missingness at random (MAR) assumption. Solutions for verification bias are available under MAR using, for example, the inverse of the propensity of verification conditional on test results and other predictors of verification (de Groot et al. 2011; Braga et al. 2012; Bruni et al. 2014; Kosinski and Barnhart 2003). Verification bias often happens in studies in which it is not feasible to obtain diagnostic results from the "gold standard" on subjects thought to be at low risk. Thompson et al. (2005) studied the operating characteristics of prostate-specific antigen (PSA), in which prostate biopsy, the gold standard, was only recommended to men with PSA greater than 4.0 ng/ml or abnormal rectal examination results (Thompson et al. 2005). Harel and Zhou (2006) found that multiple imputations could help correct the verification bias by assuming that the missing information of prostate biopsy would not relate to the true prostate cancer status, but may depend on the values of PSA or rectal examination among some other variables (Harel and Zhou 2006). As such, under the MAR assumption, we can still obtain asymptotic unbiased estimates of diagnostic test performance results (e.g., sensitivity and specificity) with full information maximum likelihood.

Comparing Diagnostic Accuracy of Multiple Tests

Often a diagnostic trial is initiated to compare a promising new diagnostic procedure with an existing one, with the hypothesis that the new procedure is expected to be more accurate and can replace the standard procedure. Study designs used for such assessment of *comparative diagnostic accuracy* are the *randomized controlled trial (RCT)* and the *paired trial*. The distinction lies in the methods of assigning the diagnostic procedures to trial participants.

Randomized Controlled Trial (RCT)

RCTs are recommended to avoid various biases in the assessment of diagnostic accuracy when comparing an experimental diagnostic procedure with the reference procedure. In the uncontrolled setting, patients may undergo one of the two procedures due to a variety of reasons, such as lower cost, higher comorbidity, or hospital policy. These reasons might not be documented if the study is of observational nature, hampering the necessary adjustment for confounding. Yet, even if a diagnostic test is considered accurate in such a study after controlling for confounding, it will not be clear whether the result is influenced by unobserved confounders. In RCTs, patients undergo diagnostic procedures (i.e., experimental vs. reference) according to the results of randomization. The randomization mechanism rules out the potential impact of unmeasured confounders and thus helps to protect the conclusion from biases (Braga et al. 2012).

For example, cervical cancer is one of the leading causes of cancer-related mortality in sub-Saharan Africa. Visual inspection with acetic acid (VIA) is the standard test in this setting, but visual inspection with Lugol's iodine (VILI) is also a commonly recommended diagnostic technique for detecting cervical cancer. Huchko et al. (2015) conducted a randomized clinical trial to compare the diagnostic accuracy of VILI with VIA among HIV-infected women in western Kenya (Huchko et al. 2015). The trial enrolled 654 women, who were randomized to undergo either VILI or VIA with colposcopy (1:1 ratio). Any lesion suspicious for cervical intraepithelial neoplasia 2 or greater (CIN2+) was then biopsied as the gold standard for determining true disease status. To maximize the statistical power in a two-arm RCT, the randomization ratio is usually set as 1:1, so the numbers of patients undergoing different procedures are equal. However, a formulation for ratios other than 1:1 could also be used and might be preferred for some practical reasons, such as reducing the costs, and enhancing the feasibility of recruitment into or execution of a RCT.

Paired Trial

When diagnostic tests do not interfere with each other and can be done in the same study subject, a trial with a paired design might provide a more efficient alternative. For example, Ahmed et al. (2017) reported a diagnostic trial with a paired design comparing two imaging tests for prostate cancer (Ahmed et al. 2017). Men with high serum prostate-specific antigen (PSA) usually undergo transrectal ultrasound-guided prostate biopsy (TRUS-biopsy), which can cause side effects such as bleeding, pain, and infection. Multi-parametric magnetic resonance imaging (MP-MRI) might allow avoiding these side effects and improve diagnostic accuracy. To test this idea, 576 men were enrolled and underwent an MP-MRI followed by a TRUS-biopsy. At the end of the study, a template prostate mapping (TPM) biopsy was conducted for each patient, and the result was adopted as true disease status (gold standard). Diagnostic comparison was made on the paired results for the competing tests.

Definitions of Accuracy

A binary outcome, defined as presence (positive) or absence (negative) of a certain disease, is frequently used as the gold standard. The data can be typically presented in a 2X2 table (Table 1) with columns representing the true disease status, usually

Table 1 Underlying statistics for evaluation of a diagnostic test with binary outcomes

		True disease (golden standard)	
		Disease	No disease
Test results	Positive	True positive	False positive
	Negative	False negative	True negative

defined by the gold standard (e.g., TPM biopsy) and rows indicating the results of either experimental or reference procedure (e.g., MP-MRI or TRUS-biopsy). A diagnostic test that leads to a high proportion of positive results among patients with true disease, and a high proportion of negative results among patients without true disease, indicates good or better diagnostic accuracy.

Sensitivity and Specificity

A pair of measures, sensitivity and specificity, are commonly used in discussing diagnostic trials. *Sensitivity* answers the question "How likely is it that a patient with the true disease can be correctly identified as having a positive result under a diagnostic procedure?" The value of sensitivity varies from 0 to 1, with one indicating a perfect test. A diagnostic procedure with high sensitivity is important for identifying a serious and treatable disease. However, having a high sensitivity is not always sufficient for a diagnostic procedure to be clinically useful, because calculation of sensitivity only focuses on patients with the true disease. A diagnostic test with high sensitivity generally also leads to a high proportion of positive results in patients without the true disease. Thus, achieving balance requires also considering *specificity*, which answers the question "How likely is it that a patient without the true disease can be correctly identified as negative under a diagnostic procedure?" In a disease for which treatment is burdensome and costly, incorrectly claiming that someone has the disease may lead to unnecessary treatment. Similar to sensitivity, the value of specificity varies from 0 to 1; a procedure with specificity equal to 1 correctly identifies all patients without the true disease.

Table 2 gives the diagnostic results of MP-MRI. All 576 men in the trial underwent MP-MRI; 418 were diagnosed as positive for prostate cancer and 158 were diagnosed as negative. Based on the gold standard, there were 230 patients with true prostate cancer. Thus, the sensitivity was 0.93 (=213/230). On the other hand, there were 346 patients without true prostate cancer; thus, the specificity was 0.41 (=141/346).

Ideally, a perfect diagnostic procedure would have both sensitivity and specificity equal to 1, such that all patients with and without the true disease can be correctly identified. However, in practice, a clinician often needs to choose between a procedure with high sensitivity and low specificity, versus one with low sensitivity and high specificity. Values of sensitivity and specificity are not directly affected by the prevalence of the target disease (Table 2).

Table 2 Diagnostic results of MP-MRI and impact of change in disease prevalence: PROMIS trial

(A) Original MP-MRI with 40% prevalence					(B) Prevalence rate increase from 40% to 60%			
	Disease	No disease	Total			Disease	No disease	Total
Negative	17	141	158	→	Negative	24	94	118
Positive	213	205	418	→	Positive	322	136	458
Total	230	346	576		Total	346	230	576

Positive and Negative Predictive Values

Two other measures of accuracy commonly used in diagnostic trials are positive and negative predictive values. *Positive predictive value* (PPV) answers the question "How likely is it that a patient has the true disease given a positive result?" *Negative predictive value* (NPV) answers the question "How likely is it that a patient does not have the disease given a negative result?" In the example, 418 and 158 patients were diagnosed as positive and negative, respectively, based on MR-MRI results. Thus, the PPV was 0.51 (=213/418) and the NPV was 0.89 (=141/158). Unlike sensitivity and specificity, PPV and NPV are affected by disease prevalence. It is more likely to find positive test results in a high-prevalence population compared to a low-prevalence population (Trevethan 2019). If the disease prevalence of prostate cancer increases from 40% to 60%, for the same diagnostic procedure with a sensitivity of 0.93 and a specificity of 0.41, the PPV would increase from 0.51 to 0.7 (=322/346) and the NPV would decrease from 0.89 to 0.80 (=94/118). On the contrary, when disease prevalence decreases, the PPV of a diagnostic procedure will decrease and NPV will increase, while the sensitivity and specificity remain constant (Table 2). PPV and NPV are important because posttest probabilities eventually determine the clinical impact of subsequent treatment and the test-treatment strategy as a whole. When the PPV of a diagnostic procedure is high, more benefit can be expected from an efficacious treatment, whereas when the NPV is high, less harm can be expected from foregoing treatment.

Receiver Operating Characteristics Curve

When the diagnostic test has a continuous scale, researchers may face multiple possible cutoff points, and each cutoff point leads to a pair of sensitivity and specificity values. For example, Park et al. (2004) reported a study in which 70 patients with solitary pulmonary nodules underwent plain chest radiography to determine whether the nodules were benign or malignant. Chest radiographs were interpreted according to a five-point scale: 1-definitely benign, 2-probably benign, 3-possibly malignant, 4-probably malignant, and 5-definitely malignant. Thus, a positive result in this study was based on four possible cutoff points: ≥ 2, ≥ 3, ≥ 4, and 5, and vice versa. Note that sometimes a low score relates to a positive test, for example, lower cycle threshold (Ct)

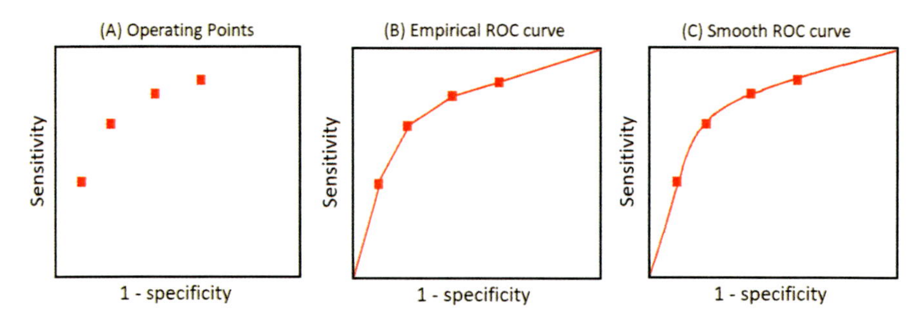

Fig. 1 Operating points, empirical and smooth ROC curves in the radiograph study

values in reverse transcription polymerase chain reaction (RT-PCR) tests. Consequently, we can define four diagnostic tests, each of which corresponds to a particular cutoff point, and thus followed by a pair of sensitivity and specificity. A diagnostic test with lower cutoff point leads to more patients with true disease diagnosed as positive (i.e., higher value of sensitivity) and less patients without true disease diagnosed as negative (i.e., lower value of specificity). Therefore, when the cutoff point moves from 5 to 2, the sensitivity of the diagnostic test will increase and the specificity will decrease, and vice versa. Note that sometimes a low score relates to a positive test, for example, lower cycle threshold (Ct) values in reverse transcription polymerase chain reaction (RT-PCR) tests.

A *receiver operating characteristics (ROC) curve* is an effective tool for summarizing the accuracy of a diagnostic procedure with a continuous measure when there is the potential for multiple cutoff points. It is a two-dimensional probabilistic measurement curve of sensitivity versus specificity that discloses how a true positive rate (TPR) varies with the change in false positive rate (FPR) across all the possible cutoff points. ROC curves can be drawn using either parametric or empirical methods (Hajian-Tilaki et al. 1997). To draw an *empirical ROC curve* for the data in the above example, the four pairs of sensitivities and 1-specificities are plotted as discrete points, called *operating points,* as shown in Fig. 1a. These operating points and the two endpoints can be connected at (0, 0) and (1, 1) (Fig. 1b) by assuming a linear relationship between sensitivity and 1-specificity between two nearby operating points. A smooth ROC curve can be fit using the parametric method by assuming the diagnostic accuracy measurement follows a particular probabilistic distribution (Fig. 1c). Distributions of ROC curves include binomial, Poisson, chi-squared, gamma, and logistic distributions (Pepe 2003; Ogilvie and Douglas Creelman 1968; Swets 1986; Walsh 1997). Faraggi and Reiser (2002) provide an excellent review of these details (Faraggi and Reiser 2002).

The Area Under the ROC Curve (AUC)

In clinical trials aiming to evaluate the overall performance of diagnostic procedures that classify patients into with and without the disease based on a particular threshold of a continuous measure, it is common to use the ROC curve as the primary outcome due to its advantage in summarizing the variation of TPR and FPR across different possible cutoff points. The accuracy of a diagnostic procedure in the ROC context is widely measured by area under the ROC curve (AUC). The AUC provides the average value of TPR given all the possible values of FPR. Considering both the ranges of TPR and FPR are (0, 1), the AUC can take any value between 0 and 1. The practical value of the AUC is reflected by a value that ranges from 0.5 (area under the chance diagonal) to 1 (area under a ROC with perfect diagnostic ability). A higher value of the AUC indicates better overall diagnostic performance. As with TPR and FPR, the AUC is independent of disease prevalence. Considering that the AUC of a diagnostic procedure from a trial is estimated based on a random sample, appropriate statistical inference is necessary for making a conclusion, and the uncertainty around the AUC is typically handled by a certain level of confidence interval (e.g., 95%). We can estimate the AUC by using parametric (McClish 1989; Metz 1978) and empirical methods (McClish 1989; Metz 1978; Obuchowski and Bullen 2018). Zhou et al. (2009) reviewed the performances of both parametric and empirical estimators of AUC (Zhou et al. 2009). When diagnostic procedures are evaluated based on continuous (e.g., biomarker) or quasi-continuous (e.g., a percent-confidence scale with range 0–100%) measurements, both empirical and parametric estimators perform well, and the bias is negligible. When considering discrete outcomes (e.g., radiography in the study) by the empirical method sometimes underestimates the AUC. On the other hand, parametric methods rely on the distributional assumption and sometimes have poor performance in small diagnostic trials.

Sample Size Calculation

Determination of sample size plays an important role in designing a trial for assessment of diagnostic accuracy. Too small samples may lead to imprecise estimation (i.e., a wider confidence interval), whereas obtaining a large sample size is costly and could require that patients undergo potentially unnecessary subsequent testing with an unknown risk from subsequent treatments (e.g., adverse events). Depending on the study setting and analytical plan, sample size calculations can be considered using two concepts: estimation and comparison. To determine the sample size for a diagnostic trial that seeks to estimate the sensitivity (or specificity) of a single diagnostic test, four essential elements must be considered: (1) a predetermined value of sensitivity; (2) the confidence level ($1 - \alpha$); (3) the precision of estimation, or the maximal marginal error, which is the maximum difference between estimated sensitivity and the true value; and (4) disease prevalence. The sample size calculation of a diagnostic trial based on a comparison of test accuracies is hypothesis driven. It is applied to either a single-arm trial for comparing the accuracy of a diagnostic procedure with a historical control, or a randomized trial for comparing the accuracy between the experimental procedure versus an appropriate control. In this situation, the targeted statistical power (i.e., 1- type II error) and the significance level of hypothesis test (i.e., type I error) also need to be specified.

Simel et al. (1991) provide a sample size formula based on the likelihood ratio, defined as the ratio between sensitivity and (1-specificity). Beam (1992) provided a

Table 3 Statistical software for sample size calculation under a specific design

Software procedure	Design of diagnostic trial
PASS: Proportions/test for one sample sensitivity and specificity	Observational study design for comparing sensitivity and specificity of a new diagnostic procedure to an existing standard procedure
PASS: Proportions/test for paired sensitivities and specificities	Match-paired design for comparing sensitivities/specificities of two diagnostic procedures
PASS: Proportions/test for two independent sensitivities and specificities	Observational study design or RCT for comparing sensitivities/specificities of two diagnostic procedures between two independent samples
PASS: Proportion/confidence intervals for one-sample sensitivity	Observational study design for estimating a single sensitivity using confidence intervals
PASS: Proportion/confidence intervals for one-sample specificity	Observational study design for estimating a single specificity confidence interval
PASS: Proportion/confidence intervals for one-sample sensitivity and specificity	Observational study design for estimating both sensitivity and specificity confidence intervals, based on a specified sensitivity and specificity, interval width, confidence level, and prevalence
PASS: AUC-based test for one ROC curve	Observational study design for comparing ROC curve of a new diagnostic procedure to a standard procedure
PASS: ROC/test for two ROC curve	Match-paired design for comparing the AUCs of two diagnostic procedures
PASS: ROC/confidence intervals for the AUC	Observational study design for estimating a specified width of a confidence interval for AUC

AUC area under the curve, *RCT* randomized clinical trial, *ROC* receiver operated characteristics. Observational study includes cohort and case-control designs

sample size formula that can be applied to trials with a paired design (Simel et al. 1991; Beam 1992). A variety of formulation for different settings and improved efficiency are provided by many authors (Flahault et al. 2005; Fosgate 2009; Kumar and Indrayan 2011; Li and Fine 2004; Liu et al. 2005; Obuchowski 1998; Steinberg et al. 2009). The statistical software, PASS, implements most of these methods and is easy to use. Table 3 summarizes these procedures and the design corresponding to each procedure.

Reporting Diagnostic Trials for Accuracy

Several surveys have shown that studies evaluating diagnostic accuracy often fail to transparently describe core elements of design and analysis, including how the cohort was selected and what design parameters the sample size was based on, as well as to comprehensively describe the study findings and how they will impact clinical practice (Korevaar et al. 2014, 2015; Lijmer et al. 1999). They also find that the recommendations from these studies are often unnecessarily generous and optimistic. The Standards for Reporting of Diagnostic Accuracy Studies (STARD) statement was developed to facilitate complete and transparent reporting. STARD recommends a checklist of items that should be reported for diagnostic accuracy studies. Although quite a few journals have adopted STARD into their instruction to authors, uptake remains low (Korevaar et al. 2014; NCSS 2018).

Failures in reporting fall in many categories and can jeopardize the decision-making on which diagnostic test should be used in clinical practice. For example, Hu (2016) noted that in their systematic review of diagnostic studies of osteopontin for ovarian cancer, few publications did not report research results in accordance with the STARD guideline (Hu 2016). This hindered their overall ability in estimating the risk of bias and applicability concerns of included studies remained unresolved. They furthermore found that in some of the studies, the inclusion and exclusion criteria for subject enrollment were not reported, and only the disease spectrum sample size were reported (Hu et al. 2015). Therefore, the authors performing the systematic review did not know whether the prevalence of the target disease in the study cohorts was consistent with the real word. Knowledge of the prevalence of the target disease is vital because it can greatly affect estimates of test performance in the presence of spectrum bias (Whiting et al. 2004). In summary, without knowledge of inclusion/exclusion criteria and prevalence, it is difficult to decide under which condition the diagnostic test should be adopted.

Many other types of reporting failures have been found that may prevent the appropriate translation of research into clinical practice, and these also apply to diagnostic research. How to improve reporting has however remained a vexing problem despite many efforts. Reporting guidelines were first published simultaneously in a number of high-impact journals hoping wide adoption. In addition, interventions have been attempted including convincing journal publishers to make the use of reporting guidelines a requirement for the authors and reviewers, educating them on how to use reporting guidelines, and training them on how to evaluate quality of a manuscript through guideline-based scoring etc. However, most evaluations show that a continued effort for further improvement is needed. One of the most robust efforts so far is the development of the Enhancing the QUAlity and Transparency Of health Research (EQUATOR) Network. The EQUATOR network, established in 2006, is a global initiative that has brought together researchers and journal editors with the aim of achieving accurate, complete, and transparent reporting of health research studies to support research reproducibility and usefulness (Network, Equator 2017). Their work aims to increase the value of health research and minimize avoidable waste of financial and human investments in health research projects. The work of the EQUATOR investigators has already been bestowed with an award from the Council of Science Editors for improvement of scientific communication through the pursuit of high standards in reporting (Majeed and Amir 2018). This kind of high-level recognition, regular publication of commentaries on this topic, and making reporting guidelines part of regular training in the medical school curriculum are bound to make a favorable impact.

Diagnostic Trial Type II: Diagnostic Randomized Clinical Trials for Assessment of Clinical Effectiveness

There are circumstances when diagnostic accuracy results from *type 1 diagnostic trials* are considered sufficient to extrapolate about net health benefits. Yet, further empirical evidence is often needed about how the test affects longer-term outcomes. One way to better evaluate the potential utility of diagnostic tests is to investigate how well test results match with future patient outcomes by determining the *prognostic value* and/or the ability to modify treatment effects (*predictive value*). The latter should be generally assessed in a randomized setting with testing performed at baseline in all patients prior to the randomization to treatment(s) (Lijmer and Bossuyt 2009). However, diagnostic tests are seldom used on their own, independent of treatment. Test results generally guide or determine treatment decisions as part of a broader management strategy. Thus, differences in diagnostic accuracy will likely result in differences in delivery of treatment, which will ultimately affect disease prognosis and patient outcomes. As such, the downstream consequences of tests followed by treatment decisions should be evaluated together. The *diagnostic randomized clinical trial* or the so-called *test-treatment trial* design is considered the gold standard to provide such proof for the *clinical effectiveness or clinical utility* of diagnostic tests (Ferrante di Ruffano et al. 2012, 2017). Sometimes consequences beyond those for the health of patients need to be considered as well, including those for use of resources in the healthcare sector and/or society. The goal is then for the *test-treatment trial* to also provide evidence for changes in efficiency of care by evaluation of economic outcomes, i.e., *cost-effectiveness* or *cost-utility analysis*. In this chapter, a clinical perspective is taken for discussing the concepts of designing *test-treatment trials*, although the broader healthcare sector and societal perspectives are briefly discussed as well.

Test-Treatment Trial Designs

Optimizing the design of *test-treatment trials* requires a good prior understanding of how the application of diagnostic tests may change outcomes in the target patient population by conceptualizing potential underlying pathways. Figure 2 illustrates a pathway showing how diagnostic tests in comparison with comparator strategies (strategies of alternative diagnostic tests, recommended care or the current practice) may affect health outcomes (Ferrante di Ruffano et al. 2012).

For an initial conceptualization of a test-treatment trial, researchers should start by defining which alternative diagnostic and management pathways need to be compared, while specifying where differences can be expected. These steps will allow them to select mechanisms underlying the outcomes of interest (Mustafa et al. 2017). A helpful method to conceptualize a trial is using care pathway algorithms or flow diagrams based on the components depicted in Fig. 2. Different test-treatment applications can be defined depending on the medical decision problem based on single, replacement, triage, add-on, and parallel or combined testing. The optimal

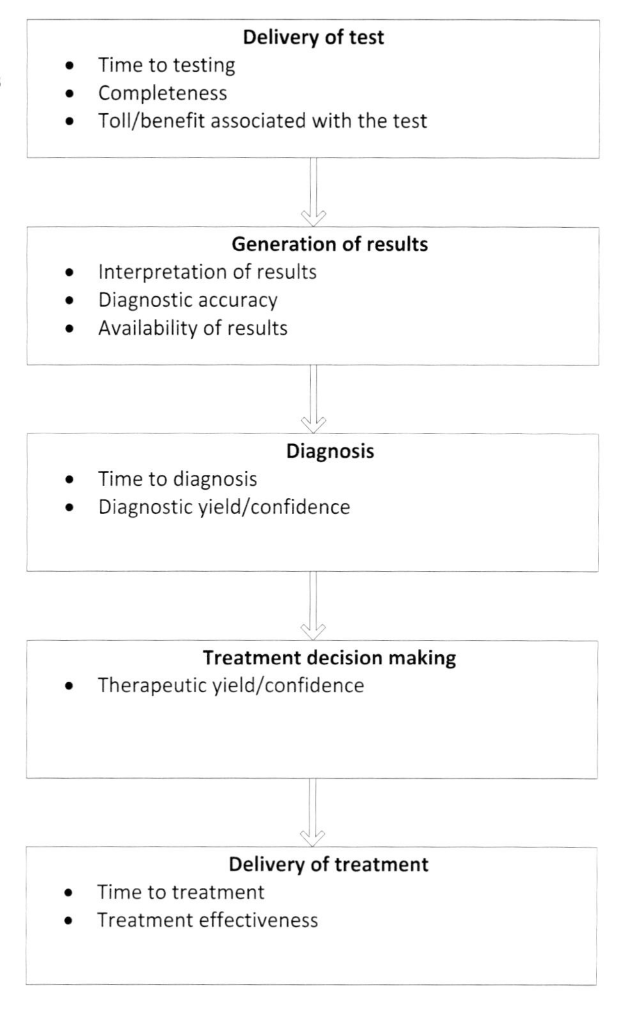

Fig. 2 Simplified test-treatment pathway showing each component of a patient's management that can affect health outcomes (Ferrante di Ruffano et al. 2012)

design of the trial depends on the application type and the certainty about the diagnostic accuracy of the test(s), as well as the added value of disclosing test results, and treatment effectiveness.

Evaluating a Single Test

Randomized Controlled Trial (RCT) of Testing

This design can be used for comparing health outcomes following a new or established diagnostic test to health outcomes from a comparator *no test* strategy, in the most extreme case defined as *treat all* or *treat none*). As the comparator strategy does not rely on testing, the randomization concerns the decision whether to perform the testing or not. This trial can answer the question whether it would be beneficial to avoid treatment in those who test negative, when the comparator is a *treat all* strategy, or to offer treatment to those who test positive, when the comparator is a *treat none* strategy. This scenario is illustrated in Fig. 3. The *no test* strategy is oftentimes defined as *usual care* in which diagnostic and therapeutic interventions following randomization are not protocolized by the investigators. For example, a randomized trial was conducted in low-risk pregnant women to evaluate whether routine ultrasonography in the third trimester improves severe adverse perinatal outcomes compared with *usual care* (Henrichs et al. 2019). Routine ultrasonography was associated with a higher antenatal detection of small for gestational age fetuses, higher incidence of induction of labor, and lower incidence of augmentation of labor. However, it did not significantly improve severe adverse perinatal and maternal peripartum outcomes.

Random Disclosure Trial

Sometimes the medical decision problem pertains to understanding whether *communication* of test results would affect treatment decisions and subsequent health outcomes. If there are no ethical constrains about delaying the communication of test results, the randomization point can occur *after* performance of the diagnostic test (Fig. 4). Patients are thus randomized to disclosure of test results versus no (or delayed) disclosure. In this trial design, randomization can be stratified by test results to ensure more balanced groups. The random disclosure design has also the option of studying the prognostic value of the diagnostic test by statistical modeling of patient outcomes observed conditional on test results in the non-disclosed arm. For example, Modic et al. used a random disclosure design to investigate the effect of disclosing imaging findings on outcome in patients with acute low back pain or radiculopathy, as well as to determine the prognostic role of MR imaging for physical disability due to low back pain and patient satisfaction (Modic et al.

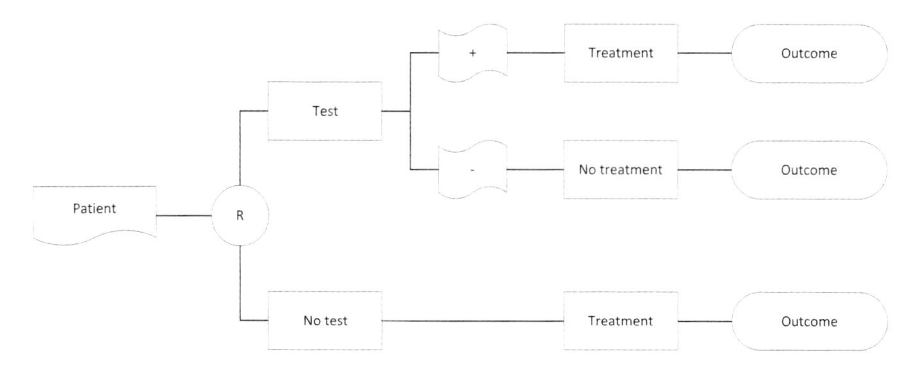

Fig. 3 Trial of testing with treatment as comparator, modify fig (Lijmer and Bossuyt 2009)

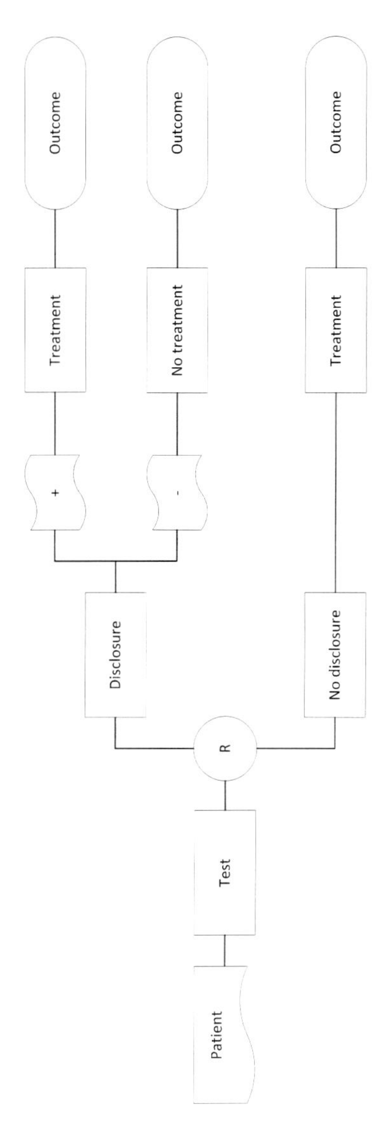

Fig. 4 Random disclosure trial, with treatment as comparator, modify fig (Lijmer and Bossuyt 2009)

2005). Patients underwent MR imaging at presentation and were then randomized to either an early information arm (results provided to referring physician and patient within 48 hours) or a blinded arm (both patient and physician were blinded to MR imaging results). Improvement in function and other patient reported outcomes at 6-weeks were similar in unblinded and blinded patients. Multivariable modeling of imaging results did not reveal any relationship between herniation type, size, and behavior over time with physical disability and patient satisfaction.

Evaluating Multiple Tests

For many medical decision problems, the question is not whether *to test* or *not to test*, but *which* test or *which combination* of tests to use. Conceptually, the trial design concerning such research questions is equivalent to designing a trial for a single test as outlined above, with some modifications.

Comparative Test RCT

When the test-treatment strategies concerning two or more tests are intrinsically different (e.g., because delivery of the tests and/or the process of achieving test results vary), the optimal randomization point is when the decision is made about which test to use (Fig. 5). An example of such a *head-to-head* or *two-arm* comparison is the Prospective Multicenter Imaging Study for Evaluation of Chest Pain (PROMISE) trial (Douglas et al. 2015). In this trial, patients with symptoms of coronary heart disease were randomized to an initial strategy of coronary computed tomographic angiography (CTA) or a diagnostic strategy using functional testing (exercise electrocardiography, nuclear stress testing, or stress echocardiography). Although, the CTA strategy was associated with a lower incidence of invasive catheterization showing no obstructive coronary artery disease at 90-days, the composite endpoint of mortality and coronary outcomes did not differ between groups over a median follow-up of 2 years. However, the PROMISE trial was not designed to incorporate subsequent additional diagnostic tests or revascularization procedures.

Discordant Test Results RCT

When two or more competing, mutually exclusive test-treatment strategies are compared, usually one test is considered as standard practice. In some occasions, the competing tests have a similar delivery and process for generation of test results. It can then be assumed that when the tests being compared have the same result (either all positive or all negative), the subsequent management should be the same and expected outcomes would be identical. When these conditions are satisfied and it is feasible to perform both tests in all patients, the *discordant test results* trial design or *paired design* (Fig. 6), in which only the patients with discordant test results are randomized to treatment(s) and followed up, is the most efficient design (Lijmer and Bossuyt 2009). This design, however, only allows for estimation of an absolute risk difference between the test-treatment strategies and not a relative risk measure, and it

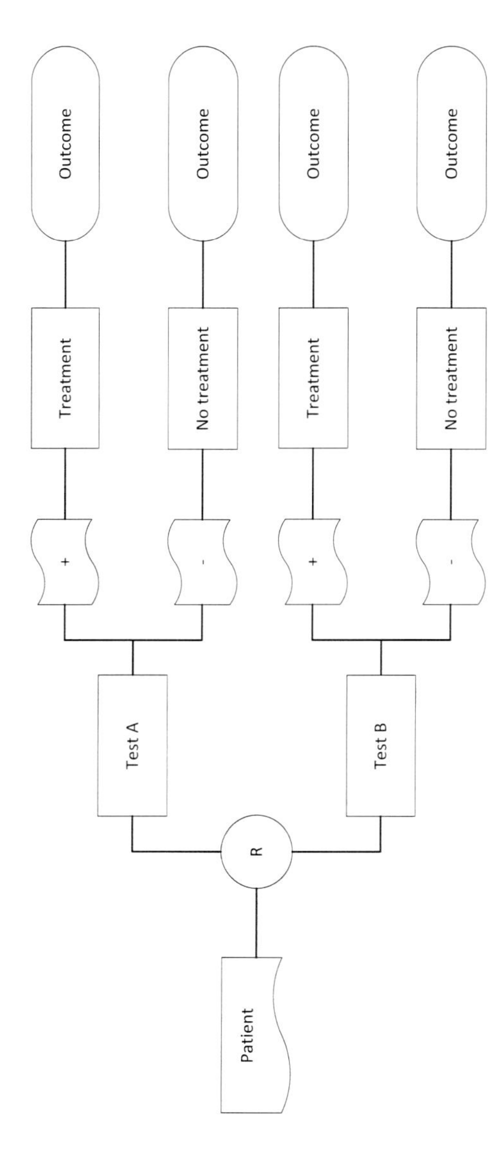

Fig. 5 Trial comparing two different tests (Lijmer and Bossuyt 2009)

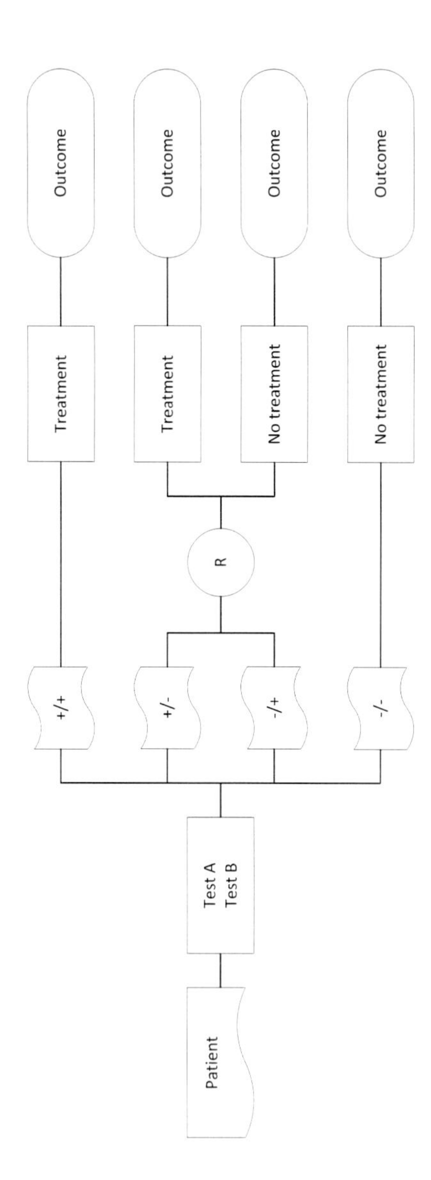

Fig. 6 Discordant test results trial

is rarely implemented in practice. Hooper et al. (Hooper et al. 2013), however, describe a good decision analytic example based on the MINDACT trial, a trial comparing a 70-gene expression profile with standard clinicopathologic criteria for determining which patients with node-negative breast cancer should receive adjuvant chemotherapy (Cardoso et al. 2007). A *discordant test results* trial was found to be ~four times more efficient than the conventional *head-to-head* trial in terms of required sample size and only around a third of the sample needed to be followed up, thus rendering follow-up 12 times more efficient.

Random Disclosure Trial

Similar to extension of the trial design for an RCT investigating a single test-treatment strategy versus no testing, the random disclosure trial as explained above and depicted in Fig. 4 can be extended for multiple tests as well. However, in this situation, both diagnostic tests will need to be performed in all patients. In the next step, patients are randomized to disclosure of one test only in each arm. The subsequent management or treatment is solely done in that arm based on the results of the disclosed test. The flowchart of such a trial with randomization after testing is depicted in Fig. 7 for two tests. Note that randomization can also be conducted prior to the testing, which may be preferable in case test results could affect clinical equipoise.

Add-On, Triage, and Parallel or Combined Testing

Test-treatment strategies often consist of a series or combinations of multiple tests, instead of a single test followed by patient management. There are clinical scenarios in which a decision should be made about whether using the results of a new test would provide useful additional information. For example, the Scottish Computed Tomography of the Heart (SCOT-HEART) trial investigated the use of CTA in addition to standard noninvasive stress testing (electrocardiography, radionuclide scintigraphy, echocardiography, or MR imaging) versus noninvasive stress testing alone for patients with stable chest pain (Newby et al. 2018). Adding CTA resulted in a significantly lower rate of coronary events at 5 years by improving the use of subsequent tests and treatments. For such *add-on tests*, the designs as presented for the single test (Figs. 3 and 4) can be used and need only minor modification.

Another frequent clinical application is using results from a new (perhaps less invasive) test to select patients for an established, more invasive test (*triage*). Lastly, a new test may be used independently and in parallel with a conventional test, after which results of both tests are interpreted simultaneously for the diagnosis. New *triage* or *parallel testing* strategies can be compared to the established test-treatment strategy in a randomized fashion, similar to the design depicted in Fig. 5. However, alternative trial designs exist for evaluating new triage strategies to improve efficiency. For example, a triage test could be performed in all patients, followed by randomization of patients to the established test only when management based on the established test seems questionable. Another option is to perform both the triage and established tests in all patients, and then randomize only those for whom the established test is negative, but the new test for triage is positive (Lijmer and Bossuyt

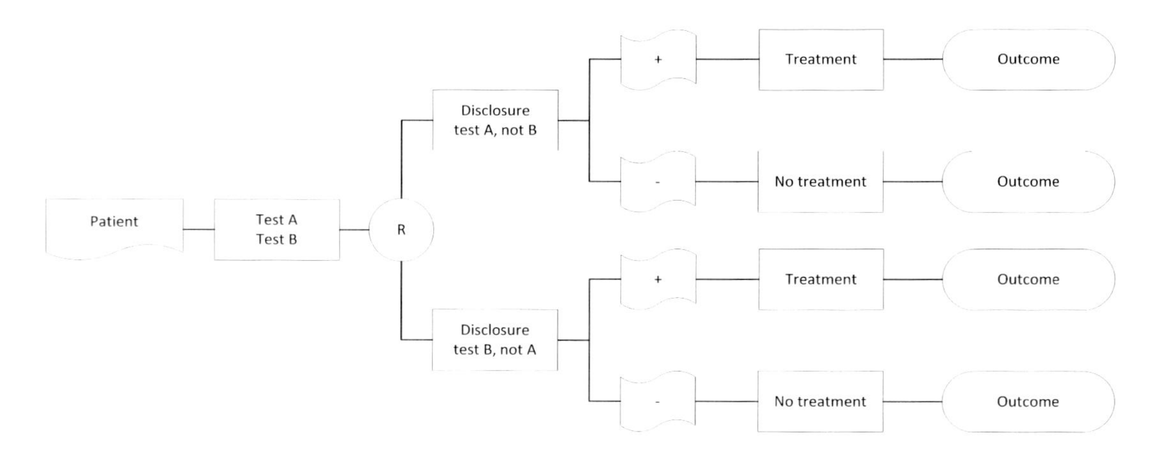

Fig. 7 Random disclosure trial

2009). The Canadian Pulmonary Embolism Diagnosis Study (CANPEDS) Group, for example, investigated if additional diagnostic testing can be safely withheld in patients with suspected pulmonary embolism in those who have negative erythrocyte agglutination D-dimer test results. Four hundred and fifty-six patients with negative erythrocyte agglutination D-dimer test results out of 1126 patients with suspected pulmonary embolism were randomly assigned to no further diagnostic testing or a ventilation-perfusion lung scan followed by ultrasonography of the proximal deep veins of the legs. Results showed that additional diagnostic testing can be safely withheld without increasing the frequency of venous thromboembolism during follow-up (Kearon et al. 2006).

Explanatory Versus Pragmatic Approaches for Test-Treatment Trials

In general, results from pragmatic trials are considered more generalizable to current practice than those from explanatory trials. Pragmatic test-treatment trials enroll patients within a standard care setting and allow both clinical decision-making at the discretion of the clinician and patient nonadherence to recommended care (Ferrante di Ruffano et al. 2017). The PROMISE trial enrolled patients with stable chest pain who were predominantly at high cardiovascular risk and for whom noninvasive cardiovascular testing was considered necessary in an outpatient setting (Douglas et al. 2015). The data coordinating center ensured all study sites had experienced staff and used diagnostic procedures in agreement with guidelines. Local physicians made all clinical management decisions at their discretion based on the test results in both the functional testing as CTA study arm. Follow-up visits were scheduled at 60 days and at 6-month intervals after randomization. Clinical events were adjudicated in a blinded fashion by an independent committee.

Likewise, the SCOT-HEART trial was conducted within a standard care outpatient setting and management following diagnostic testing was done at the discretion of the clinician in both study arms (Newby et al. 2018). There were, however, no trial-specific visits planned, and routinely collected data on events were used from the Information and Statistics Division and the electronic Data Research and Innovation Service of the National Health Service (NHS) Scotland. There was no formal event adjudication committee involved in the study, and study end points were classified using diagnostic codes and procedural codes from discharge records. Thus, both the PROMISE and SCOT-HEART trial can be considered pragmatic trials, although the SCOT-HEART trial may be considered more so.

Reporting of Test-Treatment Trials

Nonetheless, findings from any trial (pragmatic or less pragmatic of nature) are more likely to be translated into clinical practice when the protocol is published and provides transparent and detailed information on all test-treatment pathways that should be followed (e.g., decision trees or flow diagrams). Results should include data on the diagnoses that were made, as well as data on how the test results may have impacted subsequent clinical decision-making and outcomes. For example, treatment decisions should be reported with stratification by test results to show the extent which clinical decisions were guided by the recommended test-treatment protocols (Ferrante di Ruffano et al. 2017). The Template for Intervention Description and Replication (TIDieR) checklist and guide can be used to improve the reporting of test-treatment trials.

Statistical Analysis and Sample Size Calculations

Statistical analysis plans and sample size estimations depend on the design of test-treatment trials and outcome type (e.g., binary, continuous, time-to-event). For *two-arm* designs, as in *single test* and *comparative test* trials, the statistical analysis is relatively straightforward and preferably performed using the intention-to-treat principle. Sample size and power formulas depend on disease prevalence, sensitivities, and specificities of test(s), and response rate of the treatment(s). For the *paired* design used in *discordant test results* trials, formulas are more complicated, because overall treatment response rates depend on how many patients had discordant test results. This in turn is a function of the total number of patients, disease prevalence, sensitivities, and specificities (Hooper et al. 2013; Lu and Gatsonis 2013).

Economic Analysis in Test-Treatment Trials and Decision Models

Usually when new tests are being evaluated against conventional tests or standard care, it is critical for decision-makers to consider whether replacing existing care by implementing the new test strategy would be cost-effective. Contemporary clinical trials therefore frequently include a secondary economic analysis or analysis that integrates clinical effectiveness and cost implications, i.e., *cost-utility* or *cost-effectiveness analysis*. For example, the PROMISE trialists conducted an economic sub-study in which costs of the initial outpatient testing strategies were estimated from administrative data, costs of hospitalizations were estimated from uniform billing claims data, and physician fees were assessed based on reimbursement rates (Mark et al. 2016).

The preferred health outcome used in a more comprehensive *cost-effectiveness analysis* is the quality-adjusted life year (QALY), which combines morbidity and mortality by considering both generic health-related quality of life and survival time. When the cost-effectiveness analysis is conducted alongside an RCT, average cumulative QALYs can be estimated by the integral of quality of life utility repeatedly scored at a scale from 0 (death) to 1 (perfect health) for each participant during the trial follow-up period (Glasziou et al. 1998). Utility scores are generally derived from generic quality of life questionnaires that can be mapped to community preference weights obtained by standard gamble or time trade-off methods. Costs can be estimated using a micro-costing approach or a more indirect gross-costing

Table 4 Key differences between test-treatment trials and decision models for evaluating utility of medical tests (Adapted from Bossuyt et al. (2012), PMID 22730450)

Test-treatment trial	Decision model
Can compare few competing test-treatment strategies	Can compare multiple competing test-treatment strategies
Can evaluate a limited number of effectiveness and safety outcomes	Can evaluate all relevant effectiveness and safety outcomes based on multiple sources
Restricted by a limited time horizon	Lifetime horizon is possible
User empirical data and correlations can be observed and accounted for	Assumptions about model structure and parameters need to be made

approach, like done in the PROMISE trial. For example, in the Netherlands, a cost-utility analysis was performed parallel to a randomized controlled trial to determine the cost-effectiveness of early referral for MR imaging by general practitioners versus *usual care* alone in patients with traumatic knee symptoms. QALYs and costs were estimated over the trial duration from a healthcare and societal perspective. Results from this analysis showed that MR imaging referral was more costly (mean costs €1109 vs €837) and less effective (mean QALYS 0.888 vs 0.899). Thus, *usual care* was deemed the dominant strategy for patients with traumatic knee symptoms (van Oudenaarde et al. 2018).

Test-treatment trials are, however, often limited by the number of strategies that can be evaluated, follow-up duration, and ability to evaluate outcomes with low event rates (e.g., radiation risk) or large variability (cost data). For these reasons, decision models are increasingly used to assess the cost-effectiveness of diagnostic tests by combining and linking data from multiple sources. These sources can include evidence regarding diagnostic accuracy, disease prevalence, immediate and future adverse event rates, treatment efficacy, and quality of life. Similar to a cost-effectiveness analysis conducted alongside the trial, decision models generally analyze outcomes relevant to the healthcare sector and society. As such, preference weights and costs from multiple components (formal and informal health care, and non-health care sectors) are assigned to the modeled tests, treatments, events, and health states. Key differences in characteristics of empirical test-treatment trials and decision models are listed in Table 4.

Decision models can also be used to extrapolate cost-effectiveness outcomes beyond the trial duration, when it is expected that the trial follow-up is too short to capture all potential future benefits and harms. For example, in the economic analysis of the PROMISE trial, a parametric model was used to extrapolate costs from 90 days to 3 years (Mark et al. 2016). The analysis showed that CTA and conventional diagnostic testing resulted in similar costs through 3 years of follow-up.

Summary and Conclusions

In summary, the usefulness of diagnostic tests firstly depends on making an accurate diagnosis and/or determining disease severity. However, diagnostic data are generally sought for a broader set of reasons, including improvement of health outcomes in the target patient population. Key questions to ask are how good is a diagnostic test at providing the desired answers concerning these outcomes, and what rules of evidence should be used to judge the value of new tests. The ultimate determinant is whether the clinical intervention imposed based on the diagnostic test result truly helped improving a relevant clinical metric for patients. The encompassing field of diagnostic trials helps addressing these questions through the various designs presented in this chapter. Researchers must weigh the strengths and weaknesses of each of these designs, compute sample sizes with an eye toward feasibility, and report all results transparently to ensure that the new information obtained is useful for clinical practice and future studies.

Key Facts

- The field of diagnostic trials has grown tremendously in the last 40 years. Two types of diagnostic trials have emerged: (I) studies that estimate and compare accuracy of diagnostic procedures and (II) studies that estimate and compare effectiveness of a treatment pathway triggered by specific results of diagnostic tests.
- Each type of diagnostic trial has a variety of design options, and related sample size computation and software tools are now available.
- Guidelines for reporting designs and results of diagnostic trials remain underused.

Cross-References

▸ Bayesian Adaptive Designs for Phase I Trials
▸ Biomarker-Driven Adaptive Phase III Clinical Trials
▸ Cluster Randomized Trials
▸ Introduction to Meta-Analysis
▸ Monte Carlo Simulation for Trial Design Tool
▸ Power and Sample Size
▸ Principles of Clinical Trials: Bias and Precision Control
▸ Pragmatic Randomized Trials Using Claims or Electronic Health Record Data
▸ Sequential, Multiple Assignment, Randomized Trials (SMART)

References

Ahmed HU, El-Shater Bosaily A, Brown LC, Gabe R, Kaplan R, Parmar MK, Collaco-Moraes Y et al (2017) Diagnostic accuracy of multi-parametric MRI and TRUS biopsy in prostate cancer (PROMIS): a paired validating confirmatory study. Lancet 389(10071):815–822. https://doi.org/10.1016/s0140-6736(16)32401-1

Beam CA (1992) Strategies for improving power in diagnostic radiology research. AJR Am J Roentgenol 159(3):631–637. https://doi.org/10.2214/ajr.159.3.1503041

Begg CB, Greenes RA (1983) Assessment of diagnostic tests when disease verification is subject to selection bias. Biometrics 39(1):207–215

Bossuyt PM, Reitsma JB, Linnet K, Moons KG (2012) Beyond diagnostic accuracy: the clinical utility of diagnostic tests. Clin Chem 58(12):1636–1643. https://doi.org/10.1373/clinchem.2012.182576

Braga LH, Farrokhyar F, Bhandari M (2012) Confounding: what is it and how do we deal with it? Can J Surg 55(2):132–138. https://doi.org/10.1503/cjs.036311

Bruni L, Barrionuevo-Rosas L, Albero G, Serrano B, Mena M, Gómez D, Muñoz J, Bosch FX, de Sanjosé S (2014) Human papillomavirus and related diseases report. L'Hospitalet de Llobregat: ICO Information Centre on HPV and Cancer

Cardoso F, Piccart-Gebhart M, Van't Veer L, Rutgers E (2007) The MINDACT trial: the first prospective clinical validation of a genomic tool. Mol Oncol 1(3):246–251. https://doi.org/10.1016/j.molonc.2007.10.004

Colli A, Fraquelli M, Casazza G, Conte D, Nikolova D, Duca P, Thorlund K, Gluud C (2014) The architecture of diagnostic research: from bench to bedside–research guidelines using liver stiffness as an example. Hepatology 60(1):408–418. https://doi.org/10.1002/hep.26948

de Groot JA, Bossuyt PM, Reitsma JB, Rutjes AW, Dendukuri N, Janssen KJ, Moons KG (2011) Verification problems in diagnostic accuracy studies: consequences and solutions. BMJ 343: d4770. https://doi.org/10.1136/bmj.d4770

Douglas PS, Hoffmann U, Patel MR, Mark DB, Al-Khalidi HR, Cavanaugh B, Cole J et al (2015) Outcomes of anatomical versus functional testing for coronary artery disease. N Engl J Med 372 (14):1291–1300. https://doi.org/10.1056/NEJMoa1415516

Faraggi D, Reiser B (2002) Estimation of the area under the ROC curve. Stat Med 21(20):3093–3106. https://doi.org/10.1002/sim.1228

Ferrante di Ruffano L, Dinnes J, Taylor-Phillips S, Davenport C, Hyde C, Deeks JJ (2017) Research waste in diagnostic trials: a methods review evaluating the reporting of test-treatment interventions. BMC Med Res Methodol 17(1):32. https://doi.org/10.1186/s12874-016-0286-0

Ferrante di Ruffano L, Hyde CJ, McCaffery KJ, Bossuyt PM, Deeks JJ (2012) Assessing the value of diagnostic tests: a framework for designing and evaluating trials. BMJ 344:e686. https://doi.org/10.1136/bmj.e686

Fosgate GT (2009) Practical sample size calculations for surveillance and diagnostic investigations. J Vet Diagn Investig 21(1):3–14. https://doi.org/10.1177/104063870902100102

Flahault A, Cadilhac M, Thomas G (2005) Sample size calculation should be performed for design accuracy in diagnostic test studies. J Clin Epidemiol 58(8):859–862. https://doi.org/10.1016/j.jclinepi.2004.12.009

Glasziou PP, Cole BF, Gelber RD, Hilden J, Simes RJ (1998) Quality adjusted survival analysis with repeated quality of life measures. Stat Med 17(11):1215–1229. https://doi.org/10.1002/(sici)1097-0258(19980615)17:11<1215::aid-sim844>3.0.co;2-y

Gluud C, Gluud LL (2005) Evidence based diagnostics. BMJ 330(7493):724–726

Hajian-Tilaki KO, Hanley JA, Joseph L, Collet JP (1997) A comparison of parametric and nonparametric approaches to ROC analysis of quantitative diagnostic tests. Med Decis Mak 17(1):94–102. https://doi.org/10.1177/0272989x9701700111

Harel O, Zhou XH (2006) Multiple imputation for correcting verification bias. Stat Med 25(22): 3769–3786. https://doi.org/10.1002/sim.2494

Henrichs J, Verfaille V, Jellema P, Viester L, Pajkrt E, Wilschut J, van der Horst HE, Franx A, de Jonge A (2019) Effectiveness of routine third trimester ultrasonography to reduce adverse perinatal outcomes in low risk pregnancy (the IRIS study): nationwide, pragmatic, multicentre, stepped wedge cluster randomised trial. BMJ 367:l5517. https://doi.org/10.1136/bmj.l5517

Hooper R, Díaz-Ordaz K, Takeda A, Khan K (2013) Comparing diagnostic tests: trials in people with discordant test results. Stat Med 32(14):2443–2456. https://doi.org/10.1002/sim.5676

Huchko MJ, Sneden J, Zakaras JM, Smith-McCune K, Sawaya G, Maloba M, Bukusi EA, Cohen CR (2015) A randomized trial comparing the diagnostic accuracy of visual inspection with acetic acid to visual inspection with Lugol's iodine for cervical cancer screening in HIV-infected women. PLoS One 10(4):e0118568. https://doi.org/10.1371/journal.pone.0118568

Huang EP, Lin FI, Shankar LK (2017) Beyond correlations, sensitivities, and specificities: a roadmap for demonstrating utility of advanced imaging in oncology treatment and clinical trial design. Acad Radiol 24(8):1036–1049. https://doi.org/10.1016/j.acra.2017.03.002

Hu ZD (2016) STARD guideline in diagnostic accuracy tests: perspective from a systematic reviewer. Ann Transl Med 4(3):46. https://doi.org/10.3978/j.issn.2305-5839.2016.01.03

Hu ZD, Wei TT, Yang M, Ma N, Tang QQ, Qin BD, Fu HT, Zhong RQ (2015) Diagnostic value of osteopontin in ovarian cancer: a meta-analysis and systematic review. PLoS One 10(5): e0126444. https://doi.org/10.1371/journal.pone.0126444

Kearon C, Ginsberg JS, Douketis J, Turpie AG, Bates SM, Lee AY, Crowther MA et al (2006) An evaluation of D-dimer in the diagnosis of pulmonary embolism: a randomized trial. Ann Intern Med 144(11):812–821. https://doi.org/10.7326/0003-4819-144-11-200606060-00007

Kosinski AS, Barnhart HX (2003) A global sensitivity analysis of performance of a medical diagnostic test when verification bias is present. Stat Med 22(17):2711–2721. https://doi.org/10.1002/sim.1517

Korevaar DA, van Enst WA, Spijker R, Bossuyt PM, Hooft L (2014) Reporting quality of diagnostic accuracy studies: a systematic review and meta-analysis of investigations on adherence to STARD. Evid Based Med 19(2):47–54. https://doi.org/10.1136/eb-2013-101637

Korevaar DA, Wang J, van Enst WA, Leeflang MM, Hooft L, Smidt N, Bossuyt PM (2015) Reporting diagnostic accuracy studies: some improvements after 10 years of STARD. Radiology 274(3):781–789. https://doi.org/10.1148/radiol.14141160

Kumar R, Indrayan A (2011) Receiver operating characteristic (ROC) curve for medical researchers. Indian Pediatr 48(4):277–287. https://doi.org/10.1007/s13312-011-0055-4

Li J, Fine J (2004) On sample size for sensitivity and specificity in prospective diagnostic accuracy studies. Stat Med 23(16):2537–2550. https://doi.org/10.1002/sim.1836

Liu A, Schisterman EF, Mazumdar M, Hu J (2005) Power and sample size calculation of comparative diagnostic accuracy studies with multiple correlated test results. Biom J 47(2):140–150. https://doi.org/10.1002/bimj.200410094

Lijmer JG, Mol BW, Heisterkamp S, Bonsel GJ, Prins MH, van der Meulen JH, Bossuyt PM (1999) Empirical evidence of design-related bias in studies of diagnostic tests. JAMA 282(11):1061–1066. https://doi.org/10.1001/jama.282.11.1061

Lijmer JG, Bossuyt PM (2009) Various randomized designs can be used to evaluate medical tests. J Clin Epidemiol 62(4):364–373. https://doi.org/10.1016/j.jclinepi.2008.06.017

Lu B, Gatsonis C (2013) Efficiency of study designs in diagnostic randomized clinical trials. Stat Med 32(9):1451–1466. https://doi.org/10.1002/sim.5655

Mark DB, Federspiel JJ, Cowper PA, Anstrom KJ, Hoffmann U, Patel MR, Davidson-Ray L et al (2016) Economic outcomes with anatomical versus functional diagnostic testing for coronary artery disease. Ann Intern Med 165(2):94–102. https://doi.org/10.7326/m15-2639

McClish DK (1989) Analyzing a portion of the ROC curve. Med Decis Mak 9(3):190–195. https://doi.org/10.1177/0272989x8900900307

Metz CE (1978) Basic principles of ROC analysis. Semin Nucl Med 8(4):283–298. https://doi.org/10.1016/s0001-2998(78)80014-2

Majeed H, Amir E (2018) EQUATOR-Oncology: reducing the latitude of cancer trial design and reporting: Nature Publishing Group

Mustafa RA, Wiercioch W, Cheung A, Prediger B, Brozek J, Bossuyt P, Garg AX, Lelgemann M, Büehler D, Schünemann HJ (2017) Decision making about healthcare-related tests and diagnostic test strategies. Paper 2: a review of methodological and practical challenges. J Clin Epidemiol 92:18–28. https://doi.org/10.1016/j.jclinepi.2017.09.003

Modic MT, Obuchowski NA, Ross JS, Brant-Zawadzki MN, Grooff PN, Mazanec DJ, Benzel EC (2005) Acute low back pain and radiculopathy: MR imaging findings and their prognostic role and effect on outcome. Radiology 237(2):597–604. https://doi.org/10.1148/radiol.2372041509

NCSS. PASS (Power Analysis and Sample Size) Software 2018

Network, Equator (2017) EQUATOR Network: what we do and how we are organised 2016

Newby DE, Adamson PD, Berry C, Boon NA, Dweck MR, Flather M, Forbes J et al (2018) Coronary CT angiography and 5-year risk of myocardial infarction. N Engl J Med 379(10):924–933. https://doi.org/10.1056/NEJMoa1805971

Obuchowski NA (1998) Sample size calculations in studies of test accuracy. Stat Methods Med Res 7(4):371–392. https://doi.org/10.1177/096228029800700405

Ogilvie JC, Douglas Creelman C (1968) Maximum-likelihood estimation of receiver operating characteristic curve parameters. J Math Psychol 5(3):377–391

Obuchowski NA, Bullen JA (2018) Receiver operating characteristic (ROC) curves: review of methods with applications in diagnostic medicine. Phys Med Biol 63(7):07tr01. https://doi.org/10.1088/1361-6560/aab4b1

Park SH, Goo JM, Jo CH (2004). Receiver operating characteristic (ROC) curve: practical review for radiologists. Korean J Radiol 5(1):11–18. https://doi.org/10.3348/kjr.2004.5.1.11

Pepe MS (2003) The statistical evaluation of medical tests for classification and prediction. Medicine

Sackett DL, Haynes RB (2002) The architecture of diagnostic research. BMJ 324(7336):539–541. https://doi.org/10.1136/bmj.324.7336.539

Simel DL, Samsa GP, Matchar DB (1991) Likelihood ratios with confidence: sample size estimation for diagnostic test studies. J Clin Epidemiol 44(8):763–770. https://doi.org/10.1016/0895-4356(91)90128-v

Steinberg DM, Fine J, Chappell R (2009) Sample size for positive and negative predictive value in diagnostic research using case-control designs. Biostatistics 10(1):94–105. https://doi.org/10.1093/biostatistics/kxn018

Sun F, Schoelles KM, Coates VH (2013) Assessing the utility of genetic tests. J Ambul Care Manage 36(3):222–232. https://doi.org/10.1097/JAC.0b013e318295d7e3

Swets JA (1986) Indices of discrimination or diagnostic accuracy: their ROCs and implied models. Psychol Bull 99(1):100–117

Thompson IM, Ankerst DP, Chen C, Scott Lucia M, Goodman PJ, Crowley JJ, Parnes HL, Coltman CA (2005) Operating characteristics of prostate-specific antigen in men with an initial PSA level of 3.0 ng/ml or lower. JAMA 294(1):66–70

Trevethan R (2019) Response: commentary: sensitivity, specificity, and predictive values: foundations, Pliabilities, and pitfalls in research and practice. Front Public Health 7:408. https://doi.org/10.3389/fpubh.2019.00408

van Oudenaarde K, Swart NM, Bloem JL, Bierma-Zeinstra SMA, Algra PR, Bindels PJE, Koes BW et al (2018) General practitioners referring adults to MR imaging for knee pain: a randomized controlled trial to assess cost-effectiveness. Radiology 288(1):170–176. https://doi.org/10.1148/radiol.2018171383

Whiting P, Rutjes AW, Reitsma JB, Glas AS, Bossuyt PM, Kleijnen J (2004) Sources of variation and bias in studies of diagnostic accuracy: a systematic review. Ann Intern Med 140(3):189–202. https://doi.org/10.7326/0003-4819-140-3-200402030-00010

Walsh SJ (1997) Limitations to the robustness of binormal ROC curves: effects of model misspecification and location of decision thresholds on bias, precision, size and power. Stat Med 16(6):669–679. https://doi.org/10.1002/(sici)1097-0258(19970330)16:6<669::aid-sim489>3.0.co;2-q

Zhou X-H, McClish DK, Obuchowski NA (2009) Statistical methods in diagnostic medicine. John Wiley & Sons

Designs to Detect Disease Modification

64

Michael P. McDermott

Contents

Abstract

Designing a trial to determine whether or not an intervention has modified the underlying course of the disease is straightforward for certain conditions, such as cancer, in which it is possible to directly measure the disease course. For many other diseases, the disease course is latent, and one must rely on indirect measures such as clinical symptoms to quantify the effects of interventions. In this case, it is difficult with conventional trial designs to determine the extent to which the treatment is modifying the disease course as opposed to merely alleviating the symptoms of the disease. This distinction has become critically important in

M. P. McDermott (✉)
Department of Biostatistics and Computational Biology, University of Rochester Medical Center, Rochester, NY, USA
e-mail: Michael_McDermott@urmc.rochester.edu

© Springer Nature Switzerland AG 2022

S. Piantadosi, C. L. Meinert (eds.), *Principles and Practice of Clinical Trials*,
https://doi.org/10.1007/978-3-319-52636-2_93

the study of treatments for neurodegenerative diseases such as Alzheimer's disease and Parkinson's disease, but it applies to many other diseases as well.

This chapter discusses proposed strategies for trial design to attempt to distinguish between the disease-modifying and symptomatic effects of a treatment in diseases with a latent disease course. Two-period designs, such as the withdrawal design and the delayed start design, are being used for this purpose, most commonly in neurodegenerative disease. In these designs, the first period involves a standard randomization of participants to active and placebo treatments. In the second period, those in the active treatment group are switched to placebo (withdrawal design), or those in the placebo group are switched to active treatment (delayed start design). These designs are reviewed in detail in terms of their underlying assumptions, limitations, and strategies for statistical analysis.

Keywords

Two-period design · Withdrawal design · Delayed start design · Disease-modifying effect · Symptomatic effect · Alzheimer's disease · Parkinson's disease · Missing data · Noninferiority

Introduction

For many diseases, it is not possible to directly observe the underlying disease process. Instead, clinical symptoms and/or function or, in some cases, even laboratory or biological markers might serve as indirect measures of this process. Examples of such conditions include diabetic peripheral neuropathy, depression, anemia, osteoporosis, and neurodegenerative disease (e.g., Alzheimer's disease, Parkinson's disease, and Huntington's disease). In recent years, interest has increased substantially in the problem of designing clinical trials to determine whether a treatment has modified the underlying course of the disease or has merely exerted its effect on disease symptoms.

This heightened interest in trial designs that can detect disease modification has been most prominent in the area of neurodegenerative disease, specifically in Alzheimer's disease (AD) and Parkinson's disease (PD). Although a wide variety of effective treatments have been developed for these conditions, none have been conclusively shown to modify the underlying course of the disease, and most are believed to only alleviate disease symptoms. The discovery of a treatment that either slows, halts, or even reverses underlying disease progression has been termed "the highest priority in PD research" (Olanow et al. 2008). The aging of the population has raised grave concerns regarding the global public health crisis posed by AD (Cummings 2017) and PD (Dorsey and Bloem 2018), exacerbating the need for disease-modifying treatments.

The term *disease modification* implies that the treatment has an enduring effect on the course of the underlying disease. Modifications of a key pathological feature of the disease, such as tau and β-amyloid protein levels in the brain in AD (Kaye 2000)

or the rate of loss of catecholaminergic neurons (primarily the dopaminergic projection from the substantia nigra to the striatum) in PD (Clarke 2004), are examples of this. For a disease-modifying effect to be important, however, a clear benefit with respect to the clinical course of the disease would also be required (Cummings 2009). Treatments that merely ameliorate the symptoms of the disease without affecting the underlying disease process, on the other hand, would be expected to lose their benefit relatively soon upon discontinuation.

Designing a trial to determine whether a treatment has an impact on the underlying disease is straightforward when a valid measure of the underlying disease is available (e.g., tumor size in cancer or viral load in HIV infection). Some success has been realized in establishing disease modification for treatments on the basis of a combination of clinical and imaging markers. One example is in relapsing-remitting multiple sclerosis, where several treatments are considered to be disease-modifying on the basis of reductions in relapse rates and the appearance of new brain lesions detected by magnetic resonance imaging, and of slowing of the accumulation of disability (Sormani and Bruzzi 2013). Another example is in rheumatoid arthritis, for which disease-modifying antirheumatic drugs (DMARDs) have been shown to improve clinical, laboratory, and radiologic endpoints; see Emery et al. (2008) for an example. Although a considerable amount of research has been (and continues to be) devoted to establishing valid markers of underlying disease progression in neurodegenerative disease, these efforts, so far, have been unsuccessful (Athauda and Foltynie 2016; Cummings 2009; Cummings 2017; Vellas et al. 2008). In the absence of such a measure, there are difficult challenges in designing a clinical trial that can clearly distinguish between the symptomatic and disease-modifying effects of the treatment.

In response to these challenges, special trial designs termed *two-period designs* (McDermott et al. 2002), including the withdrawal and delayed start designs, have been developed that attempt to distinguish between the symptomatic and disease-modifying effects of treatment using clinical outcome measures. This chapter outlines the rationale for these designs and their specific features and assumptions. Issues related to implementation, statistical considerations, and important limitations of the designs are also discussed. Although these designs have been used mainly in the context of neurodegenerative diseases such as AD and PD, they are more broadly applicable.

Standard Single-Period Designs

It has been suggested by some that standard parallel group designs can be used to infer a disease-modifying effect of an intervention by examining whether the pattern of group differences in mean responses on a suitable clinical rating scale diverges over time (Guimaraes et al. 2005; Vellas et al. 2008). For example, if the pattern of change over time is linear in each treatment group, a group difference in the rate of change (slope) would indicate an effect of treatment on the underlying progression of the disease. The trouble with this interpretation is that such results are also compatible with the interpretation of a very slow-onset symptomatic effect (Ploeger and Holford 2009). They are also compatible with the interpretation that the symptomatic effect of the treatment increases over time. It is quite plausible in a neurodegenerative disease, for example, for the magnitude of the symptomatic effect in a participant to increase as the underlying disease worsens or as the score on the clinical rating scale worsens.

Some trials attempting to discern the disease-modifying effects of an intervention have relied on milestone endpoints in their design. The Deprenyl and Tocopherol Antioxidative Therapy of Parkinsonism (DATATOP) trial was one of the earliest trials to explicitly test a hypothesis concerning the disease-modifying effects of an intervention, in this case two interventions, selegiline and vitamin E (The Parkinson Study Group 1989; The Parkinson Study Group 1993). At the time the trial was designed, it was believed that neither selegiline nor vitamin E had symptomatic effects. The trial randomly assigned 800 participants with early, untreated PD in a 2×2 factorial design to receive selegiline, vitamin E, both treatments in combination, or placebo, with the primary outcome variable being the time from randomization until the development of disability sufficient to require treatment with dopaminergic therapy, as judged by the enrolling investigator. A substantial beneficial effect of selegiline was observed in terms of delaying the need for dopaminergic therapy. On the other hand, an unanticipated short-term effect of selegiline thought to be indicative of a symptomatic benefit was also apparent (The Parkinson Study Group 1989), making the results difficult to interpret with respect to mechanism. A very similar design was employed in a trial of the same interventions in AD in which the primary outcome variable was the time from randomization until death, institutionalization, loss of basic activities of daily living, or a diagnosis of severe dementia, whichever occurred first (Sano et al. 1997). The problem with this strategy is that such endpoints can be influenced by symptomatic effects as well as disease-modifying effects. Ideally, one would employ an endpoint that is not influenced by a treatment with symptomatic benefit and that can be ascertained in a reasonably short period of time.

An alternative approach to evaluating the disease-modifying effects of an intervention is to combine a model for disease progression with a pharmacodynamic model for drug effects, the latter facilitating inference concerning the mechanisms of the drug effect (Holford 2015). These methods are analytically complex and rely on several modeling assumptions, but they might overcome some of the limitations of two-period designs discussed below and might facilitate understanding of the mechanisms of drug benefit (Holford and Nutt 2011).

Two-Period Designs

Withdrawal Design

In a seminal paper, Leber (1996) formally proposed the use of two-period designs to attempt to distinguish between the symptomatic and disease-modifying effects of an intervention. In the *withdrawal design*, participants are randomly assigned to receive either active treatment or placebo in the first period (Period 1) and followed for a fixed length of time. In the second period (Period 2), those who were receiving active treatment are switched to placebo (A/P group), and those who were receiving placebo remain on placebo (P/P group) (Fig. 1). Period 1 is chosen to be sufficiently long to permit the emergence of a measurable disease-modifying effect of the treatment. Period 2 is chosen to be long enough to eliminate (or "wash out") any symptomatic effect of the treatment from Period 1; the two periods do not have to be of equal length. The purpose of the withdrawal maneuver is to determine whether any portion of the treatment effect that is apparent at the end of Period 1 persists after withdrawal of treatment, i.e., to distinguish between the short-term symptomatic effect and the long-term disease-modifying effect. In theory, any difference in mean response at the end of Period 2 in favor of the A/P group can be attributed to a disease-modifying effect of the treatment.

A key assumption of the withdrawal design is the adequacy of the length of the withdrawal period (Period 2). Consider, for example, the Early vs. Late L-dopa in

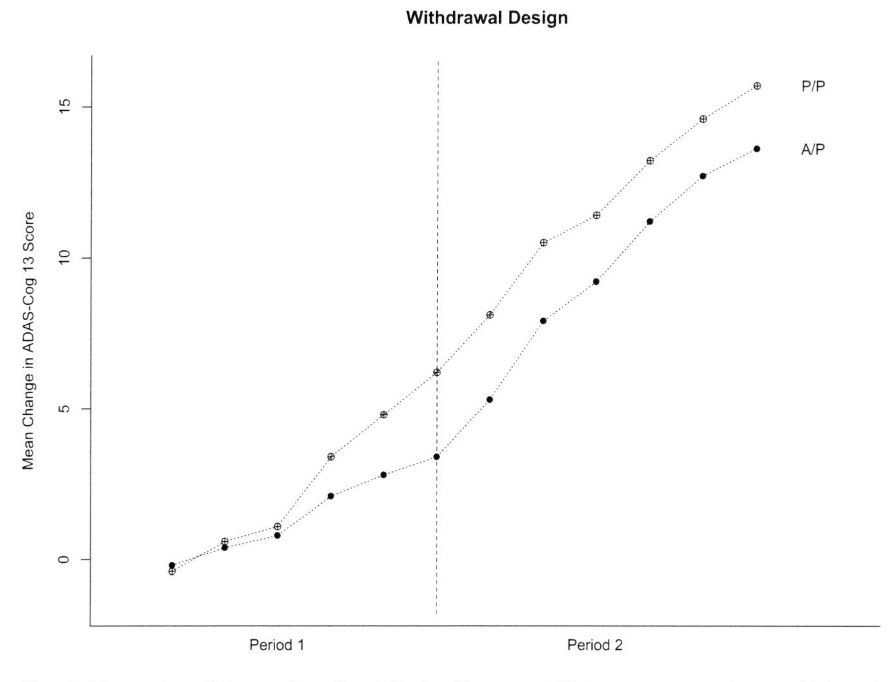

Fig. 1 Illustration of the results of a trial of a disease-modifying treatment using a withdrawal design. In this design, participants are randomly assigned to receive either active (A) or placebo (P) treatment in Period 1 followed by placebo treatment for all participants in Period 2. The notation "A/P" indicates the group that received active treatment in Period 1 followed by placebo treatment in Period 2. The plotted points are mean changes from baseline in the 13-item Alzheimer's Disease Assessment Scale-Cognitive Subscale (ADAS-Cog 13) score, where positive changes indicate worsening. Disease modification is supported by a persisting difference in mean response between the A/P and P/P groups at the end of Period 2, with evidence that the group difference in mean response is not continuing to decrease over time near the end of this period

Parkinson Disease (ELLDOPA) trial in which participants were randomly assigned to receive one of three dosages of levodopa or matching placebo and followed for 40 weeks. At the conclusion of the 40-week treatment period, participants underwent a 2-week withdrawal of study medication and were reevaluated (The Parkinson Study Group 2004). Participants receiving levodopa in Period 1, regardless of dosage, continued to have substantially better mean scores on the Unified Parkinson's Disease Rating Scale (UPDRS) than those receiving placebo after the withdrawal period, but it is not clear if the duration of the withdrawal period was sufficient to completely eliminate the symptomatic effects of levodopa. It is interesting to note that the underlying hypothesis being tested in the ELLDOPA trial was that levodopa would be associated with a *worsening* of PD progression.

One problem with the withdrawal design is that there is no blinding with respect to the treatment received during the withdrawal period (Period 2), which can result in bias. In addition, participant retention during Period 2 might become a problem depending on its duration since participants will be aware that they are not receiving active treatment. A solution would be to add a third randomized group to the study in which participants remain on active treatment in both periods (A/A), enabling the blind to be maintained throughout the trial. Since the A/A group would have no value in distinguishing between the disease-modifying and symptomatic effects of the treatment (McDermott et al. 2002), it would be wise to assign relatively few participants to this group to minimize the loss of efficiency.

Delayed Start Design

The withdrawal design is associated with concerns regarding participant recruitment and retention; this motivated Leber (1996) to propose an alternative two-period design that he termed the *randomized start design*, now commonly known as the *delayed start design*. The design is identical to that of the withdrawal design in Period 1, but in Period 2 those who were receiving placebo are switched to active treatment (P/A group), and those who were receiving active treatment remain on active treatment (A/A group) (Fig. 2). Period 1 is chosen to be sufficiently long to permit the emergence of a measurable disease-modifying effect of the treatment. Period 2 is chosen to be long enough for the treatment to fully exert its symptomatic effect; again, these periods do not have to be of equal length. The inference would be that any difference in mean response at the end of Period 2 in favor of the A/A group can be attributed to a disease-modifying effect of the treatment.

An important assumption of the delayed start design is that Period 2 is sufficiently long to ensure that the P/A group will not continue to "catch up" to the A/A group. For example, in the Attenuation of Disease Progression with Azilect Given Once-Daily (ADAGIO) trial of rasagiline (Olanow et al. 2008; Olanow et al. 2009), participants were randomly assigned with equal allocation to one of four groups: (1) rasagiline 1 mg/day for 72 weeks, (2) placebo for 36 weeks followed by rasagiline 1 mg/day for 36 weeks, (3) rasagiline 2 mg/day for 72 weeks, and (4) placebo for 36 weeks followed by rasagiline 2 mg/day for 36 weeks. The design, therefore, included two delayed start

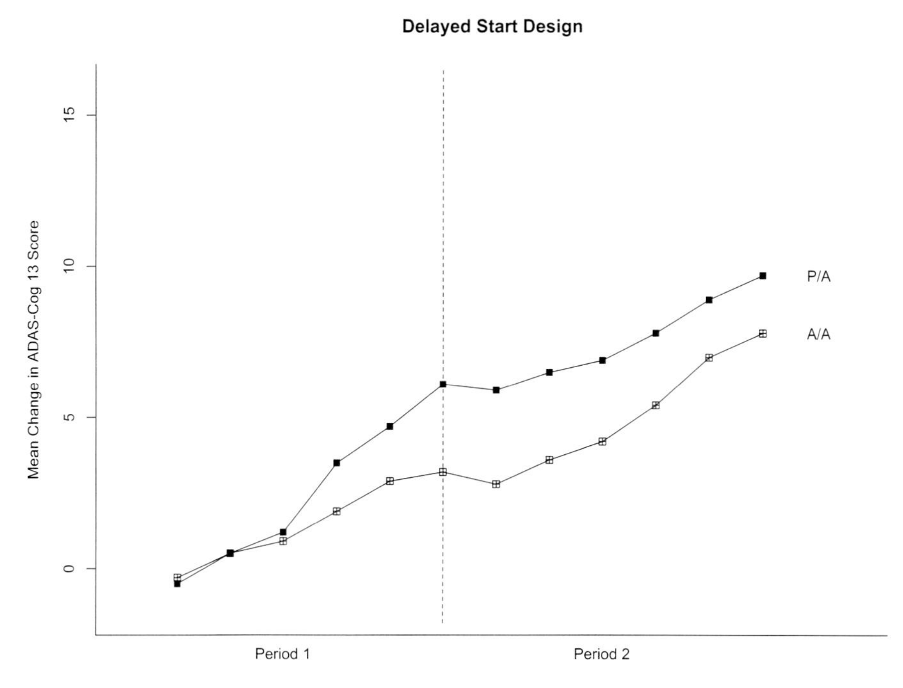

Fig. 2 Illustration of the results of a trial of a disease-modifying treatment using a delayed start design. In this design, participants are randomly assigned to receive either active (A) or placebo (P) treatment in Period 1 followed by active treatment for all participants in Period 2. The notation "P/A" indicates the group that received placebo treatment in Period 1 followed by active treatment in Period 2. The plotted points are mean changes from baseline in the 13-item Alzheimer's Disease Assessment Scale-Cognitive Subscale (ADAS-Cog 13) score, where positive changes indicate worsening. Disease modification is supported by a persisting difference in mean response between the P/A and A/A groups at the end of Period 2, with evidence that the group difference in mean response is not continuing to decrease over time near the end of this period

trials, one for the 1 mg/day dosage and one for the 2 mg/day dosage of rasagiline. The trial unexpectedly produced conflicting results (Olanow et al. 2009). While the 1 mg/day dosage yielded a pattern of mean UPDRS total scores over time that would be expected from a drug that had at least a partial disease-modifying effect, the 2 mg/day dosage did not demonstrate evidence of a disease-modifying effect as the delayed start (P/A) group "caught up" to the early start (A/A) group in terms of mean response during Period 2, as measured by the UPDRS total score.

Like the withdrawal design, the delayed start design has the problem that there is no blinding with respect to the treatment received during Period 2. Again, one could add a third randomized group to the study in which participants remain on placebo throughout the trial (P/P) to address this problem, with relatively few participants assigned to this group since it would have no value in distinguishing between the disease-modifying and symptomatic effects of the treatment (McDermott et al. 2002). The addition of this third group, which would never receive active treatment, might make it more difficult to recruit participants in the trial.

Assumptions

Simplified statistical models for the withdrawal and delayed start designs can be used to illustrate the assumptions that each of these designs requires. Suppose that a normally distributed outcome variable Y is measured on each participant at the end of Period 1 (Y_1) and at the end of Period 2 (Y_2). A typical analysis of data from this design would incorporate the additional longitudinal data collected and would likely include certain covariates such as enrolling center and the baseline value of the outcome variable, but these will be ignored here for simplicity. Additional details regarding these models are described elsewhere (McDermott et al. 2002).

The models for the mean responses at the end of each period for the withdrawal and delayed start designs are provided in Table 1. At the end of Period 1, participants receiving placebo (i.e., those in the P/P and P/A groups) have a mean response μ_1, but participants receiving active treatment (i.e., those in the A/P and A/A groups) have a mean response that also includes a treatment effect that is assumed to be a sum of two components: a symptomatic effect (θ_S) and a disease-modifying effect (θ_D). The data at the end of Period 1 can only be used to estimate the total treatment effect, $\theta_S + \theta_D$, in that period; they cannot distinguish between these two components. In the withdrawal design, for example, the difference in mean response between the A/P and P/P groups would estimate $\theta_S + \theta_D$. Similarly, in the delayed start design, the difference in mean response between the A/A and P/A groups would also estimate $\theta_S + \theta_D$. The data from Period 2 are used to attempt to distinguish between the symptomatic and disease-modifying components of that effect.

In the withdrawal design, participants who received placebo in both periods (P/P) have a mean response μ_2 at the end of Period 2. For the A/P group, which had active treatment withdrawn in Period 2, it is assumed that the disease-modifying effect acquired from active treatment during Period 1 is retained at the end of Period 2, but that any symptomatic effect acquired during Period 1 disappears by the end of Period 2. The mean response in this group at the end of Period 2 is, therefore, $\mu_2 + \theta_D$.

In the delayed start design, the P/A group receives active treatment in Period 2; therefore, the mean response in this group at the end of Period 2 is $\mu_2 + \lambda_T$, i.e.,

Table 1 Statistical models for mean responses in the withdrawal and delayed start designs

Design	Group	End of Period 1	End of Period 2
Withdrawal	P/P	μ_1	μ_2
	A/P	$\mu_1 + \theta_S + \theta_D$	$\mu_2 + \theta_D$
	Difference (A/P – P/P)	$\theta_S + \theta_D$	θ_D
Delayed start	P/A	μ_1	$\mu_2 + \lambda_T$
	A/A	$\mu_1 + \theta_S + \theta_D$	$\mu_2 + \theta_D + \delta_T$
	Difference (A/A – P/A)	$\theta_S + \theta_D$	$\theta_D + \delta_T - \lambda_T$

Group indicates the Period 1/Period 2 treatment assignments, with P = placebo and A = active
θ_S = Symptomatic effect acquired during Period 1
θ_D = Disease-modifying effect acquired during Period 1
λ_T = Total treatment effect (symptomatic + disease-modifying) acquired during Period 2
δ_T = Total treatment effect (symptomatic + disease-modifying) acquired during Period 2

is augmented by a total treatment effect λ_T acquired during this period that could consist of both symptomatic and disease-modifying components. Note, however, that λ_T is not necessarily equal to $\theta_S + \theta_D$ since the total treatment effect acquired during Period 2 might not be the same as that acquired during Period 1. In the A/A group, the mean response at the end of Period 2 is $\mu_2 + \theta_D + \delta_T$; it is assumed that this group retains the disease-modifying effect (θ_D) and loses the symptomatic effect (θ_S) acquired during Period 1 but also acquires a total treatment effect δ_T during Period 2 that might differ from that acquired by the P/A group.

The important assumptions of the withdrawal and delayed start designs are illustrated by this simple model for the mean responses: (1) Period 1 is of sufficient duration to permit the emergence of a measurable disease-modifying effect θ_D; (2) the disease-modifying effect θ_D acquired during Period 1 persists at least through the end of Period 2, but presumably longer; (3) Period 2 is of sufficient duration for the symptomatic effect from Period 1 (θ_S) to completely disappear by the end of Period 2; and (4) withdrawal of active treatment does not modify (e.g., hasten) the disease process in some way.

It can be seen from Table 1 that in the withdrawal design, the difference in observed mean response between the A/P and P/P groups at the end of Period 2 will be an unbiased estimate of θ_D, the disease-modifying effect, under the assumed statistical model. In the delayed start design, however, the difference in observed mean response between the A/A and P/A groups at the end of Period 2 will not be an unbiased estimate of θ_D under this model unless $\lambda_T = \delta_T$, i.e., unless the total treatment effect acquired during Period 2 is the same for the P/A and A/A groups. The assumption, therefore, is that the total (symptomatic + disease-modifying) effect of treatment received in Period 2 is the same regardless of whether or not the participant received treatment during Period 1. Because of this assumption, it is important to ensure that the duration of Period 2 is sufficient to allow the symptomatic effect of the treatment to become fully apparent in the P/A group.

Although the assumption that $\lambda_T = \delta_T$ is necessary in the delayed start design to interpret the difference in observed mean response between the A/A and P/A groups at the end of Period 2 as the magnitude of the disease-modifying effect of the treatment, it is not a testable assumption in this design. The assumption could be tested, however, using data from a *complete two-period design* (McDermott et al. 2002), i.e., a combination of the withdrawal and delayed start designs that includes all four treatment arms (P/P, P/A, A/P, P/P) (Fig. 3). In this design, an unbiased estimate of λ_T is the difference in observed mean response between the P/A and P/P groups at the end of Period 2 (Table 1). Similarly, an unbiased estimate of δ_T is the difference in observed mean response between the A/A and A/P groups at the end of Period 2 (Table 1). A test of the null hypothesis $\lambda_T = \delta_T$, then, could be based on the difference between these estimates. If one were comfortable with the assumption of $\lambda_T = \delta_T$, a pooled estimate of θ_D could be formed from the withdrawal and delayed start components of the design (McDermott et al. 2002). Such a design would also promote blinding. Issues regarding allocation of participants to the different treatment arms of a complete two-period design, including recruitment, dropout, and statistical efficiency, are discussed in detail elsewhere (McDermott et al. 2002). A

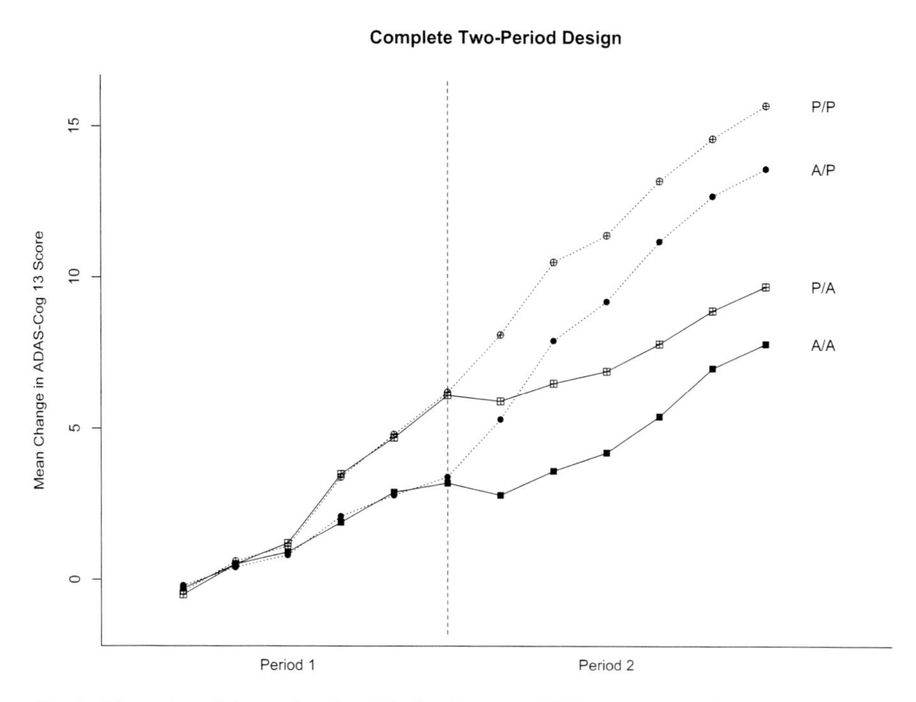

Fig. 3 Illustration of the results of a trial of a disease-modifying treatment using a complete two-period design, which can be viewed as the combination of the withdrawal and delayed start designs. In this design, participants are randomly assigned to receive either active (A) or placebo (P) treatment in Period 1 followed by either active or placebo treatment during Period 2. The notation "A/P" indicates the group that received active treatment in Period 1 followed by placebo treatment in Period 2; similar notation is used for the other three groups

slight variation on this design was used in two randomized trials of pegaptanib sodium for the treatment of age-related macular degeneration (Mills et al. 2007). The complete two-period design was also presented for a trial of propentofylline in AD (Whitehouse et al. 1998), although the results of this trial do not seem to have been published.

Eligibility Criteria

Depending on the disease in question, it might be helpful to enroll trial participants as soon as possible after disease diagnosis, with the thought that a disease-modifying treatment might be more effective if given earlier in the disease course. This is especially a concern in neurodegenerative diseases such as AD or PD. For example, trials with a delayed start design in PD have restricted enrollment to participants who were diagnosed within the past 18–24 months and do not yet require treatment with dopaminergic therapy (Olanow et al. 2008; Schapira et al. 2010). Such considerations have motivated the idea of investigating potential disease-modifying treatments in participants with "pre-manifest" disease. This concept would be easier to apply in diseases where the genetic defect is known, such as Huntington's disease; for other conditions, identifying a population at high risk of developing manifest disease within a relatively short period of time is a major challenge. Also, more research is needed on identifying appropriate outcome measures before such trials can be recommended (Kieburtz 2006; Vellas et al. 2007). In addition, there are practical challenges in the design and execution of trials of potentially toxic treatments in individuals who have pre-manifest disease (Kieburtz 2006).

Because trials attempting to distinguish between the disease-modifying and symptomatic effects of an intervention have explanatory or mechanistic aims rather than pragmatic aims, it is important to minimize the use of, or changes in, concomitant treatments during the trial. This is especially important for concomitant treatments that might themselves have disease-modifying effects. For example, the ADAGIO trial prohibited the use of levodopa, dopamine agonists, selegiline, rasagiline, and coenzyme Q_{10} (> 300 mg/day) within 4 months of randomization. Retention is another critical issue that must be considered in terms of eligibility criteria. Exclusion of patients who have certain comorbid conditions or who will likely need ancillary treatment during the trial might be indicated. In the ADAGIO trial, for example, eligibility was restricted to patients who were judged by the site investigator to not likely require symptomatic treatment in the subsequent 9 months. A potential concern with this criterion is that it might yield a cohort of participants with a slower underlying disease progression in whom a disease-modifying effect might be more difficult to detect (Ahlskog and Uitti 2010; Clarke 2008). Such restrictions on eligibility criteria need to be balanced with the ability to recruit potentially large numbers of participants and considerations related to generalizing the trial results (Clarke 2008).

Duration of Follow-up Periods

As noted above, in a two-period design, Period 1 should be chosen to be sufficiently long to allow a measurable disease-modifying effect to emerge. Also, convincing support for the hypothesis of a disease-modifying effect of a treatment using either a withdrawal design or a delayed start design would have to include evidence that the group differences in mean response near the end of Period 2 are no longer decreasing over time. For this reason, Period 2 should be chosen to be sufficiently long for the symptomatic effect from Period 1 to completely disappear by the end of Period 2 and, in the delayed start design, for the symptomatic effect of the treatment to fully emerge in Period 2. Clearly the duration of these periods will depend on the nature of the treatment being studied, but practical aspects of study execution such as recruitment and retention will also have to be considered.

In the ADAGIO delayed start study, Periods 1 and 2 were each 9 months in duration. In the setting of inexorable progression of PD and the availability of effective symptomatic treatments, 9 months might be the longest duration for Period 1 that would be considered practical. For the same reason, withdrawal designs in PD might not be feasible unless any symptomatic effect associated with the treatment is expected to disappear rapidly. In AD, a duration of 18 months is typically used for Period 1 (Liu-Seifert et al. 2015). In diseases that are not progressive or have no known effective treatment, Huntington's disease being an example of the latter, longer period durations might be feasible.

Statistical Considerations for Two-Period Designs

Primary Analyses

The primary analyses for withdrawal and delayed start designs aim to address three scientific hypotheses in support of disease modification: (1) that there is an overall effect of the treatment during Period 1; (2) that there remains a difference between the groups (the A/P and P/P arms in the withdrawal design or the P/A and A/A arms in the delayed start design) in Period 2; and (3) that the group differences in mean responses near the end of Period 2 are not continuing to decrease over time.

Several authors have advocated for a comparison of the mean responses at the end of Period 1 between those receiving active treatment and those receiving placebo to address the first hypothesis (Liu-Seifert et al. 2015; McDermott et al. 2002; Zhang et al. 2011); others have suggested a comparison of average slopes during this period, perhaps including only time points after which the symptomatic effect or any placebo effects are thought to have fully emerged (Bhattaram et al. 2009; Xiong et al. 2014). For example, in the ADAGIO trial, the analyses involved comparisons of the average slopes between the rasagiline and placebo groups in Period 1, where the slopes were based on data from Week 12 to Week 36 (Olanow et al. 2008; Olanow et al. 2009). The rationale for this strategy seems to be that increasing separation of the active treatment and placebo groups over time with respect to mean response would be expected in a trial of a disease-modifying agent. Although this strategy might be more powerful if the assumption of a linear trajectory of response over time holds, it should only be of interest in Period 1 to determine whether or not the treatment groups differ with regard to mean response at the end of this period and not to speculate about the mechanism of the treatment effect; the latter is addressed in the second hypothesis. Also, this strategy requires strong assumptions concerning the time point after which the symptomatic effect of the treatment has fully emerged (Week 12 in ADAGIO) and linearity of the trajectory of response over time, which might be problematic (Holford and Nutt 2011) and ended up being a main point of contention as rasagiline was being considered for a disease-modification claim by the Food and Drug Administration (Li and Barlas 2017).

There is consensus in the literature concerning the key analyses to address the second hypothesis, namely, that these should involve group comparisons of the mean responses at the end of Period 2 (Bhattaram et al. 2009; Liu-Seifert et al. 2015; McDermott et al. 2002; Zhang et al. 2011). The analyses for the third hypothesis should address the issue of whether or not the group differences in mean response near the end of Period 2 are continuing to decrease over time. Decisions are required as to how to quantify the evolution of the group difference in mean response over time as well as which time points to include in the analysis. In the ADAGIO trial, the investigators followed the recommendation of Bhattaram et al. (2009) to compare the slopes of the two groups during Period 2, assuming a linear trajectory of response over time in each group. They used the data from Weeks 48–72 in this comparison because it was thought that the symptomatic effect of rasagiline would appear within 12 weeks of its initiation in the delayed start group at Week 36 (Olanow et al. 2009).

Evidence for disease modification would be supported by a finding that the group differences in mean response are *not* continuing to decrease over time. Therefore, it is appropriate to formulate the hypothesis testing problem as one involving *non-inferiority*. Let $\beta_{P/A}$ be the slope (Weeks 48–72) in the delayed start (P/A) group, and let $\beta_{A/A}$ be the corresponding slope in the early start (A/A) group. The following statistical hypotheses were specified in the ADAGIO trial:

$$H_0 : \beta_{P/A} - \beta_{A/A} > \delta \text{ vs.} H_1 : \beta_{P/A} - \beta_{A/A} \leq \delta,$$

where δ is the *noninferiority margin*. If H_0 is rejected, the conclusion would be that the slope in the P/A group is not meaningfully larger than the slope in the A/A group, as measured by the noninferiority margin δ. Convincing evidence of disease modification would require that δ be chosen to be quite small. The choice of $\delta = 0.15$ UPDRS points/week in ADAGIO was not justified in the trial publications (Olanow et al. 2008; Olanow et al. 2009) and was much too large, being consistent with the group difference in mean responses shrinking by as much as 3.6 points (0.15×24) over the 24-week time period (Weeks 48–72), *a value greater than the treatment effect observed during Period 1*. Considering such a large difference to be non-decreasing over time would be clearly inappropriate. The estimate of $\beta_{P/A} - \beta_{A/A}$ was 0.00 for the 1 mg/day dosage, with a 95% confidence interval of −0.04–0.04 (Olanow et al. 2009), indicating that the data are consistent with a group difference between the slopes of no more than 0.04 UPDRS points/week or with convergence of the group means by no more than approximately 1 UPDRS point (0.04×24) over the 24-week period. One then has to decide whether this evidence is sufficient to declare that the group difference in mean responses is not continuing to decrease appreciably over time.

A slightly different approach to assessing the hypothesis that the group differences in mean response are not decreasing over time was proposed by Li and Barlas (2017). They suggested a noninferiority test for a linear trend over time in the group differences, which does not assume a linear trajectory over time in the mean responses in each group. Liu-Seifert et al. (2015) suggested testing a noninferiority hypothesis using only the differences in the group means at the end of Periods 1 and 2:

$$H_0 : \Delta_2 - 0.5\,\Delta_1 \leq 0 \text{ vs.} H_1 : \Delta_2 - 0.5\,\Delta_1 > 0,$$

where Δ_1 and Δ_2 are the group differences in mean response at the end of Period 1 and at the end of Period 2, respectively. Rejection of H_0 would imply that at least

50% of the total treatment effect observed during Period 1 is preserved after Period 2. A problem with this approach is that it does not address the issue of whether the group differences in mean response are decreasing over time.

To adequately test the hypothesis that the group differences in mean response are not decreasing over time, more frequent evaluations might be required in the latter part of Period 2. The frequency of evaluations will depend on the disease and treatment being studied. In the context of AD, Zhang et al. (2011) suggested monthly evaluations in the final 3 months of Period 2; however, evaluations so close together in time might not allow the slopes during this period to be estimated with sufficient precision, and there could be problems with feasibility as well (Liu-Seifert et al. 2015).

Both Bhattaram et al. (2009) and Zhang et al. (2011) propose testing the three null hypotheses of interest in sequence: (1) no group difference in average slopes (or mean responses) in Period 1; (2) no group difference in mean response at the end of Period 2; and (3) group differences in mean response are decreasing over time at a rate that is greater than the specified noninferiority margin. Each hypothesis is tested at a pre-specified significance level (say 5%), and one proceeds to test the next hypothesis in the sequence if and only if the previous hypothesis is rejected. If one takes the position, however, that all three null hypotheses would have to be rejected in order for the treatment to be considered disease-modifying, then this would be an example of *reverse multiplicity* (Offen et al. 2007) whereby the overall probability of a false-positive result will be *less* than the significance level used for each of the three tests, so correction for multiple testing would not be required. Of course, if it is desired to make an efficacy claim about the treatment using data from Period 1 alone, regardless of the mechanism of this effect, then an appropriate adjustment for multiplicity would be necessary (D'Agostino Sr 2009).

Strategies for Accommodating Missing Data

Compared to standard clinical trial designs, the problem of missing data can be exacerbated in two-period designs due to the long duration of follow-up and the fact that the evidence concerning potential disease modification is derived from the data acquired during Period 2. The 2010 National Research Council (NRC) report on *The Prevention and Treatment of Missing Data in Clinical Trials* (National Research Council 2010) has led to increased attention to how missing data are handled in clinical trials. In particular, the report highlighted the shortcomings of simplistic methods such as carrying forward the last available observation (LOCF) and so-called complete case analyses that omit cases with missing data (Mallinckrodt et al. 2017; National Research Council 2010) and promoted the use of more principled methods such as those based on direct likelihood, multiple imputation, and inverse probability weighting (Molenberghs and Kenward 2007).

Most of the literature on the analysis of data from two-period designs favors the use of so-called "mixed model repeated measures" (MMRM) analyses (Mallinckrodt et al. 2008) that treat time as a categorical variable and use maximum likelihood to estimate model parameters (e.g., mean treatment group responses at each individual time point) using all available data, including all observed data from participants who prematurely withdraw from the trial (Li and Barlas 2017; Liu-Seifert et al. 2015; Zhang et al. 2011). Linear or nonlinear mixed effects models (Molenberghs et al. 2004) that specify a functional form for the relationship between response and time can also be used for this purpose and might be more efficient than the MMRM strategy if the specified functional form is (approximately) correct, but this could be a strong assumption in practice. Multiple imputation can also be a useful strategy in this setting (Little and Yau 1996; Schafer 1997).

These methods all rely on the "missing at random" (MAR) assumption concerning the missing data mechanism, namely, that the missingness depends only on observed outcomes in addition to covariates, but not on unobserved outcomes (Little and Rubin 2002). The reasonableness of this untestable assumption depends on the clinical setting but also on the estimand of interest (International Conference on Harmonization 2017; National Research Council 2010). The estimand is the population quantity to be estimated in the trial and requires specification of four elements: the target population, the outcome variable, the handling of post-randomization (intercurrent) events, and the population-level summary for the outcome variable. Key among these elements in the context of missing data is the handling of intercurrent events such as discontinuation of study medication, use of rescue medication, and use of an out-of-protocol treatment. The need for additional treatment is particularly important for trials in PD, for which there are many available effective treatments, but applies to AD and other conditions as well. There are a number of options for dealing with this issue, including (1) withdrawing the participant from the trial; (2) moving the participant directly into Period 2; and (3) allowing the participant to receive additional treatment while continuing participation in the trial. The second of these options only applies to participants who require treatment in Period 1 and would not apply in the case of a withdrawal design. The third option is consistent with strict adherence to the intention-to-treat principle and might be sensible in a trial with a pragmatic aim, but it is not appealing in a trial that aims to evaluate the disease-modifying effect of a treatment using a two-period design, an aim that is explanatory or mechanistic.

In the ADAGIO trial, participants who were followed for at least 24 of the scheduled 36 weeks in Period 1 were allowed to proceed directly into Period 2 if judged by the enrolling investigator to require additional anti-parkinsonian medication. While this allows information to be obtained in these participants on the mechanism of the effect of the treatment, the time scale for follow-up becomes compressed for these participants, the implications of which are not entirely clear. Also, if the active treatment has a beneficial effect regardless of its mechanism, the early initiation of Period 2 might occur preferentially in those receiving placebo during Period 1, which could complicate interpretation of the results. ADAGIO participants who required additional treatment in Period 2 were withdrawn from the trial at that time. Only participants who had at least one follow-up evaluation after the start of Period 2 were included in the primary analyses of Period 2 data. Even though participant retention in ADAGIO was quite good (Olanow et al. 2009), exclusion of randomized participants from these analyses has the potential to introduce bias of unknown magnitude and direction. Methods such as propensity score adjustment (D'Agostino Jr 1998) can be useful in reducing the bias resulting from such participant exclusion (D'Agostino Sr 2009). The ADAGIO trial used the MMRM strategy to deal with missing data in Period 2.

Given the explanatory aim of a trial with a two-period design, the strategy of excluding data from participants after the introduction of required additional treatment, or withdrawing participants from follow-up at that time, is arguably a reasonable one. This would be consistent with specification of the disease modification estimand as the group difference in mean response for all randomized participants at the end of Period 2 that would have been obtained if all participants tolerated and complied with treatment (Mallinckrodt et al. 2012; National Research Council 2010), a *de jure* estimand (Carpenter et al. 2013). An MMRM analysis, for example, could yield an appropriate estimator for this quantity. Because the MAR assumption is not testable, however, it would be important to perform analyses that examine the sensitivity of the results to the assumptions that are made concerning the missingness mechanism (Carpenter et al. 2013; Liu and Pang 2017; O'Kelly and Ratitch 2014; Tang 2017). This was an emphasis of the NRC report (National Research Council 2010) and the draft addendum to the International Conference on Harmonization guidance on *Statistical Principles for Clinical Trials* (International Conference on Harmonization 2017) in the context of clinical trials in general.

Sample Size Determination

The considerations for sample size determination that are unique to two-period designs are the specification of the effect size for disease modification (θ_D) to be detected at the end of Period 2 and the noninferiority margin for the third hypothesis that the group differences in mean response are not decreasing over time. The effect size specified for sample size determination in ADAGIO was chosen to be 1.8 points for the UPDRS total score (Olanow et al. 2009), which was criticized by some to not represent a clinically important effect (Clarke 2008). This group difference, however, must be interpreted in the proper context: it is the benefit attributable to disease modification that would accrue over the duration of Period 1, i.e., 36 weeks. This is a very short time period relative to the expected duration of the disease. If this effect is truly due to disease modification, it would be expected to continue to accrue over time, possibly over many years. The observed effect of the 1 mg/day dosage of rasagiline (1.7 points over 36 weeks) represents a 38% reduction in the change from baseline (Olanow et al. 2009); if this truly represents disease modification, an effect of this magnitude would arguably be of major clinical importance. In a two-period design, the choice of effect size for sample size determination should be based on a realistic expectation of the magnitude of a disease-modifying effect that could accrue over a follow-up period that is brief relative to the disease course and might not be very large.

The sample size required to determine whether the group difference in mean responses is not continuing to decrease appreciably over time near the end of Period

2 could be quite large depending on the choice for the noninferiority margin; considerations for choosing this margin are discussed in the ADAGIO example above. Assumptions such as the time points included in this analysis and the residual variability around the slopes would have to be carefully considered in the calculation. Additional factors that need to be considered in the sample size calculation include intercurrent events (e.g., participant withdrawal and noncompliance) and misdiagnosis (if applicable). Given the complexities that these considerations introduce, the technique of simulation can be highly useful in assessing the required sample size under a variety of design assumptions.

Summary and Conclusion

There is great interest in developing interventions that can modify the course of neurodegenerative diseases and other diseases in a meaningful way. The development of reliable and valid methods to measure the underlying course of these diseases is urgently needed, and this is a highly active area of research. In the meantime, clinical trials in these conditions have to rely on rating scales, functional measures, or other instruments to indirectly measure disease status. In this setting, two-period designs represent a potentially attractive option to distinguish between effects of interventions that are enduring (disease-modifying) vs. those that are short-term/reversible (symptomatic).

Two-period designs are associated with several limitations, including uncertainty regarding the required durations of the two periods; the assumption in the delayed start design that the total (symptomatic + disease-modifying) effect of treatment received in Period 2 is independent of whether or not the participant received treatment during Period 1; potential difficulties with recruitment and retention, particularly for the withdrawal design; potential compromise of blinding; requirements of large sample sizes; the need for effective ancillary treatments in some cases; and the problem of how to address the issue of missing data from subjects who cease participation in the trial. Another limitation, in the context of enrolling trial participants with relatively mild disease, is that the outcome measure might lack sensitivity to assess disease-modifying effects, especially if there is a large symptomatic component to the effect of the intervention (Olanow et al. 2009).

As discussed above, many of the assumptions of two-period designs cannot be verified directly and need to be informed by knowledge of the intervention acquired outside of the trial. Also, it will likely be difficult with a two-period design to discern the mechanisms of interventions with a very slow onset and/or offset of a symptomatic effect (Holford and Nutt 2011; Ploeger and Holford 2009).

So far, the withdrawal and delayed start designs to detect disease modification have been used mainly in the context of neurodegenerative disease. Definitive demonstration of the disease-modifying effect of an intervention has not been achieved to date with these designs, and the experience in the ADAGIO trial illustrates some of the difficulties in achieving this goal. Additional experience with these designs and the development of strategies to address their limitations will eventually determine their usefulness in detecting the disease-modifying effects of interventions.

Cross-References

▶ Estimands and Sensitivity Analyses
▶ Missing Data

References

Ahlskog JE, Uitti RJ (2010) Rasagiline, Parkinson neuroprotection, and delayed-start trials: still no satisfaction? Neurology 74:1143–1148
Athauda D, Foltynie T (2016) Challenges in detecting disease modification in Parkinson's disease clinical trials. Parkinsonism Relat Disord 32:1–11
Bhattaram VA, Siddiqui O, Kapcala LP, Gobburu JV (2009) Endpoints and analyses to discern disease-modifying drug effects in early Parkinson's disease. AAPS J 11:456–464
Carpenter JR, Roger JH, Kenward MG (2013) Analysis of longitudinal trials with protocol deviation: a framework for relevant, accessible assumptions, and inference via multiple imputation. J Biopharm Stat 23:1352–1371
Clarke CE (2004) A "cure" for Parkinson's disease: can neuroprotection be proven with current trial designs? Mov Disord 19:491–498
Clarke CE (2008) Are delayed-start design trials to show neuroprotection in Parkinson's disease fundamentally flawed? Mov Disord 23:784–789
Cummings JL (2009) Defining and labeling disease-modifying treatments for Alzheimer's disease. Alzheimers Dement 5:406–418
Cummings J (2017) Disease modification and neuroprotection in neurodegenerative disorders. Transl Neurodegener 6:25. https://doi.org/10.1186/s40035-017-0096-2
D'Agostino RB Jr (1998) Propensity score methods for bias reduction in the comparison of a treatment to a non-randomized control group. Stat Med 17:2265–2281
D'Agostino RB Sr (2009) The delayed-start study design. N Engl J Med 361:1304–1306
Dorsey ER, Bloem BR (2018) The Parkinson pandemic – a call to action. JAMA Neurol 75:9–10
Emery P, Breedveld FC, Hall S, Durez P, Chang DJ, Robertson D, Singh A, Pedersen RD, Koenig AS, Freundlich B (2008) Comparison of methotrexate monotherapy with a combination of methotrexate and etanercept in active, early, moderate to severe rheumatoid arthritis (COMET): a randomised, double-blind, parallel treatment trial. Lancet 372:375–382
Guimaraes P, Kieburtz K, Goetz CG, Elm JJ, Palesch YY, Huang P, Ravina B, Tanner CM, Tilley BC (2005) Non-linearity of Parkinson's disease progression: implications for sample size calculations in clinical trials. Clin Trials 2:509–518
Holford N (2015) Clinical pharmacology = disease progression + drug action. Br J Clin Pharmacol 79:18–27
Holford NHG, Nutt JG (2011) Interpreting the results of Parkinson's disease clinical trials: time for a change. Mov Disord 26:569–577
International Conference on Harmonization (2017) ICH E9 (R1) addendum on estimands and sensitivity analysis in clinical trials to the guideline on statistical principles for clinical trials: Step 2b, 16 June 2017
Kaye JA (2000) Methods for discerning disease-modifying effects in Alzheimer disease treatment trials. Arch Neurol 57:312–314

Kieburtz K (2006) Issues in neuroprotection clinical trials in Parkinson's disease. Neurology 66(Suppl 4):S50–S57
Leber P (1996) Observations and suggestions on antidementia drug development. Alzheimer Dis Assoc Disord 10(Suppl 1):31–35
Li JD, Barlas S (2017) Divergence effect analysis in disease-modifying trials. Statist Biopharm Res 9:390–398
Little RJA, Rubin DB (2002) Statistical analysis with missing data. John Wiley and Sons, Hoboken
Little R, Yau L (1996) Intent-to-treat analysis for longitudinal studies with drop-outs. Biometrics 52:1324–1333
Liu GF, Pang L (2017) Control-based imputation and delta-adjustment stress test for missing data analysis in longitudinal clinical trials. Statist Biopharm Res 9:186–194
Liu-Seifert H, Andersen SW, Lipkovich I, Holdridge KC, Siemers E (2015) A novel approach to delayed-start analyses for demonstrating disease-modifying effects in Alzheimer's disease. PLoS One 10(3):e0119632. https://doi.org/10.1371/journal.pone.0119632
Mallinckrodt CH, Lane PW, Schnell D, Peng Y, Mancuso JP (2008) Recommendations for the primary analysis of continuous endpoints in longitudinal clinical trials. Drug Inf J 42:303–319
Mallinckrodt CH, Lin Q, Lipkovich I, Molenberghs G (2012) A structured approach to choosing estimands and estimators in longitudinal clinical trials. Pharm Stat 11:456–461
Mallinckrodt C, Molenberghs G, Rathmann S (2017) Choosing estimands in clinical trials with missing data. Pharm Stat 16:29–36
McDermott MP, Hall WJ, Oakes D, Eberly S (2002) Design and analysis of two-period studies of potentially disease-modifying treatments. Control Clin Trials 23:635–649
Mills E, Heels-Ansdell D, Kelly S, Guyatt G (2007) A randomized trial of pegaptanib sodium for age-related macular degeneration used an innovative design to explore disease-modifying effects. J Clin Epidemiol 60:456–460
Molenberghs G, Kenward MG (2007) Missing data in clinical studies. John Wiley and Sons, Chichester
Molenberghs G, Thijs H, Jansen I, Beunckens C, Kenward MG, Mallinckrodt C, Carroll RJ (2004) Analyzing incomplete longitudinal clinical trial data. Biostatistics 5:445–464
National Research Council (2010) The prevention and treatment of missing data in clinical trials. National Academies Press, Washington, DC
O'Kelly M, Ratitch B (2014) Clinical trials with missing data: a guide for practitioners. John Wiley and Sons, Chichester
Offen W, Chuang-Stein C, Dmitrienko A, Littman G, Maca J, Meyerson L, Muirhead R, Stryszak P, Baddy A, Chen K, Copley-Merriman K, Dere W, Givens S, Hall D, Henry D, Jackson JD, Krishen A, Liu T, Ryder S, Sankoh AJ, Wang J, Yeh C-H (2007) Multiple co-primary endpoints: medical and statistical solutions. Drug Inf J 41:31–46
Olanow CW, Hauser RA, Jankovic J, Langston W, Lang A, Poewe W, Tolosa E, Stocchi F, Melamed E, Eyal E, Rascol O (2008) A randomized, double-blind, placebo-controlled, delayed start study to assess rasagiline as a disease modifying therapy in Parkinson's disease (the ADAGIO study): rationale, design, and baseline characteristics. Mov Disord 15:2194–2201
Olanow CW, Rascol O, Hauser R, Feigin PD, Jankovic J, Lang A, Langston W, Melamed E, Poewe W, Stocchi F, Tolosa E, the ADAGIO Study Investigators (2009) A double-blind, delayed-start trial of rasagiline in Parkinson's disease. N Engl J Med 361:1268–1278
Ploeger BA, Holford NHG (2009) Washout and delayed start designs for identifying disease modifying effects in slowly progressive diseases using disease progression analysis. Pharm Stat 8:225–238
Sano M, Ernesto C, Thomas RG, Klauber MR, Schafer K, Grundman M, Woodbury P, Growdon J, Cotman CW, Pfeiffer E, Schneider LS, Thal LJ (1997) A controlled trial of selegiline, alpha-tocopherol, or both as treatment for Alzheimer's disease. N Engl J Med 336:1216–1222
Schafer JL (1997) Analysis of incomplete multivariate data. Chapman and Hall/CRC, Boca Raton
Schapira AHV, Albrecht S, Barone P, Comella CL, McDermott MP, Mizuno Y, Poewe W, Rascol O, Marek K (2010) Rationale for delayed-start study of pramipexole in Parkinson's disease: the PROUD study. Mov Disord 25:1627–1632

Sormani MP, Bruzzi P (2013) MRI lesions as a surrogate for relapses in multiple sclerosis: a meta-analysis of randomised trials. Lancet Neurol 12:669–676
Tang Y (2017) An efficient multiple imputation algorithm for control-based and delta-adjusted pattern mixture models using SAS. Statist Biopharm Res 9:116–125
The Parkinson Study Group (1989) Effect of deprenyl on the progression of disability in early Parkinson's disease. N Engl J Med 321:1364–1371
The Parkinson Study Group (1993) Effects of tocopherol and deprenyl on the progression of disability in early Parkinson's disease. N Engl J Med 328:176–183
The Parkinson Study Group (2004) Levodopa and the progression of Parkinson's disease. N Engl J Med 351:2498–2508
Vellas B, Andrieu S, Sampaio C, Wilcock G, the European Task Force Group (2007) Disease-modifying trials in Alzheimer's disease: a European task force consensus. Lancet Neurol 6:56–62
Vellas B, Andrieu S, Sampaio C, Coley N, Wilcock G, the European Task Force Group (2008) Endpoints for trials in Alzheimer's disease: a European task force consensus. Lancet Neurol 7:436–450
Whitehouse PJ, Kittner B, Roessner M, Rossor M, Sano M, Thal L, Winblad B (1998) Clinical trial designs for demonstrating disease-course-altering effects in dementia. Alzheimer Dis Assoc Disord 12:281–294
Xiong C, Luo J, Gao F, Morris JC (2014) Optimizing parameters in clinical trials with a randomized start or withdrawal design. Comput Statist Data Anal 69:101–113
Zhang RY, Leon AC, Chuang-Stein C, Romano SJ (2011) A new proposal for randomized start design to investigate disease-modifying therapies for Alzheimer disease. Clin Trials 8:5–14

Screening Trials

65

Philip C. Prorok

Contents

Abstract

The most rigorous approach to evaluating screening interventions for the early detection of disease is the randomized controlled trial (RCT). RCTs are major undertakings requiring substantial resources to enroll and follow large populations over long time periods. Consequently, it is important that such trials be carefully conducted to ensure high quality information and scientifically valid results. The purpose of this chapter is to discuss some of the intricacies of

P. C. Prorok (✉)
Division of Cancer Prevention, National Cancer Institute, Bethesda, MD, USA
e-mail: prorokp@mail.nih.gov

© Springer Nature Switzerland AG 2022

S. Piantadosi, C. L. Meinert (eds.), *Principles and Practice of Clinical Trials*,
https://doi.org/10.1007/978-3-319-52636-2_95

screening trial design, analysis, and monitoring. General design considerations include the choice of interval between screens, the number of screening rounds, and duration of follow-up. A crucial issue in screening trials is choice of the proper outcome measure. This should reflect the impact of the intervention on the clinical outcome for the disease of interest. In cancer screening, the most valid endpoint is the trial population cause-specific mortality. Concerns about lead time bias, length bias and overdiagnosis bias that render other endpoints questionable are discussed. Following presentation of an approach to sample-size calculation for these trials, there is a discussion of commonly employed data analysis methods, including comparison of cause-specific mortality rates between screened and control arms as the primary analysis. Lastly there is a discussion of topics to address in monitoring an evolving screening trial. Examples from completed or ongoing cancer screening trials are used throughout the presentation.

Keywords

Screening · Early detection · Lead time · Length bias · Cancer

Introduction

Screening for the early detection of disease is considered by many to be an obvious intervention strategy to help alleviate the burden of various diseases, particularly cancer. However, it is not always recognized that screening interventions are not automatically beneficial and that there are real or potential harms and costs associated with screening. Therefore, before screening is introduced into a population it is important that a screening test and associated screening program be carefully evaluated to ensure the benefits outweigh the harms. It is widely recognized that the randomized controlled trial (RCT) is the most scientifically valid approach to accomplish this. This chapter is a discussion of issues in the design, analysis, and monitoring of such trials to evaluate disease screening, with examples drawn from the cancer screening literature.

Design Issues

The term clinical trial often brings to mind the concept of an investigation aimed at testing a clinical intervention or treatment in a group of individuals. The trial participants are patients who have been diagnosed with some disease and have sought treatment to alleviate their condition. Such therapy trials typically involve a few hundred to perhaps a few thousand patients, last for perhaps a few years, and seek to improve a clinical outcome such as reduced recurrence rate or improved survival rate. Many such trials have been performed by cooperative groups and other organizations in various countries. In contrast, relatively few screening trials have been conducted due to their size, cost and duration. They generally involve thousands of ostensibly healthy participants followed for many years to determine if the screening intervention reduces the disease related death rate in the screened population. Given these contrasting features of screening trials compared to therapy trials, and acknowledging many well-known requirements of clinical trials in general, it is important to give careful thought to a number of key considerations in designing screening trials.

Informed consent is an initial consideration in screening trial design. Both pre and post randomization consent have been used. In post randomization consent, participants are chosen from nationwide or regional registration rolls, for example, and randomly assigned to the trial arms. Those in the control arm receive their usual medical care, and sometimes are not informed that they are in a trial. Those in the intervention arm are asked to consent to screening after being randomized (e.g., Bretthauer et al. 2016). This approach has the advantage of being population based, and the participants in the control arm are less likely to undergo the screening procedure since they are not aware of the study. One disadvantage is that intervention arm participants have to choose to be screened after they are already in the trial, and invariably some do not, thereby reducing compliance and diluting any effect of the screening. Further, it may be difficult to obtain information other than vital status about control arm individuals because they have not agreed to participate. There might also be ethical concerns about entering individuals into a study which they do not know about.

Prerandomization consent, on the other hand, requires informed consent from all participants before randomization into study and control arms (e.g., NLST Research Team 2011; Prorok et al. 2000). This method may lead to greater compliance in the screening arm and allows the collection of similar detailed information from both the study and control arms because all participants agree to be part of the study. A disadvantage is that it may be more difficult to recruit participants because many may refuse randomization. There may also be substantial contamination in the control arm because the controls are aware of the screening tests being used and could, in theory, seek them elsewhere. This would also dilute any screening effect.

A major issue is the question of whether an available test is ready for evaluation in a large scale randomized trial, and/or how to choose among several candidate tests. There are no straightforward scientific answers since a standard set of criteria does not exist. Hopefully there are preliminary data providing estimates of the key process measures of the test: sensitivity (the probability of being test positive when disease is present), specificity (the probability of being test negative when disease is absent), and positive predictive value (the probability of having disease when the test is positive). However, these data often emanate from studies involving small numbers of individuals in a clinical setting, few of whom have preclinical disease that is the target of a population screening program. Even when appropriate data exist, agreed-upon threshold values for these parameters that would trigger the decision to undertake a trial do not exist. It seems clear, however, that for population screening, particularly for a relatively rare disease such as cancer, there is a requirement for very high specificity (on the order of 95% or higher) because of low disease prevalence, while sensitivity need not be so high, although a value of at least 80% is often deemed preferable.

The issue also arises as to the number of screens or screening rounds and the interval between screens to be used in a trial. The interval between screens is typically chosen to be 1 or 2 years (e.g., Prorok 1995), although irregular intervals have been used, but these may be more difficult to implement in practice in terms of participant compliance. The number of screening rounds depends on the tradeoff between a sufficient number to produce a statistically valid effect on the primary outcome measure, if there is one, and the cost of adding additional rounds. Although some cancer screening trials have involved screening for essentially the entire follow-up period (Tabar et al. 1992), most have employed an abbreviated screening period typically involving four or five screening rounds, with a subsequent follow-up period devoid of screening (e.g., Miller et al. 1981; Shapiro et al. 1988). These issues can be addressed using mathematical modeling (e.g., NLST Research Team 2011).

As an example, in the Prostate, Lung, Colorectal and Ovarian (PLCO) cancer screening trial, the initial choice of four annual screens, at baseline plus three annual re-examinations, was later expanded to six annual screens for PSA testing for prostate cancer and CA125 testing for ovarian cancer. This was a trade-off between enough screens to produce an effect versus anticipated resources (Prorok et al. 2000) Three or four screening rounds were sufficient in some breast cancer screening trials (e.g., Shapiro et al. 1988; Tabar et al. 1992). The annual interval between screens was chosen as the most frequent yet practical interval if screening is shown to be effective. Compared to less frequent screening, an annual interval also increases the likelihood of detection of a broad spectrum of the preclinical conditions in the natural history of the cancers under study. A longer interval might allow some rapidly growing lesions, which might be a source of mortality but which could be cured if found early, to escape detection.

Another design consideration involves the relationship between study duration, sample size, and the expected timing of any effect or achievement of a maximal effect. Sample size and study duration are inversely related. If only these two parameters were involved, the relationship between follow-up cost versus recruitment and screening cost would determine the design. For example, if follow-up costs were substantial compared with those of recruitment and screening, a relatively larger population would be recruited that would be screened and followed for a shorter period to achieve the desired statistical validity. However, the issue of the time at which the screening effect (reduction in mortality, see below) may occur must also be considered. For those cancer screening trials that have demonstrated an effect, a separation in the mortality rates between the screened and control groups has often not begun to occur until 4–5 years or more into the study (e.g., Mandel et al. 1993; Shapiro et al. 1988). Thus, even with a very large sample size, follow-up may have to continue for many years to observe the full effect of the screening. A follow-up period of at least 10 years is common (Prorok and Marcus. 2010).

For example, in the PLCO trial a minimum of 10 years of follow-up was initially decided upon to allow sufficient time for any mortality reduction from screening to emerge. Follow-up intervals of 7 years or more were typically required in breast cancer screening trials (e.g., Shapiro et al. 1988; Tabar et al. 1992), and it was assumed in designing PLCO that the longer natural history of prostate cancer, and perhaps other cancers under study, warranted a longer follow-up period. In the National Lung Screening Trial (NLST), modeling of the disease and screening processes resulted in the decision to capture endpoint events over an approximately 7 year period (NLST Research Team 2011). It must be recognized that these and other design parameter choices were based on the best information at the time. In some circumstances the value of a design parameter is found to be inaccurate once a trial is underway. One particularly important parameter in this regard is the control arm event rate. In the Minnesota trial of fecal occult blood testing for colorectal cancer, the initially estimated screening and follow-up periods were both extended to provide the opportunity for valid findings to emerge (Mandel et al. 1993).

Endpoints

The appropriate and most meaningful endpoint in a screening study is the clinical event that the screening is aimed at preventing. For major chronic diseases such as diabetes or cancer the intent of screening is to find the disease in an early phase so that treatment can be initiated sooner, thereby preventing the most consequential clinical outcome of such diseases, which is death (e.g., Echouffo-Tcheugui and Prorok 2014; Prorok 1995). Particularly in cancer screening, the most valid endpoint is the trial population cancer-specific mortality rate. This is the number of deaths from the target cancer per unit time per unit population at risk (e.g., Prorok 1995). The mortality rate provides a combined assessment of the impact of early detection plus therapy. The unequivocal demonstration of reduction in the cancer mortality rate for a population offered screening is justification for the cost of a screening program and fulfills the implicit promise of benefit to those who elect to participate in the program.

Careful study design and long-term follow-up of large populations are generally required to obtain an accurate estimate of a mortality reduction. Consequently, intermediate or surrogate outcome measures have been proposed. There are, however, critical shortcomings associated with these end points (Prorok 1995). The shortcomings are a consequence of well-known biases that occur in screening programs: lead time bias, length bias, and overdiagnosis bias.

If an individual participates in a screening program, his or her disease may be detected earlier than it would have been in the absence of screening. The amount of time by which the diagnosis is advanced as a result of screening is called the lead time. Because of the lead time, the point of diagnosis is advanced and survival as measured from diagnosis is automatically lengthened for cases detected by screening even if length of life is not increased. This is referred to as lead-time bias and renders the case survival endpoint invalid (Prorok 1995).

Length bias is the phenomenon that cases of disease detected by a screening program are not a random sample from the general distribution of cases of preclinical disease in the screened population. Instead, cases with longer duration preclinical disease are overrepresented among the detected cases (Kafadar and Prorok 2009; Prorok 1995). If, as seems reasonable, disease with long preclinical duration is slow-growing preclinical disease that then progresses to slow-growing clinical disease, it follows that cases of disease with more favorable progression rates are the ones more likely to be detected by screening. Therefore, screen-detected cases will tend to have characteristics of good prognosis, such as lack of involvement of regional lymph nodes or longer survival from diagnosis. These good-prognosis cases have a more favorable outcome even in the absence of screening.

Overdiagnosis bias is related to the concepts of lead-time bias and length bias, and can be considered an extreme form of length bias. One can postulate the existence of a nonprogressive or regressive preclinical disease state in which cases of the disease are detectable by the screening test but would not progress to clinical disease during the person's lifetime in the absence of screening. This is a major concern in screening for several cancers including prostate cancer and breast cancer (e.g., Andriole et al. 2012; Welch et al. 2016). The detection of such cases cannot benefit the individual, but such cases remain preclinical over a long time and, with repeated screenings, are therefore more likely to be detected. The counterparts to these cases never surface clinically in the control arm of a trial. Thus, there will be a higher proportion of early-stage cases in the screened arm even if there is no mortality effect from screening.

Three often proposed alternative endpoints are case-finding rate or yield, case survival, and stage of disease. The case finding rate or incidence rate can be an early clue as to whether screening might be having an effect, as more cases should be detected in the presence than in the absence of screening. However, this rate generally yields little information on the effect of the screening program on disease outcome (but see discussion below on incidence rate). Case finding should increase in a screened population, at least initially, relative to an unscreened population, because of lead-time bias. This can happen whether or not there is a mortality effect. Furthermore, some borderline lesions found by modern screening modalities may not be progressive disease. This results in overdiagnosis bias, as noted above. If this occurs, individuals are treated unnecessarily and exposed to other possible risks of screening. Thus, an increased disease rate in a screening program, in and of itself, is only an indication of increased cost.

In contrast to mortality, which is a population measure, the case survival rate (see ▶ Chap. 89, "Survival Analysis II") refers only to cases of the target disease within a population. The N-year survival rate is defined as the number of cases alive after N years of observation divided by the number of cases diagnosed at the beginning of the time period. Because there are losses to follow-up, this measure is ordinarily calculated using life table methods. Survival does address the final outcome of disease and suggests that screening could be effective. However, it may not accurately reflect mortality because of lead time and length biases.

If screening is effective, this should be reflected in an increased case survival rate as well as a reduction in the population mortality rate. However, any observed increase in survival from time of diagnosis is, at least in part, a reflection of lead time. For any case of disease that is screen detected, it is impossible to distinguish between a true increase in survival time and an artificial increase due to lead time because lead time cannot be directly observed for ethical reasons. Further, there is no universally accepted procedure to estimate lead time or to adjust survival for lead time. Thus case survival is not a valid measure of screening effectiveness.

Furthermore, even if one could adjust for lead time, length bias could still confound survival comparisons. In comparing survival of cases in two groups, for example between two subgroups of cases detected by different screening modalities, cases in one subgroup may have a different distribution of natural histories than the cases in another subgroup because of a modality-dependent sampling effect. Even if one could adjust for lead time, any remaining survival difference could simply be a consequence of the difference in disease natural history between the two subgroups caused by differing sampling bias. Methodology has been developed to explore the length bias effect on survival (e.g., Kafadar and Prorok 2009), but no general methodology exists to either estimate the magnitude of a length bias effect or to adjust survival for length bias. Approaches to separating the effects of treatment, lead time, and length bias in certain circumstances have been proposed (Duffy et al. 2008; Morrison 1982).

Stage of disease at diagnosis, or a related prognostic categorization, can also be used as an early indicator of screening effect, but it can be misleading and is unsatisfactory as a final end point. The relationship between the magnitude of a shift in the stage distribution of cases as a result of screening and the magnitude of a reduction in mortality is not usually known. The detection of in situ or borderline lesions can also affect the stage distribution but should have little impact if any on mortality. The problem is most pronounced for stage I or localized cases where lead time and length bias can lead to slow-growing, even nonprogressive, cases being detected in stage I in a screened arm to a greater extent than in a control arm. Some counterpart cases in the control arm may never surface clinically. As a result, the screened arm will contain a higher proportion of stage I cases even if screening has no effect on mortality. Or, the magnitude of a real mortality effect could be exaggerated by focusing on stage of disease. Thus, a proportional stage shift in a screened arm can be a sign of early detection, but it is insufficient evidence to conclude that there is an improvement in disease outcome.

A related measure that can be a reasonable surrogate endpoint in some screening circumstances is the population incidence rate of advanced-stage disease. The overall incidence rate or the rate of early-stage disease should increase with screening, as discussed above, rendering these measures invalid as endpoints. However, if screening reduces the rate of advanced disease, disease that has metastasized and/or is likely to lead to death, then it is reasonable to expect that the death rate from the disease will also be reduced. Whether this is a valid substitute for mortality must be established in a given setting. Advanced-stage disease must first be defined, then the relationship between advanced disease and mortality must be established in properly designed studies. Advanced stage rate is the primary endpoint in a breast cancer screening trial comparing digital mammography with tomosynthesis (Pisano 2018).

Some screening tests for cancer, such as tests for cervical cancer and colorectal cancer, do detect true precursor lesions. The subsequent removal of these lesions then prevents the cancer from ever being clinically diagnosed, and consequently the incidence rate of the cancer is reduced. The incidence rate is a meaningful endpoint in such circumstances, but it is important to monitor the mortality rate as well, since it is possible that cancers that are eliminated are not a major source of cancer deaths, and so there may not be a direct correspondence between incidence effect and mortality effect.

Sample Size Calculation

A crucial element of trial design is calculation of the number of participants required for the trial. There are well known clinical trial sample size calculation methods (see other chapter in this book) that could potentially be adapted to screening trials. Also, statistical formulas can be supplemented with modeling to tailor the calculations to a specific trial (e.g., NLST Research Team 2011). Whatever the approach, in screening there are several key issues that must be addressed. In particular, since screening trial participants are ostensibly healthy, despite informed consent, they may be inclined not to undergo the screening test. Alternatively, those assigned to a control arm might become aware of the intervention and get tested outside the trial protocol. Thus noncompliance in both arms is an issue. Further, it is well known that individuals who volunteer to participate in screening trials are not typical of the general population, generally being healthier (e.g., Pinsky et al. 2007; Shapiro et al. 1988). This healthy screenee bias must be accounted for in sample size calculations.

One relatively straightforward approach to screening trial sample size calculation is that used in the PLCO trial (Prorok et al. 2000). Let N_C be the number of individuals randomized to the control arm and N_S be the number randomized to the screened arm, with $N_S = f\,N_C$. The trial is designed to detect a $(1-r) \times 100\%$ reduction $(0 < r < 1)$ in the cumulative disease-specific death rate over the duration of the trial. Further, let P_C be the proportion of individuals in the control arm who comply with the usual-care protocol and P_S be the proportion of individuals in the screened arm who comply with the screening protocol. The total number of disease-specific deaths needed for a one-sided a-level significance test with power $1-b$ is given by

$$D = \frac{\left\{(Q_C + f\,Q_S)\,Z_{1-a} - \sqrt{Q_C.Q_S\,(1+f)}\,Z_b\right\}^2}{f\,(Q_C - Q_S)^2}$$

where $Q_C = r + (1-r)P_C$ and $Q_S = 1 - (1-r)P_S$. The number of participants in the control arm is given by

$$N_C = \frac{D}{(Q_C + f\,Q_S)\,R_C Y}$$

where Y is the duration of the trial from entry to end of follow-up in years and R_C is the average annual disease-specific death rate in the control arm expressed in deaths per person per year, adjusted for healthy screenee bias.

Screening Trial Design Options

Standard or Traditional Two Arm Design

Most screening trials have used a traditional or standard two arm design targeting one disease and aimed at addressing the basic question of whether the screening intervention results in a reduction in cause-specific mortality. Participants in one arm receive the screening test for a given disease and those in the other arm serve as a control (unscreened or usual care) (e.g., Shapiro et al. 1988; Schroder et al. 2014; Yousaf-Khan et al. 2017). Other standard trials have addressed the effect of adding one screening modality to another (e.g., Miller et al. 1981). A related three arm design has been used to compare different frequencies of screening (Mandel et al. 1993). Several variants of this standard design are now discussed (Etzioni et al. 1995).

Continuous Screen Design

A natural design approach is to randomize individuals to an intervention or a control arm and offer periodic screening in the intervention arm throughout the trial. If the trial is of very long duration, the screening intervention in this design approximates population screening over a long age range, such as might happen in a national public health program. However, a drawback of this design is the potentially prohibitive cost of screening all intervention group participants for the duration of the trial.

Stop Screen Design

The Stop Screen design is similar to the Continuous Screen design, except that screening is offered for only a limited time in the intervention arm while follow-up continues. Both arms are followed for the mortality endpoint until the end of the trial. This is the design of choice when it is anticipated that a long time will be required before a reduction in mortality can be expected to emerge, and when it would be expensive or difficult to continue the periodic screening for the entire trial period. Examples of this design are the Health Insurance Plan (HIP) of Greater New York Breast Cancer Screening Study (Shapiro et al. 1988), the PLCO trial (Prorok et al. 2000), and the European prostate cancer screening trial (Schroder et al. 2014). As an illustration, the HIP trial randomized 62,000 women aged 40–64. The intervention arm was offered four annual screens consisting of two-view mammography and clinical breast examinations. The screens were offered at entry and for the next 3 years. Women in the control arm followed their usual medical practices. Although screening ended after 3 years, follow-up continued to year 15. By restricting the screening period, the Stop Screen design can result in a considerable saving in cost and effort relative to the Continuous Screen design. Importantly, the Stop Screen design is the only one that allows a direct assessment of overdiagnosis, provided compliance is high and follow-up is complete. However, analysis of the Stop Screen design can be more complex than that of the Continuous Screen design. This is because the difference in disease-specific mortality between the two arms may be diluted by deaths that arise from cancers that develop in the intervention arm after screening stops. (See Analysis section below).

Split Screen or Close Out Screen Design

The Split Screen design is related to the Stop Screen design. The difference is that at the time the last screen is offered to the intervention arm, a screen is also offered to all participants in the control arm. The Stockholm Breast Cancer screening trial is an example of this design. (Friskell et al. 1991) Women were randomized to intervention or control arms. The intervention was single-view mammography at an initial round then two succeeding rounds performed 24–28 months apart. The control group was offered a single screen, at approximately 4.5 years after study entry. One potential advantage of this design is that comparable groups of cancer cases in the two trial arms can theoretically be identified, which can potentially enhance the analysis (See Analysis section). A downside is that some of the control arm cancers detected by screening may benefit, and if so, any screening benefit in the intervention arm will be diluted.

Delayed Screen Design

In the Delayed Screen design, periodic screening is offered to control arm participants starting at some time after the start of the study, then screening continues in both arms until the end of the intervention period. The UK Breast Cancer Screening Age Trial followed this design (Moss et al. 2015). Women in the intervention arm were offered annual screening starting at age 39–41 and continuing to age 47–48, then at age 50–52 all women in both arms were offered periodic screening as part of the National Health Care Program. Thus one can assess the impact of starting periodic screening at age 39–41 relative to waiting until age 50–52. This design is well suited for the situation where screening is the standard of care beginning at a certain age, and the research question centers on the marginal benefit of introducing screening at an earlier age.

Designs Targeting More Than One Intervention and Disease

As noted, RCTs to assess early detection interventions face several challenges. It is necessary to recruit large numbers of healthy participants and follow them for many years, with consequent expenditure of substantial resources. There is therefore interest in exploring more efficient ways to conduct trials so as to share resources and participant pools. A study design that can answer multiple questions in a single study is one possible approach. Options include factorial, reciprocal control, and all-versus-none designs (Freedman and Green 1990). These designs have rarely been considered in screening, but the latter was used in the PLCO trial.

A major design issue for the PLCO trial was whether to undertake separate trials for each of the four cancer sites and corresponding screening modalities under investigation or combine them. An examination of the costs and logistics of separate trials resulted in the decision to conduct one combined trial. The reciprocal control and all-versus-none designs were the primary options (Prorok et al. 2000). The reciprocal control design would have had three arms: one devoted to screening for prostate or ovarian cancer, the second to colorectal cancer screening, and the third to lung cancer screening. Since screening would be undertaken for only one cancer site per gender in any given arm, the other two arms combined would serve as controls. This design was not deemed feasible because of the cost of bringing all participants in for screening and the anticipated substantial levels of contamination, because all participants would be aware that participants in the other arms were receiving other screening tests, that they would then request. A two arm all-versus-none design was chosen instead. One arm served as a control, while screening for all cancers was done in the other arm, in the spirit of a multiphasic screening endeavor. Use of the all-versus-none design required the reasonable assumptions for the cancers and screening tests in PLCO that the tests for each cancer do not detect any of the other cancers, and that the endpoints, death from each of the four cancers, are not related. In other circumstances these assumptions might not be as tenable.

Analysis Methods

Follow-Up Analysis

As discussed above (Endpoint section), for a screening RCT targeting a chronic disease the only generally valid end point is mortality. Specifically, some appropriate measure of the target disease mortality from entry to the end of follow-up in the population randomized to the intervention group is compared with that in the population randomized to the control group. All deaths from the target disease that occur throughout the trial in both arms are analyzed, including all that occur after screening ceases if the trial does not use a Continuous Screen design. This has been termed a follow-up analysis (Nystrom et al. 1993). This approach includes all endpoint events that occur after randomization and is therefore consistent with the intent-to-screen principle. This analysis should be done and reported for any screening trial.

Mortality in a particular trial arm can be measured by several quantities, including (1) the average annual or cumulative mortality, which is the ratio of the number of deaths from the disease of interest to the number of individuals randomized, (2) the average annual or cumulative mortality rate, which is the ratio of the number of deaths from the disease of interest to the number of person-years at risk of dying of the disease, and (3) the survival distribution of the population using death from the disease of interest as the endpoint, with the time of entry into the trial as the time origin. To assess whether or not the screening intervention is of benefit, either the difference or the ratio of the intervention and control group mortalities can be used. The former is a measure of the absolute change in mortality due to the screening, while the latter is a measure of the relative mortality change due to the screening. Rate ratios, rate differences, and their confidence intervals can readily be calculated (e.g., Ahlbom 1993).

Various statistical procedures can be used to test formally for a difference in the mortality experience between the randomized arms. For the first measure, standard procedures for comparing two proportions are available, such as Fisher's exact test. The cumulative mortality rates can be tested using Poisson methods for comparing two groups. A test statistic is

$$Z = (PY_S\, D_C - PY_C D_S)/\{PY_C\ \ PY_S\ \ (D_C + D_S)\}^{1/2},$$

where D_C is the number of deaths from the disease of interest in the control arm through the time of analysis, D_S is the corresponding number of deaths in the screened arm, PY_C = the number of person-years at risk of death from the disease of interest in the control arm through the time of analysis and PY_S = the corresponding number of person-years in the screened arm. This statistic has an approximately standard normal distribution. For comparing the survival distributions, nonparametric tests such as the logrank test are used. It is important to note that these analyses involve all individuals randomized to the respective trial arms.

Additional approaches that have been used are Cox proportional hazards regression and Poisson regression. These methods offer the possibility of a more thorough exploration of screening trial data. Further, with the availability of modern computing power, randomization tests are an option that should be considered since these avoid the assumptions required for other procedures (see ▶ Chap. 94, "Randomization and Permutation Tests").

Related testing and modeling techniques have been suggested to address the problem of the optimal timing of a screening trial analysis relative to the appearance of an effect (e.g., Baker et al. 2002). For several cancer screening trials that have reported a benefit, a pattern was exhibited where the endpoint rates in the two arms were roughly equivalent for some random period after the start of the trial, after which they separated gradually leading to a statistically significant difference (e.g., Shapiro et al. 1988; Schroder et al. 2014; Tabar et al. 1992). This implies that the proportional hazards assumption often invoked in survival analysis does not hold and other methods of analysis are required. One possibility would be a method that in a sense ignores the period where there is no difference in the rates and uses only data from the period where there is a difference. However, such an approach must account for multiplicity in the choice of the time point when separation of the rates begins, and must be done with appropriate statistical methods to obtain the correct variance of the test statistic (Prorok 1995).

Evaluation Analysis

The follow-up analysis is generally the preferred choice, but the method is subject to bias in the relative effect of the screening if the effect is diluted (described below) during follow-up. Evaluation analysis is an attempt to adjust for this.

There are many screening trials in which the intervention arm is offered screening for a limited time only, with the follow-up continuing thereafter to the end of the study (e.g., see Stop Screen design above). During the period of follow-up after screening ceases, those in the intervention arm, as is the case for those in the control arm throughout the study, follow their usual medical care practices. If the post screening follow-up period is lengthy, the mortality comparison will be subject to error relative to a study in which screening continues.

The primary problem is that there can be a dilution of the effect in that the mortality in both arms will become more alike as time from the end of screening increases. The dilution can occur when some of those dying of the disease are individuals whose disease was diagnosed during the post screening period. For such deaths in the intervention arm, it is unlikely that screening could have any beneficial impact on their mortality. Hence, their inclusion in the analysis dilutes the screening effect. However, in the control arm, some cases may correspond to cases in the intervention arm that were screen-detected and that did benefit from the screening. If, hypothetically, deaths among these control arm cases of the disease were to be excluded from the analysis, the screening effect is diluted in that the control arm's mortality will be underestimated. Thus, deaths from the disease of interest that occur among cases diagnosed after screening stops, incorrectly included or excluded, can result in the observed mortalities of the two randomized arms appearing to be more similar or dissimilar than they should. This can lead to erroneous conclusions about the effectiveness of the screening program.

An approach to countering this problem is evaluation analysis (Nystrom et al. 1993). This applies to the Split Screen design. Recall in this design participants in the control arm are screened once at the time of the last screen in the intervention arm. The evaluation analysis then includes deaths that occur from randomization through the end of follow-up, but only those deaths from the target disease that occur among cases diagnosed from the time of randomization through and including the last screen, in each arm. If the sensitivity of the screening test is very high, this can create two groups of cases, one in each arm, that are comparable in terms of their natural history distributions, and hence their expected mortality outcomes in the absence of screening. Thus, analysis of the deaths confined only to those arising from the comparable case groups can theoretically provide an unbiased analysis and eliminate the dilution. A concern, however, is that most screening tests do not possess very high sensitivity. Further, it is crucial that the control arm screen be done exactly at the same time as the last screen in the intervention arm, a circumstance unlikely to arise in practice. Otherwise, the case groups will likely not be comparable and the inference about a mortality effect can be biased (Berry 1998).

In some circumstances comparable case groups can arise naturally. This can happen in a Stop Screen design when the number of cases in the control arm "catches up" to that in the screened arm at some point during follow-up after screening stops. Cases in the comparable groups up to the "catch up" point are then the source of deaths for the mortality analysis. Deaths among cases diagnosed after this point are excluded thereby mitigating dilution. This situation occurred in the HIP trial, where at about 5 or 6 years after randomization the cumulative numbers of breast cancer cases were very similar in the two arms (Shapiro et al. 1988). The mortality measures and statistical methods used in the follow-up analysis, appropriately modified, can be used for this analysis (Prorok 1995). However, successfully determining the appropriate "catch up" point to identify case groups for this analysis can be problematic. Of additional concern is that with modern screening tests, there is the likelihood of overdiagnosis, so that the control arm will never catch up to the screened arm.

Monitoring an Ongoing Screening Trial

Several categories of data and information are anticipated at various stages of a screening trial. These relate to the population under study, acceptance of the screening test by the population, results and characteristics of the screening test, harms of the intervention, and intermediate and final endpoints. These variables should be examined on a regular basis for evidence to alter the protocol or stop the trial. They are valuable in assessing the consistency of findings and can be examined within important strata defined by age, gender, and other risk factors. Categories for consideration (with particular reference to cancer trials) include:

1. Population Characteristics
   The demographic, socioeconomic, and risk characteristics of the study participants, possibly including dietary and occupational histories. These data are useful for describing the study population and assessing the comparability of the screened and control arms and may be used in statistical adjustment procedures.
2. Coverage and Compliance
   Determination of the proportion offered screening who actually undergo the initial screening. This can inform the acceptability of the screening procedures and indicate whether the level is consistent with that assumed in the trial design. Compliance with each scheduled repeat screen should also be recorded.
3. Test Yield in the Screened Arm
   The number of cases found at each screen should be recorded and related to the interval cases not discovered by screening. This is important for gauging how successful the screening test is in finding the disease.
4. Contamination
   The amount of screening in the control arm outside the trial protocol should be assessed. This is crucial for ascertaining the potential level of dilution of any intervention effect. Ideally this would be ascertained at the individual level, but sometimes sampling of the controls is used. Approaches aimed at minimizing contamination include cluster rather than individual randomization and post randomization consent, and methods exist to adjust for contamination in the analysis (Baker et al. 2002; Cuzick et al. 1997).

5. Screening Test Characteristics
   Determination of the detection capabilities of the screening test by estimating sensitivity, specificity, and predictive value.
6. Diagnostic Follow-Up
   Collection of medical records and related information on diagnostic procedures subsequent to every positive screening test. The diagnostic process is also tracked in both the screened and control arms for cases diagnosed as a result of signs or symptoms. For cancer screening trials, the biopsy rate can be calculated relative to each screen and for the program as a whole, and the biopsy yield of cancers can be determined.
7. Disease Case Characteristics
   Key histologic and prognostic variables should be determined for every case of disease in both the screened and control arms. In cancer, these include histological type and grade, lesion size, nodal involvement, and perhaps genetic or other biomarkers. This information can be used for comparing cancer case subgroups and in survival and other case-based analyses. Comparison between screen detected and interval cancers is also of interest.
8. Stage of Disease
   This should be ascertained for every cancer case in the trial population. This information is used to compare the stage distribution of screen detected cases versus other case subsets to suggest whether screening might have an impact on mortality, and is necessary for defining stage-specific incidence rates.
9. Case Survival
   When sufficient follow-up time accrues, survival of individuals in whom disease is observed can be investigated. Although potentially biased as noted above (Endpoint section), the survival distributions of all cases in the screened arm and of screen-detected cases can be compared with the distributions of other case subgroups to provide a suggestion of whether screening might have an effect on disease outcome. Of interest is an order relationship in the survival rates where it would be expected that the survival of screen-detected cases would exceed that of control arm cases, which in turn would exceed that of interval cases.
10. Incidence Rate
    Calculation of the disease incidence rate requires information on the time of diagnosis of each case as well as the number of person-years at risk of disease incidence in each time interval of follow-up. These data are of interest, particularly in a Stop Screen design, because a higher total incidence in the screened arm relative to the control arm is expected until some point after screening stops. If the rates do not equalize, this is evidence of overdiagnosis.
11. Advanced Stage Rate
    For cancer screening trials, the incidence rate of advanced-stage cancer can be calculated yearly and cumulatively for each randomized arm. This rate is often considered to be a reasonable surrogate for mortality.
12. Mortality Rate
    As noted, mortality rates are the basis for the primary inference regarding the effectiveness of screening. Calculation of these rates requires the date and cause of every death in the population as well as the number of person-years at risk of

death during each follow-up interval. Mortality rates should be compared between the screened arm and the control arm. In addition, the death rates from other causes should be scrutinized to assess the comparability of the randomized populations, and all-cause mortality should be reported.

13. Therapy
    The specific therapy used for every case of disease should be recorded. At a minimum, this should be the initial therapy, but adjuvant therapy or treatment for recurrence is valuable as well. This information is crucial for separating the early detection component from the therapy component of any screening effect. That is, within each stage of disease, the therapy distribution should be comparable for each randomized group to eliminate any confounding effect of therapy in assessing the impact of the screening.
14. Harms
    Harms of screening include overdiagnosis, false positives, and complications of the screening, diagnostic, and treatment procedures administered to trial participants. Complications include any adverse medical events and any mortality potentially related to trial procedures, notably any procedures that follow a positive screen.
15. Procedures and Costs
    The ultimate decision whether to implement a screening program in a population rests on a tradeoff between costs and benefits. To facilitate assessment of cost and cost-effectiveness of the screening program, data can be collected on the costs of all phases of the program in an evaluation trial. An alternative is to record the procedures done in each phase so that costs can be assigned at a later date. Included are efforts to recruit the population, the screening tests, diagnostic procedures, treatment procedures, and efforts used to follow the population.
16. Sequential Monitoring and Interim Analysis
    A process for regular, formal monitoring of safety issues and accumulating data should be established early in the course of a screening trial. This is best accomplished by the creation of a data and safety monitoring board (DSMB). This board is comprised of experts not associated with the trial who can therefore provide an independent assessment of trial progress. A DSMB typically uses statistical monitoring methods to examine emerging data. Accruing mortality and secondary endpoints are examined regularly to determine if and when a protocol change is warranted that would result in early termination of the trial. Formal statistical procedures are available (e.g., Proschan et al. 2006).

Conclusion

As in other areas of research, much has been learned over time from completed and ongoing screening trials. This chapter is an attempt to convey some of this knowledge. Hopefully this will lead to improved trial design and analysis in the future. Some additional insights are the following:

1. New screening tests can rapidly become widely used, especially in the U.S., often without valid scientific evidence of benefit nor proper assessment of harm. It is therefore important to undertake rigorous trials as soon as possible when a new test becomes available to take advantage of a window of opportunity, before widespread use precludes establishment of a proper control;
2. Over-diagnosis has been indicated repeatedly, particularly in cancer screening. This should be expected and accounted for in study design, analysis, and interpretation;
3. A pilot phase prior to or at the beginning of a trial can be extremely valuable for testing operational components and evaluating study centers. Although not discussed in this chapter, pilot studies have been instrumental in several cancer screening trials (e.g., NLST Research Team 2011; Prorok et al. 2000);
4. Quality assurance of all trial operations is crucial.

As has been stated previously, a screening trial is a major endeavor requiring a long-term commitment by participants, investigators and funding organizations. If a decision is made to do a such a trial, necessary resources must be provided for the full study duration. To accomplish this in the usual climate of resource competition and peer review can be difficult. One strategy is full commitment sequentially to the primary phases of such a trial; ie, pilot, recruitment, screening, and follow-up, with funding for each successive phase contingent on successful completion of the previous phase.

What is clear however is that such trials have been successfully conducted, and that screening interventions for chronic diseases can and should be evaluated rigorously.

Cross-References

▶ Randomization and Permutation Tests
▶ Survival Analysis II

References

Ahlbom A (1993) Biostatistics for epidemiologists. Lewis Publishers, Boca Raton, pp 61–66

Andriole GL et al (2012) Prostate cancer screening in the randomized prostate, lung, colorectal and ovarian cancer screening trial: mortality results after 13 years of follow-up. J Natl Cancer Inst 104:125–132

Baker SG et al (2002) Statistical issues in randomized trials of cancer screening. BMC Med Res Methodol 2:11. (19 September 2002)

Berry DA (1998) Benefits and risks of screening mammography for women in their forties: a statistical appraisal. J Natl Cancer Inst 90:1431–1439

Bretthauer M et al (2016) Population-based colonoscopy screening for colorectal cancer: a randomized trial. JAMA Intern Med 176:894–902

Cuzick J et al (1997) Adjusting for non-compliance and contamination in randomized clinical trials. Stat Med 16:1017–1029

Duffy SW et al (2008) Correcting for lead time and length bias in estimating the effect of screen detection on cancer survival. Am J Epidemiol 168:98–104

Echouffo-Tcheugui JB, Prorok PC (2014) Considerations in the design of randomized trials to screen for type 2 diabetes. Clin Trials 11:284–291

Etzioni RD et al (1995) Design and analysis of cancer screening trials. Stat Meth Med Res 4:3–17

Freedman LS, Green SB (1990) Statistical designs for investigating several interventions in the same study: methods for cancer prevention trials. J Natl Cancer Inst 82:910–914

Friskell J et al (1991) Randomized study of mammography screening – preliminary report on mortality in the Stockholm trial. Breast Cancer Res Treat 18:49–56

Kafadar K, Prorok PC (2009) Effect of length biased sampling of unobserved sojourn times on the survival distribution when disease is screen detected. Stat Med 28(16):2116–2146

Mandel JS et al (1993) Reducing mortality from colorectal cancer by screening for fecal occult blood. New Engl J Med 328:1365–1371

Miller AB et al (1981) The national study of breast cancer screening. Clin Invest Med 4:227–258

Morrison AS (1982) The effects of early treatment, lead time and length bias on the mortality experienced by cases detected by screening. Int J Epidemiol 11:261–267

Moss SM et al (2015) Effect of mammographic screening from age 40 years on breast cancer mortality in the UK age trial at 17 years follow-up: a randomized controlled trial. Lancet Oncol 16:1123–1132

NLST Research Team (2011) The national lung screening trial: overview and study design. Radiology 258:243–253

Nystrom L et al (1993) Breast cancer screening with mammography: overview of Swedish randomized trials. Lancet 341:973–978

Pinsky PF et al (2007) Evidence of a healthy volunteer effect in the prostate, lung, colorectal and ovarian cancer screening trial. Am J Epidemiol 165:874–881

Pisano ED (2018) Is tomosynthesis the future of breast cancer screening? Radiology 287:47–48

Prorok PC (1995) Screening studies. In: Greenwald P, Kramer BS, Weed DL (eds) Cancer prevention and control. Marcel Dekker, New York, pp 225–242

Prorok PC, Marcus PM (2010) Cancer screening trials: nuts and bolts. Semin Oncol 37:216–223

Prorok PC et al (2000) Design of the prostate, lung, colorectal and ovarian (PLCO) cancer screening trial. Conrolled Clin Trials Suppl 21(6S):273S–309S

Proschan MA et al (2006) Statistical monitoring of clinical trials. Springer, New York

Schroder FH et al (2014) Screening and prostate cancer mortality: results of the european randomized study of screening for prostate cancer (ERSPC) at 13 years follow-up. Lancet 384:2027–2035

Shapiro et al (1988) Periodic screening for breast cancer: the health insurance plan project and its sequelae, 1963–1986. The Johns Hopkins University Press, Baltimore

Tabar L et al (1992) Update of the Swedish two-county program of mammographic screening for breast cancer. Radiol Clin N Am 30:187–210

Welch HG et al (2016) Breast cancer tumor size, overdiagnosis, and mammography screening effectiveness. NEJM 375:1438–1414

Yousaf-Khan U et al (2017) Final screening round of the NELSON lung cancer screening trial: the effect of a 2.5 year screening interval. Thorax 72:48–56

Biosimilar Drug Development

66

Johanna Mielke and Byron Jones

Contents

Abstract

Biologics are innovative, complex large molecule drugs that have brought life-changing improvements to patients in various disease areas like cancer, diabetes, or psoriasis. Biosimilars are copies of innovative biologics. Their development is currently a focus of attention because the patents of several important biologics have expired, making it possible for competing companies to produce their own biosimilar version of the drug. Although, at first sight, there seems to be some similarity with the development of generics, which are copies of simple small molecule drugs, there is an important distinction because of the complexity and

J. Mielke · B. Jones (✉)
Novartis Pharma AG, Basel, Switzerland
e-mail: johanna.mielke@udo.edu; byron.jones@novartis.com

© Springer Nature Switzerland AG 2022

S. Piantadosi, C. L. Meinert (eds.), *Principles and Practice of Clinical Trials*,
https://doi.org/10.1007/978-3-319-52636-2_272

the variability inherent in the development of biologics. This chapter introduces the studies and analyses required to obtain regulatory approval for marketing a biosimilar and reviews several important regulatory concepts. In addition, several important statistical challenges are highlighted and discussed.

Keywords

Follow-on biologics · Equivalence testing · Totality of the evidence · Biosimilarity · Extrapolation · Biologics · Comparability · Analytics · Switchability · Historical information

Introduction

Biologics (or large molecule drugs) have revolutionized the treatment of various diseases and dramatically improved the life of many patients. However, they suffer from the disadvantage that their costs are very high: it is estimated that the costs of treatment with biologics are 22 times higher than that of a nonbiological drug (Health Affairs Health Policy Brief 2013). That is why the question as to whether biologics should be used as the first line treatment is still controversial in many disease areas (e.g., see Finckh et al. (2009) for a discussion in rheumatoid arthritis) and the access of patients to these life-changing products if often limited.

Previous experience with (small-molecule) nonbiological drugs showed that the introduction of generics, that is, copies of the originator small-molecule drug, substantially lowered drug prices and thus improved the access of patients to these products. Generics are usually developed and produced by a competing company and can be marketed after the patent of the original drug has expired. The analogue to generics for biologics are the so-called biosimilars (also known as follow-on biologics). These medical products are developed and approved as copies of already marketed biologics.

However, while the concepts of generics and biosimilars are comparable, it is important to note that small molecule drugs and biologics differ substantially (Crommelin et al. 2005). While small molecules tend to have a well-defined and stable chemical structure which can be easily identified, biologics are more complex proteins with heterogeneous structures. In addition, small molecule drugs are chemically engineered, but biologics are grown in living cells: this makes the manufacture of biologics extremely sensitive to environmental changes (e.g., a small change of temperature in the manufacturing site might influence the therapeutic effect of the product). The high complexity of the molecule and the sensitive manufacturing process makes it, even for the manufacturer of the originator, impossible to produce an exact copy. That is why, in contrast to generics, which are chemically identical to the original small molecule drug, biosimilars are only expected to be *similar* to the originator product. The high complexity and the difficult characterization of the molecules combined with the fact that biosimilars are only similar, but not identical to the originator product, lead to a higher uncertainty if the therapeutic effect of the biosimilar is comparable to that of the originator product. Therefore, the limited evidence which is required for gaining approval for a generic is not considered sufficient for biosimilars. It should also be noted that the objectives of a biosimilar development program are not entirely the same as that of the original product, since the aim is to demonstrate comparability of the biosimilar and originator and not to establish efficacy de novo (Christl et al. 2017). Indeed, regulatory agencies, for example, the Food and Drug Administration (FDA) in the USA, have implemented a separate regulatory pathway for biosimilars.

In this chapter, we discuss some of the most important concepts, statistical challenges, and regulations of biosimilar development with a focus on the FDA's point of view. However, it should be noted that these are comparable to other highly regulated markets (Cazap et al. 2018).

The foundation of biosimilar development in the USA lies in the Biologics Price and Competition (BPCI) Act (FDA 2009) where the legal framework for approval of biosimilars has been written into law. The FDA defines a biosimilar as "a biological product that is highly similar to and has no clinically meaningful differences from an existing FDA-approved reference [i.e., original] product" (FDA 2017a). Therefore, for getting approval as a biosimilar, a sponsor (the developer of the biosimilar) needs to demonstrate that patients who are taking the biosimilar can expect the same efficacy and safety profile as patients who are taking the originator product.

For the showing of biosimilarity, the FDA recommends a stepwise approach which is introduced in detail in section "The Stepwise Approach to Biosimilarity." Before that, two fundamental concepts for biosimilar development are introduced. The most important concept in the biosimilar pathway in the USA is the idea of the "totality of the evidence" (Christl et al. 2017): not one study in the development program is considered pivotal, but all provided evidence (the results of all steps) is considered important. When the decision is made on whether to approve or to reject a biosimilar, all evidence is taken into account.

Another important concept is "extrapolation" (Weise et al. 2014). This relates to the fact that the clinical trials, which are performed as part of the stepwise approach (see section "The Stepwise Approach to Biosimilarity"), are only conducted in selected indications. In contrast, the originator is normally approved for a wide range of indications and the aim of the sponsor of a biosimilar is usually to gain approval in all the same indications as the originator product. However, since the clinical evidence is, in the context of the "totality of the evidence," not pivotal, a so-called extrapolation of the provided evidence to indications which were not explicitly studied in clinical trials is possible by appealing to scientific judgment. It should be noted that the use of extrapolation is still a topic of debate, especially for products for which the mechanism of action is not fully understood in all indications (Schellekens and Moors 2015). Nonetheless, extrapolation has been used in all biosimilar applications in the USA so far.

The rest of this chapter is structured as follows: after the introduction of the stepwise approach in the section "The Stepwise Approach to Biosimilarity," the section "Testing for Equivalence in Biosimilar Trials" gives an overview of the statistical methodology for testing for equivalence. Section "Case Study" gives a case study that illustrates the stepwise approach using the development program of the biosimilar Zarxio. Then, in section "Selected Challenges in Biosimilar Development" selected challenges related to the design and analysis of biosimilar clinical trials are discussed. Conclusions are presented in section "Summary and Conclusion."

The Stepwise Approach to Biosimilarity

In this section, the stepwise approach to biosimilarity is introduced with a focus on the FDA's terminology and regulations. However, it should be emphasized that the way of thinking is comparable also to other highly regulated markets (e.g., in the EU). The FDA's proposed biosimilar development strategy consists of three main steps which are illustrated in Fig. 1: analytical studies (Step 1), nonclinical studies (Step 2), and clinical studies (Step 3) which are split (a) into pharmacokinetic (PK) and pharmacodynamic (PD) studies and (b) therapeutic equivalence studies. It is recommended that after each step the already obtained evidence is considered and any residual uncertainty is identified before it is decided which additional studies are necessary for the establishment of biosimilarity (FDA 2015b). The FDA's expectations for each step are described in the overarching guideline on scientific questions related to biosimilar development (FDA 2015b) and further outlined in topic-specific guidelines on pharmacological data (FDA 2016).

Even though, in line with the idea of the "totality of the evidence," all provided evidence is important, the analytical studies (Step 1) are often considered the foundation of biosimilar development. The aim of the analytical studies is to establish comparability of the biosimilar and its originator at the molecular level, that is, it should be confirmed that the biosimilar molecule and the originator molecule are "highly" similar. However, due to the complexity of the molecule, it is, with the current state-of-the-art technologies, not possible to characterize the molecules sufficiently well enough with one single tool, as it is done for small

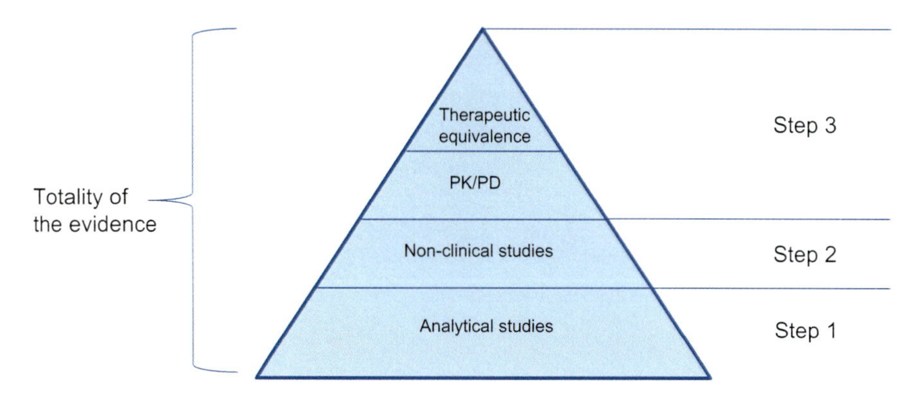

Fig. 1 Steps of biosimilar development (*PK* pharmacokinetic, *PD* pharmacodynamic)

molecule drugs. In fact, several assessments are performed in order to check different characteristics of the molecule (so-called quality attributes) and it is assumed that if all of these assessments indicate equivalence, then the molecules themselves are also sufficiently similar. The structural characteristics, for example, the identity of the primary sequence of amino acids, are analyzed with techniques like peptide mapping or mass spectrometry. Also the biological activity needs to be comparable and, for that, often bioassays are used which can assess comparability in terms of binding and functionality (Schiestl et al. 2014). The way statistics can support the comparability claims in analytical studies is still highly controversial: the FDA published (and subsequently withdrew) a draft guideline (FDA 2018) that discussed the value of statistics for the establishing of comparability. The FDA suggested using a risk-based approach where the type of statistical methodology depends on the criticality of the quality attribute. That is, for an attribute which is assumed to be strongly related to the clinical outcome (e.g., the results of a bioassay which is assessing the binding of the molecule to a target which is imitating the mechanism of action), stricter criteria for comparability are applied compared to a quality attribute which is assumed not to be critical for the therapeutic effect.

After all analytical studies are conducted, the FDA recommends classifying the obtained comparability into one of four categories (FDA 2016): (1) insufficient analytical similarity, (2) analytical similarity with residual uncertainty, (3) tentative analytical similarity, and (4) fingerprint-like analytical similarity. In categories (1) and (2), the sponsor needs to conduct additional analytical studies and/or to adjust the manufacturing process. Categories (3) and (4) allow a sponsor to proceed to the next step of biosimilar development. Dependent on the amount of residual uncertainty, selective animal and clinical studies might be sufficient. Therefore, providing a higher level of evidence (e.g., fingerprint-like analytical similarity instead of tentative analytical similarity) might reduce the amount of required studies in the following steps. On the other hand, demonstrating fingerprint-like similarity might be challenging or even not possible in some cases.

In Step 2, studies in animals are conducted. The main aim of the animal studies is to establish the toxicology profile of the proposed biosimilar. In some cases, also the PK and PD profiles in animals of the biosimilar are compared to the originator. However, it is clearly emphasized that the inclusion of animal PK and PD studies does not lead to a negation of the need for clinical studies in humans. If there is no relevant animal species, additional in vitro studies might be appropriate, for example, with human cells. The extent of the required studies highly depends on the success of the analytical studies which were performed in Step 1. This is stated in the regulatory document issued by the FDA (2015b): "If comparative structural and functional data using the proposed product provide strong support for analytical similarity to a reference [originator] product, then limited animal toxicity data may be sufficient to support initial clinical use of the proposed product."

After Step 2 is completed successfully, the proposed biosimilar is used for the first time in humans (Step 3). The "FDA expects a sponsor to conduct comparative human PK and PD studies (if there is a relevant PD measure(s)) and a clinical immunogenicity assessment" and, if these evidences are not sufficient for removing residual uncertainties, also comparative clinical trials are required (FDA 2015b). The aim of PK and PD equivalence studies is to confirm comparable exposure (PK) of the proposed biosimilar and the originator and, if possible, to show that the way the drug affects the body is sufficiently similar (PD). The results of PD studies can only be considered an important piece of evidence if there exists a well-established PD marker which can serve as a surrogate for the clinical outcome. In these cases, the PK/PD studies may be seen as a more sensitive step for detecting potential differences between the biosimilar and the originator than clinical comparability studies. For example, for the approval of Zarxio (Sandoz) the pharmacology studies reduced the need for clinical comparability studies (Holzmann et al. 2016, see for details also section "Case Study").

The design and analysis of PK/PD studies are comparable to the studies which are conducted for the showing of bioequivalence of generics. The preferred study design (FDA 2016) for products with a short half-life (the time until half of the drug is eliminated from the body) is a crossover design. Often two-period, two-treatment crossover designs are used where subjects first take the biosimilar and then the originator or vice versa. These studies have the advantage that each subject acts as his or her own control, which reduces the variability and allows for smaller sample sizes (Jones and Kenward 2014). In the case of a long half-life, parallel groups designs are also acceptable (FDA 2016). The study population should consist of healthy volunteers, if possible. This is expected to reduce the variability since patients often have confounding factors (e.g., comorbidity). However, if this is not feasible due to ethical reasons (e.g., known toxicology) or if a PD marker can only be assessed in patients (e.g., in diabetes), then patients are preferred.

The analysis of PK/PD data is, compared to the other steps in biosimilar development, standardized and leaves only a small degree of flexibility for the sponsor: a response of the drug in the blood over time is measured after the drug is injected. For PK analysis, the response of interest is the concentration of the drug in the blood, for PD, it might be a well-established PD marker. Measures like the area under the response vs. time curve (AUC) and the maximum response over time (Cmax) are reported for each subject. The aim is to show that the ratio of the mean values of the originator product and the proposed biosimilar for each of these measures as a percentage lies within 80% and 125% with a prespecified confidence level $1 - \alpha$ where commonly $\alpha = 0.1$ is used. This confidence level corresponds to a one-sided significance level of 5% which is typically used for testing for superiority.

An assessment of immunogenicity (e.g., the potential to induce an immune response, as for example anaphylaxis) is required since, with the current understanding of highly complex molecules, it is not possible to reliably predict the immunogenicity purely based on analytical studies. Since immune responses might influence the treatment effect and the safety profile, it is important to confirm similar immunogenicity. Immunogenicity is mostly assessed as part of the clinical studies (Christl et al. 2017) and the amount and type of immunogenicity assessment depends on the active substance.

If the comparability of the products at the PK/PD level has been established, but there still exists residual uncertainties, then clinical comparability studies in patients are conducted. These studies should be carefully chosen to target the residual uncertainty. The selection of endpoints, study population, study duration, and study design need to be scientifically justified. In general, the approach should be selected which is expected to be most sensitive to detect potential differences between the proposed biosimilar and the originator (FDA 2015b). Therapeutic equivalence is typically assessed at one chosen point in time using an equivalence testing approach (see section "Testing for Equivalence in Biosimilar Trials"), that is, it is confirmed that the characteristic of interest of the treatment response, for example, the mean value of a chosen endpoint, after taking the biosimilar is neither smaller nor larger than after taking the originator. A non-inferiority-type test, that is, the showing that a chosen characteristic under treatment with the biosimilar is not larger or smaller, respectively, than under treatment with the originator, might be acceptable in specific cases. For example, one might consider a noninferiority design if a higher response can be ruled out due to scientific reasons (e.g., saturation of the target with a specific dose, see Schoergenhofer et al. (2018)). In terms of the study design, mostly parallel groups designs are conducted which often are combined with an extension period in which the effect of a single switch from the originator to the biosimilar is studied and the safety and immunogenicity profile is compared between the switching and nonswitching group. This type of assessment is explicitly required in the respective guideline (FDA 2015b). Safety and immunogenicity are usually assessed descriptively.

Taking all results into account, by referring to the concept of "totality of the evidence" (see section "Introduction"), regulators make a decision if biosimilarity is established or not. Consequently, this means that the failing of one analysis does necessarily lead to the failing of the biosimilar development program, as long as a scientific justification is provided (for an example of approval with failed "components of evidence," see Mielke et al. 2016). It is important to note that the overall assessment of biosimilarity is made by appealing to scientific judgment and not by a quantitative decision making approach. This makes the decision whether as to approve a biosimilar a subjective one. In the recent past, some strategies were published on how to formalize the decision making process (e.g., the biosimilarity index by Hsieh et al. 2013), but these suggestions have not yet made it into practice.

Information regarding the provision of clinical evidence for biosimilar approval in practice can be found in Hung et al. (2017) for the USA, in Mielke et al. (2016, 2018a) for the European Union and in Arato (2016) for Japan.

Testing for Equivalence in Biosimilar Trials

Usually, the aim of a study in biosimilar development is to establish equivalence, that is, it is necessary to confirm that a characteristic of interest measured after treatment with the biosimilar is *similar* to the same characteristic of interest measured after treatment with the originator. As a simplification, it is assumed that the aim is to establish equivalence in the difference of the measurements, that is, to show that the difference between two mean values is sufficiently small. However, ratios can usually be transformed into differences with a logarithmic transformation so that the same type of hypothesis can be assessed. More formally, let τ_B be a characteristic of interest of the biosimilar (e.g., the mean value of log(AUC)) and τ_O be the same characteristic of interest of the originator. Then, the aim is to test the hypotheses (Wellek 2010):

$$H_0 : |\tau_B - \tau_O| \geq \Delta \text{ vs.} H_1 : |\tau_B - \tau_O| < \Delta,$$

where Δ is a positive value and called the equivalence margin. The choice of the equivalence margin is discussed in more detail in section "The Choice of Equivalence Margins in Efficacy Trials" and for the time being, it is assumed that an equivalence margin Δ is provided.

There exists two common ways to test the above mentioned hypotheses: first, one can split the equivalence hypothesis into two one-sided hypotheses. This approach is commonly known as the two-one-sided-test (TOST) approach (Schuirmann 1987). The two sets of hypotheses are given by:

$$H_0^{(1)} : \tau_B - \tau_O \leq -\Delta thickmathspace vs. H_1^{(1)} : \tau_B - \tau_O > -\Delta,$$
$$H_0^{(2)} : \tau_B - \tau_O \geq \Delta thickmathspace vs. H_1^{(2)} : \tau_B - \tau_O < \Delta.$$

If both $H_0^{(1)}$ and $H_0^{(2)}$ are rejected, the overarching hypotheses H_0 is also rejected and equivalence can be claimed. In the following, the test statistics and decision rules for the hypotheses $H_0^{(1)}$ and $H_0^{(2)}$ are illustrated using the example of a normally distributed endpoint. For that, let τ_B be the expected value of the biosimilar and τ_O be the expected value of originator. The standard deviation of the originator is denoted by σ_O, whereas the standard deviation of the biosimilar is denoted by σ_B. We assume that both standard deviations are equal, that is, $\sigma_B = \sigma_O$. In addition, we assume a parallel groups design with n subjects per group. Let $\bar{y}_O$ and $\bar{y}_B$ be the observed mean values of the originator and the biosimilar, respectively. The estimated standard deviations are denoted by σ_O and $\hat{\sigma}_B$. The corresponding test statistics are then

$$Z_1 = \frac{(\bar{y}_B - \bar{y}_O) + \Delta}{\sqrt{\frac{\hat{\sigma}_B^2}{n} + \frac{\hat{\sigma}_O^2}{n}}} \text{and} Z_2 = \frac{(\bar{y}_O - \bar{y}_B) + \Delta}{\sqrt{\frac{\hat{\sigma}_B^2}{n} + \frac{\hat{\sigma}_O^2}{n}}}.$$

Both test statistics follow, under the null hypotheses, a t-distribution with $2n - 2$ degrees of freedom. Therefore, the null hypothesis is rejected if both realizations are larger than the $(1 - \alpha)$-quantile of a t-distribution with $2n - 2$ degrees of freedom. A typical choice for the significance level α is $\alpha = 0.05$.

The second strategy is based on a confidence interval approach: a $(1 - 2\alpha)$-confidence interval for the difference of the mean value is calculated. If this confidence interval fully lies within

$$[-\Delta, \Delta],$$

the null hypothesis H_0 is rejected and equivalence is claimed. In the case of a normally distributed endpoint, the $(1 - 2\alpha)$-confidence interval is given by

$$\left[\bar{y}_B - \bar{y}_O - t_{1-\alpha,2n-2}\sqrt{\frac{\hat{\sigma}_B^2}{n} + \frac{\hat{\sigma}_O^2}{n}}, \bar{y}_B - \bar{y}_O + t_{1-\alpha,2n-2}\sqrt{\frac{\hat{\sigma}_B^2}{n} + \frac{\hat{\sigma}_O^2}{n}}\right],$$

where $t_{\beta,k}$ is the β-quantile of the t-distribution with k degrees of freedom.

Comparing the confidence interval approach with the TOST-approach in this example, one quickly realizes that both approaches lead to the same result. A more detailed discussion on the connection between the TOST approach and the confidence interval approach can be found in Hsu et al. (1994).

For normally distributed endpoints, typically the mean values are compared. However, also more complex approaches have previously been proposed: For example, Chow et al. (2009) proposed comparing the probability that the two characteristics of interest do not differ by more than a prespecified value and Tsou et al. (2013) discussed a consistency approach. These approaches have the advantage that the focus is not exclusively on the mean value, but also takes into account the variability of the products. However, so far, the simple comparison of mean values, if necessary adjusted for relevant covariates, is still the standard approach for establishing equivalence in a biosimilar development program.

Case Study

In 2015, Sandoz Inc., a Novartis Company, gained approval from the FDA to market Zarxio, its biosimilar version of the reference biologic, Neupogen (active substance: filgrastim). Neupogen is used to treat neutropenia (an abnormally low level of neutrophils in the blood) which can occur, for example, in cancer patients undergoing chemotherapy. This case study gives a brief description of some of the information presented by Sandoz Inc. in its submission to the FDA to gain approval to market Zarxio. This information is publically available online (FDA 2015a) and the summary given below is based directly on that text. The following subsections briefly describe the contributions to the steps that were illustrated in Fig. 1 and described in detail in section "The Stepwise Approach to Biosimilarity."

Step 1: Analytical Similarity

Analytical similarity was assessed using multiple quality attributes, and some of them are listed in Table 1. In total, it was concluded that the proposed biosimilar is "highly similar" to Neupogen.

Step 2: Nonclinical Studies

EP2006 was compared to Neupogen in animal studies for assessing the pharmacodynamics (PD), toxicity, toxicokinetics, and local tolerance of the products. Of these

Table 1 Quality attributes and methods used to evaluate analytical similarity of EP2006 and US-Licensed Neupogen (partial list, for illustration)

Quality attribute	Method
Primary structure	N-terminal sequencing
	Peptide mapping with ultraviolet (UV) and mass spectrometry detection
	Protein molecular mass by electrospray mass spectrometry (ESI MS)
	Protein molecular mass by matrix-assisted laser desorption ionization mass spectrometry (MALDI-TOFMS)
	DNA sequencing of the EP2006 construct cassette
	Peptide mapping coupled with tandem mass spectrometry (MS/MS)
Bioactivity	Proliferation of murine myelogenous leukemia cells (NFS-60 cell line)
Receptor binding	Surface Plasmon Resonance
Protein content	RP-HPLC

studies, one was a single dose tolerance study in rabbits and the other was a 28-day multiple, repeat dose toxicology study in rats. According to Bewesdorff (2016), these two studies used, respectively, a single group of 24 rabbits and two groups of 60 rats.

Step 3: Clinical Studies

To assess PK and PD, four studies were reported, labeled as EP06-109, EP06-103, EP06-105, and EP06-101. Each of these was a 2 × 2 cross-over trial and involved between 24 and 32 healthy subjects. For the PK assessment, the usual PK parameters, for example, AUC and Cmax, were used and for the PD assessment, the endpoints were the absolute neutrophil count (ANC) and the increase in CD34+ cell count.

For establishing equivalence of the PK profiles, equivalence was tested using the usual criteria that the 90% confidence interval for the geometric ratios of the AUC and Cmax parameters should lie within (80%, 125%), except for study EP06-101 which used the wider margin of (75%, 133%) for Cmax.

In the PD studies, equivalence was assessed using the criterion that the 95% confidence interval for the ratio of geometric means for AUEC (area under the effect curve over time) and the maximum ANC should lie within the (80%, 125%) interval, except for study EP06-103 where the interval was (87.25%, 114.61%) for the 2.5 mcg/kg dose and (86.5%, 115.61%) for the 5 mcg/kg dose. According to the publicly available information, there were no predefined equivalence criteria for CD35+ and 95% and 90% confidence intervals for the ratio of the parameters (AUEC and maximum CD34+ count) were reported. It is notable that, in general, the choice of equivalence margins, especially for the PD parameters, is not fixed, but may depend on the chosen endpoint. This is taken up in subsection "The Choice of Equivalence Margins in Efficacy Trials" where the choice of margins is discussed.

For the clinical assessment of efficacy and safety, data from two trials were used: EP06-301 and EP06-302. The latter trial was a double-blind parallel groups trial in women with histologically proven breast cancer and the treatments were administered over six cycles of chemotherapy. The study had four arms: (1) EP006 (E) given repeatedly for all cycles, (2) Neupogen (N) given repeatedly for all cycles, (3) E and N were alternated over the cycles in the order (N,E,N,E,N,E), and (4) E and N were alternated over the cycles in the order (E,N,E,N,E,N). This design was planned to not only assess similarity but also interchangeability. The concept of interchangeability is discussed in subsection "Interchangeability of Biosimilars." The endpoint in this study was the duration of severe neutropenia. Study EP06-301 was a non-comparative single arm study in which patients with breast cancer were treated with chemotherapy and then one day later were given daily EP2006 until neutrophil recovery.

In January, 2015, the expert panel reviewing the Sandoz Inc. application unanimously recommended its approval and in March 2015, the FDA gave approval for the biosimilar to be marketed for all five of the indications approved for Neupogen.

Selected Challenges in Biosimilar Development

In this section, selected challenges in biosimilar development are presented with a focus on statistical issues. First, the choice of the equivalence margin Δ in theory and practice is discussed before the assessment of interchangeability and strategies for including additional information in the Phase III efficacy trials are described.

The Choice of Equivalence Margins in Efficacy Trials

Equivalent efficacy has to be established during biosimilar development. As described in section "The Stepwise Approach to Biosimilarity," typically one efficacy endpoint is selected and compared under treatment with the biosimilar and with the originator. Only if the selected endpoint is "similar" in both treatment groups, therapeutic comparability is established. However, it is often not straightforward what "similar" means. The degree of acceptable differences between the biosimilar and the originator is reflected in the equivalence margin Δ (see section "Testing for Equivalence in Biosimilar Trials") which is supposed to give the maximal value such that the difference in the endpoint is not considered relevant from a clinical point of view. That is, if the null hypothesis of an equivalence test is rejected, this means that differences larger than the equivalence margins Δ can be excluded with a pre-specified probability $1 - \alpha$. This clearly shows that the choice of the equivalence margin has a major influence on the test decision.

In PK (average) bioequivalence studies for generics, a standardized approach is used for selecting the equivalence margins: typically, the equivalence margins for the difference of the PK parameters on the log-scale are set to $\pm$ log (1.25) independently of the active substance (Jones and Kenward 2014). For efficacy endpoints in biosimilar development, this is, however, not possible because the acceptable difference (the degree of similarity) in the endpoints highly depends on the active substance, the indication and the chosen endpoint. That is why a case-by-case decision has to be made for each active substance and endpoint and the margins are typically determined by negotiation with the regulatory agencies. In the following, we discuss experiences with the choice of equivalence margins in applications to the European Medicines Agency (EMA) instead of experience with the FDA since the EMA has already approved more than 40 biosimilars and therefore allows for a broader overview of current practice.

In their respective guidelines (CHMP 2014a), the EMA only states that "comparability margins should be prespecified and justified on both statistical and clinical grounds by using the data of the reference [original] product" and refers to a related guideline on the choice of non-inferiority margins (CHMP 2005). The EMA aims at being transparent in their decision making and that is why they publish so-called European public assessment reports (EPARs) which give detailed information on the provided evidence for approved biosimilars and are accessible by the general public. Thus, it is possible to analyze the choice of margins in practice where, indeed, the equivalence margins for the clinical comparability studies were usually prespecified and only in a few cases were post hoc decisions made (Mielke et al. 2018a). However, the information on the derivation provided in the EPARs was only in a few cases reported in enough detail so that a reproduction of the equivalence margins would be possible. In addition, there does not seem to be a standardized strategy for the determination of equivalence margins. This is illustrated by using the regulatory applications for Benepali (active substance: etanercept) and Rixathon (active substance: rituximab).

For Benepali, the chosen endpoint was the ACR20 responder rates (CHMP 2016): a subject is classified as an ACR20 responder if the relative improvement in percentage according to the American College of Rheumatology (ACR) criterion (Felson et al. 1993) when compared to baseline is larger than 20%. Three historical studies were identified and combined using a random-effects meta-analysis and a 95% confidence interval for the difference in response rates of the originator vs. placebo was obtained and is reported as (0.3103, 0.4996). The sponsor decided to aim for a preservation of 50% of the effect of the originator vs. placebo and chose $\Delta = 0.15$. For Rixathon, in contrast, the overall response rate to the treatment was the chosen endpoint. The sponsor used only a single historical trial in a comparable study population for deriving the equivalence margin. A 95% confidence interval for the observed add-on effect of the originator was estimated and is given by (0.14, 0.34). The sponsor decided for an equivalence margin of $\Delta = 0.12$ which preserves only 15% of the add-on effect of the originator.

It is acknowledged that the richness of historical data was different in the two situations: while for Benepali three comparable studies were used with, in total, 460 patients enrolled, for Rixathon only one single study with 320 subjects was analyzed. If only limited data are available, this leads to a wider confidence interval and that generally lowers the equivalence margin for a fixed percent of effect to be preserved. A lower equivalence margin Δ makes it finally more difficult to claim equivalence. Nonetheless, this example shows that the statistical approach for the choice of the equivalence margins is not standardized yet. Due to the close connection between the equivalence margin and the test result, it would be beneficial if more concrete guidance was provided by regulatory agencies, specifically on the percentage of effect to be preserved.

Negotiation of the equivalence margin with the regulatory authorities by seeking Scientific Advice is not mandatory in Europe. This is evident in some of the EPARs in which it is explicitly stated that the EMA did not agree with the chosen margin. One example is the application of Amgevita (active substance: adalimumab). There, the sponsor decided to use a margin of (0.738, 1.355) for the risk ratio of ACR20 responders. The EMA (CHMP 2017) was concerned that this margin was too wide because it "would correspond to an absolute margin of more than –16% on the additive scale." It was concluded that "however, in light of the results observed this does not represent an issue that could compromise the reliability of the study." It is unclear how the EMA would have decided if the study results would not have supported also the tighter margins. Therefore, an early discussion with regulatory authorities on an acceptable choice of equivalence margins is recommended.

Interchangeability of Biosimilars

The primary efficacy endpoint in therapeutic equivalence studies (see section "The Stepwise Approach to Biosimilarity") is usually compared in a parallel groups design, that is, it is confirmed that patients who are taking repeatedly the biosimilar and patients who are taking repeatedly the originator respond comparably to the treatment. The focus is typically on treatment-naive patients, that is, patients without any relevant pre-treatment prior to the start of the study (FDA 2015b). In practice, since biosimilars are often developed for chronic diseases, patients might want or need to switch between the biosimilar and its originator once or even multiple times during the duration of the treatment. While for the approval as a biosimilar in Europe, no data on transition from the originator to the biosimilar or vice versa is required, the FDA recommends assessing the impact on immunogenicity of a single transition from the originator to the biosimilar (FDA 2015b). However, also in the USA, usually no data are provided in the biosimilar application by the sponsor on the impact of multiple switches and single crossovers from the biosimilar to the originator.

To fill this gap, the FDA has the legal option to approve biosimilars as "interchangeable biosimilars." According to BPCI Act (FDA 2009), a proposed product is considered to be interchangeable, if (1) the proposed product is biosimilar to its originator, (2) it "can be expected to produce the same clinical result as the reference [originator] product in any given patient" and (3) "for a biological product that is administered more than once to an individual, the risk in terms of safety or diminished efficacy of alternating or switching between use of the biological product and the reference [originator] product is not greater than the risk of using the reference product without such alternation or switch" where alternating relates to multiple switches (e.g., biosimilar to originator back to biosimilar). It is important to note that there is a clear hierarchy between "biosimilarity" and "interchangeability": a product which is interchangeable is also biosimilar; however, biosimilarity is only one part of the showing of interchangeability.

In the past, it was not known with certainty what data and analysis are required for the showing of interchangeability. However, in 2017, the FDA published a first draft guidance (FDA 2017b) which outlined their expectation on studies for approval as an interchangeable biosimilar. Since biosimilars are diverse, there is "no one-size-fits-all approach across the product landscape to the data needed to demonstrate biosimilarity. It follows that the data needed to demonstrate interchangeability are also determined on a case-by-case basis depending on considerations such as the complexity of the product, the reference [originator] product's indications and the potential for immune system complications." (Christl 2018). Generally, the FDA expects that applications will include data from clinical studies in which specifically the effect of switching is studied for assessing its impact on efficacy and safety of the product. For the study design, the FDA recommends (FDA 2017b) including so-called switching (patients switch from the biosimilar to the originator and vice versa) and non-switching sequences (continuous treatment with the biosimilar or the originator). An example of the FDA's proposed study design for a study with the focus on interchangeability is outlined in Fig. 2. It should consists of a lead-in period which needs to be sufficiently long enough for patients to reach steady state PK (i.e., the rate of drug input is equal to the rate of elimination) before the first switch occurs. A minimum of three switches is required and the last switch needs to be a switch from the originator back to the biosimilar. After the last switch, a wash-out period of at least three half-lives needs to be included. Following this wash-out, intensive PK sampling is performed and Cmax and AUC of these PK profiles are compared by calculating a 90% confidence interval (see section "Testing for Equivalence in Biosimilar Trials") for the ratio of the means of the biosimilar and originator for both endpoints. If these intervals are both fully contained with 80–125%, the study is considered to be successful. It should be noted that the interchangeability study may be combined with the therapeutic equivalence study, which is performed for the application for getting approval as a biosimilar, if the study is planned to appropriately address both goals. In addition to the clinical studies, human factor studies

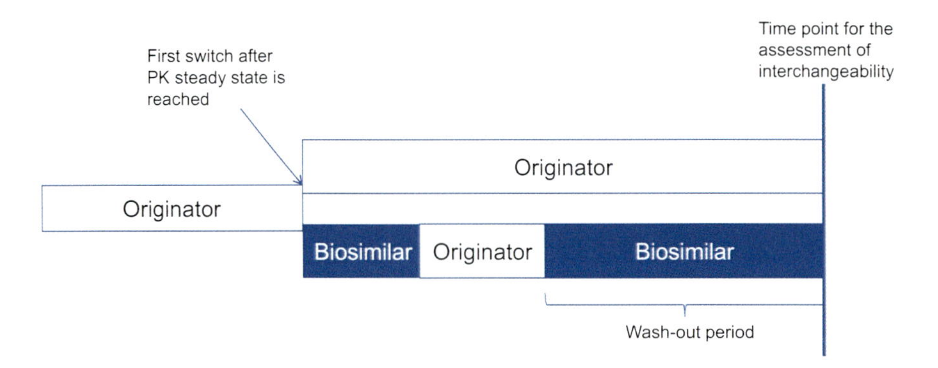

Fig. 2 FDA's proposed study design for a separate trial for establishing interchangeability

might be required which focus on the question if the patients are able to use the biosimilar device without any additional training.

In discussion among stakeholders, it can be seen that the above guidance is controversial opinions (Barlas 2017). Independently of the guidelines, a collection of statistical methodologies for the assessment of interchangeability has evolved. Compared to the recommended approach in the guideline, some of these methodologies are less focused on the mean value and are also sensitive to detect changes in variability (e.g., Li and Chow 2017) or make better use of all measured data by using the longitudinal assessments of the patients (e.g., Mielke et al. 2018d).

So far, no interchangeable biosimilar has gained approval. It is important to note that, so far, no results of any study have been published which revealed that biosimilars cannot be used interchangeably. In contrast, there exist several publications indicating that switching is not problematic (e.g., Jørgensen et al. 2017; Benucci et al. 2017). Therefore, it is unclear if the concerns related to interchangeability will diminish when more experience with biosimilars in practice is gained or if the complex clinical studies dedicated to the assessment of interchangeability will be required in the future.

It should be noted that interchangeability is not a regulatory topic in Europe since the EMA (2012) clearly states that "the Agency's evaluations do not include recommendations on whether a biosimilar should be used interchangeably with its reference [originator] medicine" and recommends that "for questions related to switching from one biological medicine to another, patients should speak to their doctor or pharmacist." The member states in Europe handle switching and alternating of biosimilars differently and no joint position is expected to evolve in the near future (Moorkens et al. 2017).

Incorporating Additional Data in Clinical Efficacy Studies

Typically when clinical efficacy studies are conducted, already rich information on the biosimilar and its originator has been gathered. The proposed biosimilar has already been evaluated in analytical, animal, and human PK (and possibly PD) studies. Even more information is available on the originator since this product is already an established medical product: the sponsor of the originator conducted several clinical efficacy studies for gaining market authorization and often the product has additionally been assessed in postmarketing studies. Furthermore, also academic institutes or health care providers might have conducted separate trials. Therefore, it seems natural to include all available information into the showing of similar efficacy. In the following, it is first assumed that historical information is available for the originator only and the information is of same type, that is, the focus is on the incorporation of results from historical clinical trials (same endpoint) in the showing of equivalent efficacy of the biosimilar and the originator. It should be noted that historical information in biosimilar trials was already used in practice by comparing the efficacy outcomes of a single-arm trial to a historical control trial, for example, in the application for Zarzio in 2008 (CHMP 2008).

In general, the aim of the inclusion of historical data is the lowering of the required sample size or, in other words, the increase of the power (the probability of claiming equivalence) of the study. However, one also needs to consider the disadvantages of including all available knowledge in the assessment of equivalent efficacy: clearly the statistical approach is more complicated, making it more difficult to analyze the study and communicate the results to a nonstatistical audience. In addition, in case the data in the new study follows a different distribution than the data in the historical trials (a so-called prior-data conflict), the Type I error rate (the probability of false positive decisions) might be higher than the acceptable nominal level. Especially the potential of an inflation of the Type I error rate, which is the patient's risk that a nonequivalent product will be called equivalent, is of concern for regulatory agencies. The use of historical information is common practice in some disease areas: for example, in rare diseases where it is challenging to recruit a sufficient number of patients in randomized trials, the use of prior information might be required so that the development is feasible at all. Also in situations in which it is unethical to include a placebo group, a comparison of the active treatment to historical placebo data has already been used for regulatory approval. In these situations, a moderate inflation of the Type I error rate is considered acceptable.

In biosimilar development, the situation is quite different (Mielke et al. 2018c): biosimilars are not developed for rare diseases; therefore, a sufficient number of subjects are available. In addition, the randomization of patients to the control group is not unethical since the control group receives the originator which is often still the standard of care. Nonetheless, even though the necessity for the inclusion of all available information is weaker for biosimilars, it is still important to emphasize that the inclusion of all available data is desirable from a scientific point of view, especially in the context of "totality of the evidence," and can also speed up the development and bring the product earlier to the patient. Therefore, the use of all information is desirable both for the sponsor and the general public. However, due to the reasons outlined above, it is expected that the regulatory expectations in terms of control of the Type I error rate are stricter.

Several approaches for the incorporation of historical information have already been proposed and an overview can be found in van Rosmalen et al. (2017). For most approaches, it is possible to adjust the methodology to make it more robust against a potential prior-data conflict and for limiting the overall Type I error rate. In the context of biosimilar development, Pan et al. (2017) developed a methodology which features some tuning parameters for an improved control of the Type I error rate. Mielke et al. (2018c) proposed not to aim for control of the Type I error rate over the whole parameter space (e.g., for response rates between 0 and 1 for a binary endpoint), but to focus instead on scenarios which are realistic in practice (e.g., true response rates between 0.2 and 0.3). This idea is displayed in Fig. 3: the Type I error rate and the power are displayed dependent on the rate of a binary characteristic of interest of the originator in the new study for two hypothetical approaches. One of these approaches is making use of the historical data (solid lines, via a prior distribution, for example), while the other (dotted horizontal line) is not

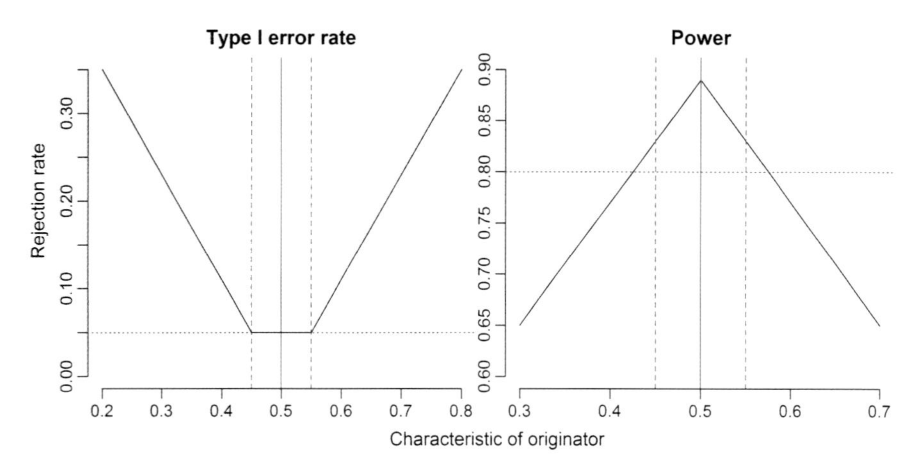

Fig. 3 Acceptable operating characteristics dependent on a characteristic of interest of the originator: the vertical solid line indicates the center of the historical data, the dotted horizontal lines are the operating characteristics for an hypothetical approach which is not using the historical data. The non-constant solid lines correspond to an hypothetical approach which incorporates the historical data. The vertical dashed lines give the interval in which the Type I error rate has to be controlled

incorporating the historical data. The vertical solid line gives the center of the historical data (e.g., the mean of the prior distribution): an observed rate on the x-axis close to this line shows the Type I error rate and the power for situations in which the data on the original in the new study approximately match the historical data. In contrast, if the observed rate of the characteristic of interest is, for example, at a position on the x-axis of 0.8, this refers to the operating characteristics for a scenario with a clear prior-data conflict. The proposal of Mielke et al. (2018c) is to control the Type I error rate only for scenarios with a good to moderate fit of historical data and data in a new study which is displayed in Fig. 3 as within the dashed vertical lines. This idea is motivated by the understanding that since the originator is already an established product, there exists a rich collection of knowledge about the originator which can be used for planning a study which might not be identical, but at least would provide results similar to those from previous studies. Outside of the chosen interval, an increased Type I error rate and a lower power are acceptable since one is certain that the true estimates will not lie outside of the chosen interval. Mielke et al. (2018c) proposed a hybrid Bayes-frequentist methodology for binary endpoints which has the above-described operating characteristics.

The incorporation of information gathered during early development (preclinic, animal, and human PK and PD) is less straightforward. Combest et al. (2014) proposed constructing an informative prior for the efficacy assessment based on preclinical data. However, the proposal is rather vague and does not give any detailed information on the underlying methodology. The main challenge for an approach like this will, most likely, be the connection of the preclinical assessment with the clinical result: in contrast to the previously discussed examples where the same endpoint was measured in the historical study as in the new efficacy study, it is here necessary to combine completely different pieces of evidence. For example, the preclinical result may be the result of a bioassay, but the clinical endpoint is a binary endpoint (responder, nonresponder). Then, one needs to establish a link between the different measurements, that is, how does a difference of, for example 0.2 from the bioassay, relate to the chance of being a responder or nonresponder. Often, the connection between preclinical and clinical results is not known and therefore even the establishing of equivalence margins for the most critical quality attributes is not straightforward. That is why the aim to include information from early development into the clinical efficacy studies is interesting, but ambitious and more research is required.

Operational Challenges in Biosimilar Development

In the previous sections, challenges related to the design and analysis of biosimilar trials were described. However, it is important to emphasize that there exists also multiple challenges which are not related to these aspects. In the following, some of these aspects are briefly discussed.

Due to the complex nature of the processes needed to manufacture a biologic, the batches of the drug that are produced over a given time period may vary in terms of their exact analytical properties. This is understood by regulators and manufacturers are expected to run so-called comparability studies at regular intervals to ensure that critical quality attributes of the biologic are maintained within agreed limits (ICH 2004). Over time, the manufacturer builds up a history of how batches vary over time, but this knowledge is not available to the developer of a biosimilar. The only knowledge that the biosimilar developer has comes from analysis of batches of the original biologic that are purchased on the open market. So, in some sense, the biosimilar developer is having to chase a moving target in terms of showing analytical similarity (Step 1 in Fig. 1). See Schiestl et al. (2011) and Mielke et al. (2019) for examples and further discussion on this. See Berkowitz (2017) for a more complete discussion of issues related to the structural assessment of biosimilarity.

As some biologics have a long half-life, this may preclude the use of cross-over trials to show equivalence of PK and PD markers for certain active substances. Therefore, parallel groups trials have to be used and these typically have much larger sample size requirements compared to those needed for providing evidence of equivalence of a nonbiologic (generic) drug with its reference using a cross-over trial.

Another challenge related to recruitment, mentioned by Weschler (2016), is that experienced clinical investigators might prefer to be involved in the development of innovative drugs rather than in the development of copies of existing drugs. This might limit the number of research centers that are available to take part in a biosimilar study.

Once the biosimilar has gained regulatory approval and is on the market, a further challenge is to convince physicians to prescribe the new drug. In addition, patients need to agree to use the biosimilar instead of the originator product. Surveys studying the level of awareness of physicians and patients regarding biosimilars indicated that the understanding of the concept of biosimilarity still needs to be improved (Cohen et al. 2016; Jacobs et al. 2016). See Blackstone and Fuhr Jr (2017), for example, for further discussion on issues related to competition in the biologic and biosimilar market.

Summary and Conclusion

This chapter provided an overview of the necessary steps of a biosimilar development program: in contrast to the development of generics, biosimilar development is a complex, expensive, and time-consuming procedure which consists of analytical, nonclinical, and clinical studies. All evidence is combined using the concept of "totality of the evidence" which means that there is not one pivotal study, but all steps in the development program are considered important. The final decision as to whether approve or reject a proposed biosimilar is based on scientific judgment by taking into account all provided evidence. Clearly, this requires a multidisciplinary team which is able to weight the very different pieces of evidence. Due to the lack of experience with biosimilars, the FDA announced that there will be an advisory committee for the first biosimilar for each originator (Brennan 2016).

Biosimilar development worldwide is not harmonized yet and each regulatory authority has its own regulations and guidelines. The main hurdles for global biosimilar development are, however, not the different regulatory requirements, but that regulatory agencies usually prefer studies which give a head-to-head comparison of the originator product (one that is approved in the respective region) and the proposed biosimilar. Nonetheless, many sponsors are not keen on conducting several separate biosimilar development programs (one per region), but one global development program and to use this global development program for approval worldwide (e.g., Webster and Woollett 2017). The key to global biosimilar development is the idea of bridging: one or several studies are conducted which establish the comparability between the biosimilar, the originator which is used in most studies (e.g., the EU-sourced originator) and the local originator (e.g., the USA-sourced product). The focus is then not only on establishing similarity between biosimilar and originator, but also on the showing of comparability of the two originator products. This approach is compatible with the FDA's requirement to compare (if not justified that any of these is not necessary) using "analytical studies and at least one clinical PK study and, if appropriate, at least one PD study" (FDA 2015b) directly against the FDA approved originator product. Animal and therapeutic equivalence studies might be performed using a non-USA-licensed originator product if the bridge between this originator product and the USA originator product has been established. The European regulations are slightly different: the comparability exercise on the analytical level needs to be conducted against an originator which is authorized in the EU. In contrast, it is explicitly stated that the clinical and in vivo nonclinical studies may be conducted with a non-EU originator if the relevance of this non-EU originator has been demonstrated in bridging studies (CHMP 2014b).

In practice, global development programs are becoming more common. From the recently approved applications in Europe, many used a strategy with bridging at the PK level (Mielke et al. 2018a). Herzuma (Celltrion Healthcare, active substance: trastuzumab) was the first approved product in Europe where bridging studies were only conducted at the analytical level and no head-to-head comparisons of the EU-approved originator to the proposed biosimilar in human subjects were performed (i. e., no PK, PD, clinical comparability, and safety studies were conducted).

In this chapter, also some key statistical challenges were highlighted (the choice of equivalence margins, the establishing of interchangeability, and the formal incorporation of additional information into the analysis of efficacy endpoints). These key challenges can certainly only be seen as a short introduction to statistical issues in biosimilar development and there exists several other important topics to be considered, for example, the handling of multiplicity (e.g., Mielke et al. 2018b), the use of statistics in preclinical development (e.g. Tsong et al. 2017; Mielke et al. 2019), or the application of advanced statistical tools like network meta-analysis for an improved efficacy assessment (e.g., Messori et al. 2017). With the increasing number of approved biosimilars, the number of tailored statistical methodologies developed specific for biosimilar development is expected to further increase in the near future.

Key Facts

Biosimilars are developed as copies of already approved, innovative, large-molecule drugs which can be sold after the patent of the originator has expired. The development and approval of biosimilars differs substantially from the development of generics (copies of small-molecule drugs). Regulators recommend a step-wise approach which consists of comparisons of structural and functional characteristics of the molecules, nonclinical studies, and clinical studies. The data from these studies is in most cases analyzed with an equivalence testing approach. Since biosimilars are a fairly new concept, there exists still many open questions; not only in terms of tailored statistical methodology, but also in terms of regulatory guidance. More research is required to make biosimilar development more efficient.

Cross-References

▶ Cross-over Trials
▶ Essential Statistical Tests
▶ Introduction to Meta-Analysis
▶ Pharmacokinetic and Pharmacodynamic Modeling
▶ Use of Historical Data in Design

Acknowledgements The authors gratefully acknowledge the funding from the European Union's Horizon 2020 research and innovation programme under the Marie Sklodowska-Curie grant agreement No 633567 and from the Swiss State Secretariat for Education, Research and Innovation (SERI) under contract number 999754557. The opinions expressed and arguments employed herein do not necessarily reflect the official views of the Swiss Government.

References

Arato T (2016) Japanese regulation of biosimilar products: past experience and current challenges. Br J Clin Pharmacol 82(1):30–40

Barlas S (2017) FDA guidance on biosimilar interchangeability elicits diverse views: current and potential marketers complain about too-high hurdles. Pharm Ther 42(8):509

Benucci M, Gobbi FL, Bandinelli F, Damiani A, Infantino M, Grossi V, Manfredi M, Parisi S, Fusaro E, Batticciotto A et al (2017) Safety, efficacy and immunogenicity of switching from innovator to biosimilar infliximab in patients with spondyloarthritis: a 6-month real-life observational study. Immunol Res 65(1):419–422

Berkowitz SA (2017) Analytical characterization: structural assessment of biosimilarity, Chap 2. In: Endrenyi L, Declerck P, Chow SC (eds) Biosimilar drug product development. CRC Press, Boca Raton, pp 15–82

Bewesdorff M (2016) Biosimilars in the U.S. – the long way to their first approval. Master of drug regulatory affairs, Rheinischen Friedrich-Wilhelms-Universitat Bonn

Blackstone E, Fuhr JP Jr (2017) Biosimilars and biologics. The prospect for competition, Chap 16. In: Endrenyi L, Declerck P, Chow SC (eds) Biosimilar drug product development. CRC Press, Boca Raton, pp 413–438

Brennan Z (2016) FDA to hold one advisory committee for each initial biosimilar. https://www.raps.org/regulatory-focus%E2%84%A2/news-articles/2016/9/fda-to-hold-one-advisory-committee-for-each-initial-biosimilar. Accessed 07 June 2018

Cazap E, Jacobs I, McBride A, Popovian R, Sikora K (2018) Global acceptance of biosimilars: importance of regulatory consistency, education, and trust. Oncologist 23:1188

CHMP (2005) Guideline on the choice of non-inferiority margins. http://www.ema.europa.eu/docs/en_GB/document_library/Scientific_guideline/2009/09/WC500003636.pdf. Accessed 07 June 2018

CHMP (2008) Zarzio: EPAR public assessment report. http://www.ema.europa.eu/docs/en_GB/document_library/EPAR_-_Public_assessment_report/human/000917/WC500046528.pdf. Accessed 26 Oct 2015

CHMP (2014a) Guideline on similar biological medicinal products containing biotechnology-derived proteins as active substance: non-clinical and clinical issues (revision 1). http://www.ema.europa.eu/docs/en_GB/document_library/Scientific_guideline/2015/01/WC500180219.pdf. Accessed 22 Feb 2018

CHMP (2014b) Guideline on similar biological medicinal products (revision 1). http://www.ema.europa.eu/docs/en_GB/document_library/Scientific_guideline/2014/10/WC500176768.pdf. Accessed 22 Feb 2018

CHMP (2016) Benepali: EPAR – public assessment report. http://www.ema.europa.eu/docs/en_GB/document_library/EPAR_-_Public_assessment_report/human/004007/WC500200380.pdf. Accessed 07 June 2018

CHMP (2017) Amgevita: EPAR – public assessment report. http://www.ema.europa.eu/docs/en_GB/document_library/EPAR_-_Public_assessment_report/human/004212/WC500225231.pdf. Accessed 07 June 2018

Chow SC, Hsieh TC, Chi E, Yang J (2009) A comparison of moment-based and probability-based criteria for assessment of follow-on biologics. J Biopharm Stat 20(1):31–45

Christl LA (2018) From our perspective: interchangeable biological products. https://www.fda.gov/Drugs/NewsEvents/ucm536528.htm. Accessed 22 Feb 2018

Christl LA, Woodcock J, Kozlowski S (2017) Biosimilars: the US regulatory framework. Annu Rev Med 68(1):243–254

Cohen H, Beydoun D, Chien D, Lessor T, McCabe D, Muenzberg M, Popovian R, Uy J (2016) Awareness, knowledge, and perceptions of biosimilars among specialty physicians. Adv Ther 33(12):2160–2172

Combest A, Wang S, Healey B, Reitsma DJ (2014) Alternative statistical strategies for biosimilar drug development. GaBI J 3(1):13–20

Crommelin D, Bermejo T, Bissig M, Damiaans J, Krämer I, Rambourg P, Scroccaro G, Strukelj B, Tredree R (2005) Pharmaceutical evaluation of biosimilars: important differences from generic low-molecularweight pharmaceuticals. Eur J Hosp Pharm Sci 11(1):11–17

EMA (2012) Questions and answers on biosimilar medicines (similar biological medicinal products). http://www.medicinesforeurope.com/2012/09/27/ema-questions-and-answers-on-biosimilar-medicines-similar-biological-medicinal. Accessed 22 Feb 2018

FDA (2009) Biologics price competition and innovation act. http://www.fda.gov/downloads/Drugs/GuidanceComplianceRegulatoryInformation/ucm216146.pdf. Accessed 22 Feb 2018

FDA (2015a) Sandoz briefing book for application to market zarxio. https://patentdocs.typepad.com/files/briefing-document.pdf. Accessed 11 Jan 2019

FDA (2015b) Scientific considerations in demonstrating biosimilarity to a reference product. https://www.fda.gov/downloads/Drugs/GuidanceComplianceRegulatoryInformation/Guidances/UCM291128.pdf. Accessed 05 June 2018

FDA (2016) Clinical pharmacology data to support a demonstration of biosimilarity to a reference product. https://www.fda.gov/downloads/Drugs/GuidanceComplianceRegulatoryInformation/Guidances/UCM397017.pdf. Accessed 05 June 2018

FDA (2017a) Biological product definitions. https://www.fda.gov/downloads/Drugs/DevelopmentApprovalProcess/HowDrugsareDevelopedandApproved/ApprovalApplications/TherapeuticBiologicApplications/Biosimilars/UCM581282.pdf. Accessed 05 June 2018

FDA (2017b) Considerations in demonstrating interchangeability with a reference product. https://www.fda.gov/downloads/Drugs/GuidanceComplianceRegulatoryInformation/Guidances/UCM537135.pdf. Accessed 22 Feb 2018

FDA (2018) FDA withdraws draft guidance for industry: statistical approaches to evaluate analytical similarity. https://www.fda.gov/Drugs/DrugSafety/ucm611398.htm. Accessed 17 Jul 2018

Felson DT, Anderson JJ, Boers M, Bombardier C, Chernoff M, Fried B, Furst D, Goldsmith C, Kieszak S, Lightfoot R et al (1993) The American College of Rheumatology preliminary core set of disease activity measures for rheumatoid arthritis clinical trials. Arthritis Rheumatol 36(6):729–740

Finckh A, Bansback N, Marra CA, Anis AH, Michaud K, Lubin S, White M, Sizto S, Liang MH (2009) Treatment of very early rheumatoid arthritis with symptomatic therapy, disease-modifying antirheumatic drugs, or biologic agents: a cost-effectiveness analysis. Ann Intern Med 151 (9):612–621

Health Affairs Health Policy Brief (2013) Biosimilars. https://www.healthaffairs.org/do/10.1377/hpb20131010.6409/full/. Accessed 05 June 2018

Holzmann J, Balser S, Windisch J (2016) Totality of the evidence at work: the first U.S. biosimilar. Expert Opin Biol Ther 16(2):137–142

Hsieh TC, Chow SC, Yang LY, Chi E (2013) The evaluation of biosimilarity index based on reproducibility probability for assessing follow-on biologics. Stat Med 32(3):406–414

Hsu JC, Hwang JTG, Liu HK, Ruberg SJ (1994) Confidence intervals associated with tests for bioequivalence. Biometrika 81(1):103–114

Hung A, Vu Q, Mostovoy L (2017) A systematic review of US biosimilar approvals: what evidence does the FDA require and how are manufacturers responding? J Manag Care Spec Pharm 23(12):1234–1244

ICH (2004) Comparability of biotechnological/biological products subject to changes in their manufacturing process, Q5E

Jacobs I, Singh E, Sewell KL, Al-Sabbagh A, Shane LG (2016) Patient attitudes and understanding about biosimilars: an international cross-sectional survey. Patient Prefer Adherence 10:937–948

Jones B, Kenward M (2014) Design and analysis of cross-over trials, 3rd edn. Chapman & Hall/ CRC monographs on statistics & applied probability. Taylor & Francis. https://books.google.ch/ books?id=tuisBAAAQBAJ

Jørgensen KK, Olsen IC, Goll GL, Lorentzen M, Bolstad N, Haavardsholm EA, Lundin KE, Mørk C, Jahnsen J, Kvien TK et al (2017) Switching from originator infliximab to biosimilar CT-P13 compared with maintained treatment with originator infliximab (NOR-SWITCH): a 52-week, randomised, double-blind, noninferiority trial. Lancet 389(10086):2304–2316

Li J, Chow SC (2017) Statistical evaluation of the scaled criterion for drug interchangeability. J Biopharm Stat 27(2):282–292

Messori A, Trippoli S, Marinai C (2017) Network meta-analysis as a tool for improving the effectiveness assessment of biosimilars based on both direct and indirect evidence: application to infliximab in rheumatoid arthritis. Eur J Clin Pharmacol 73(4):513. https://doi.org/10.1007/ s00228-016-2177-z

Mielke J, Jilma B, Koenig F, Jones B (2016) Clinical trials for authorized biosimilars in the European Union: a systematic review. Br Clin Pharmacol 82(6):1444–1457

Mielke J, Jilma B, Jones B, Koenig F (2018a) An update on the clinical evidence that supports biosimilar approvals in Europe. Br Clin Pharmacol 84(7):1415–1431

Mielke J, Jones B, Jilma B, König F (2018b) Sample size for multiple hypothesis testing in biosimilar development. Stat Biopharm Res 10(1):39–49

Mielke J, Schmidli H, Jones B (2018c) Incorporating historical information in biosimilar trials: challenges and a hybrid Bayesian-frequentist approach. Biom J 60(3):564–582

Mielke J, Woehling H, Jones B (2018d) Longitudinal assessment of the impact of multiple switches between a biosimilar and its reference product on efficacy parameters. Pharm Stat 17(3):231–247

Mielke J, Innerbichler F, Schiestl M, Ballarini NM, Jones B (2019) The assessment of quality attributes for biosimilars: a statistical perspective on current practice and a proposal. AAPS J 21:7

Moorkens E, Vulto AG, Huys I, Dylst P, Godman B, Keuerleber S, Claus B, Dimitrova M, Petrova G, Sović-Brkičić L et al (2017) Policies for biosimilar uptake in Europe: an overview. PLoS One 12(12):e0190147

Pan H, Yuan Y, Xia J (2017) A calibrated power prior approach to borrow information from historical data with application to biosimilar clinical trials. J R Stat Soc Ser C Appl Stat 66(5):979–996

Schellekens H, Moors E (2015) Biosimilars or semi-similars? Nat Biotechnol 33(1):19–20

Schiestl M, Stangler T, Torella C, Cepeljnik T, Toll H, Grau R (2011) Acceptable changes in quality attributes of glycosylated biopharmaceuticals. Nat Biotechnol 29:310–312

Schiestl M, Li J, Abas A, Vallin A, Millband J, Gao K, Joung J, Pluschkell S, Go T, Kang HN (2014) The role of the quality assessment in the determination of overall biosimilarity: a simulated case study exercise. Biologicals 42(2):128–132

Schoergenhofer C, Schwameis M, Firbas C, Bartko J, Derhaschnig U, Mader RM, Plaßmann RS, Jilma-Stohlawetz P, Desai K, Misra P et al (2018) Single, very low rituximab doses in healthy volunteers-a pilot and a randomized trial: implications for dosing and biosimilarity testing. Sci Rep 8(1):124

Schuirmann DJ (1987) A comparison of the two one-sided tests procedure and the power approach for assessing the equivalence of average bioavailability. J Pharmacokinet Biopharm 15(6):657–680

Tsong Y, Dong X, Shen M (2017) Development of statistical methods for analytical similarity assessment. J Biopharm Stat 27(2):197–205

Tsou HH, Chang WJ, Hwang WS, Lai YH (2013) A consistency approach for evaluation of biosimilar products. J Biopharm Stat 23(5):1054–1066 van Rosmalen J, Dejardin D, van Norden Y, Lwenberg B, Lesaffre E (2017) Including historical data in the analysis of clinical trials: is it worth the effort? Statistical methods in medical research. https://www.ncbi.nlm.nih.gov/pubmed/28322129

Webster CJ, Woollett GR (2017) A 'global reference' comparator for biosimilar development. BioDrugs 31(4):279–286

Weise M, Kurki P, Wolff-Holz E, Bielsky MC, Schneider CK (2014) Biosimilars: the science of extrapolation. Blood 124(22):3191–3196

Wellek S (2010) Testing statistical hypotheses of equivalence and noninferiority, 2nd edn. CRC Press, London

Weschler B (2016) Biosimilar trials differ notably from innovator studies. Appl Clin Trials. http://www.appliedclinicaltrialsonline.com/biosimilar-trials-differ-notably-innovator-studies

Prevention Trials: Challenges in Design, Analysis, and Interpretation of Prevention Trials

67

Shu Jiang and Graham A. Colditz

Contents

Abstract

Designing a prevention trial requires understanding the natural history of the disease, and the likely length of intervention required to achieve a reduction in incidence. The population suitable to contribute meaningful information to the outcomes under study, the intervention is appropriate and likely will generate a balance of risks and benefits for the typically disease free population, and the primary outcome is biologically plausible and clinically relevant. Given the

S. Jiang · G. A. Colditz (✉)
Division of Public Health Sciences, Department of Surgery, Washington University School of Medicine, Saint Louis, MO, USA
e-mail: jiang.shu@wustl.edu; colditzg@wustl.edu

© Springer Nature Switzerland AG 2022

S. Piantadosi, C. L. Meinert (eds.), *Principles and Practice of Clinical Trials*,
https://doi.org/10.1007/978-3-319-52636-2_96

relatively long evolution of chronic diseases, prevention trials bring extra pressures on two fundamental issues in the design of the trial: adherence to the preventive intervention among participants who are otherwise healthy, and sustained follow-up of trial participants. With growing emphasis on the composition of the trial participant population reflecting the overall population for ultimate application of the results, there is the need for additional attention to recruitment and retention of participants. This is fundamental to planning a prevention trial. Planning for follow-up after the intervention is completed helps place the intervention and outcomes in the context of the disease process but adds complexity to recruitment. Never the less this adds to insights from prevention trials. Improving risk stratification for identification of eligible participants for recruitment to prevention trials can improve efficiency of the trials and fit prevention trials in the context of precision prevention.

Keywords

Participants · Baseline risk · Diversity: natural history · Sustainability · Intervention timing · Adherence

Introduction

The majority of chronic diseases can be prevented through a combination of lifestyle and preventive medications, and in some settings vaccines and screening or early detection. In 2002 the leading chronic diseases were cardiovascular disease, cancer, chronic respiratory disease, and diabetes accounting for a combined 29 million deaths (Yach et al. 2004). Yet effective interventions to prevent these chronic diseases are often lacking. One central challenge for understanding the impact of prevention strategies for chronic disease is the placing of change in exposure in the time course of disease development. The level and sources of evidence supporting change in individual exposure to reduce disease risk, or to prevent chronic illnesses, vary substantially across both lifestyle exposures and chronic diseases that are a focus of prevention interventions. We focus on design and interpretation trials of such interventions here. We do not address the design issues in screening trials (see ▶ Chap. 65, "Screening Trials"), nor do we tackle cluster randomized trials (see ▶ Chap. 77, "Cluster Randomized Trials") which are increasingly used in implementation science studies, where the intervention such as changes in provider and patient behaviors (in clinical settings or schools, for example) may cluster study subjects with the clinic or classroom, and these may also be clustered within health systems for school districts, leading to multiple levels of clustering with implications for design, size, intervention delivery and outcome evaluation as well as analysis.

In this chapter, we consider several key factors that bear on the design and interpretation of prevention trials. These factors include (1) the population in which the intervention can be evaluated efficiently; (2) the underlying disease process; (3) key components of the intervention and comparison/control intervention; and (4) the outcome. For interventions we consider (a) sustainability of the behavior change, (b) the time course of the intervention within the disease process, (c) the dose, (d) the duration of "exposure" needed to effect risk reduction, and (e) the durability of the impact of the intervention after it has stopped. Issues of adherence to the intervention and approaches to analysis also impact the inference from prevention trials when informing changes in policy and practice.

Trial Population

A key assumption for enrolling participants in a trial is that they will contribute meaningful information to the outcome measures and that they are likely to engage in the intervention for the duration of the study. Participant recruitment for prevention trials brings added challenges beyond enrolling patients facing acute disease or major catastrophic outcomes in the near term. The setting of disease treatment adds to issues when enrolling participants as likely adherence is high to treatment options and the balance of risks and benefits can be conveyed in time frames that relate to the patient situation at hand. For primary prevention trials, however, we begin enrolling healthy individuals who may be at risk of future disease and engage them for longer term adherence to prevention strategies (pills, behaviors, or combinations) to observed endpoints off in the future. This challenge of recruitment to prevention trials has resulted in a number of trials where the prevalence of baseline behaviors results in population not ideally selected to evaluate the intervention (see Physicians Health Study of aspirin to prevent cardiovascular death, and very low cardiovascular disease incidence (Cairns et al. 1991)) or calcium and vitamin D in the Women's Health Initiative where baseline calcium was above the threshold of benefit as determined from observational studies(Martinez et al. 2008). On the other hand, the trials evaluating Tamoxifen for breast cancer prevention used a baseline estimate of breast cancer risk to identify women at elevated risk and so shift the balance of risks and benefits for those randomized (Fisher et al. 1998). Similar issues are discussed in ▶ Chap. 112, "Trials Can Inform or Misinform: "The Story of Vitamin A Deficiency and Childhood Mortality"").

Eligibility and enrollment of the study population may also limit the application of results beyond the trial. This issue is not limited to primary prevention of course, but is also demonstrated with exclusion based on older age, or presence of major comorbidities, that limit generalizability and application of results (see Stoll et al. (2019), and pragmatic trials (Ware and Hamel 2011)).

Beyond disease severity, risk factor profiles and the like, many clinical trials are underpopulated with minority participants (Chen et al. 2014). This is due, in part, to eligibility criteria, and lack of engagement strategies tailored to minorities. Evidence shows that concerted efforts to modify eligibility to include broader populations of patients, and use of culturally tailored materials and processes, result in increased research and trial accruals of minorities and their retention through the duration of the trial (Warner et al. 2013). Thus, to generate results applicable to the broader population, design of trials should increase eligibility to populations with multiple comorbidities as experienced by populations with cancer disparities, and promote the development of patient engagement approaches tailored to minority and underserved populations.

The Disease Process and Identifying a Population at Risk Who Can Benefit from a Preventive Intervention

Epidemiologic and natural history studies often define risk factors and provide input to models that classify risk of chronic disease. In defining the population for recruitment to a prevention trial, the aim is to identify those with sufficiently high risk of disease based on a combination of risk factors so that the benefit from a preventive intervention will outweigh any possible adverse effects of the intervention. Thus, selection of participants is in part driven by baseline disease risk being sufficient to generate a research answer in a short funding time frame. For example, after numerous meetings convened by NIH to discuss trial design for weight loss to prevent chronic disease, NIDDK choose to move forward with a prevention trial of intensive lifestyle intervention to prevent or delay development of diabetes (Knowler et al. 2002).

Numerous examples from prior trials show that healthy volunteers are not necessarily at sufficient risk to generate endpoints from the intervention. Improving risk classification for entry to prevention trials is a major imperative. Much work is ongoing in this area to more precisely define at risk groups whether by combing questionnaire risk factors, polygenic risk scores, or metabolomic profiles to differentiate those who might respond to a prevention intervention and those who will not.

Take for example breast cancer where chemoprevention shows marked differences between prevention receptor positive and negative breast cancer. Overall selective estrogen receptor modulators (SERMs) such as Tamoxifen and Raloxifene have been shown in randomized controlled prevention trials to reduce risk of preinvasive and invasive breast cancer (Fisher et al. 1998; Martino et al. 2004). The separation of incidence curves is dramatic and clear within 2 years of initiating therapy. Like aspirin, SERMs also raise the challenge of risks and benefits of therapies as well as the limitation of randomized trials to quantify potential harms that are much less frequent than the primary trial end point. Tamoxifen increases risk of uterine cancer, a finding confirmed by epidemiologic studies; Raloxifene, which looks to have a safer profile, does not (Chen et al. 2007). Yet the protection is limited to receptor positive disease. Thus, either identifying and enrolling those who are at highest risk of receptor positive but not receptor negative breast cancer could maximize benefits and reduce potential harms.

The emerging field of personalized medicine has been offering possibilities for improving risk prediction and stratification based on patient-specific demographic, clinical factors, medical histories, and genetic profile. Models that are tailored for patients have provided high-quality recommendations for screening accounting for individualized heterogeneity (Sargent et al. 2005). Traditional approaches usually aim to investigate evidence of treatment differences by conducting subgroup analysis based on prior data to gain insights on markers that can better stratify patients according to their risk level. Other approaches include regression models which usually include interaction terms between treatments and the covariates in order to examine whether these interactions are statistically significant as well as estimating the true (undiluted) benefit of the intervention. Effective classification of patients can thus be translated into statistical models which aim to minimize the prediction error, where the optimal risk classifier can lead to the best predicted outcome.

Components of Intervention

Interventions for prevention range from a one (or two) time events (some vaccines), to longer term use of preventive drugs such as aspirin, nutritional supplements, or the polypill for cardiovascular diseases (Yusuf et al. 2021), and lifestyle changes (components of diet, physical activity, sun exposure) (Knowler et al. 2002). The components of the intervention have major implications for the design and cost of prevention trials and the ultimate interpretation of the results as discussed in the next sections.

The control or comparison intervention generates similar challenges for designing and implementing a trial. If usual care is the comparison such as the Hypertension Detection Follow-up Program in the 1970s (1979), or Health Insurance Plan of New York mammography trial (Shapiro et al. 1985), the control arm may seek out the intervention and dilute the comparison. Similar issues arose in the Women's Health Initiative trial discussed below.

Sustainability of the Behavior Change

For lifestyle intervention to change diet, physical activity, or other aspects of our lifestyle such as transportation and commuting, many issues arise related to sustainability of the intervention and its associated lifestyle changes, and use of approaches to document adherence.

Adherence to interventions has not been high in long-term primary prevention trials. The Tamoxifen breast cancer prevention trial (P1) was designed allowing 10% of women/year to discontinue Tamoxifen therapy, though the observed noncompliance was lower 23.7% of women randomized to Tamoxifen stopped their therapy during the trial vs 19.7% of the placebo group (Fisher et al. 1998). In the Women's Health Initiative evaluation of menopausal hormone therapy, drop out was 42% for estrogen plus progestin and 38% for placebo. This exceeded the design projections. Of note, women in the placebo group initiated hormone use through their own clinical providers (10.7% by the sixth year) (Rossouw et al. 2002). Similar adherence issues apply for diet interventions. In the low-fat diet intervention in the Women's' Health Initiative a total of 48,835 postmenopausal women were randomized to the dietary intervention (40%) or the comparison group (60%). The intervention promoted dietary change with a goal of reducing intake of total fat to 20% of energy. Concomitant with this the participants would increase consumption of vegetables and fruit to at least five servings daily, and also increase their intake of grains to six servings daily. Estimated adherence in the intervention group was 57% at year 3, 31% at year 6, and 19% at year 9, substantially lower than the adherence in the comparison group (Prentice et al. 2006). Given the challenges of sustained behavior change in otherwise healthy trial participants, adaptations of technology such as text messaging and more real time feedback have been studied as adjuncts to motivating and sustaining lifestyle changes (Wolin et al. 2015). There is much research ongoing to identify the most effective strategies to motivate and sustain participation and adherence for different populations based on gender, age, and race/ethnicity. As technology continues to evolve, and access increases, additional insights should improve the design and interpretation of prevention trials.

One strategy that has been used to improved adherence in trial participants is the active run-in phase before randomization. For example, in the physicians health study, a randomized trial of aspirin and beta carotene to prevent heart disease and cancer, and active run in facilitated identification of those with an adverse tolerance of every other day aspirin.

Beyond examples such as these, and the continuing research to adapt and improve approaches to enroll and sustain adherence to interventions over prolonged time periods, adherence in prevention trials has major implications for design, analysis and interpretation of trial results as discussed below.

The Time Course of the Intervention Within the Disease Process

Interpreting null results in prevention trials begs the question of whether the intervention was delivered at an appropriate time in the disease process, or whether dose and duration of the intervention were chosen correctly. First, we consider the timing of the intervention.

The null RCTs of fiber and fruit and vegetables for prevention of polyp recurrence amply illustrate Zelen's concerns about the timing of the preventive intervention in the disease process. Randomized trials of fiber and fruit and vegetables in the prevention of colon polyp recurrence have not shown any benefit from increased intake (Alberts et al. 2000; Schatzkin et al. 2000). Furthermore, in prevention trials addressing recurrence of polyps, the extent of DNA damage accumulated across the colonic mucosa at the time the eligibility polyp is detected certainly is not limited to only the removed polyp. Thus we must ask of RCTs, at what stage in the disease process may fiber play a role in protecting against colon cancer? Constraints of design in RCTs usually limit to a narrow time point and defined dose of exposure (and specific duration), which contrast with the richness of epidemiologic studies that can address exposure over the life course and relate such exposure to disease risk.

Other nutritional agents have also been tested in chemoprevention trials in the developed world and in China (Greenwald et al. 2007). Based on evidence documenting that people in Linxian, China, had low intakes of several nutrients, a randomized trial comparing combinations of retinol, zinc, riboflavin, niacin, vitamin C and molybdenum, beta-carotene, vitamin E, and selenium was undertaken (Blot et al. 1993). Significant reductions in mortality were observed for those who received the combination of beta-carotene, vitamin E, and selenium (factor D), and the reduction was greater for those who began the therapy at a younger age. These results again emphasize the importance of the timing of exposure in the disease process.

Stratification of the results by sex and age was planned a priori. There were no statistically significant interactions with sex. However, when stratified by age, factor D had a strong protective effect in individuals under age 55 but demonstrated almost no effect in subjects aged 55 years or older (Qiao et al. 2009). This pattern was seen consistently for total mortality, total cancer mortality, gastric cancer mortality, and esophageal cancer mortality. Indeed, the effect of factor D on esophageal cancer was reversed by age, showing a protective effect for younger individuals but a harmful effect for older individuals. Further insight into the timing in the carcinogenic process is provided by a separate RCT in Linxian (Limburg et al. 2005), which gave further support for a preventive effect of selenium in subjects with preexisting esophageal squamous dysplasia, the precursor lesion of esophageal squamous cell carcinoma. Compared with control subjects, those with mild dysplasia who received 10 months of daily supplementation with 200 μg of selenomethionine were more likely to have regression and less likely to have progression of their esophageal squamous dysplasia.

Clear a priori definition of an analytic framework to address possible mis-specification of timing in the natural history of the disease is an essential step to position the trial analysis to address this issue of the underlying disease process.

The Dose

Often investigators move from treatment trials showing efficacy for an agent on disease outcomes to then apply the agent for prevention. This sequence has been followed in examples such as aspirin and CHD; tamoxifen and breast cancer prevention, to name a few. In both heart disease and breast cancer prevention lower doses have been chosen for prevention in part to avoid potential adverse events that accumulate in the healthy population taking a drug to prevent future disease onset.

In breast cancer prevention the dose of Tamoxifen has been reduced to minimize menopausal symptoms and now shows significant benefits with reduction in breast cancer events (DeCensi et al. 2019) and also in breast density a marker of breast cancer risk (Eriksson et al. 2021). If we have more markers of response, we might shorten the time frame from development of these trials to endpoint ascertainment. Prevention trials typically are large, expensive, and of long duration, because we are interrupting a slow disease process – e.g., chronic disease.

The initial Tamoxifen P1 breast cancer prevention trial screened 98,018 women identifying 57,641 risk eligible women and randomized 13,388 participants to determine the worth of Tamoxifen in preventing breast cancer in women with 5-year risk above 1.66%. Cumulative incidence through 69 months was 43.4/1000 women in placebo group and 22.0/1000 in the Tamoxifen group (total 175 invasive cases). This trail cost $64 million (without costs for participant enrolment, follow-up visits, or drug/placebo). Subsequent trials compared Raloxifene and Tamoxifen (Martino et al. 2004), costing $134 million, and investigators secured drug and $30 million from Novartis for the STELLAR trial (study to evaluate Letrozole and Raloxifene but NCI withdrew support at the level of $55 million (The Lancet 2007; Parker-Pope 2007).

The need to balance benefits against adverse effects from interventions in otherwise healthy populations places emphasis on determining the lowest possible does to achieve benefit and reduce risk of adverse side effects. An earlier exploration of response at lower doses of possible preventive agents may speed the move to large scale prevention or phase 3 trials. Lower dose reduces risk of adverse events in many settings, but a sufficient framework for evaluation of response by dose, including biomarkers or risk profiles would speed the path to efficient prevention trials. Promising options in precision-based approaches include prostaglandin pathways, BRAF and HLA class 1 antigen expression, among others (Jaffee et al. 2017).

The Duration of "Exposure/Intervention" Needed to Produce Risk Reduction

Dose and duration of intervention are typically informed a priori by observational data. Given the complexity of implementing a primary prevention RCT, the importance of choosing the correct dose and duration for the intervention is imperative. Two factors interplay here contributing to the cumulative exposure and the lag from the exposure to the observed benefit. This determination again requires consideration of risks and benefits because adverse effects of most therapeutic interventions cannot be completely avoided.

Trials for prevention have often focused on enrolling high-risk participants – often defined by family history of high penetrance genetic markers of risk. Such restriction to high-risk populations increases the incidence of the outcome of interest and so shortens the required duration (and cost) of the trial through improving power for a finite number of participants screened for eligibility, recruited, randomized and followed (when costs per participant are largely fixed). Largely due to the increase in contrast between the high-risk group and the control group in an RCT, fewer patients are usually required to reach the prespecified statistical power. This of course will be dependent on the actual context of the trial. On the other hand, the higher risk eligibility criteria may then limit the generalizability and applicability of the trial results. For broader prevention effectiveness consideration of the disease process and duration of "prevention" to achieve an observable reduction in incidence is essential to power a trial and use its results to estimate population benefit.

The Durability of the Impact of the Intervention After It Has Stopped

Drawing on examples from the breast cancer prevention trials and the China/Linxian trial – we see that to address the persistence of a prevention benefit after the cessation of the intervention requires planned additional follow-up beyond the primary hypothesis of the trial. If clearly defined as secondary hypothesis and analyses, then continued follow-up of trial participants can answer key questions of duration for the trial intervention, and further inform evaluation of risks and benefits for prevention.

The additional insight on prevention gained from the precise knowledge of exposure recorded in the randomized trial includes the added understanding of the disease process after cessation of a precisely measured intervention. Continued follow-up of trial participants has shown the durability of the effect of a prevention agent. In the Linxian trial, factor D, which included selenium, vitamin E, and beta-carotene, statistically significantly reduced total mortality, total cancer mortality, and mortality from gastric cancer (Blot et al. 1993). An important question remained, however: whether the preventive effects of factor D would last beyond the trial period. The results of the continued follow-up showed that hazard ratios (HRs), as indicated by moving HR curves, remained less than 1.0 for each of these end points for most of the follow-up period; 10 years after completion of the trial, the group that received factor D still showed a 5% reduction in total mortality and an 11% reduction in gastric cancer mortality (Qiao et al. 2009).

Similar insight on the duration of protection has been provided from continued follow-up of three tamoxifen trials, which showed benefit after the conclusion of active therapy (Fisher et al. 2005). The calcium polyp prevention trial also reported that the protection observed during the trial persisted for up to 5 years after supplementation ended and may, in fact, have been stronger after, rather than during, active intervention (Grau et al. 2007). With the exception of smoking cessation, cessation of exposure to occupational carcinogens, and termination of drug use, lifestyle factors (diet, energy balance, physical activity, sleep pattern or sun exposure) rarely have a clearly demarcated cessation, thus requiring observational studies to provide insight on the durability of effects and lag from exposure to disease. For pharmacologic interventions, on the other hand, long term follow-up is essential to fully determine risks and benefits (Cuzick 2010).

Outcomes for Prevention Trials

While the gold standard in prevention of chronic diseases may historically be reduction in mortality, evolving technologies, changes in detection, and treatment can bias estimates of prevention benefits. The initial community treatment of blood pressure was assessed in the hypertension detection and follow-up study, which screened over 150,000 adult 30–69 years of age to identify community living adults with hypertension. Randomization to stepped care treatment of hypertension or community care (usual care) showed 5-year mortality from all causes was significantly lower in the stepped care treatment arm compared to community care (1979). Evolving trial design and scientific agreement on more proximate endpoints reflects the evolution of understanding of the underlying disease processes and the priority for interventions that show benefits exceeding harms.

Debate regarding endpoints has included the focus on mortality reduction vs a reduction in incidence of disease. For example, the UK Doctors Study were designed to test whether aspirin 500 mg daily reduced incidence and mortality from stroke, myocardial infarction, or other vascular condition (Peto et al. 1988). The US Physicians Health Study evaluated second daily aspirin (325 mg) vs placebo randomizing 22,071 participants and following them for an average of 57 months (Steering Committee of the Physicians' Health Study Research 1988). Incident myocardial infarction was significantly reduced but mortality was equivalent in each arm (44 cardiovascular deaths). Subsequent reporting from the Data Monitoring Board demonstrated the futility of continuing the trial for a mortality benefit (Cairns et al. 1991). They present data on the substantially lower cardiovascular mortality than expected from age comparable population rates, consistent with baseline prevalence of current smoking at 12% (Glynn et al. 1994). Treatment of nonfatal myocardial infarction further complicated interpretation as demonstrated by Cook et al. (2002). While disease incidence is the primary endpoint for most prevention trials, design features and clinical diagnosis and treatment must be carefully monitored to avoid inducing bias in endpoint ascertainment.

The US FDA defines endpoints for drugs and biologics to be assessed as safe and effective. They consider clinical outcomes and surrogate endpoints. Surrogate endpoints are used when clinical outcomes might take a long time to study (think prevention trials of stroke, or cervical cancer, for example). The FDA now publishes a list of acceptable surrogate endpoints for both adult and childhood diseases (US Food and Drug Administration 2021). These are typically very strict surrogacy criteria to avoid apparent benefit for reduced clinical disease incidence when none is present. Across prevention trials the importance of outcome choice and rigor of confirmation applies in similar manner to the more general issues (see ▶ Chap. 47, "Ascertainment and Classification of Outcomes").

Analysis ITT and Adherence in Prevention Trials

Zelen considered the challenges of primary prevention trials in the 1980s and addressed both compliance and models of carcinogenesis as major impediments to the use of RCTs to evaluate cancer prevention strategies (Zelen 1988). It is important to contrast these issues in treatment trials and prevention trials. In treatment trials, we typically take recently diagnosed patients and offer them, often in a life-threatening situation, the option to participate in a trial of a new therapy compared with standard therapy or placebo. Compliance or adherence to therapy is usually very high among these highly motivated patients and outcomes are generally in a short to mid-term time frame. In contrast, prevention trials recruit large numbers of healthy participants, offer them a therapy, and then follow them over many years, since the chronic diseases being prevented are relatively rare. With substantial nonadherence – often in the range of 20–40% over the duration of the trial – an intention-to-treat analysis is no longer unbiased.

Issues in analysis using the a priori intention to treat plan (ITT) (see ▶ Chap. 82, "Intention to Treat and Alternative Approaches") and detailed approaches to modeling adherence over time in the prevention trial setting calls for rigorous details in the study protocol. Additional challenges that recur in the prevention trial setting include drop out and loss to follow-up that may be nondifferential, particularly in settings such as weight loss trials (Ware 2003). When endpoints such as weight loss or quality of life may reflect both engagement with the trial and adherence to the intervention, maximizing strategies to obtain endpoint data and retain participants in the study are fundamental to integrity of the trial results.

Many of the design issues, population, intervention and control arm, adherence and cost constraints come together to be balanced in the design of the trial. The protocol for most trial in the last 10 years have been posted online when the primary trials results are published. For older prevention trials, access to a full protocol, sample size considerations and so forth may be harder to locate. The Women's Health Initiative published their protocol (Writing Group 1998), and the Diabetes Prevention Program web site at the NIH (NIDDK) provides access to the study protocol with extensive details of a less complicate but still three arm design. The principle objective of the trial was to prevent or delay development of Non-Insulin Dependent Diabetes Mellitus (Type 2 diabetes) in persons at high risk with impaired glucose tolerance (Knowler et al. 2002; The Diabetes Prevention Program Research Group 1999). The protocol is available http://www.bsc.gwu.edu/dpp.

Biomarkers and Other Emerging Areas

The nature of many chronic disease prevention/interception interventions requires a very long timeline for assessment of effectiveness. Validated biomarkers to improve risk assessment, for example, to characterize "premalignancy" and to predict tumor aggressiveness remain active areas of research. In Alzheimer's disease (AD), for example, susceptibility to AD is determined by both monogenic and polygenic risk factors as well as environmental exposures. The evaluation of efficacy of interventions to treat AD is highly dependent on the selection of cognitively normal individuals years before the onset of AD. The need for biomarkers to predict responsiveness to various interventions, to serve as surrogate endpoints for intervention trials and to predict toxicities of prevention interventions also remain essential for progress in cancer prevention.

Artificial intelligence, analytics and applied statistics, engineering, and data science bring opportunities to speed precision medicine and precision prevention. A recent report from the National Academy of Medicine (NAM) reviews and highlights opportunities, promises, and perils in application of AI in health care (Matheny et al. 2019).

For prevention trials the challenge is to harness these resources to better stratify or classify underlying disease risk. An increasing array of technologies allows non-invasive imaging with increasing precision. Imaging is spatially defined, adaptable to a variety of instruments, minimally invasive, and sensitive to capturing detailed information, and it supports the use of contrast agents. For primary prevention of cancer – including prevention trials – imaging provides information on organ health, such as sun damage to skin, liver fat or fibrosis, and breast density. For secondary prevention, imaging identifies early disease in high-risk populations through such screenings as mammography, colonoscopy, colposcopy, lung computed tomography (CT), dermoscopy, and in prostate cancer, where better stratification of patients who may be able to forego biopsy if MRI shows evidence of indolent disease. For tertiary prevention, imaging is used to monitor a primary tumor or metastasis. Advanced imaging techniques enable digital pathomics analyses of cell shape, nucleus texture, stroma patterns, and tissue architecture arrangement.

Much of this is coupled with AI and ML to speed discovery and translation of applications. The ultimate goal is often delivery of results at point of care, with immediate decision-making and action. Importantly, point of care can increasingly be used in under-resourced settings to potentially bridge access gaps and reduce cancer health disparities. AI/ML methods are good if the data set is sufficiently large, often requiring huge data sets for training in order for them to perform optimally. Bringing these technologies to point of care for evaluation of patient eligibility for prevention trials is rapidly emerging area of study with much potential to increase efficiency of prevention trials.

Interfaces with data science and machine learning in -omics and other applications beyond imaging are rapidly expanding. Opportunities for application in precision prevention include development of conventional analysis as well as AI/ML to handle disparate data types from imaging, omics, demographic, lifestyle, environmental exposure and generate actionable information.

Multidimensional data typically combines several lines of evidence, such as whole-genome sequencing, gene expression, copy number variation, and methylation, to produce plots that can predict patient outcomes. These multidimensional data can also vary over time (e.g., time-varying factors, markers, and images). The approach with high dimensional baseline covariates is being used in the ongoing NCI Precancer Atlas (PCA) and other advances in applications require novel analytic strategies and methods to verify the robust AI and ML approaches. Bringing these approaches to risk classification will transform eligibility assessment for prevention trials with precision approaches in the coming years.

There is great promise in the integration of multidimensional data into cancer risk prediction. Risk stratification algorithms will be required. This work will build on the record of methods development and application in cancer prevention for risk models (both classic statistical models and Bayesian approaches) (Steyerberg 2009). Strategies to bring multidimensional data to point of care for risk stratification and precision prevention decision making will need integrated studies of communication of these approaches and their interpretation (Klein and Stefanek 2007). At the same time, coverage of populations regardless of socioeconomic status and race/ethnicity is essential to eliminate disparities and provide complete population application for the multidimensional data studies. The underlying importance of cohort data for model development and validation is well established and remains a priority for precision prevention (Moons et al. 2012a, b).

For chemoprevention trials, there are particular challenges. These include:

a) Efforts to improve risk stratification of at-risk populations to permit better defined study populations.
b) Novel trial designs that may support different models of chemoprevention, will further change the landscape of prevention trials. Such changes as intermittent exposures to agents otherwise too toxic for long duration use (this could enable adoption of targeted agents that might remove early cancer cells, for example), or long term evaluation of interventions that modulate the immune systems for unanticipated effects.

Interpreting Prevention Trials

Prevention trials may offer a range of stress-tests for the design and interpretation of randomized trials. Not only are these often longer in duration as they aim to reduce the incidence or onset of disease, but the challenges of volunteers or participants willing to enroll not reflecting the distribution of risk factors on the broader population that may have motivated the scientific questions being addressed add to the challenges of interpreting and applying results. Sommer reviews some case studies in the chapter in Vitamin A deficiency (see ▶ Chap. 112, "Trials Can Inform or Misinform: "The Story of Vitamin A Deficiency and Childhood Mortality"") and many have written critiques on other prevention trials when results do not "hold up" as expected from the motivation for the trial (Martinez et al. 2008; Tanvetyanon and Bepler 2008).

Recent experience with vaccines against COVID-19 demonstrate increasing public focus on trial design, protocol access, and almost real time reporting of the race/ethnic and age composition of participants to hold trialist accountable for enrolling study populations reflecting the at risk population. Despite these advances in the face of pandemic COVDI-19, there remains much room for improvement in recruitment of broader and more diverse populations of participants for prevention trials in general, and the application of advancing methods in design of trials to bring timely results for prevention of chronic diseases.

Conclusion

Prevention trials allow the investigator to evaluate the magnitude of benefit for a preventive intervention in the context of the natural history of disease develop. Through randomization prevention trials avoid self-selection to new uses of therapies or potentially preventive lifestyle patterns that can be confounded in observational settings by socioeconomic status, education, and access to prevention and diagnostic health services. Control selection is important to be realistic and practical, given the usually long duration of prevention trials. Appropriate selection of study population must balance a group with sufficiently high risk to generate endpoints and yet broad enough to support generalizability of the findings. Timing in the disease process is under the control of the investigator, more so than in the setting of treatment trials where the diagnosis of disease may set the timing for initiation of therapy. Choosing when the intervention should start, and for how long, should be grounded in the natural history of disease development and progression to clinical endpoints. Adherence to therapies (intervention and control) in prevention trials can have major impact on the interpretation of the findings and the adequacy of the contrast between intervention and control arms to support a meaningful contrast. This adds some complexity to design as illustrated through the Women's Health Initiative. Planned long-term follow-up can help maximize the value of prevention trials bringing additional information to bear on the risks and benefits of the preventive intervention. Despite their cost, prevention trials add much evidence to strategies for risk reduction across many chronic conditions.

Key Facts

- Prevention trials offer results that remove self-selection bias to evaluation prevention approaches for chronic diseases.
- Choosing population for inclusion in the trial balances level of risk, duration of trial needed for sufficient endpoints to test the intervention, and the generalizability of the findings for prevention.
- Long durational may exacerbate challenges for adherence by otherwise healthy populations.
- Extended follow-up beyond the planned trail intervention may add important details trade-offs on risk and benefits.

Cross-References

▶ Ascertainment and Classification of Outcomes
▶ Cluster Randomized Trials
▶ Intention to Treat and Alternative Approaches
▶ Screening Trials
▶ Trials Can Inform or Misinform: "The Story of Vitamin A Deficiency and Childhood Mortality"

References

Alberts DS, Martinez ME, Roe DJ, Guillen-Rodriguez JM, Marshall JR, van Leeuwen JB, Reid ME, Ritenbaugh C, Vargas PA, Bhattacharyya AB, Earnest DL, Sampliner RE (2000) Lack of effect of a high-fiber cereal supplement on the recurrence of colorectal adenomas. Phoenix Colon Cancer Prevention Physicians' Network. N Engl J Med 342(16):1156–1162. https://doi.org/10.1056/NEJM200004203421602

Blot WJ, Li JY, Taylor PR, Guo W, Dawsey S, Wang GQ, Yang CS, Zheng SF, Gail M, Li GY et al (1993) Nutrition intervention trials in Linxian, China: supplementation with specific vitamin/mineral combinations, cancer incidence, and disease-specific mortality in the general population. J Natl Cancer Inst 85(18):1483–1492. https://doi.org/10.1093/jnci/85.18.1483

Cairns J, Cohen L, Colton T, DeMets DL, Deykin D, Friedman L, Greenwald P, Hutchison GB, Rosner B (1991) Issues in the early termination of the aspirin component of the Physicians' Health Study. Data Monitoring Board of the Physicians' Health Study. Ann Epidemiol 1(5):395–405. https://doi.org/10.1016/1047-2797(91)90009-2

Chen MS Jr, Lara PN, Dang JH, Paterniti DA, Kelly K (2014) Twenty years post-NIH Revitalization Act: enhancing minority participation in clinical trials (EMPaCT): laying the groundwork for improving minority clinical trial accrual: renewing the case for enhancing minority participation in cancer clinical trials. Cancer 120(Suppl 7):1091–1096. https://doi.org/10.1002/cncr.28575

Chen WY, Rosner B, Colditz GA (2007) Moving forward with breast cancer prevention. Cancer 109(12):2387–2391. https://doi.org/10.1002/cncr.22711

Cook NR, Cole SR, Hennekens CH (2002) Use of a marginal structural model to determine the effect of aspirin on cardiovascular mortality in the Physicians' Health Study. Am J Epidemiol 155(11):1045–1053. https://doi.org/10.1093/aje/155.11.1045

Cuzick J (2010) Long-term follow-up in cancer prevention trials (it ain't over 'til it's over). Cancer Prev Res 3(6):689–691. https://doi.org/10.1158/1940-6207.CAPR-10-0096

DeCensi A, Puntoni M, Guerrieri-Gonzaga A, Caviglia S, Avino F, Cortesi L, Taverniti C, Pacquola MG, Falcini F, Gulisano M, Digennaro M, Cariello A, Cagossi K, Pinotti G, Lazzeroni M, Serrano D, Branchi D, Campora S, Petrera M, Buttiron Webber T, Boni L, Bonanni B (2019) Randomized placebo controlled trial of low-dose tamoxifen to prevent local and contralateral recurrence in breast intraepithelial neoplasia. J Clin Oncol 37(19):1629–1637. https://doi.org/10.1200/JCO.18.01779

Eriksson M, Eklund M, Borgquist S, Hellgren R, Margolin S, Thoren L, Rosendahl A, Lang K, Tapia J, Backlund M, Discacciati A, Crippa A, Gabrielson M, Hammarstrom M, Wengstrom Y, Czene K, Hall P (2021) Low-dose tamoxifen for mammographic density reduction: a randomized controlled trial. J Clin Oncol 2021:JCO2002598. https://doi.org/10.1200/JCO.20.02598

Fisher B, Costantino J, Wickerham D, Redmond C, Kavanah M, Cronin W, Vogel V, Robidoux A, Dimitrov N, Atkins J, Daly M, Wieand S, Tan-Chiu E, Ford L, Wolmark N, Other National Surgical Adjuvant Breast and Bowel Project Investigators (1998) Tamoxifen for prevention of breast cancer: report of the National Surgical Adjuvant Breast and Bowel Project P-1 study. J Natl Cancer Inst 90:1371–1388

Fisher B, Costantino JP, Wickerham DL, Cecchini RS, Cronin WM, Robidoux A, Bevers TB, Kavanah MT, Atkins JN, Margolese RG, Runowicz CD, James JM, Ford LG, Wolmark N (2005) Tamoxifen for the prevention of breast cancer: current status of the National Surgical Adjuvant Breast and Bowel Project P-1 study. J Natl Cancer Inst 97(22):1652–1662

Glynn RJ, Buring JE, Manson JE, LaMotte F, Hennekens CH (1994) Adherence to aspirin in the prevention of myocardial infarction. The Physicians' Health Study. Arch Intern Med 154(23):2649–2657. https://doi.org/10.1001/archinte.1994.00420230032005

Grau MV, Baron JA, Sandler RS, Wallace K, Haile RW, Church TR, Beck GJ, Summers RW, Barry EL, Cole BF, Snover DC, Rothstein R, Mandel JS (2007) Prolonged effect of calcium supplementation on risk of colorectal adenomas in a randomized trial. J Natl Cancer Inst 99(2):129–136

Greenwald P, Anderson D, Nelson SA, Taylor PR (2007) Clinical trials of vitamin and mineral supplements for cancer prevention. Am J Clin Nutr 85(1):314S–317S

Jaffee EM, Dang CV, Agus DB, Alexander BM, Anderson KC, Ashworth A, Barker AD, Bastani R, Bhatia S, Bluestone JA, Brawley O, Butte AJ, Coit DG, Davidson NE, Davis M, DePinho RA, Diasio RB, Draetta G, Frazier AL, Futreal A, Gambhir SS, Ganz PA, Garraway L, Gerson S, Gupta S, Heath J, Hoffman RI, Hudis C, Hughes-Halbert C, Ibrahim R, Jadvar H, Kavanagh B,

Kittles R, Le QT, Lippman SM, Mankoff D, Mardis ER, Mayer DK, McMasters K, Meropol NJ, Mitchell B, Naredi P, Ornish D, Pawlik TM, Peppercorn J, Pomper MG, Raghavan D, Ritchie C, Schwarz SW, Sullivan R, Wahl R, Wolchok JD, Wong SL, Yung A (2017) Future cancer research priorities in the USA: a Lancet Oncology Commission. Lancet Oncol 18(11):e653–e706. https://doi.org/10.1016/S1470-2045(17)30698-8

Klein WM, Stefanek ME (2007) Cancer risk elicitation and communication: lessons from the psychology of risk perception. CA Cancer J Clin 57(3):147–167. https://doi.org/10.3322/canjclin.57.3.147

Knowler WC, Barrett-Connor E, Fowler SE, Hamman RF, Lachin JM, Walker EA, Nathan DM, Diabetes Prevention Program Research Group (2002) Reduction in the incidence of type 2 diabetes with lifestyle intervention or metformin. N Engl J Med 346(6):393–403. https://doi.org/10.1056/NEJMoa012512

Limburg PJ, Wei W, Ahnen DJ, Qiao Y, Hawk ET, Wang G, Giffen CA, Wang G, Roth MJ, Lu N, Korn EL, Ma Y, Caldwell KL, Dong Z, Taylor PR, Dawsey SM (2005) Randomized, placebo-controlled, esophageal squamous cell cancer chemoprevention trial of selenomethionine and celecoxib. Gastroenterology 129(3):863–873

Martinez ME, Marshall JR, Giovannucci E (2008) Diet and cancer prevention: the roles of observation and experimentation. Nat Rev Cancer 8(9):694–703

Martino S, Cauley JA, Barrett-Connor E, Powles TJ, Mershon J, Disch D, Secrest RJ, Cummings SR (2004) Continuing outcomes relevant to Evista: breast cancer incidence in postmenopausal osteoporotic women in a randomized trial of raloxifene. J Natl Cancer Inst 96(23):1751–1761

Matheny M, Israni S, Ahmed M, Whicher D (2019) Artificial intelligence in health care: the hope, the hype, the promise, the peril, NAM special publication. National Academy of Medicine, Washington, DC

Moons KG, Kengne AP, Grobbee DE, Royston P, Vergouwe Y, Altman DG, Woodward M (2012a) Risk prediction models: II. External validation, model updating, and impact assessment. Heart 98(9):691–698. https://doi.org/10.1136/heartjnl-2011-301247

Moons KG, Kengne AP, Woodward M, Royston P, Vergouwe Y, Altman DG, Grobbee DE (2012b) Risk prediction models: I. Development, internal validation, and assessing the incremental value of a new (bio)marker. Heart 98(9):683–690. https://doi.org/10.1136/heartjnl-2011-301246

Parker-Pope T (2007) Do pills have a place in cancer prevention? Wall Street J 2007:D1

Peto R, Gray R, Collins R, Wheatley K, Hennekens C, Jamrozik K, Warlow C, Hafner B, Thompson E, Norton S et al (1988) Randomised trial of prophylactic daily aspirin in British male doctors. Br Med J 296(6618):313–316. https://doi.org/10.1136/bmj.296.6618.313

Prentice RL, Caan B, Chlebowski RT, Patterson R, Kuller LH, Ockene JK, Margolis KL, Limacher MC, Manson JE, Parker LM, Paskett E, Phillips L, Robbins J, Rossouw JE, Sarto GE, Shikany JM, Stefanick ML, Thomson CA, Van Horn L, Vitolins MZ, Wactawski-Wende J, Wallace RB, Wassertheil-Smoller S, Whitlock E, Yano K, Adams-Campbell L, Anderson GL, Assaf AR, Beresford SA, Black HR, Brunner RL, Brzyski RG, Ford L, Gass M, Hays J, Heber D, Heiss G, Hendrix SL, Hsia J, Hubbell FA, Jackson RD, Johnson KC, Kotchen JM, LaCroix AZ, Lane DS, Langer RD, Lasser NL, Henderson MM (2006) Low-fat dietary pattern and risk of invasive breast cancer: the Women's Health Initiative Randomized Controlled Dietary Modification Trial. JAMA 295(6):629–642

Qiao YL, Dawsey SM, Kamangar F, Fan JH, Abnet CC, Sun XD, Johnson LL, Gail MH, Dong ZW, Yu B, Mark SD, Taylor PR (2009) Total and cancer mortality after supplementation with vitamins and minerals: follow-up of the Linxian General Population Nutrition Intervention Trial. J Natl Cancer Inst 101(7):507–518

Rossouw JE, Anderson GL, Prentice RL, LaCroix AZ, Kooperberg C, Stefanick ML, Jackson RD, Beresford SA, Howard BV, Johnson KC, Kotchen JM, Ockene J (2002) Risks and benefits of estrogen plus progestin in healthy postmenopausal women: principal results from the Women's Health Initiative randomized controlled trial. JAMA 288(3):321–333

Sargent DJ, Conley BA, Allegra C, Collette L (2005) Clinical trial designs for predictive marker validation in cancer treatment trials. J Clin Oncol 23(9):2020–2027

Schatzkin A, Lanza E, Corle D, Lance P, Iber F, Caan B, Shike M, Weissfeld J, Burt R, Cooper MR, Kikendall JW, Cahill J (2000) Lack of effect of a low-fat, high-fiber diet on the recurrence of

colorectal adenomas. Polyp Prevention Trial Study Group. N Engl J Med 342(16):1149–1155. https://doi.org/10.1056/NEJM200004203421601
Shapiro S, Venet W, Strax P, Venet L, Roeser R (1985) Selection, follow-up, and analysis in the Health Insurance Plan Study: a randomized trial with breast cancer screening. Natl Cancer Inst Monogr 67:65–74
Steering Committee of the Physicians' Health Study Research Group (1988) Preliminary report: findings from the aspirin component of the ongoing Physicians' Health Study. N Engl J Med 318(4):262–264. https://doi.org/10.1056/NEJM198801283180431
Steyerberg EW (2009) Clinical prediction models. A practical approach to development, validation, and updating, Statistics for biology and health. Springer, New York. https://doi.org/10.1007/978-0-387-77244-8
Stoll CRT, Izadi S, Fowler S, Philpott-Streiff S, Green P, Suls J, Winter AC, Colditz GA (2019) Multimorbidity in randomized controlled trials of behavioral interventions: a systematic review. Health Psychol 38(9):831–839. https://doi.org/10.1037/hea0000726
Tanvetyanon T, Bepler G (2008) Beta-carotene in multivitamins and the possible risk of lung cancer among smokers versus former smokers: a meta-analysis and evaluation of national brands. Cancer 113(1):150–157. https://doi.org/10.1002/cncr.23527
The Diabetes Prevention Program Research Group (1999) The Diabetes Prevention Program. Design and methods for a clinical trial in the prevention of type 2 diabetes. Diabetes Care 22(4):623–634. https://doi.org/10.2337/diacare.22.4.623
The Lancet (2007) NCI and the STELLAR trial. Lancet 369(9580):2134. https://doi.org/10.1016/S0140-6736(07)60987-8
US Food and Drug Administration (2021) Table of surrogate endpoints that were the basis of drug approval or licensure. https://www.fda.gov/drugs/development-resources/table-surrogate-endpoints-were-basis-drug-approval-or-licensure
Ware JH (2003) Interpreting incomplete data in studies of diet and weight loss. N Engl J Med 348(21):2136–2137. https://doi.org/10.1056/NEJMe030054
Ware JH, Hamel MB (2011) Pragmatic trials – guides to better patient care? N Engl J Med 364(18):1685–1687. https://doi.org/10.1056/NEJMp1103502
Warner ET, Glasgow RE, Emmons KM, Bennett GG, Askew S, Rosner B, Colditz GA (2013) Recruitment and retention of participants in a pragmatic randomized intervention trial at three community health clinics: results and lessons learned. BMC Public Health 13:192. https://doi.org/10.1186/1471-2458-13-192
Wolin KY, Steinberg DM, Lane IB, Askew S, Greaney ML, Colditz GA, Bennett GG (2015) Engagement with eHealth self-monitoring in a primary care-based weight management intervention. PLoS One 10(10):e0140455. https://doi.org/10.1371/journal.pone.0140455
Writing Group (1979) Five-year findings of the hypertension detection and follow-up program. I. Reduction in mortality of persons with high blood pressure, including mild hypertension. Hypertension Detection and Follow-up Program Cooperative Group. JAMA 242(23):2562–2571
Writing Group (1998) Design of the Women's Health Initiative clinical trial and observational study. The Women's Health Initiative Study Group. Control Clin Trials 19(1):61–109. https://doi.org/10.1016/s0197-2456(97)00078-0
Yach D, Hawkes C, Gould CL, Hofman KJ (2004) The global burden of chronic diseases: overcoming impediments to prevention and control. JAMA 291(21):2616–2622. https://doi.org/10.1001/jama.291.21.2616
Yusuf S, Joseph P, Dans A, Gao P, Teo K, Xavier D, Lopez-Jaramillo P, Yusoff K, Santoso A, Gamra H, Talukder S, Christou C, Girish P, Yeates K, Xavier F, Dagenais G, Rocha C, McCready T, Tyrwhitt J, Bosch J, Pais P, International Polycap Study 3 Investigators (2021) Polypill with or without aspirin in persons without cardiovascular disease. N Engl J Med 384(3):216–228. https://doi.org/10.1056/NEJMoa2028220
Zelen M (1988) Are primary cancer prevention trials feasible? J Natl Cancer Inst 80:1442–1444

N-of-1 Randomized Trials

68

Reza D. Mirza, Sunita Vohra, Richard Kravitz, and Gordon H. Guyatt

Contents

R. D. Mirza
Department of Medicine, McMaster University, Hamilton, ON, Canada
e-mail: mirzard@mcmaster.ca

S. Vohra
University of Alberta, Edmonton, AB, Canada
e-mail: svohra@ualberta.ca

R. Kravitz
University of California Davis, Davis, CA, USA
e-mail: rikravitz@ucdavis.edu

G. H. Guyatt (✉)
McMaster University, Hamilton, ON, Canada
e-mail: guyatt@mcmaster.ca

© Springer Nature Switzerland AG 2022

S. Piantadosi, C. L. Meinert (eds.), *Principles and Practice of Clinical Trials*,
https://doi.org/10.1007/978-3-319-52636-2_97

Abstract

Single-subject trials have a rich history in the behavioral sciences, but a much more limited history in clinical medicine. This chapter deals with a particular single-subject design, the N-of-1 randomized control trial (RCT). N-of-1 RCTs are single-patient multiple crossover studies of an intervention and usually one comparator. Typically, patients undergo pairs of treatment periods; random allocation determines the order of intervention and comparator arms within each pair and patients and clinicians are ideally blind to allocation. Patients and clinicians repeat pairs of treatment periods as necessary to achieve a convincing result. In the medical sciences, N-of-1 RCTs have seen limited use, in part due to lack of familiarity and feasibility concerns that arise in day-to-day clinical practice. Investigators may carry out a number of N-of-1 RCTs of the same intervention and comparator as part of a formal research study, aggregating across N-of-1 RCTs to develop population estimates. N-of-1 RCTs have demonstrated their utility in clarifying whether a clinical intervention is effective or not. Although N-of-1 trials have the potential for improving patient outcomes, the few small randomized trials comparing N-of-1 to conventional care have not demonstrated important benefits.

Keywords

N-of-1 · Single-patient trial · Randomized controlled trial · Crossover trial · Personalized medicine

Definition

This chapter deals with a particular type of single-participant experiment, the N-of-1 randomized control trial (RCT). N-of-1 RCTs are prospective, single-patient trials with repeated pairs of intervention and comparator periods in which the order is randomized and patients and clinicians are ideally blinded with respect to allocation. We will describe the history of N-of-1 RCTs, as well as the indications, design, interpretation, reporting, and associated ethical issues.

History

Psychologists pioneered the use and development of single-subject designs, including N-of-1 trials (Kazdin 2011; Kratochwill 2013). Its debut in medicine came in a 1986 issue of the *New England Journal of Medicine* (Guyatt et al. 1986). Clinician-scientists from McMaster University presented a patient with severe asthma who was poorly controlled despite inhaled beta-agonist, anti-cholinergic (ipratropium), theophylline, and oral prednisone. They conducted an N-of-1 RCT that demonstrated that theophylline, far from improving the symptoms, made them considerably worse. A second N-of-1 trial convinced the patient his ipratropium did in fact provide benefit. Discontinuation of the theophylline and regular use of ipratropium markedly improved symptoms and allowed gradual discontinuation of prednisone.

In that same chapter, the authors announced the creation of an N-of-1 clinical service allowing local physicians to refer patients with a therapeutic question. Over 3 years, the service completed 57 N-of-1 RCTs that provided a definite answer for 50 patients; in 15 (39%) of whom the results led to a change referring physicians' planned management. Given this success, other clinicians established N-of-1 services formed in their centers including the University of Washington (Dr. Eric Larson), the University of Alberta (Dr. Sunita Vohra), and a national Australian N-of-1 service based out of the University of Queensland (Dr. Geoff Mitchell) (Mirza et al. 2017).

As of 2021, N-of-1 services are minimally active. The N-of-1 RCT remains useful for addressing clinical questions that meet certain criteria – see the next section – but most clinicians remain unaware of its existence. As clinical research embraces patient-centerd research and moves to the era of personalized medicine, there appears to be a resurgence of interest in N-of-1 RCTs (Kravitz et al. 2014; Shamseer et al. 2015; Mirza et al. 2017).

Introduction: Why Conduct an N-of-1 RCTs?

N-of-1 randomized control trials (RCTs) can be broken down into two major categories depending on the underlying purpose. In one, the purpose is to improve the care of individual patients by carrying out rigorous trials that leave patients and clinicians confident that a particular treatment is, or is not, beneficial or harmful. By ensuring applicability to the individual, N-of-1 RCTs represent the highest quality of evidence.

The second reason for conducting N-of-1 RCTs is to determine the effect of an intervention in a population. Conducting a series of N-of-1 RCTs allows investigators to provide an estimate of the proportion of patients who achieve an important benefit, or who suffer troubling adverse effects, and thus establish the extent of heterogeneity of response (Stunnenberg et al. 2018). Many patients and clinicians considering the impact of a treatment are likely to find such a result more informative than, for example, a mean effect.

Limitations of Informal Trials of Therapy

In routine practice, clinicians typically conduct informal trials of therapy. This entails starting a treatment and monitoring a patient's response. For a number of reasons, this approach is prone to false-positive, and less frequently false-negative, results.

First, patients may have been destined to get better (or worse) as a function of natural history, in which case patients and clinicians may deem the treatment responsible when improvement or worsening would have occurred without the intervention. Second, both patients and clinicians may desire to meet each other's expectations; thereby, each is more likely to infer the success of a treatment. Third, an apparent response may be due to a placebo rather than the intended biological effect. Similarly, patients who expect an adverse effect of treatment may experience that adverse effect even if the biological effect of treatment is not responsible – the so-called nocebo effect (Barsky et al. 2002). Finally, an exposure other than the treatment may have been responsible for an apparent response – for instance a week of cloudy days with minimal sun exposure may be responsible for a decrease in symptoms in a patient with systematic lupus erythematous.

How N-of-1 RCTs Address the Limitations of Informal Trials of Therapy

N-of-1 RCTs involve protecting against risk of bias that bedevils informal trials of therapy. Choosing chronic, stable diseases attenuates the risk of conflating treatment benefit and natural history. Blinding patients and clinicians to allocation to treatment versus comparator minimizes biases related to expectation and placebo effects. Multiple crossover periods control the risk of the misleading impact of transient third variables, as well as effectively addressing natural history effects (i.e., it is very unlikely that natural history will correspond closely to the institution and withdrawal of a beneficial treatment).

Five Reasons for Conducting N-of-1 RCTs to Improve Patient Care

Treatments, even if beneficial in a population, will seldom if ever achieve an important benefit in every individual in that population: In other words, treatment response is often, perhaps usually, heterogenous. N-of-1 RCTs can sort out whether an individual who would have been eligible for an RCT that has reported a positive result is one of the fortunate responders to treatment, or unfortunate nonresponders. Indeed, the N-of-1 trial can quantify treatment effect estimates specific to that individual.

A second reason for conducting an N-of-1 RCT is for patients who would, because of age restrictions, comorbidity, or concurrent therapy, have been excluded from existing parallel group RCTs. A particular strength of N-of-1 RCTs is that they can address the question of whether benefits extend to such individuals.

Third, some patients have symptoms that lack evidence-based management options, or are refractory to standard medical management. Determined clinicians may be tempted to trial off-label interventions to alleviate their patient's suffering. In these cases, an N-of-1 RCT allows for objective assessment of untested therapeutic strategies.

Fourth, patients using a therapy with anticipated benefits may be experiencing troubling symptoms for which the treatment they are using may, or may not, be responsible. N-of-1 RCTs can provide definitive evidence confirming the culpability, or exoneration, of the particular treatment (Joy et al. 2014).

Fifth, sometimes patients remain on a treatment for extended periods and it is unclear whether there is any ongoing benefit. Given the rise of polypharmacy and the increased recognition of its risks, the importance of reevaluating medications is increasingly clear. RCTs often provided only limited data on the long-term efficacy of a treatment. N-of-1 RCTs can clarify whether a medication is providing ongoing benefit, or is not. A good use case for this is chronic PPI therapy in an asymptomatic patient with a history of gastroesophageal reflux disease.

N-of-1 RCTs Addressing Treatment Effects in a Group of Patients

Soon after their introduction into medicine, proponents suggested N-of-1 RCTs may hold promise as a tool for efficient early drug development. The proposal addressed three major questions faced by drug developers before engaging in large, costly parallel group RCTs. First, does the drug in question show sufficient promise to justify drug development? Second, what patient population will be most responsive to the drug? Third, what is the optimal dose to maximize benefit and minimize adverse effects?

In drug development, these questions are managed by using a combination of small efficacy studies in conjunction with small studies using nonrepresentative healthy volunteers examining safety, tolerance, pharmacology, and drug disposition. The efficacy studies are often unblinded and uncontrolled, instead using historical reference groups. The data from these studies are of limited value due to bias and limited power. The problem manifests when trying to use the data during the design of the first large parallel group RCT. Investigators are forced to gamble on the most efficacious dose (or doses if they opt for multiple treatment arms) and which population is most likely to benefit (Guyatt et al. 1990b).

N-of-1 RCTs allow for methodologically robust small-scale studies that can address whether a drug shows promise (Phase 3), which patient populations are most responsive, and which doses are optimal (Phase 1). These principles are demonstrated in an early N-of-1 RCT examining the role of amitriptyline in fibromyalgia (Guyatt et al. 1988). Low-dose amitriptyline is currently a first-line agent for the treatment of fibromyalgia, but at the time of this N-of-1 RCT series – reported in 1988 – there was only one parallel group RCT suggesting benefit.

Table 1 Benefits of N-of-1 RCTs depending on purpose

Improving patient care	Drug development
Reliably answer clinical questions for patients regarding the efficacy of interventions	Identify if a drug shows promise to justify drug development
Patients will directly benefit from their participation	Identify patient population that will be most responsive
Patients are guaranteed an intervention arm	Identify optimal dose to maximize benefit and minimize adverse effects
Evidence can be generated for patients who would not qualify for clinical trials, due to age, comorbidity, or concurrent therapies	Low cost compared to large parallel group RCTs
	Accelerated timeline compared to large parallel group RCTs

A group at McMaster group conducted 23 N-of-1 RCTs that demonstrated rapid onset of beneficial effect in a number of patients, strongly supporting the efficacy of low-dose amitriptyline for fibromyalgia. The group went on to conduct similar studies assessing tetrahydroaminoacridine in Alzheimer's patients (no important benefit at all) (Molloy et al. 1991), and the efficacy of home oxygen in reducing symptoms in patients with chronic obstructive pulmonary disorder with exertional hypoxemia (beneficial in very few patients) (Nonoyama et al. 2007).

These success stories demonstrate how N-of-1 RCTs can address treatment efficacy in a group of patients. Almost 30 years after the publication of the paper suggesting their possible use in drug development, their implementation in this arena remains an idea waiting to be tested (Table 1).

Determining Appropriateness for an N-of-1 RCT

For a patient to be deemed appropriate for an N-of-1 RCT, the clinical circumstances must meet particular requirements. N-of-1 RCTs are useful when uncertainty exists regarding treatment effect (either benefit or harm). Earlier in this chapter, we provided examples of circumstances in which such uncertainty is likely to exist.

The N of RCT requires that specific clinical circumstances be met.

1. *The outcome of interest (typically symptoms) should occur frequently, ideally daily.*
   Intervention period lengths must be tailored to outcome frequency. If the outcome is infrequent, the requirement for treatment periods sufficiently long for the outcome to be manifest may make the N-of-1 RCT excessively burdensome for both patient and clinician. One exception is when treatments are unusually expensive, in which case clinicians and patients may be particularly motivated to complete the trial (Kravitz et al. 2008).
2. *The condition should be chronic and stable.*
   Acute symptoms may represent transient conditions that are likely to resolve spontaneously. By choosing a stable condition in terms of severity and symptoms, clinicians reduce the random error that may make true treatment effects very

difficult to detect. Stability does not preclude frequently episodic conditions, such as a child with multiple seizures a day.

3. *Interventions should have rapid onset and termination of effect.*

   Rapid onset ensures that intervention periods can be a reasonable length. An N-of-1 RCT with selective serotonin reuptake inhibitors would, for instance, be prohibitively cumbersome given the 4–6 weeks required at a minimum for treatment effect, and several weeks for tapering to discontinuation. If each intervention period was 8 weeks in length, and there are three crossovers periods, the total trial length would be at least 48 weeks (sufficient time for spontaneous resolution of the condition).

   Rapid termination of action ensures that treatments effects do not influence comparator periods, without requiring washout periods. Typically, if there are residual effects, the treatment periods are lengthened and the patient/physician team considers only the data after resolution of effects. For instance, if one expects treatment effects to persist for a week, treatment periods can continue for 2 weeks, and one can use data only from the second week. Alternatively, a washout period can be used as a buffer between periods to prevent carryover effects.

Designing an N-of-1 RCT

N-of-1 RCTs represent multiple crossover trials of an intervention and one or more comparators that, to minimize risk of bias, include randomization in terms of sequence order. Interventions are typically drugs – but may be nonpharmacologic or complementary and alternative medicine – compared in one of three ways: drug versus placebo, drug versus comparator drug, or high dose versus low dose of the same drug. For optimal rigor, clinicians and patients must be blind to allocation. Blinding is not always possible (e.g., physical therapy). N-of-1 trials are particularly amenable to being codesigned by patient and clinician, including with regards to outcome measure selection. Typically outcomes are symptoms monitored daily. Some researchers choose to use physiologic and biochemical variables as outcomes, but the value of such surrogates for inferring patient-important benefit is limited. The number of pairs – each pair including one period of each treatment and comparator – continue until both patient and clinician are satisfied that superiority or equivalence have been demonstrated. A run-in period may be employed for the same reason as in other trials: establishing dose tolerability and compliance.

Choosing an Outcome

Outcomes can be a measure of symptoms or physiologic outcomes. A 2016 systematic survey of 100 N-of-1 RCTs conducted between 1950 and 2013 using an ABAB design and assessing a health intervention for a medical condition identified measures of symptoms as most common: Likert scales (55% of trials), visual analogue scales (30%), patient diaries (26%), and patient-generated questionnaires (18%).

Physiologic outcomes were used in 35% trials, including clinical tests such as blood pressure or laboratory tests such as erythrocyte sedimentation rate (Punja et al. 2016). A single N-of-1 RCT can address more than one outcome. Regardless of the outcome(s) chosen, clinicians should work with patients to identify patient-important targets prior to starting the trial.

As mentioned earlier in the chapter, the outcome measure is ideally one that can be measured frequently (e.g., daily) to ensure that there is enough data to analyze within an intervention period (typically 5–14 days). Physiologic parameters should be one that patients can measure themselves at their convenience, such as blood pressure or blood sugar concentrations. Automated tracking using cell phones and other monitoring devices are likely to prove increasingly useful for outcome monitoring (Ryu 2012; Kravitz et al. 2018).

Likert scales are widely used outside of N-of-1 research for their simplicity, allowing for patient familiarity, ease in understanding, and ease in interpretation. There is evidence to suggest that seven-point scales are more sensitive in detecting small differences in comparison to fewer response options, and are more convenient than visual analogue scales (Guyatt et al. 1987; Girard and Ely 2008). If using a Likert scale to assess symptoms, clinicians should consider including items specifically assessing symptom interference with daily activities. An example of how one might phrase this is presented below.

Please indicate how much your pain interferes with your everyday activities of daily living, such as cooking, cleaning, and getting dressed:

1. No interference at all
2. A little interference
3. Some interference
4. Moderate interference
5. Much interference
6. Severe interference
7. I am unable to do carry out these activities as a result of the interference

Trial Length

The duration of an N-of-1 RCT will depend on the number of days in each treatment period, and the number of pairs of periods undertaken. Most often the trial addresses a single intervention and a single comparator. Typically each treatment period will range between 5 and 14 days (median: 10 days), the interquartile range of all captured N-of-1 RCTs in the aforementioned systematic survey by Punja and colleagues (Punja et al. 2016). In terms of the number of pairs of treatment periods – one period in which the patient receives the intervention and one period with the comparator, in Punja's survey 75% of trials required between 2 and 5 pairs of treatment periods (median: 3 pairs).

Based on these numbers, a typical N-of-1 RCT with a pair of treatment periods will take 20 days (10 days for each of the two arms); with 3 such pairs, the total duration would be 60 days.

Randomization

Within an N-of-1 trial, the order of treatments is subject to randomization in contrast to a randomized crossover trial where the patient is the unit of randomization. Randomization is an essential component of N-of-1 RCTs as it will control for factors that may influence outcome and vary over time, and by facilitating blinding of the clinician and patient. Clinicians can conduct randomization by tossing a coin, utilizing a computer algorithm, or consulting a randomization table, and can randomize the order in each pair separately.

Collaboration with Pharmacy

N-of-1 RCTs at their most rigorous are blinded to protect against the bias of patient and clinician expectations, co-interventions, and placebo effects. To blind effectively and efficiently, physicians should and often do collaborate with a local pharmacy to prepare treatments and comparators that are identical in appearance, taste, texture, and smell. Pharmacists can achieve this goal by crushing the active drugs and repackaging in capsules. Placebos can be filled with an inert substance.

Pharmacists can also play a number of other important roles in N-of-1 RCTs. They can provide input in terms of drug half-life and thus determining whether and how long each treatment period need be. Certainly, with increased scope of practice, Doctors of Pharmacy in particular can design, conduct, and interpret the N-of-1 trial. Pharmacist technicians can also help, particularly with monitoring drug compliance by conducting pill counts and assessing whether patients are refilling their medications at the correct time.

Advanced Techniques

Advanced techniques existing in terms of trial design allow for adaptive features. Adaptive arms allow for crossover, dose change, or discontinuation of an intervention based on patient preference or preset outcomes, such as adverse effects or response. An example of such a design is establishing a predetermined stopping rule that minimizes patient exposure to an inferior treatment. This is particularly valuable when comparing several treatments arms (Duan et al. 2013).

Interpreting the Data

There are a number of options in interpreting the data that depend on the goals of the trial, the trial design, and the data generated. Broadly this can be broken down into statistical methods, which were used in 84% of the trials that Punja reported; in the other 16%, clinicians and patients use visual inspection alone (Punja et al. 2016).

Visual Inspection

Using visual inspection of the data, clinicians and patients examine a graph displaying repeated measures of the outcome of interest with specification of intervention and control arms. The features to suggest an arm is effective include: 1) minimal variability within periods; 2) the magnitude and direction of difference between the arm of interest and comparator arm is consistent; and 3) the difference between the arm of interest and its comparator is large in comparison to the variability within periods. Review of the evidence collected after 2 or more pairs of periods can help determine whether to conduct further pairs.

The rationale for visual inspection is that both clinician and patient can intuitively assess the components of efficacy – direction, magnitude, and consistency of effect – in a straightforward manner that may satisfy both and simplify decision-making. The limitation is the subjective nature of the assessment that can lead to inconsistent and incorrect inferences. This methodology is appropriate only for individual patient clinical decision-making rather than using the N-of-1 methodology to make inferences about treatment effects in a population.

Nonparametric Statistical Tests

Broadly speaking, nonparametric tests refer to those that do not assume the data is normally distributed; this makes them a more conservative test. There are a number of nonparametric statistical tests available. We will focus on the Wilcoxon signed rank test, and a quantitative randomization test.

Wilcoxon Signed Rank Test

The Wilcoxon signed rank test incorporates the size of the treatment difference, but fails to take the absolute value of difference into account. To conduct a Wilcoxon signed rank test, the absolute difference within treatment cycles is ranked by absolute difference from smallest to largest (i.e., independent of direction). The sum of the ranks in favor of the treatment are compared to the sum of the ranks in favor of the comparator. The null hypothesis would expect the sums to be equivalent.

More sophisticated than either of two previous tests is a pure quantitative randomization test. This approach assesses not only the direction and size in comparing arms, but also the mean treatment difference. The probability of a given mean treatment difference is calculated by determining the proportion of randomizations that would lead to the given outcome over the denominator of all possible randomizations. The null hypothesis for this test states the expected mean treatment difference is zero.

Parametric Statistical Tests

Parametric statistical tests, by contrast, assume the data are normally distributed. The two most commonly used tests are the analysis of variance (ANOVA) and student's t-test, which is a special case of the ANOVA model. There are two factors that will help guide which test to use. First, if the trial under consideration is comparing three or more treatment arms, then the ANOVA is the preferred approach. ANOVA allows for a single analysis (F-test) across arms which the t-test does not.

Student's T-Test

The t-test is only appropriate for N-of-1 RCTs comparing two arms, regardless of whether the comparator is placebo or alternative treatment. In the general case, the student's t-test can be either paired or unpaired, but in the case of N-of-1 RCTs each intervention arm is paired by design, and therefore the paired t-test constitutes the appropriate approach. To conduct the paired t-test one calculates a single value for each treatment period. So, for instance, if the patient has completed a daily diary for 7 days, and each day has answered three questions, the score for that period will be the mean of 21 observations. One then makes the same calculation for the paired control period and examines the difference in means which the t-test addresses. The degrees of freedom for the test is the number of blocks of treatment periods minus one. The t-test is routinely used for N-of-1 RCTs, and is universally included in statistical packages.

ANOVA

Often the student's t-test functions as an extension of the ANOVA model and will provide the same result. There is at least one case in which this is not true. ANOVA may provide a different result when there is no dependency between one observation and the next. Under such circumstances the ANOVA can use each individual observation (in the example above, 7 instead of one observation per period). Unfortunately, independence of observations will rarely if ever be the case. For most illnesses, good days tend to run together, as do bad ones.

Aggregation of N-of-1 RCTs

The results of individual N-of-1 RCTs can be aggregated to estimate population effects with power comparable to conventional RCTs, and using similar analytic techniques. There are three common approaches to aggregation of N-of-1 data. The first method is analyzing as a traditional multipatient crossover trial. The analysis should be planned prospectively but can be done retrospectively. It is important that the analysis should consider the possibility of carryover of treatment effect between periods. This is true of any crossover trial analysis.

The second method is using conventional meta-analysis techniques. (See Chap. 8.11 to learn more about meta-analysis.) There are at least two benefits in meta-analyzing N-of-1 RCTs. The first is to generate a more precise estimates of treatment effects, and predictors of patient response versus nonresponse, sustained response, and susceptibility to side effects (Lillie et al. 2011). Second, in trials where N-of-1 methodology is compared to standard of care, meta-analysis can assess whether the N-of-1 methodology provides benefit over traditional clinical care.

The third method is Bayesian analysis that has been adapted specifically for use in N-of-1 RCTs (Zucker et al. 2010). What distinguishes Bayesian analysis from other forms of aggregation is the requisite incorporation of preexisting estimates into the analysis. Typically analyses require prespecification of population mean effect and variance. This serves as a liability in the many cases where this information is neither available in the literature nor easily estimated.

Reporting for N-of-1 RCT

The previous sections have focused on the use of N-of-1 RCTs for either clinical practice or as part of a research endeavor. If the latter, the issue of how one reports N-of-1 RCTs for a wider audience (typically in a publication) arises.

Similar to other types of trials, reporting standards for N-of-1 RCTs maintained by the Consolidated Standards of Reporting Trials (CONSORT) exist. To ensure optimal reporting for N-of-1 RCTs, CONSORT has published a standardized 25-item checklist (CENT), most recently updated in 2015 (Vohra et al. 2015). The recommendations were based on CONSORT recommendations for parallel group RCTs, and address reporting expectations of title and abstract, specifying rationale and objectives in the introduction, trial design, patient selection, intervention, outcomes, sample size, randomization, allocation concealment, randomization, results, analyses, discussion, protocol registration, and funding.

Ethics

In addition to the ethical principles of everyday clinical care – autonomy, beneficence, and nonmaleficence – those required for an N-of-1 trial depend on the purpose of the trial. Broadly, N-of-1 trials can be conducted to improve the care of an individual patient, to produce generalized knowledge, or as a blend of the two goals.

No additional scrutiny, including research ethics board (REB) approval, is required if the N-of-1 RCTs is done as a part of clinical care. The use of randomization and blinding does not, in and of itself, determine whether a therapeutic model is research. Similarly when the stated goal of the trial is quality improvement of care, there is no need for additional scrutiny. The way to conceptualize this is appreciating that the physician is engaging in the practice of confirming his or her clinical hypothesis. In this case the hypothesis is whether an intervention is effective. The key prerequisite is informed consent from the patient. This approach is sensible when one considers that N-of-1 RCTs patients do not pose any increased risk compared to informal trials of therapy, or prescription without monitoring for effectiveness. Indeed, the added rigor of close monitoring of benefits and adverse effects for a particular patient support the position that N-of-1 RCTs represent optimal clinical care (Guyatt et al. 1990a; Molloy et al. 1991; Irwig et al. 1995; Nonoyama et al. 2007).

When the purpose is a blend of clinical care with a secondary research interest in analyzing the data to inform future care, the clinical component represents the same low risk as conducting N-of-1 RCTs for clinical care or quality assurance. Given the additional intention of research, however, the project should undergo research ethics board assessment to evaluate the risk of analysis of anonymized data. This is typically an expedited review given the low-risk nature, and should be considered equivalent to a chart review.

When investigators conduct trials to create generalized knowledge, ethical standards for other research apply. One purpose in formal research is investigating the impact of N-of-1 methodology on patient outcomes. The alternative is the classic research-oriented N-of-1 RCT with the goal of producing generalizable insights regarding a therapeutic intervention in a population. These models must meet the standards for clinical research, including full REB approval and federal regulatory oversight, as appropriate (Punja et al. 2014).

An Example of an N-of-1 RCT

The following is an example of one of the early N-of-1 RCTs conducted as part of McMaster's clinical service. A 34-year-old female with a past medical history significant for scleroderma was referred for evaluation of treatment for persistent weakness, in the context of possible myasthenia gravis. Two separate encounters with specialists revealed electromyographical findings atypical for the disease, and so the question of whether treatment with pyridostigmine would benefit remained uncertain. This trial meets our criteria: she experienced symptoms daily, her disease is chronic and stable, there is uncertainty about therapeutic benefit, and pyridostigmine has rapid onset and termination of effect.

The intervention was pyridostigmine 30 mg by mouth twice daily and was placebo controlled. Each treatment period was 7 days, and the outcome measure was daily ratings of weakness and energy levels.

Figure 1 represents the patient's reported data using a seven-point Likert scale, where 7 represents the highest level of function, and 1 represents the lowest level of function. There were four pairs of treatment periods. Unsurprisingly, the patient did not have 100% adherence to symptom charting.

Visual inspection reveals that the treatment seems to be consistent better than the placebo. This is particularly clear in Figs. 2 and 3, which reveal the mean symptom score in each treatment period, and differences in each pair, respectively.

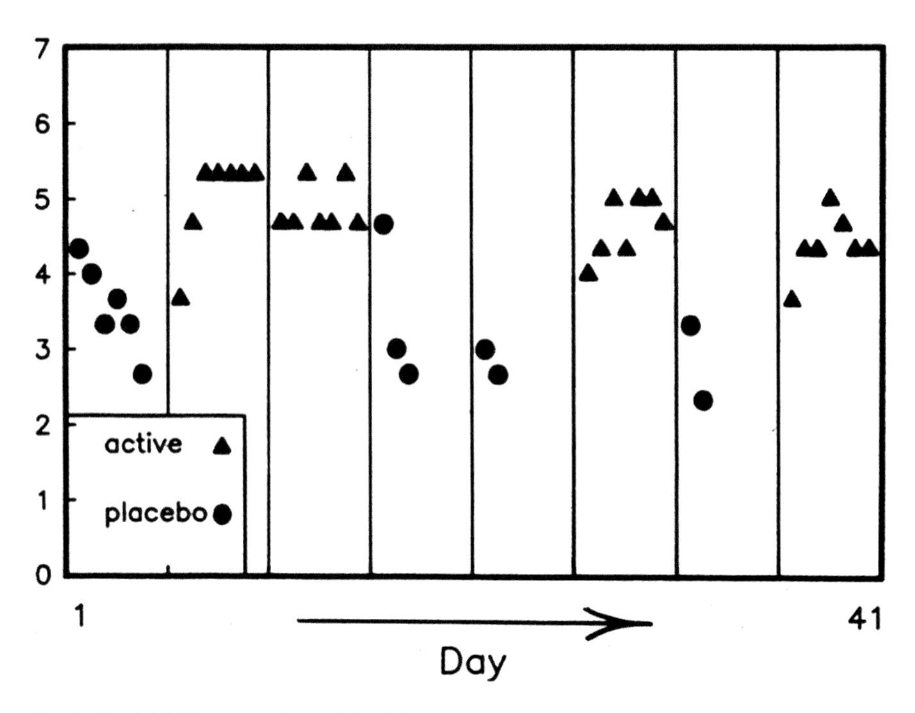

Fig. 1 N-of-1 RCT results: Mean daily Likert score

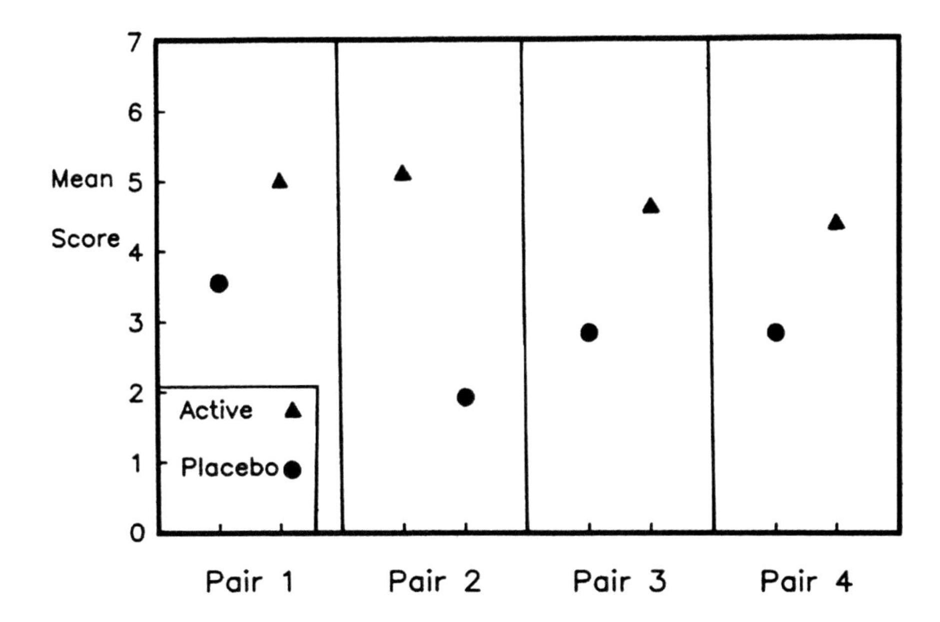

Fig. 2 N-of-1 RCT mean period score

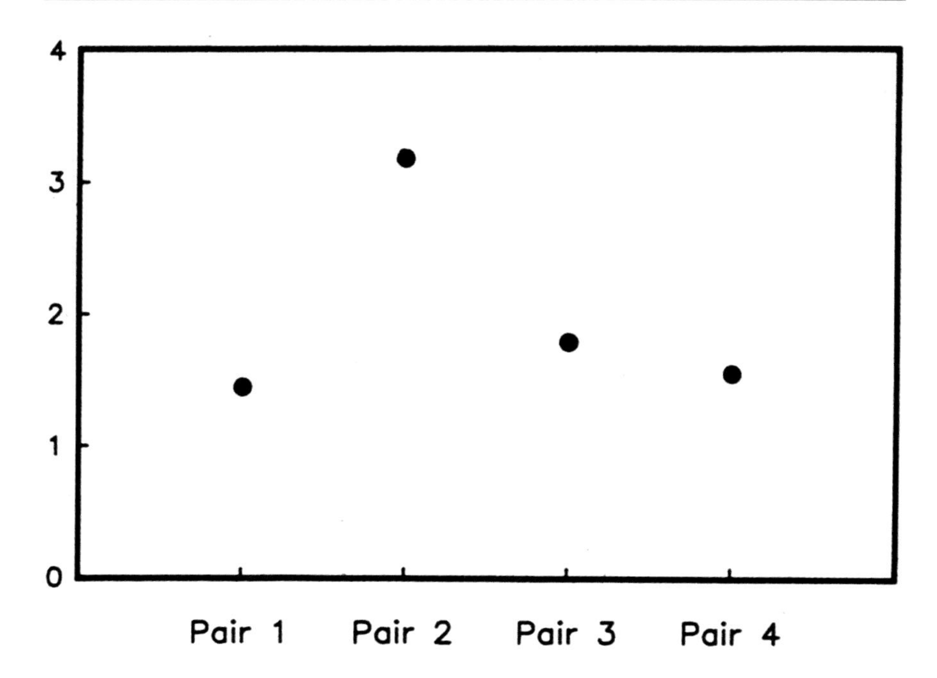

Fig. 3 N-of-1 RCT treatment and placebo difference scores

A two-tailed paired t-test comparing the differences in symptom scores across the four periods was conducted to confirm the visual inspection. The results revealed in Fig. 4 confirm a clear benefit in treatment.

Summary and Conclusion

N-of-1 RCTs are unique among experimental studies in giving physicians the ability to answer clinical questions for individual patients in a methodologically rigorous way. Other trials – including parallel group RCTs, observational trials, and meta-analyses – are all limited to answering questions at the population level. For this reason, N-of-1 trials have been suggested as the pinnacle of the evidence pyramid. Aggregation of N-of-1 RCTs by meta-analysis and Bayesian techniques allow for treatment effect estimates at the population level. By conducting an N-of-1 RCT, physicians are afforded the opportunity to offer optimal care to the individual patients whom they serve.

Key Facts

- N-of-1 RCTs are single-patient multiple crossover trials that seek to answer a clinical question and improve patient care. Multiple N-of-1 RCTs can also inform treatment effects in a population.

N of 1 RCT - Ms. A.D.

- Targets
  (data--symptom means)

	Pair 1	Pair 2	Pair 3	Pair 4
Active	5.00	5.095	4.62	4.38
Placebo	3.56	1.98	2.83	2.83
Diff.	1.44	3.18	1.79	1.55

- Analysis (2 tailed paired t-test)

	Symptoms
$\bar{D}$	1.99
t	4.94
P	0.016
C.I. (90%)	(1.041, 2.937)

Fig. 4 N-of-1 RCT t-test results

- N-of-1 RCTs constitute the highest quality evidence for a particular patient's care, because the evidence is specific to the individual patient (OCEBM Levels of Evidence Working Group 2011).
- Varied analytic techniques can inform the interpretation of N-of-1 RCTs including nonstatistical techniques (i.e., visual inspection) and statistical techniques including both nonparametric and parametric tests.

Cross-References

▶ Introduction to Meta-Analysis

References

Barsky AJ, Saintfort R, Rogers MP, Borus JF (2002) Nonspecific medication side effects and the nocebo phenomenon. JAMA 287:622–627

Duan N, Kravitz RL, Schmid CH (2013) Single-patient (n-of-1) trials: a pragmatic clinical decision methodology for patient-centered comparative effectiveness research. J Clin Epidemiol 66:S21–S28. https://doi.org/10.1016/j.jclinepi.2013.04.006
Girard TD, Ely EW (2008) Delirium in the critically ill patient. Handb Clin Neurol 90:39–56. https://doi.org/10.1016/S0072-9752(07)01703-4
Guyatt G, Sackett D, Taylor DW et al (1986) Determining optimal therapy — randomized trials in individual patients. N Engl J Med 314:889–892. https://doi.org/10.1056/NEJM198604033141406
Guyatt GH, Townsend M, Berman LB, Keller JL (1987) A comparison of Likert and visual analogue scales for measuring change in function. J Chronic Dis 40:1129–1133
Guyatt G, Sackett D, Adachi J, Roberts R, Chong J, Rosenbloom D, Keller J (1988) A clinician's guide for conducting randomized trials in individual patients. CMAJ: Canadian Medical Association Journal 139(6):497–503
Guyatt GH, Keller JL, Jaeschke R, Rosenbloom D, Adachi JD, Newhouse MT (1990a) The n-of-1 randomized controlled trial: clinical usefulness: our three-year experience. Annals of Internal Medicine 112(4):293–299
Guyatt GH, Heyting A, Jaeschke R et al (1990b) N of 1 randomized trials for investigating new drugs. Control Clin Trials 11:88–100
Irwig L, Glasziou P, March L (1995) Ethics of n-of-1 trials. Lancet (Lond) 345:469
Joy TR, Monjed A, Zou GY et al (2014) N-of-1 (single-patient) trials for statin-related myalgia. Ann Intern Med 160:301–310. https://doi.org/10.7326/M13-1921
Kazdin A (2011) Single-case research designs: Methods for clinical and applied settings. Second Edition. New York, NY: Oxford University Press
Kratochwill TR (Ed) (2013) Single subject research: Strategies for evaluating change. Academic Press
Kravitz RL, Duan N, White RH (2008) N-of-1 trials of expensive biological therapies: a third way? Arch Intern Med 168:1030–1033. https://doi.org/10.1001/archinte.168.10.1030
Kravitz R, Duan N, Eslick I et al (2014) Design and implementation of N-of-1 trials: a user's guide. Agency for Healthcare Research and Quality, US Department of Health and Human Services (2014). 540 Gaither Road. Rockville, MD 20850 www.ahrq.gov
Kravitz RL, Schmid CH, Marois M et al (2018) Effect of mobile device–supported single-patient multi-crossover trials on treatment of chronic musculoskeletal pain. JAMA Intern Med. https://doi.org/10.1001/jamainternmed.2018.3981
Lillie EO, Patay B, Diamant J et al (2011) The n-of-1 clinical trial: the ultimate strategy for individualizing medicine? Per Med 8:161–173. https://doi.org/10.2217/pme.11.7
Mirza RD, Punja S, Vohra S, Guyatt G (2017) The history and development of N-of-1 trials. J R Soc Med 110:330–340. https://doi.org/10.1177/0141076817721131
Molloy DW, Guyatt GH, Wilson DB et al (1991) Effect of tetrahydroaminoacridine on cognition, function and behaviour in Alzheimer's disease. CMAJ 144:29–34
Nonoyama ML, Brooks D, Guyatt GH, Goldstein RS (2007) Effect of oxygen on health quality of life in patients with chronic obstructive pulmonary disease with transient exertional hypoxemia. Am J Respir Crit Care Med 176:343–349. https://doi.org/10.1164/rccm.200702-308OC
OCEBM Levels of Evidence Working Group (2011) The Oxford 2011 Levels of Evidence. Oxford Centre for Evidence-Based Medicine. https://www.cebm.net/index.aspx?o=5653
Punja S, Eslick I, Duan N, Vohra S, the DEcIDE Methods Center N-of-1 Guidance Panel (2014) An ethical framework for N-of-1 trials: clinical care, quality improvement, or human subjects research? In: Kravitz RL, Duan N (eds), and the DEcIDE Methods Center N-of-1 Guidance Panel (Duan N, Eslick I, Gabler NB, Kaplan HC, Kravitz RL, Larson EB, Pace WD, Schmid CH, Sim I, Vohra S). Design and implementation of N-of-1 trials: a user's guide. AHRQ Publication No. 13(14)-EHC122-EF. Agency for Healthcare Research and Quality, Rockville, Chapter 2, pp. 13–22, January 2014. http://www.effectivehealthcare.ahrq.gov/N-1-Trials.cfm
Punja S, Bukutu C, Shamseer L et al (2016) N-of-1 trials are a tapestry of heterogeneity. J Clin Epidemiol 76:47–56. https://doi.org/10.1016/j.jclinepi.2016.03.023
Ryu S (2012) Book review: mHealth: new horizons for health through Mobile technologies: based on the findings of the second global survey on eHealth (global observatory for eHealth series, volume 3). Healthc Inform Res 18:231. https://doi.org/10.4258/hir.2012.18.3.231

Shamseer L, Sampson M, Bukutu C, Schmid C (2015) CONSORT extension for reporting N-of-1 trials (CENT) 2015: explanation and elaboration. BMJ 76:18–46

Stunnenberg BC, Raaphorst J, Groenewoud HM et al (2018) Effect of Mexiletine on muscle stiffness in patients with nondystrophic Myotonia evaluated using aggregated N-of-1 trials. JAMA 320:2344. https://doi.org/10.1001/jama.2018.18020

Vohra S, Shamseer L, Sampson M et al (2015) CONSORT extension for reporting N-of-1 trials (CENT) 2015 statement. BMJ 350:h1738. https://doi.org/10.1136/BMJ.H1738

Zucker DR, Ruthazer R, Schmid CH (2010) Individual (N-of-1) trials can be combined to give population comparative treatment effect estimates: methodologic considerations. J Clin Epidemiol 63:1312–1323. https://doi.org/10.1016/j.jclinepi.2010.04.020

Noninferiority Trials

69

Patrick P. J. Phillips and David V. Glidden

Contents

P. P. J. Phillips (✉)
UCSF Center for Tuberculosis, University of California San Francisco, San Francisco, CA, USA

Department of Epidemiology and Biostatistics, University of California San Francisco, San Francisco, CA, USA
e-mail: Patrick.Phillips@ucsf.edu

D. V. Glidden
Department of Epidemiology and Biostatistics, University of California San Francisco, San Francisco, CA, USA
e-mail: David.Glidden@ucsf.edu

© Springer Nature Switzerland AG 2022

S. Piantadosi, C. L. Meinert (eds.), *Principles and Practice of Clinical Trials*,
https://doi.org/10.1007/978-3-319-52636-2_98

Abstract

In this chapter we provide an overview of non-inferiority trials. We first introduce two motivating examples and describe scenarios for when a non-inferiority trial is appropriate. We next describe the procedures for defining the margin of non-inferiority from both regulatory and public health perspectives and then provide practical guidance for how to design a non-inferiority trial and analyze the resulting data, paying particular attention to regulatory and other published guidelines. We go on to discuss particular challenges unique to non-inferiority trials including the importance of assay sensitivity, the enigma of effect preservation, switching between non-inferiority and superiority, the interpretation of results when event rate assumptions are incorrect, and the place of interim analyses and safety monitoring. We conclude the chapter by addressing alternative methodologies and innovative perspectives on non-inferiority trials that have been proposed in an attempt to mitigate these challenges, including Bayesian approaches, alternative three-arm and pragmatic designs, and methods that address different treatment durations and the averted infections ratio.

Keywords

Noninferiority · Margin of noninferiority · Assay sensitivity · Effect preservation · Active control trial · Biocreep

Introduction

The objective of a superiority randomized clinical trial is to evaluate whether the investigational intervention has superior efficacy (or effectiveness, or safety, depending on the specific trial objectives) as compared to the control arm. The objective of a noninferiority (NI) trial, in contrast, is to evaluate whether the investigational intervention has efficacy that is not much worse than, or noninferior to, that of the control intervention. Critical to this determination of NI, is how to quantitatively describe "not much worse," and this is called the margin of NI, which is the largest reduction in efficacy that is still considered to be consistent with a finding of NI and must be prespecified prior to trial start. If there is sufficient evidence that the reduction in efficacy observed in the trial is no more than the margin of NI, then a conclusion of NI is appropriate.

Historically, NI trials were a subset of equivalence trials which had the objective of showing that an investigational intervention was not much worse *and* not much better than a control intervention (Wellek 2010). In practice, the dual objectives of equivalence are less relevant to randomized clinical trials of interventions to improve human health, apart from studies to demonstrate the bioequivalence of two pharmaceutical agents, and this chapter therefore relates exclusively to the NI trial design. This chapter describes aspects related to the design, conduct, analysis, and interpretation of NI trials, although one could extend many of these ideas to equivalence trials if needed.

The most common NI trial design is a two-arm trial where the internal comparator is an active control intervention which usually reflects a standard of care treatment, and the focus of this chapter is therefore on this two-arm design; other variations on this design are addressed in section "Alternative Analyses and Designs and Innovative Perspectives on NI Trials."

Hypotheses and Notation

The most common primary efficacy outcome of a clinical trial relates to the occurrence or nonoccurrence of an event of interest, e.g., death, failure, cure, or stable culture conversion. We therefore consider a treatment effect of the form $\theta_{EC} = p_E - p_C$, where θ_{EC} is the true treatment effect, and where p_E and p_C are the proportions of participants with the event on the investigational and control arms, respectively (the former is sometimes called the experimental arm), and where the difference might be calculated on the linear scale (for a risk difference) or the log scale (for a risk ratio). Although this convention is used here, the discussion in this chapter can easily be extended to NI trials with other types of primary outcomes, such as continuous or ordinal.

The one-sided null and alternative hypotheses for a superiority and NI trial are shown in Table 1. For simplicity, and without loss of generality, we consider a negative θ_{EC} corresponds to a beneficial effect of the investigational intervention on the outcome of interest (e.g., a reduction in mortality or an increase in cure) and therefore $\delta > 0$; we will use this convention throughout the chapter.

In setting the hypotheses of a NI trial alongside those of a superiority trial, the only difference is in changing the number on the right-hand side of the equations from 0 to δ; the hypotheses otherwise stay the same. In superiority trials, a minimum treatment effect that has some analogy to the margin of noninferiority is used for sample size and power calculations but not for hypothesis testing (see section "Two Sides of the Same Coin: Superiority Versus NI").

Table 1 A comparison of null and alternative hypotheses for superiority and NI trials

	Superiority comparison	NI comparison
Treatment effect measure	$p_E - p_C = \theta_{EC}$	$p_E - p_C = \theta_{EC}$
Null hypothesis	$H_0 : \theta_{EC} = 0$	$H_0 : \theta_{EC} = \delta \ (\delta > 0)$
Alternative hypothesis	$H_1 : \theta_{EC} < 0$	$H_1 : \theta_{EC} < \delta$

Since interpretation of a NI trial necessarily involves consideration of historical trial data (see section "Defining Margin of NI" below), we will use θ_{EP} to denote the estimate of the effect of the investigational arm as compared to no treatment (placebo) and θ_{CP} to denote the estimate of the effect of the active control arm as compared to no treatment.

Motivation for NI

NI trials arise as an option in settings where there are one or more effective treatments for a condition. Typically, a new product is being developed because there is some hope that it offers superior efficacy, a better safety profile, simpler administration, lower cost, or other advantages. This new product should be evaluated in a randomized clinical trial. If there is an established treatment for the condition, it is usually unethical to randomize trial participants to no treatment (placebo), and an active control design must be adopted. There may be settings where the condition under study is transient and not serious and a placebo could be justified.

In either case, the candidate regimen needs to be evaluated in the context of other effective regimens. The FDA guidance (Food and Drug Administration Center for Drug Evaluation and Research (CDER) 2016) for such settings lays out three major alternatives: a study which examines the incremental value of the new therapy combined with established standard of care compared to standard of care alone, a placebo-controlled trial of the new therapy among those who are not candidates for the current standard of care, or an active controlled trial which randomizes participants among the standard of care regimen and the candidate intervention. When the first two options are not feasible or ethical, then the third option, the NI trial, is used.

Because the new regimen may offer substantial advantages over the current standard of care, it would be enough to show that the current regimen is effective. However, it may not be superior, but we would want to avoid the situation of introducing the new drug if it is unacceptably worse than the standard of care. This study objective gives rise to the NI trial design. Specifically, our trial would have two objectives: to support our claim that the new regimen is superior to the withholding of the standard of care and that it is not meaningfully less effective than the standard of care. A major issue here is the choice of the standard of care arm.

NI studies formalize these standards by establishing a margin of NI in a formal statistical framework to determine when these two objectives are met.

Case Studies

Two cases studies are used to illustrate various aspects of NI trials throughout this chapter and are introduced here.

DISCOVER

Nearly 1.7 million people are infected with HIV yearly, and no vaccine is currently available. However, there are abundant safe and potent medications which can suppress HIV replication. In this context, the paradigm of HIV pre-exposure prophylaxis (PrEP) developed. PrEP involves using anti-HIV medication to prevent HIV acquisition in an HIV negative person. Several randomized trials showed that daily use of emtricitabine and tenofovir disoproxil fumarate (F/TDF) was a highly effective PrEP regimen. There is a vigorous pipeline for the development of anti-HIV drugs and/or delivery systems (e.g., long-acting injection) as candidates for PrEP.

The DISCOVER study (Mayer et al. 2020) was a randomized double blind active controlled trial evaluating the efficacy of daily oral emtricitabine and tenofovir alafenamide (F/TAF) for PrEP. The trial's primary objective was to show that, among adults at high risk of acquiring HIV, F/TAF was effective in preventing incident HIV infection. With a proven safe effective and available regimen (F/TDF), it is no longer ethical to evaluate future PrEP candidates in trials with a placebo control. Given that F/TDF is highly effective, it was considered unlikely that F/TAF would be superior in preventing HIV infections. Instead, the major motivation for the adoption of F/TAF is that the reformulation should have less subclinical effects of tenofovir on kidney and bone density. This led the investigators to adopt a NI objective.

Participants took two pills daily: F/TAF (or matching placebo) and F/TDF (or matching placebo). HIV infection was diagnosed in 7 and 15 participants on the F/TAF and F/TDF arms, respectively, yielding a relative incidence of 0.47 (95% CI: 0.19–1.15). Since the 95% confidence interval excluded the prespecified NI margin of 1.62, NI was concluded.

STREAM

Tuberculosis kills more people than any other single pathogen. 1.2 million people died from tuberculosis with 10 million new cases in 2019 (World Health Organization 2020). When the bacteria develop resistance to the main drug, rifampicin, there are few treatment options, although new drugs are in development. STREAM Stage 1 was a phase III trial conducted to evaluate a novel 9–11-month regimen for the treatment of rifampicin-resistant TB and was the first phase III trial to specifically evaluate any regimen for rifampicin-resistant TB (Nunn et al. 2014). A second stage of the trial was conducted including regimens with new drugs; for the purposes of this chapter, we refer to STREAM Stage 1 when referring to the STREAM trial. At the time that the trial was designed, the standard of care, as recommended in WHO 2011 guidelines (World Health Organization 2011), included a cocktail of 4–7 drugs given for at least 18 months. A series of nonrandomized interventional cohort studies in Bangladesh (Van Deun et al. 2010) had identified this 9–11-month regimen resulted in low rates of treatment failures and relapses with adequate safety. It was calculated that just the cost of drugs for this regimen was approximately USD $270 (Van Deun et al. 2010), only one-tenth of the cost of drugs in the WHO-recommended regimen (Floyd et al. 2012). Given these and other benefits to patients and the health system of reducing treatment duration by half, STREAM was designed as a NI trial. The primary efficacy outcome was a favorable status at 132 weeks, defined by cultures negative for *Mycobacterium tuberculosis* at 132 weeks and at a previous occasion, with no intervening positive culture or previous unfavorable outcome. The margin of NI was 10%, with the primary analysis being a calculation of the absolute risk difference in proportion favorable. There were 424 participants randomized into the trial (Nunn et al. 2019), with twice as many allocated to the intervention regimen in order to collect more safety data on the intervention regimen. NI was demonstrated in both coprimary modified intention to treat (mITT) and per protocol (PP) analysis populations. WHO guidelines for the treatment of rifampicin-resistant TB were changed to include the STREAM regimen while the trial was ongoing based on external observational cohort data but were subsequently changed to remove this regimen as a recommended regimen, despite the trial results, due to concerns with the injectable agent included in the regimen (World Health Organization 2019).

Defining Margin of NI

The testing framework for NI requires specification of a NI margin, $\delta > 0$. Ideally, this could be defined as the smallest clinically meaningful difference between the standard and investigational regimens based purely on subject matter grounds. However, this is difficult enough to define for planning a superiority trial and would seem to be even harder in the context of NI.

A major approach has been to define the NI margin by statistical criteria. The approach aims to define a margin which meets two criteria: (i) that the trial would establish that the investigational arm is superior to no treatment; and (ii) that is not unacceptably worse than the control arm. These two objectives are met by using a pair of margins which are typically referred to as the “M1” and “M2” margins, respectively. Some regulatory guidance encourages that trials be adequately powered to refute effects outside the M1 and M2 margins.

The 95/95 Method

Translating a difference between the investigational and control arms into a statement about the former’s effect against no treatment requires a working estimate ,θ^*_{CP}, of the control effectiveness compared to no treatment in the current trial.

The 95/95 method (Rothmann and Tsou 2003) uses a meta-analysis of studies of the control regimen as the starting point for such an estimate – ideally randomized placebo-controlled trials of the control. From the meta-analysis, θ^*_{CP} is taken as the upper bound of a two-sided 95% confidence interval (in a setting where $\theta^*{}_{CP} > 0$ indicates a treatment benefit of the control, the lower bound would be taken). Taking the value closer to the null than the point estimate, so-called discounting, introduces a conservatism. For example, the DISCOVER trial needed to estimate the effectiveness of F/TDF compared to placebo and used a meta-analysis of three placebo-controlled trials in similar populations to derive a meta-analysis of (log) relative hazards with upper bound of the 95% confidence interval $\theta^*{}_{CP} = -0.96$.

The M1 margin is synonymous with a test $H_0 : \theta_{EP} = 0$ which translates to $H_0 : \theta_{EC} + \theta^*{}_{CP} = 0$. Thus, the M1 margin is a comparison of the treatment contrast between investigational and control against a null of $-\theta^*{}_{CP}$. In the case of DISCOVER, the M1 margin would be ruling out a log-relative hazard of F/TAF compared to F/TDF > 0.96 (HR > 2.62).

The M2 margin is derived as a tighter (more conservative) margin which ensures that some proportion of the control treatment effect ($\rho : 0 < \rho < 1$) is preserved by the investigational agent. This functions as a standard of how much worse it can be compared to the effect of the control agent. The M2 margin is then a comparison against $-\rho\theta^*{}_{CP}$. Note that this margin is closer to the null and thus requires more evidence to refute. The 95/95 method typically choses 50% effect preservation which corresponds to $\rho = 0.5$ In the case of DISCOVER, the M2 margin with 50% requires ruling out a log-relative hazard of F/TAF compared to F/TDF $> 0.96*0.5 = 0.48$ (HR > 1.62).

An alternative approach, known as the synthesis method, derives M1/M2 margins using the uncertainty in completed trials without applying discounting.

Sample sizes for NI trials would be smaller than 95/95 if there were no discounting and/or they were powered on a M1 margin alone.

Discounting is motivated as a hedge against: (i) selection of a nonoptimal control therapy, (ii) changes in background treatment, and (iii) publication bias in the meta-analysis. These are particular concerns in mature fields where many randomized controlled trials have been conducted and where there are many estimates of the effectiveness and many possible control comparators. While discounting is clearly sensible in many settings, the 95% confidence interval has been shown to be highly conservative (Sankoh 2008; Holmgren 1999; James Hung et al. 2003). It uses a statistical criterion to handle an unquantifiable uncertainty about the control treatment effect which would have been observed if the NI trial included a putative no treatment arm. The effect preservation criterion, used to develop the M2 margin, ensures that the conclusion of NI will only be made if a high proportion of the control treatment effect is retained by the investigational regimen. The value of the "effect preservation" standards is further discussed in section "Trial Designs to Evaluate Different Treatment Durations."

Combination Therapies

The M1/M2 approach is further complicated when the intervention under evaluation is not just a single agent but is a combination, as is increasingly common in many disease areas. Where the candidate intervention and standard of care regimen have common components, the calculation of M1 and derivation of the minimum margin of NI will be less than if there are no common components.

An example of this is seen in tuberculosis which is usually treated with a combination regimen with two drugs (rifampicin and isoniazid) given for 6 months supplemented by two additional drugs (pyrazinamide and ethambutol) in the first 2 months. NI trials have been conducted to evaluate regimens that have one or two drugs replaced with novel compounds and are given for shorter durations, commonly 4 months instead of 6.

The objective of these trials can be reframed as an evaluation of whether the effect of the new drug (s) has noninferior efficacy to the combined effect of the last 2 months of therapy *and* the effect of drugs that were replaced, *where* each is added to a standard background therapy of the drugs that are common to both combination regimens in the first 4 months of treatment.

The FDA draft guidance for developing drugs for the treatment of pulmonary tuberculosis (Food and Drug Administration Center for Drug Evaluation and Research (CDER) 2013) provides a worked example where the effect of the last 2 months of therapy (for rifampicin-sensitive disease) is shown to be an absolute difference of M1 (θ_{CP}) of 8.4% (95% CI 4.8%, 12.1%) from two previous trials of 4-month regimens, providing support for a margin of NI of 4.8% using this 95/95 approach for NI trials evaluating one- or two-drug substitution trials. A comparable approach has been used to derive margins of 6% or 6.6% in recent drug-substitution trials (Dorman et al. 2020; Gillespie et al. 2014; Jindani et al. 2014), using the M1-type approach, without consideration of the M2.

In contrast, the M1 of the full effect of the entire standard of care regimen is more like an absolute difference of 50–60% given the high effectiveness of 80–90% of the standard 6-month regimen compared to an expected 30% cure from untreated tuberculosis (Tiemersma et al. 2011). For this reason, in trials of *new regimens* with only minor or no drugs in common with the standard of care, the M1/M2 approach can be used to justify margins of up to 12%, and consequently much smaller sample sizes, and still be described as preserving more than 75% (1–12%/50% = 0.76) of the treatment effect of the standard of care regimen (Tweed et al. 2021). This incongruity can discourage sponsors from including existing drugs in novel combination regimens that are more readily available with an established safety profile in favor of only new drugs that are more expensive with less data on drug safety, often to the detriment of patients and health systems.

Public Health Clinical Criteria

In some contexts, the regulatory statistical criteria are not desirable or feasible, and the margin of NI has been set on substantive grounds. For instance, the US FDA has defined a SARS-CoV-2 vaccine to be noninferior (Food and Drug Administration Center for Biologics Evaluation and Research (CBER) 2020) if $\theta_{EC} < 0.1$ where the parameters represent the vaccine efficacy of the new vaccine relative to a control.

This selection is based entirely on substantive grounds in guidance which defines an acceptable vaccine efficacy (VE) as 0.50 with a study design that could rule out a VE of 0.30 or less.

Another example occurs in the STREAM trial. When the trial was started, WHO guidelines for the treatment of rifampicin-resistance TB were based exclusively on evidence from nonrandomized clinical studies (unfortunately, this is largely still the case (World Health Organization 2019)), and it was therefore not possible to construct the M1 from previous studies. A 10% margin in the absolute difference was chosen based on discussions with trial investigators and clinicians and consequently "considered to be an acceptable difference in efficacy, given the shorter treatment duration" (Nunn et al. 2019). The regulatory guidance is somewhat inconsistent in such settings. For example, ICH E10 states "The NI trial design is appropriate and reliable only when the historical estimate of drug effect size can be well supported by reference to the results of previous studies of the control drug" (International Conference on Harmonisation of Technical Requirements for Registration of Pharmaceuticals For Human Use 2000) which seems to rule out a trial like STREAM despite the urgent and obvious public health need for such a trial.

A third example of note is the BLISTER NI trial evaluating doxycycline as a treatment of bullous pemphigoid compared to the much more toxic standard of care of prednisolone. To derive the margin of NI, the investigators conducted "a survey of dermatologists participating in the UK Dermatology Clinical Trials Network, where participants were asked their opinion on various scenarios of possible gains in safety" (Bratton et al. 2012). The chosen margin of 37% is large and "reflects the fact that the majority of dermatologists would accept a substantial reduction in treatment efficacy in exchange for a significant reduction in long-term adverse events, including mortality" (Bratton et al. 2012).

Design and Analysis

Sample Size

Sample size formulae for NI trials are similar to those for superiority trials (see ▶ Chap. 41, "Power and Sample Size") with a few differences. In addition to specifying the event rate (for a time to event end point) or proportion of events (for a binary end point) expected in the control, a key difference is that, instead of specifying a minimum clinically important difference between arms that the trial will be powered to detect, one must specify both the margin of NI and the expected event rate, or proportion of events, in the intervention arm. It is usually assumed that this event rate is the same as the control arm (namely that both arms have true comparable efficacy). If there is compelling evidence to believe that the intervention arm will have slightly better efficacy than the control, then this will result in a smaller sample size, as was done in the STREAM trial, although investigators then run the risk that the trial will be underpowered if this assumption is incorrect. On the other hand, it might be prudent to assume that the intervention arm will have slightly lower efficacy than the control (although within the acceptable margin of NI), although the disadvantage is that this will greatly inflate the sample size. Considerations for the choice of type I error rate and power are the same for NI trials as for superiority trials.

An oft repeated myth is that NI trials are larger than superiority trials. As a broad statement, this is incorrect – NI trials can be larger or smaller than comparable superiority trials, depending on the sample size assumptions. It is, however, true that the sample size of a trial designed to show superiority to placebo, via the indirect comparison in a NI trial design, is always larger than a superiority trial comparing the intervention directly with placebo as noted below in section "Effect Preservation in Determining the NI Margin."

For a trial comparing proportions, the most commonly used formulae for sample size calculations come from Farrington and Manning (1990) (using their formula based on "maximum likelihood" which is more accurate than the approximate formula based on "observed values"), and this is implemented in many statistical software packages for sample size calculations and used in the latest editions of the fourth edition of a popular sample size formulae textbook (Machin et al. 2018), although earlier editions used the less accurate approximate formula.

How to Design a NI Trial

After careful selection and justification of the margin of NI (section "Defining Margin of NI") and consideration of sample size requirements (section "Sample Size"), there are several further design aspects that must be addressed. Many of the considerations informing design aspects of NI trials are the same as those for superiority trials including level of blinding, choice of sites, and length of follow-up (see Chapters 4.5, 2.2, and 2.11). Considerations regarding interim analyses are addressed in section "Interim Analyses and Data and Safety Monitoring."

In recognition of the particular complexities in NI trials, many NI design considerations are addressed in the myriad guideline documents developed by regulators and other international groups specific to NI trials.

Regulatory Guidelines

The ICH efficacy guidelines (numbered E1 through E20) provide guidelines on various aspects of the design, conduct, and reporting of clinical trials, a selection of which specifically addresses NI trials. Of note, many of the documents were finalized more than 20 years ago when NI trials were less common and consequently less well described and understood.

Aside from ICH E3 "Clinical Study Reports" (finalized November 1995) which briefly notes that the evidence in suport of assay sensitivityis important in the NI clinical study report, ICH E9 "Statistical Principles for Clinical Trials" (finalized February 1998) addresses NI trials in several areas. The document notes "well known difficulties" associated with NI trials which include the "lack of any measure of internal validity... thus making external validation necessary," and that "many flaws in the design and conduct of the trial will tend to bias the results towards a conclusion of equivalence." A major source of controversy in the interpretation of NI trials is the choice of a less effective control regimen that can maximize differences between the arms and increase the chance of showing NI but complicating the relative benefits of the investigational regimen versus an optimal control regimen.

The document states that the active control should ideally be a "widely used therapy whose efficacy... has been clearly established and quantified in well designed and well documented superiority trial(s)" and notes that the new NI trial "should have the same important design features" as these previous superiority trial(s).

The document stresses that the trial protocol should "contain a clear statement that this [NI] is its explicit intention" and should specify the margin of NI which should be "justified clinically." The document recognizes that, while the full analysis set should be primary for a superiority trial, it is "generally not conservative" in a NI trial and therefore "its role should be considered very carefully" as it "may be biased towards demonstrating equivalence [NI]" in the presence of participants that withdraw or are lost to follow-up.

In addition to adopting the ICH guidelines described above, the US FDA has published the guidance for industry document "NI Clinical Trials to Establish Effectiveness" (Food and Drug Administration Center for Drug Evaluation and Research (CDER) 2016) (finalized November 2016), and the EMA committee for medicinal products for human use (CHMP) has published the "Guidelines on the choice of the NI margin" (Committee for Proprietary Medicinal Products 2006) (implemented January 2006); other international regulatory agencies also have other guidance documents on NI trials.

Both documents from the US FDA and the EMA provide broad guidance on the design and conduct of NI trials. It is notable that the FDA document is 56 pages as compared to the 11 pages of the EMA document, although it was also finalized 10 years later and likely reflects the increased knowledge and controversy surrounding with these trials. Both documents state that the margin of NI should be justified on statistical and clinical grounds, and the FDA document provides extensive guidance on the former.

Other Guidelines

The CONSORT statement was developed to improve the quality and adequacy of reporting of the results of randomized clinical trials and has undergone regular updates in addition to extensions to specific types of trials, including NI trials in 2006 (Piaggio et al. 2006) and most recently in 2012 (Piaggio et al. 2012). This CONSORT statement provides guidelines exclusively for the reporting of NI, and compliance is broadly required by most major medical journals prior to publication of trial results (http://www.icmje.org/recommendations/browse/manuscript-preparation/preparing-for-submission.html). It was noted that the reporting of NI trials is particularly poor (Piaggio et al. 2006), and more recent reviews have also come to the same conclusion (Rehal et al. 2016).

Key aspects of trial reporting of NI trials in the CONSORT statement include particular rationale for the NI design, statement and justification of the margin of NI, description of how eligibility criteria and choice of control compare to previous superiority trials that established efficacy of the control, and clear description of which among the primary and secondary efficacy and safety outcomes have NI hypotheses and which have superiority hypotheses.

Other widely accepted guidelines of note are the SPIRIT statement defining standard protocol items for clinical trials (Chan et al. 2013) and the guidance document for the content of statistical analysis plans for clinical trials (Gamble et al. 2017). Extensions of the SPIRIT guidelines for certain types of trials have been developed, but there is, currently, no extension specifically for NI trials – this is clearly a document that should be developed, if development is not already underway. Neither SPIRIT nor SAP guidance documents directly address NI trials beyond instructions in the elaboration documents stating that the protocol and the SAP for a NI trial should describe the framework (superiority or NI) for the primary and secondary outcomes.

The EQUATOR network (https://www.equator-network.org/) provides an online repository of guidelines and reference documents related to the reporting of health research (equator-network.org). A search on their database (May 2021) for the words "inferiority" or "equivalence" yields only the CONSORT extension for NI trials (described above).

There are three textbooks addressing the methodology of the design, conduct, and analysis of NI trials published in 2010 (Wellek 2010), 2012 (Rothmann et al. 2012), and 2015 (Ng 2015), curiously all by the same publisher; we are not aware of others. Additional review articles relating to NI trials include a guidance document on how to handle NI trials in the context of systematic reviews (Treadwell et al. 2012) and some general guidelines on the reporting of NI trials that predate the CONSORT extension (Gomberg-Maitland et al. 2003).

Analysis

In general, the methods of analysis for NI trials do not significantly depart from those used for superiority trials. The approach is to calculate a point estimate and confidence interval for the treatment effect, using appropriate methods depending on the type of outcome and study objectives ensuring that the analysis is reflective of the trial design, and desired level of significance for the confidence interval. Figure 1 shows a plot of confidence intervals against a margin of NI to demonstrate different outcomes of NI clinical trials with the upper bound denoted by a square since this is the bound that is the focus of the hypothesis tests. In a superiority trial, if the upper bound of the confidence interval of the treatment effect is lower than the null value (0.0 for a difference or log ratio), then this is evidence for superiority; in a NI trial, if the upper bound of the confidence interval is less than the margin of NI, then this is evidence for NI. If this condition is *not* met for a NI trial, the conclusion must be that there is *no evidence of NI*, that is, the investigational arm is *not noninferior*. This is a somewhat confusing double negative which is sometimes *wrongly* interpreted as evidence of inferiority. No evidence of NI is comparable to the situation in a superiority trial with no evidence of superiority which is not the same as evidence that the two arms in comparison are equivalent. It is universally true across

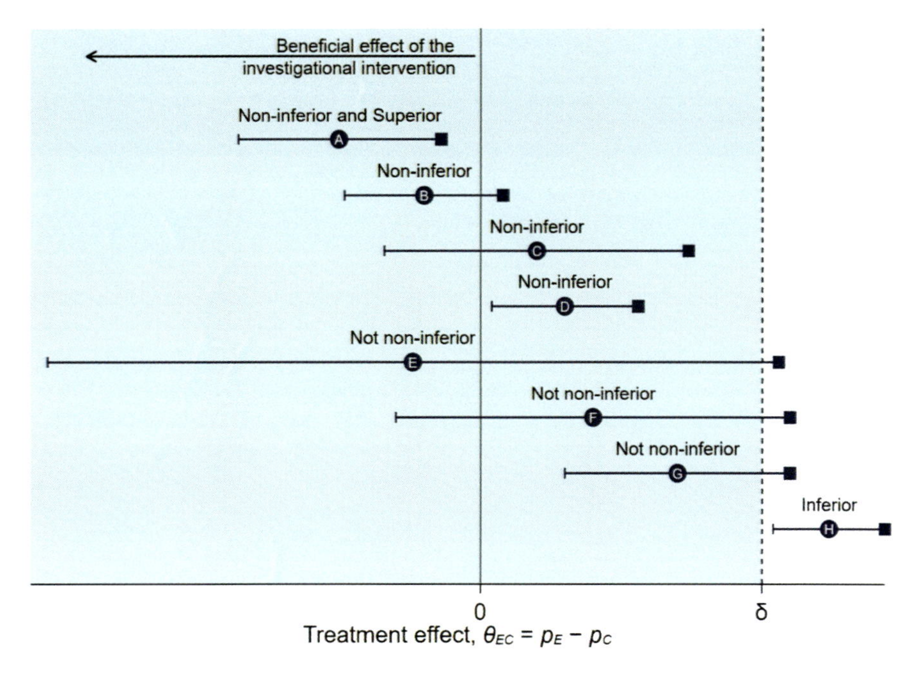

Fig. 1 Examples of potential outcomes from NI trials labeled with interpretation. The upper bound is denoted by a square to show that this is the bound used for determination of NI

superiority and NI trials that absence of evidence should never be interpreted as evidence of absence.

In the STREAM trial, the upper bound of the 95% confidence intervals for the absolute difference in the proportion with a favorable status for the coprimary mITT and PP analysis populations were 9.5% and 9.1%, respectively, both lower than the NI margin of 10% therefore leading to a conclusion of NI. In the DISCOVER trial, the upper bound of the 95% confidence interval for the HIV incidence rate ratio was 1.15 which was lower than the NI margin of 1.62 therefore also leading to a conclusion of NI.

Inferiority and NI

Although the conclusion of NI relates only to the upper bound of the confidence interval (denoted with a square in Fig. 1) since the alternative hypothesis is one-sided, nevertheless, the role of lower bound of the confidence interval can be a source of confusion. The interpretation of the results of a NI trial needs careful consideration when the lower bound of the confidence interval exceeds zero. This would normally be interpreted as evidence that the intervention has inferior efficacy as compared to the control, although this interpretation is inappropriate in a NI trial. The margin of NI defines an acceptable margin of reduction in efficacy, and so the interpretation must be no evidence of NI if the upper bound is not less than the margin (scenario G), or actual evidence of NI if the upper bound is less than the margin (scenario D).

This latter case is somewhat paradoxical and rare, although it is sometimes observed. An interesting example is provided by the BLISTER trial (Williams et al. 2017) (described in section "Public Health Clinical Criteria") where the difference in the primary outcome was 18.6% (90% CI 11.1%, 26.1%) and 18.7% (90% CI 9.8%, 27.6%) in the modified intention to treat and per protocol analyses, respectively. A large margin of NI of 37%, coupled with the finding of clear evidence of improved safety, led the investigators to appropriately conclude that the intervention was noninferior to standard treatment.

Strictly speaking, a conclusion of inferiority can only be made if the lower bound exceeds the margin of NI (scenario H). To avoid this confusion regarding the lower bound, confidence intervals for the results of NI trials are sometimes presented as one-sided confidence intervals; see this approach in JAMA (where the direction of the comparison has been switched from our example), (Kaji and Lewis 2015). ICH E9 also recommends "only the lower margin [upper bound using our convention] is needed for the active control NI trial" (International Conference on Harmonisation of Technical Requirements for Registration of Pharmaceuticals For Human Use 1998).

Choice of Analysis Populations and Estimands

For a superiority trial, it is widely recommended that the primary analysis should include all randomized participants in the treatment groups to which they were allocated; this is regarded as an "intention-to-treat" (ITT) analysis (International Conference on Harmonisation of Technical Requirements for Registration of Pharmaceuticals For Human Use 1998). This "Full Analysis Set," as it is also sometimes described, is preferred for superiority trials not only as it yields "estimates of treatment effects which are more likely to mirror those observed in subsequent practice" (International Conference on Harmonisation of Technical Requirements for Registration of Pharmaceuticals For Human Use 1998) but also because it provides a conservative or protective analysis strategy whereby misclassification of outcomes from participants that have had protocol violations is likely to dilute the treatment effect thereby reducing the chance of falsely demonstrating superiority. For exactly this reason, this ITT analysis set may actually increase the chance of demonstrating NI and is therefore not uniformly accepted as the default choice for the primary analysis for a NI trial, or as noted in ICH E9 (R1): "its role in such [NI] trials should be considered very seriously" (International Conference on Harmonisation of Technical Requirements for Registration of Pharmaceuticals For Human Use 2019).

An alternative analysis population is the modified-ITT (mITT) population with limited exclusions of randomized participants, usually those that violated eligibility criteria but were erroneously randomized, provided entry criteria were measured prior to randomization and all participants recruited undergo equal scrutiny for eligibility violations (International Conference on Harmonisation of Technical Requirements for Registration of Pharmaceuticals For Human Use 1998). A more common alternative is the "Per-Protocol" (PP) population where participants that did not adequately adhere to the treatments under evaluation or other important aspects of the trial protocol are excluded from the analysis. This is sometimes described as an "As-treated" analysis population, although the latter also implies the additional criterion of analyzing participants according to the treatment they actually received. How a PP analysis is defined varies greatly between guidelines and published NI trials (Rehal et al. 2016), and some recommend a limited interpretation and put an emphasis on causal inference methodology for analysis to overcome limitations of postrandomization exclusions (Hernan and Robins 2017). A full discussion of different analysis sets for clinical trials is outside the scope of this chapter; readers should look at chapter 7.2.

In the past, many have recommended that the (m)ITT and PP analysis populations should be coprimary (Piaggio et al. 2006; International Conference on Harmonisation of Technical Requirements for Registration of Pharmaceuticals For Human Use 1998; Jones et al. 1996; D'Agostino et al. 2003; Committee for Proprietary Medicinal Products 2002) for NI trials such that it is necessary to demonstrate NI in both analysis populations in order to declare NI of the regimen. A more recent commentary also supports this approach (Mauri and D'Agostino 2017). Other authors, however, recommend relegating a PP analysis to a secondary analysis (Wiens and Zhao 2007). There is no mention, for example, of a PP analysis in the 2016 FDA guidance on NI (Food and Drug Administration Center for Drug Evaluation and Research (CDER) 2016), although an "as-treated" analysis had been included in the earlier 2010 draft. Much of the discussion of different analysis populations has been replaced by the emphasis on a clear specification of the estimand of interest in the ICH E9 (R1) Addendum (International Conference on Harmonisation of Technical Requirements for Registration of Pharmaceuticals For Human Use 2019) (see ▶ Chap. 84, "Estimands and Sensitivity Analyses") which includes attributes specifying choice of analysis populations and also how intercurrent events (events such as treatment switching or discontinuation that affect or prevent observation of the primary outcome) are handled in analysis. In this regard, the ICH E9 (R1) addendum providing regulatory guidelines on specification of estimands addresses this controversy (International Conference on Harmonisation of Technical Requirements for Registration of Pharmaceuticals For Human Use 2019): "estimands that are constructed with one or more intercurrent events accounted for using the treatment policy strategy present similar issues for NI and equivalence trials as those related to analysis of the Full Analysis Set under the ITT principle." The addendum also recognizes the importance of the PP-type analyses: "An estimand can be constructed to target a treatment effect that prioritizes sensitivity to detect differences between treatments, if appropriate for regulatory decision making."

Further Challenges Unique to NI

Assay Sensitivity

A concern with any NI trial is the concept of "assay sensitivity." A trial is said to have "assay sensitivity" if it would detect the inferiority of an investigational intervention if it were truly inferior. This is an issue of trial conduct and aligning the trial context with assumptions. For instance, in the DISCOVER trial, if adherence to F/TDF was poor, then effectiveness of F/TDF would be expected to be low. In that setting, similarity of HIV incidence between F/TAF and F/TDF would not be evidence of substantial effectiveness of F/TAF.

The assay sensitivity also depends on trial conduct. The poor quality of conduct and design of a NI trial can directly affect whether the proportion of participants experiencing the primary event of interest is estimated with error thereby inducing bias in the estimate of the treatment effect. Quality issues such as high rates of loss to follow-up or low specificity of outcome assessment can result in underestimation of the true proportion of events and issues such as laboratory contamination, unnecessary use of rescue medication, and poor treatment adherence which can result in overestimation of the true proportion of events. Even if these errors are equally distributed between arms, such quality issues can adversely increase the chance of falsely declaring NI (a Type I error). If the true treatment effect, the difference in proportion of events between arms, is larger than the margin of noninferiority but there is underestimation of the proportion of events in each arm, the observed difference between arms will be less than the true difference, and there is a chance of falsely demonstrating noninferiority if the confidence interval is sufficiently narrow. This is in contrast to the chance of falsely declaring superiority which is not increased in this scenario of quality issues that are equally distributed between arms when an ITT analysis is used (White et al. 2012). For these reasons, quality of trial conduct is even more important in a NI trial than in a superiority trial.

ICH E10 "Choice of control group and related issues in clinical trials" (finalized July 2000) also addresses this issue of assay sensitivity. There must be consistency in aspects of trial design between the current NI trial and historical trials evaluating the active control to provide a "fair effectiveness comparison with the control" to support assay sensitivity, and the document specifically notes the choice of dose, patient population, and choice and timing of outcomes. Two approaches to collectively determine assay sensitivity are proposed: (1) historical evidence of sensitivity to drug effects and (2) appropriate trial conduct, the former being evaluated before the trial starts (as part of the derivation of the margin, see section "Defining Margin of NI" above) and the latter once the trial is completed showing that the study population was similar to that in previous trials and that the trial was "conducted with high quality (e.g., good compliance, few losses to follow-up)." The document highlights a number of specific aspects of this "appropriate trial conduct" that can dilute the observed difference between treatments thus reducing the assay sensitivity of the trial including poor adherence to therapy, use of nonprotocol medications, a selective participant population that has a lower response rate, poorly applied diagnostic criteria, and conscious or unconscious underreporting of end points.

Effect Preservation in Determining the NI Margin

A major reason that the sample size of a NI trial can be large is the required tightness of an M2 margin when the 95/95 method is used. Snappin and Jiang (2008) gave an insightful critique of M2 (preservation of effect) criterion and constructed hypothetical scenarios where an investigational therapy was truly more effective than the standard of care. They demonstrated scenarios whereby the standard was evaluated in a randomized trial compared to placebo and "approved"; however, a NI trial of the investigational therapy with the sample size, though more effective, could not exclude the M2 margin, and the investigational therapy was therefore "not approved." Simply by being second, the investigational therapy was judged to be a failure even though it would have been approved if it was first in class. Hence, under effect preservation, the new agent is held to a higher standard. Stronger evidence is required for approval, and the NI trial with an M2 margin is necessarily larger than the original superiority trials of the first agent.

The rationale for effect preservation is compelling, however, in some situations. Consider, for example, the situation when the relevant clinical question is "should the standard of care change from use of the established control as the recommended therapy to use of the investigational intervention as recommended therapy?" This would be a setting in which the objective is to substitute one therapy for another. If so, it is sensible to demand more from the new drug. For instance, the old drug might have an extensive safety record having been shown over time that it is safe and effective in unselected nontrial populations. It might be generic or about to go generic (likely resulting in considerable reductions in cost). Substituting a new drug implies losing some intangibles (demonstrated long-term safety, generics, and the access they can bring), and it is sensible to demand an additional assurance that not much efficacy is lost. If the overall clinical objective is to evaluate a substitute, then effectiveness standards should be high.

In other cases, effect preservation would be considerably less relevant. For instance, the FDA guidance suggests a placebo-controlled superiority trial among those who have contraindication for approved therapies, which implicitly only require an M1 type margin. However, in some cases, the new agent may more subtly lead to a greater therapeutic impact because it may be more acceptable through its simplicity, convenience, or acceptability, a shorter course of TB treatment, for example. An M2 margin, with its criterion of effect preservation, is a poor match for preference-sensitive decisions. It would seem to be a poor fit for contexts where many people who could benefit from the standard therapy cannot or will not use it.

Two Sides of the Same Coin: Superiority Versus NI

Some authors have pointed out that the distinction between NI and "superiority" trials is artificial in many contexts. Dunn et al. (2018a) notes that in nonregulatory situations, it can be unclear which regimen is the "control." Even if one is identified, the smallest clinically significant difference should govern the choice of the NI margin and the alternative for superiority. This yields identical sample sizes for both types of studies. Further, if the data analysis de-emphasizes null hypothesis significance testing in favor of estimation of treatment contrast with the associated confidence intervals, then the analysis and conclusions should be identical for NI and superiority questions. Hence, in many active controlled trials, the distinctions between NI and superiority are not evident. This critique is not strictly relevant when a regulatory-derived margin is used or when one regimen has such clear ancillary advantages that the comparison between the arms is greatly asymmetric.

Testing for Noninferiority and Superiority in the Same Trial

Related to this issue is a document published by the EMA CHMP "Points to consider on switching between superiority and NI" (Committee for Proprietary Medicinal Products 2000) that is focused on the relationship between superiority and NI hypotheses within a single trial. The document is clear that it is acceptable to test for superiority in a NI trial: "there is no multiplicity argument that affects this interpretation because... it corresponds to a simple closed test procedure," with the proviso that "the intention-to-treat principle is given greatest emphasis" in the superiority analysis which is likely to be different for the NI comparison. In any case, every analysis plan for a NI trial should include a plan for a superiority test.

The document also notes that it can be appropriate to test for NI in a superiority trial where superiority has not been demonstrated, provided a margin of NI has been prespecified in the protocol and that the trial was "properly designed and carried out in accordance with the strict requirements of a NI trial." This includes the notion that "in a NI trial the full analysis set and the PP [per protocol] analysis set have equal importance and their use should lead to similar conclusions for a robust interpretation," which is a departure from what is described in the FDA document which recognizes the challenges with the ITT analysis, but does not go so far as to describe a per protocol analysis as of equal importance (see section "Choice of Analysis Populations and Estimands" above).

Sensitivity of Trial Results to Arbitrary Margin and Control Arm Event Rate

A complication of NI trials is the centrality of the NI margin that must be prespecified before the trial starts in inference that occurs after the trial has been completed. For instance, trials with the same control group may derive different margins. For instance, a NI trial of an injectable PrEP agent (cabotegravir) versus F/TDF used the 95/95 method to justify a margin of 1.23 hazard ratio for cabotegravir versus F/TDF. In the same population, the DISCOVER trial specified a much wider margin of 1.62. It is awkward to have trials of products for the same population and indication yet with differing NI margins. Meeting the prespecified margin is often required by regulators, and large inconsistencies in margins give the product with a wider margin a greater chance at regulatory approval. They also further contribute to confusion among colleagues who are not deeply immersed in NI methods about the meaning of and standards for NI. By the 95/95 paradigm, a different margin could be justified in the DISCOVER trial since a stronger control efficacy was expected than in the other trial. This illustrates that fuller evaluation of the evidence for NI should consider a variety of factors including consideration of margins used in similar trials.

Further complications can arise when the observed proportion of events in the control arm deviates from that assumed in sample size calculations. This will severely affect the power of both superiority and NI trials. Such a scenario can also severely affect the interpretation of the results of a NI trial and increase the risk of a false positive (Type I) error since the margin of NI is defined in relation to the expected proportion of events in the control arm (see section "Defining Margin of NI" above). For example, in the ISAR-safe trial, fewer events were observed on the control arm than expected providing supposed strong evidence for NI based on the prespecified margin (on the absolute difference in proportions scale), but a NI conclusion was not accepted by the investigators (Mauri and D'Agostino 2017). This limitation with a fixed margin of NI has been recognized, and aside from Bayesian methods described below, alternative approaches for a flexible margin of NI have been proposed including the use NI frontier (Quartagno et al. 2020). This frontier is "a curve defining the most appropriate NI margin for each possible value of control event risk" which is proposed as a fixed arcsine difference frontier which is "power-stabilizing" and has good properties particularly in that its asymptotic variance is independent of the control arm event rate.

Justification of Margin in Practice

Reporting of NI trials frequently lacks a rigorous justification for their conclusions. A systematic review of NI trials reporting in high-impact medical journals (Rehal et al. 2016) have found that nearly half present no justification for NI margin, and margins frequently were not chosen to show that the investigational regimen was effective compared to no treatment and rarely could ensure at least 50% preservation of the control arm treatment effect (Tsui et al. 2019). Additional frequent problems include a lack of clarity on the type I error of the NI comparison and its direction and whether results are consistent between ITT and PP analyses (Aberegg et al. 2018). Most surprisingly, in 11% of cases, no clear secondary benefit of the investigational regimen was discernable or reported.

As recognized by the extension to the CONSORT guidelines specifically for NI trials (Piaggio et al. 2012), the special consideration of NI trials compels the clear reporting of methods and justification for the margin, type I error rate, and primary analysis. In addition, they should include a rationale for the NI design and the effect of sensitivity analyses such as the mITT and/or per protocol analysis.

Interim Analyses and Data and Safety Monitoring

In randomized clinical trials of untested interventions, an independent Data Monitoring Committee (DMC) will review the results of interim analyses of safety and efficacy data at regular intervals (see ▶ Chap. 37, "Data and Safety Monitoring and Reporting"). Aside from adaptive trial designs where any number of features of a clinical trial could be modified, and review of data quality and trial procedures, a main task of the DMC will be to recommend whether the trial can continue or whether it should be stopped before the scheduled end. This latter recommendation is usually only made when there is sufficient evidence for one of the following: (1) unacceptable harm to trial participants, (2) overwhelming benefit for one arm, or (3) lack of benefit of the investigational intervention. In a NI trial, the consideration of stopping guidelines should be different to those for superiority trials.

It is unlikely to be appropriate to stop a NI trial early for overwhelming evidence of NI since the margin of NI is somewhat subjective, and it would normally be better to continue the trial to get a better estimate of the treatment effect and also to determine whether the intervention might actually be superior. For this reason, a superiority comparison is recommended when evaluating evidence for overwhelming benefit, and one might consider a conditional power approach (Bratton et al. 2012), even in a NI trial (Korn and Freidlin 2018).

It will also be inappropriate to stop a NI trial for lack of benefit since lack of benefit may still be consistent with a finding of NI. When evaluating evidence for lack of benefit in a NI trial, the comparison should be against the margin of NI (effectively evaluating sufficient *lack of evidence for NI*) rather than against a null finding as would be usual in a superiority trial (Bratton et al. 2012).

Alternative Analyses and Designs and Innovative Perspectives on NI Trials

Due to the complexities and challenges in design, conduct, and interpretation of NI trials, several alternative designs or new analyses have been proposed in recent years. We highlight important developments here.

Bayesian Approaches to NI

Bayesian approaches are particularly compelling for NI trials and have been adapted in a variety of ways (Simon 1999; Gamalo-Siebers et al. 2016).

In any NI study, margins are derived directly or indirectly based on historical data. A Bayesian framework provides an intuitive and formal way to incorporate these data through prior distributions. A key source of uncertainty is the value of θ_{CP} about which there might be expert opinion or preliminary data – an ideal setting for the use of prior distributions. Bayesian methods can allow for discounting historical data through shifting the prior toward a null distribution by using skeptical prior distributions (Kirby et al. 2012) or through power priors (Ibrahim and Chen 2000) which allow development of priors which depend the historical data with a flexible weighting index. A lack of constancy can be handled by explicitly modeling variation in the standard treatment effect by using a hyperprior on heterogeneity of treatment effects (Neuenschwander et al. 2010).

This framework allows considerable flexibility in its use of prior information but also allows more flexible statements about treatment effects through the posterior distributions after the trial has been completed. For instance, what is the posterior probability that the investigational regimen is superior to no treatment or to the standard treatment (Spiegelhalter et al. 1994)? Similarly, the posterior probability that the difference between the treatment and the standard exceeds a given margin can be calculated (as was done as a secondary analysis in the STREAM trial (Nunn et al. 2019), see supplementary appendix). This allows for a more rich and nuanced examination than just the binary conclusion of the frequentist fixed margin paradigm where the confidence interval falls within the NI margin or it does not.

Trial Designs to Evaluate Different Treatment Durations

The evocatively named DOOR/RADAR approach (Evans et al. 2015) was proposed as "a new paradigm in assessing the risks and benefits of new strategies to optimize antibiotic use," particularly to avoid the "complexities of non-inferiority trials" and consequent large sample sizes when evaluating whether the duration of antibiotic use can be reduced without a reduction in effectiveness. The idea is to prespecify an ordinal clinical outcome that combines measures of efficacy and safety and then rank trial participants by this clinical outcome measure, where those with a similar clinical outcome are ordered by duration of antibiotic use with shorter duration given a higher rank. This "Desirability of outcome ranking (DOOR)" is compared between different antibiotic strategies in a "Response adjusted for duration of antibiotic risk (RADAR)" superiority comparison, and mean sample sizes needed are much smaller than comparable trials powered for NI.

There has been some uptake of this methodology, but it suffers from replacing the complexities of NI trials with a host of new complexities and a number of substantial limitations (Phillips et al. 2016). These include the introduction of a new metric "the probability of a better DOOR for a randomly selected participant" with no clinical interpretation, the same tendency with NI trials where poor quality may increase the chance of a false positive, and the obscuring of important clinical differences if an important clinical outcome occurs in only a few trial participants. This latter point was illustrated by applying DOOR/RADAR to the results of three NI comparisons from two TB trials that resulted in conclusions of an absence of NI (that were widely accepted by the clinical community) yet counterintuitively showed clear superiority in DOOR with $p < 0.001$ in each case.

A more attractive alternative design for trials evaluating different durations of therapy involves explicit modeling of the duration-response relationship and selection of the duration that achieves the desired cure proportion (Quartagno et al. 2018; Horsburgh et al. 2013).

Three-Arm NI Design

One design that can overcome many of the challenges inherent in NI trials is a three-arm trial with a single investigational intervention arm compared to an active control intervention in a NI comparison, and compared to a different control of no treatment in a superiority comparison. This three-arm trial allows for simultaneous demonstration that the investigational intervention is superior to no treatment and is noninferior to the active control standard of care. This trial design is not possible in many settings with established treatments where it would be inappropriate to withhold treatment.

A risk with NI trials designed after a first investigational intervention has been shown to be noninferior which is the phenomenon of biocreep (D'Agostino et al. 2003; Nunn et al. 2008). If a subsequent successful NI trial results in investigational interventions "not much worse" than the previous investigational interventions, this leads to an intervention that is considerably worse than the original standard of care control and consequently not much better than placebo. A three-arm design is useful to avoid the problem of biocreep. A three-arm NI trial of a second investigational intervention would include both the first intervention shown to be noninferior as well as the original standard of care control. The objective would be to demonstrate NI of the second investigational intervention compared to the original standard of care control, also allowing an internal randomized comparison between the two investigational interventions to support decision-making and facilitate informed patient choice.

Pragmatic Superiority Strategy Trial

If the investigational intervention has expected benefits that mitigate no improvement in efficacy, an alternative to conducting the much maligned NI trial is to conduct a pragmatic trial to evaluate the strategy of implementing the investigational intervention. This pragmatic strategy trial would be designed to evaluate superiority in patient-relevant outcomes in the intended clinical setting of the intervention, thereby avoiding the limitations with NI (defining the margin, assay sensitivity, etc.) altogether. This approach is likely to result in a larger sample size due to the heterogeneity in trial participants and outcomes introduced by the pragmatic design elements, but the additional cost of a larger trial may be offset by reduced complexities in a pragmatic design. Where an investigational intervention has limited safety data, this sort of design is likely to be less appropriate.

As an example of a potential pragmatic design, consider the BLISTER trial described above. When the trial was designed, it was recognized that the investigational intervention could be used in future clinical practice as a first-line therapy to be followed by the standard of care steroid treatment as second-line therapy, even if it was less effective than steroid treatment, without much additional risk to the patient due to its better safety profile. A pragmatic strategy trial that more directly addresses this question than the NI design could be a two-arm trial comparing the strategy of doxycycline as first-line therapy followed by steroid as rescue medication compared with the alternative standard of care strategy of steroid medication as first-line therapy and evaluating superiority on a major clinical outcome such as death, or severe life-threatening adverse events.

An implicit assumption in the objective of shortening treatment for the treatment for tuberculosis (in the STREAM trial, for example) is that shorter duration of treatment results in a variety of benefits to the patient, the health system, and the community. A follow-up trial to any treatment shortening TB trial to evaluate this could therefore be a pragmatic strategy trial to compare the implementation of a short regimen with the standard of care longer regimen to determine whether there are community-level benefits such as reduced TB-related (or all-cause) mortality and reduced health system and/or patient costs. Such a trial may need to be designed as a cluster-randomized or stepped-wedge trial to properly account for the pragmatic nature of the strategy, but randomization would be important, as compared to an interventional cohort study, to improve the strength of evidence generated. The BEAT Tuberculosis trial (https://clinicaltrials.gov/ct2/show/NCT04062201) is a pragmatic superiority strategy trial evaluating the strategy of treatment shortening coupled with standardized regimens based on drug-resistant profile to see whether the investigational strategy improves TB treatment outcomes about individuals with a variety of types of drug-resistance TB in South Africa.

Averted Infections Ratio

In the regulatory framework, the M2 margin plays a major role. The M2 margin is based on some fraction, typically 50%, of effect preservation. While this may seem conceptually straightforward, measures of effect preservation involve subtle choices; they depend on the estimands for the control and investigational arms (whether multiplicative or additive) as well as on what scale effect preservation is judged. Recent work in the HIV prevention context (Dunn et al. 2018b) has shown this scale dependency. This work has reinforced that effect preservation is based on a "meta estimand" and that in some contexts novel meta estimands are both useful and interpretable, providing information beyond whether a M2 margin has been crossed. In the context of HIV prevention trials, an alternative measure of effectiveness, the Averted Infections Ratio (AIR), has been proposed based on the comparison of the number of averted infections between treatment arms (Dunn et al. 2018b). This measure is simple to interpret with both clinical and public health relevance and overcomes limitations of scale dependency.

Conclusions and Recommendations for Design/Conduct/Reporting

NI trials are most compelling when there is an investigational intervention which has theoretical or known advantages over a control intervention. These might include safety, simplicity, cost, or other desirable features for patients or health systems. The key issue in the NI design is that the investigational intervention is a compelling choice provided it is not much worse than the control intervention. The NI margin quantifies this magnitude and is the key design parameter in NI trials. The choice of margin should be prespecified and transparent. In developing it, consideration should be given to the public health context and may be developed using data on historic control intervention effects (when available). If such data is used, consideration must be given to how applicable they will be to the current trial. At a minimum, margins are chosen to exclude the possibility of declaring NI if the investigational treatment effect is not superior to no treatment. Proper trial conduct (avoiding missing/mismeasured data and loss to follow-up) is essential to preserve assay sensitivity. In addition, sensitivity analyses can also be useful. Bayesian analyses have numerous advantages for importing historic knowledge and summarizing conclusions. Clear and complete reporting of key design choices is lacking in the medical literature of NI trials.

Key Facts

- NI trials are most compelling when there is an investigational intervention which has theoretical or known advantages over control interventions such as safety, simplicity, or cost.
- The key issue in the NI design is that the investigational intervention is a compelling choice provided it is not much worse than the control intervention.
- The NI margin quantifies this magnitude and is the key design parameter in NI trials. The choice of margin should be prespecified with a transparent justification.
- Proper trial conduct (avoiding missing/mismeasured data, loss to follow-up) is essential to preserve assay sensitivity.
- Clear and complete reporting of key design choices is lacking in the medical literature of NI trials.

Cross-References

▶ Data and Safety Monitoring and Reporting
▶ Estimands and Sensitivity Analyses
▶ Interim Analysis in Clinical Trials
▶ Masking of Trial Investigators
▶ Masking Study Participants
▶ Platform Trial Designs
▶ Power and Sample Size
▶ Pragmatic Randomized Trials Using Claims or Electronic Health Record Data

References

Aberegg SK, Hersh AM, Samore MH (2018) Empirical consequences of current recommendations for the design and interpretation of noninferiority trials. J Gen Intern Med 33(1):88–96

Bratton DJ, Williams HC, Kahan BC, Phillips PP, Nunn AJ (2012) When inferiority meets non-inferiority: implications for interim analyses. Clin Trials 9(5):605–609

Chan AW, Tetzlaff JM, Gotzsche PC, Altman DG, Mann H, Berlin JA et al (2013) SPIRIT 2013 explanation and elaboration: guidance for protocols of clinical trials. BMJ 346:e7586

Committee for Proprietary Medicinal Products (2000) Points to consider on switching between superiority and non-inferiority. https://www.ema.europa.eu/en/documents/scientific-guideline/points-consider-switching-between-superiority-non-inferiority_en.pdf

Committee for Proprietary Medicinal Products (2002) Points to consider on multiplicity issues in clinical trials. https://www.ema.europa.eu/en/documents/scientific-guideline/points-consider-multiplicity-issues-clinical-trials_en.pdf

Committee for Proprietary Medicinal Products (2006) Guideline on the choice of the non-inferiority margin. https://www.ema.europa.eu/en/documents/scientific-guideline/guideline-choice-non-inferiority-margin_en.pdf

D'Agostino RB Sr, Massaro JM, Sullivan LM (2003) Non-inferiority trials: design concepts and issues - the encounters of academic consultants in statistics. Stat Med 22(2):169–186

Dorman SE, Nahid P, Kurbatova EV, Goldberg SV, Bozeman L, Burman WJ et al (2020) High-dose rifapentine with or without moxifloxacin for shortening treatment of pulmonary tuberculosis: study protocol for TBTC study 31/ACTG A5349 phase 3 clinical trial. Contemp Clin Trials 90: 105938

Dunn DT, Copas AJ, Brocklehurst P (2018a) Superiority and non-inferiority: two sides of the same coin? Trials 19(1):499

Dunn DT, Glidden DV, Stirrup OT, McCormack S (2018b) The averted infections ratio: a novel measure of effectiveness of experimental HIV pre-exposure prophylaxis agents. Lancet HIV 5 (6):e329–e334

Evans SR, Rubin D, Follmann D, Pennello G, Huskins WC, Powers JH et al (2015) Desirability of outcome ranking (DOOR) and response adjusted for duration of antibiotic risk (RADAR). Clin Infect Dis 61(5):800–806

Farrington CP, Manning G (1990) Test statistics and sample size formulae for comparative binomial trials with null hypothesis of non-zero risk difference or non-unity relative risk. Stat Med 9(12): 1447–1454

Floyd K, Hutubessy R, Kliiman K, Centis R, Khurieva N, Jakobowiak W et al (2012) Cost and cost-effectiveness of multidrug-resistant tuberculosis treatment in Estonia and Russia. Eur Respir J 40(1):133–142

Food and Drug Administration Center for Biologics Evaluation and Research (CBER) (2020) Guidance for industry. Development and licensure of vaccines to prevent COVID-19. U.S. Department of Health and Human Services. https://www.fda.gov/media/139638/download

Food and Drug Administration Center for Drug Evaluation and Research (CDER) (2013) Guidance for industry. Pulmonary tuberculosis: developing drugs for treatment, draft guidance. U.S. Department of Health and Human Services. https://www.fda.gov/media/87194/download

Food and Drug Administration Center for Drug Evaluation and Research (CDER) (2016) Guidance for Industry. Non-inferiority clinical trials to establish effectiveness. U.S. Department of Health and Human Services. https://www.fda.gov/media/78504/download

Gamalo-Siebers M, Gao A, Lakshminarayanan M, Liu G, Natanegara F, Railkar R et al (2016) Bayesian methods for the design and analysis of noninferiority trials. J Biopharm Stat 26(5): 823–841

Gamble C, Krishan A, Stocken D, Lewis S, Juszczak E, Dore C et al (2017) Guidelines for the content of statistical analysis plans in clinical trials. JAMA 318(23):2337–2343

Gillespie SH, Crook AM, McHugh TD, Mendel CM, Meredith SK, Murray SR et al (2014) Four-month moxifloxacin-based regimens for drug-sensitive tuberculosis. N Engl J Med 371(17): 1577–1587

Gomberg-Maitland M, Frison L, Halperin JL (2003) Active-control clinical trials to establish equivalence or noninferiority: methodological and statistical concepts linked to quality. Am Heart J 146(3):398–403

Hernan MA, Robins JM (2017) Per-protocol analyses of pragmatic trials. N Engl J Med 377(14): 1391–1398
Holmgren EB (1999) Establishing equivalence by showing that a specified percentage of the effect of the active control over placebo is maintained. J Biopharm Stat 9(4):651–659
Horsburgh CR, Shea KM, Phillips P, Lavalley M (2013) Randomized clinical trials to identify optimal antibiotic treatment duration. Trials 14(1):88
Ibrahim JG, Chen M-H (2000) Power prior distributions for regression models. Stat Sci 15(1):46–60
International Conference on Harmonisation of Technical Requirements for Registration of Pharmaceuticals For Human Use (1998) Statistical principles for clinical trials (E9). https://database.ich.org/sites/default/files/E9_Guideline.pdf
International Conference on Harmonisation of Technical Requirements for Registration of Pharmaceuticals For Human Use (2000) Choice of control group and related issues in clinical trials (E10). https://database.ich.org/sites/default/files/E10_Guideline.pdf
International Conference on Harmonisation of Technical Requirements for Registration of Pharmaceuticals For Human Use (2019) Estimands and sensitivity analysis in clinical trials. E9(R1). https://database.ich.org/sites/default/files/E9-R1_Step4_Guideline_2019_1203.pdf
James Hung HM, Wang SJ, Tsong Y, Lawrence J, O'Neil RT (2003) Some fundamental issues with non-inferiority testing in active controlled trials. Stat Med 22(2):213–225
Jindani A, Harrison TS, Nunn AJ, Phillips PP, Churchyard GJ, Charalambous S et al (2014) High-dose rifapentine with moxifloxacin for pulmonary tuberculosis. N Engl J Med 371(17):1599–1608
Jones B, Jarvis P, Lewis JA, Ebbutt AF (1996) Trials to assess equivalence: the importance of rigorous methods. BMJ 313(7048):36–39
Kaji AH, Lewis RJ (2015) Noninferiority trials: is a new treatment almost as effective as another? JAMA 313(23):2371–2372
Kirby S, Burke J, Chuang-Stein C, Sin C (2012) Discounting phase 2 results when planning phase 3 clinical trials. Pharm Stat 11(5):373–385
Korn EL, Freidlin B (2018) Interim monitoring for non-inferiority trials: minimizing patient exposure to inferior therapies. Ann Oncol 29(3):573–577
Machin D, Campbell MJ, Tan SB, Tan SH (2018) Sample size tables for clinical, laboratory and epidemiology studies, 4th edn. Wiley, Hoboken
Mauri L, D'Agostino RB Sr (2017) Challenges in the design and interpretation of noninferiority trials. N Engl J Med 377(14):1357–1367
Mayer KH, Molina JM, Thompson MA, Anderson PL, Mounzer KC, De Wet JJ et al (2020) Emtricitabine and tenofovir alafenamide vs emtricitabine and tenofovir disoproxil fumarate for HIV pre-exposure prophylaxis (DISCOVER): primary results from a randomised, double-blind, multicentre, active-controlled, phase 3, non-inferiority trial. Lancet 396(10246):239–254
Neuenschwander B, Capkun-Niggli G, Branson M, Spiegelhalter DJ (2010) Summarizing historical information on controls in clinical trials. Clin Trials 7(1):5–18
Ng T-H (2015) Noninferiority testing in clinical trials: issues and challenges. Taylor & Francis/CRC Press, Boca Raton, xvii, 190 p
Nunn AJ, Phillips PPJ, Gillespie SH (2008) Design issues in pivotal drug trials for drug sensitive tuberculosis (TB). Tuberculosis 88:S85–S92
Nunn AJ, Rusen I, Van Deun A, Torrea G, Phillips PP, Chiang CY et al (2014) Evaluation of a standardized treatment regimen of anti-tuberculosis drugs for patients with multi-drug-resistant tuberculosis (STREAM): study protocol for a randomized controlled trial. Trials 15(1):353
Nunn AJ, Phillips PPJ, Meredith SK, Chiang CY, Conradie F, Dalai D et al (2019) A trial of a shorter regimen for rifampin-resistant tuberculosis. N Engl J Med 380(13):1201–1213
Phillips PP, Morris TP, Walker AS (2016) DOOR/RADAR: a gateway into the unknown? Clin Infect Dis 62(6):814–815
Piaggio G, Elbourne D, Altman D, Pocock S, Evans S (2006) Reporting of noninferiority and equivalence randomized trials: an extension of the CONSORT statement. JAMA 295(10):1152
Piaggio G, Elbourne DR, Pocock SJ, Evans SJ, Altman DG, Group C (2012) Reporting of noninferiority and equivalence randomized trials: extension of the CONSORT 2010 statement. JAMA 308(24):2594–2604

Quartagno M, Walker AS, Carpenter JR, Phillips PP, Parmar MK (2018) Rethinking non-inferiority: a practical trial design for optimising treatment duration. Clin Trials 15(5):477–488. https://doi.org/10.1177/1740774518778027

Quartagno M, Walker AS, Babiker AG, Turner RM, Parmar MKB, Copas A et al (2020) Handling an uncertain control group event risk in non-inferiority trials: non-inferiority frontiers and the power-stabilising transformation. Trials 21(1):145

Rehal S, Morris TP, Fielding K, Carpenter JR, Phillips PP (2016) Non-inferiority trials: are they inferior? A systematic review of reporting in major medical journals. BMJ Open 6(10): e012594

Rothmann MD, Tsou HH (2003) On non-inferiority analysis based on delta-method confidence intervals. J Biopharm Stat 13(3):565–583

Rothmann MD, Wiens BL, Chan ISF (2012) Design and analysis of non-inferiority trials. Chapman & Hall/CRC, Boca Raton, xvi, 438 p

Sankoh AJ (2008) A note on the conservativeness of the confidence interval approach for the selection of non-inferiority margin in the two-arm active-control trial. Stat Med 27(19):3732–3742

Simon R (1999) Bayesian design and analysis of active control clinical trials. Biometrics 55(2): 484–487

Snapinn S, Jiang Q (2008) Preservation of effect and the regulatory approval of new treatments on the basis of non-inferiority trials. Stat Med 27(3):382–391

Spiegelhalter DJ, Freedman LS, Parmar MK (1994) Bayesian approaches to randomized trials. J R Stat Soc A Stat Soc 157(3):357–387

Tiemersma EW, van der Werf MJ, Borgdorff MW, Williams BG, Nagelkerke NJ (2011) Natural history of tuberculosis: duration and fatality of untreated pulmonary tuberculosis in HIV negative patients: a systematic review. PLoS One 6(4):e17601

Treadwell JR, Uhl S, Tipton K, Shamliyan T, Viswanathan M, Berkman ND et al (2012) Assessing equivalence and noninferiority. J Clin Epidemiol 65(11):1144–1149

Tsui M, Rehal S, Jairath V, Kahan BC (2019) Most noninferiority trials were not designed to preserve active comparator treatment effects. J Clin Epidemiol 110:82–89

Tweed CD, Wills GH, Crook AM, Amukoye E, Balanag V, Ban AYL et al (2021) A partially randomised trial of pretomanid, moxifloxacin and pyrazinamide for pulmonary TB. Int J Tuberc Lung Dis 25(4):305–314

Van Deun A, Maug AKJ, Salim MAH, Das PK, Sarker MR, Daru P et al (2010) Short, highly effective, and inexpensive standardized treatment of multidrug-resistant tuberculosis. Am J Respir Crit Care Med 182(5):684–692

Wellek S (2010) Testing statistical hypotheses of equivalence and noninferiority, 2nd edn. CRC Press, Boca Raton, xvi, 415 p

White IR, Carpenter J, Horton NJ (2012) Including all individuals is not enough: lessons for intention-to-treat analysis. Clin Trials 9(4):396–407

Wiens BL, Zhao W (2007) The role of intention to treat in analysis of noninferiority studies. Clin Trials 4(3):286–291

Williams HC, Wojnarowska F, Kirtschig G, Mason J, Godec TR, Schmidt E et al (2017) Doxycycline versus prednisolone as an initial treatment strategy for bullous pemphigoid: a pragmatic, non-inferiority, randomised controlled trial. Lancet 389(10079):1630–1638

World Health Organization (2011) Guidelines for the programmatic management of drug-resistant tuberculosis - 2011 update. World Health Organization

World Health Organization (2019) WHO consolidated guidelines on drug-resistant tuberculosis treatment. World Health Organization, Geneva

World Health Organization (2020) Global tuberculosis report 2020. World Health Organization, Geneva

Cross-over Trials

70

Byron Jones

Contents

Abstract

Cross-over trials have the potential to provide large reductions in sample size compared to their parallel groups counterparts. In this chapter, three different types of cross-over design and their analysis will be described. In the linear models used to analyze cross-over data, the variability due to differences between the subjects in the trial may be modeled as either fixed or random effects, and both will be illustrated. In designs of the incomplete block type, where there are more

B. Jones (✉)
Novartis Pharma AG, Basel, Switzerland
e-mail: byron.jones@novartis.com

© Springer Nature Switzerland AG 2022

S. Piantadosi, C. L. Meinert (eds.), *Principles and Practice of Clinical Trials*,
https://doi.org/10.1007/978-3-319-52636-2_243

treatments than periods, the use of random subject effects enables between-subject information on the treatment comparisons to be recovered, and how this may be done will also be illustrated. Finally, if the so-called baseline measurements have been taken at the beginning of each treatment period, these can be used as covariates to reduce the variability of the estimated treatment comparisons. The use of baselines will be illustrated using the incomplete block design.

Keywords

Crossover trials · Fixed effects · Random effects · Incomplete block · Between-subject information · Baseline information

Introduction

In a cross-over trial, each subject (i.e., a patient or a healthy volunteer) receives a sequence of treatments over a set number of time periods. At the end of each period, the clinical response of interest is measured and recorded. The effects of the different treatments are then compared using the repeated measurements on the same subject. These "within-subject" comparisons are to be contrasted with those that are obtained from a parallel groups design where each subject receives only *one* of the treatments, and comparisons between treatments are made "between-subjects." Typically, the variability of the within-subject comparisons is much smaller that the variability of the between-subject comparisons, leading to cross-over designs that may require far fewer subjects than their parallel groups counterparts to achieve the same power to detect a treatment effect of a given size (see Piantadosi (1997), Sect. 16.2.1).

Three different types of cross-over design and their analyses will be described in this chapter, and this will be done using examples based on real trials. In section "Example 1: 2 × 2 Design," two treatments are compared using two periods. In section "Williams Crossover Design," five treatments are compared using five periods, and in section "Example 3: Incomplete Block Design" the trial is of the incomplete block type and compares four treatments in three periods. Using this last design, the recovery of any useful between-subject information that is typically present in an incomplete design will be illustrated.

It is not unusual in a cross-over clinical trial to take measurements at the start of each period as well as at the end of each period. The baseline measurements taken at the beginning of the periods can sometimes be included as useful covariates to reduce the variability in the estimated treatment comparisons. The use of baseline information is illustrated in section "Use of Baseline Measurements."

In the next section, the notation used in this chapter is introduced.

Notation

When discussing trials in a generic sense, those taking part will be referred to as subjects. Depending on the actual context, these may be either patients or healthy volunteers.

In a cross-over trial, the time the trial takes to complete is divided into a sequence of time periods. Within each period, a subject receives either one of the treatments to be compared or no treatment. The periods where no treatments are received are referred to as either run-in or wash-out periods. The reason for these will be explained later. Typically, a subject receives a sequence of different treatments spaced out over all time periods. In the trial as a whole, a particular (usually small) number of different treatment sequences will be used, and an example of such a trial is given in Table 1, below. The subjects that are available for the trial are randomly assigned to the different sequences, and the group of subjects assigned to a particular sequence is referred to as a sequence group. Often, the random assignment is done in a way that ensures all sequence groups are the same (or approximately the same) size.

In the cross-over trial illustrated in Table 1, there are two treatments to be compared (A and B), over four time periods. The first time period is the "run-in" period where baseline measurements are taken and subjects get acclimatized to the trial procedures; in the second period, each subject receives one of the two treatments; the third period is a "wash-out" period, and in the fourth period each subject gets the treatment that was not administered in the second period. The trial has two sequence groups, defined by the order in which the treatments are administered: AB and BA.

In general, the number of treatments, periods, and sequence groups in the design will be denoted as t, p, and s, respectively. The number of subjects in sequence group i will be denoted as n_i, $i = 1,2, \ldots, s$. Within sequence group i, n_i, subjects receive all the treatments in the specified treatment sequence for that group. Note that the total number of subjects in the trial is the sum of the n_i, i.e., $\sum_{i=1}^{s} n_i$.

If y_{ijk} $(i = 1, 2, \ldots, s; j = 1, 2, \ldots, p; k = 1, 2, \ldots, n_i)$ denotes the response observed on the kth subject in period j of sequence group i, then a typical statistical model used to explain a continuous response is:

$$y_{ijk} = \mu + \pi_j + \tau_{d[i,j]} + s_{ik} + e_{ijk}, \tag{1}$$

where μ is a general intercept, π_j is an effect associated with period j $(j = 1, \ldots, p)$, $\tau_d[i, j]$ is the direct treatment effect associated with the treatment $d[i, j]$, applied in period j of sequence group i $(d[i, j] = 1, \ldots, t)$, s_{ik} is the effect associated with the kth subject in sequence group i $(i = 1, \ldots, s,\ k = 1, \ldots, n_i)$, and e_{ijk} is an independent random error term, with zero mean and variance σ^2. We refer to this model as Model (1).

Note that the s_{ik} represent characteristics of the subjects, not the treatments. For example, some subjects may have baseline values of the response of interest that are higher or lower than others. Including the s_{ik} in the model takes account of some of the variability in the response that is just the result of variation in baseline subject

Table 1 Typical structure of the 2 × 2 cross-over trial

	Period			
Group	Run-in	1	Wash-out	2
1(AB)	-	*A*	-	*B*
2(BA)	-	*B*	-	*A*

characteristics. The s_{ik} do not account for variation in the treatment effects over the periods: other parameters defined above account for this.

In a cross-over trial, there is the possibility that the effect observed in one period may persist into the next period. This effect is known as a carry-over effect. If there is a need to allow for carry-over effects, and these are additive to the treatment effects, then the above model can be extended to include the carry-over effect term, $\lambda_{d[i,\ j\ -\ 1]}$:

$$y_{ijk} = \mu + \pi_j + \tau_{d[i,j]} + s_{ik} + \lambda_{d[i,j-1]} + e_{ijk}. \tag{2}$$

Obviously, there can be no carry-over effect in the first period, i.e., $\lambda_{d[i,\ 0]} = 0$. We refer to this model as Model (2).

Models (1) and (2) are examples of fixed-effects models: In such models, the effects (for periods, treatments, carry-overs and subjects) are constant, but unknown values, to be estimated.

An alternative model, referred to here as the random-effects model, assumes that the s_{ik} are independent random effects with mean 0 and variance σ_s^2.

The s_{ik} have mean zero, because they represent the random relative effect of the subject characteristics on the response (some values are higher and some are lower). The amount the subject effects vary is measured by the variance parameter σ_s^2 (larger σ_s^2 implies greater variability).

In addition, the s_{ik} are assumed to be independent of the e_{ijk}. Of course, it could be argued, quite rightly, that what is being referred to here as a random-effects model is actually a mixed-effects model because it contains both random and fixed effects. However, to maintain consistency with the literature, the term random-effects model will be used in this chapter.

If not stated otherwise, it is assumed in the following that the s_{ik} in Models (1) and (2) are random variables, as defined above.

Then the responses from periods j and $j'(j \neq j')$, on the same subject, have variances $Var(y_{ijk}) = Var(y_{ij'k}) = \sigma^2 + {\sigma_s}^2$ and covariance $Cov\left(y_{ijk}, y_{ij'k}\right) = \sigma_s^2$. This means that the correlation between any two responses on the same subject is $\rho = \sigma_s^2 / \left(\sigma_s^2 + \sigma^2\right)$. As can be seen, the correlation increases as σ_s^2 increases.

More complex correlation structures can be defined by making particular assumptions regarding the correlation structure of the s_{ik} or the e_{ijk}, but we do not do this here. See Chi and Reinsel (1989) for how this may be done to produce an autoregressive correlation structure.

When any two measurements on the same subject are positively correlated, the estimate of any treatment comparison has a smaller variance than would be obtained from a parallel groups design with the same number of subjects (see Piantadosi (1997), Sect. 16.2.1). So when used appropriately, the cross-over design requires fewer subjects than a parallel groups design to achieve a desired level of power to reject the null hypothesis of no treatment difference.

When the subject effects are assumed to be random, the model parameters can be estimated using restricted maximum likelihood (REML), as introduced by Patterson and Thompson (1971).

Challenges When Designing a Cross-over Design

When designing a cross-over trial, several important questions need to be answered:

- Is the condition being treated a chronic condition for which a cross-over trial is appropriate?
- Is the effect of the treatment likely to persist into a following period, i.e., are carry-over effects expected?
- Can the carry-over effects be removed by including sufficiently long wash-out periods?
- How many treatments are to be compared?
- How many periods can be used?
- Which treatment comparisons are important?
- What is the maximum sample size, i.e., the total number of subjects required?

Assuming that a cross-over design is an appropriate choice, the answers to the above questions typically do not lead to a unique design and some way of choosing between the alternatives is required. Jones and Kenward (2014) give tables of alternative designs for up to nine treatments and nine periods. Rohmeyer (2014) has provided an R package *Crossover* to accompany Jones and Kenward (2014) that provides an easy to use graphical user interface (GUI) to locate designs for different values of $(t, p, s,)$, either from the tables provided in Chapter 4 of Jones and Kenward (2014) or by using a computer search algorithm. See Chapter 4 of Jones and Kenward (2014) for examples of using the GUI and Rohmeyer (2014) for details of the search algorithm. The *Crossover* package also allows a choice for how the carry-over effects are modeled. The criterion used to distinguish between good and bad cross-over designs is referred to as the *efficiency* of the design.

Efficiency of a Cross-over Design

An important criterion when choosing between designs, especially when all pairwise comparisons between the treatments are of equal importance, is the *efficiency* of the design. The efficiency of a particular comparison is the ratio of the variance of an estimated pairwise difference of the treatment effects in the design of interest compared to a theoretical lower bound on that variance (Patterson and Lucas (1962)).

For the calculation of these variances, it is assumed that the s_{ik} are fixed effects. This is because, when comparing designs, the main interest is in maximizing the within-subject information.

The lower bound is a technical construct that has proved very useful for calibrating how good a design is relative to the (statistically) best it could be. In this technically best design, statistical theory states that the estimator of the difference between two treatment effects that has minimum variance is the difference between the simple (unadjusted) means of those two treatments. The variance of this estimator is then the variance of the difference of these two means, which can easily be calculated for any design. For example, in most designs, the planned number of responses, r, to be recorded on each treatment (A, B, and so on) is the same. If each sequence group has size n, the planned total number of responses is $N = s \times n \times p$ and $r = N/t$. The variance of the difference of two means in this case is

$$V_{bound} = \frac{2\sigma^2}{r} \tag{3}$$

and this is the technical lower bound for the difference of two treatments in the design under consideration. For some designs, the number of responses on a particular pair of treatments, i and j, say, may not be the same, and equal r_i and r_j, respectively. In this case, the technical lower bound is

$$V_{bound} = \sigma^2/r_i + \sigma^2/r_j. \tag{4}$$

If V_d is the variance of an estimated pairwise comparison in the design of interest, then the efficiency, E, is defined as

$$E = \frac{V_{bound}}{V_d}. \tag{5}$$

Basically, E measures how large V_d is when compared to the lower bound. The larger is V_d, the smaller is E.

The value of V_d depends on the design and the model assumed for the response. It can be calculated using the formulae for the least squares estimators of the treatment comparisons in the design under consideration (see Jones and Kenward (2014), Sect. 3.5, for some examples). Although it involves the within-subject variance σ^2 as a constant multiplier, this cancels out in the ratio in Eq. (5), as V_{bound} also includes σ^2 as a constant multiplier. Therefore, it can be calculated prior to the collection of any data. As already noted, E measures how large the variance of the difference of two estimated treatment effects is in the design under consideration relative to the lower bound. In an ideal design, $E = 1$, as then $V_d = V_{bound}$. The reason why V_d may be greater than V_{bound}, and $E < 1$, is that the structure of the design is such that, even after adjusting for the period and subject effects (and possibly, carry-over effects), in the statistical analysis (i.e., after fitting Models (1) or (2)), the lower bound on the variance is still exceeded for some or all estimated pairwise comparisons.

Examples of the efficiency values for two types of design will be given in sections "Williams Crossover Design" and "Example 3: Incomplete Block Design," respectively.

Example 1: 2 × 2 Design

The simplest cross-over design, known as the 2 × 2 design, compares two treatments using two active treatment periods. The basic structure of this design is given, as previously, in Table 1. Here $s = 2, p = 2$, and $t = 2$. In this design, as illustrated, there are four periods: two active treatment periods (labeled as 1 and 2), a run-in period, and a wash-out period. The purpose of the run-in period, as already noted, may be to familiarize the subjects with the clinical trial procedures, collect baseline measurements, remove the effects of a previous treatment, or confirm that a subject is able to continue into the first period, for example. The purpose of the wash-out period is to remove the effects of the drug given in Period 1 before the second drug is given in Period 2. This should ensure that subjects are in the same clinical state at the start of Period 2 as they were at the start of Period 1. It should be noted that in some trials the wash-out period is not included. This may be because its inclusion will extend the time the trial will take to complete beyond that which is reasonable or because there is confidence that carry-over effects will not exist. Typically, to remove a pharmacological carry-over effect of a single oral dose, the wash-out period should be at least five half-lives of the drug (FDA (2013)). The half-life of a drug (see Clark and Smith (1981)) is the time it takes for the concentration of the drug in the blood (or plasma) to reduce to half of what it was at equilibrium. After one half-life, the concentration should drop by $(100 \times 1/2)\% = 50\%$, after two half-lives drop by $100(1/2 + 1/4)\% = 75\%$, and by five half-lives drop by $100(1/2 + 1/4 + 1/8 + 1/16 + 1/32)\% \approx 97\%$.

For Models (1) and (2), the fixed effects are displayed in Table 2 and Table 3, respectively.

The data that will be used to illustrate the analysis of the 2×2 design are based on actual data from a completed Phase III randomized, double-blind, placebo controlled trial to assess the effect of drug A on exercise endurance in subjects with moderate to severe chronic obstructive pulmonary disease (COPD). Drug B is a placebo treatment, i.e., a drug with no active pharmacological ingredients. Exercise endurance time in seconds was measured using a constant-load cycle ergometry test after 3 weeks of treatment.

After a 1-week run-in period, subjects were randomized to receive either A or B. After 3 weeks of treatment, the drugs were withdrawn, and there was a 3-week washout-period. Patients who began on A then crossed over to B, and those who began on B crossed over to A. Due to the presence of the wash-out periods, it is assumed that there are no carry-over effects present and Model (1) applies.

Patients who received A first belong to the AB sequence group (Group 1), and subjects who received B first belong to the BA sequence group (Group 2).

The data in Tables 4 and 5 give examples of observations similar to those collected in the actual trial. The actual data have been modified to preserve their confidentiality and to enable key ideas to be presented without too much

Table 2 The fixed effects in the model that excludes carry-over effects

Group	Period 1	Period 2
1(AB)	$\mu + \pi_1 + \tau_1$	$\mu + \pi_2 + \tau_2$
2(BA)	$\mu + \pi_1 + \tau_2$	$\mu + \pi_2 + \tau_1$

Table 3 The fixed effects in the model that includes carry-over effects

Group	Period 1	Period 2
1(AB)	$\mu + \pi_1 + \tau_1$	$\mu + \pi_2 + \tau_2 + \lambda_1$
2(BA)	$\mu + \pi_1 + \tau_2$	$\mu + \pi_2 + \tau_1 + \lambda_2$

Table 4 Example of observations from Group 1(AB) subjects (endurance time in seconds)

Subject	Period 1(A)	Period 2(B)	Difference	Sum
1	*496*	*397*	*99*	*893*
3	*405*	*228*	*177*	*633*
.	.	.	.	.
.	.	.	.	.
58	*575*	*548*	*27*	*1123*
59	*330*	*303*	*27*	*633*

Table 5 Example of observations from Group 2(BA) subjects (endurance time in seconds)

Subject number	Period 1(B)	Period 2(A)	Difference	Sum
2	*270*	*332*	*−62*	*602*
5	*465*	*700*	*−235*	*1165*
.	.	.	.	.
.	.	.	.	.
54	*308*	*236*	*72*	*544*
57	*177*	*293*	*−116*	*470*

complication. To save space, only the data for a few subjects in each group are shown. Table 4 gives the data for the subjects in the AB group (Group 1). It can be seen that there are two measurements for each subject, one for Period 1 when A was received and one for Period 2 when B was received. Table 5 gives the corresponding data for the subjects in the BA group (Group 2), where it is noted that in this group the subjects received B first and then crossed over to A.

Also given in these two tables are the within-subject differences (Period 1 – Period 2) and the sum of the two responses of each subject. These will be used to estimate the treatment difference and the carry-over difference, respectively (see sections "Two-Sample t-Test" and "Testing for a Difference in Carry-Over Effects").

By taking the difference between the Period 1 measurement and the Period 2 measurement within each subject, a within-subject comparison of A versus B is obtained in Group 1 and a within-subject comparison of B versus A is obtained in Group 2.

In the following, the complete data from the 2 × 2 trial are analyzed to decide if treatment A is superior to treatment B. Before that, however, we describe two useful plots that focus on illustrating the strength of the difference (if any) between the effects of A and B.

Plotting the Data

Before conducting formal hypothesis testing, it is always useful to plot the data that are to be analyzed. For the 2 × 2 trial, a useful plot is the *subject profiles* plot, which for this example is displayed in Fig. 1. The left-hand plot is for the AB group, and the

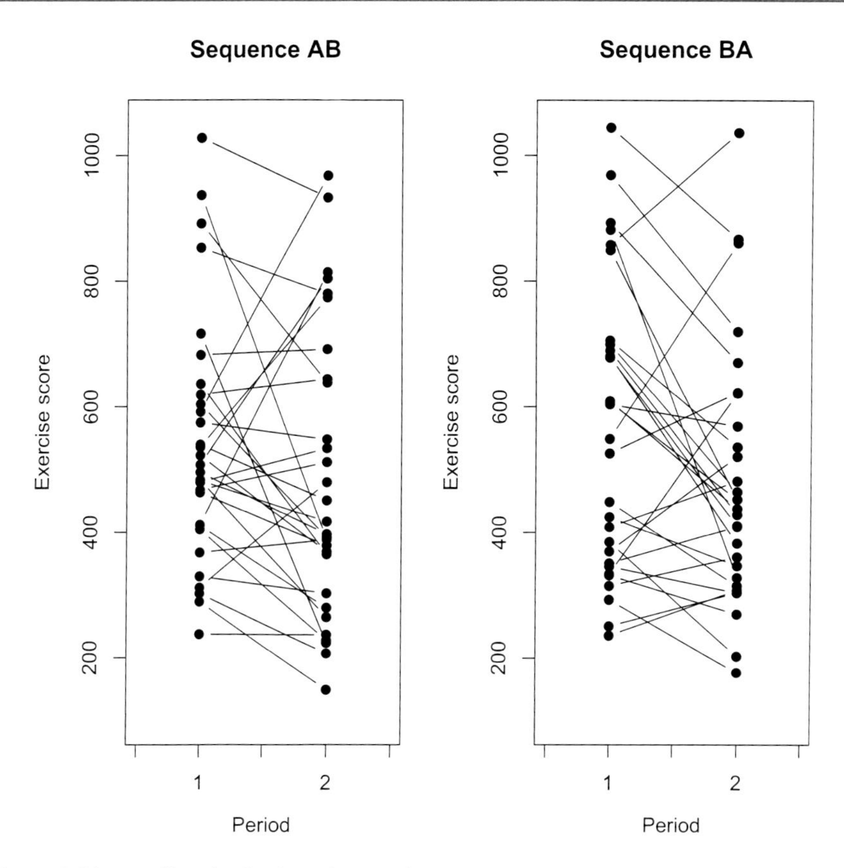

Fig. 1 Subject profiles plot for the endurance data

right-hand plot is for the BA group. Looking at the plot for the AB group, for example, it can be seen that there is a pair of points and a line connecting them for each subject. The left-hand point is the response in Period 1, and the right-hand point is the response in Period 2. It can be seen that some subjects have a much longer endurance time on A compared to B (see the second line from the top for the AB group) whereas others actually have a shorter endurance time on A compared to B (some substantially so). It is clear that the between-subject variability in the responses is large, and this is one of the situations where a cross-over trial is likely to be preferred to a parallel groups design.

However, although it might be possible to get the impression from Fig. 1 that A increases endurance time compared to B, it is not very clear and a significance test must be performed to get a definitive answer. As a preliminary to this, the mean of the responses of the subjects per group and period is calculated, as displayed in Table 6.

A very useful way to display these means is the *groups-by-periods* plot, as given in Fig. 2. The means have been joined in different ways. In the left-hand panel, the

Table 6 The means for each group and period combination

Group	Period 1	Period 2
1(AB)	*539.57*	*485.33*
2(BA)	*478.17*	*563.52*

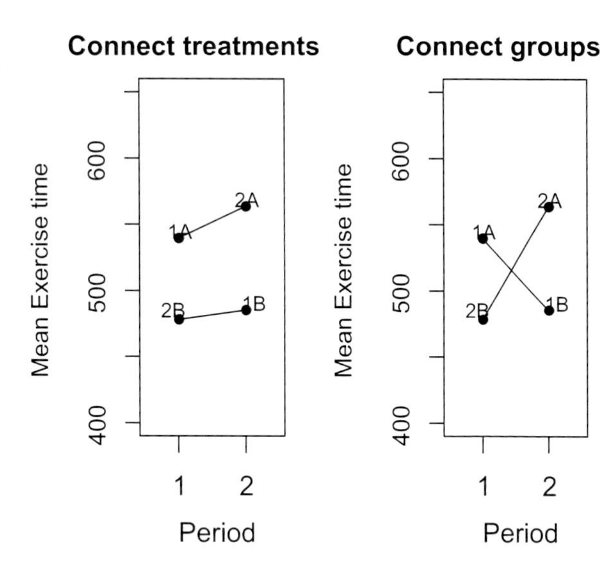

Fig. 2 Group-by-period means for the endurance data

lines connect the same treatment, and in the right-hand panel the lines connect the same group. The left-hand panel emphasizes the treatment difference in each period: It can be seen that in each period there is a consistent pattern where A is higher than B. The right-hand plot emphasizes the within-subject mean changes: In the AB group, there is a definite decline in endurance from the first period to the second, and in the BA group there is a definite increase in endurance time from the first period to the second. This displays the clearest evidence so far, that A is superior to B.

Two-Sample t-Test

Before immediately fitting Model(1), it is instructive to first see how the null hypothesis of no treatment effect can be tested using the familiar two-sample t-test. This requires the additional assumption that the within-subject differences in response are normally distributed. In the absence of an assumption of normality, the nonparametric Wilcoxon rank-sum test may be used (Jones and Kenward (2014), Sect. 2.12 and Hollander and Wolfe (1999)), although the t-test is quite robust against violations of this and other assumptions (Havliceck and Peterson (1974)).

The column headed "Difference" in both Tables 4 and 5 gives the within-subject difference for each subject in each group. Each within-subject difference in Group 1 is an unbiased estimator of $(\tau_1 - \tau_2) - (\pi_1 - \pi_2)$, where it is noted that the subject effects and the general intercept have been canceled out. Similar reasoning leads to the conclusion that the mean of the differences in Group 2 is an unbiased estimate of $(\tau_2 - \tau_1) - (\pi_1 - \pi_2)$. Consequently, the difference between the mean of the within-subject differences in Group 1 and the mean of the within-subject differences in Group 2 has expectation $2(\tau_1 - \tau_2)$. Therefore, a two-sample t-test comparing the within-subject differences of the two groups is a test of the null hypothesis of no difference between the treatments, H_0: $\tau_1 = \tau_2$.

If $d_{ik} = y_{i1k} - y_{i2k}$ denotes the within-subject difference of subject k in group i, and $\overline{d}_{i.}$ the mean of these differences in Group i, then a pooled estimator of the variance of the differences, σ_d^2, is:

$$\widehat{\sigma}_d^2 = 2\widehat{\sigma}^2 = \sum_{i=1}^{2} \sum_{k=1}^{n_i} \left(d_{ik} - \overline{d}_{i.}\right)^2 / (n_1 + n_2 - 2). \tag{6}$$

The pooled estimator of the variance is an application of a standard formula, as given, for example, in Altman (1991), Sect. 9.6.1.

The estimator of the treatment difference, $\tau_d = \tau_1 - \tau_2$, is

$$\widehat{\tau}_d = \left(\overline{d}_{1.} - \overline{d}_{2.}\right)/2 \tag{7}$$

and its standard error is

$$s_\tau = \sqrt{\widehat{\sigma}_d^2 (1/n_1 + 1/n_2)/4}. \tag{8}$$

Calculating these statistics gives: $\widehat{\sigma}_d^2 = 42393.3$, $\widehat{\tau}_d = (54.233 - (-85.345))/2 = 69.79$ and $s_\tau = 26.81$. The two-sample t-test statistic, $\widehat{\tau}_d / s_\tau$, is then 69.79/26.81 = 2.60 on 57 degrees of freedom. This gives a p-value of 0.012 (two-sided) or 0.006 (one-sided). There is clear evidence to reject the null hypothesis and to conclude that A is superior to B and increases endurance time by 69.8 seconds on average, with a 95% confidence interval for the difference of (16.10, 123.47).

Fitting a Linear Model

The analysis of variance table obtained from fitting Model (1) is given in Table 7, and the corresponding estimated treatment and period effects are given in Table 8.

Although Table 7 does not give any new information regarding the treatment effect, it does make clear that a large proportion of the total variability in the data is accounted for by the between-subject variability. By this is meant that the between-subjects SS are a large proportion of the Total SS (4,090,211/5448153 = 0.75). Also, there is no evidence of a significant period difference.

In addition, from output not shown, $\widehat{\rho} = \widehat{\sigma}_s^2 / \left(\widehat{\sigma}_s^2 + \widehat{\sigma}^2\right) = 225262/(25262 + 21197) = 0.54$.

The period difference could also have been tested using the two-sample t-test. To test for a period effect, the within-subject differences in one of the groups (e.g., Group 2)

Table 7 Analysis of variance for the endurance data [df = degrees of freedom, SS = sums of squares, MS = mean square, and F=F-ratio]

Source	df	SS	MS	F	P-value
Between-subjects	*58*	*4,090,211*	*70,521*		
Periods	*1*	*7136*	*7136*	*0.34*	*0.564*
Treatments	*1*	*143,639*	*143,639*	*6.78*	*0.012*
Residual	*57*	*1,208,209*	*21,197*		
Total	*117*	*5,448,153*			

Table 8 Estimates of the fitted effects in Model (1)

Effect	Estimate	Standard error
$\hat{\tau}_1 - \hat{\tau}_2$	*69.789*	*26.809*
$\hat{\pi}_1 - \hat{\pi}_2$	*−15.556*	*26.809*

are multiplied by -1 before the test is applied. This will change the expected value of the difference in means to $(\tau_1 - \tau_2) + (\pi_1 - \pi_2) - (\tau_1 - \tau_2) + (\pi_2 - \pi_1) = 2(\pi_1 - \pi_2)$, and hence a test of the null hypothesis H_0: $\pi_1 = \pi_2$ is obtained. Then the approach used in section "Two-Sample t-Test" can be followed, giving a t-test statistic of -0.580 and a two-sided p-value of 0.564, in agreement (as expected) with the corresponding values in Table 7.

Checking Assumptions

One advantage of fitting a linear model is that it conveniently allows the checking of assumptions made about the model.

For example, it is easy to check if the residuals from the fitted model are approximately normally distributed or if there are any outliers. The raw residual is the difference between the actual response and its prediction from the model. The standardized residual is the raw residual divided by its standard error.

Figure 3 is a quantile-quantile plot (or Q-Q plot) of the ordered standardized residuals taken from Period 1, which is a visual check for normality. In this plot, the quantiles of the sample are plotted against the theoretical quantiles of the normal distribution. The quantile for a particular value in the dataset is the percentage of data points below that value. For example, the median is the 50th quantile. It is not necessary to plot the residuals from both periods because within a subject they add up to zero and so it is only necessary to take one per subject. If the standardized residuals are normally distributed, the points in the Q-Q plot should lie on, or close to, the diagonal straight line. In Fig. 3, it can be seen that there is some deviation of the points from the line at the extremes, indicating some skewness in the distribution of the residuals. However, when some of the standard tests for normality are applied to this sample of standardized residuals, there is no evidence to reject the null hypothesis that the residuals are normally distributed. For example, the p-value for

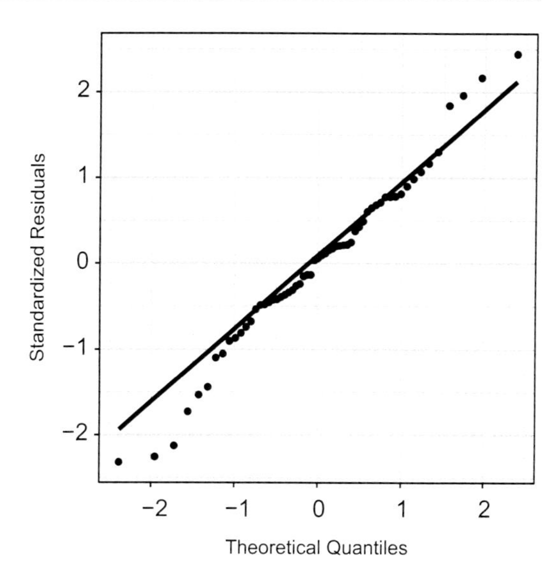

Fig. 3 Q-Q plot of the standardized residuals from Period 1

the Anderson-Darling normality test ([Anderson and Darling (1952)]) is 0.436, and the p-value for the Shapiro-Wilk test ([Shapiro and Wilk (1965)]) is 0.531.

There are five standardized residuals that are larger than 1.964 in absolute value, with values of −2.13, 2.17, 2.44, −2.25, and − 2.32, respectively. That is, 5/ 59 ≈ 8.5% of the residuals are "large," compared to the expected percentage of 5% if they were truly realizations from the standard normal distribution. However, none of the standardized residuals are excessively large (i.e., > 3), so there should be no serious concerns regarding the normality of the residuals.

As noted earlier, if the assumption of normality is not fulfilled, a nonparametric comparison of the treatment effects can be performed using the Wilcoxon rank-sum test applied to the within-period differences. For details, see Chapter 4 of Hollander and Wolfe (1999), who also note that the loss of asymptotic relative efficiency when using the Wilcoxon rank-sum test instead of the t-test is no greater than 13.6%. When the data are actually independent and normally distributed, the loss in efficiency is 4.5%.

Testing for a Difference in Carry-Over Effects

An important assumption regarding the data in this example is that carry-over effects are not present (or that they are equal and therefore do not enter into the expectation of $\widehat{\tau}_d$) and effectively Model (1) applies. Although testing for carry-over effects in the 2 × 2 design is not recommended, for reasons that will be given shortly, it can be done. For completeness, an explanation of how to do it is given below.

Suppose it is assumed that Model (2) applies. It will be recalled that the carry-over parameters for treatments A and B are denoted by λ_1 and λ_2, respectively. The difference between the carry-over effects is denoted by $\lambda_d = \lambda_1 - \lambda_2$.

In order to derive a test of the null hypothesis that $\lambda_d = 0$, it is noted that the subject totals

$$t_{1k} = y_{11k} + y_{12k} \text{ for the } k\text{th subject in Group 1}$$

and

$$t_{2k} = y_{21k} + y_{22k} \text{ for the } k\text{th subject in Group 2}$$

have expectations

$$\mathrm{E}[t_{1k}] = \mathrm{E}[2\mu + \pi_1 + \pi_2 + \tau_1 + \tau_2 + \lambda_1 + 2s_{1k} + e_{11k} + e_{12k}]$$

and

$$\mathrm{E}[t_{2k}] = \mathrm{E}[2\mu + \pi_1 + \pi_2 + \tau_1 + \tau_2 + \lambda_2 + 2s_{2k} + e_{21k} + e_{22k}].$$

As the expectations of s_{ik} and e_{ijk} are both zero, the expectations of t_{1k} and t_{2k} reduce to $\mathrm{E}[t_{1k}] = 2\mu + \pi_1 + \pi_2 + \tau_1 + \tau_2 + \lambda_1$ and $\mathrm{E}[t_{2k}] = 2\mu + \pi_1 + \pi_2 + \tau_1 + \tau_2 + \lambda_2$ respectively.

If $\lambda_1 = \lambda_2$, then these two expectations are equal. Consequently, to test if $\lambda_d = 0$, the familiar two-sample t-test can be applied to the subject totals.

The estimate of the difference in carry-over effects is $\widehat{\lambda}_d = \bar{t}_{1.} - \bar{t}_{2.}$ and has a variance of:

$$\mathrm{Var}\left[\widehat{\lambda}_d\right] = \sigma_T^2\left(\frac{1}{n_1} + \frac{1}{n_2}\right),$$

where

$$\sigma_T^2 = 2\left(2\sigma_s^2 + \sigma^2\right).$$

An estimate of σ_T^2 is

$$\widehat{\sigma}_T^2 = \sum_{i=1}^{2}\sum_{k=1}^{n_i}(t_{ik} - \bar{t}_{i.})^2/(n_1 + n_2 - 2),$$

the pooled sample variance which has $(n_1 + n_2 - 2)$ degrees of freedom.

The estimated standard error of $\widehat{\lambda}_d$ is

$$s_\lambda = \widehat{\sigma}_T\sqrt{\left(\frac{1}{n_1} + \frac{1}{n_2}\right)}.$$

On the null hypothesis that $\lambda_1 = \lambda_2$, the statistic $T_\lambda = \widehat{\lambda}_d/s_\lambda$ has a Student's t–distribution on $(n_1 + n_2 - 2)$ degrees of freedom.

The estimate of λ_d is -16.79 with a standard error of 98.63 on 57 degrees of freedom. The two-sided p-value is 0.865, indicating no evidence of a difference in carry-over effects.

While it may be informative, as a follow-up, to test if the carry-over effects are significantly different, this test should not be used as a preliminary test to decide which model to fit to the data, as advocated by Grizzle (1965). Grizzle's suggestion was to use the result of the carry-over test to decide between two strategies: (1) if the carry-over test is significant, exclude the data from the second period and base the comparison of A and B only on the data from the first period; (2) if the carry-over effect is not significant, then proceed as done above and use the data from both periods to fit Model (1). Freeman (1989) showed that Grizzle's suggestion produced a biased test and an inflated Type I error rate. See Chapter 2 of Jones and Kenward (2014) or Freeman (1989) for more details.

The best advice is to decide before the trial begins if a significant difference in carry-over effects is expected or not. If it is expected, and cannot be removed by using adequate wash-out periods, then the 2×2 design should not be used. Alternative cross-over designs are available that allow for a difference in carry-over effects, and Chapter 3 of Jones and Kenward (2014) should be consulted for more information.

Typically, when carry-over effects are included in the statistical model for the responses, the efficiency of the estimation of pairwise differences between the treatment effects is lower than when the carry-over effects are not included in the model. However, there are designs for which the efficiency of the estimators of pairwise differences between the treatment effects is the same whether or not the additive carry-over effects are included in the model. A simple example of this is the design to compare two treatments using three periods that has the two sequence groups defined by the sequences ABB and BAA. In this design, the estimators of the treatment effects are independent of the estimators of the carry-over effects (see Jones and Kenward (2014), Sect. 3.5, for more details).

Additional Use of the Random-Effects Linear Model

If the results of the trial are such that every subject provides responses in both periods, the estimates of the treatment effects and the corresponding significance tests are identical for both the fixed- and random-effects models. This is because the subject effect cancels out in any within-subject comparison. When this is not the case, the random-effects model permits the data from the single responses, provided by some subjects, to be included in the analysis.

To illustrate this, a new dataset is constructed by adding the data given in Table 9, to the previously used data that were partly shown in Tables 4 and 5. These data are for subjects who dropped out of the trial after the first period for various (treatment unrelated) reasons.

The random effects model is fitted using the Kenward-Roger adjustment [Kenward and Roger (1997)]. This adjustment is a bias correction for the variance

Table 9 Period 1 endurance time (seconds) for subjects without a second period

Group	Subject	Treatment	Time
1	*60*	*1*	*130*
1	*61*	*1*	*302*
1	*62*	*1*	*653*
1	*63*	*1*	*467*
2	*64*	*2*	*364*
2	*65*	*2*	*155*
2	*66*	*2*	*226*

of an estimator of a fixed-effects parameter in the random-effects model. See Kenward and Roger (1997) for more details.

The p-values from this analysis, for the period and treatment effects, are 0.362 and 0.010, respectively. The estimated treatment difference is 70.63 with a standard error of 26.59.

This is to be compared with the estimate (standard error) obtained from the fixed-effects model: 69.79 (26.81). Including the additional data has resulted in a slightly larger treatment difference and a slightly smaller standard error. Adding the additional data from Period 1 has made little difference to the conclusions. This is not an unusual result as the information retrieved from the additional data can only be used to compare treatments on a between-subject basis, and if the between-subject variance is large, this additional information will have a low weight compared to the within-subject information.

As noted earlier, the estimate of the within-subject correlation is estimated to be 0.54. This is not especially high, suggesting that the between-subject information may be of some use, although here, the small amount of additional data from Period 1 was probably too little to make much of a difference.

Random-effects models can also be useful when the cross-over design is of the *incomplete block* type, i.e., where each subject does not get every one of the possible treatments and therefore receives an incomplete set of treatments. An example of such a design and its analysis will be given in section "Example 3: Incomplete Block Design."

Williams Cross-over Design

Introduction

A limitation of the 2 × 2 cross-over design is that it does not permit any carry-over effects to be estimated using within-subject information. The use of adequate washout periods, of course, can remove any pharmacological carry-over effects and make redundant the need to estimate them. However, when more than two treatments are to be compared over several periods, the use of long wash-out periods can be impractical as the longer a trial takes, the greater the chance that subjects will drop out before completing all the periods. Longer trials also mean that the time a successful new drug will take to reach the patients who need it will be extended. If wash-out periods are removed, or if there is doubt that any carry-over effects can be removed using the maximum permissible length of wash-out period, then cross-over designs that allow the estimated treatment effects to be adjusted for the presence of any carry-over effects will be needed. In other words, if there are any additive carry-over effects that cannot be removed by the design of the study, suitable alternative designs will have to be used.

Fortunately, there are many such designs for two or more treatments in two or more periods. Tables of suitable designs are given in Chapter 4 of Jones and Kenward (2014), and these should be referred to for examples of designs not illustrated in this chapter. One class of designs is the *Williams design*. These designs fall into two types, depending on whether t, the number of treatments, is even or odd. If t is even, then the basic design requires t subjects and t periods. If t is odd, then the basic design requires 2 t subjects and t periods. Examples of these basic designs for $t = 3$ and $t = 4$ are given in Tables 10 and 11, respectively. The basic designs, obtained from published tables, or by computer search, can be thought of as designs with one subject allocated to each sequence group. The rows of these tables give the sequences (which define the sequence groups) to be used in the trial. In the actual trial, the available subjects are allocated at random to the sequences to form the sequence groups. Usually, the sequence groups are of the same size. Whereas, the 2×2 design has two sequence groups, the Williams design has t or 2 t sequence groups. An algorithm to determine the basic sequences in a Williams design for all values of t is given in Chapter 4 of Jones and Kenward (2014).

As with all clinical trials, at the planning stage, it is necessary to determine how many subjects in total are needed to achieve a given power, e.g., 90%, to detect a given treatment difference of interest at a specified significance level (e.g., 0.05). In

Table 10 Williams cross-over trial to compare three treatments

Group	Period 1	Period 2	Period 3
1	*A*	*B*	*C*
2	*B*	*C*	*A*
3	*C*	*A*	*B*
4	*C*	*B*	*A*
5	*A*	*C*	*B*
6	*B*	*A*	*C*

Table 11 Williams cross-over trial to compare four treatments

Group	Period 1	Period 2	Period 3	Period 4
1	*A*	*D*	*B*	*C*
2	*B*	*A*	*C*	*D*
3	*C*	*B*	*D*	*A*
4	*D*	*C*	*A*	*B*

the example that follows for $t = 5$, 80 subjects were needed, requiring, therefore, 8 subjects be assigned at random to each of the 10 sequence groups.

To calculate the sample size required to ensure a given power for a particular comparison, it is necessary to derive, for the particular design under consideration, the standard error of the estimated comparison as a function of n, the size of each sequence group (assuming equal group sizes are required). Once this has been obtained, standard formulae for sample sizes to compare two groups can then be modified to include this standard error, rather than the usual standard error for the difference of two means. How to do this is beyond the scope of this chapter and typically requires the use of purpose-written software.

The general property of a Williams design is that, if each pair of consecutive periods is considered, and the counting is over all the sequence groups in the basic design, then each treatment occurs an equal number of times before each other treatment, except itself. This ensures that each of the t possible carry-over effects occurs with each of the other $t - 1$ treatments an equal number of times. For example, in Table 10, each treatment occurs twice before each of the other two treatments. In Table 11, each treatment occurs once before each of the other three treatments. This type of design balances out the carry-over effects, and as a consequence, the estimates of the treatment comparisons adjusted for the presence of carry-over effects can be made using within-subject information. In addition, these designs typically have variances of the estimated treatment effects that are not excessively large compared to the situation where carry-over effects are assumed to be absent and are not adjusted for.

Example of a Cross-over Trial with Five Treatments

The data for this example are a simulated version of those taken from a Phase III, randomized, double-blind, placebo-controlled trial. The trial compared a novel drug at two doses (labeled here as B and C, where B is the lower dose) with a placebo drug (labeled here as A) in subjects with moderate to severe Chronic Obstructive Pulmonary Disease (COPD). Also included in the trial were two other drugs which acted as positive controls: Salbutamol and a combination of Salmeterol and Fluticasone (labeled here as D and E, respectively). The trial population consisted of 80 adult males and females (age 40 years and over) with a clinical diagnosis of moderate-to-severe COPD. The efficacy measurement of interest was the Forced Expired Volume in 1 second (FEV_1) measured in liters and taken at 5 minutes postdose. The objective of the trial was to determine if either B or C or both were superior to A (Placebo). Other pairwise comparisons were considered to be of secondary importance.

As there are five different treatments, this study was designed as a Williams design with five periods and ten sequence groups as given in Table 12. A wash-out period of 7 days was used between the treatments periods. Although, the length of the wash-out periods was considered adequate to remove any carry-over effects, there was some uncertainty about this, and so a Williams design was used to ensure that the treatment effects could be adjusted for carry-over effects. The primary

Table 12 Williams design to compare five treatments for the COPD

Group	Period 1	Period 2	Period 3	Period 4	Period 5
1	*D*	*C*	*A*	*B*	*E*
2	*E*	*A*	*B*	*D*	*C*
3	*B*	*E*	*C*	*A*	*D*
4	*C*	*B*	*D*	*E*	*A*
5	*A*	*D*	*E*	*C*	*B*
6	*E*	*B*	*A*	*C*	*D*
7	*C*	*D*	*B*	*A*	*E*
8	*D*	*A*	*C*	*E*	*B*
9	*A*	*E*	*D*	*B*	*C*
10	*B*	*C*	*E*	*D*	*A*

analysis model is therefore Model (2) and contains terms for subjects, periods, treatments, and carry-over effects.

To calculate the efficiency of this Williams design, the lower bound is calculated using, r, the number of times each treatment occurs in the basic design, i.e., $r = N/t = 50/5 = 10$. Hence, $V_{bound} = 2\sigma^2/10 = 0.2\sigma^2$. The variance of a pairwise comparison in this design, assuming a model without carry-over effects, is also $0.2\sigma^2$. Therefore, the design efficiency, in the absence of carry-over effects, is $100 \times 0.2/0.2 = 100\%$. If, as in this example, carry-over effects are included in the model, the variance of a pairwise comparison increases to $0.2111\sigma^2$, giving an efficiency of $100 \times 0.2/0.2111 = 94.74\%$.

There is clearly a price to be paid for allowing for the presence of carry-over effects, but in this case it is not high: The relative increase in sample size is less than 6% (100/94.74 = 1.055). That is, allowing for differing carry-over effects requires about 6% more subjects.

Eight subjects were randomized to each of the sequence groups. As an illustration, the data for the subjects in the first sequence group are given in Table 13.

As a first step in the analysis of these data, the raw treatment means obtained from the complete dataset are plotted in Fig. 4, where the treatments have been labeled as A = 1, B = 2, . . ., and E = 5.

It can be seen that there is evidence that treatment C (high dose of the novel drug) gives the highest mean FEV_1 response, and treatment A (Placebo) has the lowest mean.

This will be explored further by fitting Model (2) to the responses. As every subject gets every treatment, and there are no missing values, it does not matter if the subject effects are considered to be fixed or random. An example of a design where it does matter will be given in the next section.

The analysis of variance table obtained by fitting this model is given in Table 14.

From Table 14, it can be seen that the p-value for carry-over is significant at the 0.05 level, indicating that there is evidence of differences between the carry-over effects. In retrospect, therefore, it was wise that the Williams design had been used

Table 13 Group 1 treatment sequence (D C A B E) FEV_1 (liters)

Subject	Period 1	Period 2	Period 3	Period 4	Period 5
1	*1.601*	*1.493*	*1.748*	*1.795*	*1.510*
2	*1.212*	*1.395*	*1.308*	*1.250*	*1.429*
3	*2.281*	*2.358*	*2.362*	*2.376*	*2.538*
4	*1.587*	*1.904*	*1.597*	*1.485*	*1.663*
5	*1.202*	*1.373*	*1.341*	*1.328*	*1.218*
6	*1.398*	*1.708*	*1.327*	*1.506*	*1.696*
7	*1.568*	*1.677*	*1.250*	*1.321*	*1.496*
8	*1.395*	*1.259*	*1.340*	*1.245*	*1.153*

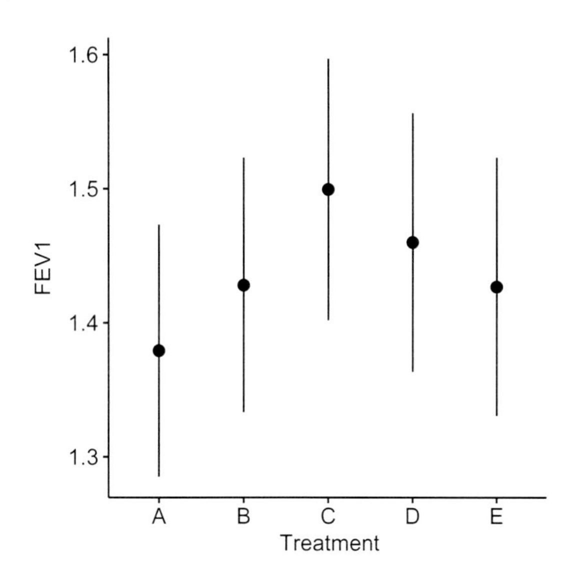

Fig. 4 Plot of raw treatment means with 95% confidence intervals

because it allows estimation of the treatment differences, even in the presence of carry-over effects.

To simplify the presentation, Table 15 shows only the comparisons between B versus A and C versus A.

As was noted in the description of this trial, the primary objective was to determine if either B or C or both are superior to A (Placebo). As there are two comparisons of interest, it is necessary to apply a multiplicity adjustment to the testing procedure in order to ensure that the family-wise error rate is not inflated above 0.05. See Bretz et al. (2016), for example, for a general coverage of approaches for dealing with multiple testing issues. One simple, although potentially conservative, way to do this is to use a Bonferroni adjustment and halve the required significance level of each test (i.e., test each one at significance level 0.025 instead of 0.05). It can be seen that both p-values are much smaller than 0.025, indicating both

Table 14 Analysis of variance for Williams design [df = degrees of freedom, SS = sums of squares, MS = mean square, and F=F-ratio]

Source	df	SS	MS	F	P-value
Between-subjects	*79*	*68.3215*	*0.8648*	*60.34*	*<0.0001*
Period	*4*	*0.0178*	*0.0044*	*0.31*	*0.8711*
Treatment	*4*	*0.6688*	*0.1672*	*11.67*	*<0.0001*
Carry-over	*4*	*0.1505*	*0.0376*	*2.63*	*0.0348*
Residual	*308*	*4.4145*	*0.0143*		
Total	*399*	*73.9643*			

Table 15 Pairwise differences in the fitted means for the Williams design

Parameter	Estimate	Standard error	One-sided p-value
B - A	*0.0470*	*0.0194*	*0.0082*
C - A	*0.1275*	*0.0194*	*<0.0001*

are significant at the overall significance level of 0.05. In summary, it can be concluded that both B and C are superior to A.

Example 3: Incomplete Block Design

Quite often it is not possible to use as many periods in a cross-over trial as there are treatments. This could be because there is a concern that subjects may not want to stay in the trial long enough to complete all t periods and will drop out before the end of the trial. Another reason could be that, with the inclusion of lengthy wash-out periods, the trial may take too long if all t periods have to be completed. In any case, trials with $p < t$ are not uncommon, and the third illustrative example has $t = 4$ and $p = 3$. Jones and Kenward (2014) give many examples of such *incomplete block* designs and their sequence groups. Their associated efficiencies can be obtained by referring to that book or by using the R package *Crossover* (Rohmeyer (2014)).

This example is also a multicenter, Phase III, cross-over trial where, for confidentiality reasons, the actual data have been replaced with simulated values. The aim of the trial was to assess the efficacy of a drug B in subjects with moderate to severe COPD. The trial also included an active control, C, another treatment of interest (labeled as A) and a placebo drug D. The main aim of the trial was to compare B with D, with the other comparisons being of secondary interest. To limit the length of the trial, the four treatments were given over three periods in an incomplete block design. The study population consisted of a representative group of adult males and females aged 40 years and over with a clinical diagnosis of moderate to severe COPD. The efficacy variable of interest was the FEV_1. The structure of the trial included a 14-day run-in period used to assess eligibility of subjects for the study. Each treatment period lasted 14 days followed by a 14-day wash-out period (after Periods 1 and 2 only).

The sequences used in this design are given in Table 16, and in the trial four subjects were allocated to each sequence group. This design is fully balanced in the sense that each estimated pairwise comparison has the same variance.

To calculate the efficiency of this incomplete block design, the lower bound is calculated using the number of times each treatment occurs in the basic design, i.e., $r = 9$. Hence, $V_{bound} = 2\sigma^2/9 = 0.2222\sigma^2$. The variance of a pairwise comparison in the basic design, assuming a model without carry-over effects, is $0.2500\sigma^2$. Therefore, the design efficiency, in the absence of carry-over effects, is $100 \times 0.2222/0.2500 = 88.89\%$. If carry-over effects are included in the model, the variance of a pairwise comparison increases to $0.3088\sigma^2$, giving a relatively low efficiency of $100 \times 0.2222/0.3088 = 71.96\%$. Fortunately, given the relatively long wash-out periods, there was no expectation in this trial that carry-over effects would be present.

As an illustration, the data from the first sequence group are given in Table 17.

The FEV_1 values obtained at the end of each period are given for each subject, along with the baseline measurement taken at the end of the run-in period and at the end of each wash-out period before the start of the following period. These baseline measurements will be ignored for now, and only the responses given in the columns that have headings Period 1, Period 2, and Period 3 will be analyzed. The analysis using baselines will be discussed in section "Use of Baseline Measurements."

Table 16 Incomplete block cross-over design to compare four treatments in three periods

Group	Period 1	Period 2	Period 3
1	*A*	*B*	*C*
2	*B*	*A*	*D*
3	*C*	*D*	*A*
4	*D*	*C*	*B*
5	*A*	*D*	*B*
6	*B*	*C*	*A*
7	*C*	*B*	*D*
8	*D*	*A*	*C*
9	*A*	*C*	*D*
10	*B*	*D*	*C*
11	*C*	*A*	*B*
12	*D*	*B*	*A*

Table 17 Group 1 (A B C) FEV_1 (mls)

Subject	Baseline 1	Baseline 2	Baseline 3	Period 1	Period 2	Period 3
1	*256.25*	*278.53*	*284.06*	*265.16*	*311.23*	*284.20*
2	*262.32*	*244.86*	*253.60*	*301.31*	*264.86*	*272.95*
3	*174.87*	*206.42*	*204.57*	*226.60*	*253.41*	*245.73*
4	*232.53*	*259.66*	*226.48*	*244.33*	*267.89*	*240.39*

As carry-over effects were not anticipated, they will not be included in the fitted model. A new feature of the analysis of an incomplete block design is that the question as to whether the subject effects s_{ik} are assumed to be fixed or random effects is now highly relevant. If they are assumed to be fixed effects, the comparison of treatments uses only the information that is available from within-subject comparisons between the responses on a subject. If the subject effects are assumed to be random, then some additional information can be obtained from the between-subject comparisons (often referred to as the inter-block information). This recovery of information is typically most advantageous when the cross-over design has low efficiency for the treatment comparisons or a low to moderate correlation between the repeated measurements on each subject and a large number of subjects. As already noted, this final example design has quite high efficiency (88.89%), so the recovery of inter-block information may not make much of a difference to the analysis of the data. Nevertheless, for the purposes of providing an illustration, the inter-block information will be recovered. The parameter estimates obtained from the fixed-subject effects model are given in Table 18. Note that the period effects are the differences compared to Period 3, and the treatment effects are the differences compared to treatment D.

When the subject effects are assumed to be random, the REML estimates of the treatment and period effects are as given in Table 19. It can be seen that the standard errors of the treatment estimates are slightly smaller when REML is used. It should be noted that the Kenward-Roger adjustment (Kenward and Roger (1997)) has been used.

As part of the output from fitting this model using standard statistical software (not shown), estimates of the variance components may also be obtained: $\widehat{\sigma}^2 = 361.35$ and $\sigma_s^2 = 1062.78$. The within-subject correlation between any pair of repeated measurements on a subject is $\rho = \left(\sigma_s^2/\left(\sigma_s^2 + \sigma^2\right)\right)$ and is estimated as $1062.78/(1062.78 + 361.35) = 0.75$. Therefore, not only does this design have a

Table 18 Parameter estimates obtained from model with fixed subject effects

Effect	Estimate	Standard error	Two-sided p-value
Period 1	*−0.4381*	*3.8798*	*0.9103*
Period 2	*0.7450*	*3.8798*	*0.8482*
Treatment A	*31.5485*	*4.7518*	*< 0.0001*
Treatment B	*29.8806*	*4.7518*	*< 0.0001*
Treatment C	*29.1396*	*4.7518*	*< 0.0001*

Table 19 Parameter estimates obtained using REML

Effect	Estimate	Standard error	Two-sided p-value
Period 1	*−0.4381*	*3.8802*	*0.9103*
Period 2	*0.7450*	*3.8802*	*0.8482*
Treatment A	*31.8566*	*4.7261*	*< 0.0001*
Treatment B	*30.5531*	*4.7261*	*< 0.0001*
Treatment C	*30.2235*	*4.7261*	*< 0.0001*

high efficiency, but the estimated within-subject correlation is also large, implying a large between-subject variance. For well-designed cross-over trials, this is often the case, and in this situation, as has been already mentioned, the recovery of inter-block information is unlikely to make much difference to the estimates of the treatment comparisons and their estimated standard errors.

Use of Baseline Measurements

When a measurement of the response is taken prior to the start of each period, these *baseline measurements* may be useful in increasing the precision of the estimated treatment effects. Whether they are useful or not depends on the degree and type of correlation structure between the response and the baseline measurements. See Chapter 5 of Jones and Kenward (2014) for more details.

Two approaches that may be considered when making use of baseline measurements are to (1) analyze the change from baseline measurements, i.e., for each subject and period replace the response by the difference between the response and the baseline value for that period or (2) include the baseline measurements as covariates. The inclusion of covariates is the recommended approach. See Senn (2006) for further discussion on this.

In this section, the data from section "Example 3: Incomplete Block Design" are reanalyzed, but now making use of the baseline measurements that were taken at the start of each treatment period. Table 17 gives these baseline values for the subjects in the first sequence group.

Typically, the analysis of the changes from baseline is only worth considering if the response and its associated baseline are close together in time, compared to the gap between periods and if the variability of the baselines is considerably less than that of the response, which may happen if the baseline is, in fact, the average over several baseline measurements, for example.

In a fixed subject effects model, it is sufficient to include the baseline (from each period) as a single covariate.

However, if a random subject effects model is used to recover between-subject information, two separate covariates must be included for each subject: Covariate (a) is the average over the p baselines, and Covariate (b) is the difference from this average of each of the p baseline measurements. See Chapter 5 of Jones and Kenward (2014) for more details.

To illustrate the construction of the covariates, Table 20 shows their values for the first subject in Table 17. For example, the value of the Covariate (a) is $(256.25 + 278.53 + 284.06)/3 = 272.9467 \approx 272.95$ and the value of Covariate (b) for Period 1 is $256.25–272.95 = -16.70$.

Assuming that there are no carry-over effects due to the inclusion of the washout periods (i.e., Model (1) is assumed), the extension of the previous analysis to include baselines is now illustrated.

Table 21 shows the estimate and its standard error for the comparison of B versus D, for a selection of models and where the subject effects are either fitted as fixed or

Table 20 Factors, response, baselines, and covariates for the first two subjects

Subject	Period	Drug	Baseline	Response	Covariate (a)	Covariate (b)
1	1	1	*256.25*	*265.16*	*272.95*	*−16.70*
1	*2*	*2*	*278.53*	*311.23*	*272.95*	*5.58*
1	*3*	*3*	*284.06*	*284.20*	*272.95*	11.11
48	1	*4*	*185.10*	*203.00*	*177.07*	*8.03*
48	*2*	*2*	*190.20*	*213.08*	*177.07*	*13.13*
48	*3*	1	*155.90*	*206.93*	*177.07*	*−21.17*

Table 21 Parameter estimates and standard errors from analyses with and without baselines (B versus D)

	Fixed subject effects		Random subject effects	
Model	Estimate	Standard error	Estimate	Standard error
(A) Response only	*29.881*	*4.752*	*30.553*	*4.726*
(B) Change from baseline	*26.196*	*3.701*	*26.820*	*3.668*
(C) Single period baseline	*27.392*	*3.500*	*27.871*	*3.324*
(D) Both baseline covariates	*27.391*	*3.500*	*28.034*	*3.323*

random effects. All models contain factors for the subjects, periods, and treatments. The fitted models are: (A) response only and no covariates; (B) the change from baseline in each period is used as the response, and no covariates are added; (C) the response is fitted with each period baseline used as the covariate; and (D) the response is fitted with Covariates (a) and (b).

It is immediately clear that making use of the baselines does increase the precision of estimation. For example, the standard error drops from 4.75 to 3.50 when one or both covariates are added to the fixed effects model. In this example, the use of the change from baseline is almost as good as using the covariates, although that may not always be the case. Because it is already known from the analysis reported in the previous section that there is little advantage in recovering the between-block information, there is not a great difference in the respective results for the fixed and random effects models. Indeed, as explained in Chapter 5 of Jones and Kenward (2014), the use of both covariates is only needed when there is some incompatibility between the within-subject and between-subject estimates. If there is little to no between-subject information on a treatment comparison, as here, then it is not necessary to fit both covariates. In fact, in such a situation, using the fixed effects model is recommended.

Summary and Conclusion

This chapter has concentrated on the design and analysis of continuous data from cross-over trials. Examples where $p = t$ and $p < t$ have been given, and the use of period baseline covariates has been illustrated. Designs also exist for $p > t$, and Jones and Kenward (2014) should be consulted for examples of these.

As a thorough treatment of the analysis of binary and categorical data from cross-over trials is beyond the scope of this chapter, the reader is referred to Chapter 6 of Jones and Kenward (2014) for a detailed coverage. However, it should be noted that for binary data from the 2×2 cross-over design, simple analyses based on 2×2 contingency tables are available. Chapter 2 of Jones and Kenward (2014) gives the details.

Key Facts

In a cross-over trial, each subject receives a series of treatments over a fixed number of periods. When used appropriately, cross-over designs require fewer subjects to achieve a given level of precision or power compared to their parallel groups counterparts. When there are more than two treatments or periods, choices between designs can be made using their efficiencies. Models used to fit data from cross-over trials may include subject effects as fixed or random variables. For designs of the incomplete block type, the use of random subject effects permits the recovery of between-subject information on treatment comparisons. The use of baseline measurements, taken before the start of each period, may be useful to increase the precision of the treatment comparisons.

Cross-References

▶ Controlling for Multiplicity, Eligibility, and Exclusions
▶ Power and Sample Size

References

Altman DG (1991) Practical statistics for medical research. London: Chapman and Hall

Anderson TW, Darling DA (1952) Asymptotic theory of certain "goodness-of-fit" criteria based on stochastic processes. Ann Math Stat 23:193–212

Bretz F, Hothorn T, Westfall P (2016) Multiple comparisons using R. Boca Raton: CRC Press

Chi EM, Reinsel GC (1989) Models for longitudinal data with random effects and AR(1) errors. J Am Stat Assoc 84:452–459

Clark B, Smith D (1981) Introduction to pharmacokinetics. Oxford: Blackwell Scientific Publications

FDA (2013) Guidance for industry: bioequivalence studies and pharmacokinetic endpoints for drugs submitted under an ANDA. Food and Drug Administration

Freeman P (1989) The performance of the two-stage analysis of two treatment, two period crossover trials. Stat Med 8:1421–1432

Grizzle JE (1965) The two-period change-over design and its use in clinical trials. Biometrics 21:467–480

Havliceck LL, Peterson NL (1974) Robustness of the t-test: a guide for researchers on the effect of violations of assumptions. Psychol Rep 34:1095–1114

Hollander M, Wolfe D (1999) Nonparametric statistical methods, 2nd edn. New York: Wiley

Jones B, Kenward MG (2014) Design and analysis of cross-over trials, 3rd edn. Boca Raton: CRC Press
Kenward MG, Roger JH (1997) Small sample inference for fixed effects estimators from restricted maximum likelihood. Biometrics 53:983–997
Patterson HD, Lucas HL (1962) Change-over designs. North Carolina Agricultural Station, Tech Bull 147
Patterson HD, Thompson R (1971) Recovery of inter-block information when block sizes are unequal. Biometrika 58:545–554
Piantadosi S (1997) Clinical Trials. A methodological perspective. New York: Wiley
Rohmeyer K (2014) Crossover. R package Crossover, Version 01-16
Senn S (2006) Change from baseline and analysis of covariance revised. Stat Med 25:4334–4344
Shapiro SS, Wilk MB (1965) An analysis of variance test for normality (complete samples). Biometrika 52:591–611

Factorial Trials

71

Steven Piantadosi and Susan Halabi

Contents

S. Piantadosi (✉)
Department of Surgery, Division of Surgical Oncology, Brigham and Women's Hospital, Harvard Medical School, Boston, MA, USA
e-mail: spiantadosi@bwh.harvard.edu

S. Halabi
Department of Biostatistics and Bioinformatics, Duke University Medical Center, Durham, NC, USA
e-mail: susan.halabi@duke.edu

© Springer Nature Switzerland AG 2022

S. Piantadosi, C. L. Meinert (eds.), *Principles and Practice of Clinical Trials*,
https://doi.org/10.1007/978-3-319-52636-2_100

Abstract

Factorial clinical trials test the effects of two or more therapies using a design that can estimate interaction between therapies (Piantadosi 2017). (This chapter revises, updates, and expands upon reference (Piantadosi 2017)) A factorial structure is the only design that can assess treatment interactions, so this type of trial is required for those important therapeutic questions. When interactions between treatments are absent, which is not a trivial requirement, a factorial design can estimate each of several treatment effects from the same data. For example, two treatments can sometimes be evaluated using the same number of subjects ordinarily used to test a single therapy. When possible, this demonstrates a striking efficiency. For these reasons, factorial designs have an important place in clinical trial methodology, and have been applied in a variety of setting, but in particular in disease prevention.

Keywords

Factorial clinical trials · Treatment interactions · Factorial designs

Introduction

Factorial clinical trials test the effects of two or more therapies using a design that can estimate interaction between therapies (Piantadosi 2017). A factorial structure is the only design that can assess treatment interactions. When interactions between treatments are absent, a factorial design can estimate each of several treatment effects from the same data. For example, two treatments can sometimes be evaluated using the same number of subjects ordinarily used to test a single therapy. For these reasons, factorial designs have an important place in clinical trial methodology, and have been applied in a variety of setting, but in particular in disease prevention.

Historically, control variables in experiments were called *factors*. For example, a *factor* can be defined by the presence or absence of a single drug. A factor can have more than one *level*, as indicated by different doses of the same drug. A factor is not strictly qualitative. The choice between treatments, A and B, is not a factor (assuming that one is not a placebo). Many factors have only two levels (present or absent) and are therefore both ordinal and qualitative. In a factorial design, all factors are varied systematically, with some groups receiving more than one treatment, and the experimental groups are arranged that may permit testing if a combination of treatments is better or worse than individual treatments, although the power is often limited.

The method of varying more than one factor or treatment in a single study was used in agricultural experiments before 1900. It was developed and popularized by R. A. Fisher (1935, 1960) and Yates (1935), and used to great advantage in both agricultural and industrial experiments. In medicine, factorial designs have been used more in prevention trials than therapeutic studies.

Factorial designs carry important assumptions that must be understood before deciding if one is the best choice for a therapeutic question. The critical issue is to distinguish between an investigation of treatment interactions versus efficient testing of multiple noninteracting individual therapies. The following section on interactions or efficiency. More complete discussions of factorial designs, especially pertaining to cancer prevention trials, can be found in (Byar and Piantadosi 1985; Byar et al. 1993). Discussion of these designs related to cardiovascular trials, particularly in the context of the ISIS-4 study (Flather et al. 1994), can be found in Lubsen and Pocock (1994) and McAlister et al. (2003).

Characteristics of Factorial Designs

Interactions or Efficiency, But Not Both Simultaneously

Factorial designs embody an essential dichotomy mentioned above that is a source of frequent misunderstanding. The same structural design can be used either to gain substantial efficiency in questions about individual treatments, or to estimate the interaction between treatments. Both objectives cannot be met in the same trial, because they require very different sample sizes. The design of a factorial trial can therefore appear conflicting or confusing unless we understand which purpose is intended.

To summarize details below, a factorial design can estimate efficacy for each of two therapies with one sample size only if the treatments are known not to interact with one another (section "Factorial Designs Can Be More Efficient"), or if any interaction between the treatments is negligible relative to the main effect of individual treatments. This two-for-one efficiency is therefore predicated on strong biological knowledge. When therapeutic interaction is the topic of inquiry, only a factorial structure can estimate it, but at the cost of a sample size that is roughly four times larger than usual (section "Factorial Designs Are the Only Way to Study Interactions"). Hence, the two possible objectives implied by a factorial structure cannot be met simultaneously. When the design is derived from the question rather than the other way around, investigators can likely to employ the factorial structure appropriately.

Factorial Designs Are Defined by Their Structure

The simplest factorial design has treatments A and B, and four treatment groups (Table 1). Assume n subjects are entered into each of the four treatment groups for a total sample size of 4n and a balanced (equal allocation) design. One group receives neither A nor B, a second receives both A and B, and the other two groups receive only one of A or B. This is called a 2×2 (two by two) factorial design. Although basic, this design illustrates many of the general features of factorial experiments. The design generates enough information to test the effects of A alone, B alone, and A plus B. The efficiencies in doing so will be presented below.

Table 1 Four treatment groups and sample size in a 2 × 2 balanced factorial design

Treatment A	Treatment B		Total
	No	Yes	
No	n	n	$2n$
Yes	n	n	$2n$
Total	$2n$	$2n$	$4n$

Table 2 Eight treatment groups and sample size in a $2 \times 2 \times 2$ balanced factorial design

Group	Treatments			Sample size
	A	B	C	
1	No	No	No	n
2	Yes	No	No	n
3	No	Yes	No	n
4	No	No	Yes	n
5	Yes	Yes	No	n
6	No	Yes	Yes	n
7	Yes	No	Yes	n
8	Yes	Yes	Yes	n

The 2×2 design generalizes to higher order designs in a straightforward manner. For example, a factorial design studying three treatments, A, B, and C is the $2 \times 2 \times 2$. Possible treatment groups for this design are shown in Table 2. The total sample size is $8n$ if all treatment groups have n subjects.

Aside from illustrating the factorial structure, these examples highlight some of the prerequisites and restrictions for using a factorial trial. First, the treatments must be amenable to being administered in combination without changing dosage in the presence of each other. For example, in Table 1, we would not want to reduce the dose of A in the lower right cell where B is present. This requirement implies that the side effects of the treatments cannot be cumulative to the point where the combination would be difficult to administer.

Second, it must be ethically acceptable to administer individual treatments or administer them at lowered doses. In some situations, this means having a no-treatment or placebo group in the trial. In other cases, A and B may be administered in addition to a standard therapy, so all groups receive some treatment. An example might be a factorial trial of chemotherapy and prophylactic brain radiotherapy in subjects with lung cancer, all of whom received chest radiotherapy. Third, we must be genuinely interested in learning about the treatment combinations or else some of the treatment groups would be unnecessary. Alternatively, to use the design to achieve greater efficiency in studying two or more treatments, we must know that some interactions do not exist.

Fourth, the therapeutic questions must be chosen appropriately. We would not use a factorial design to test treatments that have exactly the same mechanisms of action, such as two angiotensin converting enzyme (ACE) inhibitors for high blood pressure, because either agent would answer the question. Treatments acting through different mechanisms would be more appropriate for a factorial design. In some prevention factorial trials, the treatments tested may target different diseases in the same cohort.

Factorial Designs Can Be More Efficient

Although their scope is limited, factorial designs offer certain important efficiencies or advantages when they are applicable. To illustrate how this occurs, consider the 2×2 design and the estimates of treatment effects that would result using an additive model for analysis (Table 3). Assume that the responses are group averages of some normally distributed response denoted by $\overline{Y}$. The subscripts on $\overline{Y}$ indicate which treatment group it represents. Note that half the subjects receive one of the treatments. This is also true in higher order designs. For the moment, further assume that the effect of A is not influenced by the presence of B.

There are two estimates of the effect of treatment A compared with placebo in the design, $\overline{Y_A} - \overline{Y_0}$ and $\overline{Y_{AB}} - \overline{Y_B}$. If B does not modify the effect of A, it is sensible to combine or average them to estimate the overall, or main, effect of A, denoted here by β_A,

$$\beta_A = \frac{\left(\overline{Y_A} - \overline{Y_0}\right) + \left(\overline{Y_{AB}} - \overline{Y_B}\right)}{2} \tag{1}$$

Similarly,

$$\beta_B = \frac{\left(\overline{Y_B} - \overline{Y_0}\right) + \left(\overline{Y_{AB}} - \overline{Y_A}\right)}{2} \tag{2}$$

Thus, in the absence of interactions, which means the effect of A is the same with or without B, and vice versa, the design permits the full sample size to be used to estimate two treatment effects.

Now suppose that each subject's response has a variance $\sigma^2$and that it is the same in all treatment groups. We can calculate the variance of β_B to be

$$var(\beta_A) = \frac{1}{4} \times \frac{4\sigma^2}{n} = \frac{\sigma^2}{n}$$

This is exactly the same variance that would result if A were tested against placebo in a single two-armed comparative trial with $2n$ subjects in each treatment group. Similarly,

Table 3 Treatment effects in a 2×2 factorial design

	Treatment B	
Treatment A	No	Yes
No	$\overline{Y}_0$	$\overline{Y}_B$
Yes	$\overline{Y}_A$	$\overline{Y}_{AB}$

$$var(\beta_B) = \frac{\sigma^2}{n}$$

However, if we tested *A* and *B* separately, we would require *4n* subjects in each trial or a total of *8n* subjects to have the same precision obtained from half as many subjects in the factorial design. Thus, in the absence of interactions, these designs allow great efficiency in estimating main effects. In fact, in the absence of interaction, we get two trials for the price of one. Tests of both A and B can be conducted in a single factorial trial with the same precision as two single-factor trials using twice the sample size.

Design and Analysis of Factorial Trials

The literature is rich in examples of therapeutic factorial designs (Henderson et al. 2003; Sikov et al. 2015), and there are different approaches to designing factorial trials. Green (2005) provides a thorough explanation of the options in designing factorial trials and on how to interpret such trials. We focus on the design of the 2×2 factorial trials and discuss sample size computations based for a time-to-event endpoint, the most common endpoint that is utilized in phase III trials in cancer. There are two main questions that need to be addressed in designing a factorial trial. The first one pertains to whether one needs to adjust for the multiple hypotheses that are being tested. The second one is whether an interaction among the treatment arms exits. Unfortunately, there is no consensus in the literature on these two points. We present three examples of: (1) a trial designed with no interaction without adjustment for multiplicity, (2) a trial designed with no interaction and with adjustment for multiplicity, and (3) a trial designed with interaction between the two treatment arms. Moser and Halabi (2015) developed methodology for designing a factorial trial when the primary endpoint is a time-to-event endpoint. A matrix formulation was provided for calculating the required sample size to test a main effect or an interaction term for a pre-specified type I error rate and power (Moser and Halabi 2015).

Design Without Interaction

Computing the sample size for a 2×2 factorial trial assuming no interaction between the arms is straightforward. One can use the sample size formula for designing a trial comparing two treatment arms (Moser and Halabi 2015; Rubinstein et al. 1981). Suppose we are interested in testing the effect of two regimens in men with advanced prostate cancer. Patients will be randomized with equal allocation to four treatment groups: standard of care, experimental arm *A*, experimental arm *B*, or experimental arms *A*+ *B* (Table 4). Let λ_{ij} be the hazard rate of the ith factor (i = 1, 2) of treatment A and the jth factor (j = 1, 2) of treatment B. Overall survival (OS) is the primary endpoint. Similar to Rubenstein et al. (Peterson and George 1993), we make the following assumptions:

Table 4 Hazard rates of a factorial design with two factors A and B for a time-to-event endpoint

	Treatment B		
Treatment A	No	Yes	Pooled
No	λ_{11}	λ_{12}	$\lambda_{1.}$
Yes	λ_{21}	λ_{22}	$\lambda_{2.}$
Pooled	$\lambda_{.1}$	$\lambda_{.2}$	$\lambda_{..}$

(a) There is an accrual period [0, T] where T is the number of years. During this accrual period, the patients enter the clinical trial according to a Poisson process with n patients per year. The patients are randomized to k treatment groups with probability P_j $(0 < P_j < 1)$ to treatment j, where j = 1,2,...k and $\sum_{j=1}^{k} P_j = 1$.
(b) The patients are followed-up for a period of τ years. The τ is known as follow-up period. The total length of the study is T + τ years.
(c) In treatment j, the failure or death times (the times from entry into the trial to failure or death) are i.i.d exponentials with hazard λ_j. Moreover, the failure times across the treatment groups are assumed to be independent.
(d) The censored times (the times from entry into the trial to loss to follow-up) are i.i.d exponentials with common hazard Φ_c.
(e) The failure times and censored times are independent.
(f) The censoring mechanism is random censoring.
(g) Constant treatment effect for both treatments A and B over time, i.e., the proportional hazards assumption.

In designing such a 2×2 factorial trial without interaction, we are interested in testing two hypotheses concerning the main effect. Based on historical data, the median OS in men with advanced prostate cancer is 20 months in the standard of care arm. Consider the data in Table 4. For the first factor, we are interested in comparing the hazard rates for patients randomized to receive experimental treatment *A* with patients who receive standard of care, i.e., the main focus is testing the null hypothesis hazard ratio $(\Delta) = \lambda_{1.}/\lambda_{2.} = 1$ versus the alternative hypothesis $\Delta = \lambda_{1.}/\lambda_{2.} < 1$. The target total sample size is 900 patients. With 722 deaths for testing the efficacy of experimental arm *A*, the log-rank test has 85% power to detect a 20% decrease in hazard rate (equivalent to an increase in median OS from 20 months to 25 months in patients randomized to the standard of care and experimental treatment arm *A*, respectively; hazard ratio = 0.8) with a one-sided type I error rate of 0.025. We make the following assumptions in the sample size computation: equal allocation to the treatment arms, OS follows the exponential distribution, fixed sample size (no interim analysis), an accrual period rate of 30 patients/months, an accrual period of 30 months, a follow-up period of 14 months, and a trial duration of 44 months.

For testing the efficacy of treatment B (main effect), our objective is to compare the hazard rates for patients randomized to standard of care or experimental arm *B*, i.e., we focus on testing the null hypothesis $\Delta = \lambda_{.1}/\lambda_{.2} = 1$ versus the alternative hypothesis $\Delta = \lambda_{.1}/\lambda_{.2} < 1$. The target number of deaths is 434 and the total sample size is 750 patients. With 434 deaths for, the log-rank test has 85% power to detect a hazard ratio = 0.75 (assuming that the median OS = 20 months and 26.7 months in the standard of care and treatment *B*, respectively) with a one-sided type I error rate of 0.025. In designing the above trial, we base the sample size on testing the hypothesis with the smallest effect size (comparing experimental arm *A* to the standard of care) since its sample size is larger than what is required for testing the second hypothesis (comparing experimental arm *B* to the standard of care). Thus, the target sample size for this trial is 900 prostate cancer patients.

In the prostate cancer example we could adjust for the type I error rate using the Bonferroni procedure ($\alpha/2$) because we are testing two hypotheses. The required number of events is 863 deaths for testing the first hypothesis, and the log-rank test has 85% power to detect a 20% decrease in hazard rate (HR = 0.8) with a one-sided type I error rate of 0.0125. As expected, we observe that the number of events has increased drastically from a 722 to 863 deaths (approximately 20% increase). If we assume the same sample size (900 patients) and the same accrual rate of 30 patients/month, then the trial duration will be doubled from 44 months to 88 months.

Several authors have debated that there is no need to adjust for the type I error rate in designing a factorial trial when several experimental arms are compared to a control or the standard of care group (Freidlin et al. 2008; Wason et al. 2014; Proschan and Waclawiw 2000). Their rationale is that such trials are designed to answer the efficacy question for each experimental drug separately and as such the results of one comparison should not influence the results of the other hypothesis.

Design with Interaction

Peterson et al. developed the sample size required in a 2×2 factorial trial in the presence of interaction when the endpoint is time-to-event (Peterson and George 1993).

Suppose we are interested in testing the effect of the interaction of the two treatment in the prostate cancer example (Table 4) and our objective is to compare the difference in the hazard rates $\lambda_{21}/\lambda_{11}$ / $\lambda_{22}/\lambda_{12}$ (on a log-scale). Let $\Delta_1 = \lambda_{11}/\lambda_{21}$, $\Delta_2 = \lambda_{12}/\lambda_{22}$, and $\gamma = \Delta_2/\Delta_1$ be the hazard ratios for treatment effect for patients receiving treatment A versus standard of care, treatment effect for patients receiving treatments A and B versus treatment B, and the ratio of the hazard ratios (or interaction between the two treatments), respectively. The null hypothesis is that there is no interaction between the two treatment ($\gamma = 1$) versus the alternative hypothesis that there is an interaction between the treatment groups ($\gamma \neq 1$). We assume that the median OS to be $M_{11} = 19$ in patients randomized to standard of care, $M_{21} = 20$ in patients randomized to experimental arm *A*, $M_{12} = 20$ in patients randomized to experimental arm *B*, and $M_{22} = 30$ months in patients randomized to experimental arms *A* and *B* (Table 4). In order to test this hypothesis, we need to extend both the accrual period from 30 months to 48 months and the follow-up period from 14 months to 30 months. The total sample size is now 1,440 patients and the expected number of events is 1,151 at the end of the trial. The power to detect a

$\gamma = 1.5$ for the interaction between the treatment arms is 85% assuming a one-sided type I error of 0.025.

Another strategy to consider in the interaction between the treatments is to use Simon's approach (Simon and Freedman 1997), who proposed inflating the sample size by 30%. Thus, the sample size for the prostate cancer trial will be 1,170 (900*30%) and the number of deaths = 934. For the power computation, we assume an accrual of 30 patients over a 48-month period and a follow-up period of 30 months. With 1,170, the power to detect an interaction $\gamma = 1.5$ between the two factors is 77%. Including Simon's reasoning to the computation that we performed above indicates, surprisingly, that the power for testing an interaction term ($\gamma = 1.5$) is around 80% assuming a one-sided type I error of 0.025.

The main drawback to factorial trials is that often trials are not designed to test for an interaction between the treatment groups and as a result such trials are usually underpowered. While the examples above were based on testing superiority hypotheses, a factorial trial can be designed testing a superiority and a non-inferiority (or equivalence) hypothesis. For example, CALGB 80203 (NCT00077233) was originally designed as a phase III 2×2 factorial trial to test two hypotheses. The first hypothesis was to test if the addition of C225 to FOLFOX or FOLFIRI chemotherapy will improve OS in untreated metastatic colon cancer patients. The second hypothesis was to test the equivalence of FOLFOX and FOLFIRI in OS in untreated metastatic colon cancer patients. The trial was closed due to poor accrual. Recently Freidlin and Korn (2017) argued that in designing factorial trials in oncology, one needs to consider an interaction between the drugs as it is very likely that the "no interaction" assumption is not a valid one. Moreover, the authors advocate for matching the analysis with the trial design to achieve the objectives of the trial.

Designs with Biomarkers

Treatment by biomarker interaction is frequently implemented in cancer trials. Gönen (2003) considers the planning of subgroup analyses for time-to-event outcomes in a treatment by molecular marker factorial design. Factorial trials are the only design in which an investigator can test for treatment-biomarker interaction. It is important to note that testing for the treatment-biomarker interaction term (a predictive marker) is often conducted after the treatment trial has been reported. While treatment arm is defined by randomization, the biomarker status (e.g., positive or negative biomarker) is defined by observation. For a time-to-event outcome, one would use the proportional hazards model with:

$$\lambda(t|\, x_1, x_2) = \lambda_0(t)\ \exp\left(\beta_1 x_1 + \beta_2 x_2 + \beta_3 x_1 x_2\right)$$

where $\lambda_0(t)$ is the baseline hazard, $x_i = 0$ or 1 represents the treatment arm, x_2 is the biomarker level (usually measured as a continuous variable), and $x_1 x_2$ is the treatment arm-biomarker interaction term. Under the null hypothesis, $\beta_3 = 0$ indicates that there is no interaction between treatment arm-biomarker. If the interaction term between a biomarker and a treatment is statistically significant, then this is considered to be a predictive biomarker of the outcome.

We illustrate the above concept by using an example from a phase III trial of transitional cell carcinoma (Rosenberg et al. 2019) where 588 patients were randomized to one of two treatments arms: (a) gemcitabine, cisplatin, and placebo, or (b) gemcitabine, cisplatin, and bevacizumab. The investigator is interested in testing the treatment by vascular endothelial growth factor (VEGF) level interaction using a two-sided type I error rate = 0.05 to attain a power of 80%. In simplifying the power computation, we assume that the biomarker is binary (the VEGF level is dichotomized based on an established cut point with positive and negative groups) and that the prevalence of a positive VEGF marker is 30%. The primary endpoint is OS. The median survival times (months) are assumed to be: $M_{11} = 13.80$ in patients randomized to gemcitabine, cisplatin, and placebo, and have negative VEGF biomarker; $M_{21} = 15.80$ in patients randomized to gemcitabine, cisplatin, and placebo, and have positive VEGF biomarker; $M_{12} = 13.80$ in patients randomized to gemcitabine, cisplatin, and bevacizumab, and have negative VEGF biomarker; and $M_{22} = 30.40$ in patients randomized to gemcitabine, cisplatin, and bevacizumab, and have positive VEGF biomarker (Table 5). We also assumed: an accrual rate of 168 patients/year for a total accrual period of 3.5 years and a follow-up period of 1 year. Let using the methodology developed by Peterson et al. (Rubinstein et al. 1981), the null hypothesis is that there is no interaction between the treatment arm-biomarker groups ($\gamma = \Delta_2/\Delta_1 = 1$) versus the alternative hypothesis that there is an interaction between the treatment-biomarker ($\gamma \neq 1$). With 428 deaths, the power is 83% assuming two-sided test of 0.05 to detect an interaction (ratio of hazard ratios) of $\gamma = 1.92$.

The stratified biomarker trial is a powerful design that will test for the treatment arm-biomarker interaction prospectively (Liu et al. 2014). The stratified biomarker design is one where all patients regardless of their biomarker status are randomly assigned to either an experimental arm or a control (Fig. 1) (Freidlin and Korn 2014). For simplicity, we concentrate on a biomarker that is binary where patients can be classified as either having a positive or negative biomarker status. The stratified biomarker design is commonly used to test for the treatment-biomarker interaction (Liu et al. 2014). In the biomarker design, an investigator may consider testing whether the treatments differ in outcomes within a biomarker group, or test if the clinical outcome within the same treatment differ between the biomarker groups, or can test for the treatment-biomarker interaction. An example of a stratified biomarker trial is the MARVEL trial (NCT0073888) where tissues from consenting patients were to be submitted for epidermal growth factor receptor (EGFR) evaluation. In the

Table 5 Median overall survival (months) for testing a treatment-biomarker interaction

	VEFG levels	
Treatment assignment	Low VEGF	High VEGF
Gemcitabine+cisplatin	$M_{11} = 13.80$	$M_{12} = 13.80$
Gemcitabine+cisplatin+bevacizumab	$M_{21} = 15.80$	$\lambda_{22} = 30.0$

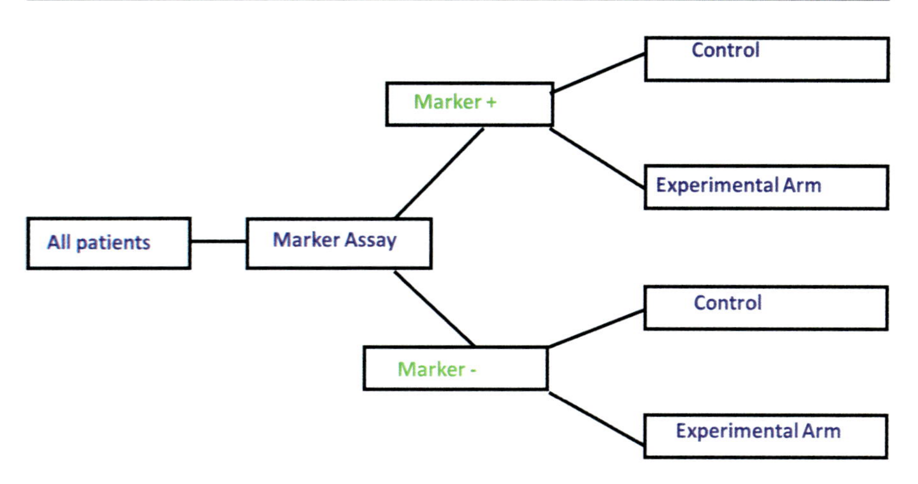

Fig. 1 Example of a stratified biomarker trial

MARVEL trial, about 1200 non-small lung cancer patients were to be randomized to either erlotinib or pemetrexed. The primary objective was to evaluate whether there are differences in progression-free survival between erlotinib and pemetrexed within the FISH positive and FISH negative subgroups. Unfortunately, the trial was closed due to slow accrual. A stratified biomarker trial often requires large sample size, that the cutoff point for the biomarker has been validated and that the prevalence of the biomarker is appropriate to allow for testing for the treatment-biomarker interaction. When biomarkers are based on tumor, the true status of the biomarker can be classified with error. Sample size formula for the stratified biomarker design to account for the misclassification error has been provided and is a hot research area (Liu et al. 2014).

Analysis of Factorial Trials

Factorial trials have been analyzed inconsistently in the literature (Freidlin and Korn 2017). Some authors maintain the view that an interaction test should be provided even if the trial was not designed to test for an interaction between the treatments (Montgomery et al. 2003; Korn and Freidlin 2016). As an example, consider the ECOG trial (E1199) 2×2 factorial trial in neoadjuvant breast cancer patients where they were randomized to: paclitaxel (administered over 3 weeks), paclitaxel (weekly), docetaxel given every 3 weeks, and docetaxel given weekly (Sparano 2008). The study was designed with 86% power using a two-sided significance level of 0.05 for testing each of the primary factors (treatment: paclitaxel vs. docetaxel; schedule: weekly vs. 3 weeks). No statistically significant differences in DFS were observed between patients randomized to paclitaxel versus docetaxel (p-value $= 0.61$) nor weekly treatment versus those who received 3 weeks treatment (p-value $= 0.33$). The authors performed a test of interaction between treatment and schedule (p-value = 0.003). Furthermore, the authors compared individual arms and demonstrated that patients receiving weekly paclitaxel had superior disease-free survival than patients who received paclitaxel over 3 weeks. The results persisted in long-term follow-up of these patients (Sparano et al. 2015).

Treatment Interactions

We now consider more general circumstances where the effect of treatment A is influenced by the presence of treatment B, and vice versa. In such cases, there is said to be a *treatment interaction*. Although the sample size efficiencies just discussed will be lost when this occurs, factorial designs become even more relevant.

Factorial Designs Are the Only Way to Study Interactions

One of the most consequential features of factorial designs is that they are the only type of trial design that permits study of treatment interactions. This is because the factorial structure has groups with all possible combinations of treatments, allowing the responses to be compared directly. Consider, again, the two estimates of the effect of A in the 2×2 design, one in the presence of B and the other in the absence of B. The definition of an interaction is that the effect of A in the absence of B is different from the effect of A in the presence of B. This difference can be estimated by comparing

$$\beta_{AB} = \left(\overline{Y_A} - \overline{Y_0}\right) - \left(\overline{Y_{AB}} - \overline{Y_B}\right) \tag{3}$$

with zero. If $\beta_{AB}$is near zero, we would conclude that no interaction is present. It is straightforward to verify that $\beta_{AB} = \beta_{BA}$.

An important principle of factorial trials is evident by examining the variance of β_{AB}. Under the same assumptions as in section “Factorial Designs Can Be More Efficient.”

$$var(\beta_{AB}) = 4\frac{\sigma^2}{n}$$

which is *four* times larger than the variance for either main effect when an interaction is known to be absent. Therefore, to have the same precision for an estimate of an interaction effect as for a main effect, the sample size has to be four times larger. This illustrates again why both the efficiency and interaction objectives cannot be simultaneously met in the same factorial study.

When there is an AB interaction, we cannot use the estimators given above for the main effects of A and B (Eqs. 1 and 2), because they assume that no interaction is present. In fact, it is not sensible to talk about an overall main effect in the presence of an interaction because Eqs. 1 or 2 would have us average over two quantities that are not expected to be equal. Instead, we could talk about the effect of A in the absence of B,

$$\beta'_A = \left(\overline{Y_A} - \overline{Y_0}\right) \tag{4}$$

or the effect of B in the absence of A,

$$\beta'_B = \left(\overline{Y_B} - \overline{Y_0}\right) \tag{5}$$

These are logically and statistically equivalent to what would be obtained from stand-alone trials.

In the $2 \times 2 \times 2$ design, there are three main effects and four interactions possible, all of which can be estimated by the design. Following the notation above, the effects are

$$\beta_A = \frac{1}{4}\left[\left(\overline{Y_A} - \overline{Y_0}\right) + \left(\overline{Y_{AB}} - \overline{Y_B}\right) + \left(\overline{Y_{AC}} - \overline{Y_C}\right) + \left(\overline{Y_{ABC}} - \overline{Y_{BC}}\right)\right] \tag{6}$$

for treatment A,

$$\beta_{AB} = \frac{1}{2}\left[\left(\left(\overline{Y_A} - \overline{Y_0}\right) - \left(\overline{Y_{AB}} - \overline{Y_B}\right)\right) + \left(\left(\overline{Y_{AC}} - \overline{Y_C}\right) + \left(\overline{Y_{ABC}} - \overline{Y_{BC}}\right)\right)\right] \tag{7}$$

for the AB interaction, and

$$\beta_{ABC} = \left[\left(\overline{Y_A} - \overline{Y_0}\right) - \left(\overline{Y_{AB}} - \overline{Y_B}\right) - \left(\overline{Y_{AC}} - \overline{Y_C}\right) - \left(\overline{Y_{ABC}} - \overline{Y_{BC}}\right)\right] \tag{8}$$

for the ABC interaction. The respective variances are $\frac{\sigma^2}{2n}$, $\frac{2\sigma^2}{n}$, and $\frac{8\sigma^2}{n}$. Thus the precision of the two-way interactions relative to the main effect is 1/4, and for the three-way interaction is 1/16.

When certain interactions are present, here again it will not be sensible to think of the straightforward main effects. But the design can yield an alternative estimator for β_A, or β_{BA},or for other effects.

Suppose that there is an ABC interaction. Then instead of β_A, an estimator of the effect of A in the absence of C would be

$$\beta'_A = \frac{1}{2}\left[\left(\overline{Y_A} - \overline{Y_0}\right) + \left(\overline{Y_{AB}} - \overline{Y_B}\right)\right]$$

which does not use β_{ABC} and implicitly assumes that there is no AB interaction. Similarly, the AB interaction would be

$$\beta'_{AB} = \left[\left(\overline{Y_A} - \overline{Y_0}\right) + \left(\overline{Y_{AB}} - \overline{Y_B}\right)\right]$$

for the same reason. Thus, when high-order interactions are present, we must modify our estimates of lower order effects, losing some efficiency. However, factorial designs are the only ones that permit treatment interactions to be studied.

Table 6 Response data from a hypothetical factorial trial showing no interaction on an additive scale of measurement

	Treatment *B*	
Treatment *A*	No	Yes
No	*5*	*10*
Yes	*10*	*15*

Table 7 Response data from a hypothetical factorial trial showing no interaction on a multiplicative scale of measurement

	Treatment *B*	
Treatment *A*	No	Yes
No	*5*	*10*
Yes	*10*	*20*

Interactions Depend on the Scale of Measurement

In the examples just given, the treatment effects and interactions have been assumed to exist on an additive scale. This is reflected in the use of sums and differences in the formulas for estimation.

In practice, other scales of measurement, particularly a multiplicative one, may be useful. As an example, consider the response data in Table 6 where the effect of treatment A is to increase the baseline response by 5 units. The same is true of B, and there is no interaction between the treatments on this scale because the joint effect of A and B is to increase the response by $5 + 5 = 10$ units.

In contrast, Table 7 shows data in which the effects of both treatments are to multiply the baseline response by 2.0. Hence, the combined effect of A and B is a fourfold increase, which is greater than the joint treatment effect for the additive case. If the analysis model were multiplicative, Table 6 would show an interaction, whereas if the analysis model were additive, Table 7 would show an interaction. Thus, to discuss interactions, we must establish the scale of measurement.

The Interpretation of Main Effects Depends on Interactions

In the presence of an interaction in the 2×2 design, there is not an overall, or main, effect of either treatment. This is because the effect of A is different depending on the presence or absence of B. In the presence of a small interaction, where all subjects benefit regardless of the use of B, we might observe that the magnitude of the overall effect of A is of some size and that therapeutic decisions are unaffected by the presence of an interaction (Fig. 2a). This is known as *quantitative interaction* because it does not affect the direction of the treatment effect. For large quantitative interactions, it may not be sensible to talk about overall effects (Kahan, 2013).

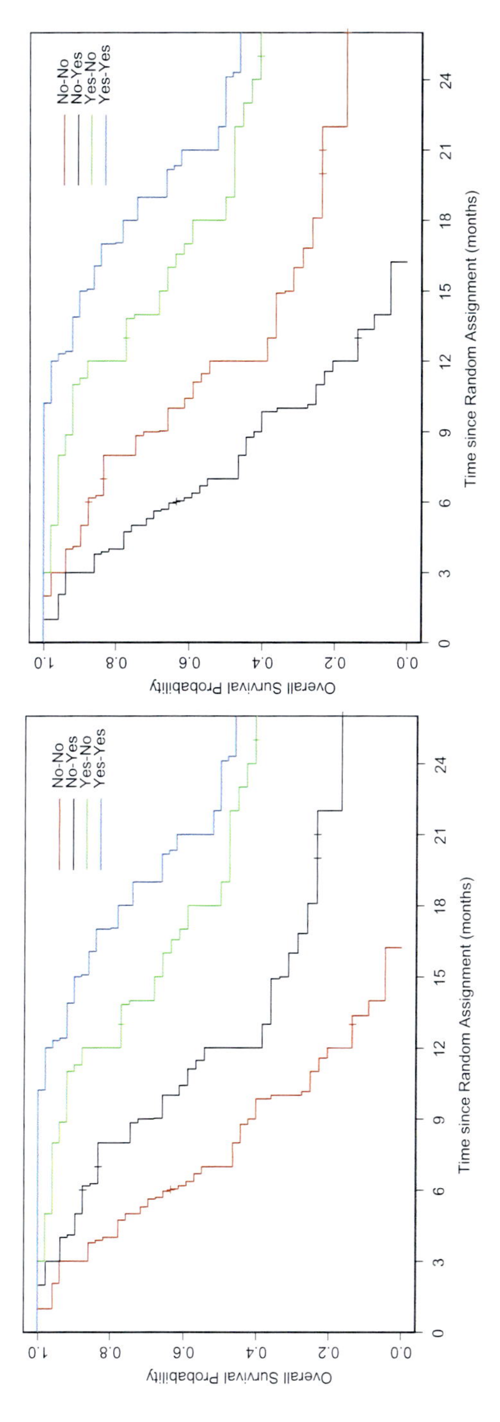

Fig. 2 Hypothetical examples of (**a**) (left) a quantitative interaction and (**b**) (right) qualitative interaction

In contrast, if the presence of B reverses the effects of A, then the interaction is *qualitative*, and treatment decisions may need to be modified (Fig. 2b). We would not talk about an overall effect of A, because it could be positive in the presence of B and negative in the absence of B and could yield an average effect near zero.

Analyses Can Employ Linear Models

Motivation for the estimators given above can be obtained using linear models. There has been little theoretical work on analyses using other models. One exception is the work by Slud (1994) describing approaches to factorial trials with survival outcomes. Suppose we have conducted a 2×2 factorial experiment with group sizes given by Table 1. We can estimate the AB interaction effect using a linear model of the form

$$E(Y) = \beta_0 + \beta_A X_A + \beta_B X_B + \beta_{AB} X_A X_B \tag{9}$$

where the X's are indicator variables for the treatment groups and β_{AB} is the interaction effect. For example,

$$X_A = \begin{cases} 1 \text{ for treatment group } A, \\ 0 \text{ otherwise.} \end{cases}$$

The design matrix has dimension $4n \times 4$ and is

$$X' = \begin{bmatrix} 1\ldots & 1\ldots & 1\ldots & 1\ldots \\ 0\ldots & 1\ldots & 0\ldots & 1\ldots \\ 0\ldots & 0\ldots & 1\ldots & 1\ldots \\ 0\ldots & 0\ldots & 0\ldots & 1\ldots \end{bmatrix},$$

where there are four blocks of n identical rows representing each treatment group and the columns represent effects for the intercept, treatment A, treatment B, and both treatments, respectively. The vector of responses has dimension $4n \times 1$ and is

$$\boldsymbol{Y}' = [Y_{01}, \ldots, Y_{A1}, \ldots, Y_{B1}, \ldots Y_{AB1}, \ldots]$$

By ordinary least squares estimation, the solution to Eq. 9 is.

$$\widehat{\beta} = (\boldsymbol{X}'\boldsymbol{X})^{-1}\boldsymbol{X}'\boldsymbol{Y}.$$

When the interaction effect is omitted, the estimates will be denoted by $\widehat{\beta}^*$. The covariance matrix of estimates is $(X'X)^{-1}\sigma^2$, where the variance of each observation is σ^2.

We have

$$\boldsymbol{X}'\boldsymbol{X} = n \times \begin{bmatrix} 4 & 2 & 2 & 1 \\ 2 & 2 & 1 & 1 \\ 2 & 1 & 2 & 1 \\ 1 & 1 & 1 & 1 \end{bmatrix}, \qquad (\boldsymbol{X}'\boldsymbol{X})^{-1} = \frac{1}{n} \times \begin{bmatrix} 1 & -1 & -1 & 1 \\ -1 & 2 & 1 & -2 \\ -1 & 1 & 2 & -2 \\ 1 & -2 & -2 & 4 \end{bmatrix},$$

and

$$\boldsymbol{X}'\boldsymbol{Y} = n \times \begin{bmatrix} \overline{Y}_0 & +\overline{Y}_A & + & \overline{Y}_B + \overline{Y}_{AB} \\ \overline{Y}_A & +\overline{Y}_{AB} & & \\ \overline{Y}_B & +\overline{Y}_{AB} & & \\ \overline{Y}_{AB} & & & \end{bmatrix},$$

where $\overline{Y}_i$ denotes the average response in the ith group. Then

$$\widehat{\beta} = \begin{bmatrix} \overline{\mathrm{Y}}_0 & & & \\ -\overline{\mathrm{Y}}_0 & +\overline{\mathrm{Y}}_\mathrm{A} & & \\ -\overline{\mathrm{Y}}_0 & +\overline{\mathrm{Y}}_\mathrm{B} & & \\ \overline{\mathrm{Y}}_0 & -\overline{\mathrm{Y}}_\mathrm{A} & -\overline{\mathrm{Y}}_\mathrm{B} & +\overline{\mathrm{Y}}_\mathrm{AB} \end{bmatrix} \quad [1] \tag{10}$$

which corresponds to the estimators given in Eqs. 3, 4, and 5. However, if the test for interaction fails to reject and the $\widehat{\beta_{AB}}$ effect is removed from the model, then

$$\widehat{\beta^*} = \begin{bmatrix} \frac{3}{4}\overline{Y}_0 & + & \frac{1}{4}\overline{Y}_A & + & \frac{1}{4}\overline{Y}_B & - & \frac{1}{4}\overline{Y}_{AB} \\ -\frac{1}{2}\overline{Y}_0 & + & \frac{1}{2}\overline{Y}_A & - & \frac{1}{2}\overline{Y}_B & + & \frac{1}{2}\overline{Y}_{AB} \\ -\frac{1}{2}\overline{Y}_0 & - & \frac{1}{2}\overline{Y}_A & + & \frac{1}{2}\overline{Y}_B & + & \frac{1}{2}\overline{Y}_{AB} \end{bmatrix} \quad [1].$$

The main effects for A and B are given above in Eqs. 1 and 2.

The covariance matrices for these estimators are

$$\widehat{cov(\beta)} = \frac{\sigma^2}{n} \times \begin{bmatrix} 1 & -1 & -1 & 1 \\ -1 & 2 & 1 & -2 \\ -1 & 1 & 2 & -2 \\ 1 & -2 & -2 & 4 \end{bmatrix} \tag{11}$$

and

$$\widehat{cov(\beta^*)} = \frac{\sigma^2}{n} \times \begin{bmatrix} \frac{3}{4} & -\frac{1}{2} & -\frac{1}{2} \\ -\frac{1}{2} & 1 & 0 \\ -\frac{1}{2} & 0 & 1 \end{bmatrix}. \tag{12}$$

In the absence of an interaction, the main effects of A and B are estimated independently and with higher precision than when an interaction is present. The interaction effect is relatively imprecisely estimated, indicating the larger sample sizes required to have a high power to detect such effects.

Examples of Factorial Designs

Factorials trials have received a lot of attention in clinical trials (Sikov et al. 2015). We list interesting examples of factorial trials in Table 8. Factorial designs are well suited to prevention trials for reasons outlined above, but many therapeutic trials have also utilized factorial designs because of the questions being addressed. One important classic study using a 2×2 factorial design is the Physicians' Health Study (Hennekens and Eberlein 1985). This trial was conducted in 22,000 physicians in the USA and was designed to test the effects of (1) aspirin on reducing cardiovascular mortality and (2) β-carotene on reducing cancer incidence. The trial is noteworthy in several ways, including its test of two interventions in unrelated diseases, use of physicians as subjects to report outcomes reliably, relatively low cost, and an all-male, high-risk study population. This last characteristic led to some criticism, which was probably unwarranted.

In January 1988, the aspirin component of the Physicians' Health Study was discontinued because evidence demonstrated convincingly that it was associated with lower rates of myocardial infarction. The question concerning the effect of β-carotene on cancer was addressed by continuation of the trial. In the absence of an interaction, the second major question of the trial was unaffected by the closure of the aspirin component and showed no benefit for β-carotene.

Another interesting example of a 2×2 factorial design is the α-tocopherol β-carotene Lung Cancer Prevention Trial, conducted in 29,133 male smokers in Finland between 1987 and 1994 (The ATBC Cancer 1994). In this study, lung cancer incidence was the sole outcome. It was thought possible that lung cancer incidence could be reduced by either or both interventions. When this trial was stopped in 1994, there were 876 new cases of lung cancer in the study population during the trial. Alpha-tocopherol was not associated with a reduction in the risk of cancer. Surprisingly, β-carotene was associated with a statistically significant *increased* incidence of lung cancer. There was no evidence of a treatment interaction. The unexpected findings of this study have been supported by the recent results of another large trial of carotene and retinol.

The Fourth International Study of Infarct Survival (ISIS-4) was a $2 \times 2 \times 2$ factorial trial assessing the efficacy of oral captopril, oral mononitrate, and intravenous magnesium sulfate in 58,050 subjects with suspected myocardial infarction (McAlister et al. 2003). No significant interactions among the treatments were found and each main effect comparison was based on approximately 29,000 treated versus 29,000 control subjects. Among the findings was demonstration that captopril was associated with a small but statistically significant reduction in 5-week mortality. The difference in mortality was 7.19% versus 7.69% (143 events out of 4,319),

Table 8 Examples of trials using factorial designs

Trial	Design	Cohort	Treatments	Outcomes
Physicians' Health Study (Hennekens and Eberlein 1985)	2 × 2	Healthy male physicians, $n = 22{,}071$	Aspirin, β-carotene	CHD, cancer
Linxian Nutrition Trial (Li et al. 1993)	2^4	4 Linxian communes, $n = 29{,}584$	Retinol + zinc Riboflavin + niacin Ascorbic acid + molybdenum Selenium + β-carotene α-tocopherol	Esophageal cancer; all-cause mortality
ISIS-4 (Flather et al. 1994)	2^3	Acute MI patients, $n = 58{,}050$	Oral captopril Oral mononitrate IV magnesium sulfate	Mortality: 5 week; 12 month
Prevention of postoperative nausea and vomiting (Apfel et al. 2004)	2^6	Patients at high risk for nausea and vomiting, $n = 5{,}199$	Ondansetron Dexamethasone Droperidol Propofol or volatile anesthetic Nitrogen or nitrous oxide Remifentanil or fentanyl	Within 24 h postoperative nausea and vomiting
Ispwich Childbirth Study (Grant et al. 2001)	2 × 2	Women needing episiotomy repair, $n = 793$	Repair: 2 stage or 3 stage Suture: polyglactin or chromic	Pain or re-suturing
Thrombosis Prevention Trial (Thrombosis prevention 1998)	2 × 2	Men at risk of ischemic heart disease, $n = 5{,}499$	Warfarin + aspirin Warfarin + placebo aspirin Placebo warfarin + aspirin Placebo + placebo	Coronary death, fatal/nonfatal MI
Women (Cook et al. 2007)	2 × 2 × 2	Women, aged 40 and over, at high risk, with a history of cardiovascular disease or three or more coronary heart disease risk factors.	Vitamin C Vitamin E Beta-carotene Folic acid/Vitamin B6/Vitamin B12	Myocardial infarction, stroke, coronary revascularization, or cardiovascular death
E1199 (Sparano et al. 2015)	2 × 2	Neoadjuvant stage II and III breast cancer	Paclitaxel vs. docetaxel Every 3 weeks vs. weekly	Disease-free survival Overall survival
EDTA chelation Trial (Lamas et al. 2014)	2 × 2	Post-MI patients ≥50 years and creatinine	EDTA chelation or placebo infusions 6 caplets daily of a 28-component	Composite of total mortality, MI, stroke, coronary revascularization,

(continued)

Table 8 (continued)

Trial	Design	Cohort	Treatments	Outcomes
		$\leq$2.0 mg/dL $n = 1{,}708$.	multivitamin or placebo	or hospitalization for angina.

Adapted from Piantadosi 2017.

illustrating the ability of large studies to detect potentially important treatment effects, even when they are small in relative magnitude. Mononitrate and magnesium therapy did not significantly reduce 5-week mortality.

Partial, Fractional, and Incomplete Factorials

Use Partial Factorial Designs When Interactions Are Absent

Partial, or fractional, factorial designs are those that omit certain treatment groups by design. A careful analysis of the objectives of an experiment, its efficiency, and the effects it can estimate may justify not using some groups. Because many cells contribute to the estimate of any effect, a design may achieve its intended purpose without some of the cells.

In the 2×2 design, all treatment groups must be present to permit estimating the interaction between A and B. However, for higher order designs, if some interactions are known biologically not to exist, certain treatment combinations can be omitted from the design and still permit estimates of other effects of interest. For example, in the $2 \times 2 \times 2$ design, if the interaction between A, B, and C is known not to exist, that treatment cell could be omitted from the design and still permit estimation of all the main effects. The efficiency would be somewhat reduced, however. Similarly, the two-way interactions could still be estimated without $\overline{Y}_{ABC}$. This can be verified from the formulas above.

Generally, partial high-order designs will produce a situation termed "aliasing" in which the estimates of certain effects are algebraically identical to completely different effects. If both are biologically possible, the design will not be able to reveal which effect is being estimated. Naturally this is undesirable unless additional information is available to the investigator to indicate that some aliased effects are zero. This can be used to advantage in improving efficiency, and one must be careful in deciding which cells to exclude. The reader is referred to Cox (1958) or Mason et al. (1989) for a discussion of this topic.

The Women's Health Initiative (WHI) clinical trial was a $2 \times 2 \times 2$ partial factorial design studying the effects of hormone replacement, dietary fat reduction, and calcium and vitamin D on coronary disease, breast cancer, and osteoporosis (Assaf and Carleton 1994; Design of the Women's 1998; Shumaker et al. 1998). The study accrued 162,000 subjects into multiple clinical trials and finished the initial study period in 2005 (Rossouw et al. 2002). The hormone therapy trials randomized 27,347 women in an estrogen plus progestin study and an estrogen alone study. The dietary component of the study randomized 48,835 women, using a 3:2 allocation ratio in favor of the control arm and 9 years of follow-up. The calcium and vitamin D component randomized 36,282 women. Such a large and complex trial was not without controversy early on (Marshall 1993), and presented logistical difficulties, questions about adherence, and sensitivity to assumptions that could only roughly be validated during design.

Incomplete Designs Present Special Problems

Treatment groups can be dropped out of factorial plans without yielding a fractional replication. The resulting trials have been called *incomplete factorial designs* (Byar et al. 1993). In incomplete designs, cells are not missing by design intent but because some treatment combinations may be infeasible. For example, in a 2×2 design it may not be ethically possible to use a placebo group. In this case, one would not be able to estimate the AB interaction. In other circumstances, unwanted aliasing may occur, or the efficiency of the design to estimate main effects may be greatly reduced. In some cases, estimators of treatment and interaction effects are biased, but there may be reasons to use a design that retains as much of the factorial structure as possible. For example, they may be the only way to estimate certain interactions.

Summary

Factorial trials are efficient under the assumption of no interaction between the treatments, and this should be considered at the design stage. Factorial designs may also be used for the purpose of detecting an interaction between the factors if the trial is powered accordingly. Therefore, factorial trial designs are useful in two circumstances. When two or more treatments do not interact, factorial designs can test the main effects of each using smaller sample sizes and greater precision than separate parallel group designs. When it is essential to study treatment interactions, factorial designs are the only effective way to do so. The precision, however, with which interaction effects are estimated is lower than that for main effects in the absence of interactions. A factorial trial designed to detect for an interaction has no advantage in terms of the required sample size compared to a multi-arm parallel trial for assessing more than one intervention.

When there are many treatments or factors, these designs require a relatively large number of treatment groups. In complex designs, if some interactions are known not to exist or are unimportant, it may be possible to omit some treatment groups, reduce the size and complexity of the experiment, and still estimate all of the effects of biological interest. Extra attention to the design properties is necessary to be certain that fractional designs will meet the intended objectives. Such fractional or partial factorial designs are of considerable use in agricultural and industrial experiments but have not been applied frequently to clinical trials.

Ethical and toxicity constraints may make it impossible to apply either a full factorial or a fractional factorial design, yielding an incomplete design. The properties of incomplete factorial designs have not been studied extensively, but they may be the best design in some circumstances.

A number of important, complex, and recent clinical trials have used factorial designs. Because of the low potential for toxicity, these designs have been more frequently applied in studies of disease prevention. Examples include the Physicians' Health Study and the Women's' Health Trial. In medical studies, the design is employed usually to achieve greater efficiency, since the treatments are unlikely to interact.

Summary and Conclusions

Factorial trials are efficient only when there is no interaction between the treatments, and this should be considered at the design stage. Factorial designs must be used when the intent is to study interactions in which case the trial must be powered accordingly. Interaction effects have roughly four times the variance of main effects and so require much larger sample sizes. If many treatments and interactions are possible, factorials designs may be impractical for therapeutic questions due to their large sample size and complexity. Other constraints may make these designs unsuitable such as the need to omit treatments or administer all therapies at full dose in some groups.

Key Facts

Factorial trials represent a structure that can test treatment by treatment interactions. In the narrow circumstance that interactions are known to be absent, the factorial structure can test the effects of two treatments using a sample size ordinarily used for a single treatment. When interactions are the focus, sample size must be increased substantially because they are estimated with less precision than "main effects." Factorial designs are often well suited to prevention questions but have been applied widely.

Cross-References

▶ Biomarker-Guided Trials
▶ Prevention Trials: Challenges in Design, Analysis, and Interpretation of Prevention Trials

References

Apfel CC, Korttila K, Abdalla M, Kerger H, Turan A, Vedder I, . . . IMPACT Investigators (2004) A factorial trial of six interventions for the prevention of postoperative nausea and vomiting. N Engl J Med 350(24):2441–2451

Assaf AR, Carleton RA (1994) The Women's Health Initiative Clinical Trial and Observational Study: history and overview. R I Med 77(12):424–427
Byar DP, Piantadosi S (1985) Factorial designs for randomized clinical trials. Cancer Treat Rep 69 (10):1055–1063
Byar DP, Herzberg AM, Tan WY (1993) Incomplete factorial designs for randomized clinical trials. Stat Med 12(17):1629–1641
Cook NR, Albert CM, Gaziano JM, Zaharris E, MacFadyen J, Danielson E, . . . Manson JE (2007) A randomized factorial trial of vitamins C and E and beta carotene in the secondary prevention of cardiovascular events in women: results from the Women's Antioxidant Cardiovascular Study. Arch Intern Med 167(15):13–27
Cox DR (1958) Planning of experiments. Wiley, New York
Design of the Women's Health Initiative clinical trial and observational study. The Women's Health Initiative Study Group. (1998) Control Clin Trials 19(1):61–109
Fisher RA (1935) The design of experiments. Oliver and Boyd, Edinburgh/London
Fisher RA (1960) The design of experiments, 8th edn. Hafner, New York
Flather M, Pipilis A, Collins R, Budaj A, Hargreaves A, Kolettis T, . . . et al (1994) Randomized controlled trial of oral captopril, of oral isosorbide mononitrate and of intravenous magnesium sulphate started early in acute myocardial infarction: safety and haemodynamic effects. ISIS-4 (Fourth international study of infarct survival) Pilot Study Investigators. Eur Heart J 15(5):608–619
Freidlin B, Korn EL (2014) Biomarker enrichment strategies: matching trial design to biomarker credentials. Nat Rev Clin Oncol 11(2):81–90
Freidlin B, Korn EL (2017) Two-by-two factorial cancer treatment trials: is sufficient attention being paid to possible interactions? J Natl Cancer Inst 109(9). https://doi.org/10.1093/jnci/djx146
Freidlin B, Korn EL, Gray R, Martin A (2008) Multi-arm clinical trials of new agents: some design considerations. Clin Cancer Res 14(14):4368–4371
Gönen M (2003) Planning for subgroup analysis: a case study of treatment-marker interaction in metastatic colorectal cancer. Control Clin Trials 24(4):355–363
Grant A, Gordon B, Mackrodat C, Fern E, Truesdale A, Ayers S (2001) The Ipswich childbirth study: one year follow up of alternative methods used in perineal repair. BJOG 108(1):34–40
Green S (2005) Factorial designs with time to event endpoints, pp 181–189
Henderson IC, Berry DA, Demetri GD, Cirrincione CT, Goldstein LJ, Martino S, . . . Norton L (2003) Improved outcomes from adding sequential paclitaxel but not from escalating doxorubicin dose in an adjuvant chemotherapy regimen for patients with node-positive primary breast cancer. J Clin Oncol 21(6):976–983
Hennekens CH, Eberlein K (1985) A randomized trial of aspirin and beta-carotene among U.S. physicians. Prev Med 14(2):165–168
Kahan BC (2013) Bias in randomised factorial trials. Stat Med 32(26):4540–4549
Korn EL, Freidlin B (2016) Non-factorial analyses of two-by-two factorial trial designs. Clin Trials 13(6):651–659
Lamas GA, Boineau R, Goertz C, Mark DB, Rosenberg Y, Stylianou M, . . . Lee KL (2014) EDTA chelation therapy alone and in combination with oral high-dose multivitamins and minerals for coronary disease: the factorial group results of the Trial to Assess Chelation Therapy. Am Heart J 168(1):37.e5–44.e5
Li B, Taylor PR, Li J-Y, Dawsey SM, Wang W, Tangrea JA, . . . Blot WJ (1993) Linxian nutrition intervention trials design, methods, participant characteristics, and compliance. Ann Epidemiol 3(6):577–585
Liu C, Liu A, Hu J, Yuan V, Halabi S (2014) Adjusting for misclassification in a stratified biomarker clinical trial. SIM Stat Med 33(18):3100–3113
Lubsen J, Pocock SJ (1994) Factorial trials in cardiology: pros and cons. Eur Heart J 15(5):585–588
Marshall E (1993) Women's health initiative draws flak. Science 262(5135):838
Mason RL, Gunst RF, Hess JL (1989) Statistical design and analysis of experiments: with applications to engineering and science. Wiley, New York
McAlister FA, Straus SE, Sackett DL, Altman DG (2003) REVIEWS – analysis and reporting of factorial trials: a systematic review. JAMA 289(19):2545

Montgomery AA, Peters TJ, Little P (2003) Design, analysis and presentation of factorial randomised controlled trials. BMC Med Res Methodol 3(26)
Moser BK, Halabi S (2015) Sample size requirements and study duration for testing main effects and interactions in completely randomized factorial designs when time to event is the outcome. Commun Stat Theory Methods 44(2):275–285
Peterson B, George SL (1993) Sample size requirements and length of study for testing interaction in a 2 x k factorial design when time-to-failure is the outcome [corrected]. Control Clin Trials 14(6):511–522
Piantadosi S (2017) Factorial designs. In: Piantadosi S (ed) Clinical trials: a methodologic perspective. Wiley, Hoboken, pp 672–687
Proschan MA, Waclawiw MA (2000) Practical guidelines for multiplicity adjustment in clinical trials. Control Clin Trials 21(6):527–539
Rosenberg J, Ballman KV, Halabi S, Watt C, Hahn O, Steen P, . . . Morris M (2019) CALGB 90601 (Alliance): randomized, double-blind, placebo-controlled phase III trial comparing gemcitabine and cisplatin with bevacizumab or placebo in patients with metastatic urothelial carcinoma. J Clin Oncol 37(15_suppl):4503–4503
Rossouw JE, Anderson GL, Prentice RL, LaCroix AZ, Kooperberg C, Stefanick ML, . . . Writing Group for the Women's Health Initiative (2002) Risks and benefits of estrogen plus progestin in healthy postmenopausal women: principal results from the Women's Health Initiative randomized controlled trial. JAMA 288(3):321–333
Rubinstein LV, Gail MH, Santner TJ (1981) Planning the duration of a comparative clinical trial with loss to follow-up and a period of continued observation. J Chronic Dis 34(9):469–479
Shumaker SA, Reboussin BA, Espeland MA, Rapp SR, McBee WL, Dailey M, . . . Jones BN (1998) The Women's Health Initiative Memory Study (WHIMS): a trial of the effect of estrogen therapy in preventing and slowing the progression of dementia. Control Clin Trials 19(6):604–621
Sikov WM, Berry DA, Perou CM, Singh B, Cirrincione CT, Tolaney SM, . . . Winer EP (2015) Impact of the addition of carboplatin and/or bevacizumab to neoadjuvant once-per-week paclitaxel followed by dose-dense doxorubicin and cyclophosphamide on pathologic complete response rates in stage II to III triple-negative breast cancer: CALGB 40603 (Alliance). J Clin Oncol 33(1):13–21
Simon R, Freedman LS (1997) Bayesian design and analysis of two x two factorial clinical trials. Biometrics 53(2):456–464
Slud EV (1994) Analysis of factorial survival experiments. Biometrics 50(1):25–38
Sparano JA (2008) Weekly paclitaxel in the adjuvant treatment of breast cancer. New Engl J Med 358(16):1663
Sparano JA, Zhao F, Martino S, Ligibel JA, Perez EA, Saphner T et al (2015) Long-term follow-up of the E1199 phase III trial evaluating the role of Taxane and schedule in operable breast cancer. J Clin Oncol 33(21):2353–2360
The ATBC Cancer Prevention Study Group, The Alpha-Tocopherol, Beta-Carotene lung cancer prevention study: design, methods, participant characteristics, and compliance. (1994) Ann Epidemiol 4(1): 1–10
Thrombosis prevention trial: randomised trial of low-intensity oral anticoagulation with warfarin and low-dose aspirin in the primary prevention of ischaemic heart disease in men at increased risk. (1998) The Lancet 351(9098):233
Wason J, Mander A, Stecher L (2014) Correcting for multiple-testing in multi-arm trials: is it necessary and is it done? Trials 15(1):1–7
Yates F (1935) Complex experiments. Suppl J R Stat Soc B2(2):181–247

Within Person Randomized Trials

72

Gui-Shuang Ying

Contents

Abstract

Within person randomized trials (e.g., trials using within subject controls) are often employed for conditions that affect paired organs or two or more body sites of a person. In within person trials, the paired organs or body sites of a person

G.-S. Ying (✉)
Center for Preventive Ophthalmology and Biostatistics, Department of Ophthalmology, Perelman School of Medicine, University of Pennsylvania, Philadelphia, PA, USA
e-mail: gsying@pennmedicine.upenn.edu

© Springer Nature Switzerland AG 2022

S. Piantadosi, C. L. Meinert (eds.), *Principles and Practice of Clinical Trials*,
https://doi.org/10.1007/978-3-319-52636-2_101

receive two competing interventions either concurrently or sequentially, and the outcome measures are taken from each of paired organs or body sites. The within person design is a useful and efficient tool because comparisons between two interventions are made within the same person, thus removing the inter-person variability. Within person trials are most commonly conducted in ophthalmology, dentistry, and dermatology. However, within person trials pose some challenges including the possible bias from the carry across effect, the difficulty in recruitment subjects with bilateral disease of similar characteristics, and the limitation in generalization of the trial results. The within person correlations in outcome measures also complicate the sample size determination and statistical analyses of trial data from within person trials.

This chapter describes the rationale and requirements for employing within person design, the considerations in designing within person trials in various disease specialty areas. The appropriate methods for sample size calculation and the statistical analysis for within person trials are also described. Real trials are used throughout the chapter to demonstrate the trial design considerations, sample size calculation, and statistical analysis of correlated data from within person trials.

Keywords

Within person trials · Within subject controls · Within person correlation · Inter-eye correlation · Paired design · Split-mouth design · Carry across effect

Introduction

Some diseases affect paired organs, body parts, or body sites of a subject (such as eyes, ears, arms, or breasts) or two sites of a single organ, body part, or body site (such as teeth or sides of the mouth). This feature provides a unique opportunity for designing efficient clinical trial by using within subject controls. Different from conventional parallel group trials where eligible persons are randomized to receive only one of the study treatments (i.e., randomization unit is per person), within person trials randomize each organ or body site to treatment (i.e., the unit of randomization is per organ or body site), and each person receives all study treatments (Paré 1575).

Within person design is efficient in that it enables the comparison between two interventions within a person, eliminates the between-person variation, and hence improves the efficiency in estimating the treatment effect. The trials using within person controls do not have a generally accepted name, although some medical specialties have their specific terms, such as "contralateral design" or "paired design" in ophthalmology, "split-mouth design" in dentistry, and "split face" or "split body" design in dermatology (ref: Machin and Fayers 2010). To encompass all possible medical specialties and to align with the terminology used in the published guidelines for Consolidated Standards of Reporting Trials (CONSORT) (Pandis et al. 2017), trials using within subject controls are called within person trials in this chapter. In ophthalmology, within person trials randomly assign treatment to one eye and another treatment (or control) to the fellow eye of the same person (CAPT Research Group 2004). In dentistry, within person trials apply one treatment to some teeth and applying another treatment to other teeth of the same person (Pandis et al. 2013).

Within person trials, in which each person receives all study treatments, should not be confused with trials in which randomization and treatment are at the person level and all the organs or body sites of a person receiving the single same treatment are in the same comparison group. For example, in the Age-Related Eye Disease Study (AREDS), the participants were randomized to one of the four treatment groups – (1) zinc alone; (2) antioxidants alone; (3) a combination of antioxidants and zinc; or (4) a placebo (The AREDS Research Group 1999) – to evaluate the effect of high doses of vitamin C, vitamin E, beta-carotene, and zinc on the progression of age-related macular degeneration (AMD) and cataract. As two eyes of each participant received the same systematic treatment (e.g., dietary supplements) and are in the same comparison group, the AREDS is not a within person trial; instead it can be viewed as a type of clustered randomized trials that are not discussed here. Although within person trials have some similarities to cross-over trials which are also not discussed here, it differs from cross-over trials in that treatment and outcome measures are at the organ level or body site level rather than at the person level.

Within person trials have been used to evaluate a variety of preventive and therapeutic treatments (Pandis et al. 2017). Pandis et al. reported that approximately 2% of published randomized clinical trials employed a within person design (Pandis et al. 2017). Within person trials are most common in ophthalmology, dentistry, and dermatology. In dentistry, a review of 413 clinical trials published in 8 high-impact oral health journals from 1992 to 2012 found 43 (10%) dental trials used split-mouth design (Koletsi et al. 2014). Another study found that 67 (24%) of 276 trials published in implant dentistry journals between 1989 and 2011 used the split-mouth design (Cairo et al. 2012). In ophthalmology, Lee CF et al. found that within person design was used in 9 (13%) of 69 ophthalmic trials published in top four general clinical ophthalmology journals (*American Journal of Ophthalmology*, *Archives of Ophthalmology*, the *British Journal of Ophthalmology*, and *Ophthalmology)* between January and December of 2009 (Lee et al. 2012).

This chapter describes the rationale and the requirements for employing within person design, the considerations in designing within person trials, the sample size/power determination, and the appropriate statistical approaches for analyzing correlated data from within person trials. The examples of real within person clinical trials are used to demonstrate the design, sample size calculation, and statistical analysis for within person trials.

Rationale for Using Within Person Design

In the parallel group trials that randomize persons to one of treatments, the treatment effect is determined through comparing outcome measure between persons randomized to one treatment and persons randomized to another treatment (i.e., through between-person comparison). The treatment outcome measures are usually affected by baseline characteristics (e.g., age, gender, disease severity, genetic factors, etc.), contributing to the variability of outcome measure for evaluating treatment effect. However, in within person trials, each person receives all study treatments (e.g., paired organs or body sites of the same person receive different treatments), and the evaluation of treatment effect is made through comparing outcomes between paired organs or body sites of the same person (i.e., through within-person comparison). Using persons as their own controls, the inter-person variability is removed; thus, the within person trials reduce variability in treatment response and improve the efficiency of the trials, leading to the smaller sample size and improved statistical power when comparing to conventional parallel group trials.

The within person design is ideal for evaluating the efficacy of a single treatment by using one organ or body site as control. In ophthalmology, as ocular diseases are usually very symmetric, affecting both eyes of a person simultaneously (Murdoch et al. 1997), ophthalmic trials often randomize one eye to study treatment, and the other eye serves as control. For example, in the US Diabetic Retinopathy Study (The Diabetic Retinopathy Study Group 1978), one eye of each eligible participant was randomly assigned to immediate photocoagulation and the other eye to follow-up without treatment. This type of paired-eye design is commonly used when the effects of treatment are localized (such as laser treatment for diabetic retinopathy) to a single eye.

As the resources available for clinical trials are usually limited and most of trials are faced with challenges of enrolling and maintaining sufficient number of subjects over the course of the trial, the reduction in the required sample size compared with the parallel group design makes the within person trials very attractive.

The Requirements for Within Person Design

No Carry Across Effect

The most important assumption underlying the use of within person design is that the treatment effect is localized, i.e., there is no spill-over effect (also called no carry across effect) from therapy in one organ or body side to another. For example, the treatment in one tooth has no effect on another tooth, or the treatment in one eye has no effect on the fellow eye. In designing a within person trial to compare surgical treatment vs. nonsurgical treatment for periodontal disease, it is desirable to demonstrate that the sections of the mouth receiving surgical treatment are not affected by the sections receiving nonsurgical therapy and vice versa. Unless this independence can be demonstrated, the treatment effect may not be surgical compared to nonsurgical therapy but the effect of surgical treatment in a section in conjunction with nonsurgical treatment in another section, and it is not possible to obtain an unbiased, independent estimate of either treatment.

The assumption of no carry across effect may not be met for some within person trials, even when the treatment is localized to an organ/body site. For example, in the initial One-eyed Trials of the Ocular Hypertension Treatment Study, the topical β-blocker was given to the eye with higher intraocular pressure (IOP) or a randomly selected eye if both eyes had the same IOP. After 2–6 weeks topical medication in the treated eye, it was found that the contralateral fellow eye had mean (± standard deviation) IOP reduction of 1.5 ± 3.0 mm Hg, as compared to the mean reduction of 5.9 ± 3.4 mm Hg in the treated eye, suggesting the topical β-blocker has contralateral effect (Piltz et al. 2000). This carry across effect is likely due to the systemic absorption of the β-blocker primarily through the nasolacrimal mucosa, resulting in the transport of the β-blocker to the contralateral eye through the blood stream (Piltz et al. 2000).

Within Person Correlation

The measures taken from paired organs or body sites of the same person are usually correlated. The within person design takes the advantage of high within person correlation that makes the within person trial more efficient than the parallel group design. Reported correlation coefficients in ophthalmology (Katz 1988), dermatology (Van et al. 2015), and orthodontics (Pandis et al. 2014) were 0.80, 0.80, and 0.50, respectively. Balk et al. (Balk et al. 2012) calculated 811 within person correlation coefficients from 123 studies. The median within person correlation value across all studies was 0.59 (interquartile range 0.40–0.81). No heterogeneity of correlation values across outcome types and clinical domains was observed (Balk et al. 2012). In ophthalmology, a wide variety of inter-eye correlation coefficients was reported for various eye diseases and outcome measures (Ying et al. 2017a, 2018; Maguire 2020). The inter-eye correlation in refractive error can be as high as 0.90 in preschoolers but is only 0.43 in patients with neovascular age-related macular degeneration (Ying 2017). The inter-eye agreement in the referral-warranted retinopathy of prematurity was reported to be 0.80 (Ying 2017). The gain in the efficiency from the within person design is positively correlated with the magnitude of within person correlation (i.e., the higher within person correlation, the more gain in the efficiency and more reduction in the sample size compared to the parallel group design).

Trial Design Considerations

In the simplest within person trials, two interventions (one of which may be a control or standard treatment) are applied to two paired organs or body sites of a person through randomization, either concurrently or sequentially, and the outcome measures are assessed at each organ or body site. For example, in the Complications of Age-Related Prevention Trials (CAPT), designed to evaluate whether prophylactic laser treatment to the retina can prevent the incidence of the advanced-stage AMD, 1052 participants with at least 10 large drusen (>125 u) in both eyes were enrolled with 1 eye randomized for laser treatment for large drusen and the contralateral eye as control (i.e., without treatment) (The CAPT Research Group 2004). Each participant was followed-up annually for at least 5 years, to compare the incidence rates of advanced-stage AMD between treated eye and the contralateral observed eye of the same participant.

Within person randomized trials present some particular challenges. When contemplating to use within person design for a clinical trial, careful considerations should be given on issues associated with bias, efficiency, and the consequences on recruitment and statistical analysis.

Bias

One potential problem of using within subject controls is the possibility of a carry across effect. For example, an intervention applied to one eye can affect the other eye systemically (Piltz et al. 2000); treatment in an area of the mouth can affect other areas of the mouth locally (Lesaffre et al. 2009; Pandis et al. 2013); success or failure of the first replacement hip in a patient requiring bilateral hip replacement can affect the success or failure of the second hip (Lie et al. 2004).

The carry across effect has been the main concern in within person trials (Piltz et al. 2000; Lesaffre et al. 2009; Lie et al. 2004). Carry across effect can bias the estimates of treatment efficacy and tend to dilute the treatment effect. However, the exact magnitude of bias due to carry across effect is difficult to estimate (Hujoel 1998); thus, the true treatment effect from intervention cannot be accurately estimated. What we can estimate is the treatment effect contaminated with the carry across effect. If the intervention is thought to have carry across effect, randomizing individual patients to treatment groups (instead of using within subject control) is preferred.

The carry across effect is similar to the temporal carry over effect in cross-over trials, in which lingering effects of the first intervention may require adjustment for different baselines before the second intervention or the use of washout periods. A within person design is not appropriate to use if a substantial carry across effect or contamination is expected. For example, in a study of oral lichen planus (Poon et al. 2006), the topical treatments applied to each side of mouth can have serious carry across effect, so the split-mouth design should not be used. Similarly, in ophthalmology, the intravitreal injection of anti-vascular endothelial growth factor (anti-VEGF) in the study eye can carry across to the contralateral eye (Acharya et al. 2011); the paired design for evaluating the efficacy of one anti-VEGF agent through randomizing one eye to treatment and contralateral eye as control or for comparing efficacy of two anti-VEGF agents within two eyes of the same subject is not ideal.

Recruitment

Within person trials require recruitment of individuals with similar disease condition that affects paired organs or body sites of a person. However, identifying such participants sometimes can be difficult, thus endangering the recruitment. In ophthalmology, a lot of eye diseases are symmetrical, such as refractive error, age-related macular degeneration and retinopathy of prematurity (Katz 1988; Quinn et al. 1995). This may not be the case in dentistry. It may be easy to find an individual with a tooth having a cavity, but it can be challenging to find individual with two teeth having cavity of similar size, particularly in two sides of the mouth. For example, for a particular periodontal disease trial, over 1500 patients were screened to find only 12 patients with symmetric periodontal lesions eligible for the study (Smith et al. 1980). This difficulty in identifying subjects with similar disease condition could be a major obstacle for achieving the sample size required by the within person trial, even though smaller sample size is required for within person trials compared to the parallel group trials. The more strict the criterion for the similarity of disease in paired organs or body sites, the more difficult the recruitment will be. Such very selective recruitment of participants for within person trials will also hurt the generalizability of trial findings.

In addition, the requirement of within person trial for each participant to receive all interventions could potentially make some patients not willing to participate the trial. Bunce et al. reported that in ophthalmic trials, some patients had very strong opinions against enrolling both eyes into within person trials because this makes patients feel like experimental units rather than people. These patients are most comfortable with enrolling only one eye into the study even though both eyes are eligible (Bunce and Wormald 2015).

Efficiency

The within person design takes the advantage of within person correlation (ρ) in outcome measures for gaining efficiency and reducing the sample size compared to the parallel group design. Assuming all the parameters for sample size calculation are the same in within person trial and parallel group trial, the ratio between the sample size (in terms of number of subjects) for the within person trial (N_{paired}) and for the parallel group trial (N_{parallel}) can be calculated using the following formula (Wang and Bakhai 2006):

$$N_{\text{paired}}/N_{\text{parallel}} = (1 - \rho)/2 \qquad (1)$$

From Eq. (1), it is clear that the higher within person correlation, the smaller the ratio in their sample size, and the more gain in efficiency. If the within person correlation is low, the gain in efficiency can be minimal, and the within person design may not be very appropriate.

Generalizability

Within person trials require each participant having similar disease in paired organs or body sites; it is uncertain whether the within person trial results from patients with bilateral disease can be generalizable to patients with unilateral disease. Bilateral disease sometimes indicates poorer clinical status than unilateral disease. For example, diabetic neuropathy is a systemic consequence of diabetes that is considered worse if multiple limbs are affected, and the need for multiple dental implants is indicative of a worse dental condition. The tendency of higher disease severity in subjects with bilateral disease than subjects with unilateral disease makes it uncertain whether the treatment effect estimated from the within person trial is generalizable to the patients with unilateral disease.

In the Early Treatment for Retinopathy of Prematurity (ETROP) Study, 269 infants with bilateral prethreshold ROP had one eye randomly assigned to treatment with peripheral retinal ablation, and the fellow eye managed conventionally, and 70 infants with unilateral prethreshold ROP were randomized to receive treatment with either peripheral retinal ablation or managed conventionally in the single eye with prethreshold ROP. It was found that the two-year structural outcome was higher in infants with bilateral prethreshold ROP than infants with unilateral prethreshold ROP. Among infants with bilateral prethreshold ROP, the rate of unfavorable structural outcome was 10.4% in eyes treated with peripheral retinal ablation and 16.7% in eyes with conventional management ($p = 0.003$), while among infants with unilateral prethreshold ROP, the rate of unfavorable structural outcome was 0% and 3.3%, respectively ($p = 0.26$) (The ETROP Cooperative Group 2006). The ETROP Study results demonstrated that within person trial results from patients with bilateral disease may not be generalizable to patients with unilateral disease.

Other Considerations

As outlined in the CONSORT guidelines for within person trials (Pandis et al. 2017), the design of within person trial also has to consider the following questions:

- What is the eligible criteria for enrollment? The within person design needs to consider two sets of eligibility criteria including the eligibility of the individual participants and the eligibility of organ (eyes) or body sites. For example, to be eligible for the CAPT study, participants had to be at least 50 years of age and free of conditions likely to preclude 5 years of follow-up (person level eligibility), each eye had to have presence of 10 or more drusen at least 125 u in diameter within 2 disc diameters of the fovea, and the standardized visual acuity had to be 20/40 or better in each eye (eye level eligibility) (The CAPT Research Group 2004).
- What is the outcome of the within person trial? The outcome of the within person trial should be specific to the organ or body site. Within person design is not appropriate for trial with outcome assessment at person level. For example, in the Dry Eye Assessment and Management (DREAM) Study (The DREAM Investigator Group 2018), although the dry eye disease is mostly bilateral (>90% participants have both eyes met the enrollment criteria), because the treatment is systematic and the outcome measure of the dry eye symptom is the Ocular

Surface Disease Index (OSDI) which was measured at the person level, it is not appropriate to use the within person design for the DREAM Study.

- Can the assessment of outcomes for efficacy and safety be adversely impacted by the decision to treat the same patients with two different treatments?
- Are the paired organs/sites for each participant similar in terms of baseline characteristics such as location, anatomy (e.g., tooth type), and severity of disease?
- Will the treatments be administered concurrently or sequentially to the same participant? If treatments are given sequentially, will baseline information be recorded at the time of randomization or at the time of treatment administration? Similarly, if the treatment were sequential, the outcome of the first intervention could affect the outcome of the second intervention, and hence the applicability of the within person trial findings to other settings can be questionable. For example, early and late loaded implants or one hip replacement at a time can potentially influence the outcome. In some cases, however, the sequential approach is standard clinical practice, such as cataract surgery (Vasavada et al. 2012).
- How will the order of treatments and allocation to paired organs/body sites be determined (e.g., right versus left)? In within person trials, randomization is needed not only to determine which intervention is applied to which organ or body site but also to determine which organ or body site is treated first (particularly if paired organs or body sites are not treated concurrently).
- Will there be any provision to monitor whether the assigned treatment is actually applied to the correct organ or body site?
- Will the outcome evaluator be masked to the treatment assignment of each organ or body site, and if so how?
- How will the blinding of treatment assignment to organs/body sites of the same subject be operated, and will accidental unblinding of treatment of one organ affect the other organ?

Concurrent Treatment Versus Sequential Treatment

When a subject is assigned to receive two treatments in a within person trial, decision needs to be made on whether two treatments given to paired organs or body sites are concurrent or sequential. In the concurrent treatment, the two treatments are delivered at the same time or within a trivial interval following a specific or random treatment order, whereas in the sequential treatment, there is a "non-trivial" time lag between the two interventions. With concurrent treatment, loss to follow-up will automatically be the same across treatment groups, but side effects (particularly systemic adverse events) from treatments may be difficult to attribute to a specific treatment. Another concern in concurrent treatment is the possible confusion as to which organ or body site receives which treatment, particularly when there is a long treatment period. The traditional methods for monitoring compliance of treatment might be insufficient in within person trials when participants are responsible for administering the treatment (e.g., topical eye drops) by themselves.

For example, in a cataract surgery trial to determine if intraocular infusion of low-molecular-weight heparin reduces postoperative inflammation in pediatric eyes undergoing cataract surgery with intraocular lens (IOL) implantation (Vasavada et al. 2012), among 20 children (40 eyes) undergoing bilateral surgery with IOL implantation, the first eye was randomly assigned to receive enoxaparin in the intraocular infusion fluid or not to receive enoxaparin, and the second eye received alternate treatment. The eye treated first was selected by a computer-generated table of random numbers. In this trial, two eyes of a child did not undergo cataract surgeries at the same time; instead the second eye underwent cataract surgery after a gap of at least 2 weeks following surgery in the first eye, as this is the clinical practice of cataract surgery.

Cautions should be executed for designing within person trials with sequential treatments, because problems can arise from carry across effects or period effects (the effect of intervention is influenced by the period of delivery) and a baseline adjustment may be required when the baseline characteristics are believed to change between two sequential treatments. For example, in a split mouth trial for comparing two types of dental implants, baseline characteristics and outcome of the second dental implants might be influenced by the time interval between the two dental implants and the status of the first implant. If the first early loaded implant results in a poor outcome or the time interval between two dental implant operations is long, or both, the patient might rely excessively on the other side of the mouth, which might have a negative impact on the outcome of the second loaded implant. Conversely, if the outcome in the first implant is good and the burden on the second implant is small, a satisfactory outcome from the second implant can be more likely (Pandis et al. 2017).

Alternatives to the Within Subject Control Design

Clinical trials for conditions that occur in multiple organs or body sites require careful consideration of study design, because it has strong implications for patient enrollment, statistical analysis, and the presentation of results. Besides the within person design, the possible alternative designs:

- Include only one organ/site per subject either through random selection, use of organ/site with the most severe disease, or at the discretion of clinician or patient. For example, in the Complications of Age-related Macular Degeneration Treatment Trials (CATT), 1185 participants with neovascular AMD were randomized to treat with intravitreal injection of ranibizumab or bevacizumab on a monthly or PRN schedule. The trial requires each study eye to have active subfoveal choroidal neovascularization (CNV) and visual acuity of between 20/25 and 20/320. The CATT only enrolled one eye per patient into the trial. When two eyes of a participant meet the enrollment criteria, the ophthalmologist and the patients decide which eye will be enrolled (The CATT Research Group 2011).

The advantage of this design is the simplicity of design and statistical analysis of the trial data, but may lead to the loss of opportunity to efficiently collect more information.

- Randomize patients to a treatment, and treat paired organs/body sites with the same treatment. This is a clustered randomized trial in which the clusters are individual patients. For example: In a multi-center randomized clinical trial to evaluate the efficacy of intravitreal injection of bevacizumab for stage 3+ ROP, 150 infants with stage 3+ ROP were randomized to receive intravitreal bevacizumab or conventional laser therapy in both eyes (ref: Mintz-Hittner et al. 2011).
- Mixture of participants with unilateral and bilateral disease. Although many diseases occur in paired organs or multiple body sites, the extent and severity of disease may not be the same. The within person design that requires similar disease condition in paired organs or body sites may significantly limit the recruitment potential and also make the results not easily generalizable to the patients with unilateral disease. In ophthalmology, some trials use hybrid design which allows both eyes to be randomized if both eyes are eligible and allows one eye to be randomized if only one eye is eligible (Lee et al. 2012; The ETROP Cooperative Group 2006; Elman et al. 2010). For example, the ETROP enrolled infants with prethreshold ROP in both eyes and also infants with prethreshold ROP in one eye only. For infants with bilateral prethreshold ROP, one eye was randomized to treatment, and the other (the control eye) was managed conventionally. For infants with unilateral prethreshold ROP, a separate randomization scheme assigned such infants to either treatment or conventional management (The ETROP Cooperative Group 2006). The Diabetic Retinopathy Clinical Research Network also used this hybrid design in several large clinical trials, as the hybrid approach can lead to faster recruitment and reduced costs considering the overall number of participants (Glassman and Melia 2015). In the Diabetic Retinopathy Clinical Research Network Protocol I (Diabetic Retinopathy Clinical Research Network, 2010), patients with one or two eligible eyes enrolled to compare four treatments for diabetic macular edema including (A) prompt laser ($N = 293$ eyes); (B) 0.5 mg ranibizumab + prompt laser ($N = 187$ eyes); (C) 0.5 mg ranibizumab + deferred laser ($N = 188$ eyes); and (D) 4 mg triamcinolone + prompt laser ($N = 186$ eyes). For 528 patients with only 1 eye eligible, they were randomized to 4 treatment groups with equal probability, while for 163 patients having both eyes eligible, the right eye was randomized to 1 of the 4 treatment groups and the left eye assigned to group A if right eye was not in group A, and the left eye was randomized to 1 of the 3 remaining treatments with equal probability if the right eye was in group A. Such hybrid design can complicate the statistical analysis for the trial data, because statistical analysis for the bilateral cases needs to adjust for the inter-eye correlation. Consistency of treatment effect among bilateral patients and unilateral patients should be checked before the assessment of overall treatment effect by combining the results from these unilateral cases and bilateral cases (The ETROP Cooperative Group 2006).

Power and Sample Size

The sample size calculation for within person trials requires an estimate of within person correlation for the primary outcome measure. This correlation estimate can be obtained from the previous studies. If such data is not available in practice, the sample size/power can be calculated assuming various degree of within person correlation (e.g., moderate correlation with correlation coefficient of 0.50 or high correlation with correlation of 0.75 etc.) to see how sensitive the sample size calculation is to assumption for the within person correlation coefficient. However, such within person correlation should not be ignored in sample size calculation, because ignoring within person correlation will result in an over-estimation of the sample size. The degree of over-estimate of sample size is dependent on the within person correlation as demonstrated in Eq. (1). The higher the within person correlation, the more over-estimation of sample size. It is a common mistake that most within person trials do not take into account the within person correlation in the calculation of sample size or statistical power (Lee et al. 2012; Lesaffre et al. 2007; Lai et al. 2007; Bryant et al. 2006).

Besides the assumption for the within person correlation, assumptions need to be made for other parameters including the expected mean and variance (σ^2) or standard deviation (SD) of continuous outcome measure and the expected event rate for binary outcome for each treatment group, the type 1 error rate (α), and the desired statistical power (1-β).

Sample Size for Continuous Outcome

Assuming for a two-arm within person trial, the expected mean is u_A for treatment A and u_B for treatment B, and their variances are the same σ^2. Their mean difference in outcome measure is $d = u_A - u_B$.

If SD for the within person difference (d) between treatment groups for the primary continuous outcome measure is available, the sample size can be calculated without need of assuming the within person correlation coefficient (ρ). However, if such data are not available, the within person correlation has to be assumed for calculating the SD of the within person difference d.

For the given within person correlation ρ, the variance for the within person difference d can be calculated as

$$\sigma_d^2 = 2\,(1-\rho)\,\sigma^2 \tag{2}$$

The required sample size N (i.e., total number subjects needed) for detecting mean difference of d in primary outcome measure with statistical power of 1-β and type I error rate of α is as follows:

$$N = \frac{\sigma_d^2\left(Z_{1-\alpha/2} + Z_{1-\beta}\right)^2}{d^2} + \frac{Z^2{}_{1-\alpha/2}}{2} \tag{3}$$

Example: A within person trial is designed with one eye randomly assigned to treatment *A* and the contralateral fellow eye assigned to treatment *B*. The primary outcome is visual acuity score (calculated as number of letters read correctly from the visual acuity chart) at one year after treatment. It is desirable to know how many patients need to be enrolled to provide 90% power for detecting five-letter difference in visual acuity score between two treatment groups at 5% type I error rate. Previous studies suggest the SD of the visual acuity score is approximately 14 letters in each treatment group.

Assuming moderate inter-eye correlation with ρ of 0.50, the variance for the mean visual acuity difference between two treatment groups calculated using Eq. (2) is $2 \times (1 - 0.50) \times 14^2 = 196$. The sample size can be calculated using Eq. (3) as:

$$N = \frac{\sigma_d^2 \left(Z_{1-\alpha/2} + Z_{1-\beta}\right)^2}{d^2} + \frac{Z^2{}_{1-\alpha/2}}{2} = \frac{196(1.96 + 1.28)^2}{25} + \frac{1.96^2}{2} = 84 \quad (4)$$

So a total of 84 patients (168 eyes) need to be enrolled. If the parallel group design is used with 1 eye per patient randomized to either treatment A or treatment B, a total of 332 patients (332 eyes) is needed to achieve the same statistical power as within person design.

To demonstrate the impact of inter-eye correlation on sample size, the sample size at various inter-eye correlations ranging from 0 to 0.9 calculated using equations (Balk et al., 2012; Bryant et al., 2006) is provided in Table 1. When comparing sample size of 332 eyes from 332 patients for the parallel group design to achieve the same statistical power as within person design, Table 1 clearly demonstrates that the gain in the efficiency from within person trial leads to the reduced sample size and the magnitude of gain in efficiency is dependent on the within person correlation, with the higher the inter-eye correlation, the smaller the sample size. For example, when the inter-eye correlation is 0.5, the percent of reduction in sample size is 75% in terms of number of patients and 50% in terms of number of eyes.

Sample Size for Binary Outcome

For a two-arm within person trial with binary outcome (e.g., treatment success or failure), the 2 × 2 table (Table 2) can be laid out to estimate the parameters needed for the sample size calculation.

The odds ratio for success between treatment *B* relative to treatment *A* is calculated as

$$\Psi = \mathrm{b}/\mathrm{c}. \quad (5)$$

The discordant proportion in response between treatment *A* and treatment *B* is calculated as

$$\pi_{\mathrm{discordant}} = (\mathrm{b} + \mathrm{c})/\mathrm{N}. \quad (6)$$

Table 1 Comparison of the sample size using within person design and parallel group design[a] under various inter-eye correlation for an ophthalmology trial

Within person correlation (ρ)	Sample size from within person trial: Number of subjects (number of eyes)[b]	% Reduction in number of subjects comparing to parallel group design[a]	% Reduction in number of eyes comparing to parallel group design[a]
0.0	166 (332)	50%	0%
0.1	150 (300)	55%	10%
0.2	134 (268)	60%	20%
0.3	117 (234)	65%	30%
0.4	101 (202)	70%	40%
0.5	84 (168)	75%	50%
0.6	68 (136)	80%	60%
0.7	51 (102)	85%	70%
0.8	35 (70)	90%	80%
0.9	18 (36)	95%	90%

[a]The parallel group design requires a total of 332 patients (332 eyes) assuming standard deviation of 14 letters, 90% power to detect mean difference of 5 letters in visual acuity between treatment A and B at type I error rate of 0.05

[b]Assume the standard deviation of 14 letters, 90% power to detect mean difference of 5 letters in visual acuity between treatment *A* and *B* at type I error rate of 0.05

Table 2 The 2 × 2 table for the comparison of paired binary outcome from within person trial with N participants

	Treatment *B*			
Treatment *A*	Failure	Success	Total	Anticipated proportions
Failure	a	b	a + b	$1 - \pi_A$
Success	c	d	c + d	π_A
Total	a + c	b + d	N = a + b + c + d	
Anticipated proportions	$1 - \pi_B$	π_B		

For the within person design, the number of subjects needed (N) with two-sided type I error rate (α) and power ($1\text{-}\beta$) can be calculated using the following formula:

$$N = \frac{\left(Z_{1-\alpha/2}(\psi+1) + Z_{1-\beta}\sqrt{\left[(\psi+1)^2 - (\psi-1)^2\pi_{\text{discordant}}\right]}\right)^2}{(\psi-1)^2\pi_{\text{discordant}}} \quad (7)$$

In order to calculate the sample size N using Eq. (7), assumptions about the expected odds ratio Ψ and the discordant percentage $\pi_{\text{discordant}}$ need to be made. If the information on Ψ and the $\pi_{\text{discordant}}$ are not available, the Ψ and the $\pi_{\text{discordant}}$ can be estimated based on anticipated treatment response rate π_A and π_B as follows:

Table 3 The pilot data from a hypothetical within person trial

	New early treatment	
Conventional treatment	Unfavorable vision	Favorable vision
Unfavorable vision	3	9
Favorable vision	6	12

$$\psi = \frac{\pi_A(1 - \pi_B)}{\pi_B(1 - \pi_A)} \tag{8}$$

$$\pi_{\text{discordant}} = \pi_A(1 - \pi_B) + \pi_B(1 - \pi_A). \tag{9}$$

Example: Suppose a large within person trial similar to the Early Treatment of Retinopathy of Prematurity (ETROP) (Good and Hardy 2001) will be designed to test the hypothesis that earlier treatment in selected high-risk cases of acute ROP results in better visual outcomes than conventional ROP management. The pilot study in 30 infants with bilateral ROP provided the following data (Table 3):

Based on this pilot data, the large multi-center within person trial is designed to provide 90% power for detecting odds ratio of $\Psi = 9/6 = 1.5$ at type I error rate of 0.05.

From the pilot data, the $\pi_{\text{discordant}} = (9 + 6)/30 = 0.5$.

Using Eq. (7), the sample size can be determined:

$$N = \frac{\left(1.96 \times (1.5 + 1) + 1.28 \times \sqrt{\left[(1.5 + 1)^2 - (1.5 - 1)^2 \times 0.5\right]}\right)^2}{(1.5 - 1)^2 \times 0.5} = 521 \tag{10}$$

So 521 infants with bilateral ROP (1042 eyes) need to be enrolled with 1 eye treated using new treatment and the fellow eye using conventional treatment.

Statistical Analysis

One of the major features of the within person trials is that comparisons of outcomes are made through within person comparison. Because outcome measures from paired organs or body sites of the same person are correlated, the appropriate statistical analysis should account for the correlation among measures from the same person. The common mistake in analysis of data from within person trials is the lack of adjustment for the within person correlation in statistical comparisons of trial outcomes, leading to the invalid conclusions (Murdoch et al. 1997; Pandis et al. 2017; Zhang and Ying 2018).

For the within person trial involving two treatments in two paired organs/body sites of each participants, the statistical methods for analyzing trial outcomes measured at the end of the trial are usually very standard, such as paired t-test for comparison of continuous outcome and McNemar test for comparison of binary outcome. Similar to the other trials, the statistical analyses of data from within person trial need to consider loss to follow-up or deal with missing data, which can occur in both organs/sites in each participant (e.g., due to missed follow-up visit) or just at a single organ/site (e.g., due to poor image quality in one eye). In within person trials with concurrent interventions, the losses to follow-up are usually equal between treatment groups, thus unlikely bias the estimate of treatment effect due to missing data from lost to follow-up, but will decrease the statistical power and limit the generalization of the trial results.

One advantage of within person trials is the elimination of confounding from person-level baseline covariates, because these person-level baseline characteristics are balanced across treatment groups. Statistical analysis and interpretation of results for treatment effect don't need to worry about the person-level confounders. However, the imbalance in the organ-specific or site-specific variables can still occur; thus, statistical analysis for comparing outcomes between treatment groups needs to account for imbalance in baseline variables at organ/site level by using the mixed effects models or marginal models (Laird and Ware 1982; Liang and Zeger 1986; Ying et al. 2017, 2018).

Analysis of Continuous Outcome Measures

For within person trials with n participants and each participant received two treatments (A and B), the outcome measure in individual i is y_i^A and y_i^B for organ/site in treatment A and treatment B, respectively. The within person difference (d) in continuous outcome measure between treatments A and B can be calculated as:

$$d_i = y_i^A - y_i^B \tag{11}$$

The mean, standard deviation (SD), and standard error (SE) for the difference between treatments A and B are

$$\overline{d} = \sum_{i=1}^{n} \frac{d_i}{n} = \overline{y_A} - \overline{y_B} \tag{12}$$

$$SD(d) = \sum_{i=i}^{n} \frac{\left(d_i - \overline{d}\right)^2}{(n-1)} \tag{13}$$

$$SE\left(\overline{d}\right) = \frac{SD(d)}{\sqrt{n}} \tag{14}$$

The corresponding paired t-test statistic for comparing continuous outcome between treatment A and B is

$$t = \frac{\overline{d}}{SE\left(\overline{d}\right)} \tag{15}$$

which follows t-distribution with degree of freedom of n-1.

If the distribution outcome measure is very skewed, nonparametric test can be used for the comparison between treatment groups using Wilcoxon signed rank test or sign test.

If the baseline covariates (at organ or body site level) need to be accounted for in the comparison of outcome between treatment groups, the model-based analysis needs to be used. However, such statistical model should account for the within person correlation by using either the mixed effects model or marginal model (Laird and Ware 1982; Liang and Zeger 1986; Ying et al. 2017a, 2018). When performing the model-based analysis for within person trials, the correlation structure for the within person correlation needs to be specified. The mis-specification of correlation can potentially impact the model results. However, in within person trials of ophthalmology (with unique feature of cluster size of 2 due to two eyes of each subject), the analyses using various specifications of correlation structure (unstructured, compound symmetry, or working correlation) provide very similar results (Ying et al. 2017, 2018).

Example: The data in Table 4 are from the 11 participants of the Choroidal Neovascularization Prevention Trial (CNVPT) (The CNVPT Research Group 1998) with equal visual acuity in their paired eyes at baseline. The primary outcome of the CNVPT is visual acuity score measured at the end of 4-year follow-up. In the CNVPT, one eye of each participant was randomized to laser treatment for drusen, and the fellow eye was observed without treatment as control. The calculation using Eqs. (11, 12, 13, 14) provided mean difference of 0.90 letters, with SD of 12.3 letters and SE of 3.7 letters. The paired t-test provided $t = 0.90/3.7 = 0.24$ with degree of freedom of 10. The two-sided p-value from paired t-test is 0.81. If nonparametric test is applied, the Wilcoxon signed rank test provided p-value of 0.85.

Statistical Comparison of Binary Outcome

When the outcome measure of the within person trial is binary (yes/no), it is not appropriate to use the standard chi-square test because it ignores the within person correlations. Instead, the McNemar test should be applied for the comparison of proportions.

A presentation using 2×2 paired tabulation format as Table 2 is desirable, as it provides the counts of concordant and discordant pairs.

Table 4 Visual acuity from 11 participants of the CNVPT

	Visual acuity score (in letters) at 4 years		
Patient ID	Laser-treated eye	Untreated eye	Difference (treated eye – untreated eye)
1	78	54	24
2	68	70	−2
3	84	83	1
4	77	77	0
5	81	82	−1
6	86	77	9
7	44	60	−16
8	63	84	−21
9	81	82	−1
10	86	76	10
11	90	83	7
Mean	76.2	75.3	0.90
SD	13.3	10.0	12.3
SE	4.0	3.0	3.7

The proportion difference for binary outcome is:

$$\Delta = \frac{b+d}{N} - \frac{c+d}{N} = \frac{b-c}{N} \tag{16}$$

Under the null hypothesis that there is no difference between treatment groups, the b and c are expected to be equal given there are a total of $b + c$ discordant pairs. When b or c is small (<5), the continuous correction is often applied using the formula:

$$\chi^2 = \frac{(|b-c|-1)^2}{b+c} \tag{17}$$

In large samples, the McNemar test is

$$\chi^2 = \frac{(b-c)^2}{b+c} \tag{18}$$

The degree of freedom for McNemar test is 1.

Example: In the CAPT Study (The CAPT Research Group 2004) designed to evaluate whether prophylactic laser treatment to the retina can prevent the development of the advanced-stage AMD, one of the analyses for the primary outcome is to compare the incidence rate of geographic atrophy (GA) between treated eye and control eye of the same participant at 4-year follow-up. The cross-tabulation for the incidence of GA among 997 participants who completed the 4-year follow-up is as follows:

	Control eye		
Laser-treated eye	No GA	GA	Total
No GA	892	32	924 (92.7%)
GA	29	44	73 (7.3%)
Total	921	76	997

The McNemar test for comparing the GA incidence rate between treated eye and untreated control eye is:

$$\chi^2 = \frac{(29 - 32)^2}{29 + 32} = 0.1475$$

with degree of freedom of 1, and the corresponding two-sided p-value is 0.70.

Summary and Conclusion

For diseases that affect paired organs or two body sites, the treatment can be either systemic or organ-specific. When treatment and outcome measure are specific to the organ or body site, within person design may be applied to improve the efficiency of the trial. Such design has been commonly used in in ophthalmology, dentistry, and dermatology. When the within person correlation is high in outcome measure, such design can substantially reduce the sample size. However, careful considerations need to be given on the possibility of carry across effect, the feasibility of recruiting sufficient patients with bilateral disease, and the limitation in the generalization of trial results to patients with unilateral disease. The sample size and statistical analysis also have to account for the within person correlation in outcome measures.

Key Facts

- The within-person design is efficient because comparisons are made within the same person.
- When within-person correlation for outcome measure is high, within-person design can substantially reduce the sample size.
- Within-person clinical trials are often used for conditions that affect paired organs or multiple body sites of a person, such as in ophthalmology, dentistry, and dermatology.
- Within-person trials pose some challenges including the possible bias from the carry across effect, the difficulty in recruitment subjects with condition affecting paired organs or multiple body sites.
- Within-person correlation should be taken into consideration in the sample size determination and statistical analyses.

References

Acharya NR, Sittivarakul W, Qian Y et al (2011) Bilateral effect of unilateral ranibizumab in patients with uveitis-related macular edema. Retina 31:1871–1876

Balk EM, Earley A, Patel K, Trikalinos TA, Dahabreh IJ (2012) Empirical assessment of within-arm correlation imputation in trials of continuous outcomes. Methods Research Report. (Prepared by the Tufts Evidence-based Practice Center under Contract No. 290-2007-10055-I.) AHRQ Publication No. 12(13)-EHC141-EF. Agency for Healthcare Research and Quality, Rockville

Bryant D, Havey TC, Roberts R, Guyatt G (2006) How many patients? How many limbs? Analysis of patients or limbs in the orthopaedic literature: a systematic review. J Bone Joint Surg Am 88: 41–45

Bunce C, Wormald R (2015) Considerations for randomizing 1 eye or 2 eyes. JAMA Ophthalmol 133:1221

Cairo F, Sanz I, Matesanz P, Nieri M, Pagliaro U (2012) Quality of reporting of randomized clinical trials in implant dentistry. A systematic review on critical aspects in design, outcome assessment and clinical relevance. J Clin Periodontol 39:81–107

Diabetic Retinopathy Clinical Research Network (2010) Randomized trial evaluating Ranibizumab plus prompt or deferred laser or triamcinolone plus prompt laser for diabetic macular edema. Ophthalmology 117:1064–1077

Elman MJ, Aiello LP, Beck RW et al (2010) Diabetic retinopathy clinical research network. Randomized trial evaluating ranibizumab plus prompt or deferred laser or triamcinolone plus prompt laser for diabetic macular edema. Ophthalmology 117:1064–1077, e35

Glassman AR, Melia M (2015) Randomizing 1 eye or 2 eyes: a missed opportunity. JAMA Ophthalmol 133:9–10

Good WV, Hardy RJ (2001) The multicenter study of early treatment for retinopathy of prematurity (ETROP). Ophthalmology 108:1013–1014

Hujoel PP (1998) Design and analysis issues in split mouth clinical trials. Community Dent Oral Epidemiol 26:85–86

Katz J (1988) Two eyes or one? The data analyst's dilemma. Ophthalmic Surg 19:585–589

Koletsi D, Fleming PS, Seehra J, Bagos PG, Pandis N (2014) Are sample sizes clear and justified in RCTs published in dental journals? PLoS One 9:e85949

Lai TYY, Wong VWY, Lam RF, Cheng AC, Lam DS, Leung GM (2007) Quality of reporting of key methodological items of randomized controlled trials in clinical ophthalmic journals. Ophthalmic Epidemiol 14:390–398

Laird NM, Ware JH (1982) Random-effects models for longitudinal data. Biometrics 38:963–974

Lee CF, Cheng AC, Fong DY (2012) Eyes or subjects: are ophthalmic randomized controlled trials properly designed and analyzed? Ophthalmology 119:869–872

Lesaffre E, Garcia Zattera M-J, Redmond C, Huber H, Needleman I, ISCB Subcommittee on Dentistry (2007) Reported methodological quality of split-mouth studies. J Clin Periodontol 34: 756–761

Lesaffre E, Philstrom B, Needleman I, Worthington H (2009) The design and analysis of split-mouth studies: what statisticians and clinicians should know. Stat Med 28:3470–3482

Liang KY, Zeger SL (1986) Longitudinal data analysis using generalized linear models. Biometrika 73:13–22

Lie SA, Engesaeter LB, Havelin LI, Gjessing HK, Vollset SE (2004) Dependency issues in survival analyses of 55,782 primary hip replacements from 47,355 patients. Stat Med 23:3227–3240. https://doi.org/10.1002/sim.1905

Machin D, Fayers PM (eds) (2010) Randomized clinical trials. Wiley-Blackwell, West Sussex

Maguire MG (2020) Assessing Intereye symmetry and its implications for study design. Invest Ophthalmol Vis Sci 61:27

Mintz-Hittner HA, Kennedy KA, Chuang AZ for BEAT-ROP Cooperative Group (2011) Efficacy of intravitreal bevacizumab for stage 3+ retinopathy of prematurity. N Engl J Med 364:603–615

Murdoch IE, Morris SS, Cousens SN (1997) People and eyes: statistical approaches in ophthalmology. Br J Ophthalmol 82:971–973

Pandis N, Walsh T, Polychronopoulou A, Katsaros C, Eliades T (2013) Split-mouth designs in orthodontics: an overview with applications to orthodontic clinical trials. Eur J Orthod 35:783–789
Pandis N, Fleming PS, Spineli LM, Salanti G (2014) Initial orthodontic alignment effectiveness with self-ligating and conventional appliances: a network meta-analysis in practice. Am J Orthod Dentofac Orthop 145(Suppl):S152–S163
Pandis N, Chung B, Scherer RW, Elbourne D, Altman DG (2017) CONSORT 2010 statement: extension checklist for reporting within person randomized trials. BMJ 357:j2835
Paré A (1575) The James Lind Library. http://www.jameslindlibrary.org/pare-a-1575. Accessed 15 Mar 2019
Piltz J, Gross R, Shin DH et al (2000) Contralateral effect of topical beta-adrenergic antagonists in initial one-eyed trials in the ocular hypertension treatment study. Am J Ophthalmol 130:441–453
Poon CY, Goh BT, Kim MJ, Rajaseharan A, Ahmed S, Thongsprasom K, Chaimusik M, Suresh S, Machin D, Wong HB, Seldrup (2006) A randomized control trial to compare steroid with cyclosporine for the topical treatment of ordal lichen planus. Oral Surg Oral Med Oral Pathol Oral Radiol Endod 102:47–55
Quinn GE, Dobson V, Biglan A et al (1995) Correlation of retinopathy of prematurity in fellow eyes in the cryotherapy for retinopathy of prematurity study. The Cryotherapy for Retinopathy of Prematurity Cooperative Group. Arch Ophthalmol 113:469–473
Smith DH, Ammons WF, Van Belle G (1980) A longitudinal study of periodontal status comparing osseous recontouring with flap curettage. J Periodontol 51:367–375
The Age-Related Eye Disease Study Research Group (1999) The age-related eye disease study (AREDS): design implications AREDS report no. 1. Control Clin Trials 20:573–600
The Choroidal Neovascularization Prevention Trial (CNVPT) Research Group (1998) Choroidal neovascularization in the choroidal neovascularization prevention trial. Ophthalmology 105: 1364–1372
The Comparisons of Age-Related Macular Degeneration Treatment Trials (CATT) Research Group (2011) Ranibizumab and bevacizumab for neovascular age-related macular degeneration. N Engl J Med 364:1897–1908
The Complication of Age-Related Macular Degeneration Prevention Trial (CAPT) Research Group (2004) The complications of age-related macular degeneration prevention trial (CAPT): rationale, design and methodology. Clin Trials 1:91–107
The Diabetic Retinopathy Study Research Group (1978) Photocoagulation treatment of proliferative diabetic retinopathy: the second report from the diabetic retinopathy study. Arch Ophthalmol 85:82–106
The Dry Eye Assessment and Management Study (DREAM) Research Group (2018) N-3 fatty acid supplementation and dry eye disease. N Engl J Med 378:1681–1690
The Early Treatment for Retinopathy of Prematurity (ETROP) Cooperative Group (2006) The early treatment for retinopathy of prematurity study: structural findings at age 2 years. Br J Ophthalmol 90:1378–1382
van Zuuren EJ, Fedorowicz Z, Carter B, Pandis N (2015) Interventions for hirsutism (excluding laser and photoepilation therapy alone). Cochrane Database Syst Rev 4:CD010334
Vasavada VA, Praveen MR, Shah SK, Trivedi RH, Vasavada AR (2012) Anti-inflammatory effect of low-molecular-weight heparin in pediatric cataract surgery: a randomized clinical trial. Am J Ophthalmol 154:252–258.e4
Wang D, Bakhai A (2006) Chapter 10, clinical trials in practice. A practical guide to design, analysis and reporting. Remedica, London
Ying GS, Maguire MG, Glynn R, Rosner B (2017a) Tutorial on biostatistics: linear regression analysis of continuous correlated eye data. Ophthalmic Epidemiol 24:130–140
Ying GS, Pan W, Quinn GE et al (2017b) Inter-eye agreement of retinopathy of prematurity from image evaluation in the telemedicine approaches to evaluating acute-phase ROP (e-ROP) study. Ophthalmol Retina 1:347–354
Ying GS, Maguire MG, Glynn R et al (2018) Tutorial on biostatistics: statistical analysis for correlated binary eye data. Ophthalmic Epidemiol 25:1–12
Zhang HG, Ying GS (2018) Statistical approaches in published ophthalmic clinical science papers: a comparison to statistical practice two decades ago. Br J Ophthalmol 102:1188–1191

Device Trials

73

Heng Li, Pamela E. Scott, and Lilly Q. Yue

Contents

H. Li (✉) · L. Q. Yue
Center for Devices and Radiological Health, U.S. Food and Drug Administration, Silver Spring, MD, USA
e-mail: heng.li@fda.hhs.gov; lilly.yue@fda.hhs.gov

P. E. Scott
Office of the Commissioner, U.S. Food and Drug Administration, Silver Spring, MD, USA

© Springer Nature Switzerland AG 2022

S. Piantadosi, C. L. Meinert (eds.), *Principles and Practice of Clinical Trials*,
https://doi.org/10.1007/978-3-319-52636-2_102

Abstract

This section provides an overview of clinical studies for medical devices. Important differences between drugs and devices are highlighted. Specific topics covered include Bayesian design and observational (nonrandomized) studies. Special considerations are given to diagnostic devices.

Keywords

Medical device · FDA · Diagnostic device · Bayesian · Nonrandomized · Propensity score

Introduction

What is a medical device? A medical device is defined by law as "*an instrument, apparatus, implement, machine, contrivance, implant, in vitro reagent, or other similar or related article, including any component, part, or accessory, which is (1) recognized in the official National Formulary, or the United States Pharmacopoeia, or any supplement to them, (2) intended for use in the diagnosis of disease or other conditions, or in the cure, mitigation, treatment, or prevention of disease in man or other animals, or (3) intended to affect the structure or any function of the body of man or other animals, and which does not achieve its primary intended purposes through chemical action within or on the body of man or other animals and which is not dependent upon being metabolized for the achievement of any of its principal intended purposes*" – [US Code, Food, Drug, and Cosmetic Act; 21 US Code 321 (h)].

A simpler definition for medical device is a definition by exclusion. A medical device is a medical product that does not have a chemical, metabolic, or biological principle of action. As such, a medical device is any medical product that is not a drug or biological product.

Medical devices range in complexity from simple products such as bedpans and tongue depressors to complex products such as heart pacemakers and laser surgical devices. The term also applies to in vitro diagnostic products and test kits for diseases, conditions, or infections such as home test kits for HIV. Electronic radiating products with medical usage and claims such as x-ray machines also meet the definition of medical devices. Certain software may be a medical device (US FDA 2016).

Drugs Versus Devices

Mechanism of Action

Medical devices do not function in the same manner as drugs. The mechanism of action of a medical device is physical and localized, whereas the mechanism of action for drugs is often chemical or biological and the effect can be localized or systemic. The process of drug development is one of discovery. Drug discovery involves the screening of candidate compounds to identify those promising enough for development, further examination, and testing in animals and humans. Once a drug is discovered, the chemical composition remains unchanged during the entire development process. Although the dose, indications for use, dosing regimen, preparation, and release of the drug can change, the chemical entity remains the same. In contrast to drugs, devices are invented and often evolve through a series of changes and improvements (Campbell and Yue 2016) during the course of development and evaluation. As a result, the device that is marketed may be different from the one that underwent testing. While any change to drug formulation may impact the safety and effectiveness profile of the drug, minor device changes may have little effect on the clinical performance or safety and effectiveness profile of the product.

Safety and Efficacy/Effectiveness Assessment

Clinical studies for medical devices are often preceded by bench/mechanical and animal testing for reliability and biocompatibility. The premarket clinical testing of investigational drugs is generally conducted in three stages or phases (I, II, and III). Phase I trials are early development trials conducted in a small number of people (e.g., 20–100) to evaluate safety issues such as adverse events and maximum tolerated dose of the drug. If this early development study demonstrates that the drug is not toxic, then clinical testing progresses to Phase II. During this middle development stage, the drug is given to up to several hundred people with the indicated condition to evaluate short-term safety and efficacy. After demonstration of short-term safety and efficacy, the comparative treatment efficacy trial (Phase III) is conducted in large numbers of people to demonstrate safety and efficacy. Typically, two Phase III trials are needed in order to market a drug.

The clinical testing of devices is generally characterized by the conduct of a feasibility (pilot) study and a pivotal study (an analog of Phase III drug trial). Pilot studies for medical devices may include only one investigator at one investigational site with a small number of patients. The main focus of those studies is on safety issues. Pilot studies are also used to obtain preliminary data to assess the learning curve for device use, to generate estimates of effect sizes and variances for sample size calculation, and to develop and refine study procedures for the pivotal trial. Generally, one pivotal study is conducted to obtain data to evaluate safety and effectiveness of devices prior to entry into the consumer marketplace. Both drugs and medical devices have post-market studies referred to as Phase IV for drugs and post-market studies for devices.

The standard for pharmaceutical drug regulation is one of substantial evidence of safety and effectiveness obtained from well-controlled investigations (21 CFR 314.126), which historically have been well-controlled Phase III trials. The statutory standard for approval and level of evidence required for devices is one of *reasonable assurance of safety and effectiveness based on valid scientific evidence*. Valid scientific evidence (21 CFR 860.7(c)(2)) is defined as "*well-controlled investigations, partially controlled studies, studies and objective trials without matched controls, well-documented case histories conducted by qualified experts, and reports of significant human experience with a marketed device*" (21 CFR 860.7). The type of study required is very device specific. It may vary depending on the indication for use and degree of experience with knowledge of the device. A reasonable assurance of safety is obtained when "it can be determined, based upon valid scientific evidence, that the probable benefits outweigh any probable risks," and can be demonstrated by establishing "the absence of unreasonable risk of illness or injury associated with the use of the device for its intended uses and conditions of use" (21 CFR 860.7(d)(1)). Similarly, a reasonable assurance of effectiveness is obtained when "it can be determined, based upon valid scientific evidence the use of the device for its intended uses will provide clinically significant results" (21 CFR 860.7(e)(1)). These criteria differ from the regulatory standards set by law for drugs and biological products in the USA, and these differences lead to a more varied approach in the studies and data required to support market approval/clearance for devices.

Skill of the User

For drugs, the influence of the physician technique or skill is very low on treatment outcome. Drugs are dispensed with instructions to the patient for medical use. It is the responsibility of the patient or caregiver to comply with these instructions. As such, the training for drug trials focuses on the protocol requirement, mechanism of action of the drug, and potential adverse effects. In contrast, for medical devices, the skill of physician or device user may play a significant role in the treatment outcome. For example, the success of the device for implants and other devices that rely on surgical technique may depend on the skill of the surgeon. The potential learning curve on the part of the surgeon may have a major impact on the performance of the product during the clinical study. The impact of the skill of the user can also be seen in diagnostic trials such as diagnostic imaging devices that rely on skilled radiologists to read and interpret the images. Consequently, training requirements for device clinical trials should include hands-on device training in addition to the protocol requirements. Studies in which patients are treated with a medical device often assess the contribution of the device user in addition to assessing contributions from the device, disease, and patient.

Implants

Since a drug is metabolized, stopping the medication often addresses many adverse effects. Devices that are implanted into the body pose a number of unique challenges. Many implantable devices cannot be easily removed once implanted in the body. Consequently, the risk of removing the implant need to be weighed against that of the device remaining in the body.

Placebo Effect and Sham Control

The use of placebo control arm is common in drug clinical trials. However, in device clinical trials it is often impractical or unethical to use a placebo (or sham) control and withhold treatment, especially when considerable risk may be associated with the sham surgery.

Blinding or Masking

Often it is not possible to blind (or mask) the treatment or implant the patient is receiving or health care provider is delivering in medical device clinical trials. Although it is possible to correctly guess the treatment in drug trials, it is more likely to correctly guess the treatment in device trials especially when the procedures reveal treatment information.

Design Considerations for Therapeutic Device Trials

Like drugs, therapeutic devices are used to treat diseases. However, due to the distinctions between drugs and devices highlighted in the previous section, certain design considerations may figure more prominently for device trials. In this section we discuss some of such considerations. The focus is on pivotal device trials. These trials are intended as the primary clinical support for a marketing application, just as Phase III drug trials.

Control Group

Medical devices may be invented for a range of purposes, from providing a therapy that is superior to those currently available to offering a less invasive treatment option for surgery. The choice of control group should reflect this purpose. Sometimes a device is meant to do both: serve as a more effective therapy than drugs for patients too frail to undergo surgery and as a less invasive option for surgery for patients who are less frail. If that is the case, then there need to be two separate trials, one with medical therapy as control and the other with surgery as control (Svensson et al. 2013). When a trial compares two different treatment modalities, patients and physicians/surgeons are impossible to blind, and therefore artifacts such as placebo effect is difficult to rule out. In such a trial the use of objective endpoints (e.g., death, stroke, etc.) as primary would be advisable.

For a trial conducted to evaluate subjective endpoints such as pain or function, one may consider using a so-called sham control when it is ethical and practical to do so. A sham control has been broadly defined as a treatment or procedure that is similar with but omits a key therapeutic element of the treatment or procedure under investigation. The riskier the sham control, the less likely it will be considered ethical. A very risky sham control that is completely without benefit is seldom justifiable. Of course, such judgment depends on the context. A recent example of a sham-controlled device trial is the ORBITA study (Al-Lamee et al. 2018). The therapy under investigation is percutaneous coronary intervention (PCI), the target population is patients with stable chronic angina, and the endpoint is the exercise time. Previously, a randomized trial of PCI (a device therapy) versus medical management had found benefit on exercise tolerance (Parisi et al. 1992). The ORBITA trial suggests that most of this apparent benefit is placebo effect, which prompts the medical community to seriously question an accepted practice.

While clinical trials for first-of-a-kind devices often use medical therapy or surgery as controls, later devices with similar indications may use other devices as control. Such trials are often noninferiority trials. Sometimes the control can even be designated as any device of the same indication that is commercially available, allowing noninferiority claim to be made to an entire class of devices.

In certain device areas randomized trials with patients as their own control are conducted. Here we are not talking about crossover trials: the treatments being compared are not separated in time. Instead, they are administered simultaneously to different parts of a patient. For example, to test an ophthalmic device, one may randomly assign one eye to treatment and the other eye to control for each patient. For such a design the experimental unit is an eye. In other device areas these within-subject designs may use a limb, a blood vessel, or some other parts of body as experimental units. The use of the subject as his/her own concurrent control allows for the advantageous use of the correlation within the subject. This design is only possible when the experimental device and control intervention effects are local and do not overlap.

Blinding

Blinding refers to keeping key persons, such as patients, health-care providers, and outcome assessors, unaware of the treatment administered. The purpose of blinding is to minimize artifacts and biases coming from various sources, such as placebo effect, performance bias (sometimes known as Hawthorne effects), and detection bias (i.e., observer, ascertainment, and assessment bias) (Mansournia et al. 2017).

Therefore, it is important to use blinding when feasible. As mentioned in the previous segment, in a device trial blinding of patients and health-care providers is not possible if the control group is medical management or surgery. When the control group is another device, it may be possible to blind patients if the control therapy is administered in a similar way as the investigational device therapy. If the control device is visually indistinguishable from the investigational device, then it may be possible to blind the health-care provider as well, which is the case with the pivotal clinical trial for the TAXUS drug-eluting stent, where the control device is a visually indistinguishable bare-metal stent (Stone et al. 2004). This is one of the few device trials in which active control is used yet double blinding is possible.

Even when blinding of patients and providers are not feasible, the blinding of outcome assessors could still be implemented in many circumstances, and it should be implemented to forestall detection bias. The evaluation of some endpoints can be conducted by examining video, audiotape, or photography, which can be sent to a blinded "core lab" for interpretation. Clinical events could be adjudicated by a blinded clinical events committee (CEC). For endpoints that need to be evaluated by directly observing patients, the blinding of outcome assessors would involve instructing the patients not to reveal the treatment they received. Of course, when patients cannot be blinded, the assessors of patient reported outcomes (PRO) cannot be blinded because they are the patients themselves.

The word blinding can also be used to refer to maintaining the confidentiality of interim data. Interested readers are referred to Fleming et al. (2008) and Fleming (2015). Yet another usage of "blinding" concerns the blinding of statisticians or data analysts to outcome data, which will be discussed later in the subsection "Observational (Nonrandomized) Clinical Studies."

Randomization

As the site-to-site variability tends to be relatively large for device therapy, it is important to balance site distributions between the treatment arms in device trials. Hence randomization is usually stratified by study site. Additional stratification on key baseline covariates is sometimes desirable but is often limited by the average number of patients per site, since this number is often relatively small given the modest sample size of most device trials.

In some trials there is a time lag between randomization and the initiation of the treatments being compared. For example, after randomization between device therapy and surgery, it takes time to schedule the procedure for a device therapy and even longer to schedule a surgery. In the meanwhile, events may happen that would complicate the analysis of trial data. A patient may die or may decide to switch treatment or drop out. Therefore, it is good practice to put a limit on this time lag in the protocol, and to eliminate it where possible, particularly in some trials in which device is compared to another device or sham procedure, such as the EchoCRT study (Ruschitzka et al. 2013). In this study, all patients underwent device implantation and was randomly assigned to have cardiac resynchronization therapy (CRT) capability turned on or off. The randomization occurred after successful implantation of the device and the adjustment of medical therapy for heart failure according to current guidelines. There was no need for any time lag between randomization and treatment initiation.

Clinical Endpoints

Pivotal device trials evaluate the safety and effectiveness of the device in the population expected to be indicated. Accordingly, primary endpoints are divided into one or more safety endpoints and one or more effectiveness endpoints. The study would be considered successful if both the safety and effectiveness endpoints are met. Occasionally, a single endpoint may play the dual role of a primary safety and effectiveness endpoint.

The specification of clinical endpoints for a device trial often involves the concept of device-related adverse events. These are events directly attributable to the device itself. Therefore, it is imperative that the investigational device is precisely defined in the protocol. The classification of whether an adverse event is device related requires careful adjudication. Distinction is made between device-related and procedure-related events. The latter are events that occur from the procedure, irrespective of the device (Ouriel et al. 2013).

Beside primary endpoints, secondary endpoints that are not part of the study success criteria are usually specified for a device trial. They may serve as the bases of additional meaningful claims or provide further insight into the device effect or mechanism of action. Sometimes it is possible to submit the primary endpoint results to the regulatory agency for device approval while data collection for a secondary endpoint is still ongoing.

Sample Size

Sample size is usually driven by study power, which is the probability of rejecting the primary endpoint null hypotheses. Sometimes a powered secondary endpoint may drive the sample size. While most device trials still adopt a fixed design, adaptive designs are more and more common where the sample size depends on outcome data. In an adaptive design the minimal sample size needs to be bigger than that required from a clinical perspective.

A recent example of a device trial using Bayesian adaptive design is the SURTAVI trial (Reardon et al. 2017). The objective of the trial is to compare the safety and efficacy of transcatheter aortic-valve replacement (TAVR) with surgical aortic-valve replacement in patients who were deemed to be at intermediate risk for surgery. It is a noninferiority trial with the primary endpoint being a composite of death from any cause or disabling stroke at 24 months and a planned sample size of 1600. A Bayesian interim analysis was prespecified when 1400 patients had reached 12-month follow-up. Through Bayesian modeling, it was possible to calculate the posterior probability of noninferiority in terms of the 24-month event rate even though at the interim analysis not every patient had had 24-month follow-up. As it turned out, this posterior probability exceeded the prespecified success threshold, thus the trial could declare success early.

Error Rate Control

Type 1 error rate and type 2 error rate (one minus power), also called operating characteristics, must be controlled in all hypothesis-driven pivotal device trials. Any valid statistical approach to error rate control applies to device trials. For complex adaptive designs, controlling the error rates is usually an iterative process. First a tentative decision rule is set up so that operating characteristics can be obtained via simulation. If the error rates are not satisfactory, then the decision rule is adjusted, and simulation is carried out again. This process continues until one arrives at a decision rule that leads to adequate error rate control. The success threshold for the posterior probability of noninferiority in the SURTAVI trial was determined in this fashion. In general, the simulation should be reasonably extensive by covering a wide range of scenarios.

Special Considerations for Diagnostics

A diagnostic device is a medical device that is used to identify or assist in identifying medical conditions of interest in a well-specified intended use population (Yu et al. 2016). Diagnostic devices can be classified into two broad categories: in vitro and in vivo. In vitro devices are laboratory tests based on tissue or blood specimens sampled from patients, such as genetic tests (Campbell et al. 2018). In vivo devices involve test procedures performed directly on the patient, such as diagnostic imaging. The data produced by a diagnostic device can be qualitative (e.g., dichotomous), quantitative, or semi-quantitative (ordinal scale). Quantitative measures can be transformed into dichotomous results via a threshold or cutoff value. Multiple cutoff points may be applied to a quantitative test to generate ordinal categories. The performance of a test producing a dichotomous result (positive or negative) is measured by its sensitivity and specificity when there is a truth standard (a gold standard test) (Pepe 2003). The diagnostic accuracy of a quantitative test can be evaluated by receiver operating characteristic (ROC) analysis. The ROC plot is a graph of the observed sensitivity versus 1 minus the observed specificity of the diagnostic test, evaluated at all possible thresholds that one could use to dichotomize the diagnostic test. One global measure of the diagnostic capability of the test is the area under the ROC plot (AUC) (Pepe 2003; Zhou et al. 2009). Some diagnostic devices are essentially instruments of measurement. Indicators of performance for such devices include systematic bias, accuracy (agreement with the true value of the measurand), imprecision (variability of repeated measurements), and limit of detection (the lowest concentration of an analyte that can be reliably distinguished from zero). The opposite of imprecision is precision.

The randomized clinical trial which is the basis of the clinical testing of drugs and some therapeutic medical devices is not generally applicable to the evaluation of diagnostic devices. It would be unethical to randomize a patient to receive an investigational device as the sole basis for diagnosis in the presence of an effective alternative method. In the area of diagnostic devices, the study design is generally observational in nature where each patient serves as his/her own control and receives both the standard diagnostic test and investigational diagnostic device. But sometimes randomized controlled trials do occur, as we will see below.

Imaging Devices

A particular type of in vivo test is diagnostic imaging. Diagnostic imaging tests often involve readings and/or interpretations by persons who may be referred to as readers (or operators, evaluators, etc.), and present unique study design problems. In the case of readers, it is often a question of what information is available and when. In a so-called sequential design, a reader is provided more information gradually to observe how their ratings change. This design is typically used for diagnostic devices that are intended to be adjunctive to the standard imaging evaluation. Alternatively, a crossover design is typically used to compare a new imaging modality with a standard modality on reader diagnostic accuracy. In a basic version of the fully crossed, multi-reader multi-case (MRMC) crossover design, cases are divided randomly into groups A and B, which are read in both modalities by all readers in two reading sessions separated by a washout period of time. A crossover design is usually used to compare a new imaging modality with a standard modality on reader diagnostic accuracy.

Companion Diagnostic Devices

Predictive biomarkers inform on likely outcomes with specific treatments. They have become increasingly important for precision (or personalized) medicine. They are the basis for an in vitro companion diagnostic device, defined by FDA as a diagnostic test essential for the safe and effective use of a corresponding therapeutic product which is identified in the product label (US FDA 2014). A companion diagnostic test often defines the intended use population of the corresponding therapeutic product. For example, patients may be considered eligible for a drug only if their companion test result is positive because only in that subpopulation have the drug's benefits been established to outweigh its risks. Restriction of the eligibility of a drug to patients with a companion test positive results can be supported by a qualitative interaction between treatment and test on the clinical outcome in an all-comers trial. However, clinical equipoise may not exist for randomly assigning the drug to test negative patients because a priori they are anticipated to not benefit from it. Thus, many drugs are evaluated with their companion diagnostics using an enrichment strategy (US FDA 2012) of enrolling just the test positive patients into a randomized trial of the drug. In an enrichment trial, a significance test for qualitative interaction is not possible; the diagnostic is evaluated only for whether it has selected a population in whom the drug's benefits outweigh its risks. For an example of a clinical trial for a companion diagnostic device, see Rosell et al. (2012).

Complementary Diagnostic Devices

In contrast, a complementary diagnostic device is not required for the use of the drug but provides information about a population who may derive greater benefit. It can help inform the discussion between prescriber and patient. A complementary diagnostic can be described as having a quantitative interaction with the drug effect (Beaver et al. 2017). The treatment is beneficial in both test negative and test positive patients, but the benefit is smaller in test negatives. Note that quantitative interactions can be an artifact of the scale of measurement of the treatment effect. Trial designs and practical considerations for clinical evaluation of predictive biomarker tests have received extensive review, including Polley et al. (2013). A general statistical framework for deciding if a treatment should be given to everyone or to just a biomarker-defined subpopulation has been proposed (Millen et al. 2012). Largely because of advances in precision medicine, subgroup analysis and its various purposes has received renewed interest (Alosh et al. 2015).

Next-Generation Sequencing

Most diagnostic in vitro medical devices are designed to test for a single analyte associated with disease. In contrast, microarray and next-generation sequencing (NGS) technologies can be used to measure large numbers of genetic analytes simultaneously, e.g., gene expressions and single-nucleotide polymorphisms (SNPs), that may confer useful diagnostic information. This creates a huge simultaneous testing problem in need of a multiplicity adjustment. The adjustment need not be as severe as the Bonferroni correction when correlation between the tests is considered. Permutation-based methods can be used to take into account the correlation (Dudoit et al. 2002). Alternatively, Bayesian approaches have also been proposed (Newton et al. 2001; Efron et al. 2001). It is worth noting that the false discovery rate (FDR) (Benjamini and Hochberg 1995) is increasingly being controlled in such large multiplicity problems, as opposed to the more traditional and more conservative familywise Type I error rate.

Bayesian Design for Device Trials

Bayesian statistical methodology has been used for well over 10 years in medical device clinical trials for premarket submissions. The Center for Devices and Radiological Health (CDRH) has published a guidance document "Guidance for the Use of

Bayesian Statistics in Medical Device Clinical Trials" (US FDA 2010). The Bayesian guidance covers many topics on study design and is an essential reference in designing Bayesian medical device clinical trials that will be reviewed by FDA.

Prior Information

The incremental steps in which improvements are made in device development make the Bayesian approach particularly suitable. Good prior information is often available from, for example, trials in other countries, earlier trials on previous device versions, or possibly bench tests or animal studies. In such situations, the natural mode of statistical inference is that of Bayesian. A Bayesian clinical trial for a medical device may include prior information for the investigational device, for the control therapy, or for both the investigational device and control therapy. Previous device studies used as sources of prior information should be recent and similar to current studies in terms of devices used, objectives, endpoints studied, protocol, patient population, investigational sites, physician training, and patient management. Covariates such as demographics and prognostic variables can be used to calibrate previous studies to the current study. The use of prior information often leads to more precise estimates enabling decision-makers to reach a decision on a device with smaller and shorter trials.

Bayesian Adaptive Design

Bayesian inference is used in medical device trials not only where there is prior information that can be incorporated into the current trial, but also where a flexible adaptive clinical trial is being considered (Berry et al. 2011; Campbell 2011, 2013). When there is no good prior information, the prior distributions used in a Bayesian adaptive design are usually relatively noninformative. One of the most prominent advantages of a Bayesian approach to adaptive design over a frequentist one is that the Bayesian approach allows for the construction of likelihood models that can use information obtained at the current time to calculate predictive distributions of observations at later time points. Predictive probabilities are widely used in medical device clinical trials and they serve many purposes. For example, at each interim analysis for sample size adaptation, one could decide whether to stop accrual, to continue enrollment, or to declare futility based on predictive probability of trial success. A possible decision rule could be: If the predictive probability of trial success given the data on the enrolled subjects exceeds a prespecified value, then stop accrual; if the probability of trial success under the maximum sample size is below a certain value, then declare futility; otherwise, enrollment will continue to the next stage unless the maximum sample size is reached. Predictions can be made only if the patients yet to be observed are exchangeable with the patients already observed. In device trials, patients enrolled later in the study may not be exchangeable with patients enrolled earlier if there is a learning curve associated with the device.

Operating Characteristics

For medical device trial designs submitted to FDA for review, including Bayesian adaptive designs, it is of paramount importance to thoroughly evaluate its operating characteristics including type I error rate, power, the distribution of sample size, and probability of stopping at each interim look. In a regulatory environment, it is necessary to control type I error rate and to maintain power at appropriate levels, just as for a frequentist design. In general, when no prior data are used, the type I error rate is controlled at the customary frequentist level. When prior data are used, the type I error rate is often controlled at a higher level, with consideration given to the credibility of the prior data and the knowledge of potential benefit-risk profile of the investigational device. Due to the inherent complexity in the design of a Bayesian clinical trial, specifically when prior data are used or a wide variety of adaptations are planned, an adequate characterization of the operating characteristics of any particular trial design usually needs extensive simulations. Simulations are performed under various more or less plausible scenarios of parameters of interest, evaluating the desirability of the operating characteristics. The process may be iterative, in the sense that sample size, any interim decision rule, study success criteria, and priors may need to be adjusted many times to achieve acceptable operating characteristics.

The advantages of Bayesian methodology have resulted in its increasing use in the medical device arena (Campbell and Yue 2016). It is the methodology of choice in situations where there is prior information that can be used to augment the current trial, or where a flexible adaptive clinical trial is desirable.

Observational (Nonrandomized) Clinical Studies

There is no standard study design or approach that is applicable to the clinical testing of all devices. As has been stated earlier, the statutory standard for approval and level of evidence required for devices is one of *reasonable assurance of safety and effectiveness based on valid scientific evidence,* and valid scientific evidence can be from *partially controlled studies or studies and objective trials without matched controls.* This is different from drugs, which require substantial evidence of safety and effectiveness obtained from well-controlled investigations. Depending on the specific device, randomized controlled trials (RCT) may be either unnecessary or unfeasible. As a result, observational (nonrandomized) studies play a substantial role in the evaluation of investigational medical devices.

Observational studies could be comparative through the explicit use of a control group or may be carried out without a control group (US FDA 2013).

Comparative Observational Study

A comparative observational study (referred to as comparative clinical outcome study in US FDA (2013)) could be conducted using an internal (but non-randomized) control, an external control, or a hybrid internal/external control. An internal control refers to a control group that is enrolled into the study concurrently with the investigational medical device group (treated group). Which treatment a patient undergoes is determined by a mechanism other than randomization, such as clinical judgment based on patient characteristics and risk factors. A key feature of this kind of design is that the patients in the treatment and control groups are enrolled prospectively and treated contemporaneously. Unlike internal control, an external control is constituted by patients treated outside the investigational study. One example is historical control, which can be formed from patients collected from earlier studies of an approved device. Another example is a control extracted from a well-designed and executed national or international patient registry database. A control group could also be constituted in part by internal control and in part by external control. In all three cases, the treatment comparison is made using data collected from the treated group and data collected from the control group.

Noncomparative Observational Study

In a noncomparative observational study (referred to as noncomparative clinical outcome study in US FDA (2013)), the medical device is evaluated by comparing the data collected from patients enrolled into the study and treated with the investigational device to information extracted from outside the study, for example, via synthesis of previously conducted studies or accumulated experience. A numerical value is currently the most common form for the extracted information on a clinical outcome of interest and such numerical values have been referred to by various names in the medical device arena, including objective performance criterion (OPC), performance goal, and target value (US FDA 2013). Statistical reasoning should be applied with judiciousness in producing such numerical values. Sometimes the comparison can also be to a standard established by clinical judgment.

Bias in Observational Studies

While observational studies could provide potential benefits, such as savings in cost or time of conducting clinical studies, statistical and regulatory challenges also arise regarding the validity of study design and the interpretability of study results. For instance, the lack of randomization in observational studies often leads to a systematic difference in the distribution of baseline covariates between investigational device group and control group, resulting in bias in treatment effect estimation. There may be more differences in baseline covariate distributions between the treatment groups in studies using external controls. Such differences lead to doubts about treatment group comparability, and hence the interpretability of study results (Li and Yue 2008). Fortunately, there exist some statistical methods that could be used to reduce bias, including traditional matching and stratification on baseline covariates, regression (covariate) analysis, and the propensity score methodology developed by Rosenbaum and Rubin (1983, 1984). However, it is important to note that all statistical methods aforementioned can only adjust for confounding covariates that are observed and incorporated in the statistical model but not for unobserved ones. Also, when there are large differences in baseline covariates between two treatment groups, these statistical methods may not be able to mitigate the bias. And, of course, none of these statistical methods can adjust for bias caused by the separation in time between a treated group and its historical control (temporal bias), or by difference in medical practice among multiregions. Therefore, it is critical that minimizing bias starts from the design stage of an investigational study.

Outcome-Free Design

In an RCT, study design and the act of outcome data analysis are clearly separated: outcome data are not available at the design phase in which their analysis is prespecified. However, traditionally this is often not the case with observational studies. It has been recognized that designing an observational study with outcome data in sight could compromise the objectivity of study design and make study result difficult to interpret (Yue 2007; Yue et al. 2014; Li et al. 2016; Yue et al. 2016). Rubin advocates objective design of observational studies, i.e., prospective study design without access to any outcome data (Rubin 2001, 2007, 2008). This outcome-free principle can be realized for propensity score design (Yue et al. 2014; Li et al. 2016) – in building a propensity score model to balance covariates between treatment groups, only baseline covariates and the treatment indicator are needed; outcome data do not need to be accessed. Propensity score design is an iterative process (Austin 2011). The aim is to derive proper propensity score estimation model and grouping or weighting method(s) such that adequate balance in covariate distributions is reached. Not accessing the outcome data eliminates the bias caused by selecting a propensity score model that favors one of the treatments. For confirmatory investigational studies, outcome-free propensity score design can be implemented via a two-stage design process (Yue et al. 2014; Li et al. 2016). Stage I occurs when the clinical protocol is being developed. Key elements of stage I include (1) selection of appropriate control group or data source for control group, (2) preliminary estimation of sample size, and (3) specification of covariates to be collected in the study and used in the second design stage. An independent statistician to perform the study design is identified at this stage. Stage II of the design starts ideally as soon as all patients are enrolled and information on all baseline covariates is available. In this stage, the independent statistician identified in the first design stage estimates propensity score, matches all patients in the investigational device group with patients in the control group according to the estimated propensity score, assesses balance in covariate distributions, and finalizes control group selection and sample size estimation as well as the statistical analysis plan for future outcome analysis. All these need to be performed without access to any outcome data (Yue et al. 2014; Li et al. 2016). The two-stage framework has been successfully applied to medical device clinical studies (Thourani et al. 2016).

Summary and Conclusion

While there are many commonalities between clinical trials for medical devices and for drugs, device trials do have some unique challenges. It is relatively straightforward to implement placebo control in a drug trial, but in many cases it is not ethical to give patients the device equivalent of a placebo, namely a sham device. Blinding or masking is often impossible to do in a device trial, especially when the treated and control arms involve different treatment modalities, such as when the comparison is between device and drug therapies. Due to the rapid pace at which innovations are made, the product life cycle of a medical device is relatively short. It is not uncommon for a newly marketed device to become obsolete and replaced by next-generation technology in a couple of years. This means that large and lengthy randomized clinical trials are often impractical in the medical device arena. A wide variety of clinical study designs and statistical methodologies, such as those overviewed in this section, have been utilized in medical device clinical trials. We believe that opportunities for clinical trial and statistical innovation will continue to expand in the future.

Key Facts

- A medical device is a medical product that does not have a chemical, metabolic, or biological principle of action. Medical device regulations are different from drug regulations.
- Due to the rapid pace at which innovations are made, the product life cycle of a medical device tends to be shorter than that of a drug.
- Bayesian design is more common in device trials than in drug trials.
- Non-randomized studies are more common in the medical device world than in the drug world.

Cross-References

▶ Bayesian Adaptive Designs for Phase I Trials
▶ Diagnostic Trials

References

Al-Lamee R, Thompson D, Hakim-Moulay D et al (2018) Percutaneous coronary intervention in stable angina (ORBITA): a double-blind, randomised controlled trial. Lancet 391:331–340

Alosh M, Fritsch K, Huque M, Mahjoob K, Pennello G, Rothmann M, Russek-Cohen E, Smith F, Wilson S, Yue LQ (2015) Statistical considerations on subgroup analysis in clinical trials. Stat Biopharm Res 7:286–304

Austin P (2011) An introduction to propensity score methods for reducing the effects of confounding in observational studies. Multivariate Behav Res 46:399–424

Beaver JA, Tzou A, Blumenthal GM, McKee AE, Kim G, Pazdur R, Philip R (2017) An FDA perspective on the regulatory implications of complex signatures to predict response to targeted therapies. Clin Cancer Res 23:1368–1372

Benjamini Y, Hochberg Y (1995) Controlling the false discovery rate: a practical and powerful approach to multiple testing. J R Stat Soc B 57:289–300

Berry SM, Carlin BP, Lee JJ, Müller P (2011) Bayesian adaptive methods for clinical trials. CRC Press, Boca Raton

Campbell G (2011) Bayesian statistics in medical devices: innovation sparked by the FDA. J Biopharm Stat 21:871–887

Campbell G (2013) Similarities and differences of Bayesian designs and adaptive designs for medical devices: a regulatory view. Stat Biopharm Res 5:356–368

Campbell G, Yue LQ (2016) Statistical innovations in the medical device world sparked by the FDA. J Biopharm Stat 26:3–16

Campbell G, Li H, Pennello G, Yue LQ (2018) Medical devices. In: Armitage P, Colton T (eds) Encyclopedia of biostatistics. Wiley, New York

Dudoit S, Yang YH, Callow MJ, Speed TP (2002) Statistical methods for identifying differentially expressed genes in replicated cDNA microarray experiments. Stat Sinica 12:111–139

Efron B, Tibshirani R, Storey JD, Tusher V (2001) Empirical Bayes analysis of a microarray experiment. J Am Stat Assoc 96:1151–1160

Fleming TR (2015) Protecting the confidentiality of interim data: addressing current challenges. Clin Trials 12(1):5–11

Fleming TR, Sharples K, McCall J (2008) Maintaining confidentiality of interim data to enhance trial integrity and credibility. Clin Trials 5(2):157–167

Li H, Yue LQ (2008) Statistical and regulatory issues in non-randomized medical device clinical studies. J Biopharm Stat 18:20–30

Li H, Mukhi V, Lu N, Xu Y, Yue LQ (2016) A note on good practice of objective propensity score design for premarket nonrandomized medical device studies with an example. Stat Biopharm Res 8:282–286

Mansournia MA, Higgins JP, Sterne JA, Hernán MA (2017) Biases in randomized trials: a conversation between trialists and epidemiologists. Epidemiology 28(1):54

Millen BA, Dmitrienko A, Ruberg S, Shen L (2012) A statistical framework for decision making in confirmatory multipopulation tailoring clinical trials. Drug Info J 46(6):647–656

Newton MA, Kendziorski CM, Richmond CS, Blattner FR, Tsui KW (2001) On differential variability of expression ratios: improving statistical inference about gene expression changes from microarray data. J Comput Biol 8:37–52

Ouriel K, Fowl RJ, Davies MG et al (2013) Reporting standards for adverse events after medical device use in the peripheral vascular system. J Vasc Surg 58:776–786

Parisi AF, Folland ED, Hartigan P et al (1992) A comparison of angioplasty with medical therapy in the treatment of single-vessel coronary artery disease. N Engl J Med 326(1):10–16

Pepe MS (2003) The evaluation of diagnostic tests and biomarkers. Oxford Press, London

Polley MY, Freidlin B, Korn EL, Conley BA, Abrams JS, McShane LM (2013) Statistical and practical considerations for clinical evaluation of predictive biomarkers. J Natl Cancer Inst 105: 1677–1683

Reardon MJ, van Mieghem NM, Popma JJ et al (2017) Surgical or transcatheter aortic-valve replacement in intermediate-risk patients. N Engl J Med 376(14):1321–1331
Rosell R, Carcereny E, Gervais R et al (2012) Erlotinib versus standard chemotherapy as first-line treatment for European patients with advanced EGFR mutationpositive non-small-cell lung cancer (EURTAC): a multicenter, open-label, randomised phase 3 trial. Lancet Oncol 13(3):239–246
Rosenbaum PR, Rubin DB (1983) The central role of the propensity score in observational studies for causal effects. Biometrika 70:41–55
Rosenbaum PR, Rubin DB (1984) Reducing bias in observational studies using subclassification on the propensity score. J Am Stat Assoc 79:516–524
Rubin DB (2001) Using propensity scores to help design observational studies: application to the tobacco litigation. Health Serv Outcomes Res Methodol 2:169–188
Rubin DB (2007) The design versus the analysis of observational studies for causal effects: parallel with the design of randomized trials. Stat Med 26:20–36
Rubin DB (2008) For objective causal inference, design trumps analysis. Ann Appl Stat 2:808–840
Ruschitzka F, Abraham WT, Singh JP et al (2013) Cardiac-resynchronization therapy in heart failure with a narrow QRS complex. N Engl J Med 369(15):1395–1405
Stone GW, Ellis SG, Cox DA et al (2004) A polymer-based, paclitaxel-eluting stent in patients with coronary artery disease. N Engl J Med 350(3):221–231
Svensson LG, Tuzcu M, Kapadia S et al (2013) A comprehensive review of the PARTNER trial. J Thorac Cardiovasc Surg 145(3S):S11–S16
Thourani VH, Kodali S, Makkar RR et al (2016) Transcatheter aortic valve replacement versus surgical valve replacement in intermediate-risk patients: a propensity score analysis. Lancet 387: 2218–2225
U.S. Food and Drug Administration (2010) Guidance for industry and FDA staff: guidance for the use of Bayesian statistics in medical device clinical trials. Available at https://www.fda.gov/downloads/medicaldevices/deviceregulationandguidance/guidancedocuments/ucm071121.pdf. Accessed 9 Feb 2018
U.S. Food and Drug Administration (2012) Draft guidance on enrichment strategies for clinical trials to support approval of human drugs and biological products. Available at https://www.fda.gov/downloads/drugs/guidancecomplianceregulatoryinformation/guidances/ucm332181.pdf. Accessed 9 Feb 2018
U.S. Food and Drug Administration (2013) Design considerations for pivotal clinical investigations for medical devices: guidance for industry, clinical investigators, institutional review boards and Food and Drug Administration Staff. Available at: https://www.fda.gov/downloads/medicaldevices/deviceregulationandguidance/guidancedocuments/ucm373766.pdf. Accessed 9 Feb 2018
U.S. Food and Drug Administration (2014) In vitro companion diagnostic devices: guidance for industry and Food and Drug Administration Staff. Available at: https://www.fda.gov/downloads/MedicalDevices/DeviceRegulationandGuidance/GuidanceDocuments/UCM262327.pdf. Accessed 9 Feb 2018
U.S. Food and Drug Administration (2016) Draft guidance: Software as a Medical Device (SAMD): clinical evaluation. Available at: https://www.fda.gov/ucm/groups/fdagov-public/@fdagov-meddev-gen/documents/document/ucm524904.pdf. Accessed 9 Feb 2018
Yu T, Li Q, Gray G, Yue LQ (2016) Statistical innovations in diagnostic device evaluation. J Biopharm Stat 26:1067–1077
Yue LQ (2007) Statistical and regulatory issues with the application of propensity score analysis to non-randomized medical device clinical studies. J Biopharm Stat 17:1–13
Yue LQ, Lu N, Xu Y (2014) Designing pre-market observational comparative studies using existing data as controls: challenges and opportunities. J Biopharm Stat 24:994–1010
Yue LQ, Campbell G, Lu N, Xu Y, Zuckerman B (2016) Utilizing national and international registries to enhance pre-market medical device regulatory evaluation. J Biopharm Stat 26: 1136–1145
Zhou X-H, Obuchowski NA, McClish DK (2009) Statistical methods in diagnostic medicine, 2nd edn. Wiley, New York

Complex Intervention Trials

74

Linda Sharples and Olympia Papachristofi

Contents

L. Sharples (✉)
London School of Hygiene and Tropical Medicine, London, UK
e-mail: Linda.Sharples@lshtm.ac.uk

O. Papachristofi
London School of Hygiene and Tropical Medicine, London, UK

Clinical Development and Analytics, Novartis Pharma AG, Basel, Switzerland
e-mail: olympia.papachristofi@novartis.com

© Springer Nature Switzerland AG 2022

S. Piantadosi, C. L. Meinert (eds.), *Principles and Practice of Clinical Trials*,
https://doi.org/10.1007/978-3-319-52636-2_245

Abstract

Clinical trial methodology was developed for pharmaceutical drug development and evaluation. In recent years, trials have expanded to an increasingly diverse range of interventions.

The term *complex intervention* describes treatments that are multicomponent and include clustering due to specific components, such as the healthcare provider, which cannot be separated from the package of treatment and influence treatment outcomes. This chapter provides an overview of the main considerations in the design and analysis of complex interventions trials.

Initial development of complex interventions is a multidisciplinary endeavor and requires rigorous qualitative and quantitative methods. Understanding both the intervention components and how they interact is crucial for successful development and evaluation of the intervention.

Published guidance on methods for feasibility, piloting, or early phase trials of complex interventions is scarce. However, there are well-established methods for phase III trials of multicomponent interventions that involve clustering. The most commonly used methods, including individually randomized trials with random effects for clusters, cluster randomized trials, and stepped-wedge cluster randomized trials, are described. Analysis focuses on generalized linear (mixed) models; methods for sample size estimation that accommodate the extra variance related to clustering are also provided for a range of designs in this setting.

With careful attention to the correlation structure induced by the chosen design, results can be analyzed in standard statistical software, although small numbers of clusters, and/or small within-cluster sizes, can cause convergence problems.

Statistical analysis results of complex interventions trials, including those relating to components of the intervention, need to be considered alongside economic, qualitative, and behavioral research to ensure that complex interventions can be successfully implemented into routine practice.

Keywords

Randomized · Cluster randomized · Clinical trial · Complex intervention · Multicomponent · Clustering · Healthcare provider · Stepped-wedge

Introduction

In recent years, clinical trial methodology has been applied in diverse healthcare settings and to a wide range of interventions beyond fixed-dose, single-drug treatments. For example, novel surgical procedures (Sharples et al. 2018), multidisciplinary packages of care for chronic diseases (education, physiotherapy, medicine) (Dickens et al. 2014), mental health coping strategies (Mohr et al. 2011), and public health interventions (Emery et al. 2017) have all been the subject of randomized controlled trials (RCTs). The interventions in these trials are generally termed *complex interventions*.

Although complex interventions have no single, universally accepted definition, there are two main issues that characterize them: (i) the multicomponent nature of the intervention itself and (ii) a level of dependency between trial participants treated by the same healthcare provider, or in a group setting, that induces *clustering* of outcome measurements. Note that, in this chapter, we use the general term *provider* for any person who delivers all or part of a complex intervention, including surgeons, physicians, therapists, nurses, physiotherapists, and so on.

In (i), what distinguishes complex from non-complex interventions is the fact that they are made up of a number of components, which may be interdependent (e.g., use of rescue treatment after failure of initial therapy) or independent (e.g., treatment packages comprising psychotherapy, physiotherapy, and health education). Some components of the intervention package may be of interest themselves and thought of as fixed effects (e.g., physiotherapy or not). Other components may not be of interest themselves (nuisance parameters), but may introduce some level of dependency between trial participants, or *clustering*. For example, two patients treated by the same surgeon may have more similar outcomes than two patients treated by different surgeons, due to differences between surgeons in experience and expertise, as well as local (to the hospital) population attributes. In general, specific surgeons are not of interest themselves, but they represent a population of surgeons who might ultimately provide the intervention of interest (see later on for an example of (ii)). In this case, providers are better defined and analyzed as random effects (e.g., surgeon performing a procedure, therapist providing group cognitive behavioral therapy). What links these (fixed and random effects) components is that they can all have an influence on the effectiveness of the package that makes up the complex intervention, and differences (between patients) in the specific treatment package received may manifest as heterogeneity in the outcome of interest. The multicomponent nature of the intervention may also mean that multiple outcomes are used to assess the success of its different components, which may complicate the choice of primary outcome (Richardson and Redden 2014).

Complex intervention trials may be further complicated due to other factors in addition to the intervention itself. The context in which interventions are delivered may be complex, an obvious example being the operating rooms in which surgical procedures are performed; these contain many instruments, machines, and devices, operated by multiple interacting clinical disciplines (Blencowe et al. 2015). Public health trials are clearly dependent on the setting in which they are conducted and on how that affects the delivery of the intervention (Emery et al. 2017). In particular, trials in hard-to-reach populations may require designs such as snowballing (index cases identifying other cases for study participation) that introduce dependency between participants (Yuen et al. 2013). Low- and middle-income countries may have diverse healthcare infrastructure, staffing, cultural, and economic factors that add to the complexity of an intervention and its evaluation (Cisse et al. 2017).

All these factors affect the way a novel intervention is developed, the amount of standardization required for each component, the assessment of treatment adherence, the fidelity to the intervention as defined, and the statistical design and analysis of the trial. In particular, any random effects or clustering inherent in the delivery of the complex intervention will increase the sample size compared to a design in which a simple intervention is applied at the patient level, as independent and identically distributed patient outcomes cannot be assumed.

General characteristics of complex interventions have been described, with the Medical Research Council (MRC) in the UK providing an early general framework for design of such trials in 2000 (Medical_Research_Council 2000), which was updated in 2008 (Medical_Research_Council 2008). Although useful, these guidelines do not provide detail on specific methods of assessment. It is generally appreciated that the design and analysis of complex intervention trials require rigorous quantitative and qualitative research methods, with collaborative work between, for example, statisticians, behavioral scientists, and clinical experts. While this chapter provides some general discussion on the use of mixed methods in this context, the focus is primarily on statistical methods in a broad sense.

Developing the Intervention

Defining the Intervention Components

Pharmaceutical interventions are manufactured under strict quality control so that the dose of active drug is known exactly (e.g., see (Pocock 1983)). Moreover, delivery of the drug rarely depends on the context, as it is typically identical across physicians and settings. In contrast, complex intervention trials are often embedded in the clinical or public health setting that they aim to address, which influences the trial design. Moreover, there may be components of the intervention that can be left to the discretion of the provider, say the type of sutures used in a surgical intervention or the number of sessions required in a psychotherapy trial. For these reasons, including differences in the way the intervention is delivered between patients, complex interventions are naturally evaluated using *pragmatic* trials (Loudon et al. 2013). Although there are exceptions (such as evaluations of new diagnostic tests), in many cases, the evaluation aims to reflect how the intervention would perform in the setting for which it is intended, rather than in a tightly controlled setting, with highly selected patients, as is the case in trials assessing drug efficacy.

Nevertheless, to maintain scientific quality and ensure that the intervention can be reproduced by other providers, a clear definition of exactly what constitutes the complex intervention, and how it will be delivered in the planned setting, is paramount. The *Template for Intervention Description and Replication* (TIDieR) checklist and guide provides general advice on the reporting of interventions (Hoffmann et al. 2014); this section provides guidance specific to complex interventions.

Focusing on surgical trial design, Blencowe et al. (2016) highlighted the importance of describing each component of a surgical procedure, as well as the level of standardization and flexibility permitted within the surgical intervention package.

For example, consider the Amaze trial of *ablation* to treat abnormal heart rhythm in patients already scheduled for cardiac surgery; the control group received the scheduled cardiac surgery alone (Sharples et al. 2018). The complete procedure involved treating 12 different sections of the heart, but because Amaze was designed to reflect the treatment as it was currently used in the UK (*pragmatic trial*), the protocol allowed surgeons to use their judgment and treat as many sections as considered necessary. In addition, surgeons were also able to use their expertise to decide whether to apply co-interventions, such as electrical stimulation (cardioversion), if the initial operation was not fully effective. All other procedure components were fixed according to protocols. The flexibility inherent in Amaze is common in surgical trials where procedure success depends heavily on the training, skill, and expertise of the surgeon; as a result, the intervention is a combination of both the operation delivered and the surgeon who performs it. Similarly, psychotherapy typically involves a set of protocols and techniques, which must be well-defined, together with a psychotherapist delivering them. The therapist will have an influence both on the content and delivery of the package, as well as on patient adherence (Walwyn and Roberts 2017).

The level of standardization to be considered when defining the intervention has been discussed in surgical (Blencowe et al. 2016), behavioral (Mars et al. 2013), and public health (Perez et al. 2018) contexts. The main factors to consider can be summarized as follows:

(i) Which intervention components are necessary and which are optional?
(ii) Under what circumstances is each component mandatory, prohibited, or optional?
(iii) For each component, what delivery methods are mandatory, prohibited, or optional?
(iv) For each component, which delivery methods have a strict definition and which can be applied flexibly?
(v) What training or competency is required for providers of each component?

Careful definition of the components of a complex intervention allows monitoring of the intervention delivery and its components. Successful intervention delivery requires both patient compliance (e.g., attendance at therapy sessions) and completion of each component of treatment according to plan by the provider, termed *fidelity*. Both are important to establish why a successful intervention worked and crucially to inform its subsequent implementation into the intended healthcare setting. Fidelity is less of an issue in traditional drug trials, where the common departure from treatment delivery is patient non-compliance to treatment, due to either side effects or lack of efficacy: see, for example, Pocock (1983).

Note that, because a complex intervention comprises multiple components and the intervention and context are difficult to separate, ensuring that its delivery will be identical in all cases is challenging. For example, in the Amaze trial (Sharples et al. 2018), almost 9% of the variation in risk-adjusted outcomes was related to differences between cardiac surgeons. Thus, no two patients can be assumed to have had an identical procedure, and the surgeon can be considered integral to the intervention package; therefore, consideration must be given to the criteria for including a surgeon in the trial. This principle is important for healthcare providers delivering complex interventions in general.

However, establishing when a provider is sufficiently experienced to be randomized in an RCT is not straightforward (discussed in detail in the next section). For instance, learning assessments are complicated because as surgeons gain experience, they are likely to undertake more high-risk cases. Their performance might seem not to improve or even to deteriorate with time, but this may be due to an increase in the risk in the cases they handle, so that the duration of their learning period (and hence when they can be randomized in an RCT) may be overestimated.

Development of the Package

Complex interventions cover such diverse areas that detailed discussion of the initial derivation of the intervention itself is beyond the scope of this chapter. General guidance on the design and evaluation of complex interventions can be found in the MRC complex intervention guidance (Medical_Research_Council. 2008); the IDEAL (Idea, Development, Exploration, Assessment, and Long-term Study) publications provide a phased development of the intervention, from conception to final evaluation, for surgical trials (Mcculloch et al. 2009), and MOST (Multiphase Optimization Strategy) describes a framework for behavioral interventions (Collins et al. 2007).

Development of the intervention package requires input from a range of clinical and research disciplines. As with all interventions, it is also important to have a comprehensive knowledge of the state of the art. This may involve some or all of the following activities:

(i) For a multicomponent intervention, systematic reviews and meta-analyses for each component will be required.
(ii) Detailed assessment of the intended healthcare setting, treatment pathways, and other contextual factors which may require both qualitative and survey work.
(iii) Understanding of the theoretical underpinnings of the intervention and its relation to behavioral change in patients and public health practice, to improve the chance of trial success and inform its implementation.
(iv) Statistical modeling using early data sets (if available) can provide estimates of the likely clinical efficacy and cost-effectiveness of the intervention.

The following section focuses on how statistical methods may contribute to the development of complex interventions; details of the use of all above methods in this context are provided in a review by Richards and Hallberg and references therein (Richards and Hallberg 2015).

Timing of Evaluation

The timing of definitive evaluation of a complex intervention is closely associated with the amount of expertise required for it to be implemented. A new treatment that is technically demanding, or depends on an in-depth understanding of its theory and practice, may require a period of training for providers to achieve satisfactory performance. Training can take a number of forms, including classroom instruction, training in individual intervention components, and mentored delivery of the intervention as a whole.

To ensure that providers have reached the required expertise level for participation in a trial, results from early cases completed during their training should be closely monitored. Moreover, treatment effects may change during the trial as the package of care is rolled out from the innovators who have initially developed it to a wider group of providers. Whether treatment effects increase or decrease during the period of evaluation may not be predictable, so that reassessment of treatment effects as the trial progresses is recommended.

Simple summary statistics can be useful in comparing the success rates for early and later recipients of the intervention during its development and evaluation. More formally, with a carefully selected clinical outcome, or a more sensitive surrogate, performance over time can be modeled as a function of the chronological order of the interventions delivered, adjusting for patient risk factors as necessary. For example, Cook et al. describe model-based methods for monitoring outcomes of a new surgical procedure during its development, focusing on three characteristics: (i) the initial level of provider performance; (ii) the learning rate, measuring how quickly performance improves; and (iii) an asymptote or plateau representing the level at which performance stabilizes (Cook et al. 2004). Papachristofi et al. demonstrate situations in which a particular surgeon has achieved the required level of performance for inclusion in an RCT (see Fig. 1); this requires setting a predetermined level of performance and monitoring results until they reach this level (1a), exceed it (1b and 1d), or are within an acceptable distance defined by the precision of the estimated performance level (1c). Papachristofi et al. also extend this work in

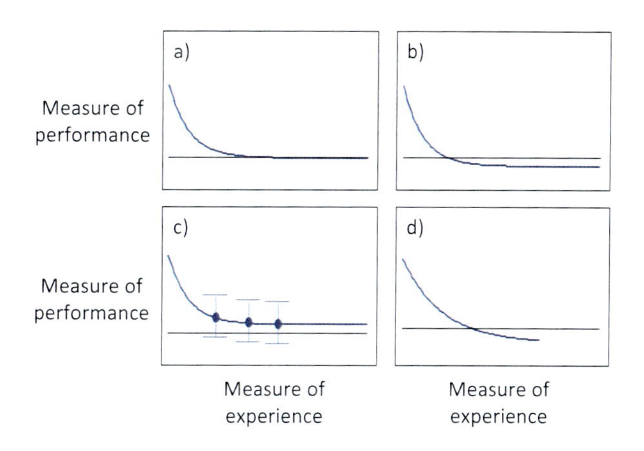

Fig. 1 Learning curve scenarios for RCT randomization (lower values on the y-axis represent superior performance)

an attempt to pinpoint the time at which performance has stabilized (Papachristofi et al. 2016a).

Such models are useful to identify the stage at which provider performance for the new intervention has stabilized, so that a phase III RCT can be initiated. Early randomization of patients and premature inclusion of providers who have not reached a stable level of performance may lead to biased estimates of treatment effects and false inference of the novel intervention's effectiveness. However, an RCT should only begin if equipoise still holds; delaying the RCT evaluation for too long carries the risk that providers form strong opinions as to the best treatment for their patients, despite the lack of scientific evidence of efficacy.

Such analyses of the intervention's development period are only possible if there is complete and rigorous data collection from the beginning of development of new interventions, documenting the timing and nature of any changes in the intervention. Trials can then begin when the intervention has been fully refined and when individual providers have reached the required level of performance.

Feasibility/Early Phase Studies

Once developed, complex interventions must go through formal evaluation. However, there are challenges in generalizing the traditional early phases of evaluation used for new drugs to the case of complex interventions, partly due to the frequent lack of surrogate endpoints for early evaluation, multiple outcomes of interest, and the inherent clustering in many complex interventions (Wilson et al. 2016). There may also be difficulty in deciding the timing of a randomized trial, particularly if the intervention requires development of new skills or competencies (Papachristofi et al. 2016a).

As a result, early evaluation of complex interventions typically addresses feasibility and piloting of a phase III trial. The aim is to finalize the finer points of the intervention delivery and inform the design of the definitive trial. Such early phase, often single-arm studies can be used to estimate patient adherence, provider fidelity, variance components, and interactions between different components of the intervention package. Variance-covariance components are a key element of trial design that captures the degree of similarity between individuals within a *cluster*. This similarity between individuals within a cluster is defined as the proportion of total variation attributable to clustering and is quantified using the intra-class correlation coefficient (ICC), denoted in this chapter by ρ.

Because some of the parameters required for designing the definitive trial are second order and above (e.g., variance components, interactions), and as useful surrogates are rarely available, the power for testing hypotheses at this early evaluation stage is low, and the emphasis is instead on estimation of parameters needed for trial design.

Recent work has provided some clear thinking around the relationship between complex interventions assessment and phase II drug trials (Wilson et al. 2016); its focus is on both hypothesis testing and Bayesian methods to inform the decision to continue to the phase III trial. Challenges that have been identified include:

(i) The small number of clusters (often defined by the few innovators who developed the intervention) at early stages
(ii) The small number of patients in each cluster
(iii) The lack of information on cluster sizes and the ICC
(iv) The number of endpoints that may be under investigation, with no clear decision about the appropriate phase III primary outcome
(v) The lack of data to inform (compound) hypothesis tests and/or Bayesian utilities when assessing multiple outcomes (e.g., both efficacy and safety)

Although this work and references therein provide some useful guidance, early phase trial statistical methodology is not yet established in the field.

Evaluation/Statistical Methods for Trial Design

The pivotal phase of evaluation is the phase III RCT assessing clinically important outcomes, usually in a large sample of patients: see, for example, Pocock (1983). As the phase III trial aims to estimate treatment efficacy or effectiveness, all aspects of the intervention package, including treatment protocols, treatment duration, and safety profiles, should have already been established. In what follows, the most commonly used designs for phase III complex intervention trials are described.

Individually Randomized Designs

Consider first trials in which randomization, treatment, and outcomes assessment are all conducted at the individual patient level. In situations where the intervention is to be evaluated as a package of care, ignoring any random effects, standard trial design, and analysis methods can be used. In order to introduce some notation, assume a generalized linear model for patient i, $i = 1, \ldots, m$, with x_i a categorical covariate representing treatment allocation:

$$g^{-1}(E[y_i]) = \beta_0 + \beta_1 x_i, \tag{1}$$

where y_i is a measure of outcome and g is an appropriate link function. For example, for continuous outcomes, the identity link is used, and the residual error terms are (usually) assumed to be independent and identically distributed as $e_i \tilde{N}(0, \sigma_e^2)$. This section focuses on generalized linear models for illustration, but methods for time-to-event outcomes are also available; further covariates can additionally be incorporated (omitted here for clarity).

Supplementary exploratory analysis of fixed components of the package can be undertaken based on subsets of package components or interactions between components. Such exploratory analyses will likely be underpowered unless the trial has been designed to accommodate them. However, paired with qualitative exploration of the reasons for differential response to the intervention, they can identify areas for further research, suggest components linked with worse outcomes that need refinement, and inform the optimum method of implementing the intervention in clinical practice.

Clustering is often inherent in complex intervention trials due to the nature of the intervention itself. For example, patients may be allocated to open surgery or minimal access (keyhole) surgery arms individually, but the well-known heterogeneity between surgeons' outcomes means that outcomes for two patients treated by the same surgeon will be more similar than outcomes for two patients treated by different surgeons; that is, there is clustering by surgeon (Papachristofi et al. 2016b). This violates the usual statistical assumption that patient outcomes are *independent and identically distributed*. The extent to which violation of this assumption affects the point estimate and precision of the treatment effect clearly depends on the degree of similarity between outcomes of patients within the same cluster.

Patient clustering within treatment providers and hospitals introduces hierarchies of care (patient within provider within hospital). Providers (clusters) can be modeled as *fixed effects*; however, this may introduce many additional parameters in the model that are not of interest in themselves, that is, *nuisance* parameters. Alternatively, providers can be modeled as random effects; these treat the clusters as a random sample from a population so that the specific treatment providers are only of interest in that they represent a population of providers, to which the results will be generalizable. In this case, accommodation of clustering during modeling using random intercept terms should reduce bias and correct the type I error in the treatment effect estimation (Papachristofi et al. 2016b; Kahan and Morris 2013).

The statistical model for patient i, $i = 1, \ldots, m$ in cluster j, $j = 1, \ldots, c$ can be written:

$$g^{-1}\left(E\left[y_{ij}\right]\right) = \beta_0 + \beta_1 x_{ij} + u_j \tag{2}$$

where $u_j \tilde{N}\left(0, \sigma_u^2\right)$ are the cluster-specific random intercepts for providers. For the case of a linear model, the residual error terms for patient i in cluster j, $e_{ij} \mid u_j \tilde{N}\left(0, \sigma_e^2\right)$ are now independent conditional on cluster occupancy. Such a model is termed a *hierarchical* or *nested* design (see Fig. 2a). Normally distributed random effects (on some scale) are almost universally used in the trials' literature for the primary analysis, with other distributional assumptions explored in sensitivity analyses.

For the simple nested model (2) the ICC is given by

$$\rho = \frac{\sigma_u^2}{\sigma_u^2 + \sigma_e^2}. \tag{3}$$

We refer to this as the *simple ICC*. The ICC can be interpreted as the proportion of the total variation that is attributable to between-cluster variance and is an important

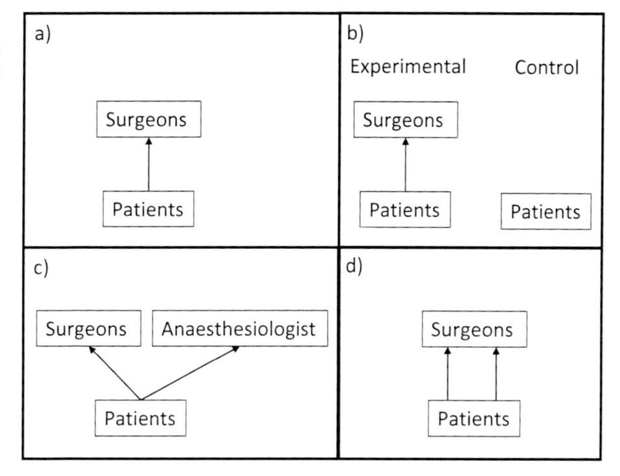

Fig. 2 Illustration of individually randomized trials with clustering in (**a**) both trial arms, (**b**) the experimental arm only, (**c**) cross-classified, and (**d**) multiple membership multiple classification

parameter for sample size estimation for phase III trials (see section "Sample Size Estimation for Trials with Clustering" below). High values for ρ indicate that intervention delivery is quite heterogeneous between clusters relative to the within-cluster variation and vice versa.

There are two main alternative scenarios to this simple design: first, the random components affect outcomes differently in the intervention and control arms, and, second, the treatment effect varies between clusters within the same arm (i.e., random coefficient for treatment).

The first scenario might arise in trials with very different treatment arms, for example, a trial of a new technically demanding surgery (high variation) compared with standard surgery (low variation) and can be modeled by

$$g^{-1}\left(E\left[y_{ij}\right]\right) = \beta_{\mathbf{0}} + \beta_{\mathbf{1}}x_{ij} + u_j\delta\left(x_{ij} = 1\right) + u_j'\delta\left(x_{ij} = 0\right) \tag{4}$$

where $u_j\tilde{N}\left(0, \sigma_u^2\right)$ and $u_j'\tilde{N}\left(0, \sigma_{u'}^2\right)$ are the cluster-specific random effects in the treatment and control arms respectively, and δ is the treatment arm indicator function; for a linear model, residual error terms are again expressed as $e_{ij} \mid u_j \sim N(0, \sigma_e^2)$. Such trials are described as *partially nested* if the control arm random effects are all zero (e.g., surgery versus medical management trial; *s*ee Fig. 2b). Assuming equal numbers of patients per cluster and equal numbers of clusters per arm, the ICC can be written as

$$\rho = \frac{0.5\left(\sigma_u^2 + \sigma_{u'}^2\right)}{0.5\left(\sigma_u^2 + \sigma_{u'}^2\right) + \sigma_e^2} \tag{5}$$

and comprises three variance terms; the two random effects variances are considered independent since they are estimated in different clusters.

The second scenario might arise in a novel surgery versus standard surgery trial, where the between-surgeon variation in outcomes manifests through heterogeneity in the treatment effect; this can be modeled by

$$g^{-1}\left(E\left[y_{ij}\right]\right) = \beta_0 + \beta_1 x_{ij} + u_j + u'_j x_{ij}, \tag{6}$$

where $u_j \tilde{N}\left(0, \sigma_u^2\right)$ and $u'_j \tilde{N}\left(0, \sigma_{u'}^2\right)$ are the cluster-specific random effects on the intercept and treatment coefficient, respectively; for a linear model, $e_{ij} \mid u_j, u_{j'} \tilde{N}\left(0, \sigma_e^2\right)$ are residual error terms. In the random coefficient model, correlation between the two random effects parameters is possible $\left(\sigma_{uu'} = r\sigma_u\sigma_{u'}\right)$ and the ICC can be written as

$$\rho = \frac{\sigma_u^2 + \sigma_{u'}^2 + 2\sigma_{uu'}}{\sigma_u^2 + \sigma_{u'}^2 + 2\sigma_{uu'} + \sigma_e^2}. \tag{7}$$

Cross-Classified Designs

Extending the single random component model to accommodate intervention packages with multiple random components is not straightforward since they are usually not fully nested; that is, the resulting structure is not fully hierarchical. For example, Papachristofi et al. (2016b) describe outcomes after surgical interventions including both surgeons and anesthesiologists as random effects, while Roberts and Walwyn (2013) consider both psychotherapists and general medical doctors as random effects in mental health trials. In both these examples, two types of provider were expected to influence outcomes, and pairs of providers were expected to share some, but not all of their patients (Fig. 2c). Such components are said to be *crossed* and can be analyzed using *cross-classification methods* (Browne et al. 2001). For illustration, consider a two-level cross-classified model for patient i treated by the j^{th}provider of type A, and the k^{th}provider of type B, with treatment x_{ijk} and outcome y_{ijk}. The corresponding cross-classified model may be written as

$$g^{-1}\left(E\left[y_{ijk}\right]\right) = \beta_0 + \beta_1 x_{ijk} + u_j + v_k, \tag{8}$$

where $u_j \tilde{N}\left(0, \sigma_u^2\right)$ and $v_k \tilde{N}\left(0, \sigma_v^2\right)$ are independent cluster-specific random effects for providers of type A and B, respectively; for a linear model, $e_{ijk} \mid u_j, v_k \tilde{N}\left(0, \sigma_e^2\right)$ are residual error terms. This model can be extended to accommodate the two alternative scenarios described above.

Assuming equal cluster sizes and independence between provider types, the ICC for this two-provider crossed design is

$$\rho = \frac{\sigma_u^2 + \sigma_v^2}{\sigma_u^2 + \sigma_v^2 + \sigma_e^2}. \tag{9}$$

When the two providers are not independent, resulting in correlated random effects ($\sigma_{uv} = r\sigma_u\sigma_v$), the ICC can be written as

$$\rho = \frac{\sigma_u^2 + \sigma_v^2 + 2\sigma_{uv}}{\sigma_u^2 + \sigma_v^2 + 2\sigma_{uv} + \sigma_e^2}. \tag{10}$$

In this case of two correlated random components, the ICC requires three variance and one covariance components; if further random effects components were to be accommodated, the number of terms in the models and the complexity of the interrelationships between components would increase. Therefore, investigation of crossed components should focus on a small number of components that have been identified as most important during trial design.

When designing complex intervention trials, it is essential to have a clear understanding of the different components of variation and how these affect the treatment effect estimates. For interventions with several components, high-level interactions between fixed and random effects are difficult to robustly estimate. Our recommendation is to rank components according to the level of clustering in the primary outcome(s) and investigate them in a stepwise manner (Papachristofi et al. 2016b)

A generalization of the cross-classified model is the multiple membership multiple classification (MMMC) model, which considers a second random component that operates across several elements of the first (see Fig. 2d). An example of this would be a surgical intervention that requires more than one surgeon to be involved, or a psychological intervention provided by more than one therapist, say in a group session. Each provider might work with a number of other providers during the trial. Details of these models can be found in Browne et al. (2001).

Cluster Randomized Trials

The parallel cluster randomized controlled trial (CRCT) is an established design for evaluating interventions that are either randomized to all patients within a predefined group (cluster) or where the intervention is delivered at a group level (Eldridge and Kerry 2012). Examples include trials involving care of dementia patients (Surr et al. 2016), primary care (Emery et al. 2017), and hospitals where interventions are applied to individual wards or clinics (Erasmus et al. 2011). CRCTs are also an attractive option when individuals within the same geographical or clinical area can access information from other trial participants, so that individual randomization may lead to contamination of treatment effects. For example, patients attending the same clinic may share educational resources or coping strategies from a multi-component intervention, despite being assigned to different treatment arms.

In the simplest CRCT, assuming common cluster size m, the statistical model for patient i, $i = 1, \ldots, m$ in cluster j, $j = 1, \ldots, c$, with x_j the categorical covariate representing treatment allocation for cluster j, can be specified as follows:

$$g^{-1}\left(E\left[y_{ij}\right]\right) = \beta_0 + \beta_1 x_j + u_j \tag{11}$$

where y_{ij} is a measure of outcome, g is an appropriate link function, and $u_j\tilde{N}\left(0, \sigma_u^2\right)$ are the cluster-specific random effects; for a linear model, $e_{ij} \mid u_j\tilde{N}\left(0, \sigma_e^2\right)$ are residual error terms. In this model, all patients in a cluster receive the same treatment, and the treatment effect is common across clusters. Note that further patient- or cluster-specific covariates have been omitted for clarity, although it is straightforward to include them in these models; generalized linear models are again used for illustration, but methods for clustered time-to-event outcomes are also available.

Model (11) reflects a trial in which the outcome is assessed at the individual participant level, but the same framework (with a suitable link function and error structure) can accommodate cluster-level outcomes, which are common in CRCTs. For example, the model in (11) is appropriate if hospitals as a whole are randomized to active treatment or control, but outcomes are assessed for each patient, perhaps so that patient-level covariates can be adjusted for. Alternatively, analysis could be based on hospital-level outcomes, such as the proportion of patients per cluster that have a successful outcome. These aggregated outcomes can be considered independent and analyzed using standard statistical methods, with the outcomes weighted by their precision or the number of cases within each cluster. While this approach results in a simple analysis, it does not allow for inclusion of patient-level covariates and thus may be less efficient than an individual patient data analysis. The associated ICC is identical to the *simple ICC* for the two-level hierarchical model in Eq. (3).

Stepped-Wedge Designs

An alternative type of CRCT that is gaining in popularity is the stepped-wedge design (SWD). In this design, all clusters of patients begin in the control group. A proportion of clusters is then randomized to the experimental treatment arm at the end of each of a number of predetermined time periods, that is, in *steps*, until all clusters are in the experimental intervention arm in the final time period (see Fig. 3) (Brown and Lilford 2006). The first period is often used to collect baseline data, and the time period at which a cluster commences the experimental intervention is determined at random. The most commonly reported SWD trials are cross-sectional,

Time period

Step	1	2	3	4	5	6
1						
2						
3						
4						
5						

Fig. 3 Illustration of a stepped-wedge cluster randomized trial. Each cell represents a cluster, and each time period after the first cell represents a step. Darker cells indicate clusters having the experimental treatment, and lighter cells represent control clusters

in that new patients are recruited in each time period, and even though they may be followed up over time for an event, the outcome is analyzed according to the period of recruitment (e.g., see the FIT trial of hand hygiene compliance (Fuller et al. 2012)). An alternative, but less frequently used, design is the cohort SWD, in which all patients are recruited in the first period and followed throughout the trial, with a proportion of the patient clusters randomized to switch to the active intervention at the end of each period. For example, Jordan et al. (2015) conducted a trial in which dementia patients in care homes were switched to nurse-led prescribing of medications in a series of steps, until all patients were in the intervention arm.

The choice between the SWD and the traditional CRCT depends on the context and nature of the intervention. The SWD is particularly suited to service delivery or healthcare policy interventions, for which traditional CRCTs are logistically difficult to implement. However, as in the SWD all clusters are exposed to the active intervention by the end of the trial. It is more difficult to revert to the control treatment if the experimental intervention proves to be ineffective. Thus, the SWD is only appropriate if the intervention has negligible side effects and if it is considered very unlikely to be less effective than the standard of care. For example, it is difficult to imagine how provision of sterile hand wash could introduce substantial risk of side effects or an increase in infectious episodes.

Because SWD trials are conducted over a series of periods, they are not appropriate for interventions requiring long-term follow-up in order to establish an effect or when treatment effects vary over time.

Analysis for a SWD uses a model with random effects for clusters, and fixed effects for time periods, i.e., for patient i in cluster j at time period k:

$$g^{-1}\left(E\left[y_{ijk}\right]\right) = \beta_0 + \beta_1 x_{ijk} + \omega_k + u_j \tag{12}$$

where y_{ijk} is a measure of outcome, g an appropriate link function, x_{ijk} a categorical covariate representing treatment allocation, ω_k the effect of time period k, and $u_j \tilde{N}\left(0, \sigma_u^2\right)$ are the cluster-specific random effects; for a linear model, $e_{ijk} \mid u_j \tilde{N}\left(0, \sigma_e^2\right)$ are residual error terms.

Although the time period effects ω_k are not of interest in themselves, their inclusion in this model is important. On average there are more control clusters at the beginning of the trial and more intervention clusters toward the end. If the period effects are omitted from the model, any contextual or intervention changes over time will result in bias in treatment effect estimates (Hemming et al. 2018).

The simple model (12) further relies on a number of assumptions that require justification including

(i) A common period effect across clusters and treatment arms
(ii) Constant period effects within a period (no smooth changes across time)
(iii) A common treatment effect across clusters and periods

Analysts may consider additional exploratory analyses that relax these assumptions using strata (groups of clusters)-by-period interactions, strata-by-treatment interactions, and treatment-by- period interactions. Although such analyses are underpowered, and their results should be interpreted cautiously, they may identify major departures from the simple model's assumptions (Hemming et al. 2018).

The ICC for model (12) is identical to the *simple ICC* in (3) for the two-level hierarchical model.

Other designs that fit into the SWD framework have been published, including CRCTs where the clusters are observed in multiple periods (Ukoumunne and Thompson 2001) and cluster randomized crossover trials (Turner et al. 2007), but these are outside the scope of this chapter.

Sample Size Estimation for Trials with Clustering

The sample size for trial designs with clustering is affected both by the cluster size and the number of clusters. Methods for sample size estimation have been published for a wide range of individually randomized trials with clustering (Walwyn and Roberts 2010), CRCTs (Eldridge and Kerry 2012), and SWDs (Hemming and Taljaard 2016). The general principles and some simple calculations based on normally distributed random effects are provided in this section.

Typically, sample size estimation for trials with clustering involves calculation of a design effect (DE), used to inflate the sample size estimate from the corresponding trial design for independent, identically distributed outcomes; the simplest version is given below.

The standard sample size estimate n for each arm of an individually randomized parallel two-group trial, with 1:1 allocation ratio and a normally distributed outcome, is given by

$$n = \frac{\left(Z_{\alpha/2} + Z_{1-\beta}\right)^2 2\sigma_e^2}{\Delta^2}, \tag{13}$$

where Δ is the target mean difference in the outcome between the two arms, Z_p is the pth percentage point of the standard $Normal(0,\ 1)$ distribution, and α and β are type I and II error probabilities, respectively.

In a similar CRCT, where all patients in a cluster receive the same treatment, and the cluster size is fixed and known, the number of patients per arm n can be calculated using

$$n = \frac{\left(Z_{\alpha/2} + Z_{1-\beta}\right)^2 2\sigma_e^2}{\Delta^2} \left(1 + (m-1)\rho\right), \tag{14}$$

where m is the fixed cluster size and ρ the ICC; the DE term $(1 + (m - 1)\rho)$ is the inflation factor due to clustering (Donner et al. 1981). In this simple case, the number of clusters required per arm would be $c = n/m$. Note that the DE increases with the number of patients per cluster and the size of the ICC. For clusters of size 1 or ICC of zero (independence between clusters), the DE reduces to one, and the sample size formula reverts to that for the independent, identically distributed outcomes design. In general, keeping the number of clusters fixed and increasing the within-cluster sample size are not efficient, in that such a strategy will require more trial participants overall than if the number of clusters were to be increased.

When the cluster sizes are unequal, as it is the case for most trials, the DE relies on knowing the mean and coefficient of variation of cluster sizes and becomes

$$DE = \left(1 + \left(\overline{m}\left(1 + cv^2\right) - 1\right)\right)\rho, \qquad (15)$$

where $\overline{m}$ is the average cluster size and cv is the coefficient of variation for the cluster sizes (see, e.g., Eldridge et al. (2006)). The number of patients required per arm is larger than for the equal cluster size case and increases as the variability between the cluster sizes increases. The DE for unequal cluster sizes given in Eq. (15) is the most commonly used; Eldridge et al. (2006) provide alternative formulations and further discussion.

Note that the above inflation factors can be applied to any sample size calculations for which the treatment effect is estimated from a generalized linear model; for example, Δ in Eq. (14) may represent the log odds ratio or log rate ratio for the treatment effect, with appropriate values for σ_e^2.

Advocates of SWD have argued that the additional time periods involved render them more efficient than parallel CRCTs, requiring fewer patients (Woertman et al. 2013). However, this does not appear to be true in all cases, with the relative efficiency of the two approaches dependent on design parameters such as the ICC, the size and number of clusters, and the number of periods (Hemming and Taljaard 2016).

Assuming that the number of time periods (steps) s, and the cluster size m have been fixed, the DE for a simple SWD has been derived as

$$DE = (s+1)\frac{1 + \rho(sm + m - 1)}{1 + \rho(sm/2 + m - 1)} \times \frac{3s(1-\rho)}{2(s^2 - 1)}. \qquad (16)$$

The sample size needed per time period can be obtained by equating this with the total sample size for a SWD ($m(s+1)c$) and solving a quadratic equation (Hemming and Taljaard 2016). Close inspection of the DE shows that this will be most efficient with large numbers of time periods, or steps, and small numbers of clusters at each step.

Model Fitting and Analysis

All models described in this chapter can be implemented in standard statistical software such as R, Stata, and SAS. Fitting requires integration over random effects distributions, which is exact if the response is normally distributed, but requires approximate methods for generalized linear and other more complex models. Papachristofi et al. provide an overview of available methods and their limitations, with detailed referencing (Papachristofi et al. 2016b).

Adaptive Gauss-Hermite quadrature has been shown to yield more accurate estimates than other approximate methods and to perform well even in the case of large clusters and high ICCs; however, it is slower than other methods (Rabe-Hesketh and Skrondal 2012). It is implemented in Stata (*gllamm* procedure) (Rabe-Hesketh and Skrondal 2012) and R (*lme4* package) (Austin 2010). Marginal (MQL) and penalized quasi-likelihood (PQL) are implemented in the general-purpose multilevel modeling software MLwiN and use a Taylor expansion approximation to transform nonlinear models. MQL is a quicker algorithm but tends to underestimate random effects terms. PQL is not suitable for cases combining small clusters with large ICCs and does not employ likelihood-based methods, so that likelihood-ratio tests and information criteria cannot be used (Goldstein and Rasbash 1996).

The restricted maximum likelihood (REML) approach involves maximizing a likelihood form based on a transformation of the data, in order to remove the effects of nuisance parameters. This method is unbiased for generalized linear models unless the random effects variance is very small (Rabe-Hesketh and Skrondal 2012).

Small numbers of clusters or clusters of small size may lead to poor estimation of variance components, and all likelihood-based approaches may encounter convergence problems in these cases. The minimum number of clusters, as well as patients per cluster, to ensure robust estimation of multilevel models has been widely studied. The literature suggests that at least ten clusters per arm will allow unbiased estimation of treatment effects, provided that the number of patients per cluster is not too small (<5) (see Papachristofi et al. and references therein for an overview (Papachristofi et al. 2016b)). Nevertheless, the decision on the model structure will depend on the context of the trial and its specific constraints.

Reporting

As the popularity of complex interventions has grown, so has the number of documents that guides the conduct and reporting of trials evaluating them. The CReDECI guidelines provide criteria for reporting the development phases of a complex intervention, including ways in which it was altered during initial testing, as well as its piloting and evaluation (Mohler et al. 2015). CReDECI aims to encompass both qualitative and quantitative research designs so that the guidelines are quite general. The TIDieR guide for the reporting of complex interventions recommends a 12-point checklist for describing the intervention itself (Hoffmann et al. 2014). Additionally, the Consolidated Standards of Reporting Trials (CONSORT) group have published extensions of their original reporting guidance (Moher et al. 2010) covering CRCTs (Campbell et al. 2012) and abstracts for non-pharmacological interventions (Boutron et al. 2017). These freely accessible tools are helpful to guide initial trial design and contribute to improvements in research reporting.

Implementation

A key element of the MRC framework for evaluation of complex interventions is the implementation of a successful treatment into routine healthcare (Medical_Research_Council. 2008). As complex interventions are often fully embedded in the healthcare setting they are intended for, and are evaluated using pragmatic trial designs (Loudon et al. 2013), generalization of results should be straightforward compared with more tightly controlled efficacy trials. The MRC guidance recommends a reporting style for trials that is accessible to healthcare decision-makers; quantitative (statistical) methods alone are unlikely to be sufficient for successful implementation. First, an understanding of the behaviors that need to change for a successful treatment to enter routine practice, including barriers and facilitators of change, is required. This information must be elicited in a formal qualitative study alongside the randomized phase III evaluation. Since the economic burden of the intervention implementation is a key driver of behavioral change, complex intervention trials should include an assessment of the costs and effects of the intervention for health providers and other related services (Drummond et al. 2015). Post trial evaluation, a monitoring phase is recommended to assess whether benefits and harms observed in the trial manifest similarly in routine practice (Medical_Research_Council. 2008). Details of these methods can be found in the review by Richard and Hallberg and references therein (Richards and Hallberg 2015).

Summary and Conclusion

Interest in complex interventions has grown substantially in recent years. They are characterized by multicomponent treatment packages and clustering due to specific components, such as the provider and implementation setting, which cannot be separated from the package of treatment and have an influence on the outcome of treatment. Development of complex interventions is a multidiscipline endeavor and requires a mixture of rigorous qualitative and quantitative methods. Although research on feasibility, piloting, and early phase trials is sparse, there are well-established methods for phase III trials of multicomponent interventions that involve clustering. The most commonly used methods are individually randomized trials with random effects for clusters, cluster randomized trials, and, more recently, stepped-wedge cluster randomized trials. Sample size estimation methods exist for a range of designs. With careful attention to the correlation structure induced by the chosen design, results can be analyzed in standard statistical software. Post-trial implementation in routine practice will depend on statistical, economic, qualitative, and behavioral analysis.

Key Facts

- Complex interventions typically have multiple components and are subject to clustering of patient outcomes.

- Both qualitative and quantitative methods are required in the development and evaluation of complex interventions.
- Timing of the definitive evaluation of a complex intervention needs careful consideration, taking into account its stage of development and treatment equipoise of both patients and healthcare providers.
- Complex interventions are usually evaluated in pragmatic trials since they are often embedded in the healthcare context they are intended for.
- A range of well-established trial designs for complex interventions are available, including clustered individually randomized trials, cluster randomized trials, and stepped-wedge designs.
- With careful definition of the correlation structure resulting from their design, trials can typically be analyzed using standard statistical software packages.

Cross-References

▶ Cluster Randomized Trials
▶ Power and Sample Size

References

Austin PC (2010) Estimating multilevel logistic regression models when the number of clusters is low: a comparison of different statistical software procedures. Int J Biostat 6

Blencowe NS, Brown JM, Cook JA, Metcalfe C, Morton DG, Nicholl J, Sharples LD, Treweek S, Blazeby JM, Members of the, M. R. C. H. F. T. M. R. N. W (2015) Interventions in randomised controlled trials in surgery: issues to consider during trial design. Trials 16:392

Blencowe NS, Mills N, Cook JA, Donovan JL, Rogers CA, Whiting P, Blazeby JM (2016) Standardizing and monitoring the delivery of surgical interventions in randomized clinical trials. Br J Surg 103:1377–1384

Boutron I, Altman DG, Moher D, Schulz KF, Ravaud P, Group, C. N (2017) CONSORT Statement for randomized trials of nonpharmacologic treatments: a 2017 update and a CONSORT extension for nonpharmacologic trial abstracts. Ann Intern Med 167:40–47

Brown CA, Lilford RJ (2006) The stepped wedge trial design: a systematic review. BMC Med Res Methodol 6:54

Browne WJ, Goldstein H, Rasbash J (2001) Multiple membership multiple classification (MMMC) models. Stat Model 1:103–124

Campbell MK, Piaggio G, Elbourne DR, Altman DG, Group, C (2012) Consort 2010 statement: extension to cluster randomised trials. BMJ 345:e5661

Cisse MBM, Sangare D, Oxborough RM, Dicko A, Dengela D, Sadou A, Mihigo J, George K, Norris L, Fornadel C (2017) A village level cluster-randomized entomological evaluation of combination long-lasting insecticidal nets containing pyrethroid plus PBO synergist in Southern Mali. Malar J 16:477

Collins LM, Murphy SA, Strecher V (2007) The multiphase optimization strategy (MOST) and the sequential multiple assignment randomized trial (SMART): new methods for more potent eHealth interventions. Am J Prev Med 32:S112–S118

Cook JA, Ramsay CR, Fayers P (2004) Statistical evaluation of learning curve effects in surgical trials. Clin Trials 1:421–427

Dickens C, Katon W, Blakemore A, Khara A, Tomenson B, Woodcock A, Fryer A, Guthrie E (2014) Complex interventions that reduce urgent care use in COPD: a systematic review with meta-regression. Respir Med 108:426–437
Donner A, Birkett N, Buck C (1981) Randomization by cluster. Sample size requirements and analysis. Am J Epidemiol 114:19
Drummond MF, Sculpher MJ, Claxton K, Stoddart GL, Torrance GW (2015) Methods for the economic evaluation of health care programmes, 4th edn. University Press, Oxford
Eldridge S, Kerry S (2012) A practical guide to cluster randomised trials in health services research. Wiley, Chichester
Eldridge SM, Ashby D, Kerry S (2006) Sample size for cluster randomized trials: effect of coefficient of variation of cluster size and analysis method. Int J Epidemiol 35:1292–1300
Emery JD, Gray V, Walter FM, Cheetham S, Croager EJ, Slevin T, Saunders C, Threlfall T, Auret K, Nowak AK, Geelhoed E, Bulsara M, Holman CDJ (2017) The Improving Rural Cancer Outcomes Trial: a cluster-randomised controlled trial of a complex intervention to reduce time to diagnosis in rural cancer patients in Western Australia. Br J Cancer 117:1459–1469
Erasmus V, Huis A, Oenema A, Van Empelen P, Boog MC, Van Beeck EH, Polinder S, Steyerberg EW, Richardus JH, Vos MC, Van Beeck EF (2011) The ACCOMPLISH study. A cluster randomised trial on the cost-effectiveness of a multicomponent intervention to improve hand hygiene compliance and reduce healthcare associated infections. BMC Public Health 11:721
Fuller C, Michie S, Savage J, Mcateer J, Besser S, Charlett A, Hayward A, Cookson BD, Cooper BS, Duckworth G, Jeanes A, Roberts J, Teare L, Stone S (2012) The Feedback Intervention Trial (FIT)–improving hand-hygiene compliance in UK healthcare workers: a stepped wedge cluster randomised controlled trial. PLoS One 7:e41617
Goldstein H, Rasbash J (1996) Improved approximations for multilevel models with binary responses. J R Stat Soc Ser A-Stat Soc 159:505–513
Hemming K, Taljaard M (2016) Sample size calculations for stepped wedge and cluster randomised trials: a unified approach. J Clin Epidemiol 69:137–146
Hemming K, Taljaard M, Forbes A (2018) Modeling clustering and treatment effect heterogeneity in parallel and stepped-wedge cluster randomized trials. Stat Med 37:883–898
Hoffmann TC, Glasziou PP, Boutron I, Milne R, Perera R, Moher D, Altman DG, Barbour V, Macdonald H, Johnston M, Lamb SE, Dixon-Woods M, Mcculloch P, Wyatt JC, Chan AW, Michie S (2014) Better reporting of interventions: template for intervention description and replication (TIDieR) checklist and guide. BMJ 348:g1687
Jordan S, Gabe-Walters ME, Watkins A, Humphreys I, Newson L, Snelgrove S, Dennis MS (2015) Nurse-led medicines' monitoring for patients with dementia in care homes: a pragmatic cohort stepped wedge cluster randomised trial. PLoS One 10:e0140203
Kahan BC, Morris TP (2013) Assessing potential sources of clustering in individually randomised trials. BMC Med Res Methodol 13:58
Loudon K, Zwarenstein M, Sullivan F, Donnan P, Treweek S (2013) Making clinical trials more relevant: improving and validating the PRECIS tool for matching trial design decisions to trial purpose. Trials 14:115
Mars T, Ellard D, Carnes D, Homer K, Underwood M, Taylor SJ (2013) Fidelity in complex behaviour change interventions: a standardised approach to evaluate intervention integrity. BMJ Open 3:e003555
Mcculloch P, Altman DG, Campbell WB, Flum DR, Glasziou P, Marshall JC, Nicholl J, Balliol C, Aronson JK, Barkun JS, Blazeby JM, Boutron IC, Campbell WB, Clavien PA, Cook JA, Ergina PL, Feldman LS, Flum DR, Maddern GJ, Nicholl J, Reeves BC, Seiler CM, Strasberg SM, Meakins JL, Ashby D, Black N, Bunker J, Burton M, Campbell M, Chalkidou K, Chalmers I, De Leval M, Deeks J, Ergina PL, Grant A, Gray M, Greenhalgh R, Jenicek M, Kehoe S, Lilford R, Littlejohns P, Loke Y, Madhock R, Mcpherson K, Meakins J, Rothwell P, Summerskill B, Taggart D, Tekkis P, Thompson M, Treasure T, Trohler U, Vandenbroucke J (2009) No surgical innovation without evaluation: the IDEAL recommendations. Lancet 374:1105–1112
Medical_Research_Council (2000) A framework for the development and evaluation of RCTs for complex interventions to improve health

Medical_Research_Council (2008) Developing and evaluating complex interventions: new guidance
Moher D, Hopewell S, Schulz KF, Montori V, Gotzsche PC, Devereaux PJ, Elbourne D, Egger M, Altman DG, Consolidated Standards of Reporting Trials, G (2010) CONSORT 2010 explanation and elaboration: updated guidelines for reporting parallel group randomised trials. J Clin Epidemiol 63:e1–e37
Mohler R, Kopke S, Meyer G (2015) Criteria for Reporting the Development and Evaluation of Complex Interventions in healthcare: revised guideline (CReDECI 2). Trials 16:204
Mohr DC, Carmody T, Erickson L, Jin L, Leader J (2011) Telephone-administered cognitive behavioral therapy for veterans served by community-based outpatient clinics. J Consult Clin Psychol 79:261–265
Papachristofi O, Jenkins D, Sharples LD (2016a) Assessment of learning curves in complex surgical interventions: a consecutive case-series study. Trials 17:266
Papachristofi O, Klein A, Sharples L (2016b) Evaluation of the effects of multiple providers in complex surgical interventions. Stat Med 35:5222–5246
Perez MC, Minoyan N, Ridde V, Sylvestre MP, Johri M (2018) Comparison of registered and published intervention fidelity assessment in cluster randomised trials of public health interventions in low- and middle-income countries: systematic review. Trials 19:410
Pocock SJ (1983) Clinical trials: a practical approach. Wiley, Chichester
Rabe-Hesketh S and Skrondal A (2012) Mulilevel and longitudinal modelling using Stata. Stata Press, Texas
Richards DA, Hallberg IR (2015) Complex interventions in health. Routledge, Oxford
Richardson E, Redden DT (2014) Moving towards multiple site outcomes in spinal cord injury pain clinical trials: an issue of clustered observations in trial design and analysis. J Spinal Cord Med 37:278–287
Roberts C, Walwyn R (2013) Design and analysis of non-pharmacological treatment trials with multiple therapists per patient. Stat Med 32:81–98
Sharples L, Everett C, Singh J, Mills C, Spyt T, Abu-Omar Y, Fynn S, Thorpe B, Stoneman V, Goddard H, Fox-Rushby J, Nashef S (2018) Amaze: a double-blind, multicentre randomised controlled trial to investigate the clinical effectiveness and cost-effectiveness of adding an ablation device-based maze procedure as an adjunct to routine cardiac surgery for patients with pre-existing atrial fibrillation. Health Technol Assess 22:1–132
Surr CA, Walwyn RE, Lilley-Kelly A, Cicero R, Meads D, Ballard C, Burton K, Chenoweth L, Corbett A, Creese B, Downs M, Farrin AJ, Fossey J, Garrod L, Graham EH, Griffiths A, Holloway I, Jones S, Malik B, Siddiqi N, Robinson L, Stokes G, Wallace D (2016) Evaluating the effectiveness and cost-effectiveness of Dementia Care Mapping to enable person-centred care for people with dementia and their carers (DCM-EPIC) in care homes: study protocol for a randomised controlled trial. Trials 17:300
Turner RM, White IR, Croudace T, Group, P. I. P. S (2007) Analysis of cluster randomized cross-over trial data: a comparison of methods. Stat Med 26:274–289
Ukoumunne OC, Thompson SG (2001) Analysis of cluster randomized trials with repeated cross-sectional binary measurements. Stat Med 20:417–433
Walwyn R, Roberts C (2010) Therapist variation within randomised trials of psychotherapy: implications for precision, internal and external validity. Stat Methods Med Res 19:291–315
Walwyn R, Roberts C (2017) Meta-analysis of standardised mean differences from randomised trials with treatment-related clustering associated with care providers. Stat Med 36:1043–1067
Wilson DT, Walwyn RE, Brown J, Farrin AJ, Brown SR (2016) Statistical challenges in assessing potential efficacy of complex interventions in pilot or feasibility studies. Stat Methods Med Res 25:997–1009
Woertman W, De Hoop E, Moerbeek M, Zuidema SU, Gerritsen DL, Teerenstra S (2013) Stepped wedge designs could reduce the required sample size in cluster randomized trials. J Clin Epidemiol 66:752–758
Yuen WW, Wong WC, Tang CS, Holroyd E, Tiwari AF, Fong DY, Chin WY (2013) Evaluating the effectiveness of personal resilience and enrichment programme (PREP) for HIV prevention among female sex workers: a randomised controlled trial. BMC Public Health 13:683

Randomized Discontinuation Trials

75

Valerii V. Fedorov

Contents

Abstract

Randomized discontinuation trials are usually considered as a special case of population enrichment trials. Most often they consist of a few stages with the early ones targeting the selection of a subpopulation that responds or may respond to an experimental treatment and allowing an early escape of patients doing poorly. The succeeding stages validate the treatment's superiority to placebo or more generally to a comparator for the selected (enriched with potential responders) subpopulation. The approach increases the trial feasibility and the chances of correct response-to-treatment detection, often at the expense of decreased ability to extrapolate results over the initially targeted population. The first randomized discontinuation trials were used exclusively to test long-term, non-curative therapies for chronic or slow evolving diseases. The development of stochastic longitudinal models combined with Bayesian ideas and

V. V. Fedorov (✉)
ICON, North Wales, PA, USA

© Springer Nature Switzerland AG 2022

S. Piantadosi, C. L. Meinert (eds.), *Principles and Practice of Clinical Trials*,
https://doi.org/10.1007/978-3-319-52636-2_104

the increase of computing power led to their acceptance in various therapeutic areas, most notably in oncology. If the statistically valid partitioning of the source population is proven, then it might be viewed as evidence of the existence of some classifiers and pave the road to precision medicine.

Keywords

Enrichment trials · Population enrichment · Randomized discontinuation trials · Screening · Subpopulation selection

Introduction

The basic idea of ***randomized discontinuation trials*** (RDTs) can be traced back to the 1970s when Amery and Dony (1975) proposed the trial design (see Fig. 1) that consists of an open-label stage with all patients exposed to the experimental treatment, while at the second stage, all responders are randomized to placebo or an experimental treatment arm. They showed that under rather mild assumptions, such designs reduce patients' exposure to placebo and mitigate the impact of placebo responders on drug efficacy evaluation. Initially, RDTs were intended for chronic and slow progressing diseases such as various types of angina, psychiatric disorders, early stages of Parkinson's and Alzheimer's diseases, pain mitigation, and

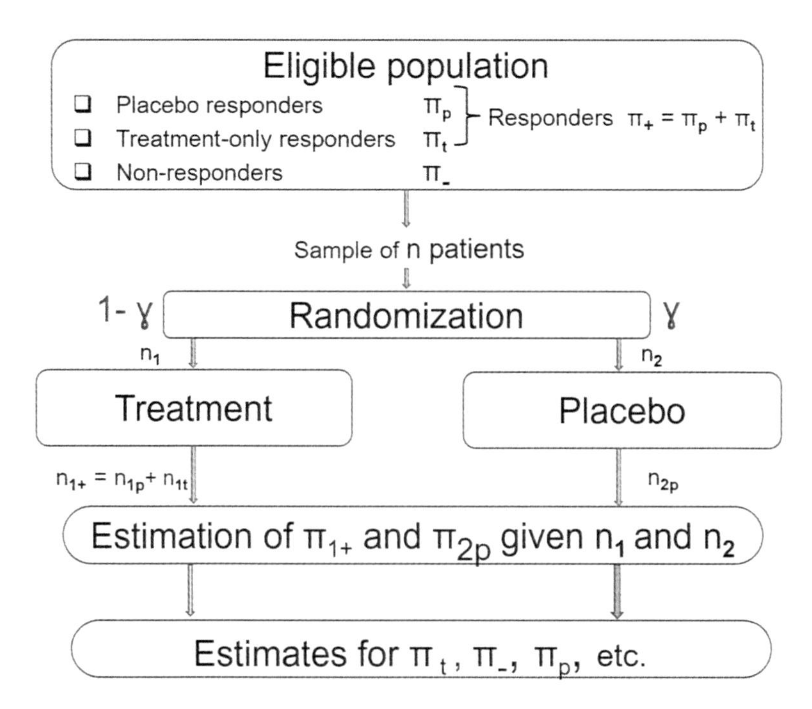

Fig. 1 Conventional two-arm design of a randomized clinical trial

hypertension treatments. Rather detailed descriptions of early examples can be found in Chiron et al. (1996), Temple (1994), Fava et al. (2003), and FDA Guidance for Industry (2019b). Among these, the trial for the validation of nifedipine as a treatment of vasospastic angina was the first one to be accepted (in 1980) by the FDA, see Temple (1994). The use of stochastic longitudinal models combined with Bayesian techniques led to the increasing popularity of RDT in other therapeutic areas, most notably in oncology, for cases when a reliable assay for selection of sensitive patients is not available (Freidlin and Simon 2005; Korn et al. 2001; Ratain et al. 2006; Rosner et al. 2002; Stadler et al. 2005; Trippa et al. 2012). In 2008, Daugherty et al. (2008) mentioned that at least two oncology studies had been completed using RDT, one with sorafenib (a positive trial) and one with carboxyaminoimidazole (a negative trial). Numerous references to the recent randomized discontinuation/withdrawal trials in various therapeutic areas can be found in the FDA Guidance for Industry (2019b) and directly on the FDA WEB site. So far the terminology is not well established, and in the publications, "RDT designs" may appear as "enrichment/re-randomization designs, postdosed designs, pre-admission qualification designs, randomized withdrawal designs, randomized relapse designs and randomized maintenance designs," cf. Grieve (2012). These variations suggest, that the purposes of the trials and their clinical settings may be quite different.

Typically, the design of an RDT relies on the following assumptions:

- The experimental treatment will not cure the condition during the open-label stage.
- The treatment effect(s) of the open-label stage will not be carried over to the second stage. This assumption can be satisfied with adding a washout period between the two stages if it is ethically admissible.
- Following Amery and Dony (1975), most publications assume that a treatment effect is binary: either there is or there is not a response to treatment. Respectively, the patients are labeled as either responders or nonresponders.

The later versions of RDT designs use slightly modified assumptions. For instance, instead of "responders and non-responders," one may consider patients with "positive response, stable disease, and negative response," or instead of stable tumor size, one may consider a stationary tumor growth rate. The introduction of longitudinal models as in Trippa et al. (2012) is a crucial part of the successful design of such RDT. The list of different settings can be continued but in all of them there are two major steps: population enrichment and treatment validation for the enriched subpopulation.

Often, the observed responses to treatment may be continuous (e.g., blood pressure, duration of anginal pain), discrete (e.g., frequency of angina), or ordinal (e.g., various scores in pain studies). Their dichotomization may lead to a significant information loss, see Fedorov, Mannino, and Zhang (2008), Uryniak et al. (2011), and may be questionable when it is based solely on "investigator's judgment of success," see Temple (1994). To minimize the impact of dichotomization, one can use dichotomized data only to guide patient assignment to different treatment arms and perform the final statistical analysis using original, non-dichotomized data.

Capra (2004) compared the power of RDT with that of RCT when the primary endpoint is time-to-disease progression. Kopec et al. (1993) evaluated the utility and efficiency of RDT when the endpoints are binary. They compared the relative sample size required for a fixed power of RDT versus RCT under different scenarios and parameter settings. The approaches are based on the outcomes solely from the second stage, treating the open-label stage as a screening process. This simplifies the statistical analysis, but the information contained in the open-label stage is mostly wasted. Examples when the statistical analysis includes the information from both the open-label and the treatment validation stages can be found in Fedorov and Liu (2005, 2014), and Ivanova, Qaqish, and Schoenfeld (2010).

The next section presents the statistical aspects of the Amery-Dony design (AD design) and its symmetric version, complimented with their comparison to conventional randomized trial designs. Both types of AD designs are very basic versions of RDT designs. However, their consideration allows illumination and discussion of major properties that are common across all RDT designs published so far, and/or currently used in clinical trials. Section "Clinical Applicability" will address the major concerns associated with RDT implementation in medical practice.

Example: AD Design Versus Two-Arm RCT

Let the eligible population consist of three basic subpopulations: ***treatment-only responders, placebo responders***, and ***nonresponders***, and let their fractions be π_t, π_p, and $\pi_- = 1 - \pi_t - \pi_p$, respectively. The variances of estimated π_t and of the ratio $R = \pi_p/\pi_+$, where $\pi_+ = \pi_t + \pi_p$ is a fraction of all responders, will be used to compare statistical efficiency of various trial designs. All trials considered here start with sampling (enrolling, accruing) n patients from the eligible population. For convenience, the major notations are repeated in Figs. 1, 2, and 3.

Notations and Major Assumptions

If the assumption of random sampling holds, then the following working model is used:

- There exist infinitely many eligible patients of three mutually exclusive types: treatment-only responders, placebo responders, and nonresponders.
- At each draw, the probabilities that a sampled patient belongs to one of these categories are π_t, π_p and $\pi_- = 1 - \pi_t - \pi_p$ respectively.
- An experiment consists of n random drawings with $n = n_t + n_p + n_-$, where n_t, n_p, and $n_- = n - n_t - n_p$ are numbers of treatment-only responders, placebo responders, and nonresponders. In what follows, the triplet $\{n, n_t, n_p\}$ will be called the "*complete data set.*"

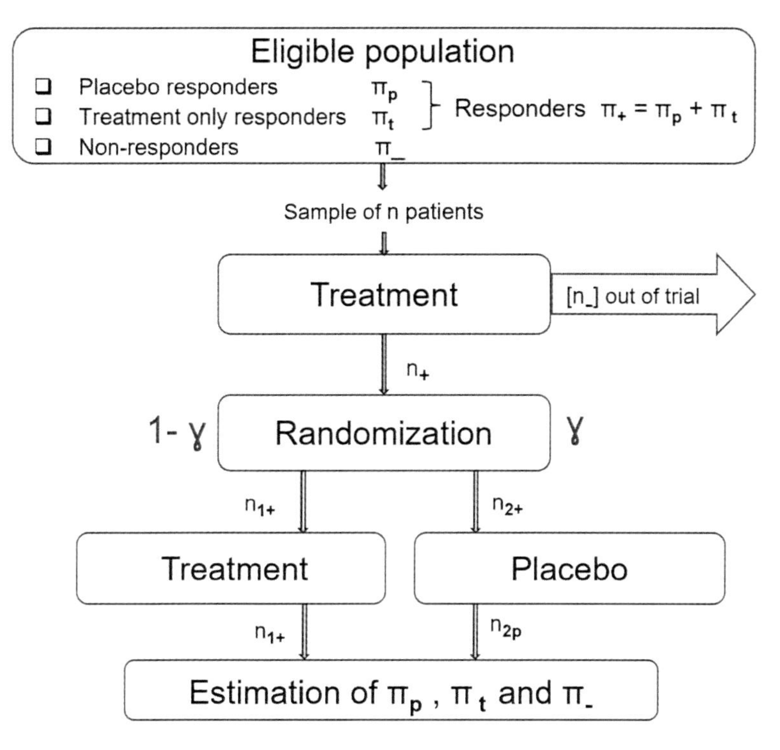

Fig. 2 Amery-Dony trial design

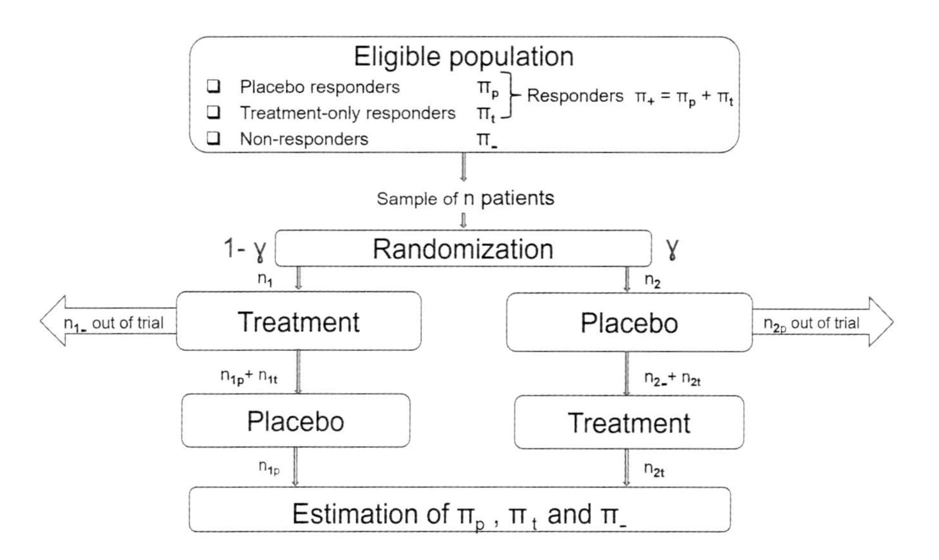

Fig. 3 Symmetric AD-design

- The sampled n_t, n_p, n_- have a trinomial distribution, see Chap. 35, Johnson, Kotz, and Balakrishnan (1997), with parameters (n, π_t, π_p, π_-).

If n_t and n_p are known ***exactly,*** then the ***maximum likelihood estimators*** (MLE) of π_t, π_p, and π_- are very simple and readily available, cf. Chap. 35.6, Johnson, Kotz, and Balakrishnan (1997):

$$\widehat{\pi}_t = \frac{n_t}{n}, \widehat{\pi}_p = \frac{n_p}{n}, \widehat{\pi}_- = \frac{1 - n_t - n_p}{n}. \tag{1}$$

The variance-covariance matrix of the first two (the third one π_- is their linear combination):

$$\mathrm{Var}\left(\widehat{\pi}_t, \widehat{\pi}_p\right) = \frac{1}{n}\begin{pmatrix} \pi_t(1-\pi_t) & -\pi_t\pi_p \\ -\pi_t\pi_p & \pi_p\left(1-\pi_p\right) \end{pmatrix}. \tag{2}$$

Given n, this matrix provides the lower bounds for the variances of any estimators of π_t, π_p, or any function of them. The latter is often called the "estimand" (cf. FDA Guidance for Industry 2019a).

If the function of interest $\psi(\pi)$, $\pi = (\pi_t, \pi_p)^{\mathrm{T}}$, is smooth enough, then the variance of its MLE $\widehat{\psi} = \psi\left(\widehat{\pi}_t, \widehat{\pi}_p\right)$ is

$$\mathrm{Var}[\widehat{\psi}] \simeq \frac{\partial \psi}{\partial \pi^{\mathrm{T}}} \mathrm{Var}(\widehat{\pi}) \frac{\partial \psi}{\partial \pi}. \tag{3}$$

For a linear function ψ, formula (3) is exact. Otherwise, it is valid asymptotically when $n \Rightarrow \infty$. For a reasonably large sample size n and moderate π_t and π_p, formula (3) serves as a good approximation and is often dubbed the "delta rule" or "delta method," cf. Oehlert (1992). For the two popular cases $\psi(\pi) = \pi_t + \pi_p = \pi_+$ and $\psi(\pi) = \pi_t/(\pi_t + \pi_p) = R_t$, the delta method readily provides that

$$\mathrm{Var}[\widehat{\pi}_+] = \frac{\pi_+(1-\pi_+)}{n} \quad \text{and} \quad \mathrm{Var}\left[\widehat{R}_t\right] = \frac{R_t(1-R_t)}{n\left(\pi_t + \pi_p\right)}. \tag{4}$$

Formulae (2), (3), and (4) will be used as benchmarks for the statistical efficiency of various trial designs when this is expressed in terms of variances or more generally covariance matrices of parameter estimators. It should be emphasized that these benchmarks are reachable when it is possible to extract the complete data set $\{n, n_t, n_p\}$ from the original data. In most cases, it is not.

Conventional Randomized Clinical Trial

The conventional two-arm RCT, see Fig. 1, is set up as follows. Suppose that n patients be randomly sampled from a legitimate population and out of them n_1 patients are randomized to the treatment arm and the rest $n_2 = n - n_1$ patients to the placebo arm.

Let n_{1+} and n_{2p} be the numbers of responders observed on the treatment arm and the placebo arm, respectively. Note that from these two outcomes, the ***exact*** values of n_t or n_p are not available and estimator (1) cannot be used. However, the MLE of π_+, π_p, and π_t together with their variances can be built using the observed n_{1+} and n_{2p}:

$$\widehat{\widehat{\pi}}_+ = \frac{n_{1+}}{n_1} \text{ and } \operatorname{Var}\left(\widehat{\widehat{\pi}}_+\right) = \frac{\pi_+(1-\pi_+)}{n_1}, \tag{5}$$

$$\widehat{\widehat{\pi}}_p = \frac{n_p}{n_2} \text{ and } \operatorname{Var}\left(\widehat{\widehat{\pi}}_p\right) = \frac{\pi_p(1-\pi_p)}{n_2}, \tag{6}$$

$$\widehat{\widehat{\pi}}_t = \widehat{\widehat{\pi}}_+ - \widehat{\widehat{\pi}}_p \text{ and } \operatorname{Var}\left(\widehat{\widehat{\pi}}_t\right) = \frac{\pi_+(1-\pi_+)}{n_1} + \frac{\pi_p(1-\pi_p)}{n_2}, \tag{7}$$

see notations in Fig. 1. As expected, the estimators presented in Eqs. (5), (6), and (7) have variances ***greater than the respective lower bounds (2) and (4) for any choice of*** n_1 ***and*** n_2, $n_1 + n_2 = n$. The validity of this statement for the first two is obvious. To verify the same statement for the treatment effect estimator $\widehat{\widehat{\pi}}_t$, one may use the following chain of inequalities:

$$\begin{aligned}\min_{n_1, n_2; n_1+n_2=n} \operatorname{Var}\left(\widehat{\widehat{\pi}}_t\right) &= \frac{1}{n}\left[\sqrt{\pi_+(1-\pi_+)} + \sqrt{\pi_p(1-\pi_p)}\right]^2 \\ &\geq \frac{1}{n}\left[\pi_+(1-\pi_+) + \pi_p(1-\pi_p)\right] \geq \frac{1}{n}\pi_t(1-\pi_t),\end{aligned} \tag{8}$$

where the optimal allocation ratio is $n_1^*/n_2^* = \sqrt{\pi_+(1-\pi_+)/\pi_p(1-\pi_p)}$, cf. Piantadosi (1997, Chap. 9.6). Note, that the lower bound $\pi_t(1 - \pi_t)/n$ is reached only when $\pi_p = 0$ and $n_1^* = n$, i.e., for a trial with all patients allocated to the treatment arm.

In a practical setting, the variance of the estimated fraction π_t of treatment responders significantly exceeds its lower bound $n^{-1}\pi_t(1 - \pi_t)$, especially in the presence of numerous placebo responders. This fact was a motivation for the development of trial designs that allow mitigation of the negative impact of placebo responders, on statistical properties of trials. Usually placebo responders and treatment nonresponders are withdrawn from the next trial stage to avoid their exposure to useless or harmful treatment(s).

Amery-Dony Design

In the Amery and Dony design (AD design) at the open-label stage, all qualified n patients are be assigned to the treatment arm, see Fig. 2. After completion of this stage, all nonresponders n_- leave the trial, while n_+ all responders, including placebo responders, are randomized between placebo and treatment arms. Let n_{1+} and $n_{2+} = n_+ - n_{1+}$ be the numbers of patients assigned to the treatment and placebo arms, respectively. It is assumed that one of the restricted randomization methods (for instance, randomization in blocks or an urn method, cf. Piantadosi (1997, Chap. 9.3) is applied to keep the ratio n_{2+}/n_{1+} as close as possible to the targeted allocation rates ratio $\gamma/(1-\gamma)$. Most statements/derivations that follow will use allocation rates ratio.

The results of the second stage are the number of placebo responders n_{2p} out of n_{2+} responders assigned to the placebo arm, the number of treatment-only responders $n_{2t} = n_{2+} - n_{2p}$, and the number of responders n_{1+} on the treatment arm, which is identical to the number of randomized patients n_{1+}, and does not provide any new information. Whence, the most informative, albeit not very ethical, AD design should be executed with $\gamma = 1$.

The straightforward application of the maximum likelihood method leads (cf. Fedorov and Liu 2014) to the following MLE of π_t:

$$\breve{\pi}_t = \frac{n_{2t}}{\gamma n} \text{ and } \mathrm{Var}(\breve{\pi}_t) = \frac{1}{n}\left[\pi_t(1-\pi_t) + \frac{1-\gamma}{\gamma}\frac{\pi_t\pi_p}{\pi_t+\pi_p}\right]. \tag{9}$$

The choice of γ defines the ***"learn-or-treat"*** aspects of the AD-design. It should be large enough to secure the validity of statistical inferences but not too large to violate ethical constraints by placing too many patients on the placebo arm. Note that for $\gamma = 1$, the variance defined in Eq. (9) coincides with its benchmark (Eq. 2), and it is always less than the variance of $\widehat{\widehat{\pi}}_t$ associated with any RCT design, see Eqs. (7) and (8). Interestingly, when $\gamma \geq 1/2$ the AD design is always superior to the conventional RCT with equal enrollment rates for treatment and placebo arms, i.e., the variances of the maximum likelihood estimators of π_t, π_p, R_t, etc. are lower for AD designs than for RCT designs.

Symmetric AD-Design

The analogy between RDT and cross-over designs opens the way to various modifications of RDT. For instance, similar to the conventional RCT, on the onset of the trial, patients can be randomized to two compound arms. The first one, ***treatment-placebo*** arm (TP arm), starts with the experimental treatment followed by discontinuation of nonresponders and by the placebo assignment for responders. The second one, the ***placebo-treatment*** arm (PT arm), starts with the placebo run-in followed with the discontinuation of placebo responders and by the experimental treatment assignment for the rest. See Fig. 3 for details and notations.

Unlike traditional cross-over design (cf. Piantadosi 1997, Chap. 16; Senn 1997, Chap. 17), the number of patients at the second stage is less than at the first stage: nonresponders leave the TP arm and placebo responders leave the PT arm. Under assumptions made in section "Notations and Major Assumptions," the withdrawal of patients (n_{1-} from the TP arm and n_{2p} from the PT arm) does not lead to any loss of information but improves the ethical profile of the respective clinical trials.

Let n_1 and n_2 patients be randomized to the TP and PT arms, respectively. As in the previous section, $n = n_p + n_t + n_-$ and only n is known before the trial. After the completion of the first stage, the numbers of nonresponders n_{1-} for the TP arm and the numbers of placebo responders n_{2p} for the PT arm will be known. These two groups leave the trial. All $n_{1+} = n_{1p} + n_{1t}$ responders to treatment are assigned to placebo and all $n_{2-} + n_{2t}$ placebo nonresponders are assigned to the experimental treatment. One can observe that

$$n_t = n_{1t} + n_{2t}, \quad n_p = n_{1p} + n_{2p}, \quad n_- = n_{1-} + n_{2-},$$

i.e., n, n_t, n_p, and n_- are known, and the MLE (Eq. 1) can be calculated:

$$\widehat{\pi}_t = \frac{n_{1t} + n_{2t}}{n_1 + n_2} = \frac{n_t}{n}, \quad \widehat{\pi}_p = \frac{n_{1p} + n_{2p}}{n_1 + n_2} = \frac{n_p}{n}, \quad \widehat{\pi}_- = \frac{n_{1-} + n_{2-}}{n_1 + n_2} = \frac{n_{1-}}{n}. \tag{10}$$

They have variances that coincide with their benchmark values, see Eq. (2). Whence, the symmetric AD design is always statistically superior to the conventional two-arm RCT design and to the original AD design except for the case with $\gamma = 1$. The symmetric AD-design assumes that all qualified patients are randomized to two compound arms (TP and PT) at the first stage, preserving most of the conventional RCT features related to blinding and operational integrity. Curiously enough the variances of all estimators in Eq. (10) do not depend on n_1, n_2, but only on the total number n of qualified patients. Consequently, a trialist may select any randomization rates to address ethical and operational constraints. This makes the symmetric AD designs very attractive.

There exist a few designs similar to the symmetric AD-design, for instance, the "sequential parallel comparison design" introduced in Fava et al. (2003). The major distinction is that in the latter treatment and placebo response rates may be different for stage 1 and 2. Otherwise, they are identical. The statistical properties of the sequential parallel comparison designs are extensively discussed in Ivanova, Qaqish, and Schoenfeld (2010) for binary responses, and with possible dropouts.

Sample Size Calculation

Required Variance

Given the sample size, the variances of estimated parameters (π_t, π_p, R_t, etc.) can be found using formulae (2), (3), (4), (5), (6), (7), (8), (9), and (10). The same equations allow calculation of sample sizes that are needed to reach a required variance V^* of the estimated parameters. For instance, for estimating π_t, the sample size is

$$n' = \frac{v'}{V^*} = \frac{1}{V^*}\left[\sqrt{\pi_+(1 - \pi_+)} + \sqrt{\pi_p(1 - \pi_p)}\right]^2, \tag{11}$$

for the optimized conventional trial design and

$$n'' = \frac{v''}{V^*} = \frac{1}{V^*}\pi_t(1 - \pi_t), \tag{12}$$

for the symmetric AD design, see Eq. (2) and comments to Eq. (10).

For an illustration, consider a toy scenario with the prior guesses for $\pi_t = 0.2$, $\pi_p = 0.2$, and the required $V^* = 0.044$, i.e., $\sqrt{V^*} = \pi_t/3$. From Eqs. (11) and (12) it follows that $v' = 0.79$, $v'' = 0.16$, and respectively $n' = 180$ and $n'' = 36$ (after rounding to the next integer).

The inverses of v' and v'' can be interpreted as the (Fisher) information values gained per one subject/observation, cf. Atkinson et al. (2014) and Fedorov (1972). Formulae (2), (3), (4), (8), and (9) provide v' and v'' for various designs and estimands by choosing $n = 1$. Note, that ratio n'/n'' depends only on v'/v'':

$$\frac{n'}{n''} = \frac{v'}{v''} = \frac{\left[\sqrt{\pi_+(1-\pi_+)} + \sqrt{\pi_p(1-\pi_p)}\right]^2}{\pi_t(1-\pi_t)} \tag{13}$$

and the design efficiency ordering is the same either in terms of variances given sample size or in terms of sample sizes given variance.

Hypotheses Testing

Let us consider testing of hypotheses and let

$$H_0 : \psi = \psi_0 \text{ and } H_A : \psi \geq \psi_A,$$

where ψ is a parameter/estimand of interest. Let α and β be the targeted type one and type two error rates, respectively. Under assumption of the asymptotic normality of estimators $\widehat{\psi}$ the required sample size for a one-sided test is

$$n \simeq v\left[\frac{Z_{1-\alpha} + Z_{1-\beta}}{\psi_A - \psi_0}\right]^2, \tag{14}$$

where, as before, v is the variance of a single observation, cf. Fedorov and Liu (2014). Let us continue with the previous example, i.e., with prior guesses $\pi_t = 0.2$, $\pi_p = 0.2$ and respectively with $v' = 0.79$ and $v'' = 0.16$. Let $\psi_0 = 0$, $\psi_A = \pi_t = 0.2$ and let $\alpha = 0.025$, $\beta = 0.1$, i.e., $Z_{1-\alpha} = 1.96$, $Z_{1-\beta} = 1.28$. Substituting all these numbers into Eq. (14) provides $n' = 208$ (the sample size for the optimized RCT design) and $n'' = 42$ (the sample size for the symmetric AD design). As in the previous subsection $n'/n'' = v'/v''$.

Clinical Applicability

Generalization of Results to the Source Population

The major concern over inferences generated by randomized discontinuation trials is their applicability to the originally targeted population. An immediate reaction to such a query is that no reasonable and scientifically sound response can be given until the ***estimands of prime interest*** and their estimators are carefully defined (cf. FDA Guidance for Industry 2019a).

For instance, if the fraction π_t of the total source population is the estimand of major interest, then the enrichment trial based on the symmetric AD design allows estimation of this quantity, see either Eq. (10) or (11). Both formulae use data from stages 1 and 2. The data from stage 2 are not sufficient to estimate π_t but the estimation of the subpopulation fraction of treatment responders $\phi_t = \pi_t/\pi_+$ is still possible. In general, the data from all stages of RDT provide information that allows scientific inferencing for the source population, often more precisely than from the RCT with the same sample size. Apparently, it is not true for the data collected from the enriched subpopulation only. The statement that RDT, like conventional RCT, may generate valid statistical inferences for the same estimands related to the source population is not equivalent to the statement that the respective estimates will be quantitatively and qualitatively close. RDT and CRT have different statistical and operational profiles. The respective estimators may have different statistical properties and different operational biases. The RCT designs were specifically developed to avoid disclosure of any information that may influence the behavior of either patients or trial staff, or both through careful randomization, double blinding, etc. to minimize operational bias (see Piantadosi 1997, Chap. 5.3; Pocock 1983, Chap. 4). At the same time, the RDT designs, which use open label run-in stages and interim analyses, are more prone to such biases, see examples in Freidlin, Korn, and Abrams (2018) and Kopec et al. (1993).

Ethical Aspects

The initial motivation for developing the RDT methodology was the very ethically sound intention to find "a clinical trial design avoiding undue placebo treatment," see Amery and Dony (1975). They managed to reduce the prolonged exposure of the patient(s) to placebo treatment, which is a typical ethical problem in conventional randomized clinical trials. Returning to Figs. 1 and 2, one can observe that with randomization rates equal for placebo and treatment arms, the total exposure times for RCT an RDT are $T_{RCT} = n/2 \times [\text{treatment duration}]_{RCT}$ and $T_{RDT+} = n_+/2 \times [\text{treatment duration at stage 2}]_{RDT}$. Usually, $n > n_+$, and therefore $T_{RCT} > T_{RDT}$.

Another ethically attractive feature of RDT is an opportunity to withdraw patients who do not benefit from the experimental treatment. However, some critics have argued that reassigning the confirmed treatment responders to the placebo arm, as in RDT, is an unethical move and unacceptable, for instance, in oncology trials. Thus, there are many pro and con aspects that need a thorough professional discussion before and during crafting a trial protocol. In general, balancing the pros and cons is and should be very specific for each therapeutic area. Interesting examples can be found, for instance, in Daugherty et al. (2008), Fava et al. (2003), FDA Guidance for Industry (2019b), Ratain et al. (2006), Sonpavde et al. (2006), Stadler (2007), Stadler et al. (2005), and Temple (1994).

Classification Hurdles

The concept of ***"responder"*** is essential for RDT, and is based on the dichotomization of continuous or discrete responses (cf. Uryniak et al. 2011; Fedorov et al. 2008). The poor selection of cutoff levels may lead to nonzero probabilities p_1 of false-negative (a "true" responder is assigned to the group of nonresponders) and p_2 of false-positive classifications (a "true" nonresponder is assigned to the group of responders). These probabilities can be appreciable for some response types: blood pressure in the cardiovascular area and scores in psychiatry are typical examples. In other therapeutic areas, it is natural to assume that the open-label stage of RDT takes a shorter time than a single stage of a conventional RCT and therefore practitioners resort to surrogate endpoints (cf. Burzykowski et al. 2005), which do not provide results identical to measurements at the end of RDT. For instance, in oncology, the tumor size change at the end of stage 1 might be used to separate responders and nonresponders, while the actual endpoint could be the tumor size change at the end of stage 2 that can be of the opposite sign. In general, false classification should be taken into account whenever within-patient variability is expected to be comparable with the population variability.

The statistical RDT superiority (lower variances of estimated parameters, smaller sample sizes in hypothesis testing) to RCT diminishes with the increase of probabilities of false classifications: the "enriched" subpopulation will miss some "responders" falsely claimed as "non-responders" and will include some pseudo "non-responders." As a result, erroneously classified patients will be assigned to the wrong treatment arms. For the relatively simple AD designs, it was shown in Fedorov and Liu (2005, 2014) that the set of scenarios where RDTs dominate RCTs decreases with the increase of p_1 and p_2.

The negative role of the false classification could be mitigated if the inferential part of data analysis were performed with original (non-dichotomized) data. The reporting component may include the post-analysis dichotomization to make conclusions more comprehensible and transparent for the larger audience.

Place of RDT Designs in the Family of Enrichment Trial Designs

As was previously pointed out, randomized discontinuation trial designs are commonly viewed as special cases of enrichment strategies, see, for instance, Fedorov and Liu (2007), FDA Guidance for Industry (2019b), Hallstrom and Friedman (1991), Pablos-Méndez et al. (1998), and Temple (1994). The difference between RDT and other types of population enrichment trials is that their design and analysis does not rely on any disease-related labels (e.g., biomarkers and social markers). All others rely on partitioning source populations into subpopulations with specific labels. This partitioning is based on prior/historic data or some intelligent guesses. The major goal of the respective enrichment strategies is the identification of the treatment responsive subpopulations and thorough validation of the respective efficacy-toxicity profiles.

RDTs pursue a seemingly easier goal, which is ***the proof of the existence of such a subpopulation***. However, it has to be reached from a more remote starting point where the disease-informative population partitioning does not exist. The proof that some patients benefit from the experimental treatment is very encouraging but not sufficient for the prediction of outcomes for future patients. Further, to move closer to precision medicine, the RDT methodology has to be complemented with statistical methods that allow the posttrial selection of disease informative markers. The situation is similar to that of unsupervised and supervised learning in artificial intelligence or, more specifically, in the machine learning paradigm. In the unsupervised case, given unlabeled/unmarked data, the algorithms try to make sense by extracting patterns (responsive subpopulations) on their own. In the supervised case, the algorithms learn on a labeled dataset (i.e., build "knowledge") and provide a prediction of what may happen to subsets with specific labels (subpopulations with specific biomarkers), followed by field verification of the validity/accuracy of this prediction on newly accrued data.

Key Facts

The idea of randomized discontinuation (withdrawal) trials was conceived to pursue two targets: to filter out the placebo effect noise while measuring the efficacy of a novel treatment and to minimize exposure of enrolled subjects to placebo. To some extend, the RDT design methodology was borrowed from the theory of cross-over designs: expose a patient to different treatments to gain more information and minimize the impact of the between patient variability. This fact was mentioned in the pioneering paper by Amery and Dony (1975) and it may help to develop more sophisticated designs that allow effective comparison of several treatments and their effects across multiple subpopulations.

It should be emphasized that the benefits RDT-s are gained at the expense of limited applicability of trial results to the general population: often they are valid only for the enriched subpopulations and, as was already mentioned, extra statistical and medical effort is needed to determine the sound identifiers that can predict which future patients will benefit from the new treatment. Without this knowledge, one has to resort to the old-fashioned "trial and error" method to select the right treatment for a given patient.

References

Amery W, Dony J (1975) Clinical trial design avoiding undue placebo treatment. J Clin Pharmacol 15:674–679

Atkinson AC, Fedorov VV, Herzberg AM, Zhang R (2014) Elemental information matrices and optimal experimental design for generalized regression models. J Statis Plan Inference 144: 81–91

Burzykowski T, Molenberghs G, Buyse M (2005) The evaluation of surrogate endpoints. Springer, New York

Capra WB (2004) Comparing the power of the discontinuation design to that of the classic randomized design on time-to-event endpoints. Control Clin Trials 25:168–177
Chiron C, Dulac O, Gram L (1996) Vigabatrin withdrawal randomized study in children. Epilepsy Res 25:209–215
Daugherty CK, Ratain MJ, Emanuel EJ, Farrell AT, Schilsky RL (2008) Ethical, scientific, and regulatory perspectives regarding the use of placebos in cancer clinical trials. J Clin Oncol 26: 1371–1378
Fava M, Eveins A, Dorer D, Schoenfeld D (2003) The problem of the placebo response in clinical trials for psychiatric disorders: culprits, possible remedies, and a novel study design approach. Psychother Psychosom 72:115–127
FDA Guidance for Industry (2019a) ICH E9 (R1) addendum on estimands and sensitivity analysis in clinical trials to the guideline on statistical principles for clinical trials. https://www.fda.gov/media/108698/download
FDA Guidance for Industry (2019b) Enrichment strategies for clinical trials to support determination of effectiveness of human drugs and biological products. https://www.fda.gov/ucm/groups/fdagov-public/@fdagov-drugs-gen/documents/document/ucm332181.pdf
Fedorov VV (1972) Theory of optimal experiments. Academic, New York
Fedorov VV, Liu T (2005) Randomized discontinuation trials: design and efficiency. GlaxoSmithKline biomedical data science technical report, 2005–3
Fedorov VV, Liu T (2007) Enrichment design. In: Wiley encyclopedia of clinical trials. Wiley, Hoboken, pp 1–8
Fedorov VV, Liu T (2014) Randomized discontinuation trials with binary outcomes. J Stat Theory Pract 8:30–45
Fedorov VV, Mannino F, Zhang R (2008) Consequences of dichotomization. Pharm Stat 8:50–61
Freidlin B, Simon R (2005) Evaluation of randomized discontinuation design. J Clin Oncol 23(22): 5094–5098
Freidlin B, Korn EL, Abrams JS (2018) Bias, operational bias, and generalizability in phase II/III trials. J Clin Oncol 36(19):1902–1904
Grieve AP (2012) Discussion: Bayesian enrichment strategies for randomized discontinuation trials. Biometrics 68:219–224
Hallstrom AP, Friedman L (1991) Randomizing responders. Control Clin Trials 12:486–503
Ivanova A, Qaqish B, Schoenfeld A (2010) Optimality, sample size, and power calculations for the sequential parallel comparison design. Stat Med 30:2793–2803
Johnson NL, Kotz S, Balakrishnan N (1997) Discrete multivariate distributions. Wiley, New York
Kopec J, Abrahamowicz M, Esdaile J (1993) Randomized discontinuation trials: utility and efficiency. J Clin Epidemiol 46:959–971
Korn EL, Arbuck SG, Pulda JM, Simon R, Kaplan RS, Christian MC (2001) Clinical trial designs for cytostatic agents: are new approaches needed? J Clin Oncol 19:265–272
Oehlert GW (1992) A note on the delta method. Am Stat 46:27–29
Pablos-Méndez A, Barr RG, Shea S (1998) Run-in periods in randomized trials. J Am Med Assoc 279:222–225
Piantadosi S (1997) Clinical trials: a methodologic perspective. Wiley, New York
Pocock SJ (1983) Clinical trials: a practical approach. Wiley, New York
Ratain MJ, Eisen T, Stadler WM, Flaherty KT, Kaye SB, Rosner GL, Gore M, Desai AA, Patnaik A, Xiong HQ, Rowin-sky E, Abbruzzese JL, Xia C, Simantov R, Schwartz B, Dwyer PJ (2006) Phase II placebo-controlled randomized discontinuation trial of sorafenib in patients with metastatic renal cell carcinoma. J Clin Oncol 24:2505–2512
Rosner GL, Stadler WM, Ratain MJ (2002) Randomized discontinuation design: application to cytostatic antineoplastic agents. J Clin Oncol 20:4478–4484
Senn SJ (1997) Statistical issues in drug development. Wiley, New York
Sonpavde G, Hutson TE, Galsky MD, Berry WR (2006) Problems with the randomized discontinuation design. J Clin Oncol 24:4669–4670

Stadler WM (2007) The randomized dicontinuation trial: a phase II design to access growth-inhibitory agents. Mol Cancer Ther 6:1180–1185
Stadler WM, Rosner G, Small E, Hollis D, Rini B, Zaentz SD, Mahoney J (2005) Successful implementation of the randomized discontinuation trial design: an application to the study of the putative antiangiogenic agent carboxyaminoimidazole in renal cell carcinoma – CALGB 69901. J Clin Oncol 23:3726–3732
Temple RJ (1994) Special study designs: early escape, enrichment, study in non-responders. Commun Stat Theory Methods 23:499–531
Trippa L, Rosner GL, Müller P (2012) Bayesian enrichment strategies for randomized discontinuation trials. Biometrics 68:203–225
Uryniak T, Chan ISF, Fedorov V, Jiang Q, Oppenheimer L, Snapinn SM, Teng CH, Zhang J (2011) Responder analyses – a PhRMA position paper. Stat Biopharm Res 3:476–487

Platform Trial Designs

76

Oleksandr Sverdlov, Ekkehard Glimm, and Peter Mesenbrink

Contents

Abstract

Modern drug development is increasingly complex and requires novel approaches to the design and analysis of clinical trials. With the precision medicine paradigm, there is a strong need to evaluate multiple experimental therapies across a spectrum of indications, in different subgroups of patients, while controlling the chance of false positive and false negative findings. The

O. Sverdlov (✉) · P. Mesenbrink
Novartis Pharmaceuticals Corporation, East Hannover, NJ, USA
e-mail: alex.sverdlov@novartis.com; peter.mesenbrink@novartis.com

E. Glimm
Novartis Pharma AG, Basel, Switzerland
e-mail: ekkehard.glimm@novartis.com

© Springer Nature Switzerland AG 2022

S. Piantadosi, C. L. Meinert (eds.), *Principles and Practice of Clinical Trials*,
https://doi.org/10.1007/978-3-319-52636-2_107

concept of *master protocols* provides a new approach to clinical trial design that can help drug developers to enhance efficiency of clinical trials by addressing multiple research questions within the same overall trial infrastructure. There are three general types of trials requiring a master protocol: basket trials, umbrella trials, and platform trials. The present chapter provides an overview of platform trial designs. We discuss operating models for implementing platform trials in practice, as well as some important statistical considerations for design and analysis of such trials. We also discuss four real-life examples of platform trials: the EPAD-PoC study in Alzheimer's disease; the I-SPY COVID-19 study for rapid screening of re-purposed and novel treatments for COVID-19; the GBM AGILE study in glioblastoma; and the FOCUS4 study in metastatic colorectal cancer.

Keywords

Master protocols · Multi-arm randomized controlled trials · Multiple comparisons

Introduction

Modern drug development is increasingly complex and requires novel approaches to the design and analysis of clinical trials. With the precision medicine paradigm, there is a strong need to evaluate multiple experimental therapies across a spectrum of indications, in different subgroups of patients, while controlling the chance of false positive and false negative findings. The concept of *master protocols* provides a new approach to clinical trial design that can help drug developers to enhance efficiency of clinical trials by addressing multiple research questions within the same overall trial infrastructure (Woodcock and LaVange 2017). There are three general types of trials requiring a master protocol: basket trials, umbrella trials, and platform trials. Basket trials evaluate a single investigational compound in different indications to find the indication(s) that can be efficiently treated with the given compound. Umbrella trials evaluate multiple investigational compounds in one indication to find the "most promising" compounds, possibly within different patient subgroups for the chosen indication. Platform trials evaluate multiple experimental treatments for a given indication in a perpetual manner, and in theory, the platform trial can continue until the intervention(s) with the desired risk/benefit profile are found.

Master protocols use a common trial infrastructure, often with a shared control group, which may help streamline clinical operations and achieve enhanced and expedited developmental decisions. At the same time, master protocols are complex, may incur higher cost, and necessitate a lot of upfront planning and early engagement with health authorities and other relevant stakeholders. Despite these challenges, the uptake of master protocols in drug development is increasing, and more applications of these designs are expected in the near future (Park et al. 2019; Meyer et al. 2020).

The present chapter provides an overview of one type of master protocols – platform trials. Two other types of master protocols, basket and umbrella trials, are beyond the scope of this chapter. For a recent book-length discussion on platform, umbrella, and basket trials, see Antonijevic and Beckman (2019). Platform trials represent a broad concept that can be applied in different stages of clinical development. However, one should keep in mind an important distinction between exploratory studies and studies with a confirmatory component. The former studies are common in phase II, where one of the objectives is to perform a screening of various candidate compounds, eliminating suboptimal ones as early as possible, and focusing research efforts on "most promising" treatment candidates. Such studies are hypothesis generating and are not intended for marketing authorization. By contrast, studies with a confirmatory component (e.g., phase II/III) should provide substantial evidence to support claims for drug effectiveness, and therefore, they should incorporate some formal considerations of control of the type I error rate. In this chapter, we intend to cover both phase II and phase II/III platform trial designs, emphasizing the distinctions between the two types where appropriate.

Section "Background on Platform Trials" presents some general background on platform trials and describes two distinct operating models – single-sponsor and multisponsor – for implementing platform trials in practice. Section "Statistical Considerations" presents some important statistical considerations for design and analysis of platform trials. Section "Examples of Platform Trials" discusses four real-life examples of platform trials – the EPAD-PoC study in Alzheimer's disease; the I-SPY COVID-19 study for rapid screening of re-purposed and novel treatments for COVID-19; the GBM AGILE study in glioblastoma; and the FOCUS4 study in metastatic colorectal cancer. Section "Concluding Remarks" provides some concluding remarks.

Background on Platform Trials

General Definitions

Using the terminology of Woodcock and LaVange (2017), the objective of a platform trial is "to study multiple targeted therapies in the context of a single disease in a perpetual manner, with therapies allowed to enter or leave the platform on the basis of a decision algorithm." Unlike standard randomized clinical trials (RCTs) that are "intervention-focused," platform trials are "disease-focused" (Berry et al. 2015; The Adaptive Platform Trial Coalition 2019; Park et al. 2020). When carefully designed and implemented, platform trials can potentially be more efficient than a sequence of two-arm RCTs (Saville and Berry 2016).

Similar to platform trials, *basket* trials involve the application of a single therapy to several subvariants of a disease and *umbrella* trials attempt several therapies on a single disease. All of these trials require a *master protocol* describing the entire trial. Typically then, per intervention, there is an *intervention specific appendix* (ISA) detailing the specifics of the single interventions. In what is to follow, we will focus on platform trials. However, many of the considerations given here also apply to basket and umbrella trials.

Several recent systematic literature searches have revealed the growing popularity and use of master protocol trials, and platform trials in particular (Siden et al. 2019; Park et al. 2019; Meyer et al. 2020). More specifically, the number of identified platform trials/total number of identified master protocols were 25/99 (Siden et al. 2019), 16/83 (Park et al. 2019), and 12/50 (Meyer et al. 2020). All of these references highlight a rapid increase in the number of master protocols over the past 5 years, and this trend is expected to continue.

Figure 1 presents an example of an open platform master protocol.

We consider a randomized, placebo-controlled, open platform trial evaluating therapeutic effects of various investigational treatments (agents) in a selected indication. Figure 1a shows the structure of the master protocol. The core part (Sections 1 to 16) describes key design elements that remain the same across all agents in the study. Section 17 details any information or procedures that are specific to a particular agent. The platform trial will enroll patients in cohorts/substudies. In our example, the study starts with Cohort 1, in which eligible patients will be randomized to TRT1 or Control (Fig. 1b). Interventions for future cohorts will become available over time, and subsequent Cohorts 2, 3, and 4 are planned to be added to the master protocol. In each cohort, there is a control group (not displayed in Fig. 1a), that is assumed to be the current standard-of-care (SOC) treatment. We assume that each subsequent cohort may include up to three investigational agents; for example, in Cohort 2, we provision for TRT2, TRT3, and TRT4. Within each cohort, eligible patients will be randomized among the available active treatment arms or control.

At some prespecified time points in the study, interim analyses (IAs) will be performed (Fig. 1b). At each interim analysis (IA1, IA2, IA3, ...), accrued data will be analyzed and a predetermined statistical decision rule will be applied. The nature of decisions will generally depend on the trial design and the study objectives. Fundamentally, both the analyses and the types of decisions should be prespecified in the protocol (not made on an ad hoc basis) to maintain the integrity and the validity of the results.

Our considered example in Fig. 1 is typical for a phase II platform trial. In this case, the following decisions can be considered for any given investigational treatment arm:

(i) Advance the arm for further development (outside of the current master protocol), if it exhibits sufficient evidence of activity. Or
(ii) Drop the arm from the study, if there is sufficient evidence of lack of activity. Or
(iii) Continue the arm in the study to the next decision point, if the results are indeterminate and the maximum sample size for this treatment arm has not been reached.

A more complex scenario is a phase II/III platform trial, which may include IAs during both phase II and phase III parts of the study. The IA decisions during a

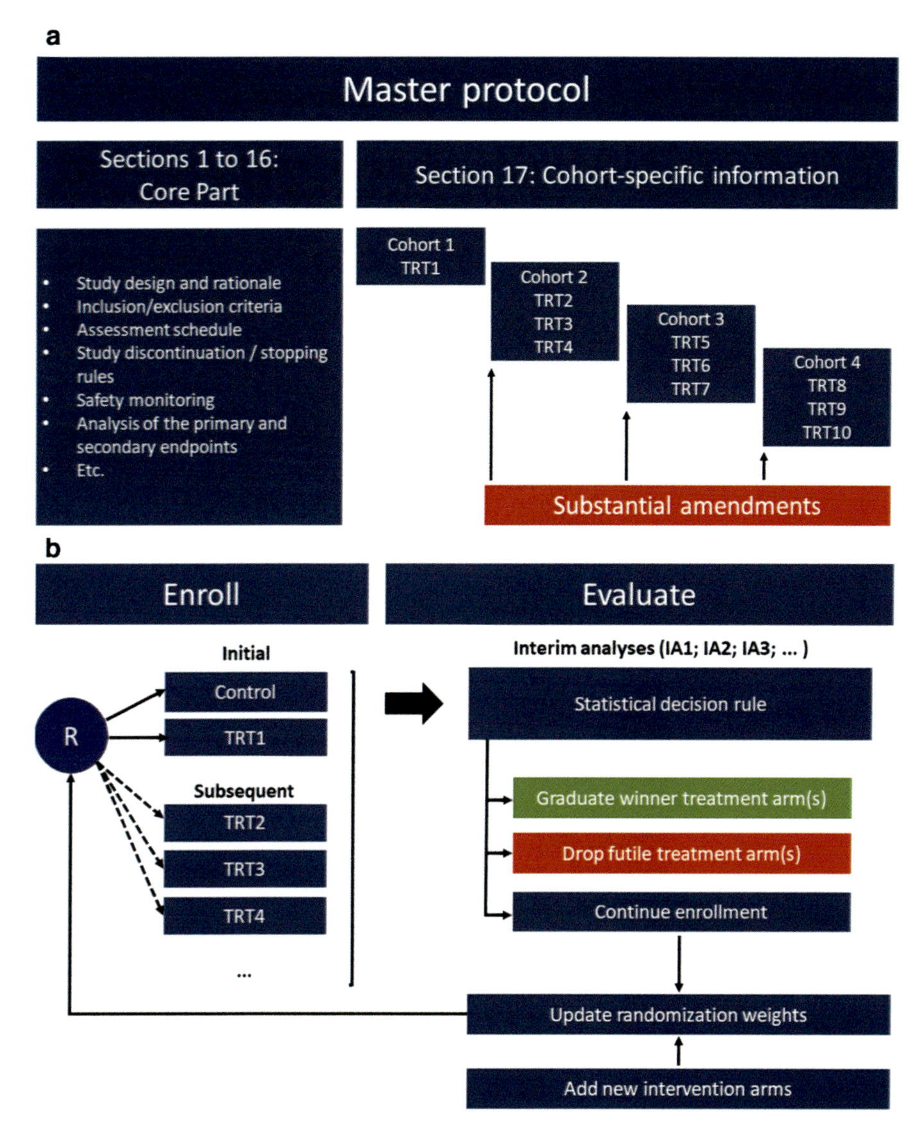

Fig. 1 An example of an open platform trial master protocol

phase II part of a phase II/III trial often would be based on a surrogate outcome measure, such as some biomarker predictive for clinical efficacy, and these decisions can be described using items (i)–(iii) above. However, additional IAs can be also considered during a confirmatory (phase III) part of the study. In this case, the interim decisions will be made based on accrued clinical outcome data, which may be the primary efficacy endpoint. For any investigational treatment arm, the decisions may be:

(iv) Declare superior efficacy of the treatment arm over the control and stop the trial early, if clinical efficacy results are outstanding for this arm. Or
(v) Terminate the treatment arm for futility, if there is sufficient evidence of lack of efficacy for this arm. Or
(vi) Continue the treatment arm to the next decision point (IA or end of study), if evidence for efficacy and futility is inconclusive and the maximum sample size for this arm has not been reached.

The efficacy decision would typically require a formal decision rule such as a statistical test with type I error control. In contrast, the futility rule - even in phase III – would typically not require the same level of formality. In addition to efficacy assessments, the usual safety monitoring rules would commonly be applied, such that interventions or the entire study may be stopped due to safety findings.

The open-endedness of the platform trial allows adding and removing of interventions as the study is ongoing. If it is decided to introduce a new arm, an additional ISA would be added to the master protocol (Fig. 1a). The randomization weights must be updated accordingly, and new eligible subjects will be randomized to a specific ISA and then to a specific treatment within the ISA (Fig. 1b). (Other approaches for implementing randomization can be considered; e.g. subjects may be randomized among all available study arms, as done in a parallel multi-arm trial.) In our example, the initial randomization in Cohort 1 is 1:1 (TRT1 or Control), and thereafter it can be modified, with potentially increased allocation ratio to novel experimental agents. The choice of a randomization algorithm (e.g., if response-adaptive randomization is utilized) should be discussed with the health authorities and it must be carefully justified in the master protocol. We shall discuss response-adaptive randomization (RAR) in more detail in section "Response-Adaptive Randomization"; for now, we just make an important remark that RAR has both merits and limitations, and it may potentially be utilized in a phase II platform trial or during the phase II screening part of a phase II/III platform trial, but not during its confirmatory stage.

Single-Sponsor Platform Trials

Platform trials can provide a valuable framework for the development of novel therapies within a biopharmaceutical company. While platform trials can be designed in both early and late clinical development, the concept may be more appealing in the early stages (e.g., phase II), where the objective is to perform a fast screening of many investigational agents, many of which are potentially not efficacious. Suppose we have an indication with an unmet medical need for treatment and assume that there are multiple potential candidate compounds for this indication within the drug development portfolio of Company X. Once the safety of a particular compound has been established (e.g., with first-in-human data and sufficient toxicology data), it is ready to be further assessed in the clinical proof-of-mechanism and clinical proof-of-concept (PoC) trials. A traditional 1:1 randomized controlled PoC trial explores whether the investigational drug is likely to achieve the desired therapeutic effect and whether it merits testing in a large-scale confirmatory trial in patients. However, given a large variety of candidate compounds and their combinations, running multiple PoC trials may be infeasible. A phase II platform trial is an attractive option, if:

- There is a strong scientific rationale (e.g., common scientific hypothesis, consistently defined population, and other design elements) for evaluating multiple therapies and possibly their combinations in the chosen indication.
- The company has multiple candidate compounds/formulations for the chosen indication.
- There is a strong need/interest in developing more than one compound in the given indication; for example, due to different mechanisms of action or due to inadequate preclinical models to make comparative assessment of compounds.

There are several options with respect to the structure of a clinical trial team (CTT) for a platform trial within a single pharmaceutical Sponsor. One approach would be to build upon some existing clinical teams in the given disease area. This will ensure that the clinical lead and key team members are the same across compounds, which helps establish consistency and efficient communication; however, it also requires considerable commitment and continuous support from the team members. Another approach is to designate an "independent" platform trial team that would collaborate with different compound teams within the company, thus providing integrated efforts to develop the master protocol and ensure that the design properly accommodates each compound. A third approach is to have an external group run the trial on behalf of the company and tap into their disease area knowledge. All of these approaches require substantial upfront planning and investment, greater than one would expect for a standard clinical development path (Schiavone et al. 2019; Hague et al. 2019; Morrell et al. 2019).

As an example, consider a Novartis-sponsored phase II open-entry platform trial evaluating efficacy and safety of novel spartalizumab combinations in previously treated unresectable or metastatic melanoma (ClinicalTrials.gov Identifier: NCT03484923). The study design is described in detail by Racine-Poon et al. (2020). The design consists of two parts: the exploratory Part 1 in which candidate treatments are evaluated for activity in a randomized manner, and the confirmatory Part 2 in which the "winner" treatment arms from Part 1 are expanded to achieve the desired level of predictive power for confirmatory statistical hypothesis testing on the objective response rate (ORR). The study core team was formed on the basis of the Novartis clinical oncology group, capitalizing on internal knowledge and relevant subject matter expertise.

Multisponsor Platform Trials

Taking a broad perspective, the overall success rates of new drug development have been disappointingly low (Scannell et al. 2012; Wong et al. 2019), despite rising developmental costs (DiMasi et al. 2016). The need for innovation and modernization of drug development through collaboration among multiple public and private entities has become apparent over the years (Woodcock and Woosley 2008). *Crowdsourcing* or multisponsor models, where different biopharmaceutical companies are working in a coordinated manner to develop new medicines for high unmet medical needs, may provide a very useful framework for modern drug development (Bentzien et al. 2015). One sensible model is when an academic research unit (or a network of several academic centers) acts as the coordinator of the platform trial activities. In this case, the academic research unit may: (i) secure funding for this research through grants, (ii) develop the master protocol, (iii) build the trial infrastructure, (iv) attract different pharma/biotech companies to participate and contribute their investigational compounds for the trial, etc.

Multisponsor platform trials are increasingly common in clinical research. Some notable examples include the I-SPY 2 trial of novel neoadjuvant therapies in breast cancer (Barker et al. 2009; Esserman et al. 2019), the I-SPY COVID-19 study of promising therapeutic agents in critically ill COVID-19 patients (https://clinicaltrials.gov/ct2/show/NCT04488081), the Systemic Therapy for Advancing or Metastatic Prostate Cancer (STAMPEDE) study (James et al. 2009), just to name a few.

Multisponsor platform trials require more upfront planning than single-sponsor trials, because of the need to build the operational platform infrastructure, obtain alignment across the stakeholders, and get all necessary authorizations from health authorities. In fact, the FDA guidance for industry "Adaptive designs for clinical trials of drugs and biologics" (Food and Drug Administration 2019) states this explicitly:

> ...Because these (adaptive platform) trials may involve investigational agents from more than one sponsor, may be conducted for an unstated length of time, and often involve complex adaptations, they should generally involve extensive discussion with FDA...

The "independent" clinical development team on a platform trial would be liaising with different companies interested in providing their investigational compounds and co-sponsoring the study. From an individual sponsor's perspective, there are both advantages and disadvantages to having an independent clinical trial team. The advantages include significant work by this independent team, which includes careful coordination of tasks, starting from the development of a master protocol and involvement in all subsequent activities as the study progresses. A major limitation is the lack of full control over the study for any participating company. The "independent" team may be less experienced in the disease area than some developers from the sponsor companies. Moreover, while each company should be able to have a comparison of the effects of their investigational assets to the shared control group, the direct between-asset comparisons would be less common (Food and Drug Administration 2018).

Statistical Considerations

The design of a platform trial poses scientific, statistical, operational, and regulatory challenges. In addition, the choice of a study design will depend on the disease area, the competitive landscape, the established industry practices, and the development phase, in particular if the study is exploratory or confirmatory. The main objective of any scientific experiment is to obtain reliable answers to the questions of interest. Keeping this in mind, various designs options should be judiciously evaluated at the study planning stage. Comparing these options through simulations under different experimental scenarios will be an essential step in selecting the design to be implemented (Mayer et al. 2019).

We discuss some important statistical considerations and key design elements that can be viewed as "building blocks" for constructing a platform trial. Our presentation here is high-level and nontechnical. The intent is to provide a succinct summary of strategic considerations for design and analysis of platform trials and, where appropriate, to provide references to relevant statistical methodology papers. Given the novelty of the topic, our review here is by no means comprehensive; many new designs and concepts are yet to emerge.

Choice of a Control Arm

The use of a control group is a fundamental principle of the design of any comparative clinical trial. The main purpose of a control group is to minimize confounding of the treatment effect with other factors (such as the natural history of the disease), thereby improving the quality of statistical inference on the treatment effect. The importance of the choice of a control group in clinical trials is well acknowledged and is documented in the ICH E10 guideline (International Conference on Harmonisation E10 2001). In platform trials, many of which are designed to evaluate the effects of various experimental treatments, considerations on the control group are particularly important. The FDA guidance on master protocols has the following statement in this regard (Food and Drug Administration 2018):

> ...FDA recommends that a sponsor use a common control arm to improve efficiency in master protocols where multiple drugs are evaluated simultaneously in a single disease (e.g., umbrella trials). FDA recommends that the control arm be the current SOC so that the trial results will be interpretable in the context of U.S. medical practice...

In a recent literature review, Meyer et al. (2020) found that among 50 identified master protocol trials, the majority (28 out of 50, 56%) had no control group. More specifically, among the 12 identified platform trials, five trials were designed using concurrent control, six trials included nonconcurrent control, and one trial had no control group. The similar numbers for nine identified umbrella trials were four (concurrent control), one (nonconcurrent control), and four (no control). Let us discuss different possibilities for the control group in more detail.

Historical Controls

Historical data (e.g., from previous clinical trials in the same indication) provides valuable information that may potentially supplement evidence from a new RCT (Pocock 1976). However, one cannot simply rely on historical controls as a basis for comparison, because there might be differences in the populations, for example, due to change in medical care over time (Byar 1980).

There are different methods to utilize historical control data both in the design and the analysis of clinical trials (Viele et al. 2014; Chen et al. 2018). Many phase II trials in oncology simply use a historical reference value of the objective response rate (ORR). For instance, a common approach to evaluate the activity of a new compound is through Simon's two-stage optimal design (Simon 1989) to test the hypotheses H_0: ORR $=p_0$ vs. H_1: ORR $=p_1$, where p_0 is the historical reference value of the ORR, and $p_1 > p_0$ is some threshold representing promising activity.

In a platform trial, one is interested in evaluating multiple candidate treatments, and so the study design may involve randomization to one of the treatment arms, but the analysis for each arm is standalone (i.e., involves no comparison against control). This approach was implemented in the platform trial in metastatic melanoma (NCT03484923; Racine-Poon et al. 2020), where no adequate SOC is currently available. In that study, the primary analysis for each "winner" arm that has been promoted from Part 1 to Part 2 involved testing H_0: ORR $=0.10$ vs. H_1: ORR $=0.30$. The lower bound of the 95% confidence interval using Clopper-Pearson's exact method for ORR was used as a criterion to decide whether a treatment warranted further investigation in pivotal studies. Alternatively, the analysis could incorporate relevant historical control data using some Bayesian borrowing technique, such as hierarchical modeling (Viele et al. 2014). Such analysis would account for uncertainty in the historical ORR, but it would also require careful assessment of assumptions necessary for a valid treatment comparison.

Concurrent Controls

In clinical settings where it is not feasible to run a series of standard adequately powered two-arm RCTs (e.g., in rare diseases), a multiarm randomized platform trial with a shared control group may be an appealing and efficient approach (Saville and Berry 2016). For instance, platform trials evaluating multiple treatments from different sponsors can benefit from borrowing of data from the pooled placebo group for individual treatment comparisons. Since platform trials evaluate novel treatments perpetually, some special considerations on the shared control are required.

For illustrative purpose, consider a hypothetical platform trial with five experimental treatment arms and Control (Fig. 2).

Suppose for each comparison of experimental vs. control, 100 patients per arm provide sufficient sample size to test treatment difference. The trial starts with randomizing initial 100 patients equally between TRT1 and Control. After that, two new arms are added, and additional 200 patients are randomized among TRT1, TRT2, TRT3, and Control (50 per arm). At that point, TRT1 achieves its target sample size, and the randomization is shifted to TRT2, TRT3, or Control such that additional 150 patients are randomized (50 per arm). Thereafter, a new arm TRT4 is added (ISA2) and the next 100 patients are randomized between TRT4 and Control (50 per arm). Finally, after TRT5 is added (ISA3), the trial continues with randomizing additional 150 patients among TRT4, TRT5, or Control, and the last

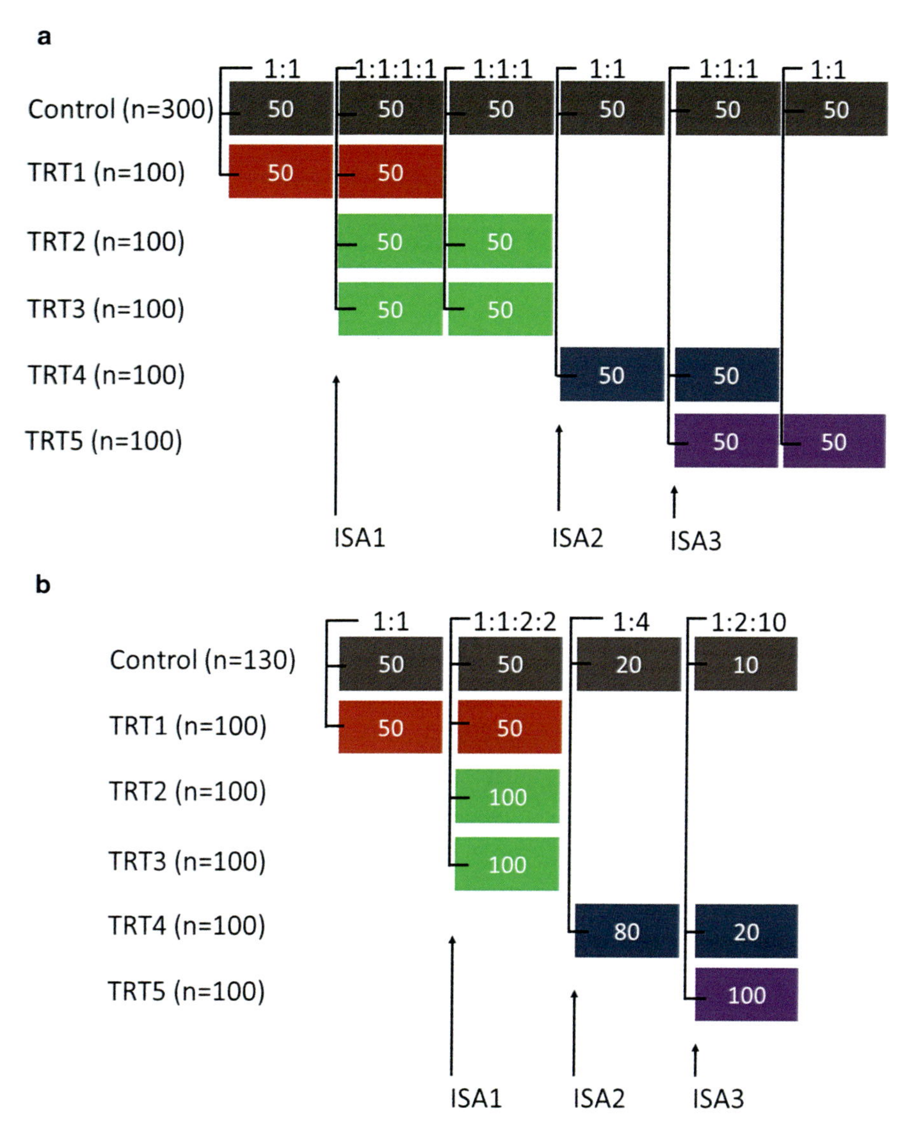

Fig. 2 A hypothetical platform trial with five experimental arms and a shared control arm

100 patients between TRT5 and Control. Overall, in this hypothetical study, each treatment arm has 100 patients, and the Control arm has 300 patients.

Assume the primary outcome is available soon after randomization, and the data analysis for each arm takes place after the target number of subjects have been randomized and treated. In the analysis, different strategies for utilizing control data are possible.

1. All accrued data in the Control arm at the time of analysis is utilized, treating all observations as if they had been concurrently obtained. In our example, the size of the control group for treatment comparison is 100 for TRT1, 150 for each of the TRT2 and TRT3, 250 for TRT4, and 300 for TRT5. A larger size for the control arm would enable more robust inference. A major assumption is that there are no hidden confounders such as a time trend.
2. Only data from the Control arm that was part of the randomization sequence concurrent with the given experimental treatment arm is utilized. The argument here is that it is difficult to justify pooling of control observations that are separated by some time interval. In our example, first 100 allocations to control are concurrent with TRT1, allocations 51–150 to control are concurrent with TRT2 and TRT3, allocations 151–250 to control are concurrent with TRT4, and allocations 201–300 to control are concurrent with TRT5. Therefore, in this case, the size of the control group for each treatment comparison is 100.
3. Pooling of data from the Control arm in the study is performed using some statistical methodology. Several recent papers discuss approaches that may be relevant in this context (Yuan et al. 2016; Galwey 2017; Hobbs et al. 2018; Jiao et al. 2019; Tang et al. 2019; Normington et al. 2020). The methods include "test-then-pool" strategy, dynamic pooling, Bayesian hierarchical modeling, to name a few. These methods can be applied not only to the shared internal control arm, but also to some historical control data or some relevant concurrent external data that may become available as the platform trial is ongoing. They provide a compromise between approaches #1 and #2 in that either historical information is down-weighted, but not entirely discarded, or is included in the analysis only if sufficiently similar to the concurrent data (which could also be interpreted as a form of down-weighting, since it is included in the analysis with a probability less than 1).

Some additional important notes should be made here. First, it may be difficult to justify upfront the analytic strategy for handling control data, and several approaches may have to be designated to ensure robust analysis. This argument applies to both phase II and phase II/III platform trials. In fact, it is increasingly recognized (even in phase III trials) that a single, albeit carefully prespecified, primary analysis may be insufficient and it is prudent to have several sensitivity analyses. For instance, the estimand framework (ICH E9(R1), 2020; Jin and Liu 2020) suggests to designate a main estimator to serve as primary analysis and several sensitivity estimators targeting the same estimand but under different assumptions for missing data and/or censoring. Second, the investigational treatments may have different mechanism of action and/or different routes of administration (e.g., oral vs. injections), in which case the concurrent placebo group may be different across experimental arms and this should be accounted for in the analysis. Third, in some platform trials, if a current active treatment shows evidence of superiority over SOC, then this treatment may become the SOC and the control group would have to be changed for subsequent cohorts. This was the case, for instance, in PREVAIL II trial in Ebola (Dodd et al. 2016; PREVAIL II Writing Group 2016) and in the currently ongoing I-SPY COVID-19 trial (NCT04488081).

Randomization

Randomization in clinical trials mitigates potential for experimental bias, promotes comparability of treatment groups, and validates the use of statistical methods in the analysis.

The choice of both the allocation ratio and the randomization procedure to implement the chosen allocation is an essential ingredient of the clinical trial design. For multiarm trials where the number of treatment arms is fixed and predetermined, an optimal allocation can be obtained according to the formulated study objectives (Sverdlov and Rosenberger 2013; Sverdlov et al. 2020). In platform trials, determining optimal allocation may be more challenging due to the open-ended nature of these trials and uncertainty in the total number of treatment arms to be tested in the study. The chosen allocation can be implemented in practice using some sequential randomization procedure with established statistical properties (Rosenberger and Lachin 2015; Hu and Rosenberger 2006). Broadly speaking, randomization procedures can be classified into two major types: fixed allocation (e.g., equal) randomization and adaptive randomization. The latter class of procedures includes covariate-adaptive, response-adaptive, and covariate-adjusted response-adaptive randomization procedures (Rosenberger et al. 2012).

Below we discuss two approaches – equal and fixed unequal allocation randomization (section "Equal and Fixed Unequal Randomization") and response-adaptive randomization (section "Response-Adaptive Randomization") – in the context of platform trials.

Equal and Fixed Unequal Randomization

Consider a platform trial that initially starts with $K \geq 1$ experimental treatment arms and a control arm. A popular design choice is the equal randomization (1:1:. . .:1) for which m patients are randomized to arm $k = 0, 1, \ldots, K$, where $k = 0$ is the control. While equal allocation are optimal for some experimental objectives, such as estimation of treatment contrasts (Sverdlov and Rosenberger 2013), unequal allocation may sometimes be preferred. For instance, if $K \geq 1$ experimental treatments are compared against the common control, the optimal allocation ratio for the pairwise comparison of experimental vs. control (assuming constant variance across all groups and assuming the same value of the mean treatment difference over control) is 1:. . .:1: $\sqrt{K}$ (Dunnett 1955). An increased allocation to the control group may be also attractive from the cost efficiency perspective, for example, if the control treatment is significantly cheaper than experimental ones (Sverdlov and Ryeznik 2019). On the other hand, there may be nonstatistical rationales for increasing the allocation proportion to the experimental arms; for example, in situations when historical control data can be utilized to supplement the concurrent control data, investigators may be interested in gaining more information on experimental treatment arms.

In platform trials, the total number of experimental treatments may be unknown at the trial start, and the allocation ratio may have to be determined adaptively. To illustrate this, consider our earlier example where the study starts with one experimental treatment and control, and more experimental arms are added over time (Fig. 2a). We assume that $m = 100$ subjects per arm provide sufficient data to test treatment difference vs. control. In Fig. 2a, the design uses equal allocation to available arms throughout the study. If at some point new experimental arms are added, the randomization scheme accommodates these arms accordingly: for example, the design starts with 1:1 randomization (50 patients to each of TRT1 and Control), then changes to 1:1:1:1 randomization (50 patients to each of TRT1, TRT2, TRT3 and Control), etc. While this ensures 100 patients per experimental arm, one may argue that we have over-allocation to the control arm. More specifically, in the described example in Fig. 2a, the size of the control group at the time of the final analysis is 100 for TRT1 comparison, 150 for each of TRT2 and TRT3 comparisons, 250 for TRT4 comparison, and 300 for TRT5 comparison. This is natural if experimental arms are added over time and we want to maintain equal randomization throughout the study.

If we can assume exchangeability of observations in the control group, then allocation to control may be gradually decreased over time. Generally speaking, this idea may be applied in both phase II and phase II/III platform settings; however, it requires careful considerations of the trial context, sample size, and other design parameters. For instance, one could apply an allocation strategy as displayed in Fig. 2b. After randomizing initial 100 patients between TRT1 and Control, TRT2 and TRT3 are added at ISA1. The randomization ratio is changed to 1:1:2:2, to have additional 50 patients assigned to each of the TRT1 and Control and 100 patients to each of the TRT2 and TRT3. By the time TRT4 is added at ISA2, the Control arm already has 100 patients. We modify the allocation ratio to 1:4, to assign additional 25 patients to Control and 100 patients to TRT4. Once this change in randomization has been applied and 100 additional assignments have been made (20 to Control and 80 to TRT4), TRT5 is added at ISA3. We decide to further amend the allocation ratio to 1:2:10 to assign extra 10 patients to Control, 20 patients to TRT4, and 100 patients to TRT5. Overall, in this example the total sample size for the Control arm is 130 (compared to 300 in Fig. 2a). In the analyses of TRT1, TRT2, and TRT3 vs. Control, the comparisons are based on 100 patients per arm, and in the analyses of TRT4 and TRT5 vs. Control, the sample size is 100 per experimental arm and it is 130 for the control arm. Such a dynamic modification of the allocation ratio may impact type I error and type II error rates. With this approach, one should exercise caution if the study has a confirmatory component. Of note, the issues of multiplicity adjustments and strategies for proper utilization of the shared control in platform trials are still emerging (Sridhara et al. 2021; Wason and Robertson 2021; Berry 2020; Parker and Weir 2020; Bretz and Koenig 2020; Stallard et al. 2019; Howard et al. 2018; Kopp-Schneider et al. 2020; Dodd et al. 2021). Some of them will be briefly discussed in section "Sample Size and Power."

Note that this example provides only one possibility of modifying the control allocation ratio over time. A major assumption was that the randomization ratios were prefixed (e.g., 1:1 up to patient 100, 1:1:2:2 for additional 300 patients, etc.) such that there is no selection bias issue. If, however, these decisions are made "pragmatically," whenever a new treatment arm is added or dropped, then it is important to ensure that the selected new randomization ratios are not dependent on the observed response data; otherwise the procedure can no longer be regarded as "fixed," but it rather becomes response-adaptive, for which special considerations are required; see section "Response-Adaptive Randomization."

To implement the chosen equal or unequal allocation ratio, the simplest and most common approach is the permuted block randomization which sequentially randomizes cohorts of study participants in the desired ratio until the target sample size is reached. Other randomization procedures with enhanced statistical properties can be considered (Kuznetsova and Tymofyeyev, 2011; Kuznetsova and Tymofyeyev 2014; Ryeznik and Sverdlov 2018).

Response-Adaptive Randomization

Response-adaptive randomization (RAR) can be applied in platform trials to increase the chance of trial participants to receive an empirically better treatment while maintaining important statistical properties of the trial design. Here, "empirically better treatment" refers to a treatment that has been more successful in a nonstochastic sense (e.g., simply has a greater observed proportion of responders) in view of the data accrued in the trial thus far. RAR has a long history in the biostatistics literature and it has been used occasionally in clinical trials (Hu and Rosenberger 2006). In platform trials, RAR can potentially increase trial efficiency in the sense that efficacious treatment arms can be identified quicker and quite reliably (Saville and Berry 2016). There are both advantages and disadvantages of RAR, and its implementation always requires careful considerations (Robertson et al. 2020). For instance, one motivation for using RAR is to maximize the expected number of successes in the trial, which may be particularly important in trials of rare and life-threatening diseases with limited patient horizon (Palmer and Rosenberger 1999). Another possibility for application of RAR is trials of highly contagious diseases such as Ebola where the hope is that the disease may be eradicated by the investigational treatment or vaccine (Berger 2015). In all, various stakeholders' perspectives should be taken into account when assessing the possibility of incorporating RAR in the design. A general consensus is that RAR may be useful in phase II exploratory settings but less so in phase III confirmatory settings. It is also instructive to quote the following recent perspective on RAR from the FDA (Food and Drug Administration 2019):

> ...Response-adaptive randomization alone does not generally increase the Type I error probability of a trial when used with appropriate statistical analysis techniques. It is important to ensure that the analysis methods appropriately take the design of the trial into account. Finally, as with many other adaptive techniques based on outcome data, response-adaptive randomization works best in trials with relatively short-term ascertainment of outcomes...

It should be noted that RAR designs rely on certain assumptions on responses (e.g., statistical model linking responses with effects of treatments and biomarkers, fast availability of individual outcome data to facilitate model updates, and modifications of randomization probabilities) and require calibration through comprehensive simulations before they are implemented in practice. It is also important to acknowledge that RAR designs may potentially have deteriorating performance if outcome data are affected by time trends (Thall et al. 2015), and special statistical techniques are required to obtain robust results in the analysis (Villar et al. 2018). However, different RAR procedures vary in the statistical properties, and some issues pertinent to particular RAR procedures, for example, high variability and potential loss in statistical power of the randomized play-the-winner rule (Wei and Durham 1978), should not be overgeneralized to all RAR procedures (Villar et al. 2020).

Several recent papers provide simulation reports on RAR for multiarm trials with and without control arm (Wathen and Thall 2017; Viele et al. 2020a, b). One sensible RAR approach is to skew allocation to the empirically best arm (if it exists) while maintaining some allocation to the control (Trippa et al. 2012; Wason and Trippa 2014; Yuan et al. 2016). This would provide sufficient power to formally compare the effects of the most successful experimental treatment against the control. One extra challenge, however, is that new experimental arms are added over time and RAR requires some burn-in period to ascertain estimates of treatment effects to facilitate adaptations. Some efficient RAR designs for multiarm controlled platform trials where experimental arms can be added/dropped during the course of the study are available; see papers by Ventz et al. (2018), Hobbs et al. (2018), Kaizer et al. (2018), Normington et al. (2020), to name a few.

An increasingly useful idea in RAR platform trials is inclusion of stratification using genetic signatures or some other predictive biomarkers. In this case, RAR probabilities for an individual participant are adjusted such that the participant has increased probability to be assigned to the treatment that is putatively most efficacious given their baseline biomarker profile. The research question is: which compound/biomarker pairs are most promising to be taken further in development to more focused confirmatory phase trials? This approach was applied, for instance, in the I-SPY 2 trial in breast cancer (Barker et al. 2009) and in the BATTLE trial in nonsmall cell lung cancer (Zhou et al. 2008; Kim et al. 2011). Both I-SPY 2 and BATTLE trials carried hypothesis-generating value and aimed at identifying targeted therapies, but not formally testing their clinical efficacy. A more elaborate design is GBM AGILE – an ongoing seamless phase II/III platform trial in glioblastoma, which combines data from promising treatments identified during a phase II multiarm Bayesian RAR part with the data for these treatments during a phase III part to formally test clinical efficacy with respect to overall survival and enable submissions (Alexander et al. 2018).

Data Monitoring and Interim Decision Rules

Platform trials involve data monitoring and various interim decisions. A key principle of any adaptive design is that adaptations must be carefully preplanned to ensure statistically valid results. The FDA guidance on master protocols states (Food and Drug Administration 2018):

> ...Master protocols evaluating multiple investigational drugs can add, expand, or discontinue treatment arms based on findings from prespecified interim analyses or external new data. Before initiating the trial, the sponsor should ensure that the master protocol and its associated SAP describe conditions that would result in adaptations such as the addition of a new experimental arm or arms to the trial, reestimation of the sample size based on the results of an interim analysis, or discontinuation of an experimental arm based on futility rules.

The guidance also emphasizes the importance of having an independent data monitoring committee (IDMC) to conduct interim analyses and make recommendations. The IDMC ensures trial integrity and mitigation of operational bias.

In a platform trial, various interim decisions can be made on ongoing investigational treatment arms; see section "General Definitions." Also, a platform trial protocol may provision for addition of new investigational arms. Some papers discuss methodology to formally justify a decision to add new arms to an ongoing trial (Elm et al. 2012; Cohen et al. 2015; Lee et al. 2019; Choodari-Oskooei et al. 2020).

Another important aspect is the timing and frequency of interim analyses (IAs). Safety monitoring is usually performed continuously throughout the study, but interim analyses of efficacy are less frequent.

Decision rules should be based on some statistical criteria and the corresponding boundary. The statistical criterion may be:

- Observed treatment effect (e.g., point estimate, confidence interval, or test statistic)
- Bayesian posterior probability of the treatment effects
- Conditional power (probability of rejecting the null hypothesis in the final analysis given current data)
- Bayesian predictive probability of success (average conditional power or "assurance")

Often, it is possible to establish a one-to-one correspondence among the decision rules, for example, a statement on Bayesian posterior probability or conditional power can be transformed into a statement on the observed treatment effect (Gallo et al. 2014). In practice, decision criteria will be considered together with other design elements such as sample size, randomization, study endpoints, etc.

It is instructive to look at the development of decision rules by example. Consider OPTIM-ARTS design for a phase II open platform trial in melanoma (Racine-Poon et al. 2020). The design consists of two parts: 1) randomized, open platform phase to screen for activity multiple targeted therapy combinations and 2) expansion phase to formally test promising treatments from the first phase. The primary efficacy endpoint is ORR at 20 weeks posttreatment initiation, and there is no control arm due to lack of adequate SOC in this indication. The study starts with three arms and randomizes patients in a 1:1:1 ratio. The first IA is planned after about 10 patients per arm contribute data for evaluation of ORR. Subsequent IAs are planned approximately every five months thereafter. The maximum number of patients per arm in Part 1 is capped at 30. To facilitate decision making in part 1, the ORR for each treatment arm is modeled using a standard Bayesian beta-binomial model with uniform prior. At a given IA, an arm can be: (i) expanded into Part 2, if $\Pr(ORR > 0.20 | \, data) > 0.70$; (ii) stopped for futility, if $\Pr(ORR < 0.15 | \, data) > 0.70$; or (iii) continued in Part 1, if neither (i) nor (ii) is met. If an arm has reached its cap of 30 patients and neither (i) nor (ii) is met, the arm is stopped and not pursued further.

If a decision to expand an arm is made, the sample size for Part 2 is determined adaptively, using Bayesian shrinkage estimation to mitigate treatment selection bias and to ensure >70% Bayesian predictive power to obtain significant final results. The final analysis for each treatment arm in Part 2 is done using standard frequentist methodology (exact binomial test), based on cumulative data from Part 1 and 2 for this arm.

All decision rules/criteria in OPTIM-ARTS design are calibrated through Monte Carlo simulation under various true values of ORR, to achieve desirable statistical characteristics, such as reasonably high correct decision probabilities in part 1, and high power and control of the type I error rate in Part 2. A combination of Bayesian monitoring in Part 1 with formal hypothesis testing for selected treatment arms in Part 2 allows flexible and statistically rigorous design.

Sample Size and Power

Sample size determination is an integral part of any clinical trial design, and the platform trial is no exception. Some important considerations for the sample size planning include the study objectives, the choice of a research hypothesis, primary endpoint, study population, control and experimental treatment groups, statistical methodology for data analysis, etc. The common statistical criteria for sample size planning are statistical power and significance level (probability of a type I error); however, additional criteria such as estimation precision, probabilities of correct go/no-go decisions may be considered as well.

At the design stage, the sample size planning will likely be an iterative process that may involve a combination of standard calculations and simulations. Suppose we have $K \geq 1$ experimental treatment arms and a control arm, and we decide to use equal randomization with m patients per arm. There are different ways to characterize power in a multi-arm setting (Marschner 2007). One way is to consider null hypotheses on individual treatment contrasts (experimental vs. control) as follows: $H_0^{(j)} : \Delta_j = 0$ vs. $H_1^{(j)} : \Delta_j > 0$, where $\Delta_j = \mu_j - \mu_0$ and $j = 1, \ldots, K$. Assuming individual responses on the kth treatment are normally distributed with mean μ_k and variance σ^2, the sample size $m = 2\sigma^2(z_{1-\alpha} + z_{1-\beta})^2/\Delta^2$ per arm (where z_u is the 100uth percentile of the standard normal distribution and $\Delta > 0$ is some clinically relevant value of the mean treatment difference) provides power of $(1 - \beta)$ for each of the K comparisons. This assumes that each hypothesis is tested at significance level α and no multiplicity adjustment is made.

Another way is to consider simultaneous testing $H_0 : \cap_{j=1}^{K} H_0^{(j)}$ vs. H_1: not H_0. In this case, an investigator may wish to control a family-wise error rate (FWER), that is, the probability of rejecting any true null hypothesis, at some prespecified level α. A conservative way of doing this would be to use a comparison-wise level of α/K (the Bonferroni approach). If the same standardized treatment effect Δ applies in all K comparisons and the correlation between all endpoints is ½, then the requisite sample size per arm is $m = 2\sigma^2(z_{1 - \alpha/K} - u_{K,\ 1/2,\ \beta})^2/\Delta^2$ where $u_{K,\ 1/2,\ u}$ is the 100uth percentile of the K-variate normal distribution with zero mean and covariance matrix that has diagonal elements equal to 1 and all off-diagonal elements equal to ½. Alternatively, Dunnett's (1955) procedure accounts for the positive correlation among contrasts with the common control. The sample size per arm to achieve power of $(1 - \beta)$ per comparison while maintaining the FWER at level α using Dunnett's test is then $m = 2\sigma^2(u_{K,\ 1/2,\ 1 - \alpha} - u_{K,\ 1/2,\ \beta})^2/\Delta^2$. More on sample size calculations for multiple tests can be found in Horn and Vollandt (2000). A recent paper (Choodari-Oskooei et al. 2020) extended Dunnett's procedure to the case of adding new research arms and platform trials, and the resulting approach was shown to be less conservative than the Bonferroni approach.

In the literature, there have been debates on whether adjustment for multiplicity is required in multiarm trials with a shared control group (Proschan and Follmann 1995; Freidlin et al. 2008; Wason et al. 2014). For instance, Freidlin et al. (2008) argued that multiarm trials that are designed with a common control group for logistical efficiency do not require multiplicity adjustments. However, in multiarm trials where the research questions of different comparisons are clinically related (e.g., experimental arms represent different dose levels of a compound, or a trial evaluates the addition of an experimental agent to several backbone regimens against the control arm), then the adjustment for multiple comparisons would be appropriate. Either way, such issues should be a part of the discussion with regulatory agencies (Collignon et al. 2020).

The sample size planning for a platform trial should also take into consideration the adaptive nature of the experiment, that is, that some arms can be stopped early for futility and/or efficacy. How many effective treatments should be identified within the platform trial before it can stop is another important part of the master protocol planning. Interim analyses may inflate probabilities of type I/type II error, and sample size planning should account for that. Many frequentist designs that provision for interim decisions, such as group sequential designs (Jennison and Turnbull 2000), are well-established for confirmatory trials, and their validity depends on adherence to the prespecified futility and/or efficacy rules. By contrast, Bayesian designs do not formally incorporate considerations of the type I error rate control; however, these designs can be fine-tuned via simulations to ensure they have desirable statistical properties across a range of plausible experimental scenarios and trial parameters. There are some examples in the literature how this can be done in practice (Quan et al. 2019; Ventz et al. 2017).

The theory of adaptive designs (see e.g., Wassmer and Brannath 2016) allows for many modifications (such as dropping or adding treatment arms, restricting recruitment to subpopulations, changing sample size or randomization ratios, in theory even changing endpoints) while maintaining the family-wise error rate. However, these methods were originally not developed for very frequent adaptations; hence, power loss can be severe when applying them in platform trials with many design adaptations.

The uncertainty on the final sample size numbers for the chosen platform trial design should always be quantified; ideally, not only the values of the expected sample size, but also the entire distribution of the sample size per arm and overall in the study should be obtained and presented via simulations. The choice of the experimental scenarios for simulations should be comprehensive but it will never be exhaustive. There are some good industry practices on simulation of adaptive trials in drug development (Mayer et al. 2019) that can be useful for sample size planning for platform trial designs.

Data Analysis Issues

The analysis of any clinical trial should be reflective of the trial design. The statistical analysis plan for a platform trial should include details of the planned analyses, both interim and final. Since many platform trials have adaptive elements, some important principles for adaptive designs naturally apply for platform trials. The FDA guidance for industry "Adaptive designs for clinical trials of drugs and biologics" (Food and Drug Administration 2019) makes the following statement that applies to all clinical trials intended to provide substantial evidence of effectiveness:

> . . .In general, the design, conduct, and analysis of an adaptive clinical trial intended to provide substantial evidence of effectiveness should satisfy four key principles: the chance of erroneous conclusions should be adequately controlled, estimation of treatment effects should be sufficiently reliable, details of the design should be completely prespecified, and trial integrity should be appropriately maintained...

The strong control of the type I error rate is a major requirement for any clinical trial with a confirmatory component. Various interim decisions can inflate the type I error rate. Thus, special statistical techniques are required to ensure the overall type I error is maintained at a prespecified level. Some design methodologies, such as group sequential designs (Jennison and Turnbull 2000) and adaptive designs (Wassmer and Brannath 2016), specifically address the issue of the type I error control by properly selecting interim stopping boundaries. Adaptive designs with treatment (or subgroup) selection at interim, known as seamless phase II/III designs (Bretz et al. 2009; Wassmer and Brannath 2016), provide ways to properly combine data from the exploratory and confirmatory parts of the trial in the analysis (i.e., *inferentially seamless* designs) while controlling the type I error. For other designs and analysis techniques, simulations can be used to evaluate the probability of false positive findings. For a platform trial with a confirmatory component, the control of the type I error rate is more complex due to uncertainty on the number of experimental treatment arms that will be tested in the study and possibly multiple registrations that may follow. Industry best practices on type I error considerations in master protocols with shared control are still emerging (Sridhara et al. 2021).

Another important aspect is estimation of treatment effects. Design adaptations such as selection of an arm that exhibits the best interim results introduce positive bias in the final estimation of treatment effect. In order to quantify this bias, bias-corrected estimates accounting for design adaptations (Bowden and Glimm 2008; Stallard and Kimani 2018) can be reported. These methods correct for the selection bias generated by specific types of selections such as "pick-the-winner" or "drop-the-loser" in multiarm situations. The insistence on unbiasedness inflates the mean squared error (MSE) which, for several of these methods, is larger than that of the corresponding maximum likelihood estimator (MLE). However, shrinkage estimation techniques (which reduce, but not entirely eliminate bias) have been proven to have lower MSE than the MLE (Carreras and Brannath 2013; Bowden et al. 2014). The magnitude of the bias is situation dependent. It generally depends on the "severity" of the selection (e.g., the number of treatment arms from which a winner is picked), the size of the study, and the similarity of the underlying true but unknown treatment effects. In a well-planned, large study with limited selection options, it will often be small. However, in studies with a wide range of potential selection decisions, it can be substantial.

In addition to point estimates, confidence intervals are of interest. Construction of confidence intervals accounting for multiple interim looks at the data and design adaptations has been discussed in the literature (Neal et al. 2011; Kimani et al. 2014; Kimani et al. 2020); however, no fully satisfactory construction method exists and applications are very diverse. Overall, it may be prudent to report both stage-wise unadjusted estimates and confidence intervals and adjusted quantities based on combined data. The assessment of data homogeneity from different stages (both baseline characteristics and the outcome data) is very important for interpretation of the study results (Gallo and Chuang-Stein 2009; Friede and Henderson 2009). This is explicitly documented in the EMA "Reflection paper on methodological issues in confirmatory clinical trials planned with an adaptive design" (European Medicines Agency 2007):

> ...Using an adaptive design implies that the statistical methods control the pre-specified type I error, that correct estimates and confidence intervals for the treatment effect are available, and that methods for the assessment of homogeneity of results from different stages are pre-planned. A thorough discussion will be required to ensure that results from different stages can be justifiably combined...

Some special considerations are required for reporting of the results of a platform trial. For instance, how should the results of completed treatment arms be reported while the main master protocol is still ongoing? In this regard, a good example is the STAMPEDE (Systemic Therapy for Advancing or Metastatic Prostate Cancer) study

(James et al. 2009), which has been ongoing since 2005 while providing periodic updates on the investigational treatments (comparisons) that have been completed in due course.

Examples of Platform Trials

EPAD-PoC Study in Alzheimer's Disease

The European Prevention of Alzheimer's Disease (EPAD) Consortium was a public-private effort funded by the EU through the Innovative Medicines Initiative (IMI) and the European Federation of Pharmaceutical Industries and Associations (EFPIA) partners, which included pharmaceutical, biotechnology and related companies. It started in January 2015 with the mission to develop improved models of Alzheimer's disease and creating a research environment for optimized testing of novel treatments for the secondary prevention of Alzheimer's dementia, and it ended in October 2020 (https://www.imi.europa.eu/projects-results/project-factsheets/epad). The EPAD project had several foundational elements, including the virtual registry of potential research participants, the longitudinal cohort study (EPAD-LCS) to provide information on disease progression in the presymptomatic phase, and the PoC study (EPAD-PoC) to test new interventions in the earliest stages of Alzheimer's disease.

The EPAD PoC study was designed as a phase II, open platform, randomized, placebo-controlled Bayesian adaptive trial (Ritchie et al. 2016). The master protocol specified a common framework for all interventions and covered the inclusion criteria, patient stratification, assessment schedule, study logistics, and other design features. The ISAs would provide additional compound-specific details. The study provisioned for a Clinical Candidate Selection Committee (CCSC) that would determine which experimental therapeutics to include for testing in the study. In general, a study compound would have already shown clinical safety and clinical proof-of-mechanism (target engagement). The clinical PoC criteria were based on the Repeatable Battery for the Assessment of Neuropsychology Status (RBANS), planned to be analyzed through a repeated measurement model with Bayesian decision criteria for futility and efficacy. The potential efficiency gains in the EPAD-PoC study were envisioned to be due to an operationally streamlined design and the use of the shared control group.

While EPAD-PoC was conceptually designed using the I-SPY2 study (Barker et al. 2009) as a prototype, it also had some unique features. The EPAD-LCS provided important observational data on subjects with a high risk to develop Alzheimer's disease, which formed the basis for development of longitudinal disease models using subjects' genetic information, biomarkers, and other risk factors. This, in turn, would help identify and stratify participants for the EPAD-PoC study that would subsequently advance most promising compounds for optimized testing in large-scale phase III trials.

By the end of 2019, EPAD-LCS recruited and deeply phenotyped more than 2000 participants; however, the PoC study (EPAD-PoC) to test new interventions did not take place due to lack of drug sponsors to run trials. The EPAD initiative finished in late 2020. Overall, this case study represents the complexity of clinical research in challenging indications such as Alzheimer's disease and reinforces the importance of lessons learned in this context.

I-SPY COVID-19 Study

The COVID-19 pandemic has been a major public emergency since February 2020. Global efforts are taken worldwide to develop effective vaccines and treatments against COVID-19 infections. Clinical development for COVID-19 treatments poses several challenges:

- Being a global pandemic causing hundreds of thousands of deaths, there is a tremendous need for the speedy development of treatments and vaccines as well as for rapid production and dissemination of these.
- The pool of candidate treatments is huge, including drugs that have been already approved for other indications, novel agents, and possibly their combinations.
- The SOC is likely to change over time, for example, due to identification of efficacious therapies.

Several platform trials for rapid testing of various re-purposed and novel treatments for COVID-19 were initiated in 2020 and are now ongoing. Here we discuss just one of them, the I-SPY COVID-19 trial (Identifier: NCT04488081). This is an open-label, randomized, multiarm, active-controlled, Bayesian adaptive phase II platform trial to rapidly screen promising agents for treatment of critically ill COVID-19 patients. Eligible patients are stratified based on their status at entry (ventilation vs. high-flow oxygen) before randomization. The primary endpoint is time to recover to a durable (at least 48 h) level of 4 or less on the WHO-recommended COVID-19 ordinal scale (WHO 2020) (time frame: up to 28 days).

The trial design (NCT04488081) describes four experimental arms (combinations of novel agents with remdesivir) and an active comparator (remdesivir plus SOC), and there is a provision to add more experimental agents to the study, depending on the recruitment and the time course of COVID-19 in the USA. The sample size per experimental arm is capped at 125 patients. The arms can be dropped early for futility after enrollment of 50 patients. The arms exhibiting strong efficacy signals can qualify for further development, in which case the enrollment to these arms will cease, and new investigational arms can be added.

The I-SPY COVID-19 trial is a massive collaborative effort that involves several university medical centers in the USA, pharma/biotech industry, and the FDA, with the estimated enrollment of up to 1500 participants and estimated primary completion date of July 2022.

GBM AGILE Study in Glioblastoma

Alexander et al. (2018) described the design of the Glioblastoma (GBM) Adaptive Global Innovative Learning Environment (AGILE) – an international, multiarm, randomized, open platform, inferentially seamless study to identify effective therapies for newly diagnosed and recurrent GBM within different biomarker-defined patient subtypes (ClinicalTrials.gov Identifier: NCT03970447).

The trial employs a master protocol that allows multiple novel experimental therapies and their combinations to be evaluated within the same trial infrastructure. The design consists of two parts:

1. Phase II screening stage, designed using Bayesian adaptive randomization, to identify effective therapies within biomarker subtypes based on overall survival, compared with a common control
2. Phase III confirmatory stage, which expands sufficiently promising treatment arms from the first part and formally tests their clinical efficacy against the control with respect to overall survival, in an inferentially seamless manner to enable registration

The GBM AGILE design has several innovative features that are worthy elaborating upon:

- Study participants are stratified into three subtypes of GBM: newly diagnosed methylated (NDM), newly diagnosed unmethylated (NDU), or recurrent disease (RD). Each experimental arm can have one enrichment biomarker, thought to be predictive to the outcome for the given arm. A combination of stratification and enrichment biomarkers creates up to six different subtypes for patient randomization. Within each subtype, different SOC control arms and different experimental drug combinations are considered.
- Bayesian adaptive randomization is applied such that within each stratum, 20% of participants are randomized to the control, and allocation to experimental arms is skewed such that greater proportions are assigned to arms with evidence of prolonged overall survival compared to the control group given the patient's subtype.
- A longitudinal model linking the effects of treatments, covariates, biomarkers, and overall survival is developed to predict the individual survival time. The model can potentially be used to "speed up" Bayesian response-adaptive randomization algorithm that otherwise relies on survival times that are observed with natural delay.
- During phase II screening part, treatment efficacy is assessed within predefined biomarker "signatures" (that may be different from the stratification subtypes), such that an experimental arm exhibiting very promising results for a particular signature will be expanded into phase III confirmatory part within this signature.

In summary, GBM AGILE study provides an open platform for clinical investigation with both exploratory and confirmatory components. It can potentially enable faster, more efficient, and more ethically appealing development of therapies for glioblastoma.

FOCUS4 Study in Metastatic Colorectal Cancer

The FOCUS4 study (ISRCTN90061546) was a phase II/III randomized, stratified, platform trial of several targeted therapies for patients with advanced or metastatic colorectal cancer. The study was sponsored by the UK Medical Research Council (MRC) and designed and conducted by the MRC Clinical Trials Unit. The FOCUS4 study used a master protocol with independent comparison-specific protocols corresponding to five different biomarker-based cohorts, with elements of multiarm multistage (MAMS) design methodology (Kaplan et al. 2013; Kaplan 2015).

Eligible patients would receive an initial 16-week period of standard first-line chemotherapy, and their tumor tissues would undergo several molecular assays to determine the appropriate biomarker stratum for the patient. Within each stratum, patients would be randomized in a 2:1 ratio to a targeted experimental treatment or placebo. The five strata defined five subtrials (comparisons): FOCUS4-A for patients with BRAF-mutant tumors; FOCUS4-B for patients with PIK3CA mutations or PTEN loss; FOCUS4-C for patients with KRAS or NRAS mutations; FOCUS4-D for patients whose tumor was wild-type for BRAF, PIK3CA, KRAS, and NRAS; and FOCUS4-N for patients who could not be classified as any of the subtypes above.

The platform nature of the FOCUS4 study provisioned for addition of new investigational therapies to the randomization process mid-trial or terminating the arms that would show evidence of futility early on. More specifically, FOCUS4 master protocol (FOCUS4 2019) specified four analysis stages for each biomarker-defined comparison of experimental treatment vs. placebo: safety (stage I), lack-of-sufficient-activity (stage II), efficacy for progression-free survival (PFS) (stage III), and efficacy for overall survival (OS) (stage IV). Interim results for each stage would be reviewed by the IDMC to guide subsequent decisions for each comparison. Importantly, different substudies of FOCUS4 had their own targeted effect sizes for PFS and OS and called for different maximum sample sizes.

Overall, FOCUS4 provided many valuable scientific and operational insights and lessons learned (Hague et al. 2019; Morrell et al. 2019; Schiavone et al. 2019). The study recruitment started in October 2014. The first full-length published results were from FOCUS4-D subtrial (Adams et al. 2018). Based on data from 32 randomized patients, 16 to AZD8931 (a HER1, 2, and 3 inhibitor) and 16 to placebo, the IDMC recommended closure of FOCUS4-D at the first preplanned interim analysis for futility as it was found that AZD8931 was unlikely to improve PFS compared to placebo in this population.

We accessed the recruitment chart of FOCUS4 (www.focus4trial.org/recruitmentoverall/). The listed numbers of randomized patients were as of November 30th, 2019; and they were as follows: $n = 6$ for FOCUS4-B (recruitment closed in August 2018); $n = 32$ for FOCUS4-D (recruitment closed in April 2016); $n = 60$ for FOCUS4-C; and $n = 246$ for FOCUS4-N. It was also mentioned at the

FOCUS4 website (www.focus4trial.org) that the recruitment into the study was suspended in March 2020 due to COVID-19 pandemic and the study closed follow-up of all patients on October 31st 2020.

Summary and Conclusion

In this chapter, we provided an overview of platform trial designs, an important type of master protocols to evaluate multiple experimental treatments in a chosen indication within a common trial infrastructure. Platform trials can be cast as open-ended randomized multiarm trial designs with or without a shared control arm, and the experimental arms may be added/dropped during the course of the study on the basis of a predefined decision algorithm. Platform trials have the potential to significantly improve efficiency of clinical drug development by screening more experimental therapies and answering more research questions in a systematic way.

Although the concepts of master protocols and platform trials are relatively new, these designs have already found broad use in practice, which is signified by an exponential growth of publications on both methodological work and real clinical trials (Park et al. 2019; Meyer et al. 2020). Amid the COVID-19 pandemic, several platform trials to evaluate re-purposed therapies, novel experimental agents, and possibly their combinations were initiated and are currently ongoing. The platform trial model makes it feasible to assess a huge number of treatment options for the pandemic in a scientifically rigorous and ethical manner.

Master protocol study designs require more upfront planning and early engagement with health authorities and other relevant stakeholders. These studies are operationally complex and require careful coordination and collaboration among various functions in the drug development enterprise. Information technology is an important ingredient and key to a successful implementation of these studies. Statistical software for simulation of design operating characteristics can help clinical investigators evaluate different design options under various experimental scenarios at the study planning stage and select the best design option for the study objectives (Meyer et al. 2021).

Finally, we would like to highlight the importance of precompetitive collaboration and broad discussions among stakeholders in industry, academia, and health authorities on master protocols, in particular on platform trials. Best industry practices on master protocols are still emerging, and we anticipate increasing interest in both the methodology and applications of these designs in the near future.

References

Adams R, Brown E, Brown L, Butler R, Falk S, Fisher D, Kaplan R, Quirke P, Richman S, Samuel L, Seligmann J, Seymour M, Shiu KK, Wasan H, Wilson R, Maughan T, FOCUS4 Trial Investigators (2018) Inhibition of EGFR, HER2, and HER3 signalling in patients with colorectal cancer wild-type for BRAF, PIK3CA, KRAS, and NRAS (FOCUS4-D): a phase 2-3 randomised trial. Lancet Gastroenterol Hepatol 3(3):162–171

Alexander BM, Ba S, Berger MS, Berry DA, Cavenee WK, Chang SM, Cloughesy TF, Jiang T, Khasraw M, Li W, Mittman R, Poste GH, Wen PY, Yung WKA, Barker AD, GBM AGILE Network (2018) Adaptive global innovative learning environment for glioblastoma: GBM AGILE. Clin Cancer Res 24(4):737–743

Antonijevic Z, Beckman RA (2019) Platform trials in drug development: umbrella trials and basket trials. CRC Press, Boca Raton

Barker AD, Sigman CC, Kelloff GJ, Hylton NM, Berry DA, Esserman LJ (2009) I-SPY 2: an adaptive breast cancer trial design in the setting of neoadjuvant chemotherapy. Clin Pharmacol Ther 86(1):97–100

Bentzien J, Bharadwaj R, Thompson DC (2015) Crowdsourcing in pharma: a strategic framework. Drug Discov Today 20(7):874–883

Berger VW (2015) Letter to the editor: a note on response-adaptive randomization. Contemp Clin Trials 40:240

Berry SM (2020) Potential statistical issues between designers and regulators in confirmatory basket, umbrella, and platform trials. Clin Pharmacol Ther 108(3):444–446

Berry SM, Connor JT, Lewis RJ (2015) The platform trial: an efficient strategy for evaluating multiple treatments. JAMA 313(16):1619–1620

Bowden J, Brannath W, Glimm E (2014) Empirical Bayes estimation of the selected treatment mean for two-stage drop-the-loser trials: a meta-analytic approach. Stat Med 33:388–400

Bowden J, Glimm E (2008) Unbiased estimation of selected treatment means in two-stage trials. Biom J 50(4):515–527

Bretz F, Koenig F (2020) Commentary on Parker and Weir. Clin Trials 17(5):567–569

Bretz F, Koenig F, Brannath W, Glimm E, Posch M (2009) Adaptive designs for confirmatory clinical trials. Stat Med 28:1181–1217

Byar DP (1980) Why data bases should not replace randomized clinical trials. Biometrics 36: 337–342

Carreras M, Brannath W (2013) Shrinkage estimation in two-stage adaptive designs with midtrial treatment selection. Stat Med 32:1677–1690

Chen N, Carlin BP, Hobbs BP (2018) Web-based statistical tools for the analysis and design of clinical trials that incorporate historical controls. Comput Stat Data Anal 127:50–68

Choodari-Oskooei B, Bratton DJ, Gannon MR, Meade AM, Sydes MR, Parmar MK (2020) Adding new experimental arms to ransomised clinical trials: impact on error rates. Clin Trials 17(3): 273–284

Cohen DR, Todd S, Gregory WM, Brown JM (2015) Adding a treatment arm to an ongoing clinical trial: a review of methodology and practice. Trials 16:179

Collignon O, Gartner C, Haidich AB, Hemmings RJ, Hofner B, Pétavy F, Posch M, Rantell K, Roes K, Schiel A (2020) Current statistical considerations and regulatory perspectives on the planning of confirmatory basket, umbrella, and platform trials. Clin Pharmacol Ther 107(5): 1059–1067

DiMasi JA, Grabowski HG, Hansen RW (2016) Innovation in the pharmaceutical industry: new estimates of R&D costs. J Health Econ 47:20–33

Dodd LE, Freidlin B, Korn EL (2021) Platform trials – beware the noncomparable control group. N Engl J Med 384(16):1572–1573

Dodd LE, Proschan MA, Neuhaus J, Koopmeiners JS, Neaton J, Beigel JD, Barrett K, Lane HC, Davey RT (2016) Design of a randomized controlled trial for ebola virus disease medical countermeasures: PREVAIL II, the Ebola MCM study. J Infect Dis 213(12): 1906–1913

Dunnett CW (1955) A multiple comparison procedure for comparing several treatments with a control. J Am Stat Assoc 50:1096–1121

Elm JJ, Palesch YY, Koch GG, Hinson V, Ravina B, Zhao W (2012) Flexible analytical methods for adding a treatment arm mid-study to an ongoing clinical trial. J Biopharm Stat 22:758–772

European Medicines Agency. Reflection paper on methodological issues in confirmatory clinical trials with an adaptive design. London, 18 October 2007. Available from https://www.ema.europa.eu/en/documents/scientific-guideline/reflection-papermethodological-issues-confirmatory-clinical-trials-planned-adaptive-design_en.pdf

Esserman L, Hylton N, Asare S, Yau C, Yee D, DeMichele A, Perlmutter J, Symmans F, van't Veer L, Matthews J, Berry DA, Barker A (2019) I-SPY2: unlocking the potential of the platform trial. In: Antonijevic Z, Beckman RA (eds) Platform trial designs in drug development: umbrella trials and basket trials. CRC Press, Boca Raton, pp 3–22

FOCUS4 master protocol (2019). http://www.focus4trial.org/media/1809/03a_focus4_master-protocol-v70_11sep2019_clean.pdf

Food and Drug Administration. Master protocols: efficient clinical trial design strategies to expedite development of oncology drugs and biologics. Guidance for industry (draft guidance). September 2018. https://www.fda.gov/media/120721/download

Food and Drug Administration. Adaptive designs for clinical trials of drugs and biologics: guidance for industry. November 2019. https://www.fda.gov/media/78495/download

Freidlin B, Korn EL, Gray R, Martin A (2008) Multi-arm clinical trials of new agents: some design considerations. Clin Cancer Res 14(14):4368–4371

Friede T, Henderson R (2009) Exploring changes in treatment effects across design stages in adaptive trials. Pharm Stat 8:62–72

Gallo P, Chuang-Stein C (2009) What should be the role of homogeneity testing in adaptive trials? Pharm Stat 8:1–4

Gallo P, Mao L, Shih VH (2014) Alternative views on setting clinical trial futility criteria. J Biopharm Stat 24(5):976–993

Galwey NW (2017) Supplementation of a clinical trial by historical control data: is the prospect of dynamic borrowing an illusion? Stat Med 36:899–916

Hague D, Townsend S, Masters L, Rauchenberger M, Van Looy N, Diaz-Montana C, Gannon M, James N, Maughan T, Parmar MK, Brown L et al (2019) Changing platforms without stopping the train: experiences of data management and data management systems when adapting platform protocols by adding and closing comparisons. Trials 20(1):294

Hobbs BP, Chen N, Lee JJ (2018) Controlled multi-arm platform design using predictive probability. Stat Methods Med Res 27:65–78

Horn M, Vollandt R (2000) A survey of sample size formulas for pairwise and many-to-one comparisons in the parametric, nonparametric and binomial case. Biom J 42(1):27–44

Howard DR, Brown JM, Todd S, Gregory WM (2018) Recommendations on multiple testing adjustment in multi-arm trials with a shared control group. Stat Methods Med Res 27(5): 1513–1530

Hu F, Rosenberger WF (2006) The theory of response-adaptive randomization in clinical trials. Wiley, New York

International Conference on Harmonisation. ICH E9(R1) Addendum on Estimands and Sensitivity Analysis in Clinical Trials to the Guideline on Statistical Principles for Clinical Trials. 17 February 2020. https://www.ema.europa.eu/en/documents/scientific-guideline/ich-e9-r1-addendum-estimands-sensitivity-analysis-clinical-trials-guideline-statistical-principles_en.pdf

International Conference on Harmonisation. E10: Choice of Control Group in Clinical Trials. January 2001. https://www.ema.europa.eu/en/ich-e10-choice-control-group-clinical-trials

James ND, Sydes MR, Clarke NW, Mason MD, Dearnaley DP, Anderson J, Popert RJ, Sanders K, Morgan RC, Stansfeld J, Dwyer J, Masters J, Parmar MK (2009) Systemic therapy for advancing or metastatic prostate cancer (STAMPEDE): a multi-arm, multistage randomized controlled trial. BJU Int 103(4):464–469

Jennison C, Turnbull BW (2000) Group sequential methods with applications to clinical trials. CRC Press, Boca Raton

Jiao F, Tu W, Jimenez S, Crentsil V, Chen YF (2019) Utilizing shared internal control arms and historical information in small-sized platform clinical trials. J Biopharm Stat 29(5):845–859

Jin M, Liu G (2020) Estimand framework: delineating what to be estimated with clinical questions of interest in clinical trials. Contemp Clin Trials 96:106093

Kaizer AM, Hobbs BP, Koopmeiners JS (2018) A multi-source adaptive platform design for testing sequential combinatorial treatment strategies. Biometrics 74(3):1082–1094

Kaplan R (2015) The FOCUS4 design for biomarker stratified trials. Chin Clin Oncol 4(3):35

Kaplan R, Maughan T, Crook A, Fisher D, Wilson R, Brown L, Parmar M (2013) Evaluating many treatments and biomarkers in oncology: a new design. J Clin Oncol 31(36):4562–4568

Kim ES, Herbst RS, Wistuba II et al (2011) The BATTLE trial: personalizing therapy for lung cancer. Cancer Discov 1:44–53

Kimani PK, Todd S, Renfro LA, Glimm E, Khan JN, Kairalla JA, Stallard N (2020) Point and interval estimation in two-stage adaptive designs with time to event data and biomarker-driven subpopulation selection. Stat Med 39(19):2568–2586

Kimani PK, Todd S, Stallard N (2014) A comparison of methods for constructing confidence intervals after phase II/III clinical trials. Biom J 56(1):107–128

Kopp-Schneider A, Calderazzo S, Wiesenfarth M (2020) Power gains by using external information in clinical trials are typically not possible when requiring strict type I error control. Biom J 62(2): 361–374

Kuznetsova OM, Tymofyeyev Y (2011) Brick tunnel randomization for unequal allocation to two or more treatment groups. Stat Med 30(8):812–824

Kuznetsova OM, Tymofyeyev Y (2014) Wide brick tunnel randomization – an unequal allocation procedure that limits the imbalance in treatment totals. Stat Med 33(9):1514–1530

Lee KM, Wason J, Stallard N (2019) To add or not to add a new treatment arm to a multi-arm study: a decision-theoretic framework. Stat Med 38:3305–3321

Marschner IC (2007) Optimal design of clinical trials comparing several treatments with a control. Pharm Stat 6:23–33

Mayer C, Perevozskaya I, Leonov S, Dragalin V, Pritchett Y, Bedding A, Hartford A, Fardipour P, Cicconetti G (2019) Simulation practices for adaptive trial designs in drug and device development. Stat Biopharm Res 11(4):325–335

Meyer EL, Mesenbrink P, Dunger-Baldauf C, Fülle HJ, Glimm E, Li Y, Posch M, König F (2020) The evolution of master protocol clinical trial designs: a systematic literature review. Clin Ther 42(7):1330–1360

Meyer EL, Mesenbrink P, Mielke T, Parke T, Evans D, König F on behalf of EU-PEARL (EU Patient-cEntric clinicAl tRial pLatforms) Consortium (2021) Systematic review of available software for multi-arm multi-stage and platform clinical trial design. Trials 22:183

Morrell L, Hordern J, Brown L, Sydes MR, Amos CL, Kaplan RS, Parmar MK, Maughan TS (2019) Mind the gap? The platform trial as a working environment. Trials 20(1):297

Neal D, Casella G, Yang MCK, Wu SS (2011) Interval estimation in two-stage, drop-the-losers clinical trials with flexible treatment selection. Stat Med 30:2804–2814

Normington J, Zhu J, Mattiello F, Sarkar S, Carlin B (2020) An efficient Bayesian platform trial design for borrowing adaptively from historical control data in lymphoma. Contemp Clin Trials 89:105890

Palmer CR, Rosenberger WF (1999) Ethics and practice: alternative designs for phase III randomized clinical trials. Control Clin Trials 20:172–186

Park JJH, Harari O, Dron L, Lester RT, Thorlund K, Mills EJ (2020) An overview of platform trials with a checklist for clinical readers. J Clin Epidemiol 125:1–8

Park JJH, Siden E, Zoratti MJ, Dron L, Harari O, Singer J, Lester RT, Thorlund K, Mills EJ (2019) Systematic review of basket trials, umbrella trials, and platform trials: a landscape analysis of master protocols. Trials 20:572

Parker RA, Weir CJ (2020) Non-adjustment for multiple testing in multi-arm trials of distinct treatments: rationale and justification. Clin Trials 17(5):562–566

Pocock SJ (1976) The combination of randomized and historical controls in clinical trials. J Chronic Dis 29:175–188

PREVAIL II Writing Group (2016) A randomized, controlled trial of Zmapp for ebola virus infection. N Engl J Med 375:1448–1456

Proschan MA, Follmann DA (1995) Multiple comparisons with control in a single experiment versus separate experiments: why do we feel differently? Am Stat 49(2):144–149

Quan H, Zhang B, Lan Y, Luo X, Chen X (2019) Bayesian hypothesis testing with frequentist characteristics in clinical trials. Contemp Clin Trials 87:105858

Racine-Poon A, D'Amelio A, Sverdlov O, Haas T (2020) OPTIM-ARTS – an adaptive phase II open platform trial design with an application to a metastatic melanoma study. Stat Biopharm Res. https://doi.org/10.1080/19466315.2020.1749722

Ritchie CW, Molinuevo JL, Truyen L, Satlin A, Van der Geyten S, Lovestone S, on behalf of the European Prevention of Alzheimer's Dementia (EPAD) Consortium (2016) Development of interventions for the secondary prevention of Alzheimer's dementia: the European Prevention of Alzheimer's Dementia (EPAD) project. Lancet Psychiatry 3(2): 179–186

Robertson DS, Lee KM, López-Kolkovska BC, Villar SS (2020) Response-adaptive randomization in clinical trials: from myths to practical considerations. https://arxiv.org/pdf/2005.00564.pdf

Rosenberger WF, Lachin J (2015) Randomization in clinical trials: theory and practice, 2nd edn. Wiley, New York

Rosenberger WF, Sverdlov O, Hu F (2012) Adaptive randomization for clinical trials. J Biopharm Stat 22(4):719–736

Ryeznik Y, Sverdlov O (2018) A comparative study of restricted randomization procedures for multiarm trials with equal or unequal treatment allocation ratios. Stat Med 37:3056–3077

Saville BR, Berry SM (2016) Efficiencies of platform clinical trials: a vision of the future. Clin Trials 13:358–366

Scannell JW, Blanckley A, Boldon H, Warrington B (2012) Diagnosing the decline in pharmaceutical R&D efficiency. Nat Rev Drug Discov 11(3):191–200

Schiavone F, Bathia R, Letchemanan K, Masters L, Amos C, Bara A, Brown L, Gilson C, Pugh C, Atako N, Hudson F et al (2019) This is a platform alteration: a trial management perspective on the operational aspects of adaptive and platform and umbrella protocols. Trials 20(1):264

Siden EG, Park JJH, Zoratti MJ, Dron L, Harari O, Thorlund K, Mills EJ (2019) Reporting of master protocols towards a standardized approach: a systematic review. Contemp Clin Trials Commun 15:100406

Simon R (1989) Optimal two-stage designs for phase II clinical trials. Control Clin Trials 10:1–10

Sridhara R, Marchenko O, Jiang Q, Pazdur R, Posch M, Redman M, Tymofyeyev Y, Li X, Theoret M, Shen YL, Gwise T, Hess L, Coory M, Raven A, Kotani N, Roes K, Josephson F, Berry S, Simon R, Binkowitz B (2021) Type I error considerations in master protocols with common control in oncology trials: report of an American Statistical Association Biopharmaceutical Section open forum discussion. Stat Biopharm Res. https://doi.org/10.1080/19466315.2021.1906743

Stallard N, Kimani P (2018) Uniformly minimum variance conditionally unbiased estimation in multi-arm multi-stage clinical trials. Biometrika 105(2):495–501

Stallard N, Todd S, Parashar D, Kimani PK, Renfro LA (2019) On the need to adjust for multiplicity in confirmatory clinical trials with master protocols. Ann Oncol 30(4):506–509

Sverdlov O, Rosenberger WF (2013) On recent advances in optimal allocation designs for clinical trials. J Stat Theory Pract 7(4):753–773

Sverdlov O, Ryeznik Y (2019) Implementing unequal randomization in clinical trials with heterogeneous treatment costs. Stat Med 38:2905–2927

Sverdlov O, Ryeznik Y, Wong WK (2020) On optimal designs for clinical trials: an updated review. J Stat Theory Pract 14:10

Tang R, Shen J, Yuan Y (2019) ComPAS: a Bayesian drug combination platform trial design with adaptive shrinkage. Stat Med 38:1120–1134

Thall PF, Fox P, Wathen JK (2015) Statistical controversies in clinical research: scientific and ethical problems with adaptive randomization in comparative clinical trials. Ann Oncol 26(8): 1621–1628

The Adaptive Platform Trials Coalition (2019) Adaptive platform trials: definition, design, conduct and reporting considerations. Nat Rev Drug Discov 18:797–807

Trippa L, Lee EQ, Wen PY, Batchelor TT, Cloughesy T, Parmigiani G, Alexander BM (2012) Bayesian adaptive randomized trial design for patients with recurrent glioblastoma. J Clin Oncol 30(26):3258–3263

Ventz S, Cellamare M, Parmigiani G, Trippa L (2018) Adding experimental arms to platform clinical trials: randomization procedures and interim analysis. Biostatistics 19(2):199–215
Ventz S, Parmigiani G, Trippa L (2017) Combining Bayesian experimental designs and frequentist data analysis: motivations and examples. Appl Stoch Model Bus Ind 33:302–313
Viele K, Berry S, Neuenschwander B, Amzal B, Chen F, Enas N, Hobbs B, Ibrahim JG, Kinnersley N, Lindborg S, Micallef S (2014) Use of historical control data for assessing treatment effects in clinical trials. Pharm Stat 13(1):41–54
Viele K, Broglio K, McGlothlin A, Saville BR (2020a) Comparison of methods for control allocation in multiple arm studies using response adaptive randomization. Clin Trials 17(1): 52–60
Viele K, Saville BR, McGlothlin A, Broglio K (2020b) Comparison of response adaptive randomization features in multiarm clinical trials with control. Pharm Stat 19:602–612
Villar SS, Bowden J, Wason J (2018) Response-adaptive designs for binary responses: how to offer patient benefit while being robust to time trends? Pharm Stat 17:182–197
Villar SS, Robertson DS, Rosenberger WF (2020) The temptation of overgeneralizing response-adaptive randomization. Clin Infect Dis ciaa1027. https://doi.org/10.1093/cid/ciaa1027
Wason JMS, Stecher L, Mander AP (2014) Correcting for multiple-testing in multi-arm trials: is it necessary and is it done? Trials 15:364
Wason JMS, Trippa L (2014) A comparison of Bayesian adaptive randomization and multi-stage designs for multi-arm clinical trials. Stat Med 33:2206–2221
Wason JMS, Robertson DS (2021) Controlling type I error rates in multi-arm clinical trials: a case for the false discovery rate. Pharm Stat 20:09–116
Wassmer G, Brannath W (2016) Group sequential and confirmatory adaptive designs in clinical trials. Springer International Publishing, Cham
Wathen JK, Thall PF (2017) A simulation study of outcome adaptive randomization in multi-arm clinical trials. Clin Trials 14(5):432–440
Wei LJ, Durham SD (1978) The randomized play-the-winner rule in medical trials. J Am Stat Assoc 73:840–843
World Health Organization. WHO R&D Blueprint Novel Coronavirus COVID-19 Therapeutic Trial Synopsis, 2020. https://www.who.int/blueprint/priority-diseases/key-action/COVID-19_Treatment_Trial_Design_Master_Protocol_synopsis_Final_18022020.pdf
Wong CH, Siah KW, Lo AW (2019) Estimation of clinical trial success rates and related parameters. Biostatistics 20(2):273–286
Woodcock J, LaVange LM (2017) Master protocols to study multiple therapies, multiple diseases, or both. N Engl J Med 377:62–70
Woodcock J, Woosley R (2008) The FDA critical path initiative and its influence on new drug development. Annu Rev Med 59:1–12
Yuan Y, Guo B, Munsell M, Lu K, Jazaeri A (2016) MIDAS: a practical Bayesian design for platform trials with molecularly targeted agents. Stat Med 35:3892–3906
Zhou X, Liu S, Kim ES, Herbst RS, Lee JJ (2008) Bayesian adaptive design for targeted therapy development in lung cancer – a step toward personalized medicine. Clin Trials 5:181–193

Cluster Randomized Trials

77

Lawrence H. Moulton and Richard J. Hayes

Contents

L. H. Moulton (✉)
Departments of International Health and Biostatistics, Johns Hopkins Bloomberg School of Public Health, Baltimore, MD, USA
e-mail: Lmoulto1@jhu.edu; LMOULTON@JHSPH.EDU

R. J. Hayes
Faculty of Epidemiology and Population Health, London School of Hygiene and Tropical Medicine, London, UK
e-mail: Richard.Hayes@lshtm.ac.uk

© Springer Nature Switzerland AG 2022

S. Piantadosi, C. L. Meinert (eds.), *Principles and Practice of Clinical Trials*,
https://doi.org/10.1007/978-3-319-52636-2_108

Abstract

In a randomized clinical or field trial, when randomization units are comprised of groups of individuals, many aspects of design and analysis differ greatly from those of an individually randomized trial. In this chapter, we highlight those features which differ the most, explaining the nature of the differences and delineating approaches to accommodate them. The focus is on design, as many readers will be familiar with the correlated data analysis techniques that are appropriate for many (although not all) cluster randomized trials (CRTs). Thus, the chapter begins by covering motivations for using a CRT design, basic correlation parameters, the variety of potential estimands, delineation and randomization of clusters, and sample size calculation. This is followed by sections on the analysis and reporting of results, which highlight ways to handle the multilevel nature of the data. Finally, ethical and monitoring considerations unique to CRTs are discussed.

Keywords

Cluster randomized trial · Group allocation · Correlated data

Definition

A *cluster randomized trial* (CRT) is a randomized controlled trial (RCT) in which the random assignment of the treatment or experimental condition is performed on sets of individuals, so that within any given set, all individuals are allocated to the same study arm.

Introduction

The vast majority of RCTs employ a randomization scheme wherein trial participants are individually randomized. A typical arrangement in a therapeutic trial is to identify eligible patients as they arrive, one by one, at a clinic or hospital, and assign them to a study arm according to a fixed randomization list. The therapy to be tested, or a control version, is then administered to each individual accordingly, and later the individual's response is recorded. In a cluster randomized trial, however, entire groups of potential participants are defined or identified, with those in a given group assigned the same experimental condition, which they may even experience simultaneously. Group membership may be determined by geography, e.g., place of residence or catchment area of a hospital, or by location where services are received: all the children in a given classroom, say, or all the patients in a hospital ward. It can also be determined by timing, with all the patients presenting on randomly selected days receiving the experimental treatment and the patients on other days receiving the standard-of-care treatment, with each day's patients constituting a group.

Perhaps the first trial that was designed and appropriately analyzed as a CRT was one of isoniazid administration to prevent tuberculosis, where randomization was performed, for administrative ease, by groupings of wards in mental institutions (Ferebee et al. 1963, as reported by Donner and Klar 2000). Still, it was not until statistical and computing advances made in the 1980s, and uptake of these methods in the 1990s, that CRTs became a common tool in the trialist's design repertoire. There are now a number of English-language books devoted to the subject (Murray 1998; Donner and Klar 2000; Hayes and Moulton 2017; Eldridge and Kerry 2012; Campbell and Walters 2014), and hundreds of related methodological articles have been published in the biostatistics and epidemiology literature.

Basic Characteristics of CRTs

The reasons for carrying out randomization at the group or cluster level are usually a combination of (with examples):

1. The intervention to be tested can only be assigned to groups of people. (A campaign to raise public awareness of a health problem might employ messages delivered by radio or newspaper.)
2. It is logistically much easier to deliver the intervention in groups. (It may be too difficult for staff in a clinic to continually switch their procedures for different patients.)
3. It is more acceptable to the study population to receive the intervention in groups. (In an indoor air pollution study where some households receive modern cook-stoves, neighbors may become jealous and hence refuse to participate as controls.)
4. An individually randomized approach might result in too much "contamination," with individuals assigned to the control arm taking up the intervention. (Materials delivered to promote exclusive breastfeeding might be shared or discussed among neighbors.)
5. It is desired to capture effects that are due to group dynamics. (Individuals in a group may communicate with each other and reinforce health messages; deployment of a vaccine throughout a geographic cluster might reduce secondary and tertiary transmissions and result in some herd protection, thereby increasing overall effectiveness at the cluster level.)

The principal drawback to CRTs is that, in general, they require greater sample size in terms of numbers of participants than do individually randomized trials. There is almost always positive within-cluster correlation, which can reduce the effective sample size to a large degree, as will be seen in the sample size section. More participants translate into larger costs for trials that perform maneuvers at the individual level, and there can be cluster-level costs as well, due to increased transportation and communications with community leaders or clinic directors.

A related feature of CRTs is that they often are comprised of relatively small numbers of clusters, say 8–50, although they may have thousands of participants. This is primarily due to the logistics and costs associated with adding each additional cluster. Small numbers of clusters can engender inferential difficulties, both in terms of small sample properties of statistical estimators and greater risks associated with clusters that in one way or another become outliers.

Variability Across Clusters

There is almost always positive correlation among members of a designated group or cluster with respect to any characteristic, measured or not, including health outcomes. This correlation may be viewed as a result of cluster-to-cluster variability of these characteristics. This point needs to be emphasized:

$$\text{Between} - \text{cluster variability} \longleftrightarrow \text{Within} - \text{cluster correlation}$$

Imagine classrooms in an elementary school. There is a large variation in children's height by grade: first graders are on average shorter than second, etc. Otherwise stated, *first graders are more like each other in height than they are like second graders*. This within-grade correlation or dependence can be thought of in another way: knowing the height of one randomly selected second grader; if a second student is randomly selected from any grade, then knowing the second student's grade gives us information about their height relative to the first student's height.

When planning or analyzing a CRT, it is important to account for within-cluster correlation (or, equivalently, between-cluster variation). The two statistical measures most often used in such circumstances are the coefficient of variation k and the intracluster correlation coefficient ρ. To help explain these, consider the example of 1-year period prevalence of tuberculosis among patients attending HIV clinics in Rio de Janeiro. Thus, the data elements are the number of patients enrolled in a clinic (the denominator of the prevalence) and the number of them who were diagnosed with tuberculosis in a given year (the numerator). There are two sources of variation to be considered: (1) binomial variability (within-clinic) and (2) extra-binomial variability (between-clinic). Each clinic has its own, intrinsic prevalence $P_j, j = 1, \ldots N$ clinics. These are assumed to vary across clinics; the distribution of these P_j has its own mean, π, and variance, σ_B^2, the between-clinic (cluster) variance. The clinics' prevalences may differ because of differences in characteristics of their catchment area populations, differences in staff skills, available diagnostic tests, etc. And for any specific clinic, there will be variability in its outcome due to year-to-year variation in exposure or detection. Then a measure of the variability of the true clinic proportions is the coefficient of variation given by $k = \sigma_B/\pi$. Thus, the standard deviation is scaled by the mean and becomes dimensionless – this makes it a fairly transferrable, or meaningful, measure that can be used in other studies or situations. The intracluster correlation coefficient is also dimensionless and can be defined as

$$\rho = \frac{\sigma_B^2}{\sigma^2} = \frac{\sigma_B^2}{\sigma_B^2 + \sigma_W^2},$$

where W stands for "within-cluster"; for proportions, this is:

$$\rho = \frac{\sigma_B^2}{\pi(1 - \pi)}.$$

A third measure, the design effect (DEff for short), is not a measure of cluster variability per se but rather a descriptive measure of the effect of within-cluster correlation in the context of a given study design. It can be designated as:

$$\begin{aligned} \text{DEff} &= \frac{\text{Sample size required when accounting for within} - \text{cluster correlation}}{\text{Sample size required when there is no such correlation}} \\ &= \text{actual sample size/effective sample size} \\ &> 1 \text{ if ICC} > 0 \text{ or if } k > 0, \text{which is the usual situation.} \end{aligned}$$

The DEff depends not only on the correlation but also on cluster size, so that it is more specific to the actual design being considered, but, hence, less generalizable or applicable to other studies.

Parameters to Be Estimated: Analysis Populations and Effects

Analysis Populations

When designing a study, it is important to think carefully about what one wishes to estimate and among whom. In individually randomized trials, several analytic populations may be specified, including intent-to-treat, as-treated, and per-protocol populations (see ▶ Chap. 82, "Intention to Treat and Alternative Approaches"). The same is true for CRTs, but there is an extra layer of complication due to randomizing clusters of people.

In a typical individually randomized trial, participants are enrolled (consented and given an identification code) and then assigned a randomized study treatment – a strict intent-to-treat approach would then analyze all data collected from that point on as if the participant then actually received the assigned treatment. In a CRT, however, there can be two levels of treatment: the treatment condition the cluster receives and the treatment received by participants. If clinics are randomized to have or not have certain educational materials about stroke in their waiting rooms, the intent-to-treat time at the clinic level may begin months before an individual patient shows up at the clinic – the individual's intent-to-treat time-at-risk for having a stroke would begin when they enter the waiting room. That would mimic the long-term effectiveness of the intervention were it ever to be adopted, as the individual would be exposed to the materials from the first time they go to the clinic.

More complications may arise depending on who is considered as having been randomized. If a cluster is defined by geographic residence, at the time of randomization, a strict approach might only follow up individuals who were resident at that moment. However, that results in a closed cohort that ages over time and might not be of as much interest as a dynamic cohort with people entering and leaving clusters. On the other hand, people may move into a cluster because they know it is receiving a treatment they want to receive. The particular nature of the intervention (e.g., applied at the cluster or at the individual level), whether it is masked, its general availability, and potential biases all need to be considered in order to determine exactly what parameters the study should try to estimate.

Effects

There are further questions regarding what events should be counted for which analyses. Halloran and Struchiner (1991) introduced a nomenclature that helps clarify how different parameters of interest may be estimated, as a function of which individuals' events are counted and compared, taking into consideration the possibility of indirect or herd effects occurring within clusters. Figure 1 indicates four possible effects and their estimation: direct, indirect, total, and overall effects. Halloran et al. (1997) may be consulted for further details.

In Fig. 1, comparing the attack rates among those enrolled in each trial arm provides an estimate of the total effect of the intervention. The total effect is a combination of the direct effect (the protection afforded to an individual enrolled in

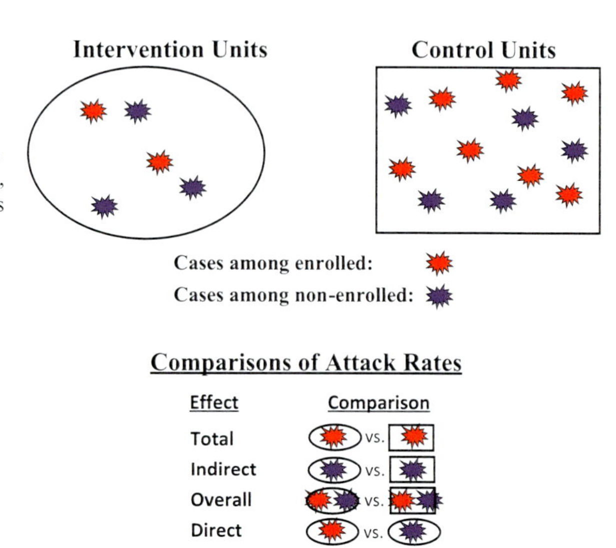

Fig. 1 Depiction of possibly estimable effects in a cluster randomized trial where a subset of individuals in a cluster (unit) are enrolled and receive a study treatment (e.g., a drug in the intervention units and a placebo in the control units), but all may have outcomes measured. Two representative, equal-sized denominator clusters are shown, with "explosion" symbols representing cases arising from the respective populations

an intervention cluster) and the indirect effect (the protection due to decreased exposure, as a result of lower secondary transmission) of an intervention. If outcomes can be measured among individuals who are not specifically enrolled in a trial, say if there are population disease registries or health-care system data available, then indirect and overall effects can be measured. In such a situation, the indirect effect can be directly estimated by comparing attack rates among those who have not been enrolled in the trial (the rates of the purple cases in Fig. 1). Note that people who enroll in a study tend to differ from those who do not; thus, it is best not to compare the non-enrolled in the intervention clusters to everyone in the control clusters. The overall effect is a combination not only of direct and indirect effects but also the degree of coverage that has been attained, i.e., the uptake of the study intervention. It compares attack rates among all those in the clusters who would have been eligible for the trial, regardless of whether they were enrolled. Finally, the direct effect can be estimated by comparing those enrolled to those not enrolled within intervention clusters but may be too biased to be of interest, as there often will be differences in the kinds of people who enter into a trial and those who do not.

Cluster Specification

It may be clear how to define the clusters in a CRT: if the intervention is the introduction of a new triage system in an emergency room, the unit of randomization would be the hospital in which the ER is located, with patients (or patients with a particular condition) arriving at its ER forming the cluster. With geographically defined clusters, however, there may be many different options, including postal codes, census tracts, towns, counties, states, or districts. In a given entire study area, in general, the more clusters there are, the greater will be the study's power, given diminishing returns with respect to cluster size (more on this below in the sample size section). However, the fewer the clusters, the less the potential for contamination occurring from control participants adopting or accessing intervention practices or from control participants introducing pathogens into intervention communities, both of which would tend to reduce observed effectiveness of an intervention. Also, with fewer clusters, there can be reduced costs due to logistics, transportation, and dealing with cluster-level communications and assent from gatekeepers. As an example, in a pneumococcal conjugate vaccine study in infants on an American Indian reservation, the randomization could have been performed at the level of the Indian Health Service administrative units, of which there were eight. Although mixing of infants in intervention areas with those in the control areas would have been minimized, there would not have been much power. There were 110 smaller, tribal organization units, but consultation with local staff indicated there might be substantial contamination across them. In the end, the 110 areas were grouped into 38 randomization units according to a number of factors including location of shopping areas and Head Start preschool program centers (Moulton et al. 2001).

If cross-cluster contamination is a risk, another strategy is to designate buffer zones around the clusters from which outcome data are not collected, although intervention or control activities might still be carried out in these zones. Note that this may increase cost of the trial through requiring setting up the trial in larger geographic areas or more clusters.

Matching and Stratification

As is often done in individually randomized trials, it can be advantageous to carry out randomization of clusters within specified strata, so that within each stratum there is a designated balance of the treatment conditions. Stratification has the dual role of reducing variance by combining similar clusters into strata and of enforcing balance according to the stratification factors so as to reduce confounding. As will be seen in the section on randomization, there are other strategies that may be employed to achieve balance with respect to possibly confounding variables, so that the main advantage of stratification is to compare like-with-like.

When there are not many clusters, we have found that placing them in just 2–4 strata is often sufficient to substantially reduce within-stratum variability in outcomes while only losing a few degrees of freedom in the analysis. Stratifying more deeply to the point of pair-matching can minimize bias and improve the inferential basis for causality but can have some limitations with respect to the statistical analyses that can be carried out, due to lack of replication within the matched pairs. In situations with potentially high variability in outcomes, pair-matching can be very efficient – in the Mwanza STD trial, there was an estimated 13-fold relative efficiency in using matched pairs as compared to an unstratified design (Hayes and Moulton 2017). But if the matching is not done on variables strongly related to the outcomes and there are fewer than ten pairs, one may gain power by ignoring the matching at the time of analysis (Diehr et al. 1995), although it is best to specify this in advance.

Randomization

Many aspects of randomization are covered in ▶ Chap. 40, "Principles of Clinical Trials: Bias and Precision Control." There are, however, two ways in which CRTs often differ from the standard clinical trial that can affect choice of randomization method. First, for most CRTs, all of the units of randomization are identified before the randomization occurs. This can facilitate the process, as complicated systems of assignment, either through distributed or centralized randomization, are not necessary for concealment or minimization of assignment bias. Usually all that is needed is a list of the geographic areas, or the clinics in a research network, a pseudo-random number generator, and 5 min in a quiet room. An exception is when units come online over time, an example of which is the randomized ring vaccination strategy employed in the Ebola ç*a suffit!* trial (Ebola ça suffit Ring Vaccination Trial Consortium 2015), in which clusters of individuals were defined as a randomization unit whenever a new Ebola case was identified. The second potentially distinguishing factor is the number of randomization units, which may be limited in a CRT. Certainly, there are many small phase I clinical trials, but these are often looking at specific biologic responses to a new drug, say, which do not vary greatly from person to person. CRTs may be investigating a combination of behavioral and biologic effects and have additional cluster-level factors that can introduce variability in the outcomes. In addition, a CRT with a small number of clusters may still have thousands of participants and thus be rather expensive. Thus, constructing a good randomization scheme can be more critical in a CRT than in an individually randomized trial with the same number of randomization units.

Stratification to enforce balance was mentioned in the previous section. In an individually randomized trial, age and gender may be the only covariates that affect an outcome, and using four strata (female/male crossed with younger/older) may suffice. But take the example of randomizing 12 census tracts in a city to a new drug harm reduction strategy versus the status quo. One can easily obtain many baseline covariates that would be desirable to have balanced: housing value, proportion of residents with a college education, median household income, population density, etc.; if there are ten such variables that are rendered dichotomous, that yields $2^{10} = 1024$ potential strata. Clearly, with 12 randomization units, a standard stratification strategy will not suffice. Any one of these covariates might end up with a post-randomization imbalance that would not look good in a "Table 1" of a research article and could lead one to question the study results. A multi-million dollar study would not want to risk this kind of imbalance.

Randomization Criteria

A recent article on randomization methods for achieving covariate balance in CRTs states there are two desirable criteria for a successful randomization: unbiasedness and covariate balance (Morgan and Rubin 2012). Covariate balance can be defined in a number of ways, depending on whether exact balance or a caliper-based near balance is required and whether univariate or multivariate functions of covariates are to be employed (e.g., achieving balance on the number of high-income recent immigrants to an area). An unbiased randomization is one in which each randomization unit has the same probability to be selected for a given treatment arm as any other unit. Stated a bit more formally, a design is unbiased if the expected value, over all possible randomization allocations, of the difference in treatment means is equal to the true difference (Bailey and Rowley 1987).

There is, however, a third criterion that is important for randomization, that of "validity." This criterion, perhaps first enunciated in R.A. Fisher's *Design of Experiments* (1947), relates to whether the assignments for different units may in some way be linked to each other. Clearly, if under all possible allocations a given geographic unit was always assigned the same treatment condition as a given neighboring unit, the number of randomization units would effectively be reduced by one. While unbiasedness is a first-moment (mean) consideration, validity is a second-moment (variance) one: a "...scheme is said to be *valid* if the expectations of the treatment mean square and the error mean square are equal in the absence of treatment effects..." (Bailey 1987). An operationally useful result is that in a completely (simple) randomized design, the design is valid if each pair of randomization units has the same probability of being allocated the same treatment (Bailey and Rowley 1987).

Highly Constrained Randomization

Standard implementations of stratified or permuted block designs are both unbiased and valid. Yet when balance is required with respect to many variables, or near-balance across treatment arms on the marginal means of a variable is desired, achieving a completely valid design becomes virtually impossible. For example, determining a valid randomization scheme in a factorial design with just one constraining variable required Bailey (1987) to use a deep knowledge of abstract algebra. For more complicated situations, many methods have been proposed, including simultaneous univariate restriction on sets of variables (Raab and Butcher 2001), Mahalanobis distance (Morgan and Rubin 2012), propensity scores (Xu and Kalbfleisch 2010), or p-values (Bruhn and McKenzie 2009). If their constraining criteria are not too strict, they will yield schemes that are nearly valid. It is easy to see how a given constraint might induce dependence of allocation outcomes among units. Suppose in the above community drug harm reduction strategy it was desired to have the total population in the intervention arm to be within 10% of the population size of the control arm. If there were one very large unit, and one very small one, then among the acceptable allocations, there might be only a few that did not have both of these units in the same study arm, as they would generally need to be in the same arm to achieve the desired marginal balance.

A given system of constraints may result in a high proportion of the total number of possible allocations being deemed unsuitable, resulting in lack of uniformity in the number of times given pairs of units could be placed in the same study arm. A "validity matrix" that consists of the numbers of times each pair of units might be included in the same arm can be constructed and inspected either from enumeration among the acceptable allocations or, if this number is too large, from a random sample of those acceptable (Moulton 2004). Simulations have shown that it takes a large departure from a uniform distribution of inclusion probabilities coupled with high correlation of responses to meaningfully affect Type I error. As with many aspects of experimental design, there is a trade-off: the tighter the constraints, the greater the possibility of inadvertent linkage in treatment assignments, thereby straying further from validity. The analyst can, after the study, perform a randomization analysis, based on the set of potential allocations, as a check, but it is convenient to have a randomization scheme that will allow the standard array of statistical analyses to be conducted. Alternatively, covariate adjustment with the constraining variables can mitigate the effects of a non-valid scheme (Li et al. 2017).

Alternative Designs

Although the focus in this chapter is on two-arm, parallel design trials, there are many possible variations in CRT design. Factorial trials are fairly common; the large cost of a CRT can be more easily justified if two interventions can be evaluated for nearly the price of one, as can be done with a 2×2 factorial design (Montgomery et al. 2003). It is rare, however, to see more than two levels of two factors used, due to the required larger number of clusters and high per-cluster costs.

An increasingly popular design is the stepped wedge design, which is a one-way crossover trial with staggered implementation, so that clusters are scheduled to go from control phase to intervention phase at randomly assigned times (steps), until all clusters have received the intervention. Choice of this design can be motivated by political considerations, when it is desirable to show a steady march toward all clusters receiving an intervention. Interpretation of results, however, can be fraught with difficulties, primarily due to secular trends and variable lengths of implementation (Kotz et al. 2012). Hussey and Hughes (2007) provide a useful framework for modeling these trials, but such models have strong assumptions regarding correlation structures and commonality of effects across clusters that need to be carefully considered (Thompson et al. 2017). It must be noted that subjecting a population to a trial that leads to inconclusive results can be ethically problematic. This design is perhaps best used in situations where an intervention is going to be rolled out in a population anyway, so that randomizing the rollout affords an opportunity to obtain a better evaluation of the program than might otherwise be possible. A useful set of articles on this design, and its many variants, may be found in *Trials* (Torgerson 2015).

Sample Size and Power

Minimum Number of Clusters

The reader may be acquainted with quasi-experimental designs of demonstration projects that randomly assign one or two clusters to each treatment arm. Although technically randomized, such studies do not provide the requisite robustness to provide statistically solid answers to research questions. With a 2 versus 2 design, one can perform a Student t-test with the four cluster means and base a statistical conclusion on it, but there are not enough clusters to get any idea as to whether the assumptions underlying the t-test are met. One cluster whose participants generate an outlying mean response can drastically affect the outcome. It is best to conduct CRTs that have a sufficient number of clusters so that at least a nonparametric check of the results can achieve “statistical significance,” usually meaning obtaining a p-value less than 0.05 from a two-sided hypothesis test. Thus, it is best to have at least eight clusters in a simple randomized design or six pairs of clusters in a matched-pair design. In the former, a rank sum test will achieve $p < 0.05$ if all four intervention clusters are superior (or all inferior) to all four control clusters ($p = 1/C_4^8 = 0.029$).

In the latter, the results of every pair must be the same (intervention clusters all do better than their matched control clusters, or vice versa; in which case $p = 2 * 2^{-6} = 0.031$). Clearly, if in one of these designs just one cluster has difficulties, perhaps withdrawing from the study, or undergoes substantial contamination due to local events, the whole experiment is jeopardized.

Sample Size Methods

The basic concepts involved in sample size determination for CRTs are the same as for individually randomized trials, except that for CRTs there are two sizes that need to be designated for a study: the number of randomization units (clusters) in each trial arm (assuming for simplicity equal numbers of clusters per arm), N, and the number of individuals in each cluster, n, or $n_j, j = 1,\ldots,N$ if the sizes vary by cluster.

Sometimes, the total number of clusters, 2 N, is fixed, say the number of convenient geopolitical units in an area, but it is possible to modify n – we may have 40 districts to randomize and plan to measure the outcome among a random sample of 200 individuals per district. In other circumstances, all individuals in a cluster can be measured easily, say from electronic records in a clinic, but one needs to decide on how many clinics to enter into the trial. It may be that both N and n are fixed, but the follow-up time can be increased to obtain more person-years at risk and hence more events. Typically, it costs less to increase cluster size than to increase the number of clusters, as there can be extra per-cluster costs associated with communication, transportation, and gatekeeper signoff. Yet, as will be seen, there are diminishing returns in terms of power with respect to increasing the size of clusters.

In individually randomized trials, a measure of response variability needs to be specified: the individual level variance. In CRTs, this is also required, as well as specification of a measure of between-cluster variability: either the coefficient of variation k or the intracluster correlation coefficient ρ may be used.

The design effect in terms of ρ may be written as $1 + (n - 1)\rho$ (Kish 1965), an increasing function of both cluster size and the ICC. Then the total number of individuals in a trial arm can be found by multiplying the usual sample size formula by this design effect:

$$Nn = \left(z_{\alpha/2} + z_\beta\right)^2 \frac{\left(\sigma_0^2 + \sigma_1^2\right)}{\left(\mu_0 - \mu_1\right)^2} [1 + (n - 1)\rho]$$

where σ_i^2 is the arm-specific variance of individuals' responses in a given cluster (these are the same as what were subscripted with W for "within," above) and μ_i is the true mean response in each arm (Donner and Klar 2000). Hence, adding one cluster to each arm as an approximate small sample correction, we can take the requisite number of clusters in each arm to be:

$$N = 1 + \left(z_{\alpha/2} + z_\beta\right)^2 \frac{\left(\sigma_0^2 + \sigma_1^2\right)}{n\left(\mu_0 - \mu_1\right)^2} [1 + (n - 1)\rho].$$

Using the coefficient of variation k to express variability across clusters yields the similar formula:

$$N = 1 + \left(z_{\alpha/2} + z_{\beta}\right)^2 \frac{\left(\sigma_0^2 + \sigma_1^2\right)/n + k^2\left(\mu_0^2 + \mu_1^2\right)}{\left(\mu_0 - \mu_1\right)^2}.$$

These formulas can be modified to allow for unequal allocation of clusters in the trial arms and to allow for differential levels of within-cluster correlation across trial arms (Hayes and Bennett 1999). Other modifications include the special case of the matched pairs design and accounting for varying cluster sizes: the greater the variance, the greater the loss of power.

The formula based on k cannot be used directly when dealing with responses that may be negative, e.g., with anthropometric Z-scores; the formula based on ρ is not appropriate for Poisson or rate (based on person-years of observation) response variables. An advantage of k is that it is easily interpretable, and reasonable values for it can be posited even in the absence of good background data. For example, it may be known that in a given district the incidence rate of rotavirus diarrhea in infants is 5 per 10 infant-years and that it is highly unlikely for this rate to vary by more than twofold (from the lowest to the highest) across subdistrict health centers. If the true rates are approximately normally distributed, it might be reasonable to assume about 95% of the rates would be between 3.33 and 6.67 per 10 infant-years, so the standard deviation would be about $(6.67 - 5)/2 = 0.835$, giving $k = 0.835/5 = 0.17$.

As already mentioned, when it comes to study power, there are greatly diminishing returns to increasing cluster sizes for a specified number of clusters. The following table gives an illustration of this for a continuous response variable, diastolic blood pressure, which in a study population has a mean of 100 mmHg, with a standard deviation of 10 mmHg. For a study design with 30 clusters in each arm, power to detect a lowering to 95 mmHg is displayed as a function of cluster size for several levels of k, with 5% Type I error.

Power to detect a 5 mmHg decrease given 30 clusters in each of the intervention and control arms, population SD = 10 mmHg, and 5% Type I error

Coefficient of variation k	Cluster size n	Power
0.050		
	10	91%
	50 500	96% 97%
0.075		
	10	67%
	50 500	72% 74%
0.100		
	10	46%
	50 500	49% 50%

There is usually little variation across clusters in biologic parameters such as blood pressure. In this situation, there is very little to be gained by increasing the sample size tenfold, from 50 to 500. For the two larger values of k, regardless of how much cluster size is increased, the trial will be infeasible, in that not even 80% power would be attainable. If k is thought to be as large as 0.075, more clusters will need to be added to the design.

Statistical Analysis

Individual-Level Regression Methods

Since the 1980s, flexible regression methods for the analysis of correlated data have been readily accessible to researchers. Maximum likelihood estimation of random effects models (Laird and Ware 1982), and generalized estimating equations (GEE) with robust variance estimation (Liang and Zeger 1986), have been the main approaches for handling longitudinal or multilevel data. These methods are also appropriate for the analysis of many CRTs, provided there are sufficient numbers of clusters, say 10–15 in each trial arm. For designs with fewer clusters, the cluster-level methods discussed in the next section may be preferable.

In general, random effects models, which have a "subject-specific" or conditional (on cluster) interpretation, are best used when there are sufficient numbers of observations and/or events in each cluster. GEE models, on the other hand, were designed for situations with small numbers of observations per cluster. GEE yields "population-averaged" (Neuhaus et al. 1991) estimates that are usually close to or identical to the marginal values obtained when ignoring clusters but corrects for over- or under-dispersion via empirical variance estimation. Several adjustments for GEE models have been devised to correct the Type I error, which can be inflated when there are relatively few clusters (Scott et al. 2017).

Because these standard approaches for analyzing correlated data have been well elaborated in the literature, we now focus on cluster-level methods.

Cluster-Level Methods

Within-cluster correlation can be handled directly by reducing the data to a single summary measure for each cluster. For example, this could be the mean height-for-age Z-score of all study children in a cluster, the number of deaths in a cluster divided by the person-years of exposure in that cluster in the time interval of interest, or the number of people with a disease condition divided by the number tested in a cluster. Once these summaries are obtained, any analysis may be performed that could be done with 2 N uncorrelated observations. A Student t-test with associated confidence interval can be applied to either these summaries or to log-transformed measures, and weights may be incorporated if desired. The t-test is fairly robust to its normality assumption, but there may be too few clusters to gauge how well the assumption is met; a Wilcoxon rank sum test can be used as a check and to downweigh undue influence of "outlying" clusters.

If there is a sufficient number of clusters, cluster summaries can be used as responses in regression models that adjust for cluster-level covariates (e.g., whether there is a tertiary care facility in a geographic cluster, or the median income of cluster residents). More often, adjustment for individual-level covariates will be required. Even with very few clusters, the following two-stage method can be employed (Bennett et al. 2002; Hayes and Moulton 2017): (1) In the first stage, ignoring clusters, a regression of the outcome variable on all the adjusting variables is fit, but with the treatment arm indicator(s) omitted; (2) in the second stage, residuals from the fit in the first stage are calculated for each cluster – then the standard analysis, say a *t*-test, is conducted on the residuals. This approach is especially useful in matched pairs designs, where individual-level regression modeling is problematic.

Effects of Correlation Structure on Analyses

In a geographically defined cluster, e.g., a village, the correlation structure of outcomes among residents can be complex. There may be stronger inter-person correlation in the center, more densely populated area, and weaker in the sparser periphery. People may talk with immediate neighbors about a behavioral intervention but also with classmates in a school. There may be repeated measures on individuals over time, inducing within-person correlation as well. One rarely knows the full extent of these correlations. Happily, accounting for correlation at the cluster level, using any of the above methods, automatically accounts for any correlation at all lower levels in the sense that the variance of estimates of treatment effects will be estimated consistently. The more accurately the correlation structure is modeled, however, the more efficient will be the analysis. Typically, an equi-correlation structure is assumed, in the absence of any other information, either through a random effects analysis or a GEE model with specified exchangeable correlation. The further the departure from exchangeability, the more additional clusters are required to achieve accurate variance estimation.

Reporting Results

Standardized reporting of trials has improved greatly with the publication of the CONSORT Statement (see chapter "Reporting guidelines") (Begg et al. 1996). A specialized version has been produced for CRTs, the most recent of which is by Campbell et al. (2012). Many checklist items are the same while calling for additional details on rationale for the cluster design, cluster definition, levels of masking, how clustering is accounted for in the analyses, and estimates of the degree of observed clustering. Not mentioned in this CONSORT, but desirable when there are not too many clusters (say less than 40), is the display in a table or figure of cluster-by-cluster outcome data, so that readers can identify the degree to which clusters varied in size or in magnitude of response.

Ethics and Data Monitoring

Of the three precepts given in the Belmont Report (The National Commission for the Protection of Human Subjects of Biomedical and Behavioral Research 1979) – respect for persons, beneficence, and justice – it is the respect, or informed consent process, that can be the most problematic for CRTs. It may not be possible to obtain informed consent on the part of individuals when the intervention is applied at the community level, say a public health information campaign. In such situations, community leaders, political figures, clinic directors, or other gatekeepers will need to be approached. This is often the case even when the intervention is delivered directly to individuals, so that consent at both the community and individual level is required. The *justice* principle also calls for special consideration, as inequitable distribution (or perception thereof) of risks and benefits may occur, perhaps with certain communities becoming stigmatized for their role in the trial. Individuals who do not partake in the trial may suffer adverse effects related to the treatment of the community in which they live – for example, a mass administration of an antibiotic to children may result in resistance to some organisms, making it difficult to cure adults who succumb to them. The Ottawa Statement (Weijer et al. 2012) addresses further ethical details specific to CRTs.

CRTs will typically have a Data Monitoring Committee (DMC), and perhaps also a Steering Committee, Safety Monitor, or Data Monitor, each of which has some role in overseeing or ensuring the ethical conduct of the study. For CRTs, the DMC has to take a broader view than is done in individually randomized trials, considering the impact on communities or clusters as a whole, which can include those not directly involved in the trial. Monitoring for early evidence of effectiveness and early stopping does not occur as frequently in CRTs as in individually randomized trials, as long-term effects are often of interest, for example, reduction in secondary or tertiary attack rates. When potential early stopping is of interest, the DMC needs to be aware that information is accrued, relatively speaking, more rapidly in a CRT, due to the diminishing returns within clusters of obtaining further information on individuals in a cluster, as described above in the section on sample size (Hayes and Moulton 2017).

Discussion

While this chapter explained some introductory statistical notions relevant to cluster randomized trials, it also concentrated on aspects of how they differ from individually randomized trials that will prove useful even to seasoned statisticians and trialists who have not worked with CRTs. In individually randomized trials, it is usually the case that the intervention is applied at the individual level and data are collected at the individual level. In CRTs, however, there may be three different levels involved in randomization, intervention, and data collection. For example, cluster, individual, and disease registry could be the levels, respectively. When crossed with differing possible analysis populations, from intent-to-treat to per-protocol, and different effects (e.g., indirect) of interest, the potential estimands become myriad. As a consequence, investigators have to think long and hard about exactly what answers a trial should be designed to provide. This will guide cluster formation and specification of inclusion/exclusion criteria for enrollment, intervention, and data collection.

By contrast, methods of analysis of CRTs are relatively straightforward. This chapter has mentioned approaches for handling the particularly problematic analytic feature of CRTs, namely, that many trials involve small numbers of clusters. That means methods relying on large-sample asymptotics may become suspect, and we need to consider alternative methods or conduct additional sensitivity analyses.

As new methods arise in the design and analysis of individually randomized trials, say for covariate specification or causal inference for handling loss to follow up, there will be parallel application of them to CRTs. Such transfer of methodology, however, needs to be done carefully, especially when accounting for within-cluster correlation and small numbers of clusters.

Cross-References

▶ Intention to Treat and Alternative Approaches
▶ Principles of Clinical Trials: Bias and Precision Control
▶ Reporting Biases

References

Bailey RA (1987) Restricted randomization: a practical example. J Am Stat Assoc 82:712–719

Bailey RA, Rowley CA (1987) Valid randomization. Proc R Soc Lond A Math Phys Sci 410:105–124

Begg C, Cho M, Eastwood S, Horton R, Moher D, Olkin I, Pitkin R, Rennie D, Schulz KF, Simel D, Stroup DF (1996) Improving the quality of reporting of randomized controlled trials. The CONSORT statement. JAMA 276:637–639

Bennett S, Parpia T, Hayes R, Cousens S (2002) Methods for the analysis of incidence rates in cluster randomized trials. Int J Epidemiol 31:839–846

Bruhn M, McKenzie D (2009) In pursuit of balance: randomization in practice in development field experiments. Am Econ J Appl Econ 1:200–232

Campbell MJ, Walters SJ (2014) How to design, analyse and report cluster randomised trials in medicine and health related research. Wiley, West Sussex

Campbell MK, Piaggio G, Elbourne DR, Altman DG, CONSORT Group (2012) Consort 2010 statement: extension to cluster randomised trials. BMJ 345. https://doi.org/10.1136/bmj.e5661

Diehr PD, Martin C, Koepsell T, Cheadle A (1995) Breaking the matches in a paired t-test for community interventions when the number of pairs is small. Stat Med 14:1491–1504

Donner A, Klar N (2000) Design and analysis of cluster randomised trials in health research. Arnold, London

Ebola ça suffit Ring Vaccination Trial Consortium (2015) The ring vaccination trial: a novel cluster randomised controlled trial design to evaluate vaccine efficacy and effectiveness during outbreaks, with special reference to Ebola. BMJ 351. https://doi.org/10.1136/bmj.h3740

Eldridge S, Kerry S (2012) A practical guide to cluster randomised trials in health services research, 1st edn. Wiley, West Sussex

Ferebee SH, Mount FW, Murray FJ, Livesay VT (1963) A controlled trial of isoniazid prophylaxis in mental institutions. Am Rev Respir Dis 88:161–175

Fisher RA (1947) The design of experiments, 4th edn. Hafner-Publishing Company, New York

Halloran ME, Struchiner CJ (1991) Study designs for dependent happenings. Epidemiology 2:331–338

Halloran ME, Struchiner CJ, Longini IM Jr (1997) Study designs for evaluating different efficacy and effectiveness aspects of vaccines. Am J Epidemiol 146:789–803

Hayes RJ, Bennett S (1999) Simple sample size calculation for cluster-randomized trials. Int J Epidemiol 28:319–326

Hayes RJ, Moulton LH (2017) Cluster randomised trials, 2nd edn. Chapman & Hall, Boca Raton

Hussey MA, Hughes JP (2007) Design and analysis of stepped wedge cluster randomized trials. Contemp Clin Trials 28:182–191

Kish L (1965) Survey sampling. Wiley, New York

Kotz D, Spigt M, Arts ICW, Crutzen R, Viechbauer W (2012) Use of the stepped wedge design cannot be recommended: a critical appraisal and comparison with the classic cluster randomized controlled trial design. J Clin Epidemiol 65:1249–1252

Laird NM, Ware JH (1982) Random-effect models for longitudinal data. Biometrics 38:963–974

Li F, Turner EL, Heagerty PJ, Murray DM, Volmer WM, Delong EL (2017) An evaluation of constrained randomization for the design and analysis of group-randomized trials with binary outcomes. Stat Med 36:3791–3806

Liang KY, Zeger SL (1986) Longitudinal data analysis using generalized linear models. Biometrika 73:13–22

Montgomery AA, Peters TJ, Little P (2003) Design, analysis and presentation of factorial randomized controlled trials. BMC Med Res Methodol 3:26. https://doi.org/10.1186/1471-2288-3-26

Morgan KL, Rubin DB (2012) Rerandomization to improve covariate balance in experiments. Ann Stat 40:1263–1282

Moulton LH (2004) Covariate-based constrained randomization of group-randomized trials. Clin Trials 1:297–305

Moulton LH, O'Brien KL, Kohberger R, Chang I, Reid R, Weatherholtz R, Hackell JG, Siber GR, Santosham M (2001) Design of a group-randomized Streptococcus pneumoniae vaccine trial. Control Clin Trials 22:438–452

Murray DM (1998) Design and analysis of group randomised trials. Oxford University Press, New York

Neuhaus JM, Kalbfleisch JD, Hauck WW (1991) A comparison of cluster-specific and population-averaged approaches for analyzing correlated binary data. Int Stat Rev 59:25–35

Raab GM, Butcher I (2001) Balance in cluster randomized trials. Stat Med 20:351–365

Scott JM, deCamp A, Juraska M, Fay MP, Gilbert PB (2017) Finite-sample corrected generalized estimating equation of population average treatment effects in stepped wedge cluster randomized trials. Stat Methods Med Res 26:583–597. https://doi.org/10.1177/0962280214552092

The National Commission for the Protection of Human Subjects of Biomedical and Behavioral Research (1979) Protection of human subjects; Belmont report: notice of report for public comment. Fed Regist 44:23191–23197

Thompson JA, Fielding KL, Davey C, Aiken AM, Hargreaves JR, Hayes RJ (2017) Bias and inference from misspecified mixed-effect models in stepped wedge trial analysis. Stat Med 36:3670–3682

Torgerson D (ed) (2015) Stepped wedge randomized controlled trials. Trials 16:351,353,354,358,352,350,359

Weijer C, Grimshaw JM, Eccles MP, McRae AD, White A, Brehaut JC, Taljaard M, Ottawa Ethics of Cluster Randomized Trials Consensus Group (2012) The Ottawa statement on the ethical design and conduct of cluster randomized trials. PLoS Med 9. https://doi.org/10.1371/journal.pmed.1001346

Xu Z, Kalbfleisch JD (2010) Propensity score matching in randomized clinical trials. Biometrics 66:813–823

Multi-arm Multi-stage (MAMS) Platform Randomized Clinical Trials 78

Babak Choodari-Oskooei, Matthew R. Sydes, Patrick Royston, and Mahesh K. B. Parmar

Contents

Abstract

Efficient clinical trial designs are needed to speed up the evaluation of new therapies. The multi-arm multi-stage (MAMS) randomized clinical trial designs have been proposed to achieve this goal. In this framework, multiple

B. Choodari-Oskooei (✉) · M. R. Sydes · P. Royston · M. K. B. Parmar
MRC Clinical Trials Unit at UCL, Institute of Clinical Trials and Methodology, London, UK
e-mail: b.choodari-oskooei@ucl.ac.uk; m.sydes@ucl.ac.uk; j.royston@ucl.ac.uk; m.parmar@ucl.ac.uk

© Springer Nature Switzerland AG 2022

S. Piantadosi, C. L. Meinert (eds.), *Principles and Practice of Clinical Trials*,
https://doi.org/10.1007/978-3-319-52636-2_110

experimental treatments are compared against a common control arm in several stages. This approach has several advantages over the more traditional designs since it obviates the need for multiple two-arm studies, and allows poorly performing experimental treatments to be discontinued during the study. To further increase efficiency, Royston and colleagues proposed a particular class of MAMS designs where an intermediate outcome can be used at the interim stages, thus allowing phases II and III of evaluation to be incorporated under one protocol. The MAMS Platform designs speed up the evaluation process even further by allowing new treatments to be introduced for assessment during the course of a MAMS trial.

In this chapter, we describe the rationale for Royston et al.'s MAMS design, and discuss their underlying principles. An example in prostate cancer is used to explain how the MAMS design can be realized in practice. We present analytical solutions for the strong control of the type I and II error rates, and show how these quantities and the required sample size can be calculated using available software. We also describe the challenges in the design and statistical analysis of such trials, and suggest how these difficulties should be addressed. The MAMS platform design has been used in a variety of disease areas, and holds considerable promise for speeding up the evaluation of new treatments where many new regimens are available for testing in the randomized phase II and phase III trials.

Keywords

Multi-arm multi-stage randomized trials · MAMS designs · Platform protocols · Adaptive clinical trials · Intermediate outcome · STAMPEDE trial · Prostate cancer

Introduction

Background

Randomized controlled trials (RCTs) are the gold-standard for testing whether a new treatment is better than the current standard of care. Recent reviews of phase III trials showed a success rate of around 40% in oncology trials, and only around 7% chance of approval from drugs starting phase I testing (Hay et al. 2014). In many disease areas such as oncology, traditional randomized trials take a long time to complete and are often expensive. Multi-arm, multi-stage (MAMS) trial designs have been proposed to overcome these challenges. The MAMS design aims to speed up the evaluation of new therapies and improve success rates in identifying effective ones (Parmar et al. 2008). In this framework, a number of experimental arms are compared against a common control arm and these pairwise comparisons can be made in several stages. The multi-stage element of the MAMS design resembles the parallel-group sequential designs, where the accumulating data are used to make a decision whether to take a certain treatment arm to the next stage.

Comparing multiple new regimens against a single, common control arm in a multi-arm approach removes the need for multiple two-arm trials with separate control arms and reduces the overall required sample size. For example, Freidlin et al. (2008) showed that comparing four experimental arms in parallel to a single control (one five-armed trial) reduces the required sample size by 37% compared to four separate two-arm trials assuming no adjustments for multiple testing are made. In general, comparing K experimental arms to a single control reduces the overall sample size by a factor of $(K - 1)/2K$ compared to K separate two-arm trials (Freidlin et al. 2008). The efficiency of the multi-arm element can be greatly increased by incorporating a multi-stage element which introduces formal interim-monitoring guidelines to allow stopping early for strong evidence of benefit of the experimental agent (efficacy) or when it seems that the experimental agent will not be better than the control treatment, that is, lack-of-benefit analysis. Figure 1 displays how a MAMS design might compare with a traditional series of separate trials evaluating the same agents.

This chapter describes the multi-arm multi-stage trial design proposed by Royston et al. (2003, 2011), with a focus on the underlying principles and concepts. We use the initial design of the STAMPEDE trial in prostate cancer to describe how the design can be realized in practice. We then explain how to calculate the operating characteristics of the design, and discuss the issues of treatment selection and adding new research arms. Finally, we describe a number of challenges in the design and

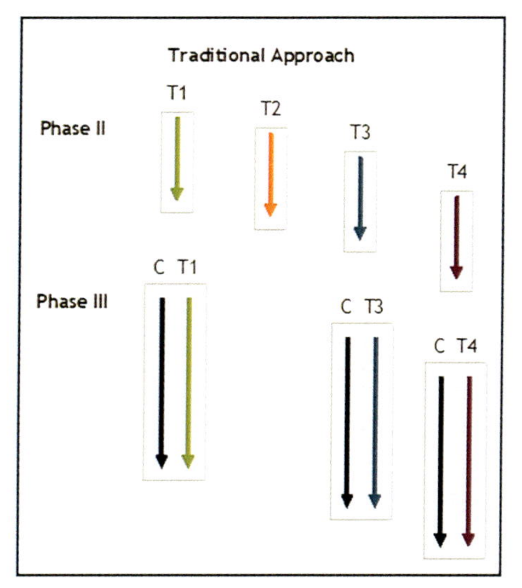

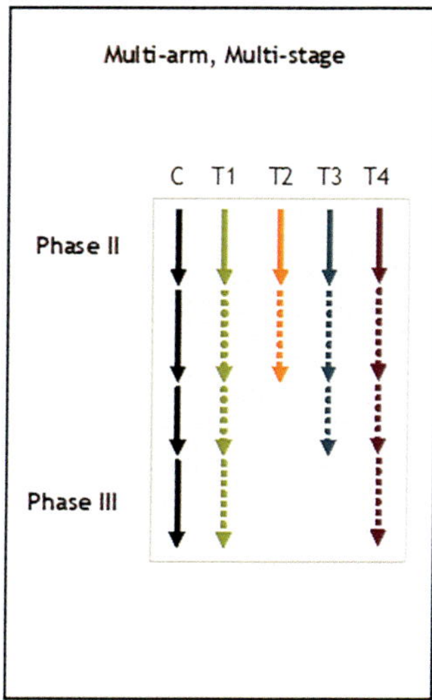

Fig. 1 Schematic representation of traditional approach (left) and a multi-arm, multi-stage design (right) of evaluating experimental treatments (T) against control (C). Traditional approach has a set of separate phase II studies (activity), some of which may not be randomized, with follow-up phase III trials (efficacy) in some interventions that pass the phase II stage. Multi-arm, multi-stage approach provides a platform in which many interventions can be assessed against the control arm simultaneously and are randomized from the phase II component onwards

analysis of MAMS trials, and make suggestions for tackling them. Throughout, we use the acronym MAMS to refer to the multi-arm, multi-stage design described by Royston et al. (2003). Other approaches to MAMS designs will be briefly discussed in "Summary."

The MAMS Approach

Royston et al. (2003) developed a framework for a multi-arm multi-stage design for time-to-event outcomes which can be applied to designs in the phase II/III settings (Royston et al. 2003). In this design, an *intermediate* (I) outcome can be used at the interim stages to further increase the efficiency of the MAMS design by stopping recruitment to treatment arms for lack-of-benefit at interim stages. Using an I outcome in this way allows interim analyses to be conducted sooner and so recruitment to poorly performing arms can be stopped much earlier than if the primary outcome of the trial was used throughout. Examples of intermediate and primary or definitive (D) outcomes are progression-free survival (PFS) and overall survival (OS) for many cancer trials, and CD4 count and disease-specific survival for HIV trials. When using an I outcome at interim stages, each of the experimental arms is compared in a pairwise manner with the control arm using the I-outcome measure, for example, the PFS (log) hazard ratio. Section "Steps to Design a MAMS Trial" outlines the steps that should be taken to design a MAMS trial. Section "Choosing Pairwise Design Significance Level and Power" explains how to choose the stagewise stopping rules and design power, and section "Intermediate and Definitive Outcomes" provides guidance on how to choose an I outcome within this framework.

This design has been extended to binary outcomes with the risk difference (Bratton et al. 2013), and can easily be extended to odds ratio as the primary effect measure (Abery and Todd 2019). The design has also been extended to include stopping boundaries for overwhelming efficacy on the definitive (D) outcome of the trial (Blenkinsop et al. 2019). It is one of the few adaptive designs being deployed both in a number of trials and across a range of diseases in the phase II and III settings, including cancer (Sydes et al. 2012), tuberculosis (TB), and surgical trials (ClinicalTrials.gov Identifier: NCT03838575) (Sydes et al. 2012; ROSSINI 2018; MRC Clinical Trials Unit at UCL). One example is the STAMPEDE trial for men with prostate cancer which is used as an example in this chapter for illustration (Sydes et al. 2012). In the remainder of this chapter, the MAMS designs that utilize the I-outcome for the lack-of-benefit analysis at the interim looks are denoted by $I \neq D$. Designs that monitor all the arms on the same definitive (D) outcome throughout the trial are denoted by $I = D$.

Advantages of MAMS

The MAMS design has several advantages. First, several primary hypotheses or treatments can be evaluated under one (master) protocol. This maximizes the chance of identifying a new treatment which is better than the current standard (Parmar et al. 2014). Second, all patients are randomized from the start which will ensure a fair and contemporaneous comparison. This ensures a seamless run through to the phase III if an early phase (phase II) element is built in the design and under the same protocol and, if at all possible, includes in the phase III evaluation the information from patients in the early evaluation. As a result, the overall trial duration will be markedly reduced compared to separate phase II and III studies since on average many fewer patients will be required in most situations.

Furthermore, a MAMS design can be part of trials with master protocols such as platform or umbrella trials. Master protocols allow major adaptations such as ceasing randomization to an experimental arm or introducing new comparisons through the addition of new experimental arms – see section "Adding New Research Arms and Comparisons." Platform trials provide notable operational efficiency since evaluation of a new treatment within an existing trial will typically be much quicker than setting up a new trial (Schiavone et al. 2019). Therefore, fewer patients tend to be exposed to insufficiently effective or harmful treatments as these treatments are eliminated quickly from the study. This shifts the focus to the more promising treatments as the trial progresses.

Finally, MAMS designs tend to be popular with patients perhaps because the increased number of active treatments means that they are more likely to receive the new treatments. Recruitment tends to markedly improve over time in MAMS trials while many traditional designs may struggle to accrue – particularly, within the context of platform trials and when new treatments are to be tested for different, often biomarker-defined, subgroups of a specific disease. In summary, MAMS platform designs are efficient because they share a control arm, allow for early stopping for lack-of-benefit and adding new research arms, and are operationally seamless.

Example: STAMPEDE Trial

STAMPEDE is a multi-arm multi-stage (MAMS) platform trial for men with prostate cancer at high risk of recurrence who are starting long-term androgen deprivation therapy (Sydes et al. 2009, 2012). In the initial 4-stage design, five experimental arms with treatment approaches previously shown to be suitable for testing in a phase II/III trial were compared to a control arm regimen. In the original design, all patients received standard of care treatment, and further treatments were added to this in the experimental arms. The primary analysis was carried out at the end of stage 4, with overall survival as the primary outcome. Stages 1 to 3 used an intermediate outcome measure of failure-free survival (FFS) to drop arms for lack-of-benefit. As a result, the corresponding hypotheses at interim stages were on lack-of-benefit on failure-free survival. Claims of efficacy could not be made on this outcome because such a claim can only be made on the primary (D) outcome of the trial.

Royston et al.'s MAMS design is constructed by specifying a one-sided significance level α_j and power ω_j for each pairwise comparison in each stage $j, j = 1,\ldots, J$, along with the target treatment effect, for example, log hazard ratio (HR), for the outcome of interest in that stage. The one-sided significance level α_j is the type I error rate to drop an arm for the accumulated trial data until the end of stage j, and ω_j is the corresponding power to continue under the target treatment effect. For sample size calculation, other stagewise design parameters are also required – see Steps 1–10 in section "Steps to Design a MAMS Trial." For example, the user should specify the accrual rate, allocation ratio, and the expected event rate in the control arm in trials with binary or time-to-event outcomes. Based on these and other design parameters, the overall operating characteristics of the design, the timing of each analysis, critical hazard ratio for continuation, and sample sizes can then be calculated using the **nstage** or **nstagebin** packages in Stata – see section "Software and Example."

Table 1 illustrates how the MAMS design was applied to the original comparisons of the STAMPEDE trial. It shows the design specification for the original treatment comparisons at each stage: the outcome measure, target hazard ratio under the alternative hypothesis for the experimental arms (HR^1), pairwise (design) power at each stage (ω_j, $j = 1,2,3,4$), one-sided pairwise significance level (α_j). Given these design parameters, the critical hazard ratio to drop arms for lack-of-benefit and control arm events required to trigger each analysis are calculated using the **nstage** program and included in Table 1. Note that the required number of control arm events in stages 2–4 are slightly higher than those previously reported in Sydes et al. (2012) and other references. These have been calculated using the latest (beta) version of the **nstage** program, to be officially released, that gives more accurate sample sizes – see section "Software and Example." The same design parameters were used for all five original comparisons. The one-sided design significance levels at interim stages (α_j, $j = 1,2,3$) can be used as the "stopping boundaries" on the P-value scale to drop arms for lack-of-benefit. At the end of each stage, if the observed P-value for a comparison is larger than α_j, recruitment (but not necessarily follow-up) to that experimental arm ceases. Recruitment to the other experimental treatments and the control arm continues to the next stage.

In the MAMS design, all P-values are one-sided for the following reasons. At the interim stages, the focus is on continuing with those experimental therapies that show a prespecified level of benefit on the outcome of interest. There would be no

Table 1 Design specification for the 6-arm 4-stage STAMPEDE trial. HR^1, ω_j, α_j are the target hazard ratio (HR) under the alternative hypothesis for the experimental arms, pairwise (design) power, and significance levels at each stage. The critical HR and the required control arm events for each stage are calculated given these design parameters

Stage (j)	Type	Outcome	HR^1	ω_j	α_j	Critical HR	Contl. arm events
1	Activity	FFS	0.75	0.95	0.50	1.00	113
2	Activity	FFS	0.75	0.95	0.25	0.92	223
3	Activity	FFS	0.75	0.95	0.10	0.88	350
4	Efficacy	OS	0.75	0.90	0.025	–	437

interest in continuing with an experimental therapy which was no better than the control regimen (including those which are detrimental). Thus, the interim decision rules are distinctly one-sided. Considering the final stage on the D-outcome, any therapy that is likely to be detrimental in terms of final outcome is very unlikely to have passed the interim stages. It therefore seems inappropriate to test for differences in both directions at the final stage.

Recruitment to the original comparisons of the STAMPEDE trial began late in 2005 and was completed early in 2013. The design parameters for the primary outcome at the final stage were a (one-sided) significance level of 0.025, power of 0.90, and the target hazard ratio of 0.75 on overall survival which requires 437 control arm deaths (i.e., events on overall survival). An allocation ratio of $A = 0.5$ was used for these original comparisons so that, over the long-term, one patient was allocated to each experimental arm for every two patients allocated to control. Proportional hazards assumptions were made in both FFS and OS outcomes.

Because distinct hypotheses were being tested in each of the five experimental arms, the emphasis in the design for STAMPEDE was on the pairwise comparisons of each experimental arm against the control arm, with emphasis on the control of the pairwise type I error rate (PWER) – see section "Operating Characteristics" for definition. Out of the initial five experimental arms, only three of them continued to recruit through to their final stage. Recruitment to the other two arms was stopped at the second interim look due to lack of sufficient activity. Since November 2011, new experimental arms have been added to the original design with five new comparisons added between 2011 and 2018.

MAMS Design

In this section, we present the MAMS design more formally and discuss how it can be realized in practice. We present the design for a variety of outcome measures. We also outline how the operating characteristics of the design can be calculated in different scenarios.

Design Specification

Consider a J–stage trial where patients are randomized between K experimental arms ($k = 1,\ldots,K$) and a single control arm ($k = 0$). The parameter θ_{jk} represents the true difference in the outcome measure between the experimental arm k and control at stage $j, j = 1,\ldots,J$.

For continuous outcomes, θ_{jk} could be the difference in the means of the two groups at stage j, $\mu_{jk} - \mu_{j0}$; for binary data difference in the proportions, $p_{jk} - p_{j0}$; for survival data a log hazard ratio, $\log(HR_{jk})$. For simplicity in notation, we outline the design specification for the case where the same definitive (D) outcome is monitored throughout the trial, that is, $I = D$ designs. Therefore, in all notations θ and

Z represent the definitive primary outcome treatment effect and the corresponding Z-test statistic comparing experimental arm $k = 1, 2\ldots,K$ to the control arm.

The test statistic comparing experimental arm k against the control arm at stage j can be defined as $Z_{jk} = \hat{\theta}_{jk}\sqrt{V_{jk}}$ where V_{jk} is the inverse of the variance of the treatment effect estimator at stage j for the pairwise comparison k – in statistical terms, V_{jk} is known as the Fisher's (observed) information. In the literature, I is used instead of V as the standard notation for Fisher's information. Since in this chapter the intermediate outcome is abbreviated as I, we use the rather nonstandard notation V for Fisher's information. A detailed discussion of information quantification in various outcome settings is provided in Lan and Zucker (1993). The Z-test statistics is (approximately) normally distributed, that is, $Z_{jk} \sim N\left(\theta_{jk}\sqrt{V_{jk}}, 1\right)$, and is assumed standard normal under the null hypothesis, $Z_{jk} \sim N(0, 1)$. For normal or binary data, V_{jk} depends on the number of subjects on the study arms. In time-to-event or survival settings, it depends on the number of events on the study arms. Table 2 presents the treatment effect measures for continuous, binary, and survival outcomes with the corresponding Fisher's (observed) information V_{jk}.

For example, in trials with continuous outcomes where the aim is to test that the outcome of n_1 individuals in experimental treatment E_1 is on average better (here better means smaller, e.g., blood pressure) than that of n_0 individuals in control group (C) at stage j, the null hypothesis ${H^0}_{j1} : \mu_{j1} \geq \mu_{j0}$ is tested against the (one-sided) alternative hypothesis ${H^1}_{j1} : \mu_{j1} < \mu_{j0}$. In this case, the one-sided type I error rate and power at stage j are α_{j1} and ω_{j1} where $\alpha_{\ j1} = \Phi\left(z_{\alpha_{\ j1}}\right)$, $\omega_{\ j1} = \Phi\left(z_{\omega_{\ j1}}\right)$, and $\Phi(.)$ is the normal probability distribution function. In the MAMS design, α_{jk} and ω_{jk} are the key stagewise design parameters, and are needed for sample size calculations – see section "Steps to Design a MAMS Trial" for the other design parameters.

Without loss of generality, assume that a negative value of θ_{jk} indicates a beneficial effect of treatment k. In trials with K experimental arms, a set of K null hypotheses are tested at each stage j,

$$H^0_{jk} : \theta_{jk} \geq {\theta^0}_j, j = 1, \ldots, J : k = 1, \ldots, K$$
$$H^1_{jk} : \theta_{jk} < {\theta^0}_j, j = 1, \ldots, J : k = 1, \ldots, K$$

for some prespecified null effects ${\theta^0}_j$. In practice, ${\theta^0}_j$ is usually taken to be 0 on a relevant scale such as the log hazard ratio for survival outcomes or the mean difference in continuous outcomes. If the same definitive (D) outcome is monitored throughout the trial ($I = D$), then the true treatment effect (θ_{jk}) and ${\theta^0}_j$ are assumed constant for all j. Otherwise, θ_{Jk} and θ^0_J correspond to the true and null effects on the definitive outcome, and θ_{jk} and ${\theta^0}_j$ correspond to the intermediate outcome for all $j < J$ and are constant. For sample size and power calculations, a minimum target treatment effect (often the minimum clinically important difference) is also required, that is, ${\theta^1}_j$. For example, in the STAMPEDE design with five experimental arms and four stages, there are up to 20 sets of null and alternative hypotheses as above. In this

Table 2 Treatment effects, statistical information, and correlation between the test statistics of pairwise comparisons in trials with continuous, binary, and survival outcomes, with common allocation ratio (A) in all pairwise comparisons. Also, see section "Software and Example" (and "Correlation Structure Between Pairwise Comparisons") for an example when an intermediate outcome is used in a MAMS design and how to calculate the between stages correlation structure in this case

Outcome	Treatment effect or outcome measure (θ)	Fisher's information (V)	Correlation structure	
			$Corr(Z_{jk}, Z_{j'k})$ for $j' > j$	$Corr(Z_{jk}, Z_{jk'})$
Continuous	$\mu_{jk} - \mu_{j0}$	$V_{jk} = \left(\frac{\sigma^2_{j0}}{n_{j0}} + \frac{\sigma^2_{jk}}{An_{j0}}\right) - 1$	$\sqrt{\frac{n_{jk}}{n_{j'k}}}$	$\frac{A}{A+1}$
Binary	$p_{jk} - p_{j0}$ $\log\left\{\frac{p_{jk}(1-p_{j0})}{p_{j0}(1-p_{jk})}\right\}$ $\log\left\{\frac{p_{jk}}{p_{j0}}\right\}$	$V_{jk} = \left(\frac{p_{j0}(1-p_{j0})}{n_{j0}} + \frac{p_{jk}(1-p_{jk})}{An_{j0}}\right) - 1$ $V_{jk} = \left(\frac{1}{n_{j0}p_{j0}(1-p_{j0})} + \frac{1}{An_{j0}p_{jk}(1-p_{jk})}\right) - 1$ $V_{jk} = \left(\frac{1-p_{j0}}{n_{j0}p_{j0}} + \frac{1-p_{jk}}{An_{j0}p_{jk}}\right)^{-1}$	$\sqrt{\frac{n_{jk}}{n_{j'k}}}$ $\sqrt{\frac{n_{jk}}{n_{j'k}}}$ $\sqrt{\frac{n_{jk}}{n_{j'k}}}$	$\frac{A}{A+1}$ $\frac{A}{A+1}$ $\frac{A}{A+1}$
Survival	$\log(HR_{jk}) = \log\left(\frac{\lambda_{jk}}{\lambda_{j0}}\right)$	$V_{jk} = \left(\frac{1}{e_{j0}} + \frac{1}{e_{jk}}\right)^{-1}$	$\sqrt{\frac{e_{jk}}{e_{j'k}}}$	$\frac{A}{A+1}$

trial, the null $\left(\theta_j^0\right)$ and target treatment effects $\left(\theta_j^1\right)$ used in all the stages (and comparisons) were 0 and log(0.75), respectively. In MAMS designs that use an intermediate (I) outcome measure at interim stages, the primary null and alternative hypotheses, H_{Jk}^0 and H_{Jk}^1, concern θ_{Jk}, with the hypotheses at stage j ($j < J$) playing a subsidiary role, mainly to calculate the interim stage sample sizes.

The joint distribution of the Z-test statistics therefore follows a multivariate normal distribution $MVN\left(\theta\sqrt{V}, \sum\right)$ where θ and V are the $J \times K$ matrices of the mean treatment effects and the corresponding Fisher's (observed) information $\left(V_{jk} = 1/\text{var}\left(\widehat{\theta}_{jk}\right)\right)$, and Σ denotes the correlation matrix between the $J \times K$ test statistics – see the last two columns of Table 2, for example in trials with time-to-event outcomes note $Corr\left(Z_{jk}, Z_{j'k}\right) = \sqrt{e_{jk}/e_{j'k}}$ for $j' > j$.

The one-sided stagewise significance level α_j plays two key roles in the MAMS design. Together with power ω_j, it is used as the design parameter to calculate the required (cumulative) sample size at the end of stage j. Further, it acts as the stopping boundary for lack-of-benefit at the end of stage j. In principle, in a MAMS design different stopping boundaries can be specified for each pairwise comparison. For simplicity, here we assume the same stopping boundaries (α_j) for all pairwise comparisons. Section "Choosing Pairwise Design Significance Level and Power" explains how to choose the stagewise stopping rules and design power. The interim lack-of-benefit stopping boundaries can also be defined on the Z-test statistic since there is a one-to-one correspondence between them – that is, $l_j = z_{\alpha_j}$ and $j = 1,\ldots, J - 1$. For simplicity in notation, let $L = (l_1, \ldots, l_{J-1})$ be the stopping boundary for lack-of-benefit prespecified for interim stages which correspond to the one-sided significance levels $\alpha_1, \ldots, \alpha_{J-1}$ in all k comparisons – see section "Choosing Pairwise Design Significance Level and Power." For example, in survival outcomes, where the treatment effect is measured by the (log) hazard ratio, L forms an upper bound because the alternative treatment effect being targeted indicates a relative reduction in (log) hazard compared to the control arm.

In designs that include interim stopping boundaries for overwhelming efficacy on the primary outcome measure, another set of $\alpha_j^{(E)}$ should be specified at the design stage. This may be desirable for both investigators and sponsors because being able to identify effective regimens earlier increases the efficiency of the design further by reducing resources allocated to these arms. It may also result in stopping the trial early to progress efficacious arms to the subsequent phase of the testing process or to seek regulatory approval and thus expedite uptake of the treatment by patients. Two popular efficacy stopping boundaries are the Haybittle-Peto and O'Brien-Fleming stopping rules. Blenkinsop et al. (2019) investigated the impact of the efficacy stopping rules on the operating characteristics of the MAMS design. Section "Software and Example" illustrates how to control the overall type I error rate in MAMS designs with both lack-of-benefit and efficacy stopping rules using the STAMPEDE trial as an example. Let $B = (b_1, b_2, \ldots, b_J)$ be the stopping boundary for overwhelming evidence of efficacy on the primary outcome at interim stages, where $b_j = z_{\alpha_j^{(E)}}$ and b_J is the threshold for assessing efficacy at the final analysis corresponding to α_J. The two stopping boundaries meet at the final stage J to ensure a conclusion can be made regarding efficacy. In $I = D$ designs, the primary outcome test statistic is compared to the stopping boundaries at each stage where one of three outcomes can occur (assuming binding boundaries – see section "Binding/Nonbinding Stopping Boundaries"):

- If $b_j < Z_{jk} < l_j$, experimental arm k continues to the next stage (recruitment and treatment k continue).
- If $Z_{jk} > l_j$, experimental arm k is "dropped" for lack of benefit (recruitment and treatment k stopped).
- If $Z_{jk} \leq b_j$, the corresponding null hypothesis can be rejected early and experimental arm k is stopped early for overwhelming efficacy.

Note that the follow-up of randomized subjects in the "dropped" experimental arms should be continued to the planned end of the trial. This has two main advantages. First, follow-up can help in capturing the relevant information on safety endpoints. Second, any potential bias in the estimated treatment effects on the definitive outcome can be markedly reduced by following all patients up to the planned end of the trial and performing analyses then, irrespective of whether recruitment was stopped early for lack of benefit (Choodari-Oskooei et al. 2013).

For the experimental treatments which pass through all interim stages without crossing the boundaries, at the final stage J, the test statistic for each experimental arm is compared with the threshold for the final stage b_J to assess for efficacy, where one of two outcomes can occur:

- If $Z_{Jk} > b_J$, the test is unable to reject the final stage null hypothesis H_{Jk}^0 at level α_J.
- If $Z_{Jk} \leq b_J$, reject H_{Jk}^0 at level α_J and conclude efficacy for experimental arm k.

In designs which include efficacy stopping boundaries on the D-outcome measure and use the I-outcome measure for the lack-of-benefit analysis, there are two (correlated) outcome measures with their respective (correlated) test statistics. The test statistic on the I outcome is used at the interim stages $j = 1,\ldots, J - 1$ for the lack-of-benefit analysis only to eliminate treatment arms that do not show the prespecified level of activity – that is, it is not used for efficacy analysis. In section "Intermediate and Definitive Outcomes," we describe the impact of the I-outcome measure on the operating characteristics of the design with guidance on how to choose the I-outcome. Also, section "Software and Example" uses the STAMPEDE trial as an example to calculate the operating characteristics of a MAMS design with an intermediate outcome as well as the correlation structure that is needed for this purpose.

Steps to Design a MAMS Trial

The following steps should be taken to design a MAMS trial with both lack-of-benefit and efficacy stopping boundaries – see section "Considerations in Design, Conduct, and Analysis of a MAMS Trial" for further guidelines on some of the points:

1. Choose the number of experimental arms, K, and stages, J – see section "Design Considerations."
2. Choose the definitive D outcome, and (optionally) I outcome – see section "Intermediate and Definitive Outcomes."
3. Choose the null values for θ – for example, the (log) hazard ratios on the intermediate $\left(\theta_I^0\right)$ and definitive $\left(\theta_D^0\right)$ outcomes – see section "Software and Example."
4. Choose the minimum clinically relevant target treatment effect size, for example, in the time-to-event setting the (log) hazard ratio on the intermediate $\left(\theta_I^0\right)$ and definitive $\left(\theta_D^1\right)$ outcomes.
5. Choose the control arm event rate (median survival) in trials with binary (survival) outcome – see section "Software and Example."
6. Choose the allocation ratio A, the number of patients allocated to each experimental arm for every patient allocated to the control arm. For a fixed-sample (1-stage) multi-arm trial, the optimal allocation ratio (i.e., the one that minimizes the sample size for a fixed power) is approximately $A = 1/\sqrt{K}$.
7. In $I \neq D$ designs, choose the correlation between the estimated treatment effects for the I and D outcomes. An estimate of the correlation can be obtained by bootstrapping relevant existing trial data – see sections "Correlation Structure Between Pairwise Comparisons" and "Software and Example," and Sect. 2.7.1 in Royston et al. (2011) for further details.
8. Choose the accrual rate per stage to calculate the trials timelines – see section "Software and Example."
9. Choose a one-sided significance level for lack-of-benefit and the target power for each stage (α_{jk}, ω_{jk}). The chosen values for α_{jk} and ω_{jk} are used to calculate the required sample sizes for each stage – see sections "Choosing Pairwise Design Significance Level and Power" and "Design Considerations."
10. Choose whether to allow early stopping for overwhelming efficacy on the primary (D) outcome. If yes, choose an appropriate efficacy stopping boundary α_{Ej} on the D-outcome measure for each stage 1,. . ., J, where $\alpha_{EJ} = \alpha_J$. Possible choices are Haybittle-Peto or O'Brien-Fleming stopping boundaries used in group sequential designs, or one based on α-spending functions (Blenkinsop et al. 2019).
11. Given the above design parameters, calculate the number of control and experimental arm (effective) samples sizes required to trigger each analysis and the operating characteristics of the design, that is, n_{jk} in trials with continuous and binary outcomes and e_{jk} in trials with time-to-event outcomes, as well as the overall type I error rate and power. If the desired (prespecified) overall type I

error rate and power have not been maintained, for instance if the overall pairwise power is smaller than the prespecified value, steps 9–11 should be repeated until success. Or, if the overall type I error rate is larger than the pre-specified value, one can choose a more stringent (lower) design alpha for the final stage, α_J, and repeat steps 9–11 until the desired overall type I error rate is achieved – see sections "Software and Example" and "Design Considerations."

Analysis at Interim and Final Stages

In a MAMS design, the end of each stage is determined when the accumulated trial data reaches the predetermined (effective) sample size for that stage. The effective sample size is the number of subjects in designs with binary and continuous outcomes (Bratton et al. 2013), and the number of required events in designs with time-to-event outcomes (Royston et al. 2011). Reaching the end of each stage triggers an interim analysis of the accumulated trial data. The outcome of analysis is a decision to discontinue recruitment to a particular experimental arm for lack-of-benefit on I (or D), to terminate the trial for efficacy on D, or to continue.

At each interim analysis, the treatment effects are estimated using an appropriate analysis method. For example, the Cox proportional hazards model can be used to estimate the log hazard ratio, and calculate the corresponding test statistic and P-values. In $I = D$ designs, the primary outcome test statistic is compared to the stopping boundaries at each stage where one of the three outcomes, set out in section "Design Specification," can occur. In $I \neq D$ designs with efficacy stopping boundaries for the D outcome which utilize an I outcome for lack-of-benefit analysis at interim stages, two sets of treatment effects $\widehat{\theta}_{jk}^{I}$ (on I) and $\widehat{\theta}_{jk}^{D}$ (on D) are calculated, together with the corresponding test statistics and P-values. The outcome of analysis is a decision to discontinue recruitment to a particular experimental arm for lack-of-benefit on I, to terminate the trial for efficacy on D, or to continue – see Sect. 2.1 in Blenkinsop and Choodari-Oskooei (2019) for the further details on these decision rules.

At the final analysis J, the treatment effect is estimated on the primary outcome for each experimental arm, and the observed P-value is compared against the final stage significance level α_{Jk}. If the P-value is smaller than α_{Jk}, we reject the null hypothesis corresponding to the definitive outcome and claim efficacy. Otherwise, the corresponding null hypothesis cannot be rejected at the α_{Jk} level. Section "Analysis Considerations" discusses the issue of analysis in more detail, particularly the potential impact of the stopping rules on the average treatment effect.

Choosing Pairwise Design Significance Level and Power

The design stagewise type I error (α_{jk}) and power (ω_{jk}) are important in realizing a MAMS design. Together with the target effect sizes, they are the main driver of the stagewise sample sizes. The choice of their values is guided by two considerations. First, it is essential to maintain a high overall pairwise power, ω_k, in Eq. (2) in section "Pairwise Type I Error Rate and Power" for each comparison in the trial. The implication is that for testing the treatment effect at the interim analysis, the design interim-stage power $\omega_{jk}(j < J)$ should be high, for example, at least 0.95. For testing the treatment effect on the definitive outcome, the design pairwise power at the final stage, ω_{Jk}, should also be high, perhaps of the order of at least 0.90 which is higher than many academic trials might select traditionally. The main cost of using a larger number of stages is a (slight) reduction in the overall pairwise power (ω_k). For example, the overall pairwise power in the STAMPEDE trial with four stages is about 0.84 under binding stopping rules for lack-of-benefit – see Table 1 for design stagewise values for α_{jk} and ω_{jk}. Under the nonbinding rules ω_k is equal to the final stage design power ω_{Jk}, that is, 0.90. In section "Software and Example," we describe how to calculate the lower bound for the overall pairwise power in cases where we do not have an estimate of the between-stage correlation structure.

Second, given the design stagewise power ω_{jk}, the values chosen for the α_{jk} largely govern the effective sample sizes required to be seen at each stage and the stage durations. Generally, larger-than-traditional (more permissive) values of α_{jk} are used at the interim stages, because a decision can be made on dropping/continuing arms reasonably early, that is, with a relatively small sample size. It is necessary to use descending values of α_{jk}, otherwise some of the stages become redundant. Royston et al. (2011) suggested a geometric descending sequence of α_{jk} values starting at $\alpha_{1k} = 0.5$ and considering $\alpha_{jk} = 0.5^j (j < J)$ and $\alpha_{Jk} = 0.025$. The latter mimics the conventional 0.05 two-sided significance level for tests on the D outcome. Further, Bratton (2015) proposed a family of α-functions and a systematic search procedure to find the stagewise (design) significance levels. They have been implemented in the **nstagebinopt** Stata program to find efficient MAMS designs (Choodari-Oskooei et al. 2022a). Section "Considerations in Design, Conduct, and Analysis of a MAMS Trial" discusses the relevant issues about the timing and frequency of interim analyses in more details, including both design and trial conduct implications. Section "Design Considerations" addresses some of challenges on the choice of the stagewise (design) power and significance levels to increase the efficiency of a MAMS design.

Intermediate and Definitive Outcomes

The MAMS framework by Royston et al. (2003) allows the use of an intermediate (I) outcome at the interim stages which can speed up the weeding out of insufficiently promising treatments. This markedly increases the efficiency of the design since recruitment to the unpromising arms will be discontinued much faster than otherwise. Choosing appropriate and valid intermediate and definitive (D) outcomes is key to the success of the MAMS design (Royston et al. 2011).

The basic assumptions are that "information" on I accrues at the same rate or faster rate than information for the D outcome, where information is defined as the inverse of the variance of the treatment effect estimator. Another assumption is that the I outcome is on the pathway between the treatments and the D outcome. If the null hypothesis is true for I, it must also hold for D. In this setting, the I outcome does not have to be a perfect or true surrogate outcome for the definitive outcome as defined by Prentice (1989). In the absence of an obvious choice for I, a rational choice of I at the interim stages might be D itself. As a result, in some settings the efficiency of the design might be reduced since the interim analyses will be delayed compared to when using I. In this case, each pairwise comparison resembles a parallel group-sequential design. In the cancer context, typical intermediate and definitive outcomes might be PFS and OS, respectively. Information on PFS is usually available sooner in a study, and in many cancer sites, the treatment effect on PFS is usually highly positively correlated with that on OS (Royston et al. 2011).

Operating Characteristics

The operating characteristics of a conventional two-arm trial are quantified using the type I error rate and power of the design. In MAMS designs, type I error can be controlled for each or a set (or *family*) of pairwise comparisons. These are quantified by the pairwise (PWER) and familywise (FWER) type I error rates. The simplest (and perhaps most useful) measure of power in a MAMS trial is the pairwise power for the comparison of each experimental arm k against control. The correlation structure between different test statistics at different stages is required to calculate these quantities. In the following subsections, we explain how the correlation structure can be estimated. We also define the pairwise/familywise type I error rates and power for a MAMS designs with (and without) an intermediate outcome measure.

Correlation Structure Between Pairwise Comparisons

In the MAMS design, correlation between treatment effect estimates, and the corresponding test statistics, is induced in different ways. First, the shared control arm induces a correlation between treatment effect estimates of pairwise comparisons at the same stage – see the last column in Table 2. Second, since patients accrued in each stage will be included in the analysis of subsequent stages, a correlation will be induced between the treatment effect estimates of different stages in each pairwise comparison – see penultimate column in Table 2.

In $I \neq D$ designs, the correlation between the Z-test statistics at interim stages and that of the final stage will decrease – which decreases the overall pairwise power, see Table 7 in Royston et al. (2011). In these cases, the formulas presented in the penultimate column of Table 2 will be multiplied by the correlation between the treatment effect on I and D outcomes, ρ, at a fixed time-point in the evolution of the trial. For example, in the STAMPEDE trial with time-to-event I and D outcomes where *FFS* is used as the I outcome at the interim stages and *OS* as the D outcome at the final analysis, the correlation between the *FFS* test statistics at the interim stages and that of the OS at the final stage will be calculated using $\rho.\sqrt{e_{jk}^{I}/e_{Jk}^{D}}, j = 1, 2, 3,$ where ρ is the correlation between the estimated log hazard ratios on the two outcomes at a fixed time-point. Note that if the I- and D-outcomes are identical then $\rho = 1$ and $\rho.\sqrt{e_{jk}^{I}/e_{Jk}^{D}}$ reduces to $\sqrt{e_{jk}^{I}/e_{Jk}^{D}}$ (Royston et al. 2011). For other outcomes a similar formula can be derived (Bratton et al. 2013 for binary outcomes and Follmann et al. 2021 for continuous outcomes). Bootstrap analysis of individual patient data from similar previous trials can be used to assess ρ in a particular setting (Barthel et al. 2009). Section "Software and Example" explains how the correlation structure can be calculated when an I outcome is used at the interim stages in the STAMPEDE trial.

Pairwise Type I Error Rate and Power

In a single stage two-arm design, there is only one way to commit a type I error at the final analysis. In trials with lack-of-benefit interim stopping boundaries, a type I error only happens if the trial passes all the interim stopping boundaries – that is, conditional on the treatment arm passing all interim stages. In designs with both lack-of-benefit and efficacy stopping boundaries there is an increased chance of a type I error since there is a further chance of committing a type I error at interim stages – that is, when the interim efficacy boundaries are crossed. For simplicity in notations, we only define the type I error rate and power for designs with lack-of-benefit interim looks.

In designs with J stages and stopping boundaries for lack-of-benefit, Royston et al. (2011) showed that the overall pairwise type I error rate (PWER), α_k, and power, ω_k, for the experimental arm k compared to control are

$$\alpha_k = \Phi_J\left(z_{\alpha_{1k}}, \ldots, z_{\alpha_{Jk}}; R_J^0\right) \text{ under } \theta_j = \theta_j^0 \text{ for all } j \quad (1)$$

$$\omega_k = \Phi_J\left(z_{\omega_{1k}}, \ldots, z_{\omega_{Jk}}; R_J^1\right) \text{ under } \theta_j = \theta_j^1 \text{ for all } j \quad (2)$$

where Φ_J is the J-dimensional multivariate normal distribution function with correlation matrix $R_J^{0/1}$ whose (j, j')th entry is the correlation between the treatment effects in stages j and j', i.e. $Corr\left(Z_{jk}, Z_{j'k}\right)$ in Table 2. The formulas for α_k and ω_k in designs with stopping boundaries for lack-of-benefit and efficacy are more complicated and can be found in Blenkinsop et al. (2019).

In trials with an I outcome, the calculation of α_k in Eq. (1) is made under the assumption that the null hypothesis H^0 is true for both I and D. However, in this case the type I error rate is maximized when the experimental treatment is highly/infinitely effective on I but the null hypothesis is true for D. Therefore, the maximum pairwise type I error rate, $\alpha_{\max}$, is equal to the final stage significance level, $\alpha_{Jk}(>\alpha_k)$ – see Bratton et al. (2016). In the STAMPEDE trial, Table 1, the overall pairwise type I error rate calculated from Eq. (1) is 0.013 as reported in Sydes et al. (2009). However, this is only when H^0 is true for both I and D. By the above argument, the maximum pairwise type I error rate for each pairwise comparison, $\alpha_{\max}$, is actually equal to the final stage significance level of the trial: $\alpha_{\max} = \alpha_J = 0.025$.

Binding/Nonbinding Stopping Boundaries

This raises important questions about the nature of the stopping boundaries for lack-of-benefit at the interim analyses. Are these boundaries strict rules which have to be adhered to, that is, binding stopping boundaries? Or, are these simply stopping guidelines and the decision to continue with the research treatment will also depend on other factors, that is, nonbinding stopping boundaries? For instance, if the treatment effect for an experimental arm has an encouraging point estimate at an interim analysis but has not crossed the corresponding stopping boundary yet it has a highly beneficial effect on an important secondary outcome (e.g., safety), then it may be desirable to continue the arm to the next stage of the study for further assessment. Ignoring interim lack-of-benefit stopping guidelines in a MAMS trial will not inflate the maximum pairwise type I error rate, $\alpha_{\max}$, since it is controlled by the final stage significance level α_J. The interim stopping boundaries could therefore be considered "nonbinding" in these scenarios.

By contrast, lack-of-benefit stopping boundaries will inflate the overall type II error rate. This decreases the overall pairwise power, ω_k, for a fixed sample size since, under the alternative hypothesis, there is a chance to stop the experimental arms that are truly effective. Therefore, it is recommended to calculate the required sample size using nonbinding stopping boundaries for the type I error rate, and binding stopping boundaries for power. This will strongly control both the overall type I and II error rates at prespecified levels. Further, in designs that include both stopping boundaries for lack-of-benefit and efficacy, the lack-of-benefit stopping boundaries interact with the efficacy boundaries. For this reason, nonbinding lack-of-benefit boundaries are often a regulatory requirement. In such designs, the efficacy stopping boundaries have the potential to increase the type I error rate with no impact on power (Blenkinsop et al. 2019).

Familywise Type I Error Rate, All-Pair/Any-Pair Power

In multi-arm trials there are multiple ways to commit a type I error. In some settings it is required to control the overall type I error rate, that is, familywise type I error rate (FWER), for a set of pairwise comparisons of the experimental arms with the control arm at a prespecified level. The FWER is the probability of incorrectly rejecting the null hypothesis for the primary outcome for at least one of the experimental arms from a set of comparisons in a multi-arm trial. Its value is higher than the PWER if no correction for multiple testing is made.

In trials with multiple experimental arms, the maximum possible FWER often needs to be calculated and known (Wason et al. 2014). In some multi-arm trials, this maximum value needs to be controlled at a predefined level. This is called a *strongly* controlled FWER as it covers all eventualities, that is, all possible hypotheses (Bratton et al. 2016). Magirr et al. (2012) showed that the FWER is maximized under the global null hypothesis, H_0^G, that is, when the null hypothesis which maximizes pairwise alpha is true for all arms.

In a family of k "independent" pairwise comparisons each with their own control group and a PWER of α_k, the overall type I error rate (FWER) is

$$\begin{aligned} FWER &= \Pr\left(\text{reject at least one } H_0^k | H_0^G\right) \\ &= \Pr\left(\text{reject } H_0^1 \text{ or } H_0^2 \ldots \text{ or } H_0^k | H_0^G\right) \\ &= 1 - \Pr\left(\text{accept } H_0^1 \text{ and } H_0^2 \ldots \text{ and } H_0^k | H_0^G\right) \\ &= 1 - \prod_{k=1}^{K} (1 - \alpha_k). \end{aligned}$$

When $\alpha_1 = \alpha_2 = \ldots = \alpha_k = \alpha$, the FWER can be calculated using Šidák formula (Sidak 1967),

$$FWER_S = 1 - (1 - \alpha)^k. \quad (3)$$

Bonferroni correction can also be used to calculate the FWER. For example, if the family includes two (independent) pairwise comparisons each with a (one-sided) PWER of $\alpha_1 = \alpha_2 = 0.025$, the $FWER_s$ is 0.0494 from Eq. (3). In this case, Bonferroni correction can also provide a good approximation, that is, $\alpha_1 + \alpha_2 = 0.05$.

To allow for the correlation between the test statistics of different pairwise comparisons, one can replace the term $(1 - \alpha)^k$ in Eq. (3) with an appropriate quantity to reduce the FWER and gain some efficiency in scenarios where the strong control of the FWER is required. Dunnett (1955) developed an analytical formula to calculate the FWER in multi-arm trials which takes care of this correlation structure. For designs with nonbinding stopping boundaries for lack-of-benefit, the maximum FWER can be computed using Dunnett probability (Bratton et al. 2016):

$$FWER = 1 - \Phi_K(z_{1-\alpha_1}, \ldots, z_{1-\alpha_K}; C) \quad (4)$$

where Φ_K is the K-dimensional multivariate normal distribution function and C is the $K \times K$ between-comparison correlation matrix with off diagonal elements equal to $A/(A + 1)$, and A is the allocation ratio. For a family of two pairwise comparisons with a shared control and PWER of $\alpha_1 = \alpha_2 = 0.025$, the $FWER$ is 0.0455 from Dunnett's formula. In this case, the FWER is calculated more accurately than that from Eq. (3) or Bonferroni correction. In designs which require the strong control of the FWER at 0.025, the simplest approach would be to choose the final stage significance level for each pairwise comparison, α_{Jk}, such that the maximum FWER from Eq. (4) is 0.025. For example, in a design with two pairwise comparisons with equal allocation to all arms (and no stopping boundary for interim efficacy analysis), the final stage significance level which controls the FWER at 0.025 is $\alpha_J = 0.0161$ for both comparisons. This is larger than the significance level obtained from other methods, that is, Bonferroni correction ($\alpha_J = 0.0125$) or Šidák formula

(0.0126) which results in lower sample size, hence increasing the efficiency of the design.

In multi-arm designs, two other types of power can be calculated: any-pair and all-pair powers. Any-pair power is the probability of showing a statistically significant effect under the targeted effects for at least one comparison, and all-pairs power is the probability of showing a statistically significant effect under the targeted effects for all comparison pairs. The three measures of power will be identical in a two-arm trial, but when considering a multi-arm design the power measure of interest may depend on the objective of the trial (Choodari-Oskooei et al. 2020). For more complex designs with both overwhelming efficacy and lack-of-benefit stopping boundaries or designs where a new experimental arm is added at a later stage, Eq. (4) can become quite complicated (Blenkinsop et al. 2019; Choodari-Oskooei et al. 2020).

MAMS Selection Designs

In a MAMS design, all experimental arms can reach their final stage of recruitment if they pass each interim analysis activity boundary. As a result, the number of experimental arms recruiting at each stage cannot be predetermined. Therefore, the actual sample size of the trial can be varied considerably with its maximum being when all the treatment arms reach the final stage. In trials with a large number of experimental arms, the maximum sample size might be too large either to achieve or for any funding agency to fund it. In these cases, it may be more appropriate to prespecify the number of experimental arms that will be taken to each stage, alongside a criterion for selecting them. One example of such designs is the ROSSINI-2 surgical trial – see Fig. 2.

The selection of research arms can be made based on ranking of treatment effects, or a combination of efficacy and safety results. Traditionally, selection of the most promising treatments has been made in phase II trials where the strict control of operating characteristics is not a particular concern. In a MAMS selection design, the selection and confirmatory stages are implemented within one trial protocol, and selection of the most promising treatments can be made in multiple stages – see Fig. 2. Patients will be randomized from the start to all the experimental and control arms, and the primary analysis of the experimental arms that reach the final stage include all randomized individuals from start. The advantages of MAMS selection designs are (lower) maximum sample sizes and simpler planning. However, the selection process might get complicated if all arms look promising at the selection stage which might affect the operating characteristics of the design (Stallard et al. 2015). However, in this case we are less interested in individual arms, but in the process of finding an appropriate treatment to the next stage of the trial.

In MAMS selection designs, the primary aim is to select the most promising treatments with high probability of correct selection where strong control of the error rates is required in the phase III setting. The probability of correct selection is driven by the underlying treatment effects, timing of selection, and the number of

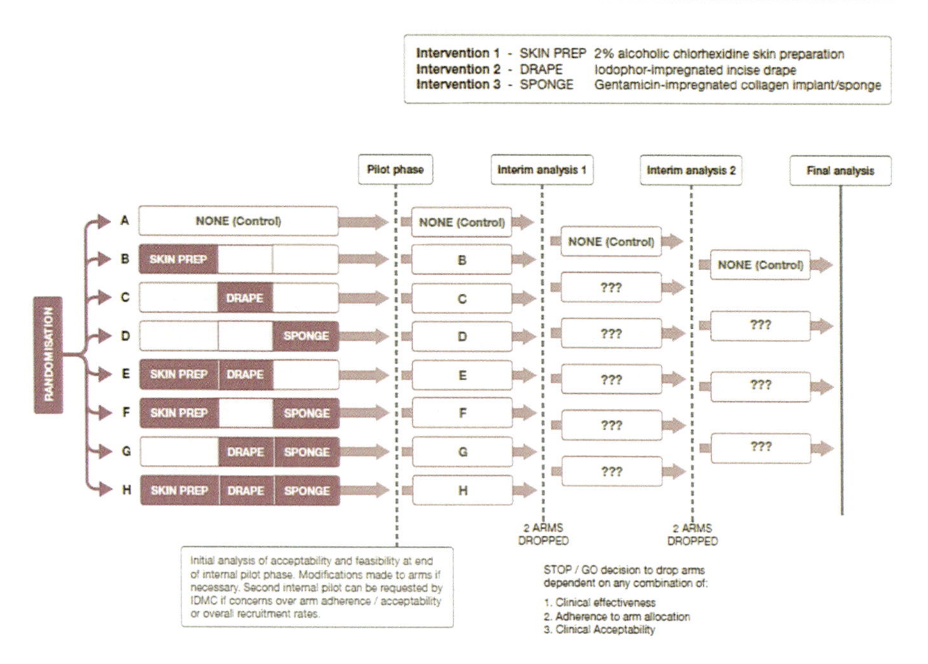

Fig. 2 Schematic representation of the ROSSINI-2 selection design with seven experimental arms and three stages. There are two prespecified subset selection stages in this trial

comparisons. Stallard et al. (2015) developed analytical derivations for the type I and II error rates in a two-stage design – more details are in Stallard and Todd (2003). Further research is needed to explore the operating characteristics of the selection designs when an *I*-outcome measure is used for the selection of best performing arms. In this case, the power of the design might be adversely affected if the rankings of treatment effects on the *I* and *D* outcomes are not similar across experimental treatments. This might also affect the average treatment effects in the arms that reach the final stage. Simulations can be done to explore the operating characteristics of the design as well as the extent of bias in the average treatment effects. Key practical issues to consider in the simulations are the timing, the selection criteria (e.g., ranking), and the number of experimental arms selected at each stage.

When there are several experimental treatments, it is sometimes more efficient to reduce the number of selected arms in multiple stages (Wason et al. 2017). Otherwise, the probability of correct selection and power of the design might be adversely affected. An example is the ROSSINI-2 design where treatment selection has been done in two stages. It has been shown that implementing treatment selection in the ROSSINI-2 trial could reduce the maximum sample size by up to 7% (by 370 patients) compared to the MAMS design with no selection imposed, without adversely affecting the operating characteristics of the trial. Simulations can be used to explore the impact of the number of treatment arms being selected at each stage on the operating characteristics of the design.

In MAMS selection designs, power is only lost under extreme selection criteria. For example in the ROSSINI-2 trial with seven research arms, at least four arms should be selected at the first interim analysis and at least three arms at the second stage to preserve power. In this case the probability of selecting truly the best arm remains above 90%. The timing of the first selection stage is also important. The probability of correct selection is generally low if the selection of treatment arms is done too early in the course of the trial – for example, earlier than 15% of information time in some settings, see Stallard and Todd (2003) and Choodari-Oskooei et al. (2022b). For a design such as ROSSINI-2, it has been suggested not selecting before a fifth of the total planned patients have been recruited.

Adding New Research Arms and Comparisons

Phase III randomized clinical trials can take several years to complete in some disease areas, requiring considerable resources. During this time, new promising treatments may emerge which warrant testing. The practical advantages of incorporating new experimental arms into an existing trial protocol have been clearly stated in previous studies, not least because it obviates the often lengthy process of initiating a new trial and competing between trials to recruit patients (Ventz et al. 2017; Schiavone et al. 2019; Hague et al. 2019). Funding bodies and scientific committees may wish to strategically encourage such collaboration. The MAMS design framework can be implemented as a platform trial. One such example is the STAMPEDE trial which has incorporated five new pairwise comparisons with more to follow, each starting accrual more quickly than the original comparisons (Sydes et al. 2012).

When adding a new experimental arm, the two major (statistical) considerations are as follows. First, the decision whether to control the type I error rate for both the existing and new comparisons should be made, that is, multiplicity adjustment and control of the FWER. The decision to focus control on the PWER or the FWER (for a set of pairwise comparisons) depends on the type of research questions being posed and whether they are related in some way, for example, testing different doses or duration of the same therapy in which case the control of the FWER is required. These are mainly practical considerations and should be determined on a case-by-case basis in the light of the rationale for the hypothesis being tested and the aims of the protocol for the trial. Second, how the type I error rate for a set of comparisons can be calculated if the strong control of the FWER is required in this setting.

Choodari-Oskooei et al. (2020) developed a set of guidelines that can be used to decide whether multiplicity adjustment is necessary when adding a new experimental arm – that is, whether to control the PWER or the FWER in a particular design, see Fig. 2 in Choodari-Oskooei et al. (2020). The emerging consensus among the broader scientific community is that in most multi-arm trials where the rationale for research treatments (or combinations) in the existing and added comparisons is derived separately, the greater focus should be on controlling each pairwise error rate (Parker and Weir 2020; O'Brien 1983; Cook and Farewell 1996). In designs where the FWER for the protocol as a whole is required to be controlled at a certain level, then the overall type I error can be split accordingly between the original and added comparisons, and each can be powered using their allocated type I error rate.

To calculate the overall type I error, the Dunnett probability in Eq. (4) can be extended to control the FWER when new experimental arms are added to a MAMS (platform) trial (Choodari-Oskooei et al. 2020). The idea is to adjust the correlated test statistics by a factor that reflects the size of the shared control group that is used in the pairwise comparisons. This allows the calculation of the operating characteristics for a set of pairwise comparisons in a platform trial setting with both planned and unplanned addition of a new experimental arm. Choodari-Oskooei et al. showed that the FWER is driven more by the number of pairwise comparisons in the family rather than by the timing of the addition of the new arms. The shared control arm information common to comparisons (i.e., shared control arm individuals in continuous and binary outcomes and shared control arm primary outcome events in time-to-event outcomes), and the allocation ratio, are required to calculate the FWER. However, the FWER can be estimated using Bonferroni correction if there is not a substantial overlap between the new comparison and those of the existing ones, or when the correlation between the test statistics of the new comparison and those of the existing comparisons is less than 0.30, that is, the correlation in last column of Table 2. Finally, in a recent review, Lee et al. (2021) addressed different statistical considerations that arise when adding a new research arm to platform trials.

Software and Example

The availability of user-friendly software is key in implementing all designs including advanced designs such as MAMS. Meyer et al. (2021) conducted a systematic literature search to identify commercial and open-source software aimed at designing platform and multi-arm and multi-stage clinical trials. The **nstage** suite in Stata and the MAMS package in R are freely available (Blenkinsop and Choodari-Oskooei 2019; Jaki et al. 2019). Two other commercial software that can be used for sample size calculations are EAST6 (http://www.cytel.com/software/east) and AddPlan (www.aptivsolutions.com/adaptive-trials/addplan6/). However, most of these programs only handle continuous outcome measures and, to our knowledge, none can yet accommodate the use of intermediate outcome measures at interim analyses. To use these packages effectively, generally a sound understanding of the underlying theory is required.

The user-written (and freely available) **nstage** and **nstagebin** programs in Stata calculate the sample size for MAMS designs with time-to-event and binary outcomes. Both of these programs are assisted with a menu and input window **nstagemenu** (Blenkinsop and Choodari-Oskooei 2019; Choodari-Oskooei et al. 2022a). They also calculate the operating characteristics of the design such as the pairwise and familywise type I error rates as well as trial timelines based on the design assumptions. Both programs can accommodate the use of an intermediate outcome measure at interim analyses. The latest versions of **nstage** and **nstagebin** can be obtained from the SSC archive, a well-known repository for user-written

Stata commands, by issuing the following command to Stata: **ssc install nstage.** Note that in this section we use a new (beta) version of **nstage** program which gives more accurate sample sizes than previously reported. The new version will also be available on the SSC archive.

We demonstrate how the **nstage** command can be used to design the STAMPEDE trial with time-to-event *I* and *D* outcomes. To illustrate the design, we follow the same steps in section "Steps to Design a MAMS Trial." The design parameters in the original comparisons of the STAMPEDE trial were as follows. In this MAMS trial, five experimental treatments were chosen to be compared against the control arm in four stages, that is, specified using **arms(6 6 6 6)** and **nstag(4)** option in **nstage** Stata command below. Each comparison was powered to detect a target hazard ratio of 0.75 on both the *I* and *D* outcome measures, **hr0 (1 1) hr1(0.75 0.75**). From previous studies, an estimate of the correlation between survival times on the *I* (excluding *D*) and *D* outcomes was available, **corr(0.60**), as well as the median survival (in years) for the *I* and *D* outcomes, **t (2 4**). Patients were allocated to the control arm with a 2:1 ratio, **aratio(0.5)**, to increase power. The accrual rate was assumed to be 500 patients per year in all stages, **accrue(500 500 500 500)**. The stopping boundaries for the lack-of-benefit were chosen as 0.5, 0.25, 0.10, and 0.025, **alpha(0.50 0.25 0.10 0.025**). The original design only included lack-of-benefit stopping boundaries – see Table 1. Here, we also include the Haybittle-Peto efficacy stopping boundary for illustration, **esb(hp**).

Given the above design parameters, **nstage** calculates the stagewise sample sizes and overall operating characteristics of the design. The first table after the **nstage** command shows the stagewise design specifications and the overall operating characteristics of the trial. The second and third columns of the operating characteristics table report the chosen stopping boundaries required for stopping for lack-of-benefit and efficacy at each interim stage. In this example, each stage requires $p \leq 0.0005$ on the definitive outcome measure to declare efficacy early, that is, Haybittle-Peto rule, shown under the column **Alpha(ESB)**. There is no efficacy boundary for the final stage, since it is equal to the final stage boundary for lack-of-benefit, denoted in the column **Alpha(LOB)**. Assuming exponential distribution (and proportional hazards) for the *FFS* and *OS*, and based on the given median survivals, the first of three interim looks is expected at 2.44 years and the final analysis at 7.16 years. Since the design includes multiple pairwise comparisons, the output also presents the maximum FWER, defined in Eq. (4), as the type I error measure of interest. The upper bound for the overall pairwise power is 0.90 because it assumes non-binding stopping boundaries for lack-of-benefit since the type I error rate is maximized under this assumption. However, if we have an estimate of the correlation between the *FFS* and *OS* (log) hazard ratios, ρ, we can calculate a lower bound for the pairwise power using Eq. (2) with correlation matrix R_4. We refer to this as the correlation between treatment effects on *I* and *D* *within the trial,* not across cognate trials. The (j, j')th entry of R_J for interim stages, that is, the correlation between the estimated *FFS* (log) hazard ratios at interim stages, can be calculated from the formula presented in Table 2 – that is, $\sqrt{e^I_{jk}/e^I_{j'k}}$ for $j^1 > j$, and $j\&\, j' =$ 1,2,3, where e^I_{jk}, is the I-outcome events at interim stage j for the kth comparison. Specifically, the correlation of the *FFS* (log) hazard ratios is time-dependent and its value depends on the accumulated numbers of events at different times. However, the correlation between the *FFS* (log) hazard ratios at the interim stages and that of the *OS* at the final stage should be calculated using $\rho.\sqrt{e^I_{jk}/e^D_{Jk}}, j = 1, 2, 3$ (Royston et al. 2011). For other outcomes a similar formula can be derived – for example $\rho.\sqrt{n_{jk}/n_{Jk}}$ in continuous outcomes, see Follmann et al. (2021). In STAMPEDE, assuming a correlation of $\rho = 0.60$ between the *FFS* and *OS* (log) hazard ratios, R_4 correlation matrix is

$$R_4 = \begin{pmatrix} 1 & 71 & 0.57 & 0.31 \\ 0.71 & 1 & 0.80 & 0.43 \\ 0.57 & 0.80 & 1 & 0.54 \\ 0.31 & 0.43 & 0.54 & 1 \end{pmatrix}$$

With this correlation structure, the lower bound for the overall pairwise power, ω, is 0.83. If we do not have an estimate of the correlation between the treatment effects on I and D, the lower bound for the overall pairwise power can be calculated assuming $\rho = 0$, that is, no correlation between the I and D outcome measures,

$$\begin{aligned} \omega_k &= \Phi_J(z_{\omega_{1k}}).\Phi_J(z_{\omega_{2k}}).\Phi_J(z_{\omega_{3k}}).\Phi_J(z_{\omega_{4k}}) \\ &= \omega_{1k}.\omega_{2k}.\omega_{3k}.\omega_{4k} \end{aligned}$$

In this case, the lower bound for the overall pairwise power is 0.77 (= 0.95 × 0.95 × 0.95 × 0.90). The all-pairs and any-pairs power can also be obtained with the **return list** command (output not shown).

nstage, nstage(4) alpha(0.5 0.25 0.1 0.025) omega(0.95 0.95 0.95 0.9) hr0(1 1) hr1(0.75 0.75) accrue(500 500 500 500) arms(6 6 6 6) t(2 4) corr(0.60) aratio(0.5) esb(hp)

Operating characteristics									
Stage	Alpha (LOB)[a]	Alpha (ESB)[a]	Power	HR|H0	HR|H1	Crit.HR (LOB)	Crit.HR (ESB)	Length[b]	Time[b]
1	0.5000	0.0005	0.950	1.000	0.750	1.000	0.439	2.436	2.436
2	0.2500	0.0005	0.950	1.000	0.750	0.920	0.512	1.189	3.625
3	0.1000	0.0005	0.950	1.000	0.750	0.882	0.553	1.161	4.786
4	0.0250		0.900	1.000	0.750	0.840		2.375	7.161
Max. Pairwise Error Rate					0.0256		Pairwise Power		0.9000
Max. Familywise Error Rate (SE)					0.1056 (0.0003)				

LOB lack of benefit, *ESB* efficacy stopping boundary
[a]All alphas are one-sided
[b]Length (duration of each stage) is expressed in periods and assumes survival times are exponentially distributed. Time is expressed in cumulative periods

Sample size and number of events							
	Stage 1				Stage 3		
	Overall	Control	Exper.		Overall	Control	Exper.
Arms	6	1	5	Arms	6	1	5
Acc. rate	500	143	357	Acc. rate	500	143	357
Patients[a]	1218	348	870	Patients[a]	2393	684	1709
Events[b]	343	113	230	Events[b]	1085	350	735
	Stage 2				Stage 4		
	Overall	Control	Exper.		Overall	Control	Exper.
Arms	6	1	5	Arms	6	1	5
Acc. rate	500	143	357	Acc. rate	500	143	357
Patients[a]	1813	518	1295	Patients[a]	3581	1023	2558
Events[b]	683	223	460	Events[b]	1332	437	895

[a] Patients are cumulative across stages
[b] Events are cumulative across stages but are only displayed for those arms to which patients are still being recruited. Events are for I-outcome at stages 1–3, D-outcome at stage 4

. . .

Although the focus of the STAMPEDE trial was on the strong control of the PWER, we demonstrate how the FWER could be controlled using this design. The following command specifies that interim analyses should assess for efficacy and the program should search for a design which controls the FWER at a maximum of 2.5%. The other design parameter inputs and options remain the same. The option for controlling the FWER identified the final stage α_J required to ensure a maximum FWER of 2.5% as 0.0043, which lengthened the time to final analysis. This could be addressed by lengthening accrual, for instance, or an additional interim analysis could be included in this case. Further simulations should be carried out to quantify the impact of such changes on the operating characteristics of the design and trial timelines, particularly on power which can be reduced marginally. Moreover, the trial timelines presented in outputs assume exponential distribution for both outcomes, which is restrictive. However, the key design quantities, that is, number of control-arm events which are needed to trigger the interim or final analysis, only assumes proportional hazards for both I and D (log) hazard ratios. So, if the exponential assumption is breached, the effect is only to reduce the accuracy of the times for each stage. In practice, it is helpful to visually represent time to analysis and accrual using diagrams.

The following output shows the sample sizes required for the final stage of the design, which has changed to achieve control of the FWER. In some settings, the interim stage stopping boundaries have to be updated to achieve control of the FWER, for example, to choose a more stringent (lower) P-value thresholds for efficacy stopping boundaries. The number of control arm D-outcome events required for the stage 4 analysis should be increased from 437 to 629 to ensure control of the FWER at 2.5%. This 44% increase in the number of events required would require substantially greater resources; for this reason investigators should consider carefully at the design stage whether control of the FWER is the focus of the design, or that of the PWER.

nstage, nstage(4) alpha(0.5 0.25 0.1 0.025) omega(0.95 0.95 0.95 0.9) hr0(1 1) hr1(0.75 0.75) accrue(500 500 500 500) arms(6 6 6 6) t(2 4) corr(0.60) aratio(0.5) esb(hp) fwercontrol(0.025)

Operating characteristics									
Stage	Alpha (LOB)[a]	Alpha (ESB)[a]	Power	HR|H0	HR|H1	Crit.HR (LOB)	Crit.HR (ESB)	Length[b]	Time[b]
1	0.5000	0.0005	0.950	1.000	0.750	1.000	0.439	2.436	2.436
2	0.2500	0.0005	0.950	1.000	0.750	0.920	0.512	1.189	3.625
3	0.1000	0.0005	0.950	1.000	0.750	0.882	0.553	1.161	4.786
4	0.0043		0.901	1.000	0.750	0.824		4.164	8.950
Max. Pairwise Error Rate					0.0054		Pairwise Power		0.8999
Max. Familywise Error Rate (SE)					0.0252	(0.0002)			

[a]All alphas are one-sided

LOB lack of benefit, *ESB* efficacy stopping boundary

[b]Length (duration of each stage) is expressed in periods and assumes survival times are exponentially distributed. Time is expressed in cumulative periods

Sample size and number of events

. . .

	Stage 4		
	Overall	Control	Exper.
Arms	6	1	5
Acc. rate	500	143	357
Patients[a]	4475	1279	3196
Events[b]	1939	629	1310

[a] Patients are cumulative across stages

[b] Events are cumulative across stages but are only displayed for those arms to which patients are still being recruited. Events are for I-outcome at stages 1–3, D-outcome at stage 4

Considerations in Design, Conduct, and Analysis of a MAMS Trial

There are a number of important considerations when designing and implementing a MAMS trial. This section addresses the challenges in design, conduct, and analysis of MAMS trials and provides guidelines on how to overcome them successfully.

Design Considerations

The number of experimental arms that can be practically included in the trial is one important consideration. There is no optimal number for this in a MAMS design as the main drivers for the number of arms are: the number of treatments that are ready and available for testing; the number of patients available; and the cost of undertaking the protocol.

Another important design consideration is the shape of the interim stopping boundaries, that is, the interim P-value thresholds for both lack-of-benefit and efficacy. In the Royston et al.'s MAMS framework, the stagewise significance levels and powers are the design parameters and chosen by the investigator. They are needed to calculate the stagewise sample sizes. However, this approach is restrictive for three reasons. First, an iterative trial-and-error approach is required in which users must continually tweak the stagewise operating characteristics until a feasible design – that is, a design with a particular (prespecified) overall type I error rate and power – is found. Second, there are likely to be many feasible designs for any pair of overall operating characteristics, some requiring smaller sample sizes than others. Therefore, the chosen design may not be the most efficient, or optimal, one for a particular true treatment effect. To address these difficulties, Bratton (2015) developed a systematic search procedure to find a large set of feasible designs and then selecting those which satisfy the Bayesian optimality criteria defined by Junge et al. (2004). These efficient designs are called admissible MAMS designs. This approach finds admissible designs under a given loss function which is a weighted sum of the expected sample size under the global null hypothesis and the hypothesis in which are experimental arms are effective. This method has been implemented in the **nstagebinopt** Stata command. Choodari-Oskooei et al. (2022a) used this approach to find the "optimal" stagewise significance levels and powers in the ROSSINI 2 design.

The timing and frequency of interim analyses are also important design considerations. Previous simulation studies found that 3-stage designs tend to provide a good trade-off between efficiency, as measured by the expected sample size (ESS), and the maximum number of interim analyses that will be required (Bratton 2015). Using four stages can reduce the ESS further when most arms are ineffective. However, in most cases there is little to no additional reductions in ESS in designs with five or more stages. The main cost of using a larger number of stages is a (slight) reduction in the overall pairwise power. Also, the results of interim analysis are, in practice, reviewed by the independent data monitoring committee (IDMC). It is, therefore, important to ensure that a meaningful amount of information accumulates so that the IDMC is not burdened with very frequent meetings except in trials where the experimental arms are thought to be toxic in which case more frequent interim analyses may be necessary to monitor safety. Traditionally, the IDMC should meet, at least, annually. They need not be presented with a formal interim analysis at every meeting. A practical overview of the establishment, purpose, and responsibilities of the IDMCs are provided by Ellenberg, Fleming, and DeMets (2019).

It should be noted that the criteria for, and implications of, stopping for lack of benefit are quite different to stopping for overwhelming benefit. In the former, the emphasis is usually on the current estimate of the "treatment effect" on an intermediate outcome measure for $I \neq D$ designs, and if it is small (or null/negative), then we may conclude the likelihood of a worthwhile treatment effect on the primary outcome measure is also likely to be small. Usually, stopping further randomizations to a research arm for lack of (sufficient) benefit has no implications for either the control arm or other experimental arms in the trial. In contrast, stopping an arm for overwhelming benefit usually focuses on the need for a small P-value for the "treatment effect" on the primary outcome measure. Furthermore, stopping for an overwhelming benefit has direct implications, for the control arm in particular, and potentially all of the other research arms since it will affect the assessment of other pairwise comparisons. If the efficacious arm is found to be unsafe, both any-pair and all-pair powers will be reduced. The reduction in power can be overcome by increasing the sample size for the other comparisons using the conditional error approach (Jaki and Magirr 2013).

In a MAMS design, the stagewise sample sizes drive the timings of the interim analyses. In trials with continuous and binary outcomes, the timing of interim analysis is typically based on observing a prespecified fraction of total sample size required for the final analysis. However, in superiority designs with time-to-event outcomes the timing of the interim analysis can be made based on the prespecified fraction of total number of events in the control arm. There are two reasons for this approach. Firstly, an event rate different to that anticipated for the trial overall, across all arms, could either arise due to a different underlying event rate in all arms or due to a hazard ratio different to that targeted initially. This level of ambiguity is removed by using the control arm event rate as the deciding factor for when to conduct the analysis. Secondly, when more than one experimental arm is recruited to, it is unlikely that we shall observe the same hazard ratio in all comparisons, giving different total numbers of events for each comparison. It is practically expedient for pairwise comparisons started at the same time to have their interim analyses at the same time. However, the calculation for the overall number of events assumes the same event rate in all comparisons in the experimental arms. Moreover, Dang et al. (2020) showed that monitoring the control arm events provides unbiased estimates of the (Fisher) "information fraction" in group sequential trials with time-to-event outcomes.

Another important design consideration is the choice between the control of the PWER or FWER. This is a major decision which drives the required patients and the cost of undertaking the protocol. Consensus is emerging that the most important consideration to decide whether to control the PWER or FWER is the relatedness of the research questions in each pairwise comparison (Choodari-Oskooei et al. 2020; Parker and Weir 2020; Proschan and Waclawiw 2000). There are cases such as examining different doses (or duration) of the same drug where the control of the FWER might be necessary to avoid offering a particular therapy an unfair advantage of showing a beneficial effect. However, in most multi-arm trials where the rationale for research treatments (or combinations) is derived separately, the greater focus should be on controlling each pairwise error rate.

Furthermore, the sample size and power calculations in trials with time-to-event outcomes assume the treatment effects follow proportional hazards (PH). In general, if the PH assumption is false, power is reduced and interpretation of the hazard ratio (HR) as the estimated treatment effect is compromised (Royston and Parmar 2020). For example, when there is an early treatment effect – where the HR is <1 in the early follow-up and increases later – the research treatment may pass the interim stage lack-of-benefit threshold. But, this may cause important lack of power at the final analysis of the *D* outcome. More serious is the late effects where lack-of-benefit is likely to appear at the intermediate stages even when there is a demonstrable treatment effect at the final stage. This is a generic problem of trials with time-to-event outcomes, and is an area of ongoing methodological research.

Finally, sample size calculations in trials with continuous and binary outcomes depend on the outcome variance and the underlying control arm event rate. The values of these parameters are generally specified based on previous studies. Departure from the assumed values can adversely affect the operating characteristics of a MAMS design. The impact on power increases with the number of stages and when the outcome variance or the control arm event rate is overestimated (Mehta and Tsiatis 2001). It is, therefore, necessary to assess these design assumptions during the trial. Several methods have been proposed in the literature (Betensky and Tierney 1997; Proschan 2005). One common approach, which has minimal impact on the operating characteristics, is to recalculate sample size using the revised values for these parameters without unblinding the treatment effect (Proschan 2005).

Conduct Considerations

Besides decisions on the statistical aspects of MAMS studies, there are a number of practical issues to consider when conducting a MAMS study which are not the focus of this chapter. They have been extensively discussed in the literature (James et al. 2008, 2012; Sydes et al. 2009, 2012; Schiavone et al. 2019; Hague et al. 2019). Such challenges include, for example, ensuring adequate supply of the treatments under investigation which is much more complex due to the stochastic nature of the demand on individual treatments; appropriately informing potential participants before the trials; updating them with new information; and setting up and managing scientific oversight committees. This highlights the need to garner large-scale collaboration bringing large parts of the research community together, to obtain significant and long-term funding, to obtain long-term commitment from the key research leaders, to ensure that responsibilities (and also acclaim) are shared as widely as possible, and to have operational structures and systems which allow the implementation of such long-term adaptive protocols. These challenges need to be addressed when the protocol is at the design stage, as they will need to be resolved before any funding is likely to be approved and released.

Analysis Considerations

A further challenge arises when estimating the treatment effects at the interim analyses or the end of the study. While it is relatively easy to define statistical bias, different definitions of an unbiased estimator are relevant in the MAMS design (Robertson et al. 2021). An estimator is unconditionally unbiased, if it is unbiased when averaged across all possible realizations of an adaptive trial. In contrast, an estimator is conditionally unbiased if it is unbiased only conditional on the occurrence of a subset of trial realizations. For example, one might be interested in an estimator only conditional on a particular experimental arm being selected at an interim analysis; as such, the focus becomes on a conditional unbiased estimator.

It has been recognized that the maximum likelihood estimate (MLE) of the treatment effect for trials with an interim selection rule can be potentially biased (Piantadosi 2005). The average treatment effect for the trials that stop at interim stages and those that reach the final stage will be different from the overall underlying treatment effect. This is known as the "selection" bias in the literature. This bias generally tends to be larger the "earlier" the selection happens, that is, when the decision to stop the treatment arm or continue to the next stage is based on a relatively small amount of information (Choodari-Oskooei et al. 2013). However, in trials with no efficacy stopping boundaries the "selection" bias in the estimate of treatment effect of comparisons that reach their final stage is a more major consideration than that of the stopped trials for lack-of-benefit. In this setting, an effective experimental arm is very likely to reach the final stage of the trial, and the results are more likely to be adopted into clinical practice.

Choodari-Oskooei et al. (2013) showed that in designs with lack-of-benefit stopping boundaries the size of the selection bias in the comparisons that reach the final stage is generally small. In fact, the bias is negligible if the experimental arm is truly effective. Furthermore, using an *I* outcome at interim stages will reduce the selection bias in the estimates of treatment effect on the primary outcome in both selected and dropped treatment arms. In this case, the degree of bias depends on the correlation between the intermediate and definitive outcome measures. This bias is markedly reduced by further patient follow-up and reanalysis at the planned "end" of the trial and performing analyses then, irrespective of whether recruitment was stopped early for lack of benefit. It has been shown that the bias will be minimal if the first interim stage is placed at a significance level of 0.30 or less (Choodari-Oskooei et al. 2013).

In designs with overwhelming efficacy stopping boundaries, the average treatment effect for the comparisons that stop for efficacy will be different from the underlying treatment effect. The difference would depend on the unknown underlying treatment effect as well as the type of efficacy stopping boundary. Haybittle-Peto and O'Brien-Fleming type boundaries are quite common in practice. In both stopping boundaries, the probability of crossing the efficacy boundaries will be very small in early stages of the trial (Freidlin and Korn 2009). For example, in a 4-stage 2-arm design with three equally spaced interim O'Brien-Fleming stopping boundaries, the chances of stopping for efficacy at the first, second, and third interim looks are 0.001%, 0.2%, and 0.8% under the null hypothesis (Freidlin and Korn 2009). With Haybittle-Peto efficacy stopping boundaries, the corresponding probabilities are about 0.1% in all stages. Even under the alternative hypothesis of a hazard ratio of 0.75, the chances of stopping for efficacy at the first interim stage are 0.3% and 7.2% for the O'Brien-Fleming and Haybittle-Peto stopping boundaries, respectively (Freidlin and Korn 2009). In all these cases, the average treatment effect for trials that cross the first interim stage efficacy boundary will be different from the underlying treatment effect. However, as we have seen, the probability of crossing the boundary will also be very small. For this reason, it can be argued that the bias in the estimate of treatment effect of trials that reach the final stage is a more major consideration than that in stopped trials.

Several unbiased estimators of the treatment effect have been proposed to correct for selection bias in these cases (Stallard and Kimani 2018; Bowden and Glimm 2008; Sill and Sampson 2007). They mostly proposed for two-stage designs with continuous, conditionally normal outcome variables. However, the proposed unbiased estimators might not be preferred to the slightly biased standard (MLE) estimator because their mean square errors are likely to be larger. Simulations should be used in these cases under different target treatment effects to assess the degree of selection bias and probability of stopping under realistic treatment effect sizes. Robertson et al. (2021) provide a comprehensive overview of proposed approaches to remove or reduce the potential bias in point estimation of treatment effects in an adaptive design, as well as illustrating how to implement them. They also propose a set of guidelines for researchers around the choice of estimators and the reporting of estimates following an adaptive design (Robertson et al. 2022). Moreover, construction of (simultaneous) appropriate confidence intervals is more complex and specialized methods need to be considered.

Finally, it is useful to note when analyzing the trial at the interim stages, power may be increased like for any trial by adjusting for covariates and stratification factors. Since the early stages of a MAMS trial will contain relatively few patients, the trial population across the arms is more likely to be unbalanced in terms of potentially confounding covariates such as age. Accounting for these known, influential covariates in the analysis may increase the robustness of the results.

Summary

This chapter focused on the underlying principles of the multi-arm multi-stage randomized platform trial designs within the Royston et al. (2003)'s framework. In general, MAMS designs are more complex than traditional designs and require sound understanding of the underlying theory and practical challenges of implementing them.

In the MAMS designs of this chapter, the stopping boundaries and selection rules are preplanned. Any data-dependent deviation from the prespecified adaptations can have an adverse effect on the operating characteristics of the design. In this framework, strong control of the operating characteristics is achieved by constructing a separate *cumulative* test statistics for each pairwise comparison and monitoring it with respect to stopping boundaries that are adjusted for multiple stages and/or testing multiple treatment arms. An alternative approach to the MAMS design is to control the operating characteristics by combining independent multiplicity adjusted P-values from the different stages of the trial in accordance with a prespecified combination function and utilizing closed testing to ensure strong control of the error rates (Posch et al. 2005). This method provides more flexibility to make data-dependent adaptive changes at the end of each stage, such as re-estimating the sample size, for the remainder of the trial. But, it is less efficient than designs based on cumulative test statistics. Mehta and Patel (2006) discussed the pros and cons of this approach and showed that more flexibility in these designs comes at the cost of large increases in expected sample sizes for these designs. Recently, Ghosh et al. (2020) extended the *cumulative* MAMS designs (with $I = D$) to permit data-dependent adaptations such as sample size re-estimation, and compared them with those based on combining independent multiplicity adjusted P-values from the different stages. They showed that the power gain from the cumulative test statistics approach can be substantial, by up to 18%, and increases with the heterogeneity of underlying treatment effects. They also showed that the power gain is larger for designs with extreme interim stopping boundaries, that is, when it is more difficult to drop arms. Their findings are consistent with results published in Koenig et al. (2008), Friede and Stallard (2008), and Magirr et al. (2014).

This chapter described a class of multi-arm multi-stage trial designs incorporating repeated tests for both lack-of-benefit and efficacy of a new treatment compared with a control regimen. Importantly, the interim lack-of-benefit analysis can be done with respect to an intermediate outcome measure at a relaxed significance level. If carefully selected, such an intermediate outcome measure can further increase the efficiency of the design compared to the other alternatives where the same primary outcome is used at the interim stages (Ghosh et al. 2020). This chapter demonstrated the mathematical calculation of the operating characteristics of the designs with/without an intermediate outcome at interim stages, and outlined advantages of the MAMS design over other alternatives. It demonstrated how the MAMS design speeds up the evaluation of new treatment regimens in phase II and III trials.

Key Facts

Multi-arm multi-stage randomized clinical trials are an efficient approach to study several treatments within one protocol. In summary, the efficiency of a MAMS trial derives from:

- Implementing a common control arm across several experimental treatments and reducing the number of competing trials
- Randomizing patients from the outset, allowing comparative testing to start sooner
- Discontinuing recruitment to unpromising arms, and consequently boosting recruitment to the arms showing promise
- Using data from all patients in a given comparison in all analyses, thus maximizing information for each stage with control arm patients contributing to multiple direct comparisons
- Increasing the probability of identifying at least one successful therapy from many research arms

Cross-References

▸ Adaptive Phase II Trials
▸ Bias Control in Randomized Controlled Clinical Trials
▸ Biomarker-Guided Trials
▸ Controlling for Multiplicity, Eligibility, and Exclusions
▸ Data and Safety Monitoring and Reporting
▸ Futility Designs
▸ Interim Analysis in Clinical Trials
▸ Monte Carlo Simulation for Trial Design Tool
▸ Platform Trial Designs
▸ Power and Sample Size

Acknowledgments We are grateful to Professor Ian White for his helpful comments on the earlier version of this chapter. This work is based on research arising from MRC grants MC_UU_00004/09 and MC_UU_12023/29.

References

Abery JE, Todd S (2019) Comparing the MAMS framework with the combination method in multi-arm adaptive trials with binary outcomes. Stat Methods Med Res 28(6):1716–1730. https://doi.org/10.1177/0962280218773546

Barthel FMS, Parmar MKB, Royston P (2009) How do multi-stage multi-arm trials compare to the traditional two-arm parallel group design – a reanalysis of 4 trials. Trials. https://doi.org/10.1186/1745-6215-10-21

Betensky RA, Tierney C (1997) An examination of methods for sample size recalculation during an experiment. Stat Med 16:2587–2598

Blenkinsop A, Choodari-Oskooei B (2019) Multiarm, multistage randomized controlled trials with stopping boundaries for efficacy and lack of benefit: an update to nstage. Stata J 19(4):782–802

Blenkinsop A, Parmar MKB, Choodari-Oskooei B (2019) Assessing the impact of efficacy stopping rules on the error rates under the MAMS framework. Clin Trials 16(2):132–142. https://doi.org/10.1177/1740774518823551

Bowden J, Glimm E (2008) Unbiased estimation of selected treatment means in two-stage trials. Biom J 50(4):515–527

Bratton DJ (2015) PhD thesis: design issues and extensions of multi-arm multi-stage clinical trials. UCL, London

Bratton DJ, Phillips PPJ, Parmar MKB (2013) A multi-arm multi-stage clinical trial design for binary outcomes with application to tuberculosis. Med Res Methodol 13:139

Bratton DJ, Parmar MKB, Phillips PPJ, Choodari-Oskooei B (2016) Type I error rates of multi-arm multi-stage clinical trials: strong control and impact of intermediate outcomes. Trials 17:309. https://doi.org/10.1186/s13063-016-1382-5

Choodari-Oskooei B, Parmar MKB, Royston P, Bowden J (2013) Impact of lack- of-benefit stopping rules on treatment effect estimates of two-arm multi-stage (TAMS) trials with time to event outcome. Trials 14:23

Choodari-Oskooei B, Bratton DJ, Gannon MR, Meade AM, Sydes MR, Parmar MK (2020) Adding new experimental arms to randomised clinical trials: impact on error rates. Clin Trials 17(3): 273–284. https://doi.org/10.1177/1740774520904346

Choodari-Oskooei B, Bratton DJ, Parmar M (2022a) Facilities for optimising and designing multi-arm multi-stage (MAMS) randomised controlled trials with binary outcomes. Stata J, submitted

Choodari-Oskooei B, Thwin S, Blenkinsop A, Widmer M, Althabe F, Parmar MKB (2022b) Treatment selection in multi-arm multi-stage (MAMS) designs: with application to a postpartum haemorrhage trial. Clinical Trials, under review.

Cook RJ, Farewell VT (1996) Multiplicity considerations in the design and analysis of clinical trials. J R Stat Soc Ser A Stat Soc 159:93–110

Dang HM, Alonzo T, Franklin M, Mack J, W., Krailo, M. D. and Eckel, S. P. (2020) Information fraction estimation based on the number of events within the standard treatment regimen. Biom J 26:1960–1972. https://doi.org/10.1002/bimj.201900236

Dunnett CW (1955) A multiple comparison procedure for comparing several treatments with a control. J Am Stat Assoc 50(272):1096–1121

Ellenberg SS, Fleming TR, DeMets DL (2019) Data monitoring committees in clinical trials: a practical perspective, 2nd edn. Wiley

Follmann D, Proschan M (2021) Two stage designs for phase III clinical trials. medRxiv. https://doi.org/10.1101/2020.07.29.20164525

Freidlin B, Korn EL (2009) Stopping clinical trials early for benefit: impact on estimation. Clin Trials 6:119–125

Freidlin B, Korn EL, Gray R, Martin A (2008) Multi-arm clinical trials of new agents: some design considerations. Clin Cancer Res 14(14):4368–4371. https://doi.org/10.1158/1078-0432.CCR-08-0325

Friede T, Stallard N (2008) A comparison of methods for adaptive treatment selection. Biom J 50(5):767–781. https://doi.org/10.1002/bimj.200710453

Ghosh P, Liu L, Mehta C (2020) Adaptive multiarm multistage clinical trials. Stat Med. https://doi.org/10.1002/sim.8464

Hague D, Townsend S, Masters L et al (2019) Changing platforms without stopping the train: experiences of data management and data management systems when adapting platform protocols by adding and closing comparisons. Trials 20:294. https://doi.org/10.1186/s13063-019-3322-7

Hay M, Thomas DW, Craighead JL, Economides C, Rosenthal J (2014) Clinical development success rates for investigational drugs. Nat Biotechnol 32(1):40–51. https://www.nature.com/articles/nbt.2786.pdf

Jaki T, Magirr D (2013) Considerations on covariates and endpoints in multi-arm multi-stage clinical trials. Stat Med 32(7):11501163. https://doi.org/10.1002/sim.5669

Jaki T, Pallmann P, Magirr D (2019) The R package MAMS for designing multi-arm multi-stage clinical trials. J Stat Softw 88:4. https://doi.org/10.18637/jss.v088.i04

James ND, Sydes MR, Clarke NW, Mason MD, Dearnaley DP, Anderson J, Popert RJ, Sanders K, Morgan RC, Stansfeld J, Dwyer J, Masters J, Parmar MK (2008) STAMPEDE: systemic therapy for advancing or metastatic prostate cancer- a multi-arm multi-stage randomised controlled trial. Clin Oncol (R Coll Radiol) 20(8):577–581

James ND, Sydes MR, Mason MD, Clarke NW, Anderson J, Dearnaley DP, Dwyer J, Jovic G, Ritchie AW, Russell JM, Sanders K, Thalmann GN, Bertelli G, Birtle AJ, O'Sullivan JM, Protheroe A, Sheehan D, Srihari N, Parmar MK (2012) Celecoxib plus hormone therapy versus hormone therapy alone for hormone-sensitive prostate cancer: first results from the stampede multiarm, multistage, randomised controlled trial. Lancet Oncol 13(5):549–558

Jung SH, Lee T, Kim K, George SL (2004) Admissible two-stage designs for phase II cancer clinical trials. Stat Med 23(4):561–569

Koenig F, Brannath W, Bretz F, Posch M (2008) Adaptive Dunnett tests for treatment selection. Stat Med 27:1612–1625. https://doi.org/10.1002/sim.3048

Lan KK, Zucker DM (1993) Sequential monitoring of clinical trials: the role of information and Brownian motion. Stat Med 12:753–765

Lee KM, Brown LC, Jaki T, Stallard N, Wason J (2021) Statistical consideration when adding new arms to ongoing clinical trials: the potentials and the caveats. Trials 22:203

Magirr D, Jaki T, Whitehead J (2012) A generalized Dunnett test for multi-arm multi-stage clinical studies with treatment selection. Biometrika 99(2):494–501

Magirr D, Stallard N, Jaki T (2014) Flexible sequential designs for multi-arm clinical trials. Stat Med 33:3269–3279
Mehta CR, Patel NR (2006) Adaptive, group sequential and decision theoretic approaches to sample size determination. Stat Med 25:3250–3269. https://doi.org/10.1002/sim.2638
Mehta C, Tsiatis A (2001) Flexible sample size considerations using information-based interim monitoring. Drug Inf J 35(4):1095–1112. https://doi.org/10.1177/009286150103500407
Meyer EL, Mesenbrink P, Mielke T, Parke T, Evans D, Konig F, EU-PEARL (EU Patient-cEntric clinicAl tRial pLatforms) Consortium (2021) Systematic review of available software for multi-arm multi-stage and platform clinical trial design. Trials 22:183. https://doi.org/10.1186/s13063-021-05130-x
MRC Clinical Trials Unit at UCL. RAMPARE Trial. https://www.rampart-trial.org/
O'Brien PC (1983) The appropriateness of analysis of variance and multiple-comparison procedures. Biometrics 39(3):787–788
Parker RA, Weir CJ (2020) Non-adjustment for multiple testing in multi-arm trials of distinct treatments: rationale and justification. Clin Trials 17(5):562–566. https://doi.org/10.1177/1740774520941419
Parmar MK, Barthel FM, Sydes M, Langley R, Kaplan R, Eisenhauer E, Brady M, James N, Bookman MA, Swart AM, Qian W, Royston P (2008) Speeding up the evaluation of new agents in cancer. J Natl Cancer Inst 100(17):1204–1214
Parmar MKB, Carpenter J, Sydes MR (2014) More multiarm randomised trials of superiority are needed. Lancet 384(9940):283–284. https://doi.org/10.1016/S0140-6736(14)61122-3
Piantadosi S (2005) Clinical trials: a methodologic perspective, 2nd edn. Wiley, New York
Posch M, Koenig F, Branson M, Brannath W, Dunger-Baldauf C, Bauer P (2005) Testing and estimation in flexible group sequential designs with adaptive treatment selection. Stat Med 24: 3697–3714. https://doi.org/10.1002/sim.2389
Prentice RL (1989) Surrogate endpoints in clinical trials: definition and operational criteria. Stat Med 8(4):431–440. https://doi.org/10.1002/sim.4780080407
Proschan MA (2005) Two-stage sample size re-estimation based on a nuisance pa-rameter: a review. J Biopharm Stat 15(4):559–574. https://doi.org/10.1081/BIP-200062852
Proschan MA, Waclawiw MA (2000) Practical guidelines for multiplicity adjustment in clinical trials. Control Clin Trials 21:527–539
Robertson DS, Choodari-Oskooei B, Dimairo M, Flight L, Pallmann P, Jaki T (2021) Point estimation for adaptive trial designs. Stat Med, under review. https://arxiv.org/abs/2105.08836
Robertson DS, Choodari-Oskooei B, Dimairo M, Flight L, Pallmann P, Jaki T (2022) Point estimation for adaptive trial designs II: practical considerations and guidance. Stat Med, under review. https://arxiv.org/abs/2105.08836
ROSSINI 2: Reduction of surgical site infection using several novel interventions trial protocol, Tech. rep (2018). https://www.birmingham.ac.uk/Documents/college-mds/trials/bctu/rossini-ii/R0SSINI-2-Protocol-V1.0-02.12.2018.pdf
Royston P, Parmar MK (2020) A simulation study comparing the power of nine tests of the treatment effect in randomized controlled trials with a time-to-event outcome. Trials 21:315. https://doi.org/10.1186/s13063-020-4153-2
Royston P, Parmar MK, Qian W (2003) Novel designs for multi-arm clinical trials with survival outcomes with an application in ovarian cancer. Stat Med 22(14):2239–2256
Royston P, Barthel FM, Parmar MK, Choodari-Oskooei B, Isham V (2011) Designs for clinical trials with time-to-event outcomes based on stopping guidelines for lack of benefit. Trials 12:81
Schiavone F, Bathia R, Letchemanan K et al (2019) This is a platform alteration: a trial management perspective on the operational aspects of adaptive and platform and umbrella protocols. Trials 20:264. https://doi.org/10.1186/s13063-019-3216-8
Sidak Z (1967) Rectangular confidence regions for the means of multivariate normal distributions. J Am Stat Assoc 62(318):626–633
Sill MW, Sampson AR (2007) Extension of a two-stage conditionally unbiased estimator of the selected population to the bivariate normal case. Commun Stat Theory Methods 36:801–813

Stallard N, Kimani PK (2018) Uniformly minimum variance conditionally unbiased estimation in multi-arm multi-stage clinical trials. Biometrika 105(2):495501. https://doi.org/10.1002/sim.3958

Stallard N, Todd S (2003) Sequential designs for phase III clinical trials incorporating treatment selection. Stat Med 22:689–703. https://doi.org/10.1002/sim.1362

Stallard N, Kunz CU, Todd S, Parsons N, Friede T (2015) Flexible selection of a single treatment incorporating shortterm endpoint information in a phase II/III clinical trial. Stat Med 34(23): 3104–3115. https://doi.org/10.1002/sim.6567

Sydes MR, Parmar MK, James ND, Clarke NW, Dearnaley DP, Mason MD, Morgan RC, Sanders K, Royston P (2009) Issues in applying multi-arm multi-stage methodology to a clinical trial in prostate cancer: the MRC STAMPEDE trial. Trials 10:39

Sydes MR, Parmar MK, Mason MD, Clarke NW, Amos C, Anderson J, de Bono JS, Dearnaley DP, Dwyer J, Green C, Jovic G, Ritchie AW, Russell JM, Sanders K, Thalmann G, James ND (2012) Flexible trial design in practice – stopping arms for lack-of-benefit and adding research arms mid-trial in STAMPEDE: a multi-arm multi-stage randomized controlled trial. Trials 13(1):168

Ventz S, Alexander BM, Parmigiani G, Gelber RD, Trippa L (2017) Designing clinical trials that accept new arms: an example in metastatic breast cancer. J Clin Oncol 35(27):3160–3168

Wason JMS, Stecher L, Mander AP (2014) Correcting for multiple-testing in multi-arm trials: is it necessary and is it done? Trials 15:364

Wason J, Stallard N, Bowden J, Jennison C (2017) A multi-stage drop-the-losers design for multi-arm clinical trials. Stat Methods Med Res 26(1):508–524. https://doi.org/10.1177/0962280214550759

Sequential, Multiple Assignment, Randomized Trials (SMART)

79

Nicholas J. Seewald, Olivia Hackworth, and Daniel Almirall

Contents

Abstract

A dynamic treatment regimen (DTR) is a prespecified set of decision rules that can be used to guide important clinical decisions about treatment planning. This includes decisions concerning how to begin treatment based on a patient's characteristics at entry, as well as how to tailor treatment over time based on the patient's changing needs. Sequential, multiple assignment, randomized trials (SMARTs) are a type of experimental design that can be used to build effective dynamic treatment regimens (DTRs). This chapter provides an introduction to DTRs, common types of scientific questions researchers may have concerning the development of a highly effective DTR, and how SMARTs can be used to address such questions. To illustrate ideas, we discuss the design of a SMART used to answer critical questions in the development of a DTR for individuals diagnosed with alcohol use disorder.

N. J. Seewald (✉) · O. Hackworth · D. Almirall
University of Michigan, Ann Arbor, MI, USA
e-mail: nseewald@umich.edu; ohackwor@umich.edu; dalmiral@umich.edu

© Springer Nature Switzerland AG 2022

S. Piantadosi, C. L. Meinert (eds.), *Principles and Practice of Clinical Trials*,
https://doi.org/10.1007/978-3-319-52636-2_280

Keywords

Dynamic treatment regimen · Adaptive intervention · Tailoring variable · Sequential randomization · Multistage randomized trial

Introduction

In clinical settings, it is often necessary to treat patients using a sequential and individually tailored approach, whereby treatment is adapted and readapted over time based on both static and changing needs of the patient (Thall et al. 2000; Lavori and Dawson 2014). A dynamic treatment regimen (DTR) is a prespecified set of decision rules that can be used to guide clinicians on how to make such sequences of treatment decisions (Murphy and Almirall 2009).

Investigators often have multiple scientific questions concerning the development of effective DTRs. These questions often involve the effectiveness of the components that make up a DTR: What is the best way to begin treatment? What is the best treatment to provide patients who respond suboptimally or who fail to adhere to an initial course of treatment? What is the best approach to monitoring patients for response to treatment? How do treatments work in sequence, with or against each other, to impact outcomes in the long term?

One type of clinical trial design that is useful for answering such questions is the sequential, multiple assignment, randomized trial, or SMART (Lavori and Dawson 2004; Murphy 2005; Collins et al. 2014). Relative to standard multiarm randomized trials, the SMART is unique in that it involves multiple stages of randomization: Participants in a SMART may be randomized more than once across multiple stages of the trial.

This chapter provides a brief introduction to DTRs (including the components that make up a DTR) and SMART designs. Throughout, we illustrate ideas using a SMART designed to answer critical questions in the development of a DTR for individuals diagnosed with alcohol use disorder.

Dynamic Treatment Regimens

A dynamic treatment regimen (DTR) is a sequence of decision rules that can be used to guide how treatment can be adapted and readapted to the individual in clinical practice settings. These treatment adaptations can be in terms of the type of treatment, mode of treatment delivery, treatment intensity or dose, or other intervention components. As with other types of manualized interventions, the decision rules that make up a DTR are prespecified and well operationalized; this helps to ensure that they can be replicated by future clinicians or evaluated by future researchers. DTRs are also referred to as adaptive interventions (Lei et al. 2012; Nahum-Shani et al. 2012b), Adaptive treatment strategies (Murphy 2005; August et al. 2016; Nahum-Shani et al. 2017), treatment policies (Lunceford et al. 2002; Wahed and Tsiatis

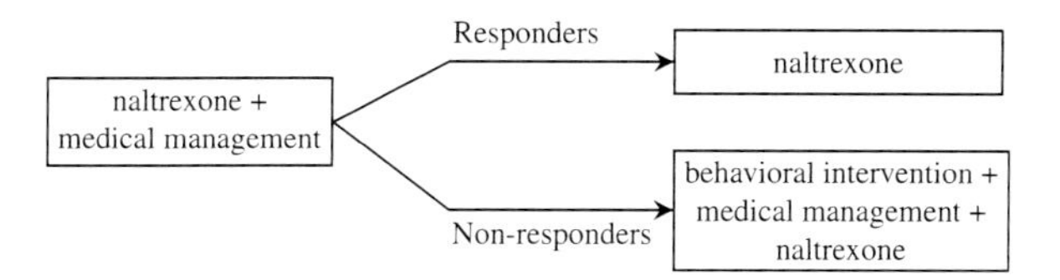

Fig. 1 Schematic of an example DTR for an adult receiving treatment for alcohol use disorder. Nonresponse to treatment is defined as two or more heavy drinking days during the 8-week initial study period

2004, 2006), multistage treatments (Thall and Kyle Wathen 2005), and multicourse treatment strategies (Thall et al. 2002).

To make the idea of a DTR more concrete, consider as an example the treatment of patients with alcohol use disorder. Naltrexone is a medication that diminishes the pleasurable effects of alcohol (Oslin et al. 2006). Response to naltrexone is heterogenous due to factors such as poor patient adherence, biological response to the medication, low social support, and poor coping skills (Nahum-Shani et al. 2017). As a result of this heterogeneity, it is important to offer a supportive intervention along with the naltrexone medication. One such intervention is medical management, a face-to-face clinical support intervention that includes monitoring for adherence to treatment. A more intensive clinical support intervention is the combined behavioral intervention, which includes components which target adherence to medication and enhance the patient's motivation for change. The intervention also involves the patient's family, when possible, and reinforces abstinence by emphasizing social support (Longabaugh et al. 2005; Lei et al. 2012). Hereafter, we refer to the combined behavioral intervention as simply "behavioral intervention."

Figure 1 illustrates an example DTR that involves the use of naltrexone, medical management, and behavioral intervention. In this example DTR, the patient is offered naltrexone alongside medical management for up to 8 weeks, with weekly check-ins with the clinician as a part of medical management. If, at any of the weekly check-ins during this 8-week period, the patient reports experiencing two or more heavy drinking days, the patient is identified as a nonresponder and is offered behavioral intervention in addition to naltrexone and medical management. If instead the patient does not experience two or more heavy drinking days during the 8-week period, then, at week 8, the patient is identified as a "durable responder" and continues treatment with naltrexone but without medical management (Lei et al. 2012).

There are four main components of a DTR, all of them prespecified: (1) decision points, (2) treatment options, (3) tailoring variables, and (4) decision rules. Decision points are times in a patient's care where a treatment decision is made. They can occur at scheduled intervals, after a specific number of clinic visits, or be event-based, such as the point at which a patient fails to respond or adhere to a treatment. The timing of decision points should be based on scientific or practical considerations which inform when treatment may need to be modified. For instance, in adolescent weight loss, clinicians typically evaluate response to treatment after about 3 months: This suggests a decision point should be placed at about this time (Naar-King et al. 2016).

The second component of a DTR is the collection of treatment options available at each decision point. This set may include aspects of treatment such as type of treatment, intensity of treatment, and/or delivery method; see Lei et al. (2012) for detailed examples. It may also include strategies for modifying treatment, such as augmenting or intensifying an intervention, or staying the course (Pelham Jr. et al. 2016). The set of possible treatment options can be different at each decision point.

The third component is the Tailoring variables which are used to individualize ("tailor") treatment at each decision point. These could be static characteristics, such as age or other demographic factors, known co-occurring conditions, or other characteristics collected at intake. Tailoring variables could also be time-varying characteristics that may change based on previous treatments, disease severity, treatment preferences, or adherence.

The fourth component in a DTR is the decision rules. At each decision point, a decision rule takes in the values of the tailoring variables and recommends a treatment option (or set of options). The collection of decision rules over all decision points is what makes up a DTR (Murphy and Almirall 2009).

In the alcohol use disorder DTR depicted in Fig. 1, there are two decision points from the perspective of the clinician. The first is when treatment begins. The second decision point is the first time the patient is identified as a nonresponder during the first 8 weeks of treatment, or when the patient is identified as a responder at week 8. In the example DTR, there is only a single treatment option at the first decision point: naltrexone with medical management. At the second decision point, there are two treatment options: naltrexone with medical management and behavioral intervention or naltrexone alone. In this example, there is a single tailoring variable, which is the number of heavy drinking days reported by the patient following the start of the initial intervention. This information is used to inform whether a patient remains a responder for 8 weeks or triggers the nonresponse criterion (two or more heavy drinking days) within the 8 weeks. The decision rule at the first decision point is to offer all patients naltrexone with medical management. The decision rule at the second decision point recommends withdrawing responders from medical management at week 8 and offering behavioral intervention in addition to existing treatment to any patient that triggers a nonresponse within the 8 weeks.

DTRs also have applications to other clinical settings, for example, in prevention medicine, implementation, or in special education. In prevention applications, DTRs could help operationalize the transition between "universal" preventive interventions, which target a large section of the population, and "selected" then "indicated" preventive interventions, which target populations at progressively higher risk of developing a disorder (August et al. 2016; Hall et al. 2019). Implementation focuses on the uptake or adoption of evidence-based practices by systems of providers (e.g., clinics); here, a DTR can be used to guide how best to adapt (potentially costly) organizational-level interventions that seek to improve the health of individuals at the organization (Kilbourne et al. 2014, 2018; Quanbeck et al. 2020). In special education, DTRs can be used to guide how best to adapt interventions designed to improve behavioral and academic outcomes in educational settings (Kasari et al. 2014; Almirall et al. 2018).

Scientific Questions about DTRS

Researchers interested in developing high-quality DTRs often have unanswered questions that cannot necessarily be answered based on the extant literature, or expert clinical opinion. These questions typically concern the relative effectiveness of different DTRs, the relative effectiveness of different DTR components at specific stages, how the intervention components at different stages work with (or against) each other, and questions related to how best to tailor treatment at different stages of intervention.

Common questions are about which treatment option the DTR should begin with, how to modify the initial treatment for nonresponders, how to best define or monitor individuals for response/nonresponse, and the timing of decision points and thus interventions.

Within the context of the alcohol use disorder example, one important question concerns the definition of nonresponse to naltrexone. In the DTR shown in Fig. 1, nonresponse is defined as a patient reporting 2 or more heavy drinking days. However, it is unclear what amount of drinking behavior corresponds to non-response to naltrexone, so researchers may have questions concerning how best to monitor a patient for nonresponse. Other scientific questions might ask which treatment options to offer as follow-up to naltrexone with medical management. For instance, should clinicians provide more intense support for nonresponders, or which treatment best maintains longer-term response for patients identified as responders at week 8.

Sequential, Multiple Assignment, Randomized Trials

A sequential, multiple assignment, randomized trial (SMART) is a type of multistage randomized trial design that aims to answer critical questions in the development of DTRs, such as those described above. In a SMART, all participants move through multiple stages of treatment. At each stage, participants may be randomized to a set of feasible treatment options. The randomizations in a SMART correspond to scientific questions about the development of an effective DTR. The treatment options to which a participant is randomized at each stage may depend on participant characteristics or prior treatment. As with other randomized trials, the randomizations at each stage allow investigators to make causal inferences about the relative effectiveness of different treatment options at each stage, without having to make unverifiable assumptions (Rubin 1974). These randomizations also allow investigators to make causal inferences about the relative effectiveness of different DTRs. As with other randomized trials, each of the randomizations in a SMART can be stratified based on factors believed to be associated with subsequent outcomes.

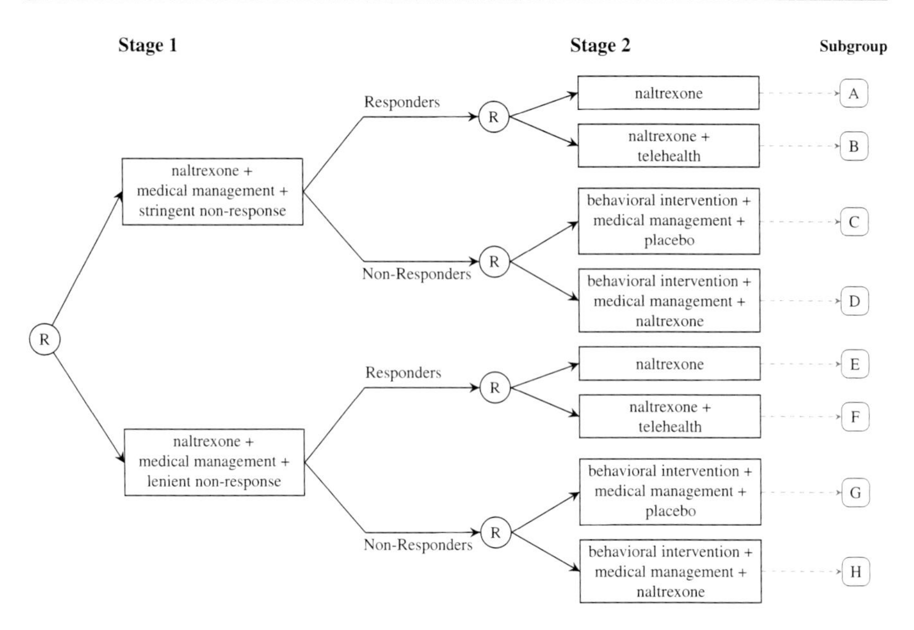

Fig. 2 Schematic of the ExTENd SMART. Circled R indicates randomization; treatments are boxed. The stringent definition of nonresponse is triggered when the participant reports 2 or more heavy drinking days in 1 week; the lenient definition, 5 or more heavy drinking days

Randomization probabilities may depend on any previously-observed covariate, as long as the probabilities are known.

As an example, consider the two-stage ExTENd SMART study, led by David Oslin, designed to inform the development of a DTR for the treatment of patients with alcohol use disorder using naltrexone and patient support (Murphy and Almirall 2009). A diagram of this SMART is shown in Fig. 2. As we describe in more detail below, the example DTR shown in Fig. 1 was drawn from this SMART. In ExTENd, all participants began by receiving naltrexone with medical management. The first randomization, which occurred at the outset of treatment, was to one of two definitions of nonresponse: a stringent definition and a more lenient one. Thus, the first randomization was designed to compare two approaches to monitoring for nonresponse. The stringent definition identifies a patient as a nonresponder if the patient reports experiencing 2 or more heavy drinking days in 1 week. The lenient definition identifies a patient as a nonresponder if the patient reports experiencing 5 or more heavy drinking days in 1 week. The participants were then assessed weekly during the 8-week first stage based on their randomly assigned definition of nonresponse. If and when a participant triggers a nonresponse, the participant is immediately rerandomized to either receive behavioral intervention in addition to naltrexone with medical management or behavioral intervention with medical management and placebo. This randomization was designed to investigate the effect of naltrexone in the context of the behavioral intervention and medical management among nonresponders to the first-stage treatment. If participants did not meet the definition of nonresponse at the end of the 8 weeks, then they were classified as responders and immediately rerandomized to either naltrexone alone or naltrexone alongside telephone disease management (medical management delivered via telephone, hereafter referred to as "telehealth"). This randomization was designed to investigate the effect of continued, lower-intensity medical management for responders to the first-stage treatment. All patients continued their second treatment for the duration of the 24-week study.

Many SMARTs are designed with an embedded tailoring variable, meaning that subsequent randomizations are restricted based on the participant's value of a tailoring variable. The ExTENd study is an example of a SMART with this feature: The second-stage treatment options for nonresponders are different from those for responders. SMARTs that include an embedded tailoring variable will, by design, include a number of DTRs embedded within it. For example, there are eight DTRs embedded in ExTENd by design (Table 1). All participants in this SMART were randomly assigned to a sequence of treatments that is consistent with recommendations made by one or more of these eight embedded DTRs. Participants who follow treatment pathways A and D in Fig. 2 are assigned treatments according to the example DTR discussed above and depicted in Fig. 1. These patients begin with naltrexone, medical management, and the stringent definition of nonresponse to treatment and are subsequently provided naltrexone alone if they respond or have behavioral intervention added to their therapy if they do not respond.

Note that within ExTENd, all participants are consistent with two of the eight embedded DTRs. This example SMART is conceptually similar to a ($2 \times 2 \times 2$) (fractional) factorial trial design (Murphy and Bingham 2009; Collins et al. 2014; Vock and Almirall 2018). The first factor is naltrexone with medical management and the stringent definition of nonresponse versus naltrexone with medical management and the lenient definition of nonresponse. The second factor is restricted to responders and is naltrexone alone versus naltrexone with telehealth among responders. The third factor, restricted to nonresponders, is naltrexone with medical management and behavioral intervention versus placebo with medical management and behavioral intervention.

Two key differences from factorial designs are the sequential nature of treatment delivery in a SMART, as well as the possible restriction of certain treatment options to participants based on their response status. Scientific questions which motivate a SMART are asked in the context of a sequence of treatments which are delivered at multiple points in time: This is not typically captured by a standard factorial design. Additionally, SMARTs which contain an embedded tailoring variable usually offer different sets of treatment options to responders and nonresponders. Similarly, first-stage treatment assignment may determine whether individuals are rerandomized, as in the SMART depicted in Fig. 4. These SMARTs are therefore not fully crossed designs (Nahum-Shani et al. 2012b).

Returning to the Scientific Questions

As stated before, the goal of SMART designs is to aid the development of DTRs. Data collected in a SMART can be used to answer questions concerning which intervention option to provide at critical decision points during care. For example, in

Table 1 Embedded dynamic treatment regimens (DTRs) in the ExTENd SMART (Fig. 2). The stringent definition of nonresponse is triggered when the participant reports 2 or more heavy drinking days in 1 week; the lenient definition, 5 or more heavy drinking days

Embedded DTR	Stage 1 treatment	Stage 2 treatment for responders	Stage 2 treatment for non responders	Subgroups in Figure 2 consistent with DTR
1	naltrexone + medical management + stringent non-response	naltrexone	behavioral intervention + medical management + placebo	A, C
2	naltrexone + medical management + stringent non-response	naltrexone	behavioral intervention + medical management + naltrexone	A, D
3	naltrexone + medical management + stringent non-response	naltrexone + telehealth	behavioral intervention + medical management + placebo	B, C
4	naltrexone + medical management + stringent non-response	naltrexone + telehealth	behavioral intervention + medical management + naltrexone	B, D
5	naltrexone + medical management + lenient non-response	naltrexone	behavioral intervention + medical management + placebo	E, G
6	naltrexone + medical management + lenient non-response	naltrexone	behavioral intervention + medical management + naltrexone	E, H
7	naltrexone + medical management + lenient non-response	naltrexone + telehealth	behavioral intervention + medical management + placebo	F, G
8	naltrexone + medical management + lenient non-response	naltrexone + telehealth	behavioral intervention + medical management + naltrexone	F, H

ExTENd, researchers were interested in the comparison of the different definitions of nonresponse to naltrexone with medical management (i.e., a comparison of first-stage treatment options), averaged over subsequent treatment. This would help to answer a question about what amount of drinking behavior corresponds with nonresponse to naltrexone in the context of a DTR designed to increase the proportion of days abstinent from alcohol. Other examples of scientific questions might be a comparison of second-stage intervention options among responders, averaged over the first-stage definition of nonresponse, similarly for nonresponders.

Questions can also focus on comparisons of the DTRs embedded in a SMART (Table 1). An example would be to compare the DTR shown in Fig. 1 (embedded DTR 2) to embedded DTR 5 based on proportion of days abstinent from alcohol at the end of the study. This type of comparison may be used to investigate the difference between, say, the most and least intensive DTRs, or the most and least expensive.

Data from a SMART can also be used to answer questions about more highly tailored DTRs beyond those included in the SMART (Laber et al. 2014; Nahum-Shani et al. 2017). Researchers can collect information about "candidate" tailoring variables and assess whether and how they could help match participants to subsequent intervention options. This could lead to more individualized DTRs. For example, ExTEND, it could be useful to investigate whether the nonresponse definition used should be further tailored to an individual's baseline years of alcohol consumption. Support for this idea is based on evidence which suggests that individuals with more severe histories of alcohol use problems are more prone to relapse which could require a more stringent definition of nonresponse to naltrexone (Heilig and Egli 2006) for some individuals. It would also be useful to explore whether the maintenance treatment for responders should be tailored based on their proportion of nonabstinence days during the initial treatment with naltrexone. This is based in the idea that although participants were categorized as responders, their failure to achieve complete abstinence suggests that they may need additional support to maintain their improvement (McKay 2005; Cable and Sacker 2007). This deeper tailoring can be investigated using Q-learning; see Nahum-Shani et al. (2012a, 2017) for details.

Other Smart Designs

The ExTENd SMART, in which all participants were randomized initially and both responders and nonresponders were rerandomized, is just one type of SMART design. The defining feature of a SMART is that at least some participants are randomized more than once; below, we introduce three additional common SMART designs. SMARTs may include more than two stages of randomizations and provide more than two interventions at each randomization. However, for simplicity, the three SMART designs described below have only two stages and two intervention options at each randomization.

Many SMARTs use a so-called "prototypical" design in which all participants are randomized in the first stage, but subsequent randomizations are restricted only to nonresponders (Sherwood et al. 2016; August et al. 2016; Gunlicks-Stoessel et al. 2016; Naar-King et al. 2016; Pelham Jr. et al. 2016; Schmitz et al. 2018). A schematic is given in Fig. 3. Note that the tailoring variable could be reversed so

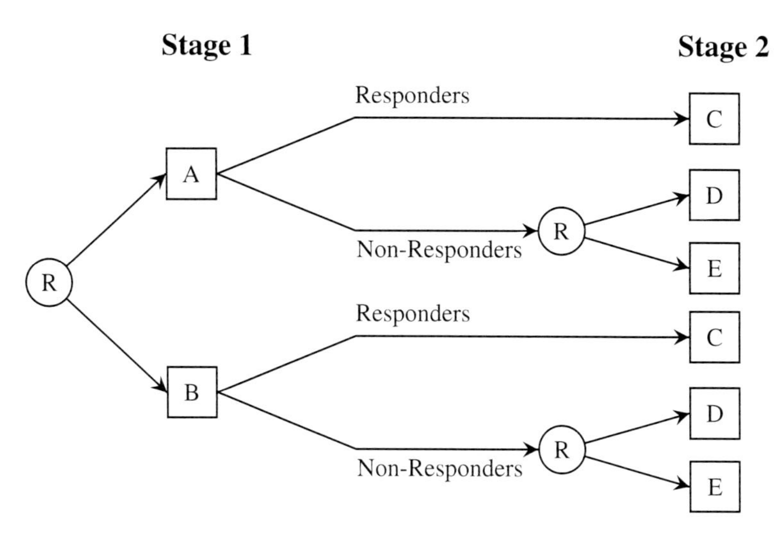

Fig. 3 "Prototypical" SMART design. All participants are randomized in the first stage; only nonresponders are rerandomized. There are four DTRs embedded in this design

that responders are the group that is rerandomized. This type of SMART design may be helpful in a scenario in which there is an open scientific question about either responders or nonresponders, but not both. For example, in the SMART described by Pelham Jr. et al. (2016), participants who responded to first-stage treatment continued on that treatment: The trial was not motivated by a question about second-stage treatment for responders. Nonresponders, however, were rerandomized between an intensified version of their first-stage intervention, or augmentation of the intervention with another component. It should be noted that it is not necessary that responders and nonresponders to different first-stage treatments be given the same second-stage intervention options: Nonresponders to B, for instance, might be rerandomized between treatments F and G.

In some contexts, scientific, practical, or ethical considerations limit the treatment options available as follow-up to a particular first-stage intervention. This type of consideration is accommodated by the SMART design described in Fig. 4, in which participant rerandomization depends on both their response status and previous treatment (Almirall et al. 2016; Kasari et al. 2014; Kilbourne et al. 2014). In Fig. 4, participants who respond to treatment A are not rerandomized, but the nonresponders are rerandomized. In the branch where participants receive treatment B as their first stage treatment, no one is rerandomized. This may be used if there are no practical or ethical treatment options available to offer nonresponders to B, for example. In the SMART described in Kasari et al. (2014), it was not feasible to rerandomize participants who did not respond to one of the initial interventions. For these participants, the only feasible option was to intensify their initial treatment. There are three DTRs embedded in this type of SMART.

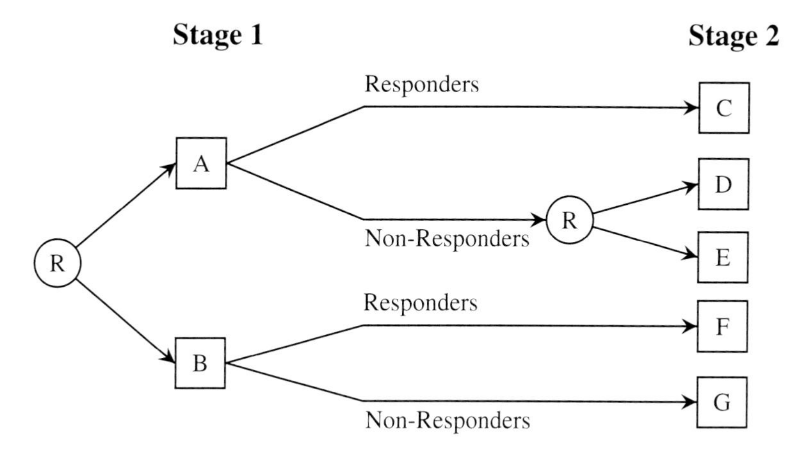

Fig. 4 A SMART design in which only nonresponders to a particular first-stage treatment are rerandomized. There are three DTRs embedded in this design

Not all SMARTs involve restricted randomization: In some designs, all participants are rerandomized regardless of their response to previous treatment (Fig. 5) (Chronis-Tuscano et al. 2016). In this scenario, investigators might collect information on one or more candidate-tailoring variables but do not use them when rerandomizing: The tailoring variable is not embedded in the design. In the SMART shown in Fig. 5, all participants are randomized to either treatment A or B, and then rerandomized to either treatment C or D regardless of their response to first-stage treatment. There are four treatment paths embedded in this design, but because there is no embedded tailoring variable, these are not DTRs per se. These so-called "unrestricted" SMARTs are sequential, fully-crossed, 2×2 factorial designs. In this case, the factors are A versus B at stage 1 for all participants, crossed with C versus D at stage 2 for all individuals. However, as above, second-stage treatment options may depend on the first randomization (i.e., individuals who receive B might be rerandomized between E and F rather than C and D).

Power Considerations and Analytic Methods for Primary Aims

Like any other randomized trial, a SMART should be powered based on the primary aim of the study. Here, we revisit three common primary aims for a SMART and discuss power considerations and analysis for each. For simplicity, we restrict our focus to two-stage studies with an outcome observed at the end of the trial and in which all randomizations occur between two treatment options with equal probability. More general situations are described by, e.g., Ogbagaber et al. (2016).

A common primary aim is the comparison of initial treatment options, averaged over subsequent treatment. This is a two-group comparison: In the context of Fig. 2,

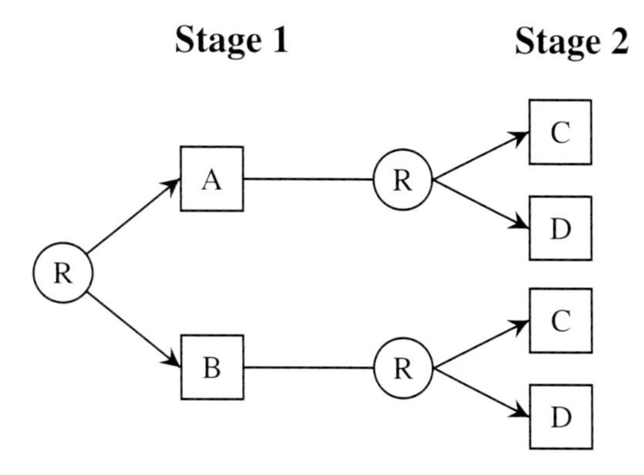

Fig. 5 An unrestricted SMART. All participants are randomized twice without regard to a tailoring variable. There are four nonadaptive treatment paths embedded in this design

for example, this compares the mean outcome across subgroups A, B, C, and D to the mean outcome across subgroups E, F, G, and H. As such, standard two-group comparison methods can be used for both analysis and power considerations. In the continuous-outcome case, linear regression with an indicator for first-stage treatment along with any prognostic baseline (prior to first-stage randomization) covariates can be used; the minimum sample size can be calculated using the standard formula

$$N \geq \frac{4\left(z_{1-\alpha/2} + z_{1-\beta}\right)^2}{\delta^2}$$

where δ is the smallest clinically relevant standardized effect size the investigator wishes to detect using a test with type-I error rate $\alpha/2$ with power $1 - \beta$. We use z_p to denote the p-th quantile of the standard normal distribution.

A second common primary aim is the comparison of second-stage treatment options among responders or nonresponders, averaged over initial treatment assignment. In a prototypical SMART (Fig. 3), this involves comparing nonresponders who received treatment D to those who received treatment E in stage 2. Again, this is simply a two-group comparison among nonresponders, so we can use standard methods for analysis restricted to the nonresponders. The formula for the total sample size for the SMART is the same as above, upweighted by nonresponse probabilities:

$$N \geq \frac{2\left(z_{1-\alpha/2} + z_{1-\beta}\right)^2}{\delta^2} \cdot \left(\frac{1}{1 - P(R_A = 1)} + \frac{1}{1 - P(R_B = 1)}\right)$$

where R_X is an indicator for whether a participant responded to first-stage treatment X ($R_X = 1$) or not ($R_X = 0$).

Investigators may also be interested in powering a SMART for a comparison of two embedded DTRs which recommend different first-stage treatments. For example, in a prototypical SMART such as the one shown in Fig. 3, this might be a comparison of individuals who are consistent with the DTR which recommends A then C for responders and D for nonresponders against those consistent with the DTR which recommends B initially, then F for responders and G for nonresponders. This comparison is often done using a regression model which allows for the simultaneous estimation of mean outcomes under each of the embedded DTRs and accounts for the facts that (1) some participants may be consistent with more than one DTR, and (2) not all participants are randomized more than once. This can be achieved using a so-called "weighted and recycled" approach (Nahum-Shani et al. 2012b).

In a prototypical SMART, responders are randomized only once whereas nonresponders are randomized twice. Therefore, there is imbalance by design in the numbers of responders and nonresponders consistent with each embedded DTR. We can correct for this imbalance with inverse-probability-of-treatment weights: Assuming equal randomization, responders receive a weight of $(1/2)^{-1} = 2$ and nonresponders receive a weight of $(1/2 \times 1/2)^{-1} = 4$. Furthermore, responders to treatment A are consistent with two embedded DTRs: The first recommends A, C for responders, and D for nonresponders; the second recommends A, C for responders, and E for nonresponders. The same holds for responders to treatment B. Regression approaches which simultaneously estimate mean outcomes for all embedded DTRs must account for this; see Appendix A of Nahum-Shani et al. (2012b) for additional details.

Sample size formulae for a comparison of two embedded DTRs are surprisingly straightforward and build on the standard formulae given above. The total sample size for the SMART is

$$N \geq \frac{4\left(z_{1-\alpha/2} + z_{1-\beta}\right)^2}{\delta^2} \cdot \mathrm{DE}$$

where DE is a "design effect" that accounts for differential randomization of responders and nonresponders in the second stage. In a prototypical SMART, $\mathrm{DE} = 2 - P(R = 1)$ assuming a common response rate across first-stage treatments. In the SMART shown in Fig. 4, $\mathrm{DE} = (3 - P(R = 1))/2$; in an ExTENd-style SMART in which all participants are rerandomized (Fig. 1), $DE = 2$ (Oetting et al. 2011).

Additional Considerations for Designing and Implementing a Smart

The SMART designs discussed above are representative of most of the SMARTs that have been implemented to date. To our knowledge, most SMARTs in the field have two stages with randomizations limited to two treatment options. However, as mentioned above, SMART designs may include more than two stages of randomization, or more than two treatment options after a randomization. As with any randomized trial, the design of a SMART is ultimately dictated by the scientific questions the investigator seeks to answer.

Each of the SMART designs discussed in this chapter is motivated by a different set of scientific questions at *multiple* stages of a DTR. Because each randomization in a SMART corresponds to an open question about subsequent treatment recommendations, and the defining characteristic of a SMART is that some or all participants are randomized more than once, questions that do not involve multiple stages of treatment do not, by themselves, motivate a SMART. Almirall et al. (2018) describe several "singly-randomized" alternatives to SMARTs in the context of research on DTRs.

SMARTs often include standard-of-care control groups. Most commonly, this is done by embedding a standard-of-care intervention as one of the DTRs. For instance, in Fig. 3, one of the embedded DTRs may be a DTR that is commonly used in practice or could recommend standard-of-care throughout. This type of SMART would allow for comparisons of the other embedded DTRs against this standard-of-care DTR.

An important consideration in the design of a SMART is the choice of embedded tailoring variable, if included. Embedding a tailoring variable into the trial also embeds it into any DTRs the trial is able to study, so its inclusion should be well justified based on scientific, ethical, or practical considerations. The tailoring variable is a component of the DTR. As such, its operating characteristics are part of the *intervention* as well as the trial. Therefore, tailoring variables should be relatively easily measured in a clinical setting and reliably identify responders and nonresponders. A variable which may "misclassify" individuals is not a good choice of tailoring variable, as it may make assignment to subsequent treatment unsystematic. This is an issue that should be anticipated and designed around, rather than corrected post hoc.

In a SMART, the same cohort of individuals participates in all stages of treatment, and a single study consent process is used for all these individuals (prior to the first stage randomization). SMARTs should not employ multiple consents (e.g., one at each randomization point); doing so could severely limit the ability to make inferences about the relative effects of the DTRs embedded in a SMART. Rather, the single consent process should inform participants of all possible treatment sequences to which they may be assigned during the study. Because the goal of a SMART is to develop a high-quality DTR, participants in the trial should experience the DTR as close to a real-world implementation as possible; a reconsent process would detract from this goal. Should they wish, investigators could randomize participants to DTRs at the start of the trial, though this should be carefully blinded to avoid expectancy effects: Participants should not have knowledge of their future treatment assignments.

Importantly, SMARTs are typically not adaptive trial designs despite having similar terminology (Meurer et al. 2012). An adaptive trial design is a multistage study in which data is used to modify characteristics of the trial as it is collected (Dragalin 2006). In contrast, in a SMART, typically all participants move through every stage of the trial and the trial design remains fixed; the goal is to learn how best to adapt treatment to the changing needs of the individual. In adaptive trials, the *trial* is adaptive; in SMARTs, the focus is on developing an adaptive *treatment strategy* (a DTR). More recently, statisticians have begun to develop randomized trial designs that are both sequentially randomized and adaptive (Cheung et al. 2015).

Readers interested in more in-depth information about SMARTs and DTRs might see the books by Chakraborty and Moodie (2013), Kosorok and Moodie (2015), or Tsiatis et al. (2019). In addition, Nahum-Shani et al. (2012b) and Ogbagaber et al. (2016) provide tutorials on analytic strategies for comparing embedded DTRs in a SMART with a continuous, end-of-study outcome. Nahum-Shani et al. (2020) also provide a tutorial for analyzing SMARTs with longitudinal outcomes. For analytic and sample size considerations for SMARTs with binary outcomes, see Kidwell et al. (2018); survival outcomes, Feng and Wahed (2009), Li and Murphy (2011); and continuous longitudinal outcomes, Lu et al. (2016), Li (2017), Dziak et al. (2019), and Seewald et al. (2020). Recently, methods have been developed for clustered SMARTs for developing clustered DTRs (NeCamp et al. 2017). Finally, for information on estimating optimal DTRs from a SMART see Moodie et al. (2007), Murphy (2003), Nahum-Shani et al. (2012a), or Zhao and Laber (2014).

Summary and Conclusion

Dynamic treatment regimens provide a guide for the type of sequential intervention decision-making that arises naturally in clinical settings (Lavori and Dawson 2014). Sequential, multiple assignment, randomized trials (SMARTs) are one type of experimental design that can be used by researchers for developing DTRs. This chapter discussed the components that make up DTRs, and scientific questions that researchers may have about them. It then described how a SMART can be used to address these scientific questions. The ExTENd SMART study – designed to develop a DTR for adults with alcohol use disorder – was used to illustrate these ideas.

For clinical trial researchers interested in developing efficient and effective DTRs, the SMART may be a useful design to consider. As discussed in the chapter, there are different types of SMART designs. Ultimately, for researchers who choose to use a SMART, the type of SMART design they choose should be grounded in the scientific questions they are seeking to answer.

Key Facts

Sequential, multiple-assignment randomized trials (SMARTs) are experimental designs which aid in the development of sequences of treatments which are able to adapt to an individual's changing needs, called dynamic treatment regimens. The key feature of a SMART is that some or all participants are randomized more than once. Like any clinical trial, the design of a SMART is motivated by specific scientific questions; for SMARTs, those questions are about dynamic treatment regimens.

Cross-References

▶ Essential Statistical Tests
▶ Estimation and Hypothesis Testing
▶ Factorial Trials
▶ Multi-arm Multi-stage (MAMS) Platform Randomized Clinical Trials
▶ Power and Sample Size
▶ Principles of Clinical Trials: Bias and Precision Control

Acknowledgments Funding was provided by the National Institutes of Health (P50DA039838, R01DA039901) and the Institute for Education Sciences (R324B180003). Funding for the ExTENd study, which was used to illustrate ideas, was provided by the National Institutes of Health (R01AA014851; PI: David Oslin).

References

Almirall D, DiStefano C, Chang Y-C, Shire S, Kaiser A, Lu X, Nahum-Shani I, Landa R, Mathy P, Kasari C (2016) "Longitudinal Effects of Adaptive Interventions With a Speech-Generating Device in Minimally Verbal Children With ASD." J Clin Child Adolesc 45 (4): 442–56. https://doi.org/10.1080/15374416.2016.1138407

Almirall D, Nahum-Shani I, Lu W, Kasari C (2018) Experimental designs for research on adaptive interventions: singly and sequentially randomized trials. In: Collins LM, Kugler KC (eds) Optimization of behavioral, biobehavioral, and biomedical interventions: advanced topics, Statistics for social and behavioral sciences. Springer International Publishing, Cham, pp 89–120. https://doi.org/10.1007/978-3-319-91776-4_4

August GJ, Piehler TF, Bloomquist ML (2016) Being 'SMART' about adolescent conduct problems prevention: executing a SMART pilot study in a juvenile diversion agency. J Clin Child Adolesc Psychol 45(4):495–509. https://doi.org/10/ghpbrn

Cable N, Sacker A (2007) Typologies of alcohol consumption in adolescence: predictors and adult outcomes. Alcohol Alcoholism 43(1):81–90. https://doi.org/10/fpmm33

Chakraborty B, Moodie EEM (2013) *Statistical Methods for Dynamic Treatment Regimes*. Statistics for biology and health. Springer New York, New York, NY. https://doi.org/10.1007/978-1-4614-7428-9

Cheung YK, Chakraborty B, Davidson KW (2015) Sequential multiple assignment randomized trial (SMART) with adaptive randomization for quality improvement in depression treatment program: SMART with adaptive randomization. Biometrics 71(2):450–459. https://doi.org/10.1111/biom.12258

Chronis-Tuscano A, Wang CH, Strickland J, Almirall D, Stein MA (2016) Personalized treatment of mothers with ADHD and their young at-risk children: a SMART pilot. J Clin Child Adolesc Psychol 45(4):510–521. https://doi.org/10/gg2h36

Collins LM, Nahum-Shani I, Almirall D (2014) Optimization of behavioral dynamic treatment regimens based on the sequential, multiple assignment, randomized trial (SMART). Clin Trials 11(4):426–434. https://doi.org/10/f6cjxm

Dragalin V (2006) Adaptive designs: terminology and classification. Drug Inf J 40(4):425–435. https://doi.org/10/ghpbrt

Dziak JJ, Yap JRT, Almirall D, McKay JR, Lynch KG, Nahum-Shani I (2019) A data analysis method for using longitudinal binary outcome data from a SMART to compare adaptive interventions. Multivar Behav Res 0(0):1–24. https://doi.org/10/gftzjg

Feng W, Wahed AS (2009) Sample size for two-stage studies with maintenance therapy. Stat Med 28(15):2028–2041. https://doi.org/10.1002/sim.3593

Gunlicks-Stoessel M, Mufson L, Westervelt A, Almirall D, Murphy SA (2016) A pilot SMART for developing an adaptive treatment strategy for adolescent depression. J Clin Child Adolesc Psychol 45(4):480–494. https://doi.org/10/ghpbrv

Hall KL, Nahum-Shani I, August GJ, Patrick ME, Murphy SA, Almirall D (2019) Adaptive intervention designs in substance use prevention. In: Sloboda Z, Petras H, Robertson E, Hingson R (eds) Prevention of substance use, Advances in prevention science. Springer International Publishing, Cham, pp 263–280. https://doi.org/10.1007/978-3-030-00627-3_17

Heilig M, Egli M (2006) Pharmacological treatment of alcohol dependence: target symptoms and target mechanisms. Pharmacol Ther 111(3):855–876. https://doi.org/10/cfs7df

Kasari C, Kaiser A, Goods K, Nietfeld J, Mathy P, Landa R, Murphy SA, Almirall D (2014) Communication interventions for minimally verbal children with autism: a sequential multiple assignment randomized trial. J Am Acad Child Adolesc Psychiatry 53(6):635–646. https://doi.org/10.1016/j.jaac.2014.01.019

Kidwell KM, Seewald NJ, Tran Q, Kasari C, Almirall D (2018) Design and analysis considerations for comparing dynamic treatment regimens with binary outcomes from sequential multiple assignment randomized trials. J Appl Stat 45(9):1628–1651. https://doi.org/10.1080/02664763.2017.1386773

Kilbourne AM, Almirall D, Eisenberg D, Waxmonsky J, Goodrich DE, Fortney JC, JoAnn E. Kirchner, et al. (2014) Protocol: adaptive implementation of effective programs trial (ADEPT): cluster randomized SMART trial comparing a standard versus enhanced implementation strategy to improve outcomes of a mood disorders program. Implement Sci 9(1):132. https://doi.org/10/f6q9fc

Kilbourne AM, Smith SN, Choi SY, Koschmann E, Liebrecht C, Rusch A, Abelson JL et al (2018) Adaptive school-based implementation of CBT (ASIC): clustered-SMART for building an optimized adaptive implementation intervention to improve uptake of mental health interventions in schools. Implement Sci 13(1):119. https://doi.org/10/gd7jt2

Kosorok MR, Moodie EEM (eds) (2015) Adaptive treatment strategies in practice: planning trials and analyzing data for personalized medicine. Society for Industrial and Applied Mathematics, Philadelphia, PA. https://doi.org/10.1137/1.9781611974188

Laber EB, Lizotte DJ, Qian M, Pelham WE, Murphy SA (2014) Dynamic treatment regimes: technical challenges and applications. Electron J Stat 8(1):1225–1272. https://doi.org/10/gg29c8

Lavori PW, Dawson R (2004) Dynamic treatment regimes: practical design considerations. Clin Trials 1(1):9–20. https://doi.org/10/cqtvnn

Lavori PW, Dawson R (2014) Introduction to dynamic treatment strategies and sequential multiple assignment randomization. Clin Trials 11(4):393–399. https://doi.org/10.1177/1740774514527651

Lei H, Nahum-Shani I, Lynch K, Oslin D, Murphy SA (2012) A 'SMART' design for building individualized treatment sequences. Annu Rev Clin Psychol 8(1):21–48. https://doi.org/10.1146/annurev-clinpsy-032511-143152

Li Z (2017) Comparison of adaptive treatment strategies based on longitudinal outcomes in sequential multiple assignment randomized trials. Stat Med 36(3):403–415. https://doi.org/10.1002/sim.7136

Li Z, Murphy SA (2011) Sample size formulae for two-stage randomized trials with survival outcomes. Biometrika 98(3):503–518. https://doi.org/10.1093/biomet/asr019

Longabaugh R, Zweben A, Locastro JS, Miller WR (2005) Origins, issues and options in the development of the combined behavioral intervention. J Stud Alcohol Suppl (15):179–187. https://doi.org/10/ghpb9f

Lu X, Nahum-Shani I, Kasari C, Lynch KG, Oslin DW, Pelham WE, Fabiano G, Almirall D (2016) Comparing dynamic treatment regimes using repeated-measures outcomes: modeling considerations in SMART studies. Stat Med 35(10):1595–1615. https://doi.org/10/gg2gxc

Lunceford JK, Davidian M, Tsiatis AA (2002) Estimation of survival distributions of treatment policies in two-stage randomization designs in clinical trials. Biometrics 58(1):48–57. https://doi.org/10/bk2dj9

McKay JR (2005) Is there a case for extended interventions for alcohol and drug use disorders? Addiction 100(11):1594–1610. https://doi.org/10/btpvtr

Meurer WJ, Lewis RJ, Berry DA (2012) Adaptive clinical trials: a partial remedy for the therapeutic misconception? JAMA-J Am Med Assoc 307(22):2377–2378. https://doi.org/10/gf3pmm

Moodie EEM, Richardson TS, Stephens DA (2007) Demystifying optimal dynamic treatment regimes. Biometrics 63(2):447–455. https://doi.org/10/ffcq8r

Murphy SA (2003) Optimal dynamic treatment regimes. J R Stat Soc B 65(2):331–355. https://doi.org/10/dmmr89

Murphy SA (2005) An experimental Design for the Development of adaptive treatment strategies. Stat Med 24(10):1455–1481. https://doi.org/10.1002/sim.2022

Murphy SA, Almirall D (2009) Dynamic treatment regimens. In: *Encyclopedia of Medical Decision Making*, 1:419–22. SAGE Publications, Thousand Oaks

Murphy SA, Bingham D (2009) Screening experiments for developing dynamic treatment regimes. J Am Stat Assoc 104(485):391–408. https://doi.org/10/dk2gpv

Naar-King S, Ellis DA, Carcone AI, Templin T, Jacques-Tiura AJ, Hartlieb KB, Cunningham P, Jen K-LC (2016) Sequential multiple assignment randomized trial (SMART) to construct weight loss interventions for African American adolescents. J Clin Child Adolesc Psychol 45(4):428–441. https://doi.org/10/gf4ks4

Nahum-Shani I, Qian M, Almirall D, Pelham WE, Gnagy B, Fabiano GA, Waxmonsky JG, Yu J, Murphy SA (2012a) Q-learning: a data analysis method for constructing adaptive interventions. Psychol Methods 17(4):478–494. https://doi.org/10.1037/a0029373

Nahum-Shani I, Qian M, Almirall D, Pelham WE, Gnagy B, Fabiano GA, Waxmonsky JG, Yu J, Murphy SA (2012b) Experimental design and primary data analysis methods for comparing adaptive interventions. Psychol Methods 17(4):457–477. https://doi.org/10.1037/a0029372

Nahum-Shani I, Ertefaie A, Xi (Lucy) Lu, Lynch KG, McKay JR, Oslin DW, Almirall D (2017) A SMART data analysis method for constructing adaptive treatment strategies for substance use disorders. Addiction 112(5):901–909. https://doi.org/10/ghpb9n

Nahum-Shani I, Almirall D, Yap JRT, McKay JR, Lynch KG, Freiheit EA, Dziak JJ (2020) SMART longitudinal analysis: a tutorial for using repeated outcome Measures from SMART studies to compare adaptive interventions. Psychol Methods 25(1):1–29. https://doi.org/10/ggttht

NeCamp T, Kilbourne A, Almirall D (2017) Comparing cluster-level dynamic treatment regimens using sequential, multiple assignment, randomized trials: regression estimation and sample size considerations. Stat Methods Med Res 26(4):1572–1589. https://doi.org/10.1177/0962280217708654

Oetting AI, Levy JA, Weiss RD, Murphy SA (2011) Statistical methodology for a SMART Design in the Development of adaptive treatment strategies. In: Shrout PE, Keyes KM, Ornstein K (eds) Causality and psychopathology: finding the determinants of disorders and their cures. Oxford University Press, New York, pp 179–205

Ogbagaber SB, Karp J, Wahed AS (2016) Design of Sequentially Randomized Trials for testing adaptive treatment strategies. Stat Med 35(6):840–858. https://doi.org/10.1002/sim.6747

Oslin DW, Berrettini WH, O'Brien CP (2006) Targeting treatments for alcohol dependence: the pharmacogenetics of naltrexone. Addict Biol 11(3–4):397–403. https://doi.org/10/fgcfbk

Pelham WE Jr, Fabiano GA, Waxmonsky JG, Greiner AR, Gnagy EM, Pelham WE III, Coxe S et al (2016) Treatment sequencing for childhood ADHD: a multiple-randomization study of adaptive medication and behavioral interventions. J Clin Child Adolesc Psychol 45(4):396–415. https://doi.org/10/gfn9xr

Quanbeck A, Almirall D, Jacobson N, Brown RT, Landeck JK, Madden L, Cohen A et al (2020) The balanced opioid initiative: protocol for a clustered, sequential, multiple-assignment randomized trial to construct an adaptive implementation strategy to improve guideline-concordant opioid prescribing in primary care. Implement Sci 15(1):26. https://doi.org/10/gjh5tx

Rubin DB (1974) Estimating causal effects of treatments in randomized and nonrandomized studies. J Educ Psychol 66(5):688–701. https://doi.org/10.1037/H0037350

Schmitz JM, Stotts AL, Vujanovic AA, Weaver MF, Yoon JH, Vincent J, Green CE (2018) A sequential multiple assignment randomized trial for cocaine cessation and relapse prevention: tailoring treatment to the individual. Contemp Clin Trials 65(February):109–115. https://doi.org/10/gc3tqr

Seewald NJ, Kidwell KM, Nahum-Shani I, Wu T, McKay JR, Almirall D (2020) Sample size considerations for comparing dynamic treatment regimens in a sequential multiple-assignment randomized trial with a continuous longitudinal outcome. Stat Methods Med Res 29(7):1891–1912. https://doi.org/10/gf85ss

Sherwood NE, Butryn ML, Forman EM, Almirall D, Seburg EM, Lauren Crain A, Kunin-Batson AS, Hayes MG, Levy RL, Jeffery RW (2016) The BestFIT trial: a SMART approach to developing individualized weight loss treatments. Contemp Clin Trials 47(March):209–216. https://doi.org/10.1016/j.cct.2016.01.011

Thall PF, Kyle Wathen J (2005) Covariate-adjusted adaptive randomization in a sarcoma trial with multi-stage treatments. Stat Med 24(13):1947–1964. https://doi.org/10/d5ztnt

Thall PF, Millikan RE, Sung H-G (2000) Evaluating multiple treatment courses in clinical trials. Stat Med 19(8):1011–1028. https://doi.org/10/bmv5jc

Thall PF, Sung H-G, Estey EH (2002) Selecting therapeutic strategies based on efficacy and death in multicourse clinical trials. J Am Stat Assoc 97(457):29–39. https://doi.org/10/dx3fkb

Tsiatis AA, Davidian M, Holloway ST, Laber EB (2019) *Dynamic Treatment Regimes: Statistical Methods for Precision Medicine*. Monographs on statistics and applied probability 164. CRC Press LLC, Milton

Vock DM, Almirall D (2018) Sequential multiple assignment randomized trial (SMART). In: Balakrishnan N, Colton T, Everitt W, Piegorsch F, Teugels JL (eds) Wiley StatsRef: statistics reference online. https://doi.org/10.1002/9781118445112.stat08073

Wahed AS, Tsiatis AA (2004) Optimal estimator for the survival distribution and related quantities for treatment policies in two-stage randomization designs in clinical trials. Biometrics 60(1): 124–133. https://doi.org/10/dc4kfb

Wahed AS, Tsiatis AA (2006) Semiparametric efficient estimation of survival distributions in two-stage randomisation designs in clinical trials with censored data. Biometrika 93(1):163–177. https://doi.org/10/cgchp6

Zhao Y-Q, Laber EB (2014) Estimation of optimal dynamic treatment regimes. Clin Trials 11(4):400–407. https://doi.org/10/f6cjrn

Monte Carlo Simulation for Trial Design Tool

80

Suresh Ankolekar, Cyrus Mehta, Rajat Mukherjee, Sam Hsiao, Jennifer Smith, and Tarek Haddad

Contents

S. Ankolekar (✉)
Cytel Inc, Cambridge, MA, USA

Maastricht School of Management, Maastricht, Netherlands
e-mail: suresh.ankolekar@cytel.com

C. Mehta
Cytel Inc, Cambridge, MA, USA

Harvard T.H. Chan School of Public Health, Boston, MA, USA
e-mail: Cyrus.Mehta@cytel.com

R. Mukherjee · S. Hsiao
Cytel Inc, Cambridge, MA, USA

J. Smith
Sunesis Pharmaceuticals Inc, San Francisco, CA, USA

T. Haddad
Medtronic Inc, Minneapolis, MN, USA

© Springer Nature Switzerland AG 2022

S. Piantadosi, C. L. Meinert (eds.), *Principles and Practice of Clinical Trials*,
https://doi.org/10.1007/978-3-319-52636-2_251

Abstract

Clinical trials often involve design issues with mathematically intractable complexity. Being part of multi-phase drug development programs, the trial designs need to incorporate prior information in terms of historical data from earlier phases and available knowledge about related trials. Some trials with inherent limits on data collection may need augmentation with simulated pseudo-data. For planning of interim looks, group sequential and adaptive trials require accurate timeline predictions of reaching clinical milestones involving complex set of operational and clinical models. In general, clinical trial design involves an interactive process involving interplay of models, data, assumptions, insights, and experiences to address specific design issues before and during the trial. This offers a rich context for simulation-centric modeling, the theme of this chapter. We will focus on practical considerations of applying simulation modeling tools and techniques to design and implementation of clinical trials. This will be achieved through two real-life case studies and relevant illustrative examples drawn from literature and our practical experience.

Keywords

Adaptive design · Bayesian discount · Sample-size re-estimation · Design simulation · Power prior · Discount function · O'Brien-Fleming efficacy

Introduction

This chapter focuses on application of Monte Carlo simulations for clinical trial design. In view of the emphasis of the book on principles and practice, we will focus on practical considerations of applying simulation modeling tools and techniques to design and implementation of clinical trials. This will primarily be achieved through two real-life case studies and relevant illustrative examples drawn from literature and our practical experience.

The chapter is organized in five sections. The next section introduces the basic simulation concepts and relates them to clinical trials. We deliberately take a simulation-centric view of clinical trials in the section and make a case for enhanced role of simulation techniques in their design and implementation. This will be followed by two detailed sections covering two real-life case studies, one completed and other currently ongoing. Finally, we conclude the chapter with a few remarks.

Monte Carlo Simulations and Trial Design

Thompson (1999) gives a notion of simulation in terms of generation of pseudo-data on the basis of a model, a database, or the use of a model in the light of a database. The generation of the pseudo-data involves pseudorandom numbers, probabilistic models, and possibly real data from historical clinical trial or currently ongoing one. For some standard probabilistic models, it could directly involve a straight forward "inverse transformation" or indirectly "Accept-Reject" methods, typically described in most simulation textbooks, such as, Robert and Casella (2010). For example, for an exponential distribution $f(X:\lambda) = \lambda e^{-\lambda X}$ with corresponding cumulative distribution $F(X:\lambda) = 1 - e^{-\lambda X}$, the pseudo-data can simply be generated by substituting uniform random variate $U \sim U[0,1]$ for $F(X:\lambda)$ and solving for X, as $X = ln(1-U)/\lambda$. A generalized inverse transformation could be applied to generate pseudo-data for related distributions, say, $Y \sim Gamma(\alpha,\beta)$ as $Y = \beta \sum_{j=1}^{\alpha} X_j$ where X_j is generated from related exponential distribution with $\lambda = \alpha/\beta$. If a cumulative distribution $F(X:\theta)$ is somehow not amenable to direct inverse transformation, then it is possible to generate the pseudo-data indirectly using "Accept-Reject" method, where a simpler distribution $g(X:\gamma)$ is used to generate $Y \sim G(X:\gamma)$ in conjunction with $U \sim U[0,1]$ and accept it as X only if $U \leq (1/M).f(Y)/g(Y)$ where M is a constant satisfying $f(x)/g(x) \leq M$ for all x. The pseudo-data can also be generated in conjunction with accumulated data of an ongoing clinical trial. For example, in a widely used Poisson-Gamma model for enrolment, λ for Poisson process is generated from a posterior $Gamma(\alpha,\beta)$ where the posterior parameters are computed as Bayesian updates of a prior $Gamma(\alpha 0,\beta 0)$ with $\alpha = \alpha 0 + n$ and $\beta = \beta 0 + \tau$ where n is the realized enrolment at time τ. More sophisticated computations could be efficiently carried out using Markov Chain Monte Carlo (MCMC) techniques with Metropolis-Hastings and Gibbs Sampler algorithms, as described in Suess and Trumbo (2010).

The purpose of this brief introduction to generation of pseudo-data was to highlight the simplicity and demystify a rather harsh traditional view that the simulation is a complex technique and to be avoided whenever an analytic solution is possible. In practice, computing environments such as R and other industry standard design tools have built-in functionality to implement the techniques. For deeper theoretical and practical insights, the reader is referred to standard textbooks on the subject, such as, Robert and Casella (2010), Suess and Trumbo (2010), and others.

Thompson (1999) further asserts that as a computational aid in dealing with and creating models of reality, the simulation could potentially be an integral part of the modeling process itself. It is a device for working with models, testing models, and building new models, a kind of paradigm for realistic evolutionary modeling, beyond simply being a mechanism for dealing with old modeling techniques, say, the numerical approximation to pointwise evaluation. This assertion is central to our simulation-centric view of clinical trials.

Thompson's assertion also resonates with an interesting "retrospective" view of clinical trial design from Evans (2010): "*Although clinical trials are conducted prospectively, one can think of them as being designed retrospectively. That is, there is a vision of the scientific claim (i.e., answer to the research question) that a project team would like to make at the end of the trial. In order to make that claim, appropriate analyses must be conducted in order to justify the claim. In order to conduct the appropriate analyses, specific data must be collected in a manner suitable to conduct the analyses. In order to collect these necessary data, a thorough plan for data collection must be developed. This sequential retrospective strategy continues until a trial design has been constructed....*" The "retrospective" view would straddle a relevant past and an imaginary future, involving relevant models/data/assumptions carried forward from previous phases and available knowledge in terms of insights/experiences and published literature, and various future design options for the protocol and statistical analysis plan (SAP). The "retrospective" strategy implies an interactive process involving interplay of models/data/assumptions/insights/experiences to address specific design issues, and offers a rich context for simulation-centric modeling.

The context for a simulation-centric clinical trial design is further reinforced by a Clinical Scenario Evaluation (CSE) approach introduced by Benda et al. (2010), and subsequently refined by Friede et al. (2010). The approach consisting of three components, data, analysis, and evaluation models, involves thorough assessment of multiple design and analysis strategies and their sensitivity to potential changes in the underlying assumptions. Dmitrienko and Pukstenis (2017) describe an implementation of the approach in open-source R package, Mediana developed by Paux and Dmitrienko (2016) and being currently maintained by representatives from multiple biopharmaceutical companies. The implementation takes a simulation-centric view of the clinical trial design. Accordingly, "*decomposition into three independent components provides a structured framework for clinical trial simulations which enables clinical trial researchers to carry out a systematic quantitative assessment of the operating characteristics of candidate designs and statistical methods to characterize their performance in multiple settings.*"

There is a clear trend in enhanced support for simulation-centric view among the industry standard tools used for clinical trial design. For example, East 6 (2018) supports extensive simulation of clinical trial designs, including conditional simulations for enrolment and clinical events predictions involving accumulated blinded and unblinded data. Some of the features have been used in the real-life case studies covered in the later sections.

The pseudo-data generated by the simulation model could be analyzed to explore specific design issues. One of the dominant themes has been power computations in the context of sample size and dose-finding studies. Chang (2011) offers wide range of simulation algorithms to generate pseudo-data for classical and adaptive designs and analyze it to compute power. Arnold et al. (2011) use a simulation study to estimate power for individual and cluster-randomized designs. Antonijevic et al. (2010) use simulation study to assess impact of Ph 2 dose selection strategy on Ph 3 probability of success.

Adaptive designs are necessarily simulation-centric by very nature of the design and range of issues involved in the continuum of design and implementation. Gao et al. (2008) use an extensive simulation experiment to establish equivalence of their proposed method of preserving type I error after an unblinded sample size reestimation with two other methods. The scope of simulation in design and implementation of clinical trial based on sample size reestimation will be elaborated in the context of a real-life case study in the next section. Muller et al. (2007) consider simulation-based methods for exploration and maximization of expected utility in sequential decision problems, such as optimal stopping problem in a clinical trial. The problem involves analytically intractable expected utility integrals at each stage. Jiang et al. (2014) use extensive simulations to evaluate their proposed Bayesian prediction model between biomarker and the clinical endpoint for dichotomous variables. Haddad et al. (2017) use a novel method for augmenting a Bayesian medical device trial by using virtual patient pseudo-data, where the extent of augmentation is controlled by a parameterized "discount function" based on similarity between pseudo-data and observed data, as described in section "Case Study 2: SPYRAL HTN OFF-MED Trial." A related simulation approach that uses historical data for augmentation instead of virtual patient pseudo-data is covered in the real-life case study presented later in the section.

Case Study 1: The VALOR Trial

Acute myelogenous leukemia (AML) is a disease of the bone marrow with poor prognosis and few available therapies, a continued area of unmet need. The VALOR study was a phase 3, double-blind, placebo-controlled trial conducted at 101 international sites in 711 patients with AML. Patients were randomized 1:1 to vosaroxin plus cytarabine (vos/cyt) or placebo plus cytarabine (pla/cyt) stratified by disease status, age, and geographic location. The primary and secondary efficacy endpoints were overall survival (OS) and complete response rate. This study is registered at clinicaltrials.gov (NCT01191801).

Motivation of Adaptive Sample Size Re-Estimation

Prior to designing the VALOR trial, Sunesis Pharmaceuticals completed a single arm Ph 2 trial in relapsed refractory AML. Observed mean OS in that trial was approximately 7 months. Assuming an expected OS of 5 months in the control arm, the VALOR trial was powered at 90% for hazard ratio (HR = 5/7 = 0.71) requiring 375 events and 450 patients. However, there can be uncertainty around Ph 2 estimates. While HR greater than 0.71 (say 0.75) could still be clinically meaningful, powering for this smaller effect size would require a large, initially unfeasible number of patients. An adaptive approach allows the sample size to be conditional on observed data accumulating in the first part of the Ph 3 trial, avoiding unnecessarily enrolling patients at the start if the true HR is close to 0.71 and allowing additional patients to be enrolled later if the effect size is smaller but still of meaningful magnitude. This flexible approach allowed the exposure of patients and the expenditure of resources to be conditional on observed results at the interim.

Statistical Methodology

VALOR was a two-arm trial with time to death as the primary endpoint. It was required to have $100 \times (1-\beta) = 90\%$ power to detect an improvement in median survival from 5 months on pla/cyt (the control arm) to 7 months on vos/cyt (the experimental arm) (HR = 0.71) using a one-sided log-rank test at the significance level $\alpha = 2.5\%$. The trial was designed with one interim analysis when 50% of the death events were observed, at which point one of the following four decisions could have been taken:

(a) Terminate for overwhelming efficacy
(b) Terminate for futility
(c) Increase the number of death events and sample size
(d) Continue the trial as planned

In trials with a time to event endpoint, the power is driven by number of events, say D, and not by sample size. Sample size plays an indirect role, however, since the larger the sample size, the earlier the required D events and the shorter will be the expected study duration. To meet the 90% power requirement, the target number of death events D is given by the formula

$$D = \left[\frac{z_\alpha + z_\beta}{\ln(HR)} \right]^2 * [IF]$$

where z_γ is the upper $(1-\gamma) \times 100\%$ percentile of the standard normal distribution and IF is an inflation factor to recover power loss due to spending some of the available α for possible early stopping at the interim analysis. Values of IF for different α-spending functions are available in Jennison and Turnull (2000). An analytical relationship between required number of events, sample size, patient enrollment rates, and study duration is available in Kim and Tsiatis (1990). Based on these considerations, the planned initial enrolment was for 450 patients and 375 events with the possibility of increasing both the planned events and sample size by 50% if the results of the interim analysis fell in the promising zone (see below). Note the total sample size was increased to allow for 5% dropouts and an effective sample size of either 450 or 676 patients. Enrolment assumptions were tested periodically by simulating the pooled study data (blinded to the treatment assignment) so that accurate assessments of dates for the interim and final analyses could be obtained. These simulations are described later in VALOR simulation.

The decision to terminate for efficacy at the interim analysis time point would be based on the O'Brien-Fleming efficacy boundary derived from the Lan and DeMets

(1983) α-spending function, invoked when 50% of the death events were observed, and the appropriate amount of α was spent to ensure that the overall one-sided type-1 error remained 0.025. This approach results in a one-sided significance level of 0.001525 for the interim analysis (with 187 of the planned 375 events) and 0.0245 for the final analysis (with 375 events). The overall significance level of this test procedure was guaranteed to be 0.025 (one-sided).

If the efficacy criterion was not met, one of the remaining three decisions would be taken based on the *conditional power* or probability of achieving statistical significance at the end of the trial conditional on the results observed at the interim analysis. Precise formulae for conditional power are available in Mehta and Pocock (2011) and Gao et al. (2008). The trial would now be modified as follows:

- Fix a maximum upper limit of 562 for the number of events and 676 for the sample size.
- Compute the conditional power with the number of events being increased to 562, based on a hazard ratio of 0.71 as specified at the design stage. If the conditional power (CP-plan-562) so computed is less than 50%, the DSMB would recommend stopping for futility. If the futility criterion was not met, continue as discussed below.
- Compute the conditional power at 187 events, with the number of events equal to 375 (CP-obs-375) at the final analysis as initially specified, based on the hazard ratio estimated at the interim analysis.
  - If CP-obs-375 $\leq$ 30%, the results are considered *unfavorable*. Continue the trial with no further change until 375 events are reached, and perform the final analysis.
  - If 30% $<$ CP-obs-375 $\leq$ 90%, the results are considered *promising*. Increase the number of events to 562 and sample size to 676.
  - If CP-obs-375 $>$ 90%, the results are considered *favorable*. Continue the trial with no further change until 375 events are reached, and perform the final analysis.

The DSMB was allowed to exercise clinical judgement, based on its access to unblinded safety and efficacy data to make minor adjustments to the sample size obtained by the above rules.

Because the number of events could potentially be increased in a data-dependent manner at the interim look, the final analysis would not use the conventional log-rank statistic to determine if statistical significance is reached. Instead it used the weighted statistic proposed by Cui et al. (1999) in which the independent log-rank statistics of the two stages are combined by prespecified weights that are equal to the planned proportion of total events at which the interim analysis would be taken if there were no change in the design. In the present case, the trial was designed for 375 events with an interim analysis at 187 events. The planned proportion was 0.5 for each stage and the log-rank statistics for the two stages were combined with weights that equal the square root of 0.5. Thus, if Z_1 and Z_2 are the standardized log-rank statistics from the data before and after the interim analysis, the combined statistic for the final analysis was

$$Z_f = \sqrt{0.5}Z_1 + \sqrt{0.5}Z_2$$

In order to ensure preservation of type-1 error, the two weights $\sqrt{0.5}$ and $\sqrt{0.5}$ for the two stages must be used even if the total number of events was increased at the interim analysis. This could result in a slight loss of efficiency, which is offset by the increase in events.

VALOR Simulations

(a) *Design-Stage Simulations*: The VALOR trial was extensively simulated to ascertain its operating characteristics at the design stage as per the following pseudocode:

```
Initialize HR for the simulation scenario (e.g. 0.71, 0.74, 0.77,
etc.)
For each of the 10000 simulations for the scenario
   Generate clinical events for each of the 450 patients
   Identify interim look dataset with earliest 187 events
   Analyze the interim dataset to compute the p-value
   If p-value < 0.001525 then
        Stop for overwhelming efficacy
   Else If p-value ≥ 0.001525
        Compute conditional power (cp-plan-562) for 562 events as
        planned at design stage
        If cp-plan-562 < 50% then
             Stop for futility
        Else If cp-plan-562 ≥ 50%
             Compute conditional power with observed HR and 375
             events (cpobs-375)
             If cp-obs-375 ≤ 30% or If cp-obs-375 > 90% then
                  Prepare and analyze dataset of 375 events for
                  450 patients
             Else If 30% < cp-obs-375 ≤ 90% then
                  Increase the sample size to 676 patients and
                  generate their events
                  Prepare and analyze dataset of 562 events for
                  676 patients
             End If [ cp-obs-375 ]
        End If [ cp-plan-562 ]
     End If [ p-value ]
End For [ 10000 simulations for the scenario ]
Summarize the results of 10000 simulations for the specified HR
scenario (e.g. 0.71, 0.74, 0.77, etc.)
```

Operating characteristics of the adaptive group sequential design under various scenarios, based on 10,000 simulations per scenario, are tabulated below in

Table 1 for hazard ratios of 0.71, 0.74, and 0.77. The operating characteristics include probabilities, conditional powers, trial durations, and sample sizes associated with unfavorable, promising, and favorable zones at the interim look. For comparison purposes the operating characteristics of the two-look nonadaptive group sequential design, with 375 maximum events, 450 patients, and no reassessment of events or sample size are also displayed. Both designs have an O'Brien-Fleming efficacy boundary and a futility boundary for terminating at the interim look if the conditional power based on HR = 0.71 is below 50%. Average power gains of 3% to 6% are obtained with the adaptive design at an average cost of 50–70 additional subjects and an average increase in study duration of 2–4 months. The real benefit of the adaptive design, however, lies in its ability to learn from the interim results and avoid an underpowered trial. This is evident from an examination of the zone-wise powers. For example, under the pessimistic scenario HR = 0.77, the study is underpowered at 71%. But if the interim results land in the promising zone, the conditional power of the adaptive designs is boosted up to 90% but remains 71% for the nonadaptive design. This gain in power does come with a cost in terms of increased sample size to 675 instead of 450 and the study duration is 38 months instead of 29. However, these additional resource commitments would have to be made only after observing the interim data, if promising. The simulation model adequately supports the sample size reestimation decision, if any, as it consistently shows

Table 1 Zone-wise operating characteristics of adaptive and non-adaptive designs

		Conditional power		Duration (months)		Sample size	
Zone	P(Zone)	Non-adaptive	Adaptive	Non-adaptive	Adaptive	Non-adaptive	Adaptive
(a) Under the design-stage scenario: HR = 0.71							
Unfavorable	0.12	56%	56%	30	30	447	447
Promising	0.27	87%	98%	30	39	375	562
Favorable	0.61	98%	99%	25	25	292	292
Average	1	91%	94%	27	29	324	373
(b) Under the moderately pessimistic scenario: HR = 0.74							
Unfavorable	0.18	44%	44%	29	29	446	445
Promising	0.32	80%	94%	30	39	450	675
Favorable	0.50	97%	97%	25	25	404	406
Average	1	82%	87%	27	30	426	499
(c) Under the pessimistic scenario: HR = 0.77							
Unfavorable	0.26	34%	33%	29	29	442	444
Promising	0.34	71%	90%	29	38	450	675
Favorable	0.40	94%	94%	26	26	412	412
Average	1	71%	77%	23	27	443	509

increased power associated with promising zone over the range of hazard ratio scenarios.

(b) *Monitoring-Stage Simulations*: In addition to the design stage, the periodic simulations were also carried out during the monitoring stage of the ongoing trial to perform blinded data reviews for enrolment and clinical events predictions. The simulations used Poisson-Gamma model with Bayesian updates based on enrolments already realized as per the following pseudocode:

```
Initialize prior site enrollment rates, hazard rates, sample size
scenarios (e.g. 450, 675)
Read dataset containing observed enrollments and clinical events
Compute posterior Gamma parameters for Poisson-Gamma model
Compute posterior parameters for hazard rates using exponential
model
Compute posterior parameters for dropouts using exponential model
For each of the 1000 simulations for the scenario
    Activate remaining sites, if any, by sampling uniform
    distribution corresponding to Site Activation Plan
    Generate posterior enrollment rates by sampling Gamma
    distribution with posterior Gamma parameters
    Generate posterior hazard rates by sampling Gamma distribution
    with posterior hazard rate parameters
    Generate posterior dropout rates by sampling Gamma
    distribution with posterior dropout parameters
    Generate remaining enrollments using Poisson-Gamma model with
    above rates
    Generate dropouts for patients-at-risk by sampling
    exponential distribution with posterior dropout rates
    Generate clinical events for patients-at-risk by sampling
    exponential distribution with posterior hazard rates
Endfor [simulations]
Analyze the simulation database to generate prediction tables and
plots
```

Figure 1 shows stochastic enrolment predictions made on the basis of 1,000 simulations of future enrolment given realized enrolment of 303 patients. Accordingly, a target enrolment of 500 patients for a sample size of 450 after dropouts is predicted to be achieved around month 24. The increased target of 750 enrolments for reestimated sample size of 676 is predicted to be achieved around month 32.

Death and dropout events were simulated in a blinded manner using an exponential distribution with prior pooled hazard rates based on design stage scenario (HR = 0.71) and initial assumed dropout with Bayesian updates based on observed death and dropout events until the review period. Figure 2 shows stochastic clinical events predictions made on the basis of 1,000 simulations of future enrolment given observed 115 events for the realized enrolment of 303 patients. Accordingly, a target

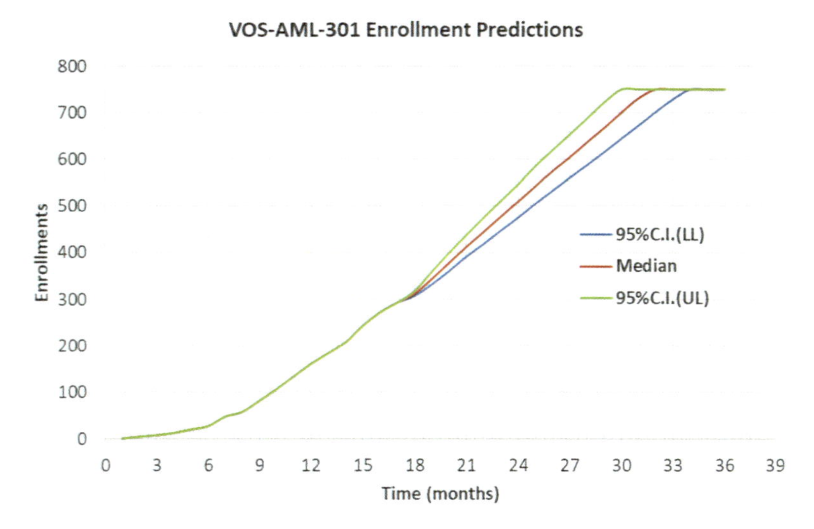

Fig. 1 Enrolment predictions after realized enrolment of 303 patients

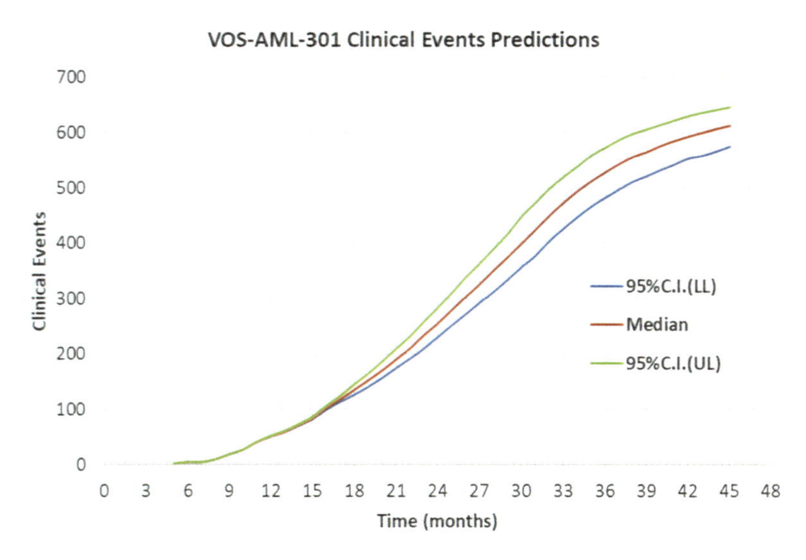

Fig. 2 Clinical events predictions after observed 115 events for realized enrolment of 303 patients

of 187 events to trigger interim analysis is predicted to be achieved around month 21 and final target of 375 events for an initial sample size of 450 is predicted to be reached around month 29. The clinical events are also predicted in the context of potential increase of sample size and target number of events at the interim analysis. Accordingly, the revised target of 562 events for reestimated sample size of 676 is predicted to be achieved around month 42.

Practicalities of Running an Adaptive Trial (With Reference to VALOR)

There are regulatory guidances on adaptive designs by both the FDA (Adaptive designs for clinical trials of drugs and biologics, draft guidance, September 2018) and EMA (Reflection paper on methodological issues in confirmatory clinical trials planned with an adaptive design, adoption by CHMP October 2007) that emphasize the need to prespecify analysis methods, minimize operational bias, and control the type I error, as well as the unbiased point estimation of treatment effect.

When there is an interim look at efficacy, as in the promising zone methodology, there are several practical considerations to minimize operational bias. First, consider strict control around the availability and communication of interim results. Decide as a sponsor what the message will be (if any) following the interim analysis. Will a change in the total sample size be announced to sites, operational entities, or investors? Various stakeholders (legal, regulatory, operational, medical, etc.) can be consulted up front to ensure that there is agreement about the planned communication strategy and an understanding of any implications. The VALOR trial made use of a special Access Control Execution System to both control and document the flow of data and reports created at the interim and shared with DSMB members. The promising zone as originally intended would increase the sample size by an amount proportionate to the observed results at the interim. The VALOR trial employed an all or nothing 50% sample size increase instead of a proportionate increase thus limiting the ability to back-calculate interim results based on the planned increase in sample size.

The promising zone methodology allows for strict control of the type I error as described in Jennison and Turnull (2000). However, there are some practical considerations that should be understood in the conduct and analysis of the trial. First, in this design, the test statistic Z_1 for the data at the interim is combined with the test statistic Z_2 for the data post-interim with prespecified weights as shown in the equation for Z_f at the end of the Statistical Methodology part of this case study. In simulation and in theory, the data supporting the interim test statistic Z_1 do not change between the time of the analysis at the interim and final analysis while in practice they may. Additional follow up (censor dates change) or data cleaning may alter the value of the test statistic computed at the time of the interim and upon which the sample size adjustment was made and the time of the final analysis. In the VALOR trial, the value of the test statistic Z_1 for the interim time point was recomputed on final data before being combined with Z_2 to produce the final adjusted statistic. Thereby the test statistic Z_1 was most representative of the final cleaned data and did not require creating and submitting data packages of the interim data to support an interim value incorporated into the final analysis. Second, a secondary analysis of OS in the VALOR trial was a stratified log rank. It was determined that the weighted Cui et al. (1999) method could also be applied to interim and post-interim test statistics after the stratification.

Case Study 2: SPYRAL HTN OFF-MED Trial

SPYRAL HTN OFF-MED is an international randomized single-blind (patient masked) study evaluating safety and efficacy of treatment with the Symplicity Spyral Multi-Node Electrode Renal Denervation System in patients with uncontrolled hypertension in the absence of antihypertensive medications (Funded by Medtronic; ClinicalTrials.gov Identifier: NCT02439749). The primary efficacy endpoint is change in systolic blood pressure (SBP) as measured by 24-h ambulatory blood pressure monitoring (ABPM) from baseline to 3 months post-procedure.

Prior studies did not find a consistent effect of renal denervation in reducing blood pressure. In particular, a large randomized study reported by Bhatt et al. (2014) in patients with resistant hypertension did not see a statistically significant benefit of renal denervation compared to a sham procedure in reducing blood pressure. Drug adherence was seen as a potentially important confounding factor in that study.

SPYRAL HTN OFF-MED was initially conceived of as a proof of concept (PoC) study to isolate the effect of renal denervation treatment (test group) versus a sham procedure (control group) in a population without resistant hypertension, where confounding by antihypertensive medications can be minimized by disallowing the use of such medications during the study. The PoC study was to be expanded to a pivotal study if a promising clinically benefits were observed.

Results of the PoC study, consisting of the first 80 consecutively randomized patients, have now been published (Townsend et al. 2017) and the study has moved into the planned pivotal phase under the same clinical investigation protocol. Because the enrollment criteria and study procedures did not change when the study moved into the pivotal phase, the sponsor plans to incorporate results from the PoC phase in the analysis of the pivotal study.

Motivation of Bayesian Design with Discount Prior Methodology

Recognizing the potential for temporal bias and other unknown factors that may impact the similarity of effect sizes in the two phases of the study, a Bayesian discount prior method is used for the primary efficacy analysis of the pivotal study as described in Haddad et al. (2017), whereby data from the PoC phase form the basis of an informative prior distribution for the pivotal study. The prior information is dynamically discounted with a factor between 0 and 1, based on the extent to which the prior data is dissimilar to the data from the pivotal study.

The pivotal study is currently ongoing, and not all details of the statistical design are publicly available at the time of writing. Our description of the design, simulations, and operating characteristics should be considered illustrative of the general approach and may not fully agree with the statistical plan of the trial.

Statistical Design

The study plans to randomize up to 433 patients total including both the PoC and pivotal phases.

The primary efficacy analysis of the pivotal trial uses a baseline adjusted comparison of change in SBP from baseline to 3 months post-procedure. Let x_i denote the baseline SBP and y_i the SBP change from baseline for the i-th patient. The linear model of interest is

$$y_i = \beta_c I_i\{\text{control}\} + \beta_t I_i\{\text{test}\} + \beta_x x_i + \epsilon_i, \epsilon_i \sim \text{Normal}\left(0, \sigma^2\right), \qquad (1)$$

where, $I_i\{\text{test}\}$ is the indicator for the test group (1 for test and 0 for control), $I_i\{\text{control}\} = 1 - I_i\{\text{test}\}$. The main parameter of interest is $\beta = \beta_t - \beta_c$, representing the baseline adjusted treatment effect. The primary efficacy hypothesis is $H_0 : \beta \geq 0$ versus $H_A : \beta < 0$.

The analysis to evaluate the efficacy hypothesis in the pivotal trial assumes separate power-prior (Ibrahim et al. 2015) normal distributions on β_c and β_t and uniform prior on log(σ), a standard choice for non-informative prior distribution on the variance term in a normal model. The prior distribution assumes zero correlation among model coefficients. The power-prior approach allows the amount of borrowing from historical data to be specified in terms of one parameter for the test group (α_t) and one parameter for the control group (α_c). The parameter values range between 0 and 1, with 0 indicating no borrowing and 1 indicating full borrowing from historical data. These power prior parameters are calculated as part of the discount prior method as described in the next section. The posterior distribution of β obtained via this approach will then be used to estimate the posterior probability that $\beta < 0$. The success criteria for this trial is that this posterior probability is greater than 0.975. This criterion aligns with the classical frequentist rule of using a one-sided test at 2.5% level of significance.

Multiple interim analyses are planned for this study. At each interim analysis, the decision to continue enrollment or stop enrollment for expected success or futility will be based on the predictive probability of success, which is derived by imputing the incomplete data from the posterior distributions of model parameters given interim data, and then recalculating the posterior probability of success. This completion process is repeated several times. The proportion of runs where the posterior probability for $\beta < 0$ achieves the success criteria (> 0.975) is the predictive probability of success. For efficacy, imputations are carried out for patients who have enrolled prior to a particular interim analysis, hence their baseline SBP values are available, but have not yet completed their 3-month follow-up. For futility, imputations are carried out for patients who have been enrolled prior to the interim analysis but completed their 3-month follow-up as well as for patients who have not yet been enrolled, up to the maximum sample size. Enrollment is stopped for expected success if the predictive probability of success with the currently enrolled patients is greater than 90%, and enrollment is stopped for futility if the predictive probability of success at the maximum sample size is less than 5%. A similar approach to interim decision-making is described in Berry (2011).

Discount Prior Methodology in the Context of the SPYRAL Trial Design

The discount prior method (Haddad et al. 2017) used in the SPYRAL trial was developed collaboratively by statisticians from the sponsor and the United States Food and Drug Administration (FDA) as part of the Medical Device Innovation Consortium (MDIC). An R package (bayesDP) developed by Musgrove and Haddad (2017) implementing this method is available. The method as it applies in the context of the trial is described here. The reader is referred to the referenced papers for details on the general methodology, and further to the R package documentation for details on implementation.

The analysis to evaluate the primary efficacy hypothesis in the pivotal trial assumes separate power-prior (Ibrahim et al. 2015) normal distributions on β_c and β_t and uniform prior on $\log(\sigma)$. The power parameter of the power-prior for the test group (α_t) and for the control group (α_c) are calculated as part of the discount prior method, which comprises four steps: compare, discount, combine, and estimate.

Compare

The test and the control group data are separately used to fit the following model, using combined data from both phases of the study in the given arm:

$$y_i = \tilde{\beta}_0 + \tilde{\beta}_1 I_i\{\text{current}\} + \tilde{\beta}_x x_i + \epsilon_i, \epsilon_i \sim \text{Normal}\left(0, \sigma^2\right),$$

where $I_i\{\text{current}\}$ equals 0 if the data is from the pivotal phase and equals 1 if the data is from the PoC phase. Here a joint uniform prior is assumed for $\log(\sigma)$ and the model coefficients. The degree of agreement between the two phases can be measured by $p = P\left(\tilde{\beta}_1 > 0|y\right)$. A value of p close to 0.5 indicates agreement while deviation from 0.5 on either side indicates lack of agreement in terms of the distribution of the response variable after adjusting for covariates. Thus, we transform p to $2p$ if $p < 0.5$ and to $2(1 - p)$ if $p \geq 0.5$, so that higher transformed values of p indicate higher levels of agreement. These calculations are carried out separately for each arm, resulting in p_c and p_t.

Discount

The similarity measures p_c and p_t are each mapped to a discount value in the interval [0, 1] by a discount function $F(p)$. Examples include the identity function $F(p) = p$

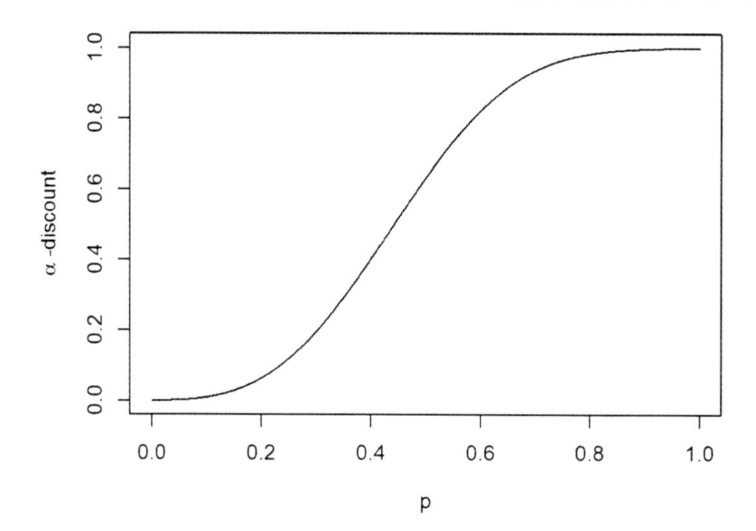

Fig. 3 Weibull discount function with shape k = 3 and scale λ = 0.5

and Weibull function $F(p) = 1 - e^{-\left(\frac{p}{\lambda}\right)^k}$. The power prior parameters for each arm are defined as $\alpha_t = \alpha_{max}F(p_t)$ and $\alpha_c = \alpha_{max}F(p_c)$, where α_{max} is a parameter between 0 and 1 defined at the beginning of the study to control the maximum level of borrowing from PoC data. The discount function and any accompanying parameters are also predefined to achieve certain operating characteristics. The same discount function is used for both arms, which may yield different levels of discount based on the values of p_t and p_c. Use of the Weibull function facilitates exploration of a wide range of discount profiles using just two parameters, the shape k and scale λ. The discount function used for one of our designs with $k = 3$ and $\lambda = 0.5$ is shown in Fig. 3.

Combine

The power prior method is used to combine the PoC and pivotal data, whereby informative normal priors based on PoC data are used for the linear model coefficients while applying a suitable level of discount according to the degree of similarity with the pivotal data. Thus, in the linear model (1), we use independent priors $\beta_c \tilde{N}\left(\widehat{\beta}_{0c}, \widehat{\tau}^2_{0c}/\alpha_c\right)$ and $\beta_t \tilde{N}\left(\widehat{\beta}_{0t}, \widehat{\tau}^2_{0t}/\alpha_t\right)$, where $\widehat{\beta}_{0c}$ ($\widehat{\beta}_{0t}$) and $\widehat{\tau}^2_{0c}$ ($\widehat{\tau}^2_{0t}$) are maximum likelihood estimates of the model parameters and their variances for the control group (test group) using PoC data. For the baseline variable, we do not apply a discount, and use $\beta_x \tilde{N}\left(\widehat{\beta}_{0x}, \widehat{\tau}^2_{0x}\right)$ where $\widehat{\beta}_{0x}$ and $\widehat{\tau}^2_{0x}$ are estimated baseline parameter and its variance using the linear model (1) fitted to the PoC data. For the variance term in (1), a flat prior on log(σ) is used. With these prior specifications, joint posterior samples for β_c and β_t are drawn conditional on pivotal trial outcomes (y), from which we generate a posterior sample for $\beta = \beta_t - \beta_c$ concerning the mean SBP change difference between the test and sham groups.

Estimate

Using the posterior distribution from the combined pivotal and PoC data, the probability of a treatment effect favoring the test group is estimated as

$$P(\beta < 0 | y, y_0, \alpha_t, \alpha_c)$$

Here y_0 denotes the PoC data, which is needed for prior specification and determination of prior discount levels α_t and α_c.

Role of Simulation

Simulations are critical in both the planning and implementation of the SPYRAL study. In the planning stage, operating characteristics are evaluated in order to optimize the design parameters and to facilitate discussion with regulatory authorities when seeking alignment on the design. The optimization process in this case was not a formal procedure involving objective functions (such an approach, while more rigorous, would have been computationally infeasible), but rather was iterative and informal, whereby simulations were performed under several combinations of realistic design parameters – such as sample size, timing and number of interim looks, discount function parameters, early stopping thresholds – under a range of plausible effect sizes including the null scenario ($\beta = 0$) and results were compared across scenarios to determine the parameter combination(s) that provided the best balance of type 1 error rate, power, and interim stopping probabilities in the judgment of the study team. One advantage of the discount prior approach is the flexibility to adjust the discount function to keep type 1 error rate at an acceptable level without needing to change the success criterion.

While the trial is ongoing, simulations are used for repeatedly imputing the incomplete data to derive estimates of the predictive probability of success for interim decision-making. Furthermore, ad hoc simulations may be requested by the Data Monitoring Committee should there be questions on how the efficacy analysis would look if the trial were to progress under particular scenarios of interest.

```
Pseudocode for Simulation Model:
For every simulation
     Simulate enrollment of all patients
     Generate baseline BP and change in BP (ΔBP) for all patients
     in treatment and control groups
     For every interim analysis (IA) with sample size Nint
          Complete data for both baseline BP and change ΔBP
          Compute Posterior of β
```

```
        Perform Nrep imputations to generate following datasets
             yimpES1 : Complete imputed dataset for Nint
             yimpES2 : Complete imputed dataset for all patients
        Compute Expected Successes, ES1 (for efficacy) and ES2
        (for futility) as follows
             ES_ = Σ I[P(β< 0 | yimpES_) > 0.975 / Nrep
        If (ES2 < 0.05) then
             Stop for futility
        Else If (ES1 > 0.9) then
             Stop for efficacy
        Else If (ES2 _ 0.05) AND ES1 _ 0.9)
             Continue to next IA
        End If
   Endfor (IA)
   Perform final Analysis
Endfor (Simulations)
Analyze simulation results to generate plots and tables
```

Programs to carry out the simulations were written in R programming language and the R package bayesDP was used to implement the discount prior analysis.

Plots showing power and type 1 error rates under two different designs are shown in Figs. 4–5. Both designs assume a maximum sample size of 400 and have two interim analyses, occurring when 280 and 320 subjects have been evaluated for 3-month SBP change. One design uses the identity discount function and the other uses a Weibull function with shape $k = 3$ and scale $\lambda = 0.5$ as shown earlier in Fig. 3. The number of simulated trials was 8,000 for estimating power, and 15,000 for estimating type 1 error. Thus, Monte Carlo standard error for power estimation is about 0.03–0.05, and for type 1 error it is about 0.01. The plots show cumulative power at each look, defined as the probability of the trial stopping at or before that look and achieving the success criterion. Using the identity discount function leads to power that is similar or marginally higher in most cases, but it also gives higher type 1 error rate (0.034) compared with the Weibull discount function (0.028). The higher type 1 error rate may be due in part to more aggressive borrowing from historical data with the identity discount function compared to the Weibull discount function when the current data are dissimilar to historical data (i.e., p_c or p_t close to 0). Additional operating characteristics of interest (not shown) may include probability of futility stopping at each look, or average percent prior information leveraged in each arm (α_c and α_t).

Validation of Simulation Tools

Validation of the programs for the Bayesian computations and trial simulations were performed so as to provide assurances to the sponsor and regulatory reviewers that the tools for design and implementation are working as intended in a manner consistent with documentation. An independent team tested specific functions from the bayesDP package that are intended to be used in the Bayesian analysis,

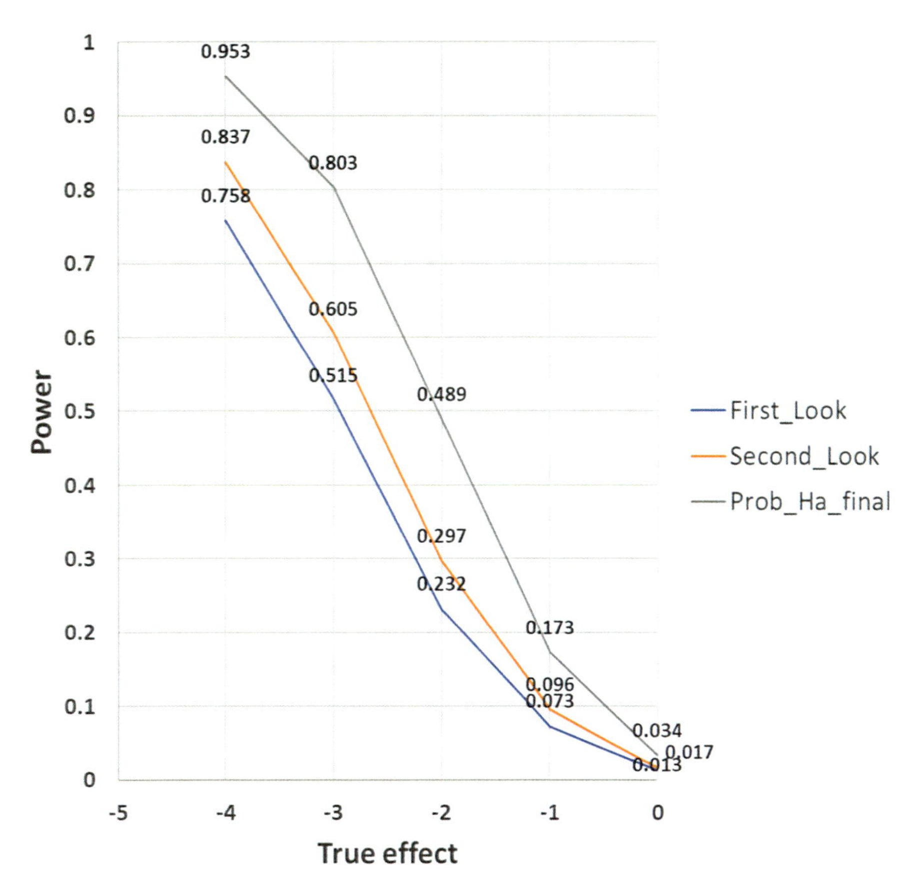

Fig. 4 Power versus treatment effect (difference in baseline adjusted SBP change at 3 months, measured in mmHg), using the identity discount function

and tested the simulation program used to establish the trial performance characteristics that are described in the statistical analysis plan.

For testing of bayesDP functions, specific test cases were derived such that the output being tested can be determined exactly using theoretical knowledge when possible. In cases where this cannot be done, outputs were compared with simulation results obtained by independent means, or evaluated for consistency with known theoretical properties.

For example, if the discount parameters are defined such that no borrowing from the prior is allowed (e.g., by setting $\alpha_{\max} = 0$), then the posterior distribution of the treatment effect β follows a scaled t-distribution, hence posterior samples generated by bayesDP were compared with their expected theoretical values. The difference (stochastic error) between the posterior sample and the theoretical distribution were quantified using the Kolmogorov-Smirnov distance, and the average and maximum distance over several runs was summarized in the validation report. On the other

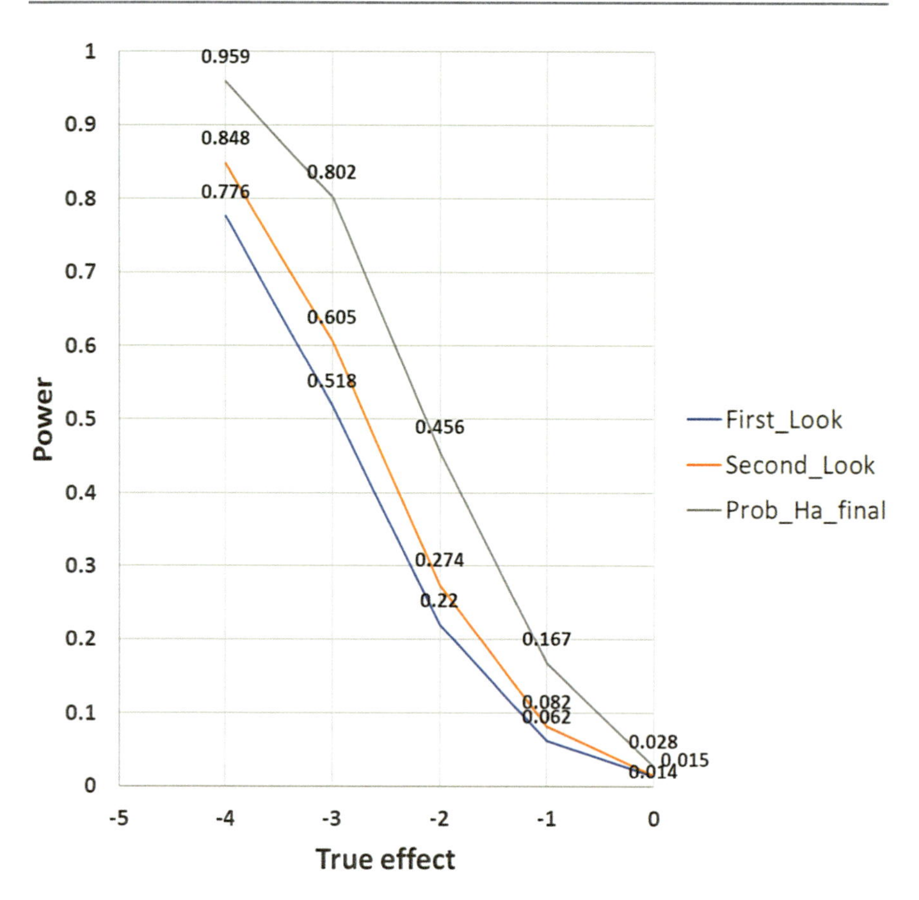

Fig. 5 Power versus treatment effect (difference in baseline adjusted SBP change at 3 months, measured in mmHg), using the Weibull discount function with shape 3 and scale 0.5

hand, if no restrictions are placed on the amount of borrowing from the prior except as dictated by the discount function ($\alpha_{\max} = 1$), then the posterior distribution of β no longer has an analytically convenient form. In this case, the posterior samples from bayesDP were compared with posterior samples obtained using Stan, a Bayesian computation tool in common use.

The strategy for validating the simulation program consisted of code review to map the logic of a single simulated trial, code review to map the logic of the execution and summary of multiple simulations, and using the program to run repeated simulations under different scenarios and ensuring operating characteristics behave as expected as the input parameters are allowed to vary. In particular, it was verified that power is a monotone function of sample size and effect size.

The simulation program, bayesDP source code (available for download from the Comprehensive R Archive Network), and validation report were made available to regulatory authorities for review.

Summary and Conclusion

In this chapter, we have taken a simulation-centric view of clinical trials with simulation as an integral part of the design and implementation of clinical trials. The simulation-centricity was guided by three related perspectives. Firstly, from a simulation perspective as a generator of pseudo-data on the basis of a model or a database and a device for working with models, testing models, and building new models, the simulation could potentially be an integral part of the modeling process itself as a kind of paradigm for realistic evolutionary modeling. Secondly, from a design perspective as an interactive process involving interplay of models, data, and assumptions, the simulation supports the process in terms of insights and experiences to address specific design issues before and during the trial. Some designs, like complex adaptive designs, are necessarily simulation-centric by very nature of the design and range of issues involved in the continuum of design and implementation. Finally, some trial design evaluation frameworks adopt simulation as a central part of their assessment of multiple design and analysis strategies and their sensitivity to potential changes in the underlying assumptions. Our two real-life case studies illustrated the critical role of simulation in adaptive trials. The scope of simulation in design and implementation of clinical trial based on sample size re-estimation was elaborated in the context of VALOR case study. A related simulation approach that uses historical data for augmentation instead of virtual patient pseudo-data was covered in the SPYRAL case study.

Key Facts

- Simulation is primarily concerned about generation of pseudo-data on the basis of a model, a database, or the use of a model in the light of a database. The generation of the pseudo-data involves pseudorandom numbers, probabilistic models, and possibly real data from historical clinical trial or currently ongoing one.
- Simulation is a mechanism for working with models, testing models, and building new models, a kind of paradigm for realistic evolutionary modeling, beyond simply being a mechanism for dealing with old modeling techniques, say, the numerical approximation to pointwise evaluation.
- Clinical trial design involves an interactive process involving interplay of models, data, assumptions, insights, and experiences to address specific design issues before and during the trial, offering a rich context for simulation-centric modeling.
- Clinical trials often involve design issues with mathematically intractable complexity. Being part of multi-phase drug development programs, the trial designs need to incorporate prior information in terms of historical data from earlier phases and available knowledge about related trials. Some trials with inherent

limits on data collection may need augmentation with simulated pseudo-data. Adaptive designs are necessarily simulation-centric by very nature of the design and range of issues involved in the continuum of design and implementation.
- For planning of interim looks, group sequential and adaptive trials require accurate timeline predictions of reaching clinical milestones involving complex set of operational and clinical models.
- The simulation-centric view is increasingly being supported by industry standard software tools used for clinical trial design and reinforced by the evaluation frameworks of the design and analysis strategies.

Cross-References

▶ Bias Control in Randomized Controlled Clinical Trials
▶ Cluster Randomized Trials
▶ Controlling for Multiplicity, Eligibility, and Exclusions
▶ Documentation: Essential Documents and Standard Operating Procedures
▶ Missing Data
▶ Power and Sample Size
▶ Statistical Analysis of Patient-Reported Outcomes in Clinical Trials
▶ Use of Resampling Procedures to Investigate Issues of Model Building and Its Stability

References

Antonijevic Z, Pinheiro J, Fardipour P, Lewis RJ (2010) Impact of dose selection strategies used in phase II on the probability of success in phase III. Stat Biopharm Res 2(4):469–486

Arnold B, Hogan D, Colford J, Hubbard A (2011) Simulation methods to estimate design power: an overview for applied research. BMC Med Res Methodol 11:94

Benda N, Branson M, Maurer W, Friede T (2010) Aspects of modernizing drug development using clinical scenario planning and evaluation. Drug Inf J 44:299–315

Berry SM (ed) (2011) Bayesian adaptive methods for clinical trials. Chapman & Hall/CRC biostatistics series. CRC Press, Boca Raton. 305 p

Bhatt DL, Kandzari DE, O'Neill WW, D'Agostino R, Flack JM, Katzen BT (2014) A controlled trial of renal denervation for resistant hypertension. N Engl J Med 370:1393–1401

Chang M (2011) Monte Carlo simulation for the pharmaceutical industry: concepts, algorithms, and case studies. Chapman & Hall/CRC biostatistics series. CRC Press, Boca Raton

Cui L, Hung HMJ, Wang S (1999) Modification of sample size in group sequential clinical trials. Biometrics 55:853–857

Dmitrienko A, Pukstenis E (2017) Clinical trial optimization using R. Chapman & Hall/CRC biostatistics series. CRC Press, Boca Raton

East 6 (2018) Statistical software for the design, simulation and monitoring clinical trials. Cytel Inc., Cambridge, MA

Evans SR (2010) Fundamentals of clinical trial design. J Exp Stroke Transl Med 3(1):19–27

Friede T, Nicholas R, Stallard N, Todd S, Parsons NR, Valdes-Marquez E, Chataway J (2010) Refinement of the clinical scenario evaluation framework for assessment of competing development strategies with an application to multiple sclerosis. Drug Inf J 44:713–718

Gao P, Ware J, Mehta C (2008) Sample size re-estimation for adaptive sequential design in clinical trials. J Biopharm Stat 18:1184–1196

Haddad T, Himes A, Thompson L, Irony T, Nair R (2017) Incorporation of stochastic engineering models as prior information in Bayesian medical device trials. J Biopharm Stat 27:1089–1103

Ibrahim JG, Chen M-H, Gwon Y, Chen F (2015) The power prior: theory and applications. Stat Med 34(28):3724–3749

Jennison C, Turnull BW (2000) Group sequential methods with applications to clinical trials. Chapman and Hall/CRC, London

Jiang Z, Song Y, Shou Q, Xia J, Wang W (2014) A Bayesian prediction model between a biomarker and clinical endpoint for dichotomous variables. Trials 15:500

Kim K, Tsiatis AA (1990) Study duration for clinical trials with survival response and early stopping rule. Biometrics 46:81–92

Lan KKG, DeMets DL (1983) Discrete sequential boundaries for clinical trials. Biometrika 70:659–663

Mehta CR, Pocock SJ (2011) Adaptive increase in sample size when interim results are promising: a practical guide with examples. Stat Med 30:3267–3284

Muller P, Berry D, Grieve A, Smith M, Krams M (2007) Simulation-based sequential Bayesian design. J Stat Plann Inference 137:3140–3150

Musgrove D, Haddad T (2017) BayesDP: tools for the Bayesian discount prior function. https://Cran.R-project.org/package=bayesDP

Paux G, Dmitrienko A (2016) Mediana: clinical trial simulations. R package version 1.0.4. http://gpaux.github.io/Mediana/

Robert C, Casella G (2010) Introducing Monte Carlo methods with R. Springer, New York

Suess E, Trumbo B (2010) Introduction to probability simulation and Gibbs sampling with R. Springer, New York

Thompson JR (1999) Simulation: a modeler's approach. Wiley, New York

Townsend RR, Mahfoud F, Kandzari DE, Kario K, Pocock S, Weber MA (2017) Catheter-based renal denervation in patients with uncontrolled hypertension in the absence of antihypertensive medications (SPYRAL HTN-OFF MED): a randomised, sham-controlled, proof-of-concept trial. Lancet 390(10108):2160–2170